P9-BBT-227

Essentials of
Cardiopulmonary
Physical
Therapy

Essentials of Cardiopulmonary Physical Therapy

ELLEN A. HILLEGASS, MMSc, PT, CCS
Assistant Professor
Department of Physical Therapy
College of Health Sciences
Georgia State University
Atlanta, Georgia

H. STEVEN SADOWSKY, MS, RRT, PT, CCS
Assistant Clinical Professor
Graduate Program in Physical Therapy
University of California, San Francisco, and
San Francisco State University
San Francisco, California

W.B. SAUNDERS COMPANY
A Division of Harcourt Brace & Company
Philadelphia   London   Toronto   Montreal   Sydney   Tokyo

W.B. SAUNDERS COMPANY
A Division of
Harcourt Brace & Company

The Curtis Center
Independence Square West
Philadelphia, Pennsylvania 19106

Library of Congress Cataloging-in-Publication Data

Essentials of cardiopulmonary physical therapy/[edited by] Ellen
   Hillegass, H. Steven Sadowsky.—1st ed.
      p. cm.
   ISBN 0-7216-3609-8
   1. Cardiopulmonary system—Physical therapy.   2. Cardiopulmonary
system—Diseases.   3. Cardiopulmonary system—Pathophysiology.
I. Hillegass, Ellen.   II. Sadowsky, H. Steven.
   [DNLM: 1. Cardiovascular Diseases—physiopathology.
2. Cardiovascular Diseases—therapy.   3. Lung Diseases—
physiopathology.   4. Lung Diseases—rehabilitation.   5. Physical
Therapy.   WG 166 E78]
RC702.E88   1993
616.1'062—dc20
DNLM/DLC   92-49848

ESSENTIALS OF CARDIOPULMONARY PHYSICAL THERAPY   ISBN 0-7216-3609-8

Printed in the United States of America.

Last digit is the print number: 9   8   7   6   5   4

To Patrick, Jamie, and Christi,
for their love, patience, and acceptance
of all the long hours I have put into this endeavor
and most especially for their "joie de vivre";
to Dan
for his love, support, and encouragement throughout this endeavor;
and to my parents, John and Norma,
who gave me a great start.

EAH

To Barbara,
for her friendship, love, and support,
as well as for her inspiration
as an ever-inquiring physical therapist;
and to Jennifer—
certainly the best of anything I was ever part of.

HSS

Contributors

RHONDA N. BARR, MA, PT
  Adjunct Associate, University of
    Iowa; Clinical Supervisor,
    Department of Physical Therapy,
    University of Iowa Hospitals and
    Clinics, Iowa City, Iowa.
  Pulmonary Rehabilitation

LAWRENCE P. CAHALIN, MA, PT,
CCS
  Assistant Instructor, Graduate
    Program in Physical Therapy,
    MGH Institute of Health
    Professions; Cardiopulmonary
    Physical Therapy Transplant
    Coordinator, Massachusetts
    General Hospital, Boston,
    Massachusetts.
  Cardiac Muscle Dysfunction;
    Pulmonary Medications

PEGGY CLOUGH, MA, PT
  Supervisor, Physical Therapy
    Division, University of Michigan
    Medical Center, Ann Arbor,
    Michigan.
  Restrictive Lung Dysfunction

MERYL COHEN, MS, PT, CCS
  Cardiopulmonary Clinical Specialist,
    Massachusetts General Hospital,
    Boston, Massachusetts.
  Cardiac Medications

SUSAN L. GARRITAN, MA, PT, CCS
  Supervisor, Cardiopulmonary
    Physical Therapy, New York
    University Medical Center, New
    York, New York.
  Chronic Obstructive Pulmonary
    Diseases

KATE GRIMES, BS, PT, CCS
  Adjunct Faculty, Massachusetts
    General Institute of Health
    Sciences, Boston, Massachusetts;
    Clinical Supervisor of Specialty
    Programs, Newton-Wellesley
    Hospital, Newton, Massachusetts.
  Cardiac Medications

ELLEN HILLEGASS, MMSc, PT, CCS
  Assistant Professor, Department of
    Physical Therapy, Georgia State
    University, Atlanta, Georgia.
  Cardiac Tests and Procedures;
    Electrocardiography;
    Cardiopulmonary Assessment;
    The Well Individual

WILLIAM T. KUNTZ, MA, PT, CCS
  Physical Therapy Coordinator,
    Cardiopulmonary Rehabilitation,
    New York University Medical
    Center, New York, New York.
  The Acute Care Setting

GENE McCOLGAN, PT, CCS
Instructor in Medicine, University of South Florida College of Medicine, Program Director for Cardiac Rehabilitation, James A. Haley Veterans Hospital, Tampa, Florida.
Ischemic Cardiac Conditions

H. STEVEN SADOWSKY, MS, RRT, PT, CCS
Assistant Clinical Professor, Graduate Program in Physical Therapy, University of California, San Francisco; Clinical Director, Center for Human Performance Testing, Education, and Research, University of California, San Francisco; Cardiopulmonary Clinical Specialist, Department of Rehabilitation Services, UCSF Hospitals and Clinics, San Francisco, California.
Anatomy of the Cardiovascular and Respiratory Systems; Cardiovascular and Respiratory Physiology; Pulmonary Diagnostic Tests and Procedures; Thoracic Surgical Procedures, Monitoring, and Support Equipment; Pulmonary Medications

WILLIAM C. TEMES, MS, PT, CCS
Owner, Oakway Therapy Clinic, Eugene, Oregon.
Cardiac Rehabilitation

JOANNE WATCHIE, MA, PT, CCS
Cardiopulmonary Clinical Consultant, San Marino, California.
Cardiopulmonary Implications of Specific Diseases

Preface

Those aspects of physical therapy commonly referred to as *cardiopulmonary physical therapy* are finally recognized as fundamental components of the knowledge and practice base of all entry-level physical therapists. Over the past 15 years, the Cardiopulmonary Section of the American Physical Therapy Association has been involved in the identification and differentiation of entry-level knowledge and skills related to the practice of cardiopulmonary physical therapy. As active participants in that process and as classroom teachers, we undertook this text in an effort to disseminate the related information that was perceived to be essential for all entry-level physical therapists. Moreover, after discussions with individuals from a variety of professional backgrounds and from numerous regions of the country, it seems that *Essentials of Cardiopulmonary Physical Therapy* could be useful to *any* practitioner working with patients suffering cardiopulmonary dysfunction as a primary or secondary diagnosis.

The book is divided into five sections: *Anatomy and Physiology, Pathophysiology, Diagnostic Tests and Procedures, Pharmacology,* and *Assessment and Treatment.* This division was chosen to present the information in what we believe is an orderly progression that will facilitate a more thorough understanding of the subject matter. It is our firm belief that the cardiac and pulmonary systems should be considered as they relate to each other, not as separate entities. Therefore, the anatomy, physiology, and assessment and treatment aspects of the cardiac and pulmonary systems are each discussed jointly, stressing their interactions; only with respect to specific pathophysiologic states have we separated the systems.

Because we believe that physical therapists should choose treatment interventions that address the specific problems identified from a thorough patient assessment (and not from a preconceived checklist of options), we have purposefully avoided the inclusion of diagnostically related "laundry lists." We have attempted to span the life cycle in all considerations.

Chapter 1 presents the developmental and maturational anatomy of the traditional cardiovascular and respiratory systems. Chapter 2 details the basic physiology underlying the "oxygen transport system." Chapters 3 through 7 examine the pathophysiology associated with cardiac ischemia (Chapter 3), myocardial dysfunction (Chapter 4), restrictive pulmonary conditions (Chapter

ix

5), obstructive pulmonary conditions (Chapter 6), and other disease processes that have cardiopulmonary implications (Chapter 7). Chapters 8 through 11 describe the diagnostic tests and procedures, surgical interventions, and monitoring and support devices commonly employed in the assessment and treatment of patients with cardiovascular and pulmonary disorders. Chapters 12 and 13 consider cardiac and pulmonary medications, respectively. Chapters 14 through 18 present information regarding the assessment (Chapter 14) and treatment of patients with cardiorespiratory disorders in acute care (Chapter 15), cardiac rehabilitation (Chapter 16), and pulmonary rehabilitation (Chapter 17) settings; Chapter 18 considers the well individual. Whenever possible, we have striven to provide case studies to exemplify the material being presented. Finally, terms that are of particular relevance or that have clinical significance have been highlighted in boldface print throughout the text; these words and abbreviations are presented in alphabetical order with a brief definition in the Glossary.

To become even a minimally competent clinician, you will have to practice physical therapy under the tutelage of an experienced clinician. *Essentials of Cardiopulmonary Physical Therapy* cannot teach everything there is to know about the assessment and treatment of cardiovascular and pulmonary disorders; but it does provide the essentials.

ELLEN A. HILLEGASS
H. STEVEN SADOWSKY

Acknowledgments

Making this book a reality required an abundance of patience, understanding, and sacrifice from our loved ones, and for this we would like to sincerely thank them. In addition, the constant support and understanding of our colleagues and co-workers—especially Gordon Cummings, Mary Lou Barnes, Carolyn Crutchfield, and Paul Andrew—as well as an exceptional office staff—including Carol Brown and Lillian Wong—allowed us to put forth this text. Likewise, our students, peers (especially Burt Prater and Joanne Watchie, who provided review and advice), and patients have contributed in many ways to the content of this book. Also, the contributors, with their knowledge and persistence, have made this text possible. We extend our sincerest thanks to them all.

In addition, we extend our heartfelt thanks to Gene Floersch, a free-lance artist, who created the majority of the line art. Finally, two special people at W.B. Saunders must be given particular thanks. They are Margaret Biblis, who first recognized that this project might be worthwhile and who kept us committed, and Shirley Kuhn, who, through her more than patient attention to the details, guided us to completion.

Contents

SECTION 2

Chapter 3

Gene McColgan

Chapter 4

Cardiac Muscle Dysfunction 123
Lawrence P. Cahalin

Chapter 5

SECTION 3

DIAGNOSTIC TESTS AND PROCEDURES, SURGICAL
INTERVENTIONS, MONITORING AND SUPPORT
EQUIPMENT 325

Chapter 8

Cardiac Tests and Procedures 327
Ellen Hillegass

Chapter **9**

Electrocardiography 355
Ellen Hillegass

Chapter 10

Pulmonary Diagnostic Tests and Procedures 403

H. Steven Sadowsky

Chapter 11

Thoracic Surgical Procedures, Monitoring, and Support Equipment 437

H. Steven Sadowsky

SECTION 4

Chapter 12

Kate Grimes and Meryl Cohen

Chapter 13

Pulmonary Medications 531

Lawrence P. Cahalin and H. Steven Sadowsky

SECTION 5

ASSESSMENT AND TREATMENT 551

Chapter 14

Cardiopulmonary Assessment 553

Ellen Hillegass

Chapter 15

Chapter **16**

Cardiac Rehabilitation 633

William C. Temes

Chapter **17**

Pulmonary Rehabilitation 677

Rhonda N. Barr

Chapter **18**

SECTION 1
ANATOMY AND PHYSIOLOGY

H. STEVEN SADOWSKY

1 ANATOMY OF THE CARDIOVASCULAR AND RESPIRATORY SYSTEMS

INTRODUCTION

This chapter reviews the structure of the cardiovascular and respiratory systems. There is no single best manner in which to describe these systems. A fundamental assumption must be made, namely, that the reader already possesses some knowledge of the material that is presented in more detail in later sections. The order of presentation that follows, therefore, is an artificial convenience for which some indulgence is requested.

DEVELOPMENT OF THE CARDIOVASCULAR AND RESPIRATORY SYSTEMS

What follows is in no way intended as a definitive discussion of the embryologic development of the cardiovascular and pulmonary systems. The reader is urged to refer to Moore,[1] Williams and Warwick,[2] Netter and colleagues,[3,4] or others for more detailed information.

The Embryonic Cardiovascular System

The cardiovascular system is the first functioning system in the embryo. Early in the third week of gestation, **angioblastic tissue** forms from the deepest layer of mesenchyme covering the yolk sac, in the body stalk, and in the chorion. The details of this process are not entirely understood, but the earliest blood vessels are formed in several separate areas. In the yolk sac and the base of the body stalk, small and essentially spherical groups of cells—the **blood islands**—develop. It is thought that the outermost cells of the islands flatten to form the vascular endothelium, and the innermost cells convert into primitive red corpuscles. These blood-containing spaces go on to form a continuous network of vessels. Typical blood islands do not form in the chorion or the chorionic end of the body stalk. Solid strands of angioblasts that contain a few rod-shaped nuclei develop instead. Each strand, in turn, develops one or two nucleated hemoglobin-containing cells, and blood vessels form as these spaces coalesce. Buds grow

3

Figure 1-1.

Ventral views of the developing heart during the fourth week of gestation. *A* and *B*, fusion of the heart tubes. *C* and *D*, bending of the single heart tube as the primitive heart grows within a confined space, finally folding on itself and forming the bulboventricular loop. (From Moore KL. Before We Are Born: Basic Embryology and Birth Defects. 3rd ed. Philadelphia, WB Saunders, 1989, p 205.)

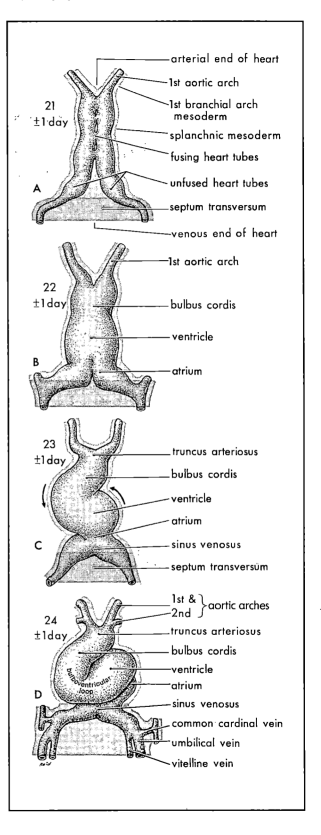

from the walls of the blood vessels that are formed initially, then become canalized, and later are converted into new vessels. These vessels join with vessels from adjacent areas to form a network.

At about the eighteenth day of development, **cardiogenic cords** in the **cardiogenic area** of the embryo are the first indications of the formation of the heart. The cardiogenic cords are soon canalized to form the **endocardial heart tubes,** which fuse together by about the twenty-first or twenty-second day, forming the pericardial cavity. At the same time, the heart elongates and develops the **truncus arteriosus, bulbous cordis, ventricle, atrium,** and **sinus venosus.** As the heart tubes fuse, a *myoepicardial mantle* is formed from a thickening of the splanchnic mesenchyme around them. At this stage, the developing heart tube is separated from the myoepicardial mantle by gelatinous connective tissue called **cardiac jelly.** The inner endocardial tube becomes the epithelial lining of the heart, called the **endocardium.** The myoepicardial mantle differentiates into the **myocardium** and the **epicardium.** The sinus venosus is a large venous sinus opening into the inferior wall of the right atrium. Initially a fairly straight tube, the heart soon bends on itself, forming a U-shaped **bulboventricular loop** (Fig. 1-1).

As may be seen in Figure 1-2, the primitive heart has only one atrium and one ventricle. Partitioning of the atrioventricular canal, atrium, and ventricle begins in the middle of the fourth week and is essentially completed by the end of the fifth week. Developing **endocardial cushions** in the dorsal and ventral walls of the atrioventricular canal grow toward each other and fuse, dividing the atrioventricular canal into *right* and *left canals.* Concurrently, a crescent-shaped membrane, the **septum primum,** grows from the dorsocranial wall of the primitive atrium. Before

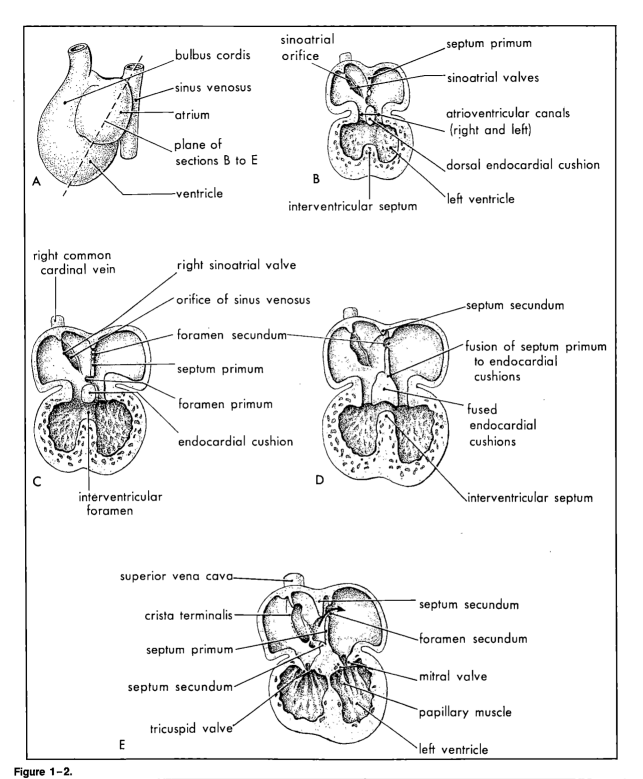

Figure 1-2.

Partitioning of the atrioventricular canal, atrium, and ventricle during the fifth to eighth weeks of gestation. *A*, plane of the frontal sections shown in *B-E*. *B*, appearance of the septum primum, interventricular septum, and dorsal endocardial cushion at about 28 days. *C*, perforations in the dorsal part of the septum at about 32 days. *D*, foramen secundum at about 35 days. *E*, four-chambered heart after completion of partitioning at about 8 weeks. (From Moore KL. *Before We Are Born: Basic Embryology and Birth Defects.* 3rd ed. Philadelphia, WB Saunders, 1989, p 209.)

the septum primum joins and fuses with the endocardial cushions, perforations form in the dorsal part of the septum and coalesce to form the **foramen secundum.**

Another crescent membrane, the **septum secundum,** grows from the ventrocranial wall of the atrium on the right side of the septum primum. This septum eventually covers the foramen secundum; the opening in the septum secundum is called the **foramen ovale.** The septum primum forms a valve for the foramen ovale. Before birth, the foramen ovale permits most of the blood entering the right atrium to pass into the left atrium. After birth, the foramen ovale normally closes, and the septum becomes a complete partition.

The left horn of the sinus venosus forms the **coronary sinus,** and the right horn becomes part of the wall of the right atrium. The remnant of the right part of the primitive atrium persists as the rough portion of the atrium and the **right auricle.** As the left atrium expands, the terminal portion of the **primitive pulmonary vein** is incorporated into the wall of the left atrium. The remnant of the left part of the primitive atrium is the **left auricle.**

During the fifth week, **bulbar ridges** form in the walls of the bulbous cordis. Similar **truncal ridges** form in the truncus arteriosus. Believed to be caused by blood streaming from the developing ventricles, these ridges have a spiral orientation that results in a spiral **aorticopulmonary septum** when the ridges fuse. This septum divides the bulbous cordis and the truncus arteriosus into the **aorta** and **pulmonary trunk.** Because of the spiral form of the aorticopulmonary septum, the pulmonary trunk twists around the ascending aorta.

The primitive ventricle begins dividing into right and left ventricles at the end of the fourth week with the development of the **interventricular septum** in the floor of the ventricle near its apex. The interventricular septum grows toward the fused endocardial cushions, closing the resultant **interventricular foramen** at about the end of the seventh week. After closure, the pulmonary trunk communicates with the right ventricle and the aorta with the left ventricle, essentially completing cardiac development.

Prenatal Circulation

Oxygenated blood returns from the placenta in the **umbilical vein.** Approximately half of this blood bypasses the liver via the **ductus venosus.** After the **inferior vena cava,** the blood enters the right atrium. Because the inferior vena cava also receives blood from the lower limbs, abdomen, and pelvis, the blood entering the right atrium is not as well oxygenated as that in the umbilical vein.

The blood from the inferior vena cava is directed primarily through the foramen ovale to the left atrium by the inferior border of the septum secundum. In the left atrium, the blood mixes with a small amount of deoxygenated blood returning from the lungs via the pulmonary veins. From the left atrium, the blood passes into the left ventricle and leaves via the ascending aorta. Therefore, the coronary arteries, the head and neck, and the upper limbs receive relatively well-oxygenated blood.

A small amount of oxygenated blood originally from the placenta remains in the right atrium and is mixed with blood from the **superior vena cava** and the coronary sinus before passing into the right ventricle. This blood exits via the pulmonary trunk, and most of it passes through the ductus arteriosus into the aorta. Very little blood passes on to the lungs before birth. The blood remaining in the aorta circulates through the inferior part of the body and eventually enters the inferior vena cava.

Postnatal Circulation

Major circulatory adjustments occur at birth with cessation of fetal blood circulation through the placenta and the beginning of function by the lungs. Occlusion of the placental circulation causes a fall in blood pressure in the inferior vena cava and right atrium. Aeration of the lungs is accompanied by a significant fall in pulmonary vascular resistance, a marked increase in pulmonary blood flow, and a thinning of the walls of the pulmonary arteries. Consequent to the increased pulmonary blood flow, the pressure in the left atrium rises above that of the right atrium. This closes the foramen ovale by pressing the septum primum against the septum secundum.

As a result of the systemic cardiovascular changes occurring at birth, the following vessels and structures are transformed:

- The intra-abdominal portion of the umbilical vein becomes the **ligamentum teres,** which passes from the umbilicus to the left branch of the portal vein.
- The ductus venosus eventually becomes the **ligamentum venosum,** which passes through the liver from the left branch of the portal vein to the inferior vena cava.
- Most intra-abdominal portions of the umbilical arteries become the **medial umbilical ligaments.** The proximal parts of these arteries persist as the **superior vesical arteries,** which supply the superior part of the urinary bladder.
- The foramen ovale normally closes functionally at birth: later anatomic closure occurs with proliferation and adhesion of the septum primum to the left margin of the septum secundum.
- The ductus arteriosus eventually becomes the **ligamentum arteriosum,** which passes from the left pulmonary artery to the arch of the aorta (anatomic closure generally occurs by the third month after birth).

The Embryonic Respiratory System

Development of the respiratory system begins during the fourth week of gestation as a **laryngotracheal groove** in the caudal end of the ventral wall of the pharyngeal floor. Shortly thereafter, a **laryngotracheal diverticulum** separates from the pharynx and grows caudally from the laryngotracheal groove, partitioning the foregut into the **esophagus** and **laryngotracheal tube.**

The **larynx** forms from the proximal endodermal lining of the laryngotracheal tube and the fourth and sixth pairs of branchial arches. The endodermal lining distal to the larynx in the central laryngotracheal tube forms the epithelium and glands of the **trachea,** and the surrounding splanchnic mesenchyme forms the tracheal cartilage, connective tissue, and muscle. The inferior

end of the laryngotracheal tube forms a **lung bud.**

The lung bud divides into two **bronchial buds,** which ultimately differentiate into the bronchi and lungs, as shown in Figure 1–3. Right and left **primary bronchi** grow from the bronchial buds and subdivide into **secondary bronchi.** Three secondary bronchi arise from the right primary bronchus: the superior secondary bronchus supplies the upper lobe of the lung; the inferior secondary bronchus continues on to supply the lower lobe but first gives off a middle secondary bronchus to the middle lobe. The left primary bronchus gives rise to two secondary bronchi, which supply the superior and inferior lobes of the left lung.

Although bursts of regular respiratory activity are interspersed with periods of apnea in the fetus, these intrauterine respiratory movements are not a necessity for normal lung development, and a regular rhythmic pattern is probably not established before birth.[5] Ensuing development of the lung may be divided into four stages.

The Pseudoglandular Period (weeks 5 to 17). As the secondary bronchi continue to develop, they progressively branch and bifurcate until, by the seventh week, there are ten segmental bronchi in the right lung and eight or nine in the left lung — the **bronchopulmonary segments.** The splanchnic mesenchyme surrounding the developing bronchi eventually gives rise to the supportive cartilaginous plates, the bronchial smooth muscle and connective tissue, and the pulmonary connective tissue and capillaries.

The Canalicular Period (weeks 16 to 25). Because the upper segments of the lung develop faster than the lower ones, this period of development overlaps the pseudoglandular period. Approximately 17 orders of branches develop, the **terminal bronchioles** each yielding two or more **respiratory bronchioles.** Each of these, in turn, divides into as many as six *alveolar ducts,* which, toward the end of the canalicular period, begin to develop *terminal sacs* complete with capillary loops.

The Terminal Sac Period (week 24 to birth). The terminal sacs — **pulmonary alveoli** — continue to develop with the attendant blood and lymphatic capillary networks. Type II alveo-

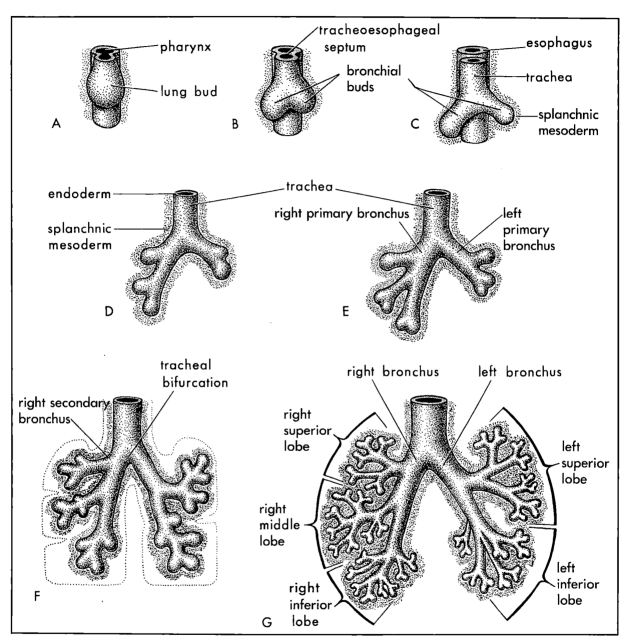

Figure 1-3.

Ventral views showing the successive stages of development of the bronchi and lungs during the fourth to eighth weeks of gestation. *A* to *D*, 4 weeks; *E*, 5 weeks; *F*, 6 weeks; *G*, 8 weeks. (From Moore KL. *Before We Are Born: Basic Embryology and Birth Defects.* 3rd ed. Philadelphia, WB Saunders, 1989, p 162.)

lar epithelial cells begin to produce **surfactant** at about 28 weeks.

The Alveolar Period (late fetal period to 7 or 8 years). The number of pulmonary alveoli continues to increase toward an adult level, about one sixth to one eighth of the adult number being present at birth.

Postnatal Respiration

The lung of the fetus is not collapsed in utero; rather, it is filled with an ultrafiltrate of plasma roughly equal in volume to the functional residual capacity of the lung in the newborn. This liquid is approximately 100 times more viscous than air and may amount to between 25% and 40% of the total lung capacity.[5] Despite the problem of viscosity imposed by the liquid in the lungs, it also keeps the radius of curvature at the air-liquid interface relatively large. As is discussed in Chapter 2, this reduces both the surface tension forces resisting inflation and the tendency of the airways toward collapse.

Obviously, the lungs must be rapidly cleared of the fluid occupying them if efficient gas exchange is to occur. About one third of the fluid is squeezed from the neonate's lungs as it passes out of the vagina. During the first few breaths approximately one half of the remaining fluid is absorbed into the capillaries, and the other half is removed by the pulmonary lymphatics. The neonate must develop a very high transpulmonary pressure to overcome the surface tension forces at the air-liquid interface in the airways and the viscosity of the liquid within the tracheobronchial tree, to move the column of liquid in the lungs, and to move air with the first breath after birth (Fig. 1-4).

No longer isolated from tactile, thermal, visual, and other stimuli, the newborn is bombarded by sensory stimuli. Additionally, placental gas exchange is impaired drastically during birth, making the fetus hypoxemic and hypercapnic, thus stimulating both the central and peripheral chemoreceptors. This combination of stimuli results in the initiation of respiration within moments of birth. The first few breaths do not expand the alveoli uniformly because airway resistance is not homogeneous, and some of the alveoli remain filled with fluid. Thus, as illustrated in Figure

Figure 1-4.

A pressure-volume graph depicting a newborn infant's first three breaths after birth. Note the significant transpulmonary pressures of the first two breaths compared with that of the third. (Redrawn from Cherniack RM, Cherniack L. Respiration in Health and Disease. 3rd ed. Philadelphia, WB Saunders, 1983, p 121.)

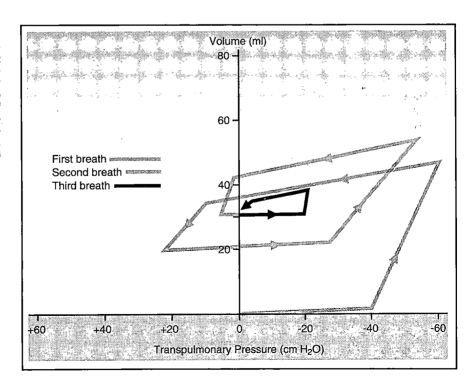

1–4, although the lungs contain a small volume of air after the first breath, subsequent inhalations require decreasing transpulmonary pressures because successively reduced impedances are encountered until normal residual volume is attained. Pulmonary surfactant is necessary for the maintenance of patent alveoli at lower transpulmonary pressures.

THE MATURE CARDIOVASCULAR AND RESPIRATORY SYSTEMS

The cardiovascular and respiratory systems are contained within and protected by the thoracic cage. The following presents a consideration of the gross anatomy of the thorax, the cardiovascular system, and the respiratory system.

The Thorax

In addition to providing a skeletal framework for the attachment of the muscles of respiration, the thorax houses the lungs and mediastinum; the mediastinum houses the heart. The thorax is intimately involved in the respiratory process.

Skeletal Framework

The thoracic cage (Fig. 1–5) is conical in its superior-inferior aspect and somewhat kidney shaped in its transverse aspect. The skeletal boundaries of the thorax are the twelve thoracic vertebrae, dorsally; the ribs, laterally; and the sternum, ventrally. The **thoracic inlet,** or upper margin of the thoracic cage, is bounded by the first thoracic vertebra posteriorly, the superior border of the manubrium anteriorly, and the first ribs laterally. The **thoracic outlet** is bounded by the twelfth thoracic vertebra posteriorly, by the seventh through tenth costal cartilages anteriorly, and the eleventh and twelfth ribs laterally. The outlet is closed by the diaphragm, which forms the floor of the thoracic cavity.

● **Thoracic vertebrae** increase in size as they descend. The anterior surfaces are highly convex, the posterior surfaces slightly concave.

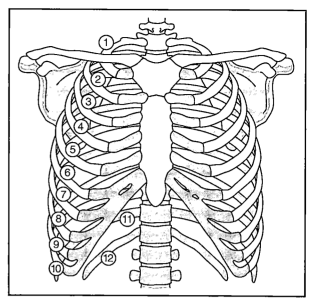

Figure 1–5.

The thoracic cage with the costal cartilages highlighted. (Modified from Evans A, Patterson P, Riley D, Sutherland S. Human Anatomy: An Illustrated Laboratory Guide. San Francisco, Regents of the University of California, 1982, Fig. 1.)

The pedicles are more toward the upper ends of the vertebral bodies. The spinous processes are typically long and directed downward enough to overlap at least the succeeding vertebra, though in the lower thoracic area they shorten and broaden more like the lumbar vertebrae. The transverse processes are long and heavy, projecting posteriorly and upward as well as laterally; at the end of each is a facet for articulation with the tubercle of a rib.

The first, ninth, tenth, eleventh, and twelfth thoracic vertebrae are not typical of the others. The body of the first thoracic vertebra is similar to that of the cervical vertebrae (being wider transversely than the typical thoracic vertebrae) and has an entire articular facet for the head of the first rib and a demifacet for the cranial half of the head of the second rib.

The ninth thoracic vertebra typically has one demifacet cranially but may occasionally have a second set of demifacets caudally. When it has two sets of demifacets, the tenth has demifacets on its cranial aspect only.

The tenth thoracic vertebra usually has one entire articular facet, which encroaches the lateral surface of the pedicle.

The eleventh thoracic vertebra begins the transition in shape toward the lumbar vertebrae. It has one entire articular facet, located principally on the pedicles, for the head of the eleventh rib. The transverse processes are rudimentary and without facets because there is no articulation with the tubercle of the eleventh rib.

The twelfth thoracic vertebra is similar to the eleventh but differs at its inferior articular surfaces, which are directed more laterally, like those of the lumbar vertebrae.

● **Ribs,** although considered "flat" bones, curve forward and downward from their posterior vertebral attachments toward their costal cartilages. The first seven ribs attach via their costal cartilages to the sternum and are called the **true ribs** (also, the vertebrosternal ribs); the lower five ribs are termed the **false ribs**—the eighth, ninth, and tenth ribs attach to the rib above by their costal cartilages (the vertebrochondral ribs), and the eleventh and twelfth ribs end freely (the vertebral ribs). The true ribs increase in length from above downward, whereas the false ribs decrease in length from above downward.

Except as noted later, each rib typically has a vertebral end separated from a sternal end by the body or shaft of the rib. The *head of the rib* (at its vertebral end) is distinguished by a twin-faceted surface for articulation with the facets on the bodies of two adjacent thoracic vertebrae. The cranial facet is smaller than the caudal facet, and a crest between these permits attachment of the interarticular ligament.

The *neck* is the 1-inch portion of the rib extending laterally from the head; it provides attachment for the anterior costotransverse ligament along its cranial border. The *tubercle* at the junction of the neck and the body of the rib consists of an articular and a nonarticular portion. The articular part of the tubercle (the more medial and inferior of the two) has a facet for articulation with the transverse process of the inferiormost vertebra to which the head is connected. The nonarticular part of the tubercle provides attachment for the ligament of the tubercle.

The *shaft* or *body* of the rib is simultaneously bent in two directions and twisted about its long axis, presenting two surfaces (internal and external) and two borders (superior and inferior). A *costal groove,* for the in-

tercostal vessels and nerve, extends along the inferior border dorsally but changes to the internal surface at the angle of the rib. The sternal end of the rib terminates in an oval depression into which the costal cartilage makes its attachment.

The first, second, tenth, eleventh, and twelfth ribs are unlike the other, typical ribs. The first rib is the shortest and most curved of all the ribs. Its head is small and rounded and has only one facet for articulation with the body of the first thoracic vertebra. The sternal end is larger and thicker than any of the other ribs.

The second rib, though longer than the first, is similarly curved. The body is not twisted. There is a short costal groove on its internal surface posteriorly.

The tenth through twelfth ribs each have only one articular facet on their heads. The eleventh and twelfth ribs have no necks or tubercles and are narrowed at their free anterior ends. The twelfth rib may sometimes be even shorter than the first rib.

● The **sternum** has three parts:
manubrium—articulates with the clavicles, the first and second ribs, and the body of the sternum
body—articulates with the second through seventh ribs, the manubrium, and the xiphoid process
xiphoid process—articulates with the seventh rib and the body of the sternum

The Mediastinum

The space between the pleurae from the vertebral surfaces to the sternum and from the thoracic inlet to the diaphragm at the thoracic outlet is occupied by the **mediastinum.** As seen in Figure 1–6, the mediastinum may be separated into superior and inferior divisions for description. The **superior division** extends from the thoracic inlet downward to a line running from the lower border of the fourth thoracic vertebra to the lower border of the manubrium; it contains the thymus, trachea, arch of the aorta, and esophagus. The **inferior division,** extending below this line downward to the diaphragmatic closure of the thoracic outlet, is further divided into anterior, middle, and posterior compartments by the

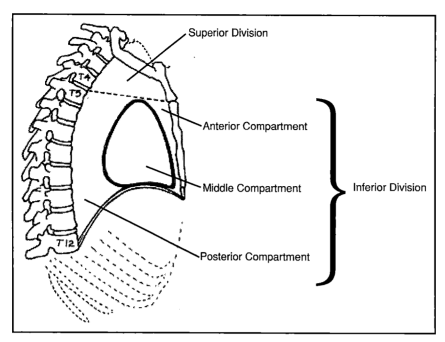

Figure 1–6.

Right lateral view of the mediastinum. The superior division contains the trachea, the arch of the aorta, the common carotid and subclavian arteries, and the upper portion of the esophagus. The inferior division is subdivided into anterior, middle, and posterior compartments. The anterior compartment contains the ascending aorta and the inferior portion of the thymus. The middle compartment contains the heart. The posterior compartment contains the thoracic aorta and the lower portion of the esophagus. (Adapted from Philo, R, Bosner MS, LeMaistre A, et al. Guide to Human Anatomy. Philadelphia, WB Saunders, 1985, p 161.)

pericardium. The pericardium is a fibroserous sac, which encloses the heart.

The *middle compartment* of the inferior division is bounded by the pericardium, containing the heart and the large vessels entering or exiting it. The *anterior compartment* lies between the sternum and the pericardium; it contains the ascending aorta. The *posterior compartment* lies posterior to the pericardium and the diaphragm and anterior to the bodies of the fifth through twelfth thoracic vertebrae; it contains the esophagus and thoracic aorta. Knowledge of the structure of the mediastinum is important to the interpretation of chest radiographs.

THE RESPIRATORY SYSTEM

The respiratory system includes the bony thorax, the muscles of respiration, the upper and the lower airways, and the pulmonary circulation. Since the thorax has already been discussed, the following section deals with the muscles of respiration, the lungs, the pulmonary vessels, and the upper and lower airways.

Intimate and exquisite interaction of these components is necessary for the accomplishment of the many respiratory and nonrespiratory functions of the respiratory system. These include gas exchange, fluid exchange, maintenance of a relatively low volume blood reservoir, filtration, and metabolism. Respiratory physiology is presented in Chapter 2.

The Muscles of Respiration

Respiration results from the coordinated interaction of the muscles of the neck, thorax, and abdomen (Fig. 1–7). The timing of specific muscular action remains debatable; the type and extent of activity probably changes with the magnitude of the respiratory effort.[6]

Primary Inspiratory Muscles

The *diaphragm:* a musculotendinous dome, forming the floor of the thorax, which arises from a tripartite (sternal, costal, and lumbar) origin to converge into a central tendon at the apex of the dome.

● *sternal portion*—arises from the posterior aspect of the xiphoid process
● *costal portion*—arises from interdigitations

with the transverse abdominal muscle and from the inner surfaces of the costal cartilages and the adjacent areas of the last six ribs bilaterally

● *lumbar portion*—arises via two aponeurotic arches, medial and lateral lumbocostal arches (arcuate ligaments), and from the lumbar vertebrae by means of a right and a left crus. The crura blend with the anterior longitudinal ligament of the vertebral column and are attached to the anterior surfaces of the lumbar vertebral bodies and intervertebral discs—first three on the right, first two on the left. The medial

lumbocostal arch extends from the body of the first or second lumbar vertebra to the front of the transverse process of the first lumbar vertebra. The lateral lumbocostal arch extends from the transverse process of the first lumbar vertebra to the tip and lower border of the twelfth rib.

During normal respiratory effort (with the lower ribs fixed), the diaphragm contracts from its crural and rib attachments to pull the central tendon down and forward. In so doing, the domed shape of the diaphragm is largely main-

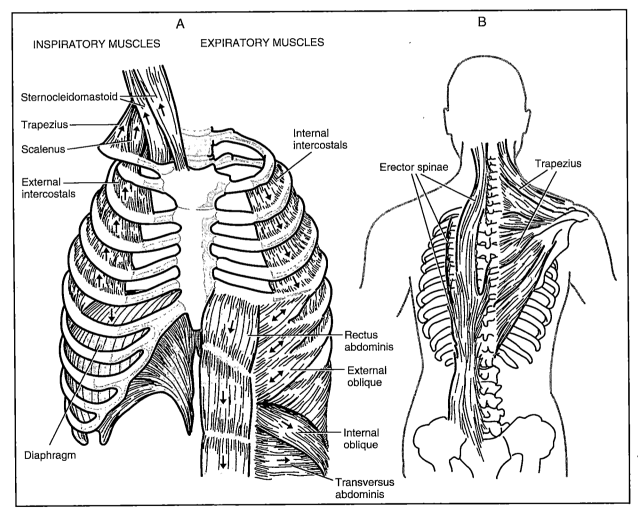

Figure 1–7.

The muscles of respiration. *A,* Anterior musculature. (Redrawn from Luce J, Culver B. Respiratory muscle function in health and disease. Chest 81:82–90, 1982.) *B,* Posterior musculature. (Redrawn from Frownfelter D. Chest Physical Therapy and Pulmonary Rehabilitation—An Interdisciplinary Approach. 2nd ed. Chicago, Mosby–Year Book, 1987, p 14.)

tained until the abdominal muscles end their extensibility, halting the downward displacement of the abdominal viscera, essentially forming a fixed platform beneath the central tendon. The central tendon then becomes a fixed point against which the muscular fibers of the diaphragm contract to elevate the lower ribs and thereby push the sternum and upper ribs forward. The right "hemidiaphragm" meets more resistance than the left (because the liver underlies the right hemidiaphragm, the stomach the left) during its descent; it is therefore more substantial than the left.

The level of the diaphragm varies considerably depending on body position and depth of respiration. In the supine position, both hemidiaphragms rest high in the thorax, and their normal inspiratory excursion is greatest. In the upright position, the level and excursion of the diaphragm is intermediate; in the sitting position the diaphragm is lower, and its excursion is smaller. In the side-lying position the hemidiaphragms are unequal in their positions: the uppermost side drops to a lower level and has less excursion than it does in the sitting position. The lowermost side rises higher in the thorax and has a greater excursion than that in the sitting position. In quiet breathing, the diaphragm normally moves about two thirds of an inch; with maximal respiratory effort the diaphragm may move from 2½ to 4 inches.[7]

Accessory Inspiratory Muscles

Eleven pairs of **intercostal muscles** occupy the intercostal spaces, connecting adjoining ribs. The actions of the intercostal muscles remain somewhat under dispute. It has been reported that as a group the intercostals act as elevators of the ribs during inspiratory effort; that the external intercostals elevate and the internal intercostals depress the ribs; that they act in concert to prevent "bulging" or "sucking in" of the intercostal spaces during respiration; that they may be primarily postural muscles.

● **External intercostals:** each muscle passes obliquely upward and backward from the upper border of one rib to the lower border of the rib above and extends forward from the tubercle of the rib nearly to the costochondral junction, where it is continued as an aponeurosis—the external intercostal membrane—to the sternum.

● **Internal intercostals:** each muscle passes obliquely upward and forward from the upper border of one rib to the floor of the costal groove of the rib above and extends backward from the sternum to the posterior costal angle, where it is continued as an aponeurosis—the internal intercostal membrane—to blend with the superior costotransverse ligament.

● **Innermost intercostals** attach to the internal aspects of two adjacent ribs, running in the same direction as the internal intercostals. They occupy the middle half of the ribs, being separated from the internal intercostals by the intercostal nerves and vessels and are not well formed in the upper thoracic level.

The **sternocleidomastoid** arises by two heads (sternal and clavicular, from the medial part of the clavicle), which unite to extend obliquely upward and laterally across the neck to the mastoid process.

The **scaleni** lie deep to the sternocleidomastoid but may be palpated in the posterior triangle of the neck (see Chapter 14).

● *anterior scalene:* arises from the anterior tubercles of the transverse processes of the third or fourth to the sixth cervical vertebra, attaching by tendinous insertion into the first rib

● *middle scalene:* arises from the transverse processes of all the cervical vertebrae to insert onto the first rib (posteromedially to the anterior scalene the brachial plexus and subclavian artery pass between anterior scalene and middle scalene)

● *posterior scalene:* arises from the posterior tubercles of the transverse processes of the fifth and sixth cervical vertebrae, passing between the middle scalene and levator scapulae, to attach onto the second or third rib

The **trapezius** (upper fibers) arises from the medial part of the superior nuchal line on the occiput and the ligamentum nuchae (from the vertebral spinous processes between the skull and the seventh cervical vertebra) to insert onto the distal third of the clavicle.

The **pectoralis major** arises from the medial third of the clavicle, from the lateral part of the anterior surface of the manubrium and body of the sternum, and from the costal cartilages of the first six ribs to insert onto the lateral lip of the crest of the greater tubercle of the humerus.

The **pectoralis minor** arises from the second to fifth or the third to sixth ribs to insert into the medial side of the coracoid process close to the tip.

The **serratus anterior** arises from the outer surfaces of the upper eight or nine ribs to attach along the costal aspect of the medial border of the scapula.

The **latissimus dorsi** arises from the spinous processes of the lower six thoracic, the lumbar, and the upper sacral vertebrae and from the posterior aspect of the iliac crest; it slips from the lower three or four ribs to attach to the intertubercular groove of the humerus.

The **serratus posterior superior** arises from the lower part of the ligamentum nuchae and the spinous processes of the seventh cervical and the first two or three thoracic vertebrae downward into the upper borders of the second to fourth or fifth ribs.

The **quadratus lumborum** arises from the iliac crest (and the transverse processes of the lumbar vertebrae between) upward to the twelfth rib.

The **iliocostalis**—the most lateral division of the erector spinae:

● *Iliocostalis lumborum:* arises from the sacrum, the iliac crest, and the spinous processes of most of the lumbar and the lower two thoracic vertebrae upward to the lower borders of the last six or seven ribs as far laterally as their angles.
● *Iliocostalis thoracis:* arises from the upper borders of the lower six ribs medial to the insertion of the iliocostalis lumborum up to the upper six ribs.
● *Iliocostalis cervicis:* arises medial to the iliocostalis thoracis from the angles of the upper six ribs to insert into the transverse processes of the fourth, fifth, and sixth cervical vertebrae.

The Pleurae

Each lung is covered by a membranous serous sac—the **pleura** (Fig. 1–8). The pleura covering the surface of each lung is called the **visceral**

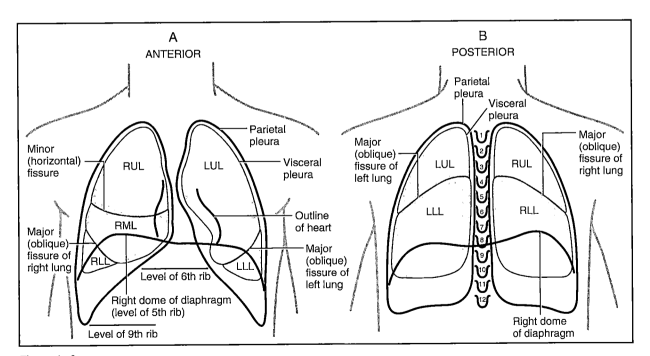

Figure 1–8.

Anterior *(A)* and posterior *(B)* views of the fissures of the lungs and the extent of the parietal pleura. (Redrawn from Kersten LD. **Comprehensive Respiratory Nursing: A Decision Making Approach. Philadelphia, WB Saunders, 1989, p 8.)**

pleura and is inseparable from the tissue of the lung, invaginating to adhere to all surfaces of the lung. The pleura covering the inner surface of the chest wall, the exposed part of the diaphragm, and the mediastinum is referred to as the **parietal pleura.** The parietal pleura is often referred to with specific names that correspond to the anatomic surfaces it covers: the portion lining the ribs and vertebrae is named the *costovertebral pleura;* the portion over the diaphragm the *diaphragmatic pleura;* the portion covering the uppermost aspect of the lung in the neck is the *cervical pleura;* and that overlying the mediastinum is called the *mediastinal pleura.* Parietal and visceral pleurae blend where they come together to enclose the root of the lung. Normally they are in intimate contact during all phases of the ventilatory cycle, being separated only by a thin serous film, the potential space between them being called the **pleural space.**

The parietal pleura receives its vascular supply from the intercostal, internal thoracic, and musculophrenic arteries. Venous return is by way of the systemic veins in the adjacent parts of the chest wall. The visceral pleura is supplied by the bronchial vessels. The parietal pleura receives somatosensory nerve fibers, but the visceral pleura does not. The costal and peripheral diaphragmatic pleura are supplied by the intercostal nerves; the mediastinal and central diaphragmatic pleura are supplied by the phrenic nerve. Thus, irritation of the intercostally innervated pleura results in the referral of pain to the thoracic or abdominal walls, whereas irritation of the phrenic-supplied pleura results in referred pain in the lower neck and shoulder.

The Lungs

The lungs are located on either side of the thoracic cavity, separated by the mediastinum. Each lung lies freely within its corresponding pleural cavity, except where it is attached to the heart and trachea by the root and pulmonary ligament. The substance of the lung — the **parenchyma** — is normally porous and spongy in nature. The surfaces of the lungs are marked by numerous intersecting lines that indicate the poly-

hedral (secondary) lobules of the lung. The lungs are basically cone shaped and are described as having a base, an apex, three borders, and two surfaces.

The apex of each lung is situated in the root of the neck, its highest point being about 1 inch above the middle third of each clavicle. The base of each lung is concave, resting on the convex surface of the diaphragm, which separates the left lung from the left lobe of the liver, the fundus of the stomach and the spleen, and the right lung from the right lobe of the liver. The costal surface of each lung conforms to the shape of the overlying chest wall. The medial surface of each lung may be divided into vertebral and mediastinal aspects. The vertebral aspect contacts the respective sides of the thoracic vertebrae and their intervertebral discs, the posterior intercostal vessels and nerves. The mediastinal aspect is notable for the **cardiac impression;** this concavity is larger on the left than on the right lung to accommodate the projection of the apex of the heart toward the left. Just posterior to the cardiac impression is the **hilus,** where the structures forming the root of the lung enter and exit the parenchyma. The extension of the pleural covering below and behind the hilus from the root of the lung forms the **pulmonary ligament.** The inferior border of the lung separates the base of the lung from its costal surface; the posterior border separates the costal surface from the vertebral aspect of the mediastinal surface; the anterior border of each lung is thin and overlaps the front of the pericardium; additionally, the anterior border of the left lung presents a **cardiac notch.**

Hila and Roots

The point at which the nerves, vessels, and primary bronchi penetrate the parenchyma of each lung is called the *hilus.* The structures entering the hila of the lungs and comprising the roots of each of the lungs are the principal bronchus, the pulmonary artery, the pulmonary veins, the bronchial arteries and veins, the pulmonary nerve plexus, and the lymph vessels (Fig. 1–9). They lie next to the vertebral bodies of the fifth, sixth, and seventh thoracic vertebrae. The

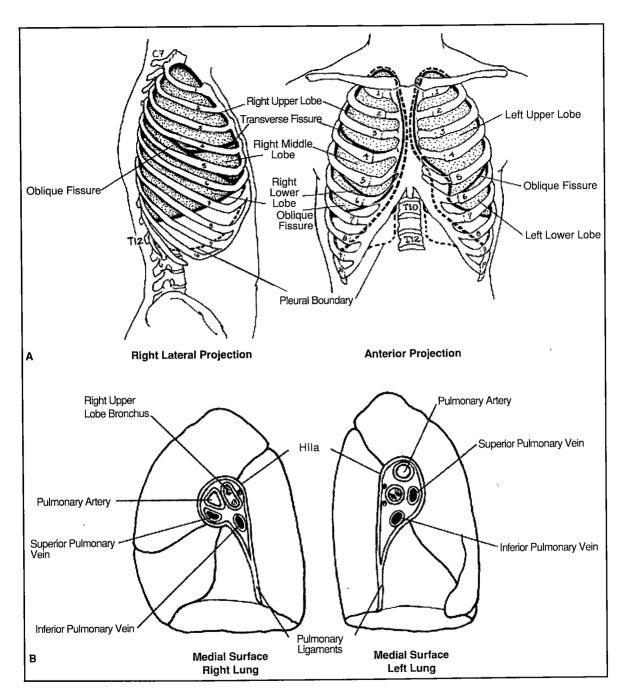

Figure 1–9.

A, Lateral and anterior views of the lungs through the rib cage at functional residual capacity, showing the extent of the pleura and the relative positions of the lungs. *B,* The medial view of the lungs demonstrates hilar structures. (Redrawn from Philo R, Bosner MS, LeMaistre A, et al. Guide to Human Anatomy. Philadelphia, WB Saunders, 1985, pp 156, 158.)

right root lies behind the superior vena cava and a portion of the right atrium, below the end of the azygos vein; the left root lies below the arch of the aorta and in front of the descending thoracic aorta. The root of each lung is formed by the mainstem bronchus, pulmonary artery, two pulmonary veins, bronchial arteries and veins, pulmonary nerve plexus, lymph vessels, and bronchopulmonary lymph nodes. The pulmonary ligament lies below the root; the phrenic nerve and the anterior pulmonary plexus lie in front of the root; the vagus nerve and posterior pulmonary plexus lie behind the root.

Fissures and Lobes

The upper and middle lobes of the right lung are separated from the lower lobe by the **oblique fissure** (see Fig. 1–8). Starting on the medial surface of the right lung at the upper posterior aspect of the hilus, the oblique fissure runs upward and backward to the posterior border at about the level of the fourth thoracic vertebra. It then descends anteroinferiorly across the anterior costal surface to intersect the lower border of the lung about 5 inches from the median plane, after which it passes posterosuperiorly to rejoin the hilus just behind and beneath to the upper pulmonary vein. The middle lobe is separated from the upper lobe by the **horizontal fissure,** which joins the oblique fissure at the midaxillary line at about the level of the fourth rib and runs horizontally across the costal surface of the lung to about the level of the fourth costal cartilage; on the medial surface, it passes backward to join the hilus near the upper right pulmonary vein. The left lung is divided into upper and lower lobes by the oblique fissure, which is somewhat more vertically oriented than that of the right lung; there is no horizontal fissure.

The Pulmonary Vessels

There are actually two vascular systems serving the lungs: the *pulmonary circulation,* which delivers deoxygenated blood to the lungs and returns oxygenated blood to the heart; and the *bronchial circulation,* which delivers the nutrient blood supply to the lungs.

The Pulmonary Circulation

The number of pulmonary arteries and veins going to and from the terminal respiratory units is complete at birth.[8] However, the number of vessels within the terminal respiratory units at birth is markedly less than the quantity after the first 10 years of life (their development paralleling that of new primary lobules).

Other changes to the pulmonary arteries occur during growth as well. During gestation, all arterial branches of the pulmonary circulation have relatively thick walls because of the large amount of smooth muscle in their medial layers. Following birth (with the normal lowering of pulmonary vascular resistance), the distal arteries rapidly become thinner, until, by the age of 4 months, they closely resemble those of adult lungs (with respect to muscular content and distribution).[9]

The *pulmonary trunk,* the *right* and *left pulmonary arteries,* and their principal branches down to the (secondary) lobular level are considered to be elastic arteries; the intralobular arteries are of the muscular type. Nonetheless, the muscular arteries have very thin muscular layers (exceeding 5% of the external diameter of the vessel only in pathologic conditions).

The *pulmonary arterioles* have a partial muscular layer near their origins, but this tapers away until the vessel wall consists of only thin endothelium and elastic lamina.[10] The *pulmonary capillaries* form an intermeshed network in the walls and septa of the alveolar ducts and alveoli. The *pulmonary veins* drain the pulmonary capillaries, from which they coalesce to form larger branches, until ultimately they come into proximity with the pulmonary arteries as two pulmonary veins from each lung. The pulmonary veins serve as a relatively low-volume reservoir for the left ventricle, normally obviating the minor fluctuations in right ventricular stroke volume that occur as a result of ventilatory effort.

The right pulmonary artery gives off a large branch to the upper lobe before entering the hilus of the right lung. The continuation of the right pulmonary artery passes between the upper lobe and continuing mainstem bronchi toward the oblique fissure where it branches to the middle and lower lobes. The left pulmonary artery crosses anterior to the left mainstem bronchus toward the posterolateral aspect of the hilus; on entering the lung, it branches first to the upper lobe segments and then to the lower lobe segments. Although the pulmonary veins and arteries closely parallel the main divisions of the bronchi, they assume different relationships at the segmental level. Generally, the pulmonary arteries accompany the bronchi in their segmental divisions. The coalescing tributaries of the pulmonary veins, however, run between the bronchopulmonary segments. In this manner, the tributaries drain adjacent segments, and each segment is drained by more than one vein. The variation in the subsegmental branching of the bronchi, arteries, and veins is considerable, the veins being most variable and the bronchi the least.

The Bronchial Circulation

The bronchial arteries vary significantly in their number and origin. There is typically one right bronchial artery, arising from the right intercostal, right subclavian, or internal mammary arteries. Two left bronchial arteries often arise directly from the upper thoracic aorta. The number of branches entering the root of each lung is variable, but on entry they distribute themselves within the connective tissue surrounding the bronchi in a peribronchial plexus that accompanies each subdivision of the airways down to the level of the terminal bronchioles. Near the terminal bronchioles, the bronchial arterioles form a network of capillaries, which anastomose readily with the capillaries of the pulmonary circulation. Total bronchial blood flow to both lungs is estimated to be approximately 1% to 2% of the cardiac output.

The bronchial veins are frequently considered in two parts: the *deep (distal) bronchial veins* and the *superficial (proximal) bronchial veins.* The deep bronchial veins begin as a network around the terminal bronchioles and form tributaries (sometimes referred to as bronchopulmonary veins)

that join the pulmonary veins. The superficial bronchial veins (true bronchial veins) are formed from tributaries originating around the segmental and lobar bronchi and from pleural branches near the hilus. These bronchial veins drain into the azygos, hemiazygos, or intercostal veins, the blood ultimately reaching the vena cava and returning to the right atrium. Although not directly measured in humans, approximately 25% to 33% of the bronchial arterial supply is returned to the right atrium via the true bronchial veins, and two thirds to three fourths is returned to the left atrium via the pulmonary arteries.[11] The relationship of the bronchial and pulmonary circulations is symbiotic; that is, if the perfusion pressure of one system changes, a concomitant oppositely directed change occurs in the other.[12] The benefit of this reciprocal relationship should be apparent immediately—preservation of viability when either circulation is impaired by disease.

A third circulatory system in the lungs—the *lymphatic circulation*—must also be considered. The lymphatic circulation drains excess fluid from the interstitial spaces and serves as a pathway for the elimination of particulate matter and microorganisms that reach the alveoli. The pulmonary lymphatics reside in the pleural, interseptal, and peribronchiovascular connective tissue spaces where lymphatic capillaries form extensive plexuses. Although further discussion of the lymphatic system is not found here, its importance should not be overlooked; for a detailed discussion, the reader should see Leak and Jamuar.[13]

The Upper Respiratory Tract

The upper respiratory tract (upper airways, Fig. 1–10) extends from the nasal and oral orifices to the false vocal cords in the larynx.

The Nose

The nose is a conglomerate of bone and hyaline cartilage. The nasal bones (right and left), the frontal processes of the maxillae, and the

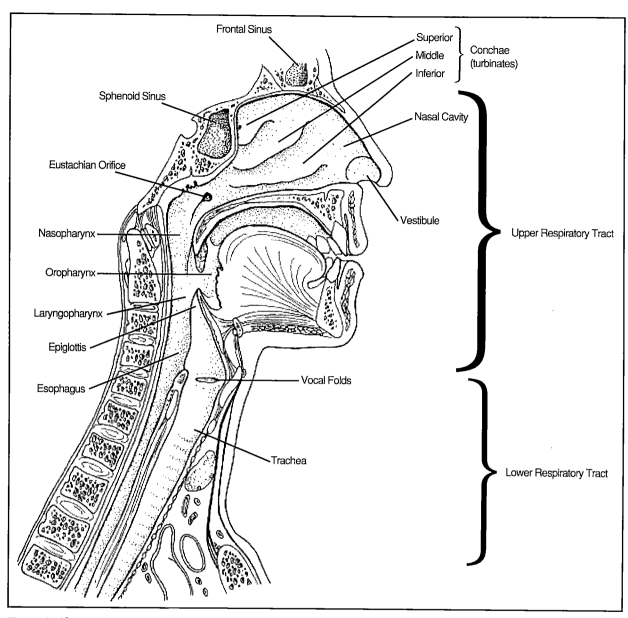

Figure 1-10.

Sagittal section through the head and neck showing the upper respiratory tract and the superior aspect of the lower respiratory tract. (Redrawn from Philo R, Bosner MS, LeMaistre A, et al. Guide to Human Anatomy. Philadelphia, WB Saunders, 1985, p 76.)

nasal part of the frontal bone combine to form the bony framework of the nose. The septal, lateral, and major and minor alar cartilages combine to form the cartilaginous framework of the nose. The periosteal and perichondral mem-branes blend to connect the bones and cartilages to one another.

A small slip of muscle (the **procerus muscle**), originating as a continuation of the occipitofron-talis, attaches to the fascia covering the lower part of the nasal bone and the upper part of the lateral nasal cartilage (this is the muscle that "wrinkles" the skin of the nose). The **nasalis muscles** (the muscles that "flare" the anterior nasal aperture) arise lateral to the nasal notch of the maxilla, spreading into an aponeurosis from its opposite-side counterpart over the bridge of the nose and an aponeurosis from the procerus (the transverse part), as well as attaching to the alar cartilages (the alar part). The **depressor muscle of the septum of the nose** runs from the maxilla above the central incisor tooth to the nasal septum; together with the nasalis, it "flares" the nostrils. Skin covers the external nose.

The Nasal Cavity

The **nasal cavity** is a wedge-shaped passageway divided vertically into right and left halves by the *nasal septum* and compartmentalized by the **paranasal sinuses** (Fig. 1–11). Opening anteriorly via the **nares** (nostrils) to the external environment, the nasal cavity blends posteriorly with the nasopharynx. The two halves are essen-

tially identical, having a floor, medial and lateral walls, and a roof divided into three regions: the *vestibule,* the *olfactory region,* and the *respiratory region.* The primary respiratory functions of the nasal cavity include air conduction, filtration, humidification, and temperature control; it also plays a role in the olfactory process.

The floor of the nasal cavity is formed by the palatine process of the maxilla (anterior three fourths) and the horizontal part of the palatine bone (posterior one fourth). The medial wall is formed by the nasal septum. Three **nasal conchae** project into the nasal cavity from the lateral wall toward the medial wall; they are named the superior, middle, and inferior conchae. The roof is made up of frontonasal, ethmoidal, and sphenoidal parts, which correspond to the bones that form each part.

The *vestibule of the nasal cavity* extends from the nares backward and upward about two thirds of an inch to the **limen nasi** (corresponding to the upper limit of the lower nasal cartilage). The vestibule is lined with skin containing many coarse hairs and sebaceous and sweat glands. Mucous membrane lines the remainder of the nasal cavity. Figure 1–12 depicts various cell

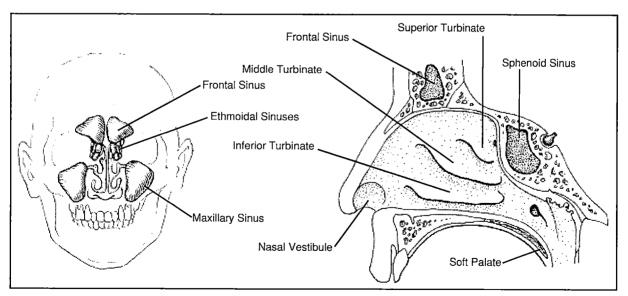

Figure 1–11.

The nasal cavity, the nasopharynx, and the paranasal sinuses. (Redrawn from Philo R, Bosner MS, LeMaistre A, et al. Guide to Human Anatomy. Philadelphia, WB Saunders, 1985, pp 77, 78.)

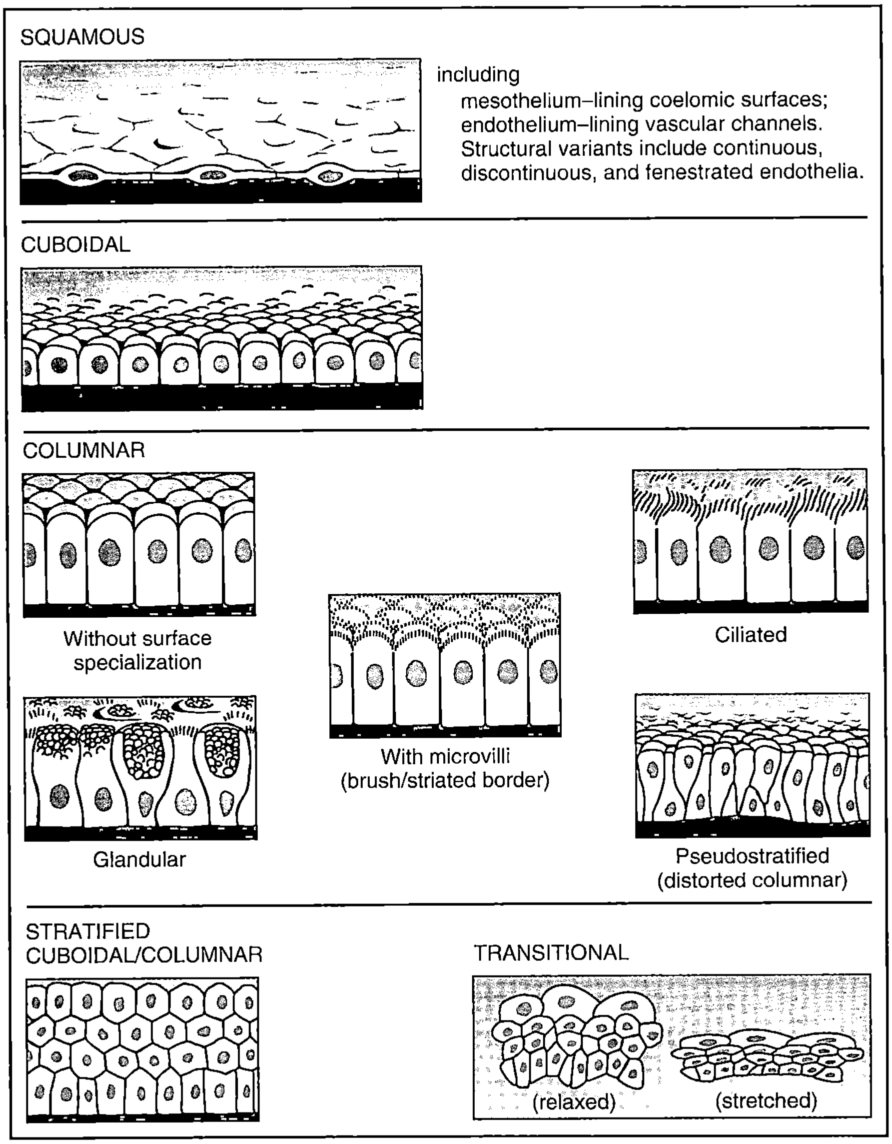

SQUAMOUS

including
mesothelium–lining coelomic surfaces;
endothelium–lining vascular channels.
Structural variants include continuous,
discontinuous, and fenestrated endothelia.

CUBOIDAL

COLUMNAR

Without surface
specialization

With microvilli
(brush/striated border)

Ciliated

Glandular

Pseudostratified
(distorted columnar)

STRATIFIED
CUBOIDAL/COLUMNAR

TRANSITIONAL

(relaxed)   (stretched)

Figure 1-12.

Types of cells comprising the mucosal lining of the upper and lower respiratory tracts. (Modified from Williams PL, Warwick R, Dyson M, Bannister LH [eds]. Gray's Anatomy. 37th ed. New York, Churchill Livingstone, 1989, p 52.)

types of the mucosa covering the upper and lower respiratory tracts.

The *olfactory region of the nasal cavity* is distinguished by the specialized mucosa overlying it in the area of the superior concha—the roof and upper aspect of the septum opposite the superior concha. This pseudostratified olfactory epithelium is thicker than the respiratory mucosa covering the respiratory region of the nasal cavity and is comprised of ciliated receptor cells, nonciliated sustentacular cells, and basal cells.

The rest of the nasal cavity is considered the *respiratory region.* This area, and the paranasal sinuses, is lined with a mixture of columnar or pseudostratified ciliated epithelial cells, goblet cells, nonciliated columnar cells with microvilli, and basal cells. Serous and mucous glands, which open to the surface via branched ducts, underlie the basal lamina of respiratory epithelium.[14]

The submucosal glands and goblet cells secrete an abundant quantity of mucus over the mucosa of the nasal cavity, making it moist and sticky. Turbulent air flow, created by the conchae, causes inhaled dust and other particulate matter larger than about 10 μm to "rain out" onto this sticky layer, which is then moved by ciliary action backward and downward out of the nasal cavity into the nasopharynx at an average rate of about 6 millimeters per minute.[15]

The paranasal sinuses—frontal, ethmoidal, sphenoidal, and maxillary—vary widely in their size and shape from person to person. Their exact function is unknown, and they are not considered further here.

The Pharynx

The pharynx is a musculomembranous tube about 5 to 6 inches long whose upper limit corresponds with the basal surface of the skull and whose lower limit corresponds with a line extending from the sixth cervical vertebra to the lower border of the cricoid cartilage. The pharynx consists of three parts: the nasopharynx, the oropharynx, and the laryngopharynx. These are described briefly, but consideration of the muscles of the pharynx exceeds the scope of this chapter.

Nasopharynx. The nasopharynx is a continuation of the nasal cavity, beginning at the posterior nasal apertures and continuing backward and downward. Its roof and posterior wall are continuous; its lateral walls are formed by the openings of the Eustachian tubes; its floor is formed by the soft palate anteriorly and the **pharyngeal isthmus** (the space between the free edge of the soft palate and the posterior wall of the pharynx), which marks the transition to the oropharynx. The epithelium of the nasopharynx is composed of ciliated columnar cells.

Oropharynx. The oropharynx extends from the soft palate and pharyngeal isthmus superiorly to the upper border of the epiglottis inferiorly. Anteriorly, it is bounded by the oropharyngeal isthmus (which opens into the mouth) and the pharyngeal part of the tongue. The posterior aspect is at the level of the body of the second and upper portion of the body of the third cervical vertebrae. The epithelium in the oropharynx is composed of stratified squamous cells.

Laryngopharynx. The laryngopharynx extends from the upper border of the epiglottis to the inferior border of the cricoid cartilage and the esophagus. The anterior aspect is formed by the laryngeal orifice and the posterior surfaces of the arytenoid and cricoid cartilages. The posterior aspect is at the level of the lower portion of the third, the bodies of the fourth and fifth, and the upper portion of the body of the sixth cervical vertebrae. The epithelium in the laryngopharynx is composed of stratified squamous cells.

The Larynx

The larynx is formed by a cartilaginous framework composed of the thyroid, cricoid, and epiglottic cartilages and the paired arytenoid, cuneiform, and corniculate cartilages. It extends anteriorly from the laryngopharynx, between the great vessels of the neck, downward to the trachea (with which it is continuous). The position of the larynx depends on the age and sex of the individual, being opposite the third to sixth cervical vertebrae in the adult male and somewhat higher in adult females and children. In infants, up to approximately 1 year of age, the highest part of the larynx is a little above the level of the upper aspect of the dens. Further consideration of the structure or the musculature of the larynx is beyond the scope of this chapter.

The cavity of the larynx, extending from the laryngeal inlet to the lower border of the cricoid cartilage, may be divided into three parts: upper, middle, and lower. The vestibular folds separate the upper and middle parts; the vocal folds separate the middle and lower parts.

The laryngeal inlet angles downward from front to back because the anterior wall of the larynx is much longer than the posterior wall; the upper edge of the epiglottis marks its anterior aspect; the **aryepiglottic folds,** formed in the mucosal tissue stretching between the sides of the epiglottis and the apex of the arytenoid cartilage, comprise its lateral borders. The posterior margin is formed by the mucous membrane stretching between the arytenoid cartilages. The laryngeal vestibule extends from the inlet to the vestibular folds. The vestibular folds are thick folds of mucous membrane covering the vestibular ligament, a fibrous band of tissue stretched between an anterior attachment at the angle of the thyroid cartilage just below the level of the epiglottic cartilage that extends to the anterolateral surface of the arytenoids posteriorly.

The middle part of the laryngeal cavity is the smallest, extending from the **rima vestibuli** (the fissure between the vestibular folds) to the **rima glottidis** (the fissure between the vocal folds, commonly called the **glottis**). A fusiform recess, the *sinus of the larynx*, lies between the vestibular and vocal folds. A small pouch—the **saccule of the larynx**—extends upward from the anterior aspect of the sinus. Many mucous glands open into the saccule, which is enclosed in a fibrous capsule receiving a few muscular fasciculi from the thyroepiglottic muscle. The muscles squeeze the sac, expelling its mucus secretions onto the surfaces of the vocal folds, lubricating and nourishing them. The vocal folds are thin folds of mucous membrane stretched between the middle angle of the thyroid cartilage to the vocal processes of the arytenoid cartilages. The epithelial covering of stratified squamous cells is so closely bound to the elastic **vocal ligament** (a continuation of the cricothyroid ligament) that there is no submucosal layer or blood vessels.

The lower part of the laryngeal cavity extends from the vocal folds to the lower border of the cricoid cartilage.

The Lower Respiratory Tract

The lower respiratory tract extends from the level of the true vocal cords in the larynx to the alveoli within the lungs (Fig. 1–13). Generally, the lower respiratory tract may be divided into two parts: the tracheobronchial tree, or conducting airways, and the acinar or terminal respiratory units (Fig. 1–14). As noted earlier, the basic structure of the cartilaginous conducting airways is complete at the time of birth; additional branching does not occur. In fact, although the extent of the process is controversial, the number of nonrespiratory bronchioles may actually decrease up to the age of 3, owing to their conversion by alveolarization into respiratory units.[16,17]

The Tracheobronchial Tree— Conducting Airways

The conducting airways are not involved directly in the exchange of gases in the lungs; they simply conduct air to and from the respiratory units. Airway diameter progressively decreases with each succeeding generation of branching from about 1 inch in diameter at the trachea to 1 millimeter or less at the terminal bronchioles. The cartilaginous "rings" of the larger airways give way to irregular cartilaginous plates, which become smaller and more widely spaced with each generation of branching until they disappear at the bronchiolar level.[18] There may be as many as 16 generations of branching in the conducting airways from the mainstem bronchi to the terminal bronchioles.[19]

Trachea. From the lower margin of the cricoid cartilage the trachea is a tube (about 4 to 4½ inches long and about 1 inch in diameter) extending downward along the midline of the body. As it enters the thorax, it passes behind the left brachiocephalic vein and artery and the arch of the aorta. At its distal end, the trachea deviates slightly to the right of midline before bifurcating into right and left mainstem bronchi. Between 16 and 20 incomplete rings of hyaline cartilage occupy the anterior two thirds of the tracheal circumference, forming a framework for the trachea. Two or more cartilages are often joined together partly or completely. The ring is completed posteriorly, by fibrous and elastic tissues and smooth muscle fibers. The first and last tracheal cartilages differ somewhat from the others, the first being broader and attached by the cricotracheal ligament to the lower border of the cricoid cartilage and the last being thicker and broader at its middle, where it projects a hook-shaped process downward and backward from its lower border—the *carina*—between the two mainstem bronchi.

Mainstem and Lobar Bronchi. The right mainstem bronchus is wider and shorter than its left counterpart and diverges at about a 25-degree angle from the trachea. It passes laterally downward behind the superior vena cava for about 1 inch before giving off its first branch—

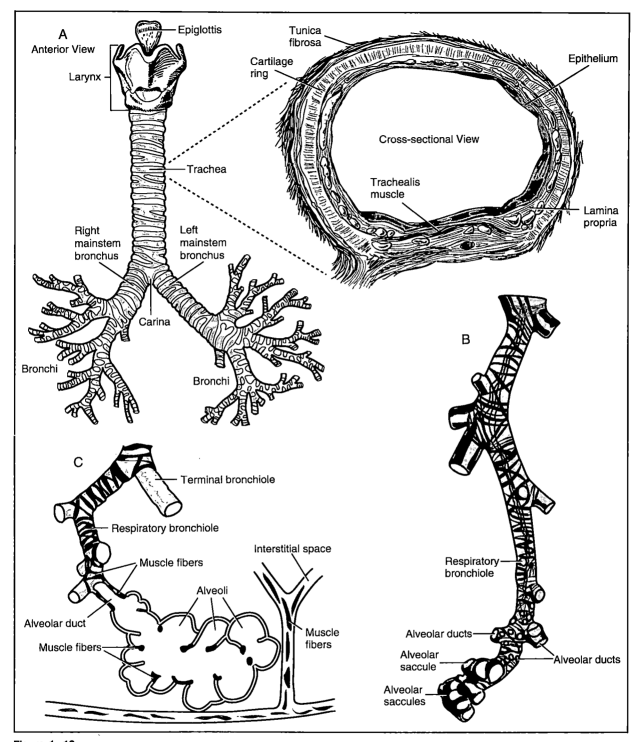

Figure 1-13.

The lower respiratory tract. *A,* The trachea in anterior and cross-sectional views. (Redrawn from Clemente CD. Gray's Anatomy. 30th ed. Philadelphia, Lea & Febiger, 1985, pp 1377, 1378. Redrawn with permission.) *B,* The general distributional scheme of the smaller airways. (Redrawn from Romanes R. Cunningham's Textbook of Anatomy. 11th ed. London, Oxford University Press, 1972, p 496.) *C,* The gross organization of the alveoli and the intimate intertwining meshwork of the capillaries, elastic fibers, and smooth muscle. (Redrawn from Nagaishi C. Functional Anatomy and Histology of the Lung. Baltimore, University Park Press, 1972, p 245.)

25

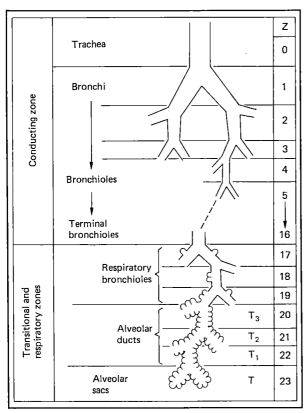

Figure 1–14.

Generational structure of the airways in the human lung. (Reproduced with permission from Weibel ER, Taylor CR. Design and structure of the human lung. In: Fishman AP [ed]. Pulmonary Diseases and Disorders. 2nd ed. New York, McGraw-Hill, 1988, p 13.)

the *upper* (superior) *lobe bronchus*—and entering the root of the right lung. About 1 inch farther, it gives off its second branch—the *middle lobe bronchus*—from within the oblique fissure. Hereafter, the remnant of the mainstem bronchus continues as the *lower* (inferior, basal) *lobe bronchus.*

The left mainstem bronchus leaves the trachea at about a 40-degree to 60-degree angle, passes below the arch of the aorta and behind the left pulmonary artery, and proceeds for little more than 2 inches where it enters the root of the left lung before giving off the *upper* (superior) *lobe bronchus* and continuing on as the *lower* (inferior, basal) *lobe bronchus.* Note that the left lung has no middle lobe: this is a major distinguishing feature in the general architecture of lungs.

Segmental and Subsegmental Bronchi. Each of the lobar bronchi gives off two or more segmental bronchi, an understanding of which is essential to the appropriate assessment and treatment of pulmonary disorders.

The right upper lobe bronchus divides into three segmental bronchi about one-half inch from its own origin. The first—the *apical segmental bronchus*—passes superolaterally toward its distribution in the apex of the lung; the second—the *posterior segmental bronchus*—proceeds slightly upward and posterolaterally to its distribution in the posteroinferior aspect of the upper lobe; the third—the *anterior segmental bronchus*—runs anteroinferiorly to its distribution in the remainder of the upper lobe. The right middle lobe bronchus divides into a *lateral segmental bronchus,* which is distributed to the lateral aspect of the middle lobe, and a *medial segmental bronchus,* which is distributed to the medial aspect of this lobe. The right lower lobe bronchus first gives off a branch from its posterior surface—the *superior segmental bronchus*—which passes posterosuperiorly to its distribution in the upper portion of the lower lobe. Then, after continuing to descend posterolaterally, the lower lobe bronchus yields the *medial basal segmental bronchus* (distributed to a small area below the hilus) from its anteromedial surface. The next offshoots from the lower lobe bronchus are the *anterior basal segmental bronchus,* which continues its descent anteriorly, and a very small trunk that almost immediately splits into the *lateral basal segmental bronchus* (distributed to the lower lateral area of lower lobe) and the *posterior basal segmental bronchus* (distributed to the lower posterior area of the lower lobe).

The left upper lobe bronchus extends laterally from the anterolateral aspect of the left mainstem before dividing into correlates of the right upper and middle lobar bronchi. However, these two branches remain within the left upper lobe, there being no left middle lobe. The uppermost branch ascends for about one third of an inch before yielding the *anterior segmental bronchus,* then continues its upward path as the *apicoposterior segmental bronchus* before subdividing further into its subsegmental distribution. The caudal branch descends anterolaterally to its distribution in the anteroinferior area of the left upper lobe —a region called the *lingula.* This lingular bronchus divides into the *superior lingular* and *inferior lingular segmental bronchi.*

The left lower lobe bronchus descends posterolaterally for about one third of an inch before giving off the superior segmental bronchus from its posterior surface (its distribution is similar to that of the right lower lobe superior segmental bronchus). After another one half to two thirds of an inch, the lower lobe bronchus splits in two. The anteromedial division is called the *anteromedial basal segmental bronchus,* and the posterolateral division immediately branches into the *lateral basal* and *posterior basal segmental bronchi.* The distributions of these segmental bronchi are similar to those of their right lung counterparts.

Many anatomists stop the naming of the segmental branches of the upper division of the left upper lobe at the apicoposterior bronchus, but many others identify its first dichotomous branches as the apical and posterior segmental bronchi. Similarly, the anteromedial basal segmental bronchus of the left lower lobe may be described as separate anterior basal and medial basal segmental bronchi arising from a common trunk. This lack of agreement should not seriously hamper an understanding of the basic segmental distribution of the conducting airways.

The segmental bronchi of both lungs ramify within self-contained, functionally independent bronchopulmonary segments (Fig. 1–15). Each of the bronchopulmonary segments is surrounded by connective tissue continuations of the visceral pleura, forming a separate respiratory unit (the importance of this compartmentalization will become clearer in later chapters that deal with pathologic states and treatment interventions). As the segmental bronchi repeatedly branch downward to bronchiolar size, a **lobular bronchiole** enters a *secondary lobule*—the smallest discrete portion of the lung surrounded by a connective tissue septum. Secondary lobules are pyramid shaped and are about one third to two thirds of an inch in size. The lobular bronchiole immediately divides into five or six terminal bronchioles, each of which in turn subdivides into one to three respiratory bronchioles, marking the transition from conducting airways to respiratory airways. Figure 1–16 depicts a secondary lobule and several terminal respiratory units. Although some disagreement exists regarding the segmental nomenclature down to the level of the terminal bronchiole, little disagreement is heard regarding the terminology used to describe the airways distal to this point. From this point, the terminal respiratory unit begins.

Bronchial Epithelium. The epithelium of the upper regions of the conducting airways is pseudostratified and, for the most part, ciliated. The epithelium of the terminal and respiratory bronchioles is single layered and more cuboidal in shape, and many of the cells are nonciliated. The lamina propria, to which the epithelial basal lamina is attached, contains, throughout the length of the tracheobronchial tree, longitudinal bands of elastin that spread into the elastin network of the terminal respiratory units. The framework thus created is responsible for much of the elastic recoil of the lungs during expiration. At least eight types of cells have been identified in the bronchial epithelium of the human lung (Fig. 1–17).

The most abundant type of cell in the bronchial epithelium is the **ciliated cell.** Ciliated cells are found in all levels of the tracheobronchial tree, down to the level of the respiratory bronchioles. As is discussed elsewhere, the cilia projecting from their luminal surfaces are intimately involved in the removal of inhaled particulate matter from the airways via the "mucociliary escalator" mechanism.

Two of the bronchial epithelial cells secrete mucus: **mucous cells** and **serous cells.** Mucous cells, formerly called goblet cells, are normally more numerous in the trachea and large airways, becoming less numerous with distal progression until they are infrequently found in the bronchioles. Serous cells are much less numerous than mucous cells, being confined predominantly to the extrapulmonary bronchi. Both types of cells are nonciliated, although both exhibit filamentous surface projections.

Ovoid undifferentiated **basal cells** are located on the basement membrane and are responsible for the characteristic pseudostratified appearance of the bronchial epithelium. They are most numerous in the epithelium of the extrapulmonary

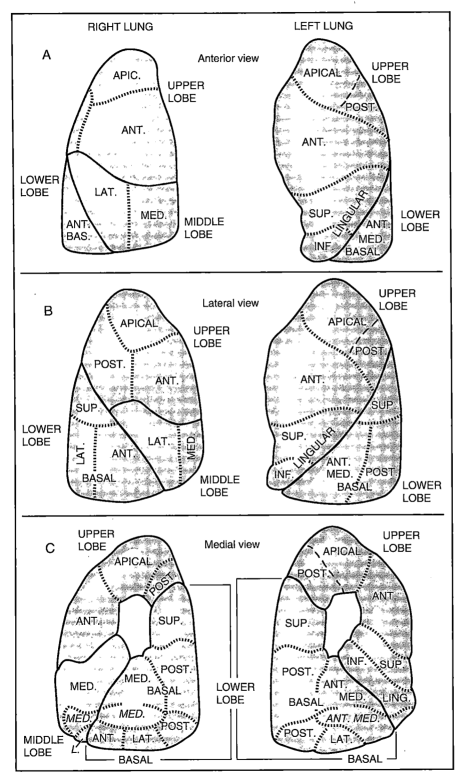

Figure 1–15.

Anterior *(A)*, lateral *(B)*, and medial *(C)* views of the bronchopulmonary segments as seen projected to the surface of the lungs. (Redrawn from Waldhausen JA, Pierce WS [eds]. Johnson's Surgery of the Chest. 5th ed. Chicago, Year Book Medical Publishers, 1985, pp 64, 65.)

Figure 1-16.

Primary lobule arising from one of the five to six terminal bronchioles that enter a secondary lobule.

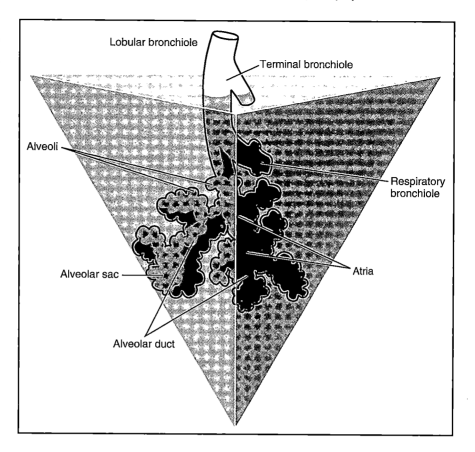

bronchi, although they may be found as far as the bronchioles. Basal cells have no specific function other than to differentiate as needed for the replacement of superficial ciliated or mucous cells. **Intermediate cells** are derived from the basal cells and form a pseudolayer over them. The intermediate cells elongate as they differentiate into ciliated or mucous cells.

Brush cells are also nonciliated but have a distinct brushlike border of microvilli on their luminal surfaces. The function of brush cells is not clearly understood. However, the presence of pinocytotic vesicles at the base of the microvilli is believed to indicate a role in liquid absorption.

Clara's cells are found mostly in the terminal airways. These are nonciliated cells that may be recognized by their cytoplasmic luminal projections, which contain secretory granules and lamellar bodies. Clara's cells have been postulated to be a source of materials present in surfac-

tant.[20] A ciliated or brush cell progenitor function has also been attributed to Clara's cells.[21]

The least abundant epithelial cell type are **Kulchitsky's cells.** These cells are similar to specialized endocrine cells of the gastro-entero-pancreatic system. Because they store and secrete amines, Kulchitsky's cells have been included in the APUD (amine precursor uptake [and] decarboxylation) category of the endocrine system.[21] A possible role in regulation of airway or capillary luminal size in response to acute hypoxia has been suggested for aggregations of apparently innervated Kulchitsky's cells — neuroepithelial bodies — in the bronchial and bronchiolar mucosa.[22]

Two additional cell types normally occur in the bronchial epithelium but are migratory in nature. The **"globular" leukocytes** have numerous filopodia and are thought to derive from mast cells. **Lymphocytes** are the second type of nonnative

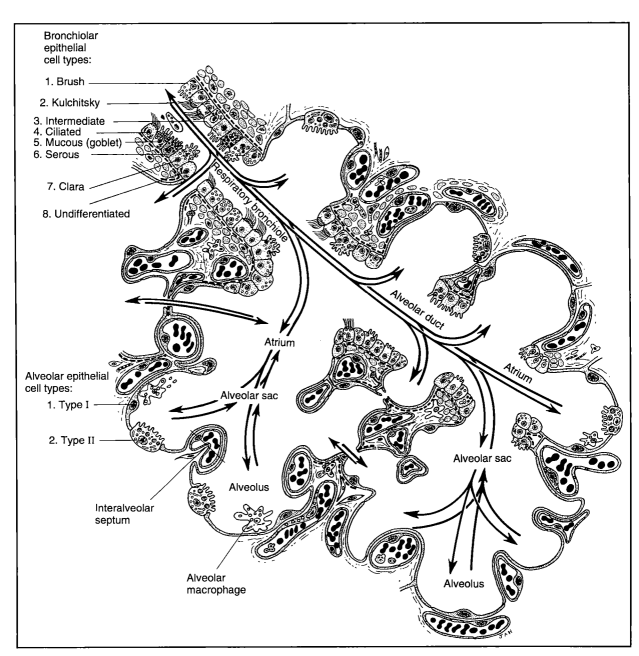

Bronchiolar
epithelial
cell types:

1. Brush
2. Kulchitsky
3. Intermediate
4. Ciliated
5. Mucous (goblet)
6. Serous
7. Clara
8. Undifferentiated

Respiratory bronchiole

Alveolar duct

Atrium

Atrium

Alveolar epithelial
cell types:
1. Type I
2. Type II

Alveolar sac

Alveolar sac

Interalveolar
septum

Alveolus

Alveolus

Alveolar
macrophage

Figure 1–17.

A cross-sectional view of the terminal respiratory unit showing the bronchiolar and alveolar epithelial cell types. (From Williams PL, Warwick R, Dyson M, Bannister LH [eds]. Gray's Anatomy. 37th ed. New York, Churchill Livingstone, 1989, p 1280.)

cell found in the mucosa. Both cell types are thought to have immunologic functions.

A characteristic feature of the submucosal layer underlying the bronchial epithelium is the presence of *bronchial glands,* which are quite numerous in the medium-sized bronchi, becoming less prevalent distally until they are absent in the bronchioles. Submucosal bronchial glands are believed to be parasympathetically innervated and are composed of several cell types, including serous cells, mucous cells, duct cells, lymphocytes, myoepithelial cells, mast cells, and Kulchitsky's cells.[23] The glands are shaped somewhat like a dual-bulbed vase with an inverted, funnellike exit duct at the top; the two "bulbs" are lined with mucous and serous cells.[24] The material that reaches the bronchial lumen from the bronchial glands is a combination of the secretions of the mucous and serous cells.

Terminal Respiratory (Acinar) Units

The respiratory bronchioles, which exhibit small lateral outpouchings — alveoli — that provide an accessory respiratory surface, open into one to three **alveolar ducts,** which lead via expanded *atria* into *alveolar sacs.* The number of alveolar outpouchings increases dramatically with distal progression into the alveolar sacs. The lung tissue supplied by a first-order alveolar duct, together with its vessels and nerves, is called by various authors the primary lobule,[25] the acinus,[26] or the terminal respiratory unit (see Fig. 1–16).[17,27] From a functional standpoint, the primary lobule may be thought of as the terminal respiratory unit because it is where gas exchange occurs. There may be as many as 50 primary lobules within a secondary lobule.

The Alveoli. The normal mature lungs contain an average of 300 million alveoli, each of which is extremely small (between 200 to 300 μm in diameter). Gehr, Bachofen, and Weibel[28] have indicated that the mean total alveolar surface area is about 143 $\pm$ 4 m². The walls of the alveoli consist of a thin epithelial layer over a connective tissue sublayer. The walls of the adjacent alveoli abut one another much like the pieces of a three-dimensional jigsaw puzzle, sandwiching the connective tissue and its associated vascula-

ture between the epithelial layers. The **interalveolar septum** thus formed is comprised of the alveolar epithelium, the capillary endothelium, and the interstitial space. Crapo and co-workers[29] analyzed the proportions of cell types comprising the parenchyma of normal adult lungs and found that alveolar epithelium accounted for approximately 24% of the cell types, capillary endothelium about 30%, macrophages about 9.5%, and interstitium the remaining 36%. The interalveolar septa are interrupted by channels called **Kohn's pores** and **Lambert's canals,** which are postulated to account for a significant collateral alveolar ventilation.[30,31,32]

Alveolar Epithelium. The alveolar epithelium consists of two primary cell types (see Fig. 1–17). **Type I (squamous) pneumocytes,** which cover about 93% of the alveolar surface and account for approximately 8.3% of the total cells of the parenchyma, have very thin, broad extensions projecting from their central bodies. Type I cells contain few cytoplasmic organelles, such as mitochondria. **Type II (granular) pneumocytes** account for approximately 16% of the total cells comprising the parenchyma but occupy only about 7% of the alveolar surface because of their small, cuboidal shape. The importance of type II cells rests in their location (in the "corners" of the alveoli) and in their function. Type II pneumocytes are believed to be the primary producers of the phospholipid film surfactant. Surfactant consists mostly of dipalmitoyl lecithin, a surface-active substance that acts to lower the surface tension of the alveoli as their size decreases during expiration and to increase the surface tension of the alveoli as their size increases during inspiration. This activity is considered further in Chapter 2. The capillary endothelium is a very thin layer of simple squamous cells. These cells perform many nonrespiratory functions (e.g., clearance of emboli and thrombi, exchange of liquids and solutes) in addition to their gas exchange role. Because the capillaries are interwoven throughout the interstitial space, a meshwork of intercommunicating capillaries is formed.

The Alveolar-Capillary Septum (Membrane). As may be seen in Figure 1–18, two distinct portions of the alveolar-capillary membrane are readily identifiable. The thin portion of the sep-

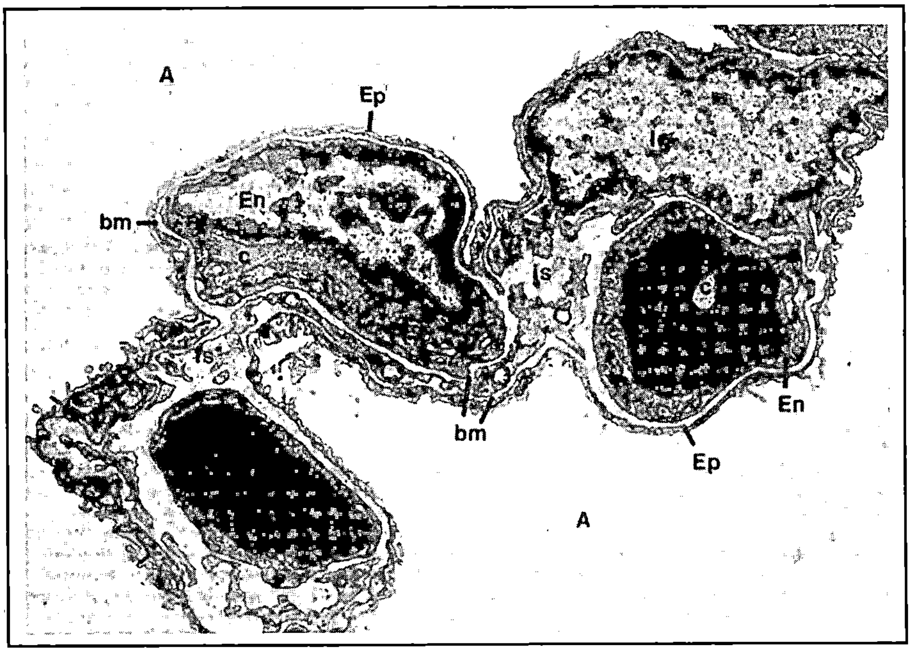

Figure 1–18.

Cross-sectional electron micrograph showing the alveolar-capillary membrane of the normal human parenchyma. Air in the alveolar lumina (A) is separated from the erythrocytes (Ec) in the capillaries (c) by epithelial cells (Ep), basement membranes (bm), endothelial cells (En), and the interstitial space (is). (From Dantzker DR. Cardiopulmonary Critical Care. 2nd ed. Philadelphia, WB Saunders, 1991, p 6. Micrograph courtesy of Theodore F. Beals, M.D., Department of Pathology, University of Michigan.)

tum is where the two basement membranes come into direct contact, giving the appearance of being fused together. This is the primary site for gas exchange, the distance across the membrane being approximately 0.5 μm. The thick portion is where the two basement membranes are separated by an interstitial space filled with fibrocollagenous fibers and rare fibroblasts. Although some gas exchange occurs here, this is the primary site for liquid and solute exchange in the lung.

Innervation of the Lungs

The lungs are invested with a rich supply of afferent and efferent nerve fibers and specialized receptors. Parasympathetic fibers are supplied by preganglionic fibers from the vagal nuclei via the vagus nerves, to ganglia around the bronchi and blood vessels. Postganglionic fibers innervate the bronchial and vascular smooth muscle as well as the mucous cells and submucosal bronchial glands. The parasympathetic postganglionic fibers from thoracic sympathetic ganglia innervate essentially the same structures. Posterior and anterior pulmonary plexuses are formed by

contributions from the postganglionic sympathetic and parasympathetic fibers at the roots of the lungs. For detailed consideration of the innervation of the lungs the reader should see Richardson[33] or Laitinen.[34] Generally, stimulation of the vagus nerve results in bronchial constriction, dilation of pulmonary arterial smooth muscle, and increased glandular secretion. Stimulation of the sympathetic nerves causes bronchial relaxation, constriction of pulmonary arterial smooth muscle, and decreased glandular secretion.[33]

Pulmonary Plexuses. The pulmonary plexuses lie anterior and posterior to the bronchial and vascular structures in the roots of the lungs; the anterior pulmonary plexus is much smaller than the posterior. Nerves from the plexuses form networks around the branches of the bronchi and the pulmonary and bronchial vessels. The *anterior pulmonary plexus* is formed by branches from the vagus nerves and the deep cardiac plexus; the left anterior plexus receives additional fibers from the superficial cardiac plexus. The *posterior pulmonary plexus* is formed by branches from the vagus nerves, the deep cardiac plexus, and the second and fifth thoracic sympathetic ganglia; the left posterior plexus also receives branches from the left recurrent laryngeal nerve.

THE CARDIOVASCULAR SYSTEM

The cardiovascular system consists of the blood vessels and the heart, the primary function of which is the transportation of extracellular fluid (blood) to all parts of the body. The blood vessels form a conduit network, and the heart provides the motive force to circulate the blood through it. Although this chapter considers only the structure of the heart and the principal blood vessels within the thorax, the reader is reminded that the peripheral vascular system comprises a major component of the total cardiovascular system.

The Blood Vessels

Certainly, the anatomic names for the vessels of particular dimension and position are familiar: *arteries, arterioles, capillaries* or *sinusoids, venules,* and *veins.* But, as depicted in Figure 1–19, a functional classification of the vessels must also be considered.

The large arteries leaving the heart and their principal branches contain a significant amount of elastic tissue in their walls (elastic arteries), which changes the intermittent contractions of the heart into a smoother, albeit pulsatile, flow of blood. The smaller arterial branches, although still exhibiting elastance, contain increasing amounts of nonstriated muscle in their walls (muscular arteries). The controlled contraction or relaxation of these muscular walls permits a variable distribution of the overall blood flow to the other organ systems in accordance with their fluctuating physiologic needs. Thus, the elastic and muscular arteries may collectively be thought of as *distributing vessels.*

The muscular walls of the arterioles and precapillary sphincters provide an even more delicate control of the flow of blood through the various tissues. These are also the primary source of the peripheral resistance to blood flow and may, therefore, be referred to as *resistance ves-*

sels. As is discussed in more detail in Chapter 2, these vessels, together with the volume of cardiac output, determine the arterial blood pressure.

Because the exchange of gases, nutrients, metabolic products, and the like occurs across the walls of the capillaries, sinusoids, and postcapillary venules they may be referred to collectively as *exchange vessels.* The larger venules and veins form a large, variable-volume and low-pressure reservoir, referred to as the *capacitance vessels.*

Structure of the Vessels

It is generally accepted that despite dimensional and ultrastructural differences in the various parts of the system, one common structural component is ubiquitous—a single layer of smooth endothelial cells. Furthermore, all vessels larger than capillaries present zones of organized tissue, which surround their endothelial lining. Although the organization of these zones varies with respect to the function of the vessels, three zones are recognized in the vessel walls. From the outside inward, they are named the **adventitia,** the **media,** and the **intima.** Figure 1–20 demonstrates the structural features of a typical blood vessel.

The outermost zone of the vessel wall—the adventitia—is a connective tissue coat with a primarily longitudinal organization. The larger vessels are supplied by their own nutrient blood vessels, the **vasa vasorum,** which permeate the adventitia to supply it and the outer part of the media. The rest of the vessel (or smaller vessels) obtains its nutritional supply by means of diffusion from the blood in the lumen of the vessel. A fenestrated **external elastic lamina** underlies the adventitia. The media, a circumferentially organized fibromuscular zone, lies between the external elastic lamina and the **internal elastic lamina.** In the coronary arteries, the internal elastic lamina is abutted by a thick layer of longitudinal muscle and fibrous tissue. This arrangement is thought to permit the vessels to accommodate to the significant length changes that occur throughout the cardiac cycle. The intima is a single layer of longitudinally oriented

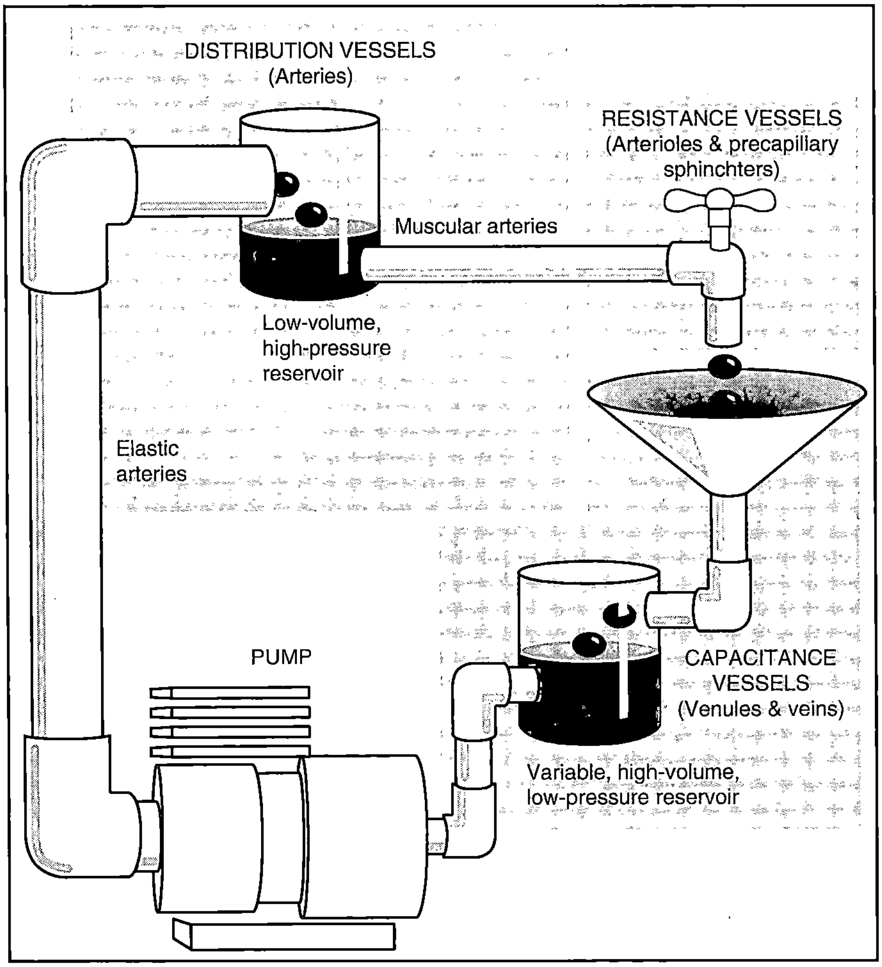

Figure 1-19.

Functional depiction of the vascular system as distribution, resistance, and capacitance vessels.

DISTRIBUTION VESSELS
(Arteries)

RESISTANCE VESSELS
(Arterioles & precapillary sphinchters)

Muscular arteries

Low-volume, high-pressure reservoir

Elastic arteries

PUMP

CAPACITANCE VESSELS
(Venules & veins)

Variable, high-volume, low-pressure reservoir

endothelial cells that rests on a delicate layer of subendothelial connective tissue.

Because venous pressure is so much lower, there are fewer muscle cells and elastic fibers in the media of the veins. Therefore, the major difference between the veins and the arteries lies in the comparative weakness of the media of the veins. Furthermore, most veins have valves that prevent the retrograde flow of blood (as shown in Fig. 1–21).

Reference is frequently made to the "great vessels." These are the vena cavae (superior and inferior), the pulmonary trunk and right and left pulmonary arteries, and the aorta.

The Heart

The relationship of the heart to the anterior thoracic wall depends on the size of the individual and the position of the body. Nonetheless, the average projections are seen in Figure 1–22. Clinically, the **base of the heart** is related to the second intercostal space, parasternally. The **apex of the heart** projects into the fifth intercostal space at the midclavicular line. A radiograph of the chest (Fig. 1–23) shows the right atrium, the superior vena cava, the aortic knob, the pulmonary artery, the left atrial appendage, and the left ventricle. Approximately one third of the heart lies to the right of the midline and two thirds to the left.

The heart is contained in a **pericardial sac** within the mediastinum. The pericardial sac actually consists of an outer sac, the *fibrous pericardium*, and a double-layered inner sac, the *serous pericardium*. The fibrous pericardium is a bag of collagenous fibrous tissue, the mouth of which blends with the adventitia of the great vessels as they enter and exit the heart. The bottom of this bag is attached to the central tendon and to a small portion of the left half of the diaphragm.

Because it is a closed sac surrounding the heart and lining the fibrous pericardium, the serous pericardium consists of a *visceral layer* and a *parietal layer.* The visceral layer, also known as the epicardium, intimately covers the heart and the great vessels from which it is reflected to form the parietal layer lining the fibrous pericardium. Where the visceral layer covers the great vessels, it forms two tubes. The aorta and the pulmonary trunk are enclosed in one of the tubes; the superior and inferior vena cavae and the pulmonary veins are enclosed in the second tube, forming a

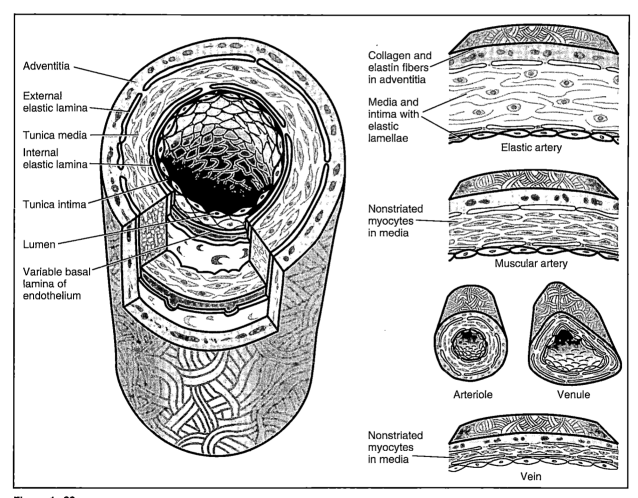

Figure 1–20.

The principal structural features of the larger blood vessels. (Redrawn from Williams PL, Warwick R, Dyson M, Bannister LH [eds]. Gray's Anatomy. 37th ed. New York, Churchill Livingstone, 1989, p 685.)

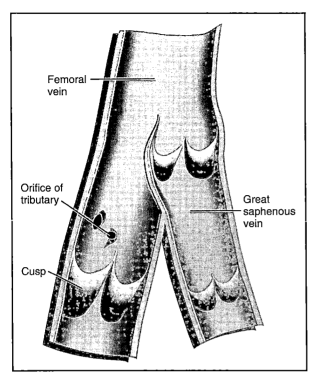

Figure 1–21.

Valves inside the upper portions of the great saphenous and femoral veins, illustrated here at approximately two thirds their natural size. (Redrawn from Williams PL, Warwick R, Dyson M, Bannister LH [eds]. Gray's Anatomy. 37th ed. New York, Churchill Livingstone, 1989, p 691.)

cul-de-sac behind the left atrium known as the **oblique sinus.** The space formed between the aorta and the pulmonary trunk is called the **transverse sinus.**

External Features

The heart is shaped like a somewhat deformed pyramid lying obliquely in the chest behind the body of the sternum and the adjoining costal cartilages and ribs. The base of the pyramid faces posteriorly and toward the right, forming the anatomic base of the heart. The apex of the pyramid points anteriorly and toward the left, forming the anatomic apex of the heart. Because of this oblique orientation and because the pyramid is distorted, precise definition of its surfaces and intervening "margins" becomes problematic. Furthermore, terminology arising from widespread

clinical usage also obfuscates the issue of nomenclature. Throughout the remainder of this description, an attempt is made to use official terminology[35] for these features and to give their common clinical correlate in parentheses. Thus, the heart may be described as having a base (posterior surface) and an apex; upper, inferior (acute), and left (obtuse) margins; and sternocostal (anterior), diaphragmatic (inferior), right, and left (pulmonary) surfaces.

Figure 1–24 illustrates the base and the diaphragmatic surface of the heart. As may be seen, all the great veins enter the heart at its base, which is formed principally by the **left atrium** but includes the **right atrium** to the right margin of the heart. (Do not confuse this anatomic base of the heart with the "clinical base" referred to during auscultation as underlying the parasternal area at the second intercostal space). The area of the heart from the base to the apex is the *diaphragmatic surface*, which consists chiefly of the

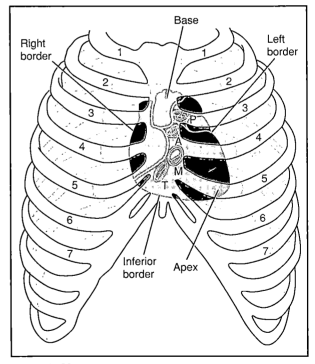

Figure 1–22.

Relationship of the heart and the principal valves to the overlying rib cage. A, aortic valve; M, mitral valve; P, pulmonary valve; T, tricuspid valve.

Figure 1–23.

A normal mediastinal profile as seen on a posteroanterior radiograph of the chest. 1, Superior vena cava as in a young adult and as in the elderly; 2, ascending aorta as in a young adult and as in the elderly; 3, right atrium; 4, inferior vena cava (not always seen); 5, left subclavian vein and artery; left common carotid artery; 6, aortic knob (arch); 7, main pulmonary artery; 8, left atrium (not always seen); 9, left ventricle; 10, cardiac fat pad (not always seen). (From Kersten LD. Comprehensive Respiratory Nursing: A Decision Making Approach. Philadelphia, WB Saunders, 1989, Fig. 15–35, p 428.)

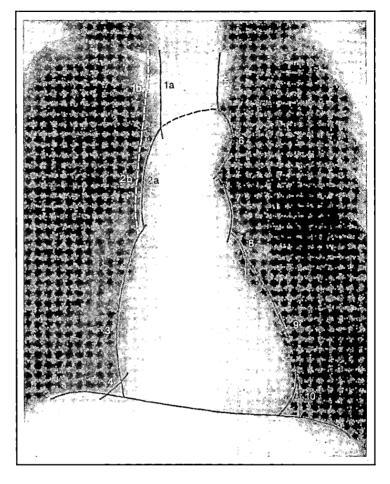

left ventricle. Passing between the inferior vena cava and the right margin of the heart, the coronary sulcus separates the left atrium from the left ventricle (where the specialized cells of the **coronary sinus** are located) as it courses upward toward the left (obtuse) margin of the heart.

Figure 1–25 illustrates the sternocostal (anterior) surface of the heart. On crossing the left (pulmonary) surface of the heart, the coronary sulcus may be seen as it passes between the *left auricle* and the left ventricle to end at the root of the pulmonary trunk. The coronary sulcus may also be seen here as it passes from the root of the aorta to separate the right atrium from the right ventricle on its way toward the inferior vena cava. The **anterior interventricular sulcus** is shown separating the right from the left ventricles.

The Cardiac Vessels. The aorta is described in sections for convenience. Within the fibrous pericardium, the **ascending aorta** begins at the base of the left ventricle and is about 2 inches long. From the lower border of the third costal cartilage at the left of the sternum, it passes upward and forward toward the right as high as the second right costal cartilage. The aorta exhibits three dilations above the attached margins of the cusps of the aortic valve at the root of the aorta: the **aortic sinuses** (of Valsalva). The sinuses extend beyond the level of the free borders of the cusps, as indicated by the **supravalvular ridge.** The coronary arteries (Fig. 1–26) open near this ridge from the sinuses of their origin, the left being typically a little lower than the right. The **arch of the aorta** continues from about the level of second costosternal articulation

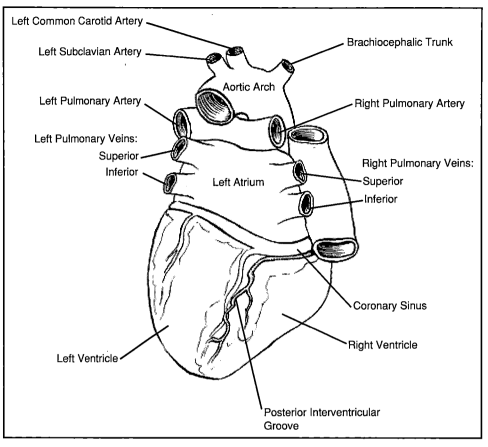

Figure 1-24.

View of the diaphragmatic (posterior) surface of the heart, illustrating the external features. (Redrawn from Philo R, Bosner MS, LeMaistre A, et al. Guide to Human Anatomy. Philadelphia, WB Saunders, 1985, p 166.)

in an upward, a backward, and a leftward orientation, arching to pass in front of the trachea on its downward turn along the left side of the fourth thoracic vertebral body and proceeding to the level of the left second costal cartilage, from which point it is known as the **descending aorta.** Three branches typically arise from the upper aspect of the arch: the **brachiocephalic trunk** (innominate artery), the **left common carotid artery,** and the **left subclavian artery.**

The **right coronary artery** arises from the right anterolateral surface of the aorta and passes between the auricular appendage of the right atrium and the pulmonary trunk, typically giving off a branch to the sinus node and yielding two

or three **right anterior ventricular rami** as it descends in the coronary sulcus to curve around the right (acute) margin of the heart into the posterior aspect of the sulcus. As the right coronary artery crosses the right margin of the heart, it gives off the **right** (acute) **marginal artery** before continuing as far as the posterior interventricular sulcus, where it usually turns to supply the diaphragmatic surfaces of the ventricles as the **posterior interventricular** (posterior descending) **artery.** In about 80% of hearts, an **atrioventricular nodal artery** is given off just before the posterior interventricular artery.[36]

The **left coronary artery** originates from the left anterolateral aspect of the aorta and generally splits into two smaller branches while still behind the pulmonary trunk, the anterior interventricular and the circumflex arteries (in about 35% of hearts, a sinuatrial artery is given off at this point[36]). The **anterior interventricular** (anterior descending) **artery** traverses the anterior interventricular groove to supply sternocostal aspects of both ventricles. In its course, the anterior interventricular artery gives off right and left anterior ventricular and anterior septal branches. The larger left anterior ventricular branches vary in number from two to nine, the first being designated the **diagonal artery.** The **circumflex artery** runs in the coronary sulcus between the left atrium and ventricle, crosses the left margin of

the heart, and usually continues to its termination, just short of the junction of the right coronary and the posterior interventricular arteries. In many instances, as the circumflex crosses the left margin of the heart it gives off a large branch — the **left marginal** (obtuse) **artery**—which supplies this area.

The right coronary artery is the primary supply route for blood to the majority of the right ventricle and the posterior portion of the left ventricle in 80% to 90% of human hearts. Less typically, instead of the right coronary artery, a continuation of the circumflex artery yields the posterior interventricular arterial branches and the branch to the atrioventricular node, consti-

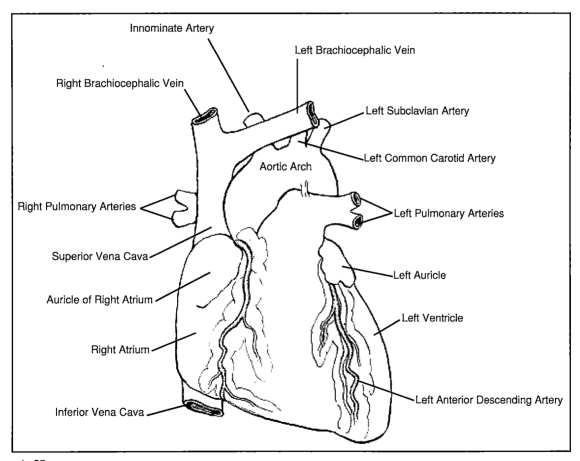

Figure 1–25.

View of the sternocostal (anterior) surface of the heart, illustrating the external features. (Redrawn from Philo R, Bosner MS, LeMaistre A, et al. Guide to Human Anatomy. Philadelphia, WB Saunders, 1985, p 165.)

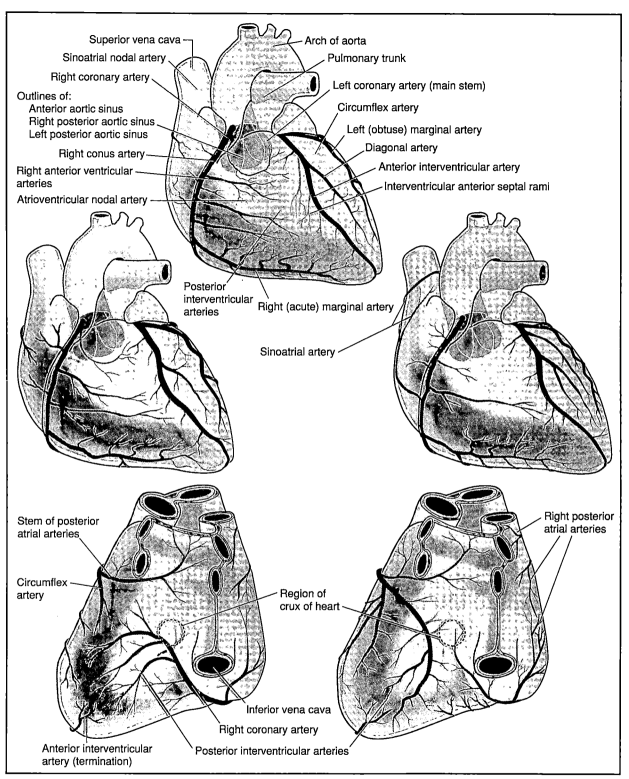

Figure 1–26.

Typical distributions of the right and left coronary arteries. (Redrawn from Williams PL, Warwick R, Dyson M, Bannister LH [eds]. Gray's Anatomy. 37th ed. New York, Churchill Livingstone, 1989, pp 728, 729.)

tuting a so-called **left dominant coronary arterial system**. Ascribing dominance to either of the coronary arteries implies that the "dominant" artery provides the majority of the blood supply to the tissues of the heart. In about 50% of hearts, there is more blood flow attributable to the right coronary artery than the left; in about 30% of hearts, the blood flow is equally distributed between the two coronary arteries; and in 20% the left coronary artery supplies the dominant blood flow.

The pulmonary trunk runs upward and backward (first in front of and then to the left of the ascending aorta) from the base of the right ventricle; it is about 2 inches in length. At the level of the fifth thoracic vertebra, it splits into right and left pulmonary arteries. The **right pulmonary artery** runs behind the ascending aorta, superior vena cava, and upper pulmonary vein but in front of the esophagus and right primary bronchus to the root of the lung. The **left pulmonary artery** runs in front of the descending aorta and the left primary bronchus to the root of the left lung. It is attached to the arch of the aorta by the ligamentum arteriosum.

The pulmonary veins, unlike the systemic veins, have no valves. They originate in the capillary networks and ultimately join together to form two veins from each lung—a **superior pulmonary vein** and an **inferior pulmonary vein**—which open separately into the left atrium.

The superior vena cava is about 3 inches long from its termination in the upper part of the right atrium opposite the third right costal cartilage to the junction of the two brachiocephalic veins. The inferior vena cava extends from the junction of the two common iliac veins, in front of the fifth lumbar vertebra, passing through the diaphragm to open into the lower portion of the right atrium. The vena cavae have no valves.

The cardiac veins are considered as three groups: the coronary sinus and its supplying veins, the anterior cardiac veins, and the thebesian veins. Most of the veins of the heart drain into the coronary sinus, which runs in the posterior aspect of the coronary sulcus and empties through the valve of the coronary sinus—a semilunar flap—into the right atrium between the opening of the inferior vena cava and the

tricuspid valve. As shown in Figure 1–27, the coronary sinus is fed by the **small cardiac vein** and the **middle cardiac vein,** the **posterior vein of the left ventricle,** the **left marginal vein,** and the **great cardiac vein.**

The **anterior cardiac veins** are fed from the anterior part of the right ventricle. They originate in the subepicardial tissue, crossing the coronary sulcus as they terminate directly into the right atrium. The **right marginal vein** runs along the right border of the heart and usually opens directly into the right atrium. Occasionally, it may join the small cardiac vein.

The **thebesian veins** (venae cordis minimae) vary greatly in their number and size. These tiny veins open into all the cavities of the heart but are most numerous in the right atrium and ventricle, occasional in the left atrium, and rare in the left ventricle.

Internal Features

The Right Atrium. The chamber of the right atrium (Fig. 1–28) consists of two parts: (1) a smooth-walled posterior part and (2) a thin-walled trabecular anterior part. A muscular ridge, the **crista terminalis,** separates the two parts as it passes in front of and along the right side of the superior vena caval orifice from the upper part of the atrial septum, extending downward to the right side of the inferior vena caval orifice, and connects to the right side of the valve of the inferior vena cava. Muscular ridges, the **pectinate muscles,** run from the crista terminalis across the anterior wall forming an interconnected network of tissue that continues into the superior part of the atrium. This upper anterior part of the chamber forms a small, muscular, conical appendage—the *auricle*—which projects toward the left to overlap the right side of the root of the ascending aorta. The trabeculated free wall of the atrium is a vestige of the embryonic right atrium.

The superior vena cava enters the right atrium, without a valve, in the upper posterior region. The inferior vena cava opens into the lowest part of the atrium near the interatrial septum, its orifice being associated with the *valve of the inferior vena cava*. The coronary sinus opens into the

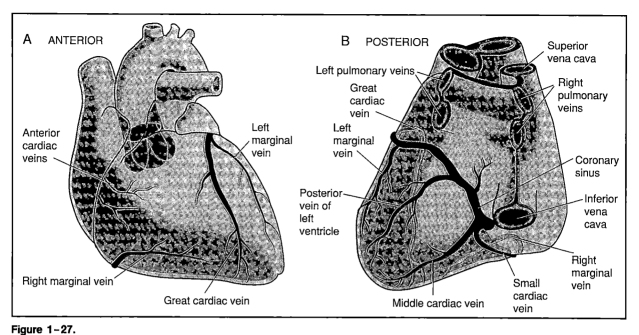

Figure 1-27.

Anterior **(A)** and posterior **(B)** view of typical distributions of the major cardiac veins.

right atrium between the inferior vena cava and the atrioventricular orifice; its orifice is also guarded by a thin *valve of the coronary sinus*. The valves of the inferior vena cava and the coronary sinus are inconsistent and are remnants of the embryonic right venous valve.

The posteromedial wall of the atrium is formed by the **interatrial septum**. Above and to the left of the inferior vena caval orifice, on the lower central portion of the septal wall, is an ovoid depression—the **fossa ovalis**.

Tricuspid Valve Apparatus. The atrioventricular valves cannot be considered as isolated structures; each is, instead, an integrated complex of structures comprised of the valvular orifice and its associated annulus, the valve leaflets, the chordae tendineae, and the papillary muscles (which are addressed with their associated ventricle).

The orifice of the tricuspid valve (see Fig. 1–28) is more a transition into the valvular leaflets than a distinct demarcation between the atrial walls and the bases of the leaflets. As such, the "orifice" is apparent only after dissection of the leaflets. To complicate matters further, the shape

of the orifice has been variously described as circular, ovoid, or almost triangular; if the naming of the valve leaflets is any indication, it would seem that the consensus tends toward the triangularity of the orifice. Clearly, the age, health status, and method of preparation of the specimen has influenced the description of the valve opening.

Some texts suggest that the orifices of the ventricular inflow and outflow tracts are surrounded by uniform collagenous rings to which the bases of the valve leaflets are attached. However, the annulus of the tricuspid valve is little more than a token of connective tissue that varies greatly in its deposition at different regions of the circumference of the orifice. The tricuspid annulus is joined, as are the annuli of the other inflow and outflow orifices, to a dense, membranous and collagenous framework of tissue—the fibroelastic "skeleton"—which lies roughly in the plane of the coronary sulcus. Although the tricuspid atrioventricular orifice and the tissues composing the annulus do not actually lie in a singular plane, their approximate orientation is almost vertical at about 45 degrees to the sagittal plane.

There are typically three **valve leaflets** (thus the name of the valve), named the *septal,* the *anterior* (posterolateral), and the *posterior,* which correspond to similarly named sectors of attachment at the orifice. The leaflets present three

distinct topographic and histologic regions: the *basal region,* extending about one tenth of an inch from the basal attachment of the leaflet, is vascularized and relatively thick and is often invested with some atrial myocardial cells; the *clear*

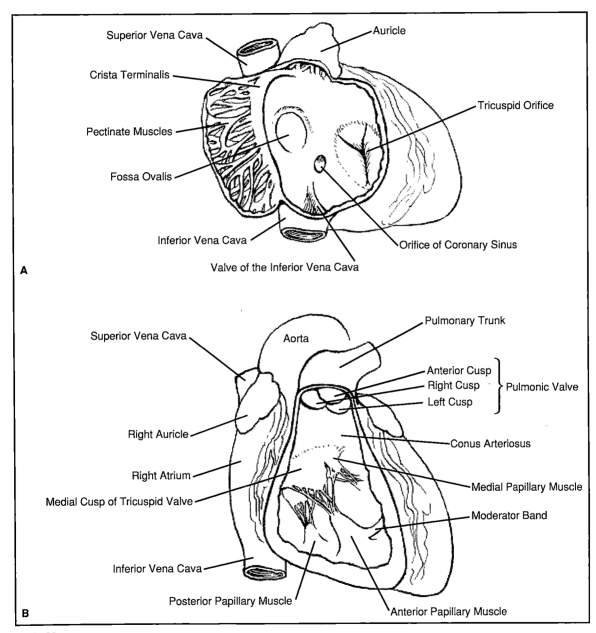

Figure 1-28.

Inside view of the right atrium *(A)* and right ventricle *(B).* **(Redrawn from Philo R, Bosner MS, LeMaistre A, et al. Guide to Human Anatomy. Philadelphia, WB Saunders, 1985, pp 166, 167.)**

region is thin and smooth, almost translucent, with few attachments of chordae; the *rough region* is thickened and roughened, especially on the ventricular side, which receives the insertions of most of the chordae tendineae.

The **chordae tendineae** are fibrous collagenous cords: the *true chordae*, spanning the gap between the papillary muscles and the valve leaflets, and the *false chordae*, passing from the papillary muscles to one another or to the ventricular walls. As may be seen in Figure 1–29, there are five primary classes of chordae: *fan-shaped, rough zone, free edge, deep,* and *basal.*[37,38] The radiating branches of the fan-shaped chordae project outward from a single stem attaching to the margins of the interleaflet commissures. Rough chordae also arise from a single stem but split into three filaments: one attaches at the free margin of the leaflet, another attaches to the ventricular aspect of the leaflet at the boundary of the rough region; the third attaches to some intermediate position. Free-edge chordae are single strands that usually arise from the papillary muscle and attach near the middle of scalloped free margin of a leaflet. The deep chordae attach to the more peripheral parts of the rough region and even to the clear region. Basal chordae arise directly from the ventricular wall to insert into the basal regions of the leaflets.

The Right Ventricle. The right ventricle (see Fig. 1–28), like the right atrium, may be considered in two parts: (1) a posteroinferior inflow tract, which contains the tricuspid valve, and (2) an anterosuperior outflow tract, from which the pulmonary trunk arises. The **supraventricular crest** marks the transition between these portions superiorly, and the **septomarginal trabecula** (also known as the *moderator band*) forms the boundary anteroinferiorly near the apex of the ventricle. The cavity of the right ventricle is crescent shaped in transverse section.

The walls of the inflow tract are heavily trabeculated, especially so at the apical aspect. These **trabeculae carneae** form irregular muscular ridges or bands of variable thickness, which project into the cavity of the ventricle. Some of the trabeculae are simple ridges; others are fixed to the septal or ventricular walls only by their

ends; and still others, the **papillary muscles,** are attached only at their bases to the walls of the ventricle, their apices extending into the ventricular cavity and becoming continuous with the chordae tendineae. The chordae tendineae are collagenous cords, which, with the papillary muscles, are part of the tricuspid valve. The *anterior papillary muscle* is fairly consistent in its origin from the inferior aspect of the moderator band. The *posterior papillary muscle* arises at the apical ventriculoseptal juncture. The *medial* or *septal papillary muscle(s)* are variable and less prominent.

The outflow tract of the right ventricle (**conus arteriosus** or **infundibulum**) has only a few trabeculae, the subpulmonic region being smooth walled. It is possible that these smooth walls increase the velocity of the ventricular stroke volume during systole. The outflow tract is a vestige of the embryonic bulbus cordis.

The Pulmonary Valve. The plane of the pulmonary valve (see Figs. 1–28 and 1–30) faces superiorly, toward the left, and slightly backward, lying somewhat anterior and superior to the other principal valves. There are three *cusps* attached at their convexities to the thickened, triple-scalloped, fibrous annulus at the junction of the pulmonary trunk and the right ventricle. The cusps of the valve are named anterior (left, left anterior), left (posterior), and right. The **Nomina Anatomica** names of the cusps relate to the embryonic positions of the cusps before the leftward rotation of the heart; the names in parentheses relate to the approximate in situ positions of the cusps in the normal adult heart.

The Left Atrium. Although the volume of the left atrium (Fig. 1–31) is smaller than that of the right, the atrial walls are much thicker. The essentially smooth cavity and walls are largely formed by the proximal parts of the pulmonary veins, which are assimilated during the development of the atrium. The pulmonary veins open into the upper aspect of the posterior surface of the left atrium, typically two on each lateral border. There may occasionally be three pulmonary veins joining on the right and sometimes only one on the left.

The generally smooth septal surface of the atrium presents an irregularly curved impression

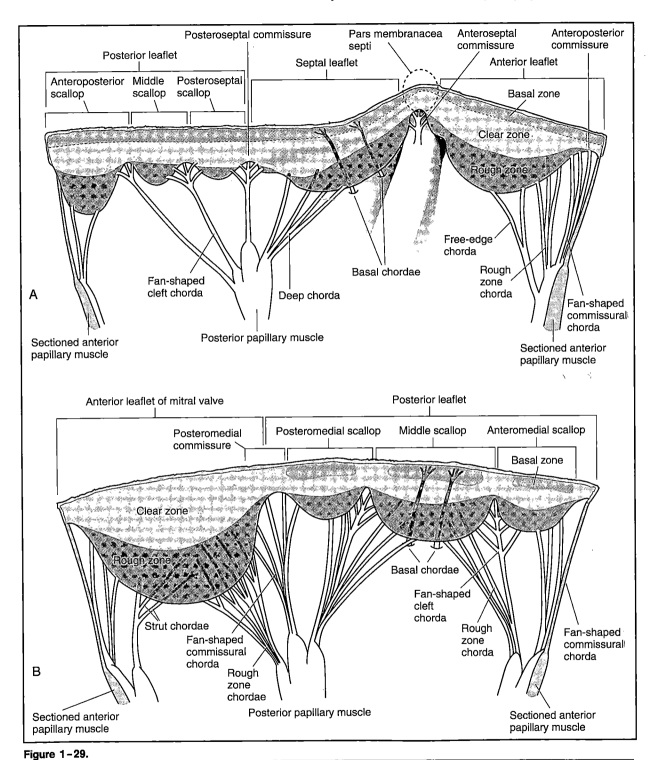

Figure 1–29.

The tricuspid *(A)* **and mitral** *(B)* **valves laid open to show the regions of the leaflets to which the five types of chordae tendineae attach. (Redrawn from Williams PL, Warwick R, Dyson M, Bannister LH [eds]. Gray's Anatomy. 37th ed. New York, Churchill Livingstone, 1989, pp 708, 709.)**

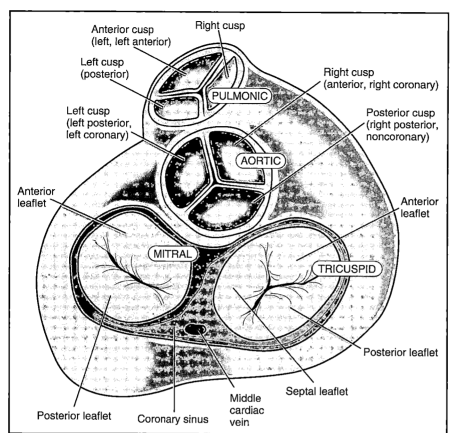

Figure 1-30.

Nomenclature for the leaflets and cusps of the principal valves of the heart.

—the *valve of the foramen ovale*—that corresponds to the embryonic septum primum, covering the ostium secundum. The left upper anterior portion of the atrium constricts slightly at its union with the *left auricle,* which is longer and narrower than the right auricle. Pectinate muscles cover the inner surface of the auricle. With careful inspection, numerous openings of the thebesian veins, which allow blood to return directly from the myocardium, may be found on the walls of the atrium.

The *left atrioventricular orifice* is smaller than that of the tricuspid orifice. It lies almost vertically in the left anteroinferior aspect of the atrium at 45 degrees to the sagittal plane. Although almost in the same plane as the tricuspid orifice, the mitral orifice lies more superiorly and posteriorly; in relation to the aortic valve, it is posteroinferior and offset to the left.

The Mitral Valve Apparatus. Much of the description of the tricuspid valve apparatus is applicable to that of the mitral valve apparatus (see Fig. 1-29 and 1-30). Like the tricuspid annulus, the mitral valve annulus is not a continuous ring of fibrous tissue; it becomes continuous with the laminae fibrosae of the valve leaflets and varies greatly in the consistency of its deposition. The annuli are discussed further in a later consideration of the fibroskeleton of the heart.

The mitral valve leaflets are typically described as being two in number.[38,39,40] However, they may be viewed more correctly as a continuous curtain, with several indentations (receiving the fan-shaped chordae) along the free edge, circumscribing the entire mitral orifice.[41] Two of the indentations are deep and typically present in consistent positions—the anterolateral and posteromedial commissures—which give the appearance of dividing the curtain into an *anterior* and a *posterior leaflet*. The anterior (anteromedial, aortic, septal) leaflet of the mitral valve has no basal zone, the clear region extending to the annulus. The posterior (ventricular, mural, posterolateral) leaflet has the same basal, clear, and rough zones as described for the tricuspid leaflets.

The chordae tendineae are generally the same as those of the tricuspid apparatus. However, the true chordae may be divided into commissural and leaflet categories. The *leaflet chordae* of the

Figure 1-31.

Inside view of the left atrium *(A)* and left ventricle *(B)*. (Redrawn from Philo R, Bosner MS, LeMaistre A, et al. Guide to Human Anatomy. Philadelphia, WB Saunders, 1985, pp 168, 169.)

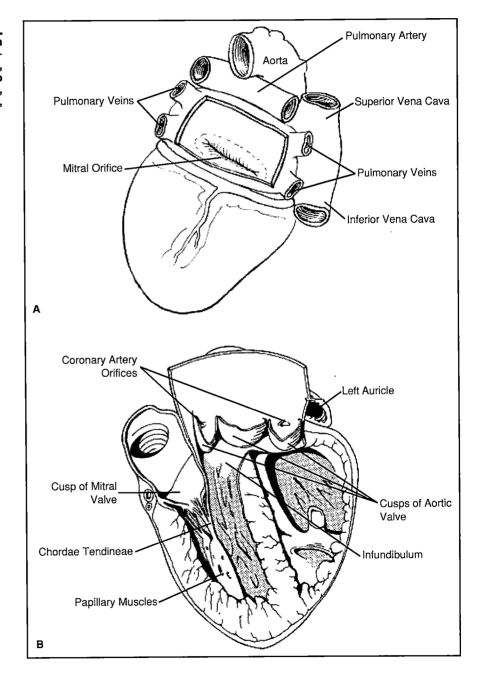

anterior leaflet are rough zone chordae with specialized variants—the *strut chordae.* The leaflet chordae of the posterior leaflet include rough zone, fan-shaped, and basal chordae. The *commissural chordae* arise from their corresponding papillary muscles. The branches of the posteromedial commissural chordae are longer and thicker than those of the anterolateral ones. The papillary muscles are considered in the discussion of the left ventricle.

The Left Ventricle. The almost conical left ventricle (see Fig. 1–31) is longer and narrower than the right ventricle. The walls of the left ventricle are about three times thicker than those of the right, and the transverse aspect of the cavity is almost circular. In contrast to the inflow and outflow orifices of the right ventricle, those of the left are located adjacent to each other, being separated only by the anterior leaflet of the mitral valve and the common fibrous ridge to which it and the left and posterior cusps of the aortic valve are attached.

The interventricular septum forms the anterolateral wall of the left ventricle and is about the same thickness as the rest of the ventricle except near the aortic valve. The **limbus marginalis** makes a clear demarcation between the muscular septum and a rounded, thin, collagenous area—the *membranous septum*—immediately below the right and posterior cusps of the aortic valve. The trabeculae carneae of the left ventricle are more stout than those of the right ventricle but present the same three types. They are particularly dense toward the apex of the ventricle.

The two papillary muscles of the left ventricle are quite variable in their appearance, being anywhere from long and thin to short and stubby, sometimes even bifurcating at their tips. The *anterior* (anterolateral) *papillary muscle* arises from the sternocostal wall of the ventricle, the *posterior* (posteromedial) *papillary muscle* from the diaphragmatic wall. The chordae tendineae have been discussed previously, but they extend from the tips and margins of the apical third of the papillary muscles to attach to the mitral leaflets. The outflow tract of the left ventricle is smooth, becoming increasingly fibrous in its terminal aspect—the **aortic vestibule.**

The Aortic Valve. The aortic valve (see Figs. 1–29 and 1–31) shares many structural features with the pulmonic valve, having three semilunar cusps attached at its base to a fibrous annulus and three dilations **(Valsalva's sinuses)** in the aortic wall that correspond to the cusps. The aortic valve lies anterosuperior and to the right of the mitral valve.

The aortic annulus is made up of three semicircular fibrocollagenous thickenings or scallops joined to encircle the junction of the aortic vestibule and the aorta like a three-pronged crown, the prongs of which are directed toward the apex of the heart. The lamina fibrosa of the semilunar valvular cusps fuses with the tissue of the luminal aspect of the arches of each of the crown points. The annular arches thus form triangular intervals between the cusps that are fused with the fibrous walls of the aortic vestibule.

The *semilunar cusps* of the aortic valve are thicker at their basal attachments than along their free edges, except that at the midpoints of the free edges there are nodular, fibrous thickenings—*Arantius's nodules.* On either side of the nodules, just inward from the free edge, the lamina fibrosa becomes quite thin—the *lunulae*—and is often fenestrated. The aortic surfaces of the cusps are rougher than the ventricular surfaces. The naming of the cusps of the aortic valve can easily confuse the reader because there are three different systems for doing so; all three names are provided in Figure 1–29.

The aortic sinuses are larger than those of the pulmonary trunk, extending upward well beyond the free edge of each cusp to terminate at the *supravalvular ridges.* As noted previously, the two coronary arteries usually open near these ridges.

The Fibroskeleton

The myocardial cells are intimately invested with, and everywhere enveloped by, connective tissue that is greatly variable in its organization in different areas of the heart. As has been alluded to in the foregoing discussions of the annuli of the principal valvular orifices, a complex framework of dense and membranous collagen—the *fibroskeleton of the heart* (Fig. 1–32)—is

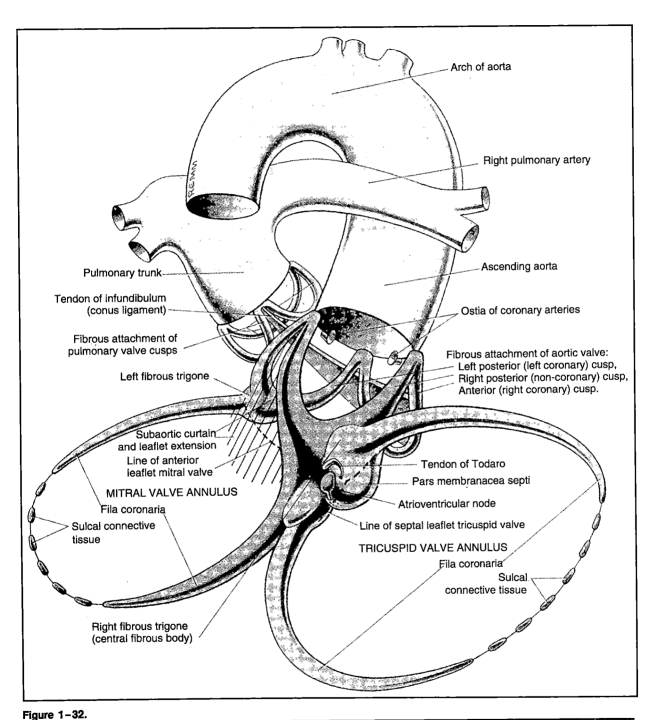

Arch of aorta

Right pulmonary artery

Ascending aorta

Ostia of coronary arteries

Pulmonary trunk

Tendon of infundibulum
(conus ligament)

Fibrous attachment of
pulmonary valve cusps

Left fibrous trigone

Fibrous attachment of aortic valve:
Left posterior (left coronary) cusp,
Right posterior (non-coronary) cusp,
Anterior (right coronary) cusp.

Subaortic curtain
and leaflet extension

Line of anterior
leaflet mitral valve

MITRAL VALVE ANNULUS

Fila coronaria

Sulcal connective
tissue

Tendon of Todaro

Pars membranacea septi

Atrioventricular node

Line of septal leaflet tricuspid valve

TRICUSPID VALVE ANNULUS

Fila coronaria

Sulcal
connective tissue

Right fibrous trigone
(central fibrous body)

Figure 1–32.

The fibroskeleton and valvular annuli of the heart. (From Williams PL, Warwick R, Dyson M, Bannister LH [eds]. Gray's Anatomy. 37th ed. New York, Churchill Livingstone, 1989, p 716.)

recognizable as an intricate, malleable, three-dimensional continuum.[42,43]

The annuli of the atrioventricular valves have already been described as essentially coplanar and at 45 degrees to the sagittal plane, facing toward the apex of the heart. Likewise, the aortic valve annulus was described as facing superiorly, to the right and somewhat anteriorly, lying anterosuperior and to the right of the mitral annulus. Not withstanding their disparate orientations, these three annuli are interconnected by a basal collagenous framework. Although situated at a distance, anterosuperior and almost at a right angle to the aortic annulus, the pulmonary annulus is connected to the aortic annulus (and thereby to the atrioventricular annuli) by a tendinous band—the *tendon of the infundibulum* (conus ligament).

The fibroskeleton maintains the position of the heart within the pericardium by providing a platform of attachment for the myocardium, valve cusps, and leaflets; it also separates (from an electrophysiologic standpoint) the atrial from the ventricular musculature. The fibroskeleton may be viewed as projecting outward from the three scallops of the "centrally" located aortic annulus. The aortic end of the tendon of the conus arteriosus blends into the tissue forming the scallop of the right (anterior) aortic cusp at its nadir. At the low point of the left (left posterior) cusp scallop the connective tissue thickens to form the *left fibrous trigone* and provides attachment for part of the anterior leaflet of the mitral valve. From its posterolateral aspect, the left fibrous trigone continues as the anterolateral arm of the mitral annulus—the *filum coronarium.* The nadir of the posterior (right posterior) scallop yields the most prominent collagenous aggregation—the *central fibrous body* (right fibrous trigone). The ellipsoid mass of the central body structurally links to the aortic, mitral, and tricuspid annuli; it continues into the second filum coronarium of the mitral annulus; it provides the base for both fila coronaria of the tricuspid annulus. Posterosuperiorly, it extends—as *Todaro's tendon*—into the right atrial wall, curving toward the medial aspect of the valve of the inferior vena cava, where it marks the position of the atrioventricular node; anteriorly, it blends with the membranous septum of the aortic vestibule.

Cardiac Muscle

The following description, a distillation of the work of many others, is by no means a definitive nor a universally accepted model. Nonetheless, it is offered in the hope that it will facilitate, rather than obfuscate, the visualization of the muscle pathways. The cardiac muscle fibers may be conveniently divided into those of the atria and those of the ventricles, these being separated by the fibrous annuli. The atrial muscle fibers are arranged in two layers: superficial fibers, which pass over both atria; and deep fibers, which are confined to each atrium.[44] The superficial fibers cross the anterior aspect of the atria most distinctly and appear as a thin sheet transversely across the bases of the atria. Looped deep fibers cross each atrium, connecting to the atrioventricular annuli. Annular deep fibers surround the auricles and encircle the vena caval orifices and the fossa ovalis.

The muscle fibers of the ventricles are more complex than those of the atria, both superficial and deep layers being described, but the deep layers are less circumscribed in the ventricles than in the atria.[45,46,47] The strata of the superficial layer include (1) fibers that pass from the conus tendon, curve across the diaphragmatic surface, then traverse leftward across the anterior interventricular groove, swirl into a vortex around the apex of the heart, and finally pass back upward into the papillary muscles of the left ventricle; (2) fibers from the tricuspid annulus that cross the diaphragmatic surface of the right ventricle to the sternocostal surface where they pass under the fibers from the conus tendon, cross the anterior interventricular groove, wind around the cardiac apex, and terminate in the posterior papillary muscle of the left ventricle; and (3) fibers that cross the posterior interventricular groove from the mitral annulus to pass into the papillary muscles of the right ventricle. The deep ventricular layers begin in the papillary muscles of one ventricle and cross the septum to end in the papillary muscles of the other ventricle, the outermost of one becoming the innermost of the other (Fig. 1–33). Beginning at the medial papillary muscle of the right ventricle, the outermost layer of deep muscle fibers circles around the right ventricle, crosses the interventricular septum (becoming the innermost layer), and blends with the superficial fibers from the tricuspid annulus to jointly form the posterior papillary muscle of the left ventricle. The second (middle) layer of deep muscle fibers spirals outward from the anterior papillary muscle to cross the septum, where it joins the superficial fibers from the anterior aspect of the conus tendon, and continues to the left ventricular side of the septal wall. The third layer of fibers, innermost of the right ventricular deep fibers, departs the posterior papillary muscle, crosses the septum (becoming the outermost layer), encircles the left ventricle to mesh with the superficial fibers from the posterior aspect of the conus tendon, together forming the anterior papillary muscle of the left ventricle.

Structure of the Cardiac Cells

Cardiac muscle is structurally and physiologically different from both skeletal and smooth muscle. It is made up of tracts of striated muscle

Figure 1–33.

The overlapping layers of the deep ventricular muscle fibers.

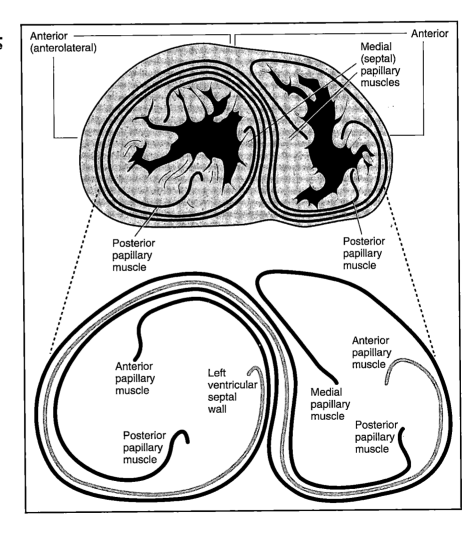

cells—**myocytes**—and intervening connective tissue. Each cell has a single, centrally located nucleus and a discrete plasma membrane separated by sarcoplasm. The individual cells may split at their ends into branches that impinge on adjacent cells, giving the appearance of a syncytial network, but this impression has been shown to be structurally incorrect. Each cardiac myocyte is striated in an organizational manner that is identical to that of skeletal muscle (although less conspicuous), with A, I, Z, and H bands (Fig. 1–34). The pattern of actin and myosin filaments is also similar to that of skeletal muscle, but they are not grouped into distinctive myofibrils. The transverse tubule system is also present, but, unlike in skeletal muscle (where it penetrates the cell at the A–I band junction), it penetrates cardiac muscle at the Z band. The sarcoplasmic reticulum is less abundant in cardiac muscle than in skeletal muscle.[48,49,50]

Each cardiac myocyte possesses an intrinsic, spontaneous rhythm—**myogenic rhythm**—that may be neurally influenced in accordance with functional demand. The rate of this rhythmic depolarization and repolarization in individual myocytes is slower than that of the heart as a whole and slower in the ventricles than in the atria. For simplicity, these cells may be thought of as *working myocytes.* Their rhythmicity is normally synchronized by other specialized "conducting myocytes." These conducting myocytes may be subdivided into *nodal, transitional,* and *Purkinje's myocytes,* accumulating in a regional network of nodes and tracts. There is general agreement regarding the principal parts of the specialized conduction system of the heart, but some aspects remain debatable.[51]

Nodal myocytes contain few myofibrils and have an atypical sacrotubular system. They are present in clusters in both the sinuatrial and atrioventricular nodes. Transitional myocytes are not as wide as regular working myocytes but are otherwise similar. They, too, are found in the nodes, extending into the atrioventricular bundle and the principal branches of the conducting system. Purkinje's myocytes are wider and shorter than regular working myocytes, contain fewer myofibrils and more mitochondria, and

have larger intercalated discs. They are found on the terminal branches of the conduction system.

The Specialized Conduction System. As mentioned earlier, the parts of the conducting system (Fig. 1–35) are the *sinuatrial* (sinus) *node,* the *atrioventricular node,* the *common atrioventricular bundle,* and *left* and *right bundle branches,* and *Purkinje's fibers.* Additional, and still debatable, components are the *interatrial, internodal,* and *accessory atrioventricular tracts or bundles.*

The sinuatrial (sinus or S-A node) node is situated in the crista terminalis at the junction of the superior vena cava and right atrium. Its name reflects its embryonic origin at the junction of the sinus venosus and the primitive atrium. The S-A node is generally described as being a flattened ellipsoid approximately 10 to 20 millimeters long, 3 millimeters wide, and 1 millimeter thick. An artery of the sinuatrial node (mentioned earlier) traverses the length of the node. Nodal myocytes occupy the central region of the S-A node, being circumferentially organized around the nodal artery. Transitional myocytes surround the nodal myocytes, and numerous Purkinje's myocytes are located around the margins of the S-A node. The sinus node is normally the "pacemaker" of the heart. James[51] contends that excitation of the atrial myocardium is initiated by the nodal myocytes and that conduction is slowed along the transitional myocytes, speeds up again along Purkinje's myocytes, and finally spreads by excitation-contraction coupling between the atrial working myocytes.

The atrioventricular (A-V node) node lies in the right atrial septal wall immediately posterior to the attachment of the septal leaflet of the tricuspid valve, just above the orifice of the coronary sinus (as noted previously, it is almost surrounded by Todaro's tendon). It, too, is shaped like a flattened ovoid, approximately 7 to 8 millimeters long, 1 millimeter wide, and 3 millimeters high. Posteriorly, the A-V node projects into the atrial septum, where it forms the nodal crest. The anteroinferior aspect of the node, which is closely associated with the central fibrous body, continues into the common atrioventricular bundle. Nodal myocytes occupy a small area inside the A-V node, especially near

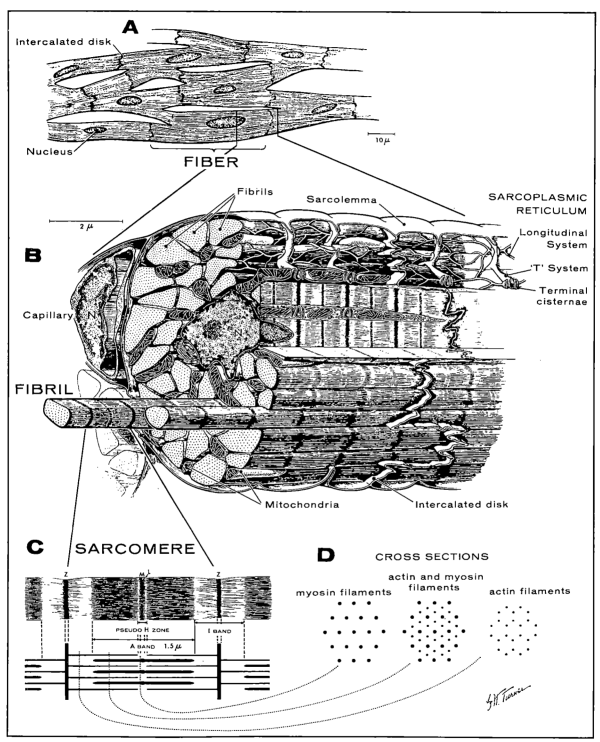

A

Intercalated disk

Nucleus

FIBER

10 μ

B

Fibrils

Sarcolemma

SARCOPLASMIC
RETICULUM

Longitudinal
System

'T' System

Terminal
cisternae

2 μ

Capillary   N

FIBRIL

N

Mitochondria

Intercalated disk

C   SARCOMERE

Z   M   Z

PSEUDO H ZONE   I BAND

A BAND   1.5 μ

D   CROSS SECTIONS

actin and myosin
filaments

myosin filaments   actin filaments

Figure 1–34.

Cardiac muscle fibers as viewed under the light microscope and the electron microscope. (From Braunwald E, Ross J, Sonnenblick EH. Mechanisms of contraction of the normal and failing heart. N Engl J Med 277:794, 1967. Reprinted by permission of the New England Journal of Medicine.)

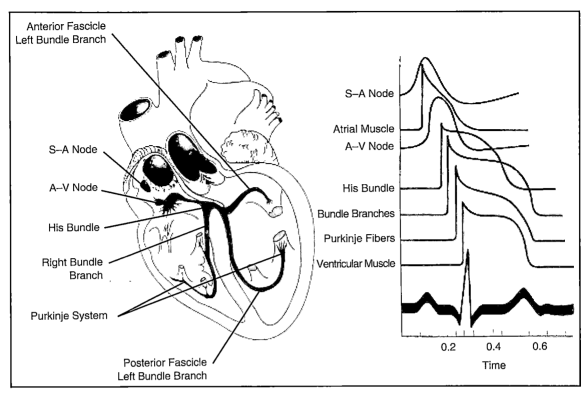

Figure 1–35.

The specialized conduction system of the heart and tracings of typical transmembrane action potentials for specific portions of the system illustrate the relative contributions made to the summated electrical activity displayed in an electrocardiogram. (Adapted from Ganong WF. Review of Medical Physiology. 15th ed. Norwalk, Conn, Appleton & Lange, 1991, p 505.)

the central fibrous body. The bulk of the node is composed of transitional myocytes, but Purkinje's myocytes cover its outer margins, receiving the terminal branchings of the internodal tracts and continuing into the atrioventricular bundle.

The atrioventricular bundle (His's bundle) rapidly narrows from its origin at the anteroinferior pole of the A-V node, enters a channel through the central fibrous body to the posteroinferior margin of the membranous septum of the aortic vestibule, and reaches the crest of the muscular interventricular septum. A narrow, rounded right bundle branch splits off at this point toward the right ventricular apex, where it enters the septomarginal trabecula and passes to the anterior papillary muscle. On reaching the anterior papillary muscle, the right bundle branch divides into

a fine network of fibers, which takes a recurrent path toward the right ventricular base (Purkinje's fibers). The left bundle branch leaves the left margin of the common bundle as a flattened sheet of fascicles that arch across the muscular septum to diverge at the left ventricular apex into anterior and posterior sheets that pass to the anterior and posterior papillary muscles, respectively. From the papillary muscles, the two sheets form complex networks of fibers, which take recurrent paths toward the left ventricular base. The common bundle is made up of mostly transitional myocytes, but as its distal aspect is approached it assumes the character of Purkinje's myocytes.

The existence of special routes of impulse transmission between the sinus and atrioventricular nodes and to distal portions of the atrial musculature has been proposed by several investigators.[51-54] These pathways are a mixture of ordinary working cells and Purkinje's cells.

The anterior internodal tract leaves the anterior aspect of the sinus node near the superior vena cava and passes posteromedially to the anterior margin of the interatrial septum. A few fibers branch off at this point to spread out into the left atrial walls (Bachmann's bundle) before the remainder continue their descent posteriorly along the right side of the septum and divide into terminal fascicles at the atrioventricular node.

The middle internodal tract (Wenckebach's bundle) leaves the S-A node from its posterosuperior aspect, passes behind the orifice of the superior vena cava, reaches and crosses the interatrial septum to finally break up around the A-V node.

The posterior internodal tract (Thorel's bundle) exits from the posteroinferior part of the S-A node, continues through the crista terminalis and the valve of the inferior vena cava, and proceeds to the posterior margin of the A-V node.

Lastly, accessory atrioventricular bundles (Kent's bundles) have been postulated as an explanation for various arrhythmias. These bundles may be present at any point around the atrioventricular annuli.

Innervation of the Heart

In addition to the specialized conducting system, the rate and strength of the cardiac rhythm is mediated by an extrinsic nerve supply. This extrinsic influence results from afferent and efferent fibers of the autonomic nervous system, the parasympathetic fibers arriving from branches of the vagus nerve and the sympathetic fibers from rami of the sympathetic trunk. Preganglionic vagal fibers arise in the medulla from the nucleus ambiguus, reticular nuclei, and possibly the dorsal nucleus of the vagus, reaching the cardiac plexuses without interruption. The preganglionic sympathetic fibers arise from neurons in the lateral grey column of the first five or six cranial segments of the thoracic spinal cord, ending in the cervical and third and fourth thoracic sympathetic ganglia, from which the post-

ganglionic fibers leave as cardiac nerves to proceed to the heart. On reaching the heart, the sympathetic cardiac nerves and the parasympathetic vagal cardiac branches form a mixed cardiac plexus.

The **cardiac plexus** is situated at the base of the heart and is divided into the closely associated superficial (ventral) and deep (dorsal) parts. The plexus contains several ganglia. The *superficial cardiac plexus* lies below the arch of the aorta, anterior to the right pulmonary artery. It is formed by the cardiac branch of the superior cervical ganglion of the left sympathetic trunk and the lower of the two cervical cardiac branches of the left vagus. The superficial part of the plexus gives branches to the deep part of the plexus, to the right coronary plexus, and to the left anterior pulmonary plexus.

The *deep cardiac plexus* lies in front of the bifurcation of the trachea above the pulmonary trunk but behind the aortic arch. It is formed by the cardiac nerves from the cervical and upper thoracic ganglia of the sympathetic trunk and the cardiac branches of the vagus and recurrent laryngeal nerves. A right half of the deep part of the plexus passes in front and behind the right pulmonary artery; those fibers passing behind the pulmonary artery give some filaments to the right atrium and then continue on to form part of the left coronary plexus; those passing in front of the pulmonary artery give a few filaments to the right anterior pulmonary plexus before going on to form a part of the right coronary plexus. The left half of the deep part of the cardiac plexus is connected with the superficial part of the plexus, giving filaments to the left atrium and to the left anterior pulmonary plexus before continuing on to form the greater portion of the left coronary plexus. The *left coronary plexus* accompanies the left coronary artery, giving branches to the left atrium and ventricle. The smaller *right coronary plexus* accompanies the right coronary artery, giving branches to the right atrium and ventricle.

References

1. Moore KL. Before We Are Born. 3rd ed. Philadelphia, WB Saunders, 1989.

2. Williams PL, Warwick R, Dyson M, Bannister LH (eds). Gray's Anatomy. 36th ed. New York, Churchill Livingstone, 1980.

3. Netter FH, Van Mierop LHS. Embryology. In: The CIBA Collection of Medical Illustrations. Vol. 5. Rochester, NY: Case-Hoyt, 1978.

4. Netter FH, Crelin ES, Huber JF, et al. Anatomy and embryology. In: The CIBA Collection of Medical Illustrations. Vol. 7. Rochester, NY: Case-Hoyt, 1979.

5. Cherniack RM, Cherniack L. Respiration in Health and Disease. 3rd ed. Philadelphia, WB Saunders, 1983.

6. Basmajian JV, De Luca CJ. Muscles Alive. 5th ed. Baltimore, Md, Williams & Wilkins, 1985.

7. Campbell EJM. The Respiratory Muscles and the Mechanics of Breathing. London, Lloyd-Luke Medical Books, 1958.

8. Hislop A, Reid L. Intra-pulmonary arterial development during fetal life—branching pattern and structure. J Anat 113:35–48, 1972.

9. Davies G, Reid L. Growth of the alveoli and pulmonary arteries in childhood. Thorax 25:669–681, 1970.

10. Heath D. Pulmonary vasculature in postnatal life and pulmonary hemodynamics. In: Emery J (ed). The Anatomy of the Developing Lung. Suffolk, England, William Heinmann Medical Books Ltd, 1969.

11. Aviado DM. The Lung Circulation. Vol. 1. Oxford, Pergamon Press, 1965:185–254.

12. Auld PA, Rudolph AM, Golinko RJ. Factors affecting bronchial collateral flow in the dog. Am J Physiol 198:1166–1170, 1960.

13. Leak LV, Jamuar MP. Ultrastructure of pulmonary lymphatic vessels. Am Rev Respir Dis 128:S59–S65, 1983.

14. Mygind N. Scanning electron microscopy of the human nasal mucosa. Rhinology 13:57–75, 1975.

15. Proctor DF. State of the art. The upper airways. I. Nasal physiology and defense of the lungs. Am Rev Respir Dis 115:97–129, 1977.

16. Thurlbeck WM. Postnatal growth and development of the lung. Am Rev Respir Dis 111:803–844, 1975.

17. Murray JF. The Normal Lung: The Basis for Diagnosis and Treatment of Pulmonary Disease. 2nd ed. Philadelphia, WB Saunders, 1986.

18. Reid L. Visceral cartilage. J Anat 122:349–355, 1976.

19. Weibel E. Design and structure of the human lung. In: Fishman A (ed). Assessment of Pulmonary Function. New York, McGraw-Hill, 1980.

20. Etherton JE, Conning DM, Corrin B. Autoradiographical and morphological evidence for apocrine secretion of dipalmitoyl lecithin in the terminal bronchiole of mouse lung. Am J Anat 138:11–35, 1973.

21. Gail DB, Lenfant CJM. Cells of the lung; biology and clinical implications. Am Rev Respir Dis 127:366–367, 1983.

22. Lauweryns JM, Van Lommel A. Morphometric analysis of hypoxia-induced synaptic activity in intrapulmonary neuroepithelial bodies. Cell Tissue Res 226:201–214, 1982.

23. Meyrick B, Reid L. Ultrastructure of cells in the human bronchial submucosal glands. J Anat 107:281–299, 1970.

24. Nadel JA, Davis B, Phipps RJ. Control of mucus secretion and ion transport in airways. Ann Rev Physiol 41:369–381, 1979.

25. Miller WS. The Lung. Springfield, Ill, Charles C Thomas, 1937.

26. Dunnill MS. Postnatal growth of the lung. Thorax 17:329–333, 1962.

27. Kersten LD. Comprehensive Respiratory Nursing: A Decision Making Approach. Philadelphia, WB Saunders, 1989.

28. Gehr P, Bachofen M, Weibel ER. The normal human lung: Ultrastructure and morphometric estimation of diffusion capacity. Respir Physiol 32:121–140, 1978.

29. Crapo FD, Barry BE, Gehr P, et al. Cell number and cell characteristics of the normal human lung. Am Rev Respir Dis 125:740–745, 1982.

30. Macklem PT. Airway obstruction and collateral ventilation. Physiol Rev 51:368–436, 1971.

31. Lambert MW. Accessory bronchiole-alveolar communications. J Pathol Bacteriol 70:311–314, 1955.

32. Raskin SP, Herman PG. Interacinar pathways in the human lung. Am Rev Respir Dis 119:425–434, 1979.

33. Richardson JB. Nerve supply to the lungs. Am Rev Respir Dis 119:785–802, 1979.

34. Laitinen A. Autonomic innervation of the human respiratory tract as revealed by histochemical and ultrastructural methods. Eur J Respir Dis 66(Suppl 140):1–42, 1985.

35. International Congress of Anatomists. Nomina Anatomica. 6th ed. New York, Churchill Livingstone, 1989.

36. Hutchinson MCE. A study of the atrial arteries in man. J Anat 125:39–54, 1978.

37. Lam JH, Ranganathan N, Wigle ED. Morphology of the human mitral valve. I. Chordae tendineae: A new classification. Circulation 41:449–458, 1970.

38. Silver MD, Lam JH, Ranganathan N, Wigle ED. Morphology of the human tricuspid valve. Circulation 43:333–348, 1971.

39. Ranganathan N, Lam JH, Wigle ED. Morphology of the human mitral valve. II. The valve leaflets: Circulation 41:459–467, 1970.

40. Walmsley R. Anatomy of the human mitral valve in the adult cadaver and comparative anatomy of the valve. Br Heart J 40:351–366, 1978.

41. Harken DE, Ellis LB, Dexter L, et al. The responsibility of the physician in selecting patients with mitral stenosis for surgical treatment. Circulation 5:349–362, 1952.

42. Walmsley R, Watson H. Clinical Anatomy of the Heart. Edinburgh, Churchill Livingstone, 1978.

43. Zimmerman J. The functional and surgical anatomy of the heart. Ann R Coll Surg Engl 39:348–366, 1966.

44. Thomas CE. The muscular architecture of the ventricles of hog and dog hearts. Am J Anat 101:17–58, 1957.

45. Mall FP. On the muscular architecture of the ventricles of the human heart. Am J Anat 11:211–278, 1911.

46. Ramon C, Streeter DD. Muscle pathway geometry in the heart wall. J Biomech Eng 105:367–373, 1983.

47. Torrent Guasp F. Estructura y Mechanica del Corazon. Barcelona, Ediciones Grass, 1987.

48. Fawcett DW, McNutt NS. The ultrastructure of the cat myocardium. I. Ventricular papillary muscle. J Cell Biol 42:1–45, 1969.

49. Forssmann WG, Girardier L. A study of the T system in rat heart. J Cell Biol 44:1–19, 1970.

50. Page E, McCallister LP. Quantitative electron microscopic description of heart muscle cells. Application to

normal, hypertrophied and thyroxin-stimulated hearts. Am J Cardiol 31:172–181, 1973.

51. James TN. Anatomy of the conducting system of the heart. In: Hurst JW (ed). The Heart, Arteries and Veins. 4th ed. New York, McGraw-Hill, 1978.

52. Wenckebach KF. Beitrage zur Kenntnis der menschlichen Herztätigkeit. Arch Anat Physiol 3:53, 1908.

53. Thorel C. Über den Aufbaum des Sinusknoten und seine Verbingdung mit der Cava superior und den Wenckenbachschen Bündeln. Munch Med Wochenschr 57:83, 1910.

54. Bachman G. The inter-auricular time interval. Am J Physiol 41:309, 1916.

2 CARDIOVASCULAR AND RESPIRATORY PHYSIOLOGY

INTRODUCTION

The principal function of the lungs is to exchange gas between the blood and the atmospheric air; that of the heart is to pump blood through the vascular system. This chapter introduces the normal physiologic considerations that underlie these vital processes. The chapter begins with a brief discussion of the basic units of measurement used to describe respiratory and cardiovascular functions. Then, because the various functions of the body are controlled by the autonomic nervous system, the second portion of this chapter reviews the components of the autonomic nervous system and discusses their function as related to the respiratory and cardiovascular systems. The last two sections of the chapter deal with the specific functions of the respiratory and cardiovascular systems, respectively.

BASIC UNITS

Throughout much of the world, the basic terminology recommended in the Systèm International to define all units of measurement has been widely adopted (Table 2–1). In the United States, however, the usage of Systèm International nomenclature is only spottily employed.

59

TABLE 2–1. Basic Units of Measurement and Examples of Some Derived Units

Basic Units	Measurement	Symbol
Mole	Amount of a substance	mol
Ampere	Electric current	A
Meter	Length	m
Candela	Luminous intensity	cd
Kilogram	Mass	kg
Kelvin	Temperature	K
Second	Time	s
Derived Units		
Square meter	Area	m^2
Cubic meter	Volume	m^3
Meter per second	Velocity	$m \cdot s^{-1}$
Meter per second per second	Acceleration	$m \cdot s^{-2}$
Newton	Force	N *or* $kg \cdot m \cdot s^{-2}$
Pascal	Pressure	Pa *or* $N \cdot m$
Joule	Work or energy	J *or* $kg \cdot m^2 \cdot s^{-2}$
Watt	Power	W *or* $J \cdot s^{-1}$ *or* $kg \cdot m^2 \cdot s^{-3}$

Consequently, the clinician is faced with several alternative units of measure, often simultaneously. For example, pressure is often reported in terms of millimeters of mercury (mm Hg) or centimeters of water (cm H_2O) instead of the Systèm International units, pascals or kilopascals (Pa and kPa, respectively; Table 2–2). For the remainder of this chapter, the units of measure common in the clinical setting are used.

THE AUTONOMIC NERVOUS SYSTEM

The **autonomic nervous system** is organized on the basis of the reflex and comprises all the

TABLE 2–2. Conversion Factors for Three Measures of Pressure

To Convert	To	Do the Following:
mm Hg	kPa	Multiply by 0.133
mm Hg	cm H_2O	Multiply by 1.36
cm H_2O	kPa	Multiply by 0.098
cm H_2O	mm Hg	Multiply by 0.735
kPa	mm Hg	Multiply by 7.519
kPa	cm H_2O	Multiply by 10.225

afferent and efferent nerves through which the viscera are innervated. In this section, the efferent pathways to the various blood vessels, heart, larynx, trachea, bronchi, and lungs are considered. Structurally, the autonomic nerves are characterized by a two-neuron chain: the cell body of the primary (preganglionic) neuron lies within the brain stem or spinal cord and sends its axon to synapse with outlying secondary (postganglionic) neurons. Autonomic efferent signals are carried to the viscera via two essentially antagonistic subdivisions: the **sympathetic** and the **parasympathetic** divisions (Fig. 2–1).

The preganglionic neuronal axons of the sympathetic nerves leave the spinal cord via the ventral roots of the spinal nerves from T1 to L3 or L4. They pass into the paravertebral sympathetic ganglion chains, with most ending on the cell bodies of the postganglionic neurons. Axons of some of the postganglionic neurons reach the viscera via various sympathetic nerves; others reenter the spinal nerves via the grey rami from the chain ganglia to be distributed in the areas supplied by those spinal nerves. The superior, middle, and stellate ganglia in the cranial extension of the sympathetic chain give off the postganglionic sympathetic nerves to the blood vessels of the head. The adrenal medulla is a sympathetic ganglion whose postganglionic neurons are specialized for secretion directly into the bloodstream.

Parasympathetic innervation of the vasculature and other viscera of the head is carried via cranial nerves III (oculomotor), VII (facial), and IX (glossopharyngeal); that of the thorax and upper abdomen via cranial nerve X (vagus); and that of the pelvic region via the second and third (occasionally also the first and fourth) sacral spinal nerves. Approximately 75% of all parasympathetic nerve fibers are in the vagus nerves. Parasympathetic preganglionic fibers end on short postganglionic neurons located on or near the targeted visceral structures.

Neurotransmitters

The sympathetic and parasympathetic nerve fibers secrete one of two transmitter substances

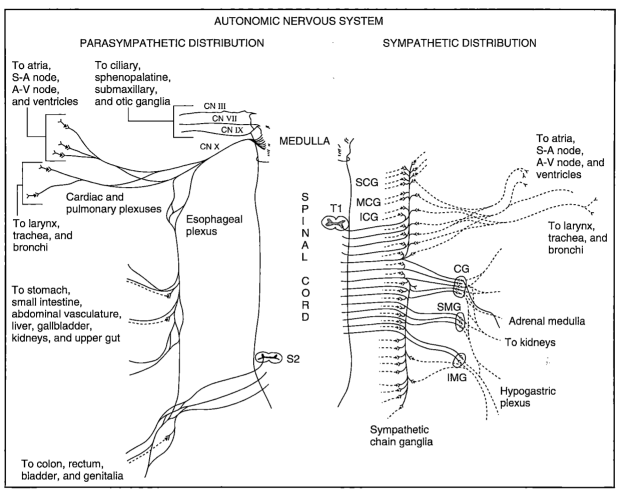

AUTONOMIC NERVOUS SYSTEM

PARASYMPATHETIC DISTRIBUTION

SYMPATHETIC DISTRIBUTION

Figure 2-1.

Sympathetic and parasympathetic efferent pathways to the cardiovascular and respiratory systems. SCG, superior cervical ganglion; MCG, middle cervical ganglion; ICG, inferior cervical ganglion; CG, celiac ganglion; SMG, superior mesenteric ganglion; IMG, inferior mesenteric ganglion.

at the various synaptic junctions: **acetylcholine** and **norepinephrine.** Acetylcholine-secreting fibers are referred to as **cholinergic;** those secreting norepinephrine are called **adrenergic.** All of the preganglionic fibers of the parasympathetic and sympathetic divisions and the postganglionic neurons of the parasympathetic division are cholinergic. Most of the postganglionic sympathetic neurons are adrenergic, although the postganglionic sympathetic fibers to the sweat glands, to the piloerector muscles, and to a few blood vessels are cholinergic. This fact is impor-

tant in later discussions of pharmacologic activity (Chapters 12 and 13).

Acetylcholine is synthesized in the terminal endings of cholinergic fibers, mostly outside of the axoplasmic vesicles in which it is ultimately stored until its release. Once it has been secreted at the cholinergic nerve ending, it is metabolized by **acetylcholinesterase**—the same process by which acetylcholine is eliminated from the neuromuscular junctions of skeletal nerves. Norepinephrine synthesis starts in the axoplasm but is completed inside the axoplasmic vesicles of the terminal nerve endings. After secretion by the terminal nerve endings, most norepinephrine is reabsorbed into the nerve endings themselves; some diffuses away from the release site into the surrounding interstitial fluid and eventually into the blood; and the remainder is metabolized by other enzymes (either **monoamine oxidase [MAO]**, at the synaptic cleft, or by **catechol-O-methyl transferase [COMT]**, which is present diffusely throughout all tissues).

Receptors

Before acetylcholine or norepinephrine can actually stimulate a response, it must first bind to specific receptor sites in the cell membranes of the effector organs. Receptors are usually portions of proteins that extend from the outer surface of the cell membrane, penetrating through it, to the interior of the cell. When the transmitter substance binds with the receptor, a conformational change in the receptor protein usually occurs that excites or inhibits the cell. It is usually achieved by changing the cell membrane permeability to one or more ions or by activating or deactivating an enzyme (second messenger) attached to the end of the receptor on the inside of the cell.

There are two primary types of postsynaptic receptors, and each of these has several subclasses. There are two categories of cholinergic receptors: **muscarinic** and **nicotinic.** Muscarinic receptors are located at the interfaces between the postganglionic neurons and the effector cells of all parasympathetic terminal synapses and some specialized sympathetic postganglionic cholinergic branches (e.g., to some blood vessels). Nicotinic receptors are found at the junctions between the preganglionic and postganglionic neurons of both branches of the autonomic nervous system and at the neuromuscular junctions of skeletal muscle fibers.

There are also two categories of adrenergic receptors: **alpha** and **beta.**[1] Based on the sensitivity of these receptors to different endogenous and exogenous agents, each adrenergic receptor subcategory is further subdivided. The alpha receptors are divided into **alpha$_1$** and **alpha$_2$** types, the beta receptors into **beta$_1$** and **beta$_2$** types.[2,3]

TABLE 2–3. The Locations and Responses of Autonomic Receptors in the Cardiovascular and Pulmonary Systems

Neurotransmitter	Type of Receptor	Location	Response
Cholinergic			
	Muscarinic	Smooth muscle of lungs and bronchioles	Contraction
		Cardiac muscle	Decreased rate of contraction
	Nicotinic	Autonomic ganglia	Mediates postganglionic neuronal transmission
Adrenergic			
	Alpha$_1$	Vascular smooth muscle	Contraction
	Alpha$_2$	Special CNS inhibitory synapses	Decreased sympathetic discharge
		Peripheral adrenergic presynaptic terminals	Modulates norepinephrine release
		Fat cells	Decreased lipolysis
	Dopaminergic	Renal arterioles	Dilation at low dosage
			Contraction at high dosage
	Beta$_1$	Cardiac muscle:	
		Atria, S-A node, A-V node	Increased rate and force of contraction
		Ventricles	Decreased rate and force of contraction
		Kidney	Increased renin secretion
		Fat cells	Increased lipolysis
	Beta$_2$	Bronchiolar smooth muscle	Dilation
		Skeletal muscle and hepatic vascular smooth muscle	Dilation
		Skeletal muscle and hepatic cells	Increased metabolic rate

CNS, central nervous system.

Alpha$_1$ receptors are located primarily on visceral and vascular smooth muscle. Alpha$_2$ receptors are located primarily on the presynaptic terminals of certain adrenergic synapses, where they modulate norepinephrine release. Norepinephrine and epinephrine have different effects in exciting the alpha and beta receptors. Beta$_1$ receptors are located principally in cardiac and renal tissues. **Dopaminergic** receptors are located on the vascular smooth muscle of the kideys. Beta$_2$ receptors are found mostly on the smooth muscle of certain vascular beds and the bronchioles. Table 2–3 summarizes the general cardiovascular and pulmonary effects of the sympathetic and parasympathetic divisions of the autonomic nervous system in accordance with the various autonomic receptor types.

THE GAS TRANSPORT SYSTEM

To satisfy the gas exchange needs of the body, the cardiovascular and respiratory systems are functionally integrated as a single **gas transport system** for the support of cellular respiration (Fig. 2–2). The respiratory system contributes to the whole by moving gas to and from the alveoli **(ventilation)** and by providing for the passage of oxygen and carbon dioxide across the alveolar-capillary interface **(diffusion)**. The cardiovascular system contributes by transporting dissolved and bound gases to and from the lungs and the cells in the blood **(perfusion)**. The various cells of the body ultimately drive the gears of the gas transport system by means of oxygen consumption

and carbon dioxide production in the utilization of metabolic substrates **(respiration).**

Ventilation

Ventilation of the lungs—the movement of air into and out of the lungs—is accomplished by a coordinated interaction of the respiratory muscles, the rib cage, and the lungs. Together, the respiratory muscles and the rib cage constitute the chest wall. Although the actions of the musculoskeletal system are generally analyzed in terms of force, length, and velocity, the force-length and force-velocity relationships of the respiratory system are inferred from measurements of pressure (implying force), volume (implying length), and flow (implying velocity).

Chest Wall Motion

The specific interactions of the diaphragm, the intercostal or accessory muscles, and abdominal muscles during inspiration remain a topic of controversy. Nonetheless, most investigators agree that the contributions of the intercostal or accessory muscles and the abdominal muscles are necessary for the proper displacement of the chest wall. For example, consider the breathing efforts of a patient with a spinal cord injury resulting in quadriplegia: on inspiration the diaphragm contracts, lifting and expanding the rib cage, thus decreasing intrathoracic pressure and initiating air flow into the lungs. However, be-

Figure 2–2.

The interdependence of the musculoskeletal, respiratory, and cardiovascular systems is well illustrated as interdigitating gears, forming a single gas transport system that supports cellular respiration. (Redrawn with permission from Wasserman K, Hansen JE, Sue DY, Whipp BJ. Principles of Exercise Testing and Interpretation. Philadelphia, Lea & Febiger, 1987, p 2.)

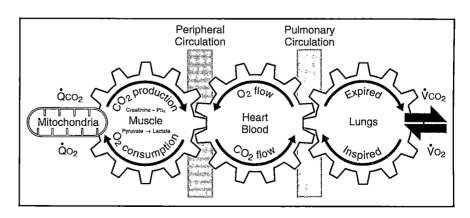

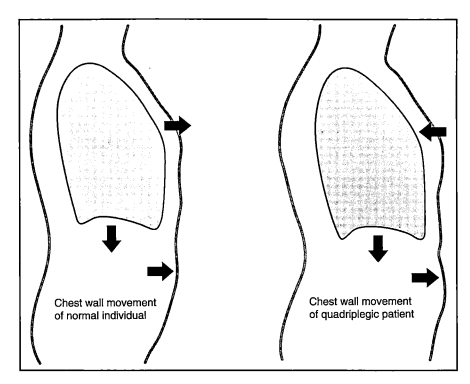

Figure 2-3.

The normal chest wall and abdominal movements during inhalation to total lung capacity are contrasted with chest wall and abdominal movements that occur as a result of quadriplegia that resulted from spinal cord injury.

Chest wall movement
of normal individual

Chest wall movement
of quadriplegic patient

cause the intercostal or accessory muscles and the abdominal muscles are paralyzed, there is no resistance to the resultant inward pull on the supra-, inter-, or subcostal tissues; likewise, there is no resistance to the downward displacement of the abdominal contents. Consequently, the supra-, inter-, and subcostal tissues are sucked inward, and the abdomen is pushed outward as the diaphragm descends. Clearly, the efficacy of the inspiratory effort is minimized. Figure 2-3 contrasts the chest wall and abdominal motions of a normal person with those of a quadriplegic patient.

The ribs normally function as levers when acted on by the respiratory muscles. The fulcrum of each rib is located just lateral to the costotransverse articulation, such that when the shaft of the rib is elevated, the neck of the rib is depressed. Small movements at the vertebral ends of the ribs result in much greater movements at the anterior ends. The anteroposterior diameter of the thorax is first increased when the anterior ends of true ribs (most especially ribs three to six) are elevated secondary to the back-

ward rotation of their necks, lifting the sternum forward and upward. This is, however, a small motion, and soon the middle part of the shaft of the ribs is elevated, increasing the transverse diameter of the thorax. The costovertebral and costotransverse joints, as well as the movements of the ribs with inspiration, are shown in Figure 2-4. The seventh through tenth ribs primarily increase the transverse diameter of the thorax because there is only slight rotation of their necks, and, therefore, their anterior ends move very little. The shaft of these ribs is elevated by an outward and a backward movement. Any distortion of this normal movement, as might occur in extreme obesity or in kyphoscoliosis, impairs chest wall mechanics. Likewise, because the diaphragm and abdominal musculature are integral parts of the thorax, any condition (e.g., elevation of the diaphragm, spasticity of the abdominal muscles) that reduces their free movement also impairs chest wall mechanics. Because the lungs normally fill the chest so that the visceral and parietal pleurae are in contact, the lungs act in unison with the chest wall and can

Figure 2–4.

An example of typical costovertebral and costotransverse joints. The "pump handle" and "bucket handle" motions of the ribs during inspiration are illustrated in *B*. (From Norkin CC, LeVangie PK. Joint Structure and Function. A Comprehensive Analysis. 2nd ed. Philadelphia, FA Davis, 1992, pp 182, 183.)

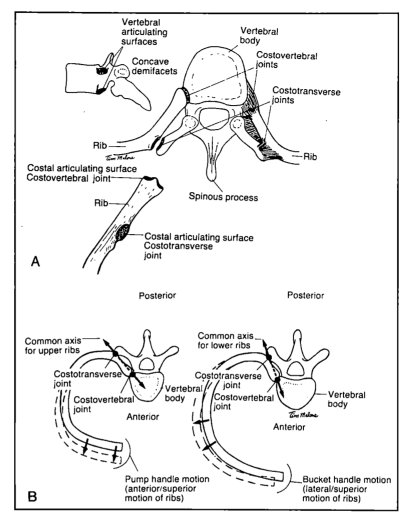

be thought of as a pump that may be characterized by its elastic, flow-resistive, and inertial properties.

Lung Volumes

Before considering the elastic, flow-resistive, or inertial properties of the lungs, the **static volumes** of the lungs should be considered (Fig. 2–5).[4–7] Spirometric and other tests of pulmonary function are discussed in Chapter 10. The volume of air normally inhaled and exhaled with each breath during quiet breathing is called the **tidal volume (V$_T$)**. The additional volume of air that can be taken into the lungs beyond the normal tidal inhalation is called the **inspiratory reserve volume (IRV)**. The additional volume of air that can be let out beyond the normal tidal exhalation is called the **expiratory reserve volume (ERV)**. The volume of air that remains in the lungs after a forceful expiratory effort is called the **residual volume (RV)**. The **inspiratory capacity (IC)** is the sum of the tidal and inspiratory reserve volumes; it is the maximum amount of air that can be inhaled after a normal tidal exhalation. The **functional residual capacity (FRC)** is the sum of the expiratory reserve and residual volumes; it is the amount of air remaining in the lungs at the end of a normal

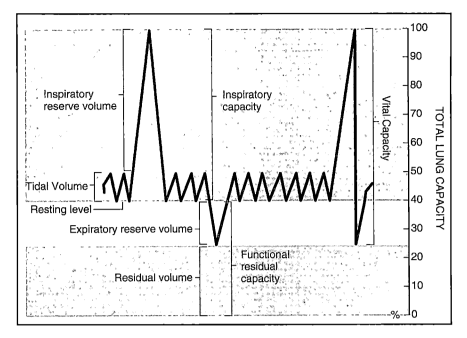

Figure 2–5.

The lung volumes and capacities, shown as percentages of total lung capacity. (Redrawn from Cherniack RM, Cherniack L. Respiration in Health and Disease. 3rd ed. Philadelphia, WB Saunders, 1983, p 12.)

tidal exhalation. The importance of the FRC cannot be overstated; it represents the point at which the forces tending to collapse the lungs are balanced against the forces tending to expand the chest wall. The **vital capacity (VC)** is the sum of the inspiratory reserve, tidal, and expiratory reserve volumes; it is the maximum amount of air that can be exhaled following a maximum inhalation. The **total lung capacity (TLC)** is the maximum volume to which the lungs can be expanded; it is the sum of all the pulmonary volumes.

The amount of air moved into or out of the lungs per unit time is called the **minute ventilation (V̇)**; it equals the product of the V_T and the respiratory rate. For example, if an individual were breathing at a frequency of 15 breaths per minute with a tidal volume of 400 ml, the in-

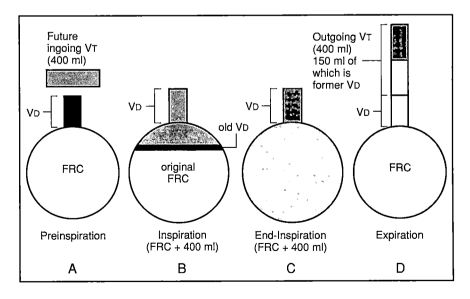

Figure 2–6.

One respiratory cycle, demonstrating the distribution of a normal tidal volume and showing the effect of dead space on alveolar ventilation.

spired minute ventilation ($\dot{V}$I) would be 6000 ml · min^{-1}. The expired minute ventilation ($\dot{V}$E) is normally slightly less than the $\dot{V}$I because the metabolic production of carbon dioxide ($\dot{V}CO_2$) is less than the metabolic consumption of oxygen ($\dot{V}O_2$).

Dead Space

Recalling the anatomic relationships of the upper and lower respiratory tracts, it is obvious that not all of the air that is inhaled reaches the alveoli. This volume of gas, which occupies the nonrespiratory conducting airways, is called the **anatomic dead space volume (VD;** normally about 150 ml). To illustrate the dead space volume, Figure 2–6 depicts the tidal nature of the respiratory cycle. In *A* is an individual at FRC; the existing VD is shown in black. In *B* and *C*, the individual inhales a volume of 400 ml; the existing VD and 250 ml of the incoming VT are mixed with the FRC, and 150 ml of the VT becomes the new VD. Then, in *D*, the ensuing exhalation pushes the VD out of the airways, along with 250 ml of the expired VT, into the environment (the last 150 ml of which remains in the airways as a new VD).

Distribution of Gas

Thus far we have assumed that all regions of the normal lung are ventilated equally. In fact, however, this is not the case.[8] Because of the weight of the lungs, the pressure near the lowermost aspects of the dependent portions is less negative than that at the uppermost aspects. Consequently, the bases of the lungs are relatively compressed at FRC and, hence, have a greater potential for expansion on inspiration than the apical portions, which are already relatively expanded. There is, therefore, a continuum of ventilation within the lungs that is position dependent. In the upright position, the bases of the lungs have a larger change in volume and a smaller resting volume than the apices, and, therefore, their ventilation is greater (Fig. 2–7). In the supine position, these differences disap-

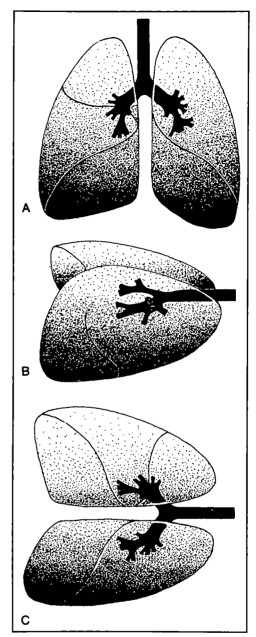

Figure 2–7.

Because of the weight of the lungs, the pressure near the lowermost aspects of the dependent portions is less negative than that at the uppermost aspects. Thus, a continuum of ventilation is created within the lungs, and gas is preferentially distributed to the dependent areas. *A*, Erect; *B*, supine; and *C*, lateral body positions. (From Shapiro BA, Harrison RA, Cane RD, Templin R. Clinical Application of Blood Gases. 4th ed. Chicago, Year Book Medical Publishers, 1989, p 24.)

pear; apical and basal ventilation becomes equal. However, the ventilation of the posterior (lowermost) aspects of the lungs becomes greater than that of the anterior (uppermost) aspects. Likewise, in the side-lying position, the dependent lung is better ventilated.

Mechanical Properties

It should be no great revelation, at this point, that the gas transport system is made of elastic materials. By its structural nature, then, its constituent parts try to pull themselves back to their original shapes whenever they are stretched. At FRC, the elastic recoil of the lungs (pulling inward) is balanced by the elastic recoil of the chest wall (pulling outward); these opposing forces generate a subatmospheric pressure of approximately 5 cm H_2O in the pleural space (the pleural pressure; Ppl). Keep in mind that the actual Ppl varies according to where it is measured, becoming more negative (subatmospheric) as the apices of the lungs are approached (in the upright position). At FRC, this negative intrapleural pressure holds the lungs inflated at a volume greater than would be observed if they were removed from the chest cavity and at the same time pulls the chest wall "down" to a volume that is less than would be observed if the chest wall were opened. If an individual with paralyzed muscles were lying at rest and receiving positive-pressure breaths from a mechanical ventilatory assistance device, it would be a simple matter to inflate the lungs to TLC and then to deflate them incrementally until RV is reached. By measuring the alveolar pressure (PA), the Ppl, and the atmospheric pressure (PB), the **transmural pressures** of the lungs, the chest wall, and the entire respiratory system could be calculated. As long as there is no movement of air into or out of the lungs, the pressure within the airways, from the mouth (P_m) or nose to the alveoli, is the same as the PB. The difference, then, between the pressure in the airways (atmospheric) and the Ppl (atmospheric—5 cm H_2O) is the pressure difference across the lung (the **transpulmonary pressure; PL**). To illustrate, consider the lungs within the chest wall as if

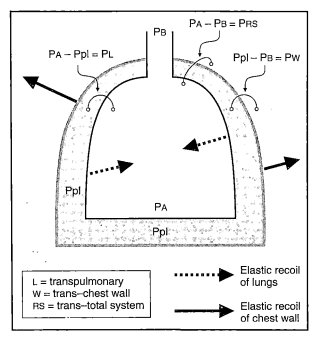

Figure 2–8.

In a simple balloon within a balloon model of the lungs and chest wall, only three transmural pressures—across the inner balloon (PL), across the outer balloon (Pw), and across both balloons (PRS)—must be considered. Imagine the complexity that arises with two lungs and 300 million alveoli. PA, alveolar pressure; PB, barometric pressure; Ppl, pleural pressure. (Adapted from Mines AH. Respiratory Physiology. 2nd ed. New York, Raven Press, 1986, p 21.)

they were one balloon inside another, as shown in Figure 2–8. In this simple balloon within a balloon model of the lungs and rib cage, there are transmural pressures across the lung (PL = PA − Ppl), across the chest wall (Pw = Ppl − PB), and across the entire respiratory system (PRS = PA − PB). Each of these pressures is crucial to the quantification of the distensibility of the respiratory system. Clearly, even this representation presents many complexities; imagine the complexity of 300 million balloons (alveoli) within the chest wall.

Compliance

The **elastance** of a material is a measure of the "stiffness" of the material. With respect to the gas transport system, the amount of stretch on the elastic walls is measured by change in volume; the force exerted by the walls as they try to return to their original volume is measured by change in pressure. Thus, the elastance of the walls of the gas transport system may be defined as the change in pressure divided by the change in volume. Clinically, however, it is the **compliance** of the heart, the blood vessels, or the lungs that is of concern. Compliance is the inverse of elastance; it is a measure of the "distensibility" of a material:

$$\text{Compliance} = \frac{\text{change of volume}}{\text{change of pressure}} = \frac{\Delta V}{\Delta P}$$

In physics, Hooke's law states that the forces acting to restore a material to its original shape are proportional to the amount of stretch applied to them. Moreover, the amount of material being stretched affects the total force that is generated. For example, if two springs, one twice as big as the other but both made from the same material, were stretched by equal amounts, the bigger spring would generate the greater force; even though the springs are made of a material having the same elastance, more of the material is in

the larger spring. Therefore, to better describe the elastance of the material, the force exerted is divided by the cross-sectional area of the object being stretched, yielding the **stress** or tension (σ). In the case of alveoli, which are essentially spherical, the tension forces ($\sigma \times$ circumference) tending to collapse the spheres must be balanced by the pressure forces inside the spheres (P $\times$ area of the sphere) tending to expand them if alveolar collapse is to be avoided. Thus, by equating the tension and pressure forces, dividing by π, and rearranging, Laplace's law for a sphere is derived: $P = 2\sigma/r$. This equation assumes that the only pressure acting on the walls is the pressure inside the sphere, but this condition is true only if no force is pushing back at the wall from the outside. Thus, the pressure calculated from this equation is actually the pressure across the wall (the transmural pressure), which is the pressure inside minus the pressure outside.

From the volume-pressure curves shown in Figure 2–9, it may be seen that the lungs have a low compliance initially (starting from TLC), but after deflating by about 17% their compliance is approximately 0.2 $L \cdot cm\ H_2O^{-1}$ until FRC is reached; below RV, their compliance is very

Figure 2–9.

Volume versus transmural pressure curves for the chest wall in isolation, the lungs in isolation, and the total system. (Redrawn from Cherniack RM, Cherniack L. Respiration in Health and Disease. 3rd ed. Philadelphia, WB Saunders, 1983, p 17.)

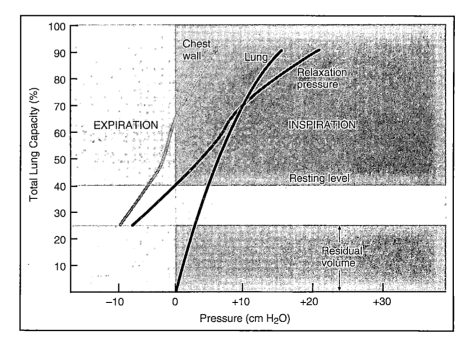

high. The compliance of the chest wall between TLC and FRC also remains fairly constant at about 0.2 L · cm H_2O^{-1}; but the chest wall gets stiffer between FRC and RV. The respiratory system as a whole has a relatively low compliance near TLC (like the lungs) and between FRC and RV (like the chest wall); but the compliance in the midrange is higher, being about 0.1 L · cm H_2O^{-1}, which indicates that the total system is about twice as stiff as either of its parts.

Surface Tension

Although the elastic characteristics of the lung tissue itself play a role in lung compliance, the surface tension at the air-liquid interface on the alveolar surface has a greater influence. Anyone who has ever attempted to separate two wet microscope slides by lifting (not sliding) the top slide from the bottom has had first-hand experience regarding the forces of surface tension. As an example of the effect of surface tension in a curved structure, consider the transmural pressures needed to maintain an alveolus open at FRC: if we assume that at FRC there is a representative alveolus with a surface tension of 75 dynes/cm and a radius of 50×10^{-4} cm, the pressure $= 2\sigma/r = 2(75$ dynes/cm$) \div (50 \times 10^{-4}$ cm$) = 30 \times 10^3$ dynes/cm². Converting dynes/cm² to cm H_2O (1 cm $H_2O = 980$ dynes/cm²), the calculated pressure needed to maintain an alveolus open at FRC is about 31 cm H_2O. This calculation suggests that the transmural pressures required to keep the alveoli open should be much greater than those actually observed (see Fig. 2–9). Something must therefore be acting to decrease the alveolar surface tension in the lungs.

For example, if we consider two alveoli of dif-

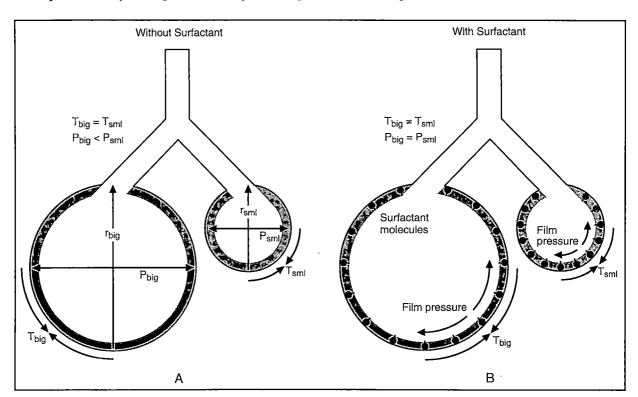

Figure 2–10.

The effect of a surface active agent is illustrated by two pairs of unequally filled alveoli arranged in parallel, one pair without surfactant (A) and the other with surfactant (B). In the alveoli without surfactant, if T_{sml} were the same as T_{big}, P_{sml} would be greater than P_{big} and the smaller alveolus would inflate the larger. In the alveoli with surfactant, T_{sml} is reduced in proportion to the radius (r) of the alveolus, which permits P_{sml} to equal P_{big}. Thus, alveoli of different radii can coexist.

ferent size, one at either end of a bifurcated respiratory bronchiole, we know that the smaller alveolus must have a higher pressure than the larger alveolus if the surface tension of each is the same (Fig. 2–10). To keep the air in the smaller alveolus from emptying into the larger, a surface-active agent that decreases the overall surface tension of the alveoli must be capable of lowering wall tension in proportion to the radius of the alveolus. Moreover, it must do so almost in anticipation of diminishing alveolar size. Only if such a surface-active agent is present can alveoli with different radii coexist in the lungs.

The surface-active agent in the human lung that performs this function is called **surfactant,** the principal active ingredient of which is *dipalmitoylphosphatidylcholine.* The structure of the surfactant molecule is such that it presents a nonpolar end of fatty acids (two palmitate residues) that is insoluble in water and a smaller, polar end (a phosphatidylcholine group) that dissolves readily in water.[9] Surfactant, therefore, orients itself perpendicularly to the surface in the alveolar fluid layer, its nonpolar end projecting toward the lumen. If surfactant were dispersed uniformly throughout the alveoli, its concentration at the air-fluid interface would vary in accordance with the surface area of any individual alveolus. Thus, the molecules would be compressed in the smaller alveoli, as depicted in Figure 2–10B. By compressing the surfactant mole-

cules, their density is increased and a "film pressure" is built up that counteracts much of the surface tension at the air-fluid interface. The rate of change in the surface tension resulting from compression of the surfactant molecules as the alveolus gets smaller is faster than the rate of change of the decreasing alveolar radius, so that a point is rapidly reached in which the pressure in the small alveolus equals the pressure in the big alveolus.

Unfortunately, if the alveolus were to remain smaller permanently, the surfactant molecules would begin to be squeezed out of the surface, and the surface tension would gradually rise. Therefore, maintenance of a constant surface area (as with constant volume breathing) could result in a gradual increase of alveolar surface tension, leading to collapse of smaller alveoli. Fortunately, we normally sigh periodically, and the result is a spreading out of the surfactant molecules (for reasons not well understood, there is also an increase in the number of surfactant molecules at the air-liquid interface).

Resistance to Gas Flow

When the respiratory muscles contract to expand the chest wall, the air in the lungs is decompressed; PA becomes subatmospheric; and PB pushes air into the lungs down a pressure gra-

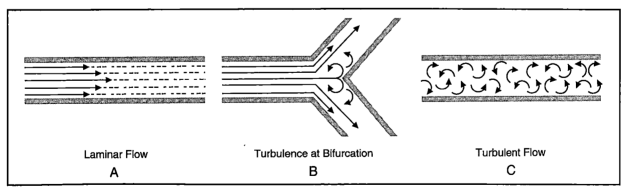

Figure 2–11.

Laminar and turbulent air flow in the airways. *A,* At low flow rates, air flows in a laminar pattern, and the resistance to air flow is proportional to the flow rate. *B,* At airway bifurcations, eddy formation creates a transitional flow pattern. *C,* At high flow rates, when a great deal of turbulence is created, the resistance to air flow is proportional to the square of the flow rate. (Redrawn from West JB. Respiratory Physiology—The Essentials. 2nd ed. © 1979, the Williams & Wilkins Co., Baltimore, p 103.)

dient. When the respiratory muscles relax, the chest wall recoils back to FRC, compressing the air in the lungs; PA is raised above PB, and air moves out of the lungs along a pressure gradient. At relatively low flow rates, gas travels parallel to the walls of the airways—a laminar flow pattern; at high flow rates, gas is disrupted, and turbulent flow results (Fig. 2–11). Generally, the pressure required to make gas flow through the airways under laminar flow conditions is proportional to the flow rate of the gas; under turbulent conditions, it is proportional to the square of the flow rate.

Thus, along with several other factors (e.g., the density of the gas, the average velocity of the gas, the radius of the airway, and the viscosity of the gas), the flow pattern of the gas in the airways dramatically influences resistance to the gas flow. Resistance to air flow (Raw) is expressed as the pressure difference between alveolar and atmospheric pressure (ΔP) divided by air flow ($\dot{V}$):

$$Raw = \frac{\Delta P}{\dot{V}}$$

Lung volume also influences Raw, because as the lungs expand during inhalation, the caliber of the bronchi and bronchioles is increased. Conversely, at low lung volumes the small airways

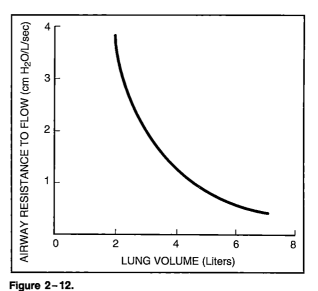

Figure 2–12.

The influence of lung volume on resistance to air flow in the lungs.

may close completely. The variation in Raw that occurs with changes in lung volume is shown in Figure 2–12.

To demonstrate the compliance, flow resistance, pressure, and volume characteristics of the lungs, consider the following scenario. Assume that the simplified respiratory system depicted in Figure 2–13 represents the lungs of an individual breathing 20 times per minute; the measured

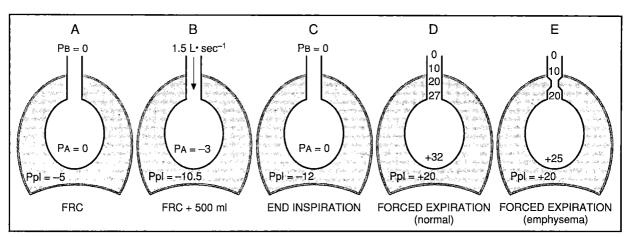

Figure 2–13.

The compliance, flow resistance, pressure, and volume characteristics of the lungs at different stages of the respiratory cycle. Refer to the text for details. PB, barometric pressure; PA, alveolar pressure; Ppl, pleural pressure; FRC, functional residual capacity.

lung compliance (C_L) is 0.2 $L \cdot cm^{-1}$ H_2O, and Raw is 2.0 $cm \cdot sec \cdot L^{-1}$ H_2O. Part A depicts FRC just before inspiration. There is no gas flow, and, therefore, $P_B = P_A$ and the intrapleural pressure is -5 cm H_2O. Part B depicts the pleural and alveolar pressures at FRC plus 500 ml with an inspiratory flow rate of 1.5 $L \cdot min^{-1}$. The values shown were derived by knowing that P_A must be lower than P_B. Thus, we can calculate that

$$P_B - P_A = V/sec \times Raw$$
$$= 1.5 \ L \cdot sec^{-1} \times 2 \ cm \cdot sec \cdot L^{-1} \ H_2O$$
$$= 3 \ cm \ H_2O$$

and therefore, P_A equals -3 cm H_2O. Also, we know that at FRC, P_L was $+5$ cm H_2O and that it increases as the lung volume is increased during inspiration. Because we know the lung compliance, we can calculate the change in transpulmonary pressure:

$$\Delta P_L = \Delta V \div C_L = 0.5 \ L \div 0.2 \ L \cdot cm^{-1} \ H_2O$$
$$= 2.5 \ cm \ H_2O$$

If the initial P_L was 5 cm H_2O, it has increased by 2.5 cm H_2O and is 7.5 cm H_2O at a volume of 500 ml. Recalling that $P_L = P_A - Ppl$, we can calculate that the new Ppl is -10.5 cm H_2O. Part C depicts end-inspiration when there is no air flow and the Ppl $= -12$ cm H_2O (can you calculate the volume at end-inspiration?). Part D demonstrates a situation of forced expiration from end-inspiration in a person with normal lungs. The expiratory muscles have generated an intrapleural pressure of $+20$ cm H_2O, which, when added to the transpulmonary pressure, yields an alveolar pressure of $+32$ cm H_2O that moves air along a pressure gradient out of the lungs. Part E presents the same situation as that depicted in Part D, but the person represented in Part E has severe emphysema. The expiratory muscles again generate an intrapleural pressure of $+20$ cm H_2O, but, because the lungs are excessively compliant, the alveolar pressure is only $+25$ cm H_2O. Air begins to flow out of the lungs, but a point is reached at which flow becomes dependent only on the lung volume, and the forced expiratory effort collapses the airways.

The significance of this obstructive effect is discussed in Chapter 6, and the pulmonary function tests that may be used to identify it are presented in Chapter 10.

Diffusion

The passive tendency of molecules to move from an area of high concentration to an area of lower concentration—*diffusion*—is responsible for the passage of oxygen and carbon dioxide between the alveoli and the pulmonary capillary blood. For oxygen molecules to get "in" and carbon dioxide molecules to get "out," they must pass through gas, tissue, and liquid.

With each breath, the linear velocity of the gas in the upper airways is very high, but it becomes less and less as the cross-sectional area of airways increases with successive branching. The magnitude of change in cross-sectional area from the trachea to the alveolar ducts is astounding, being a factor of about 5000. Airflow is effectively stopped beyond the alveolar ducts because the linear velocity of the gas molecules at that point is on the order of only about 0.4 $mm \cdot sec^{-1}$ during normal resting inspiratory effort. Therefore, gas molecules must diffuse through the gaseous medium within the alveoli to cross the small distances separating the alveolar ducts and the alveolar surface lining to effect gas exchange. The relative rates of diffusion for two gases in a gaseous medium (the air already in the lungs) varies inversely as the square root of their densities (Graham's law). More simply stated, the rate of diffusion of two gases is inversely proportional to the ratios of their molecular weights. For example, this relationship can be used to calculate relative diffusion rates for oxygen and carbon dioxide:

$$\frac{\text{Rate of diffusion of } CO_2}{\text{Rate of diffusion of } O_2} = \frac{\sqrt{M.W. \ O_2}}{\sqrt{M.W. \ CO_2}} = \frac{\sqrt{32}}{\sqrt{44}}$$
$$= 0.85$$

The gaseous diffusion of carbon dioxide is 85% as rapid as the gaseous diffusion of oxygen. The question arises, therefore, of just how much time it takes for new inhaled gas to come into equilibrium with the gas already present in the lungs. Because the average alveolar diameter is approximately 0.1 millimeter, it should take only about 0.0005 second for the gases to come into equilibrium.[10] Hence, any difference in the diffusion rates of oxygen and carbon dioxide is normally eliminated in a fraction of a second. However, if alveolar diameters are enlarged (as occurs in emphysema) and diffusion distances become greater, the diffusion times for the gas molecules are increased.

The rate of gas transfer across the alveolar-capillary membrane is proportional to the tissue area and inversely proportional to the thickness of the tissue. Moreover, the molecular weight of the gas and its solubility in liquid are factors. Therefore, the amount of gas actually diffusing through the gas-blood barrier and across the alveolar-capillary membrane is proportional to the area available for diffusion (A), a diffusibility constant that expresses the relationship of the molecular weight and the solubility of the gas (d), and the driving pressure $(P_1 - P_2)$ and is inversely proportional to the thickness of the tissues (T). These relationships are described in Fick's law:

$$\dot{V} = (d)\left(\frac{A}{T}\right)(P_1 - P_2)$$

Diffusion depends on a concentration difference. The concentration of a gas in a gaseous medium is directly proportional to the partial pressure of the gas. In a liquid medium, the concentration is directly proportional to the partial pressure of the gas times its solubility in that liquid. The partial pressure of each gas in any system may be thought of as the pressure that the gas would exert if it were alone in the system. The contribution of an individual gas to the total pressure exerted by a mixture of gases is dependent on the percentage of the total that the individual gas occupies (Dalton's law). For example, in the Earth's atmosphere nitrogen (N_2) comprises 79% of the constituent gases; oxygen (O_2) makes up 20.93%; carbon dioxide (CO_2) constitutes approximately 0.03%; and all other

gases are about 0.04%. If these atmospheric gases were at standard conditions of temperature and pressure, and dry (STPD; 0° C, a pressure of 760 mm Hg, and no water vapor pressure), the partial pressure of oxygen would simply be the product of the Pв and the fraction of O_2.

Partial Pressure of Oxygen
    = 760 mm Hg × 0.2093 = 159.06 mm Hg

However, in the real world, inspired gases are rarely completely dry. When the partial pressure of the water vapor is known, it becomes a relatively straightforward process to convert from a volume expressed in terms of STPD to ambient temperature and pressure, saturated with water vapor at ambient temperature (ATPS), or to body temperature and ambient atmospheric pressure, saturated with water vapor at body temperature (BTPS). For example, at sea level and with a typical body temperature of 37 degrees C, water vapor exerts a partial pressure of 47 mm Hg.[6,7,11] Thus, the Po_2 in the trachea would be

760 mm Hg − 47 mm Hg
    = 713 mm Hg × 0.2093 = 149 mm Hg

Henry's law allows us to calculate the concentration of a gas in a liquid if its partial pressure and solubility coefficient are known. The solubility coefficient for O_2 in a watery solution is about 0.03 ml $O_2 \cdot$ mm $Hg^{-1} \cdot L^{-1}$; for CO_2, it is about 0.7 ml $CO_2 \cdot$ mm $Hg^{-1} \cdot L^{-1}$. It is clear that carbon dioxide is approximately 23 times more soluble than oxygen. By combining Graham's and Henry's laws, we can see that oxygen diffuses about 15% more rapidly than carbon dioxide through a gas but only about 5% as rapidly through a liquid.

Oxygen Carriage

Oxygen diffuses through the pulmonary alveolar capillary membrane and is then carried to the tissues in two forms: (1) physically dissolved in the plasma, and (2) chemically bound to hemoglobin (Hb) in the erythrocytes (Fig. 2–14A).

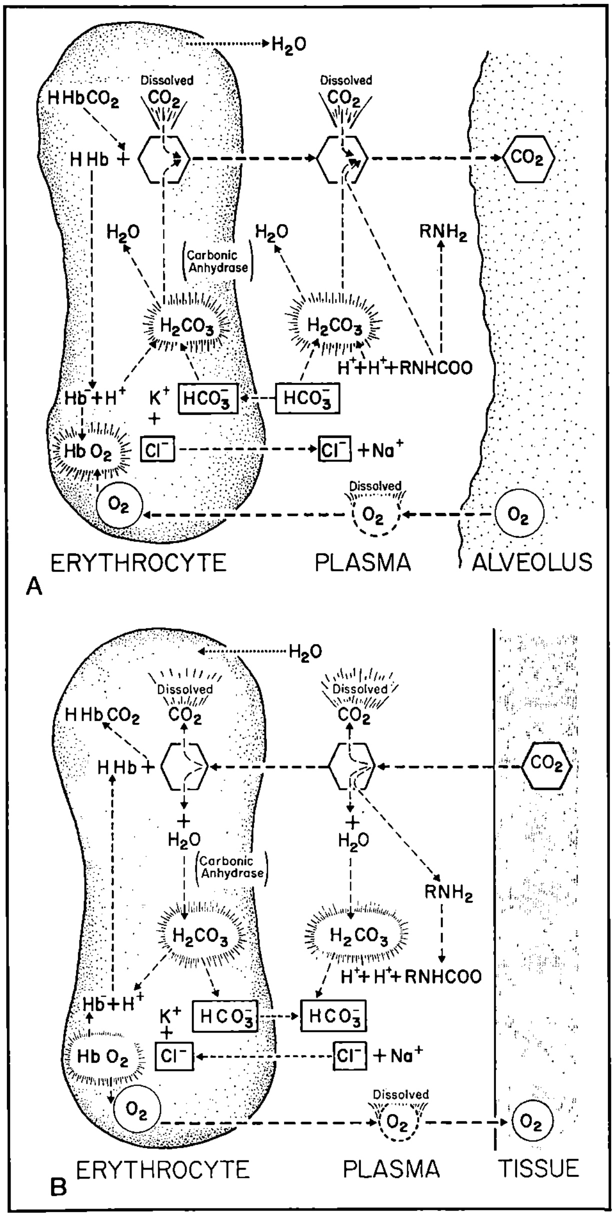

Figure 2-14.

Gas exchange at the alveolar-capillary interface *(A)* and at the capillary-tissue interface *(B)*. (Adapted from Cherniack RM, Cherniack L. Respiration in Health and Disease. 3rd ed. Philadelphia, WB Saunders, 1983, p 77.)

Dissolved Oxygen

As previously discussed, the amount of oxygen that can physically dissolve in the plasma is de-

termined by its solubility and is directly proportional to its partial pressure in the plasma. Thus, if the arterial Po_2 (Pa_{O_2}) were 100 mm Hg, there would be 3 milliliters of oxygen dissolved in each liter of the blood. If this small amount of oxygen were the only source of oxygen available to the body, a tremendous blood flow would be needed just to supply the body's resting requirements for oxygen. For example, if the body's requirement for oxygen at rest were 3.5 ml $\cdot$ kg^{-1} $\cdot$ min^{-1}, a person weighing 65 kilograms would need about 228 ml $\cdot$ min^{-1} of oxygen; with only 3 milliliters of oxygen available per liter of blood, about 76 liters of blood per minute would need to be circulated to meet the body's demand for oxygen. Clearly, another, more efficient, means of carrying oxygen to the tissues of the body must exist.

Oxygen Bound to Hemoglobin

The hemoglobin molecule is made up of four *heme* groups attached to a *globin* molecule. A heme is formed when a ferrous ion covalently binds to the four nitrogens on the pyrrole groups of a *porphyrin* ring (four pyrrole groups cyclically linked by methylene bridges). The globin molecule is formed by a combination of four amino acid chains (two alpha, two beta) that contain imidazole nitrogen groups that are capable of covalently bonding with metal ions. The heme groups are believed to bind to the globin molecule by a fifth valence bond. Thus, the ferrous ion in each heme has a sixth covalent bond available to bind with oxygen (if it is available) or with an imidazole nitrogen group in the polypeptide chains of the globin molecule (Fig. 2-15).

Because of hemoglobin's ability to reversibly bind to oxygen, the blood's carrying capacity for oxygen is increased significantly. For example, there are normally about 147 grams of hemoglobin in each liter of blood, and this amount of hemoglobin can carry approximately 197 milliliters of oxygen.[6,12] If hemoglobin were the only source for the delivery of oxygen, the 65-kilogram person from the earlier example would

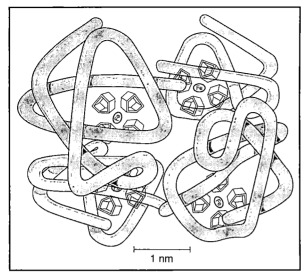

Figure 2-15.

A molecule of hemoglobin. Hemoglobin is composed of four heme molecules bound to the four polypeptide chains of a globin molecule. (Redrawn from Harper HA, et al. Physiologische Chemie. New York, Springer-Verlag, 1975.)

need to circulate only approximately 1.2 liters of blood per minute to meet the body's demand for oxygen.

Oxyhemoglobin Dissociation Curve

The oxyhemoglobin dissociation curve (Fig. 2–16) describes the relationship between the amount of oxygen bound to hemoglobin and the partial pressure of oxygen with which the hemoglobin is in equilibrium. Clinically, this is referred to as the percent saturation of hemoglobin. Under ideal conditions (blood pH = 7.4, body temperature = 37° C, [Hb] = 14.7 g · L^{-1}), less than 10% of the oxygen dissociates from the hemoglobin as Po_2 falls 40 mm Hg, from 100 to 60 mm Hg. However, nearly 60% of the oxygen is dissociated from the hemoglobin as Po_2 falls another 40 mm Hg, from 60 to 20 mm Hg. Decreasing the pH (increasing acidemia) of the blood from the normal value of 7.40 to 7.30 shifts the hemoglobin dissociation curve downward and to the right an average of approximately 7% to 8%; in contrast, alkalemia shifts the curve to the left. Increasing the concentration of carbon dioxide in the tissue capillary beds displaces oxygen from the hemoglobin, delivering the oxygen to the tissues at a higher Po_2 than would otherwise occur. In conditions of prolonged hypoxemia (longer than a few hours) the amount of 2,3-diphosphoglycerate (2,3-DPG; a phosphate compound present in the blood in varying concentrations under different conditions) in the blood is increased, resulting in a rightward shift in the hemoglobin dissociation curve. Increasing the temperature of the tissue, as happens normally in exercising muscle, also results in a shift of the hemoglobin dissociation curve to the right. The result of these rightward shifts is a decreased hemoglobin affinity for oxygen. Although these effects can be beneficial, the range of variability normally tolerated by the body is relatively narrow.

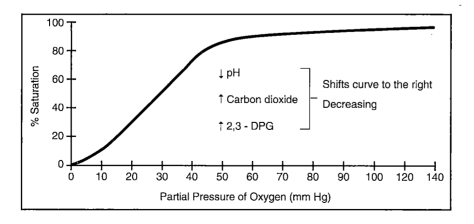

Figure 2-16.

The oxyhemoglobin dissociation curve. Note that in the "flat" portion of the curve (80 mm Hg and above), a change in Pa$_{o_2}$ of as much as 20 mm Hg does not appreciably alter the hemoglobin saturation. However, in the "steep" portion of the curve (below 60 mm Hg), relatively small changes in saturation result in large changes in the Pa$_{o_2}$.

Total Oxygen Content

The total amount of oxygen attached to hemoglobin and dissolved in plasma is represented by the arterial oxygen content (Ca_{O_2}), which is calculated as follows:

$$Ca_{O_2} = [(Pa_{O_2})(0.003)] + [(1.34)(\%Sat)(Hb)]$$
$$\text{amount dissolved} \qquad \text{amount bound}$$

where the constant, 0.003, is the Bunsen solubility coefficient for oxygen in plasma at BTPS; 1.34 (ml O_2/g Hb) represents the experimentally determined capacity of hemoglobin to carry oxygen; %Sat represents the percentage of hemoglobin actually bound with oxygen and is analytically determined; Hb represents the hemoglobin content of the blood, which, expressed as grams of hemoglobin per 100 ml blood (g%), is normally 12 g% to 16 g%.[7,12,13] The adequacy of tissue oxygenation depends on the relationship between oxygen and hemoglobin. Hence, the hematocrit is probably the single most influential component in determining the oxygen-carrying capacity of the blood.

Carbon Dioxide Carriage

Carbon dioxide diffuses through the tissue-capillary membrane and is then carried to the lungs in three forms: (1) physically dissolved, (2) bound to proteins as carbamino compounds, and (3) bicarbonate (see Fig. 2–14B).

Carbon Dioxide in the Plasma

Once carbon dioxide has diffused across the tissue-capillary membrane, some physically dissolves in the plasma; some forms carbamino compounds and hydrogen ions (H^+) by binding to the amine groups of plasma proteins; and some is hydrated to H_2CO_3, which dissociates into HCO_3^- and more H^+ ions. The hydrogen ions freed by the formation of carbamino compounds and the dissociation of H_2CO_3 are buffered to a large extent by the plasma proteins (see Acid-Base Balance). Most of the carbon dioxide, however, diffuses through the plasma and into the erythrocytes.

Carbon Dioxide in the Erythrocytes

Once carbon dioxide has diffused into the red blood cells, some is again dissolved into the cytoplasm. Some of the carbon dioxide forms carbamino hemoglobin and hydrogen ions by binding to the amine groups of hemoglobin. The remainder of the carbon dioxide is hydrated in the erythrocytes because there is an abundance of **carbonic anhydrase** to catalyze the hydration process and because there is a tremendous source of hemoglobin to buffer the hydrogen ions. Thus, as the blood passes through the tissues, the vast majority (about 90%) of the carbon dioxide taken up is converted to HCO_3^- and H^+ ions in the erythrocytes. But, because hemoglobin buffers the hydrogen ions and because the HCO_3^- ions diffuse out of the erythrocytes and into the plasma, accumulation of these by-products of the hydration process is negligible. However, owing to the influx of HCO_3^- ions into the plasma from the erythrocytes, there is a countermovement of Cl^- ions into the erythrocytes—the *chloride shift*. Additionally, the increased concentration of HCO_3^- and Cl^- ions within the erythrocytes make them hypotonic with respect to the plasma fluid. Hence, water moves into the erythrocytes, causing them to swell somewhat. For this reason, the hematocrit (the packed cell volume) of venous blood is slightly greater than that of arterial blood.

The binding of hydrogen ions and oxygen to the hemoglobin molecule is a reciprocal process. That is, the binding of hydrogen ions to hemoglobin reduces the strength of the oxygen bonds, shifting the oxyhemoglobin dissociation curve to the right (Bohr's shift); likewise, as the hemoglobin deoxygenates, it binds the hydrogen ions more strongly and becomes a weaker acid (Haldane's effect). The result of these reciprocal changes is that hemoglobin is able to change its pK (the pH at which equal amounts of acid and basic forms are present), thus minimizing the pH changes of the blood as gas exchange occurs.

Perfusion

The distribution of blood within the pulmonary circulation is dependent on three primary factors: (1) gravity, (2) amount of blood ejected from the right ventricle per unit time, and (3) pulmonary vascular resistance.

Gravity

In the normal person standing upright, the distance from the top of the lungs to the bottom of the lungs averages approximately 30 centimeters.[12] If the pulmonary artery enters each lung at its midpoint, the pulmonary artery pressure would have to be at least 15 cm H_2O to get blood flow to the top of the lungs. For this reason, blood flows with the least effort through the gravity-dependent regions of the lungs. However, because the normal mean pulmonary artery pressure is approximately 10 to 20 mm Hg, usually blood flow at the tops of the lungs is not totally absent.

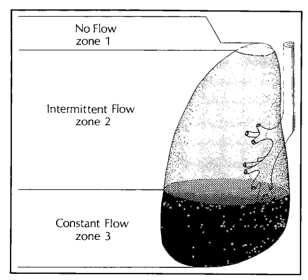

Figure 2-17.
The distribution of pulmonary blood flow is gravity dependent. In the upright lung, the lowermost portions of the lung are preferentially perfused. (From Shapiro BA, Harrison RA, Cane RD, Templin R. Clinical Application of Blood Gases. 4th ed. Chicago, Year Book Medical Publishers, 1989, p 25.)

A three-zone model is widely used to describe the effects of gravity on pulmonary perfusion (Fig. 2–17).[5,12] Zone 1, at the top of each lung, is the least gravity-dependent region and is an area of potentially no blood flow. Zone 3, at the base of each lung, is the gravity-dependent region and receives almost constant blood flow. Zone 2, the intermediate area of each lung, receives varyingly intermittent blood flow. Whether there is blood flow in zone 2 is normally determined by the difference between pulmonary arterial and alveolar pressures.

Cardiac Output

Generally, the greater the amount of blood ejected by the right ventricle per unit time (cardiac output), the greater the pulmonary artery pressure. Normally, then, as cardiac output increases, zone 3 extends farther up each lung.

Pulmonary Vascular Resistance

Unlike the systemic vascular system, the pulmonary vascular system tends to react in a passive manner to changes in pressure. Nonetheless, the pulmonary arterioles are capable of generating significant increases in resistance to pulmonary blood flow.

Ventilation-Perfusion Interactions and Shunts

The composition of the alveolar gas depends on the balanced interaction of alveolar gas flow and pulmonary capillary blood flow. The alveolar gas flow is referred to as the **alveolar ventilation** ($\dot{V}A$); the pulmonary capillary blood flow is referred to as **pulmonary perfusion** ($\dot{Q}$). Normally, the lungs receive about 4 L · min^{-1} of alveolar ventilation and about 5 L · min^{-1} of blood flow. As we already know, the $\dot{V}A$ is not equally distributed throughout the lungs, being about 2.5 times greater at the bases than at the apices. Similarly, the distribution of $\dot{Q}$ in the lungs is uneven, but $\dot{Q}$ is about six times greater at the bases than at the apices. The $\dot{V}_A$ to $\dot{Q}$ ratio, then, is approximately 2.4 times greater at the apices than at the bases of the lungs. Overall, however, the ratio of $\dot{V}_A$ to $\dot{Q}$ is 0.8. Thus, although alveolar concentrations vary during the breathing cycle, the mean $P_{A_{O_2}}$ is about 102 mm Hg and the mean $P_{A_{CO_2}}$ is about 40 mm Hg. Furthermore, because a greater amount of oxygen is taken out of the alveolar gas than carbon dioxide is added, the expired V_T is actually slightly less than the inspired V_T.

Because blood flow is not distributed evenly to all parts of the lung, some parts of the lung may actually be perfused but not ventilated. Such an excess of perfusion is called a **right-to-left shunt** because the blood passes from the right to the left side of the heart without participating in gas exchange. Likewise, it is possible that some parts of the lung may be ventilated but receive no blood flow. Such an excess of ventilation is called **physiologic dead space** because the alveolar gas cannot participate in gas exchange. Although neither of these extremes normally exists, the $\dot{V}_A$ to $\dot{Q}$ ratios of many alveoli lie above or below the obvious ratio of 0.8. For this reason, and because there is a small percentage of direct venous return to the left atrium (the bronchial and the thebesian veins), the partial pressure of oxygen in the arterial blood (Pa_{O_2}) is about 12 mm Hg less than the partial pressure of oxygen in the alveoli. Thus, a Pa_{O_2} of 90 mm Hg in a normal person breathing air at sea level is common.

Respiration

Within the cells, foodstuffs, under the influence of several enzymes, react chemically with oxygen to produce energy. Five percent or less of the overall energy metabolism of the cell occurs in the cytoplasm of the cell. The vast majority of energy is derived from the formation of **adenosine triphosphate (ATP)** within the mitochondria. Pyruvic acid, free fatty acids, and most amino acids are transformed into the intermediary compound acetylcoenzyme A (acetyl-CoA). Acetyl-CoA is, in turn, acted on by other enzymes in the **tricarboxylic acid cycle** (Krebs's cycle) and split into carbon dioxide and hydrogen ions.[14] The hydrogen ions eventually combine with oxygen to form H_2O in a process of **oxidative phosphorylation.**[15] The final step of this process is commonly referred to as the **electron transport chain.** The production of carbon dioxide and the utilization of oxygen constitutes cellular respiration.

Even when insufficient oxygen is available for the cellular oxidation of glucose to continue, small amounts of energy can still be released by the glycolytic breakdown of glucose to pyruvic acid and hydrogen ions, which are combined with NAD^+ to form NADH and H^+. These glycolytic by-products react with one another to form lactic acid, which diffuses out of the cells into the extracellular fluids, thus allowing the glycolytic reaction to continue for a short time.

Acid-Base Balance

Metabolically produced acids are largely eliminated from the body via the lungs in the form of carbon dioxide because the major blood acid, carbonic acid (H_2CO_3), is *volatile.* That is, it can chemically vary between a liquid and a gaseous state. The other blood acids (dietary acids, lactic acids, and keto acids) are regulated by the kidneys and the liver.[16] The measurement of arterial oxygen or carbon dioxide tension and hydrogen ion concentration for assessment of acid-base balance and oxygenation status is commonly accomplished by means of laboratory analysis of arterial blood gases (ABGs). Generally, an ABG report contains the pH, the Pa_{CO_2}, the Pa_{O_2}, and the HCO_3^- and base excess values for the sample analyzed. A detailed discussion of acid-base balance and arterial blood gases is presented in Chapter 10.

Control of Breathing

Unlike the muscle of the heart, the respiratory muscles are totally dependent on impulses from the brain; breathing ceases if the spinal cord is cut above the level of the phrenic nerves. Although influenced by several nonchemical mechanisms, breathing is regulated by changes in arterial Po_2, Pco_2, and hydrogen ion concentration. Moreover, although breathing is largely an automatic process, it may also be controlled voluntarily. Two separate neural mechanisms regulate breathing: (1) efferent output from the cerebral cortex to the motoneurons of the respiratory musculature carried via the corticospinal tracts effects voluntary control of breathing; (2) automatic efferent output, emanating from the pons and the medulla, to the motoneurons of the respiratory musculature is carried in the white matter of the spinal cord between the lateral and ventral corticospinal tracts. Inspiratory fibers terminate on the phrenic motoneurons in the ventral horns of the spinal cord from C3 to C5 and on the external intercostal motoneurons in the ventral horns throughout the thoracic spinal cord. Expiratory fibers terminate principally on the internal intercostal motoneurons in the ventral horns throughout the thoracic spinal cord. The motoneurons of the inspiratory and expiratory muscles are reciprocally innervated with the notable exception that the phrenic axons remain

active for a brief portion of the expiratory phase. This activity is postulated to "brake the lung's elastic recoil."[17,18]

There are two basic types of brain stem respiratory neurons: those that are active during inspiration and those that are active during expiration. Most of the inspiratory neurons increase their discharge rates during inspiration, and most of the expiratory neurons increase their rates of discharge during expiration, but some of the neurons discharge at decreasing frequencies whereas others maintain a consistently high rate of discharge during inspiration or expiration.

The classic **respiratory center** of the brain stem is actually two groups of neurons located in the medulla (Fig. 2–18).[19] A dorsal group of neurons, the dorsal respiratory group, is located in and near the nucleus of the tractus solitarius and is composed mostly of inspiratory neurons. A long, columnar ventral group of neurons, the ventral respiratory group, is located in the ventrolateral medulla extending through the nucleus ambiguus and the nucleus retroambiguus and is composed of expiratory neurons at either end

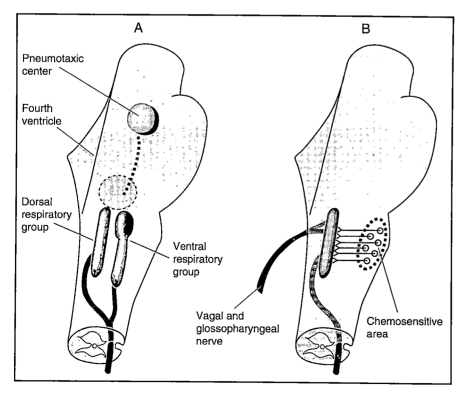

Figure 2–18.

The "respiratory center" is located bilaterally in the medulla and pons of the brain stem *(A)*. Input from the central and peripheral chemosensitive and peripheral proprioceptive receptors moderates the dorsal respiratory group of neurons *(B)*. (Redrawn from Guyton AC. Textbook of Medical Physiology. 8th ed. Philadelphia, WB Saunders, 1991, pp 445, 446.)

with inspiratory neurons interspersed centrally. At present, knowledge of the mechanism responsible for rhythmic respiratory effort is lacking. Neither the dorsal nor the ventral respiratory groups of neurons are required for the generation of automatic breathing effort, and no pacemaker cells have been identified.

Also inspiratory and expiratory neurons in the medial parabrachial and Kölliker-Fuse nuclei of the dorsolateral pons are active during both phases of breathing—the **pneumotaxic center.** The normal function of the pneumotaxic center is unknown. However, because damage to this area results in a slower rate of breathing with a greater Vt, it is believed to play a role in the alternation of inspiratory and expiratory effort. The vagi also influence the activity of the medullary neurons via afferents from receptors in the bronchi and lungs.[20]

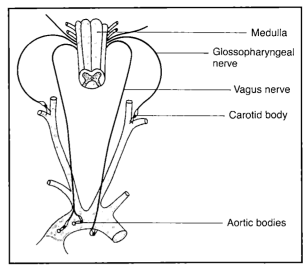

Figure 2–19.

Afferent input from the carotid and aortic bodies is carried via the glossopharyngeal and vagus nerves. (From Guyton AC. Textbook of Medical Physiology. 8th ed. Philadelphia, WB Saunders, 1991, p 448.)

Chemical and Nonchemical Mediation of Ventilation

Chemoreceptors in the carotid and aortic bodies and in the medulla are sensitive to changes in arterial Pco_2 or hydrogen ion concentration or Po_2. The carotid bodies, located near the bifurcation of the common carotid artery bilaterally, and the aortic bodies (of which there are at least two), located near the arch of the aorta, are surrounded by fenestrated sinusoidal capillaries. Studies of rats suggest that some of the cells are associated closely with glossopharyngeal afferent axons and that these cells may be responsible for sensing oxygen tension.[21] Quite possibly the aortic bodies, which are less well understood than the carotid bodies, may have a greater role in responding to hydrogen ion concentration. Afferents from the carotid bodies make their way to the medulla via the carotid sinus and the glossopharyngeal nerves, whereas afferent fibers from the aortic bodies travel in the vagi (Fig. 2–19).

Other chemoreceptors in the medulla are located near the dorsal and ventral respiratory groups of neurons (see Fig. 2–18). These chemoreceptors monitor the hydrogen ion concentration of the cerebrospinal fluid. Carbon dioxide in the cranial arteries readily passes the blood-brain barrier into the interstitium of the brain and the cerebrospinal fluid, where it is rapidly hydrated. The H_2CO_3 dissociates, and the resultant hydrogen ions elevate the local concentration, lowering the pH. This is the mechanism responsible for increasing the minute ventilation when arterial Pco_2 becomes elevated.

Both unmyelinated and myelinated vagal fibers carry impulses from receptors in the bronchi and lungs to the dorsal respiratory group of neurons in the medulla.[22] The unmyelinated fibers are C fibers; they are commonly called *J receptors* because of their juxtacapillary locations. The J receptors are stimulated by hyperinflation of the lungs and respond by causing periods of apnea interspersed with rapid breathing, bradycardia, and hypotension. The receptors supplied by myelinated fibers are further categorized as slowly adapting and rapidly adapting. The slowly adapting receptors are probably distributed in the interstitium along the airways among the smooth muscle cells. Stimulation of these receptors results in shortening of inspiration. The rapidly adapting receptors are distributed among the epithelial cells of the airways in the interstitium. Stimulation of these receptors in the trachea results in coughing, mucus secretion, and broncho-constriction; stimulation in the lung may result in hyperpnea. Additional nonchemical afferent fibers from proprioceptors, from the limbic system and hypothalamus, and from the baroreceptors have been implied from the results of experiments that studied the effects of active and passive joint movement, pain and emotional stimuli, and blood pressure on breathing.

THE CARDIOVASCULAR SYSTEM

The primary function of the cardiovascular (circulatory) system is the transportation and dis-tribution of essential substances to the tissues of the body and the removal of by-products of cellular metabolism. The heart provides the principal motive force that pushes blood through the vessels of the pulmonary and systemic circuits. However, in the case of the systemic circuit, the recoil of the arterial walls during diastole, skeletal muscle compression of veins during exercise, and negative thoracic pressure during inspiration also move the blood in a forward direction. The pulmonary circuit receives the entire output of the right ventricle with each cardiac cycle, but the systemic circuit is an arrangement of several different circuits in parallel (Fig. 2–20).

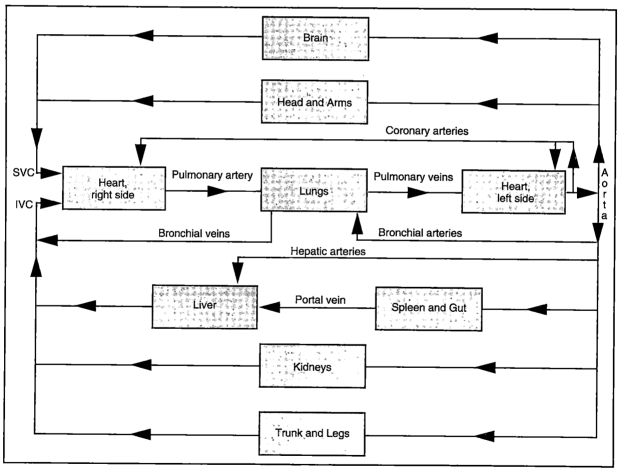

Figure 2–20.

A schematic representation of the pulmonary and systemic vascular beds. SVC, superior vena cava; IVC, inferior vena cava.

Electrical Properties of Myocytes

The unique properties of the myocardial cell membrane are responsible for differences in the ionic composition of the intracellular and interstitial fluids. Table 2-4 lists representative values for the intracellular and interstitial concentrations of the principal ions of concern.[18,23,24] Although the numbers of positively and negatively charged ions on either side of the cell membrane are almost equal, slightly more negatively charged ions are inside than are outside the cell, creating a negative charge on the inside. Thus, the **resting membrane potential** for myocardial cells is about −85 millivolts (the minus sign is used, by convention, to signify that the inside of the cell is negative relative to the outside).

Forces Acting on Ions

In very general terms, an ion moves across a cell membrane because it "wants to" and because it "can." Because the concentration of ions inside and outside the cell is different, an ion tends to move along its concentration gradient (from an area of higher concentration to one of lower concentration). Likewise, because the inside of the cell is negative with respect to the outside, an ion moves along an electrical gradient in accordance with its valence. The membrane potential at which these two forces come into equilibrium (E_{ion}) is expressed in units of millivolts and is calculated by Nernst's equation*:

$$\text{potential energy} = \\ -61.5 \log \frac{\text{concentration inside cell}}{\text{concentration outside cell}}$$

In other words, E_{ion} represents how much an ion "wants to" move. However, whether an ion "can" move across the cell membrane depends on the membrane's *permeability* (g) to the ion.

---

* In deriving the expression "−61.5," the ion in question was assumed to be univalent; in the case of multivalent ions, the expression should be divided by the valence number. Furthermore, if the ionic valence is negative, the sign of the expression becomes positive.

TABLE 2-4. Representative Intracellular and Interstitial Ionic Concentrations for Myocardial Muscle Cells

Ion	Intracellular Concentration (mM)	Interstitial Concentration (mM)
K+	147	4.5
Na+	12	145
Ca++	10^{-4}	2
Cl−	4	112

The product of these two factors is an expression of the **flux** for a given ion.

Thus far we have considered only the membrane equilibrium potential for individual ions. Of course, we must deal with a cell membrane that is actually permeable to several ions concurrently. Ions may cross the hydrophobic membrane of the myocyte only via protein-lined *channels*.[25] Although many ion-selective channels cross the myocytic cell membrane, only the most notable are mentioned here. The transmembrane potential (V_m), which depends on the intra- and extracellular [K+], [Cl−], [Ca++], and [Na+] as well as their conductances or permeability (g_K, g_{Cl}, g_{Ca}, and g_{Na}), is described by Goldman's constant-field equation:

$$V_m = -61.5 \log \frac{g_K[K^+]_{out}}{g_K[K^+]_{in}} + \frac{g_{Na}[Na^+]_{out}}{g_{Na}[Na^+]_{in}} \\ + \frac{g_{Cl}[Cl^+]_{in}}{g_{Cl}[Cl^+]_{out}} + \frac{g_{Ca}[Ca^+]_{out}}{g_{Ca}[Ca^+]_{in}}$$

The implication of this equation is that the membrane permeability plays a larger role in determining ionic flux than the concentration difference.[26]

Active transport is the means by which cells move ions against their electrochemical gradients. This process either uses ATP to supply the energy or couples the transport of one ion against its gradient with the movement of another ion down its gradient. For example, because the permeability of the cell membrane to Na+ is very low at rest, there is very little influx of Na+ into the cell. Nonetheless, it is the small inward flux of Na+ that makes the inside of the resting cell membrane slightly less negative than the predicted E_{Na}. Were it not for a metabolic pump that constantly evicts Na^+ in exchange for K^+, the steady inward leak of Na^+ would gradually depolarize the cell. However, because this **sodium-potassium pump** moves both ions against their concentration and electrostatic gradients, energy is required. The pump eliminates Na^+ and brings in K^+ in a ratio of 3 to 2, using ATP as the power source. The **sodium-calcium antiporter** uses the potential energy of Na^+ as it diffuses down its electrochemical gradient to move Ca^{++} against its gradient and out of the cell. The **calcium pump** uses ATP to pump Ca^{++} out of the cell.

As may be seen in Figure 2–21, the depolarization of fast-responding myocytes results from the controlled passage of sodium, potassium, chloride, and calcium ions across the cell membrane and lasts about 2 milliseconds. When the cell membrane potential suddenly changes to a less negative state, a sequence of ion channels

opening and closing is initiated. This sequence is called an **action potential.** But unlike the action potential of skeletal muscle, this depolarization is followed by a plateau phase that lasts about 200 milliseconds. The rapid depolarization, phase 0, is the result of rapid Na^+ influx resulting from a sudden increase in g_{Na}. When V_m is suddenly changed to the threshold level, the characteristics of the cell membrane alter dramatically. Sodium ions move into the cell via specific fast channels that are controlled by two types of "gates." One gate, the **activation gate,** opens as V_m becomes less negative; the other, the **inactivation gate,** closes the channel as V_m becomes less negative. At resting membrane potential, the activation gates are closed and the inactivation gates are open. Because anything that makes V_m less negative tends to open the activation gates, thus activating the fast Na^+ channels, they are said to be "voltage-gated" channels. The entry of Na^+ inside the cell reverses some of the internal negativity; the resultant further diminution of V_m

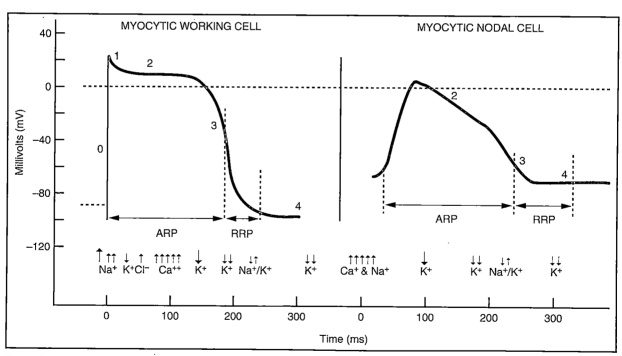

Figure 2–21.

A typical action potential in a fast response (working cell) and a slow response (nodal cell) myocyte. In addition to indicating the absolute refractory period (ARP) and the relative refractory period (RRP) for each type of cell, the relative ionic flux is also shown. (Modified from Berne RM, Levy MN. Cardiovascular Physiology. 6th ed. Chicago, Mosby–Year Book, 1992, p 6.)

augments the inward Na^+ flux and opens more activation gates. Finally, V_m passes the threshold, and the remaining activation gates open, initiating phase 0 of the action potential. As Na^+ rushes into the cell, the charge inside the cell becomes positive—the *overshoot*—and the inactivation gates start to close. Whereas the opening of the activation gates occurs in about 0.2 millisecond or less, closure of the inactivation gates takes about 1 millisecond. Once closed, the inactivation gates "inactivate" the fast Na^+ channels. The inactivation gates remain closed until about midway through phase 3 when the cell has partially repolarized.

The *initial rapid repolarization, phase 1,* occurs because of the closure of the Na^+ channels, Cl^- influx, and K^+ efflux. Transient potassium outward (K_{to}) channels are activated because the interior of the cell is positively charged and because the internal K^+ concentration gradient is so high.

The *plateau, phase 2,* is the result of the prolonged opening of voltage-gated Ca^{++} channels. There are two types of Ca^{++} channels in the cardiac cells: long lasting, or L-type, and transient, or T-type. The L-type Ca^{++} channels are abundantly more plentiful than the T-type and are activated during phase 0 when V_m reaches about -10 millivolts. The T-type Ca^{++} channels are activated at more negative potentials than the L type, and their activation duration time is very much shorter. Although their activation duration is less than L-type Ca^{++} channels, the T-type Ca^{++} channels are not blocked by calcium channel blocking drugs. The Ca^{++} entering the cell throughout phase 2 is involved in **excitation-contraction coupling.**[27-29]

The long-lasting, slow Ca^{++} influx during phase 2 is offset by a K^+ efflux. So-called *inwardly rectified K^+ current,* mediated via K_1 channels, results from a decrease in g_K for K^+ ions and serves to balance the slow inward currents of Ca^{++} and Na^+ during phase 2.

Final repolarization, phase 3, is the result of closure of the Ca^{++} channels and prolonged opening of at least three voltage-gated K^+ channels. The K_{to} channels are more prominent in the atrial myocytes than in the ventricular myocytes. They permit outward K^+ current to exceed the

slow inward Ca^{++} current early in phase 2. The delayed rectifier channels (K) are slowly activated near the end of phase 0. They allow outward K^+ current to increase gradually throughout phase 2. The K_{K1} (inwardly rectified) channels progressively increase their conductance for K^+, allowing the outward K^+ current to increase and accelerate repolarization.

Unlike fast-response action potentials, which consist of three primary components (a spike, a plateau, and a period of repolarization), slow-response action potentials lack a spike. Nodal myocytes, located principally in the S-A and A-V nodes, are typical of slow-response fibers. Depolarization in these fibers results from a slow inward Ca^{++} and Na^+ current through the Ca^{++} channels. The ionic exchanges in phases 0 and 2 in the slow-response fibers closely resemble those of phase 2 in the fast-response fibers.

Automaticity and Rhythmicity

An ability to initiate its own depolarization—**automaticity**—and the regularity with which such pacemaking activity occurs—**rhythmicity**—are intrinsic traits of the heart. Recall from Chapter 1, that there are different types of myocytes dispersed throughout the heart tissue. Typical working myocytes comprise the bulk of the tissue. The other myocytes—nodal, transitional, and Purkinje's—make up the specialized conduction system of the heart and serve as pacemaker cells having a recognized hierarchy of rhythmicity. Nodal myocytes exhibit the highest rates of rhythmicity but have the slowest impulse conduction rates. Transitional myocytes have a slower rhythmicity but conduct impulses about twice as fast as nodal cells. Purkinje's cells conduct impulses about eight times faster than nodal myocytes but have a very low rate of rhythmicity. Working myocytes have about the same conduction velocity as transitional myocytes but only exhibit the trait of rhythmicity under abnormal conditions. The proportion of nodal, transitional, and Purkinje's cells within the various regions of the specialized conduction system generally dictates the hierarchy of rhythmicity.

Under certain conditions **ectopic pacemakers,**

or **ectopic foci,** can initiate a depolarization wave. This can occur if

- the rhythmicity of the ectopic pacemaker is enhanced
- the rhythmicity of higher order pacemakers is inhibited
- the conduction path from the higher order pacemakers to the ectopic focus is blocked.

Normally, those cells with the highest intrinsic rates of rhythmicity override and pace the cells lower in the hierarchy.

In the nodal myocytes of the S-A node, the movement of at least three different ions across the cell membrane is responsible for the instability of the phase 4 membrane potential and hence for automaticity (Fig. 2–22). The movement of Na^+ into the cell, via specific channels that differ from the fast Na^+ channels, contributes to a lessening of the negativity of the cell's membrane potential. This slow Na^+ channel is activated during repolarization, as the membrane potential becomes more negative. The more negative the membrane potential becomes, the greater the activation of the slow Na^+ channels.

The second ion contributing to the phase 4 membrane potential instability is Ca^{++}. Mediated by the T-type Ca^{++} channels toward the end of phase 4, the influx of Ca^{++} destabilizes the membrane potential of the cell. These channels,

too, are activated as the membrane potential becomes more negative during repolarization.

The third ion involved in the process of diastolic depolarization is K^+. Its influence comes not from an actual influx or efflux but rather from the gradual diminution of the efflux of K^+ via the K channel throughout phase 4. As a consequence, the opposition of outward K^+ current to the depolarizing influences of the two inward-moving ions decreases.

Automaticity in the A-V node is probably mediated the same way as in the S-A node. In Purkinje's fibers, the T-type Ca^{++} channels are not involved. Thus the phase 4 membrane potential instability is mediated by the imbalance between the slow Na^+ channels and the gradually deactivating K channels. Additionally, autonomic neurotransmitters can play a role in automaticity by altering ionic currents across the cell membranes. The collective summation of the action potentials of the myocytes is graphically depicted in the electrocardiograph (ECG). The ECG, its importance, and its interpretation are discussed in Chapter 9.

Excitation-Contraction Coupling

The mechanism by which the action potential causes myofibrillar contraction is called

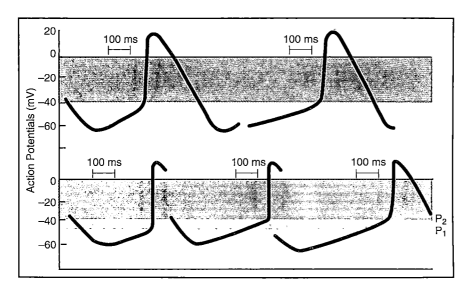

Figure 2–22.

Three mechanisms of slowing the discharge frequency of pacemaker cells. In the upper portion of the diagram, the time to onset of phase 0 in the second tracing is greater than that in the first because depolarization during phase 4 is prolonged. In the lower portion of the diagram, the threshold potential of the second tracing is less negative than that of the first. Consequently, the time to onset of phase 0 is prolonged. A similar prolongation of the time to onset of phase 0 is achieved by making the resting potential more negative for the third tracing. (Redrawn from Berne RM, Levy MN. Cardiovascular Physiology. 6th ed. Chicago, Mosby–Year Book, 1992, p 28.)

excitation-contraction coupling.[27-29] As an action potential is spread from cell to cell via the gap junctions, it is also transmitted to the innermost surfaces of the cell along the membranes of the T tubules. As noted earlier, the Ca^{++} channels are activated, and membrane permeability to Ca^{++} is increased during phase 2 of the action potential. The Ca^{++} entering the cell triggers the release of Ca^{++} ions previously bound to the sarcoplasmic reticulum. The free Ca^{++} within the cell binds to the troponin-C subunit of the troponin complex. When the Ca^{++} binds to troponin-C, the stereochemistry of the troponin complex is changed, and the troponin-I subunit is removed as a cover from the myosin binding site on the actin (thin) filament. Consequently, the crossbridges from the myosin (thick) filament are attracted to the active sites of the actin filament. It is postulated that this actin-myosin binding changes the attractive forces between the head of the crossbridge and its arm. This attraction pulls the head toward the arm, thus dragging the actin filament with it. Once the head is pulled to its arm, the actin-myosin bond is broken, and the head is free to return to its original position. Each crossbridge is independent of the others, so the more crossbridges that can bind with the actin filaments, the greater the force of contraction.

At the end of phase 2, the Ca^{++} channels close, and the sarcoplasmic reticulum reaccumulates Ca^{++} via an ATP-driven calcium pump. Simultaneously, the Na^+-Ca^{++} antiporter in the cell membrane is also removing Ca^{++} from the cell. Troponin-I is phosphorylated, and the Ca^{++} binding with troponin-C is inhibited, allowing the troponin complex to return to its original shape, thus recovering the myosin binding site on the actin filament. Muscular contraction ceases until the next action potential.

The Cardiac Cycle

The period from the beginning of one heart beat to the beginning of the next is called the **cardiac cycle.** Selected events during the cardiac cycle are depicted in Figures 2–23 and 2–24. Beginning with an action potential in the S-A node, a depolarization wave is spread through both atria to the A-V node and then, through the His-Purkinje complex, into the ventricles. However, because of the nature of the specialized conduction system, the impulse is delayed for about 0.1 second in the upper two thirds of the A-V node. This delay allows the atria to contract (a result of excitation-contraction coupling) and pump an additional volume of blood into the

Figure 2–23.

The mechanical events of the cardiac cycle shown in relation to the electrical events of the electrocardiogram. In late diastole, just prior to the P wave, the ventricles are filling passively. At about the time that the P wave ends, the atria contract to eject up to about 30% of the ventricular volume. A period of isovolumic ventricular contraction begins very shortly after the onset of the QRS complex. Ventricular ejection coincides with the early portion of the ST segment.

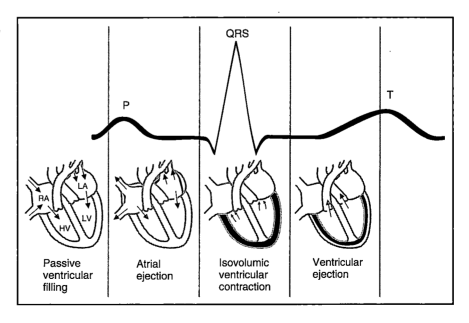

| Passive ventricular filling | Atrial ejection | Isovolumic ventricular contraction | Ventricular ejection |

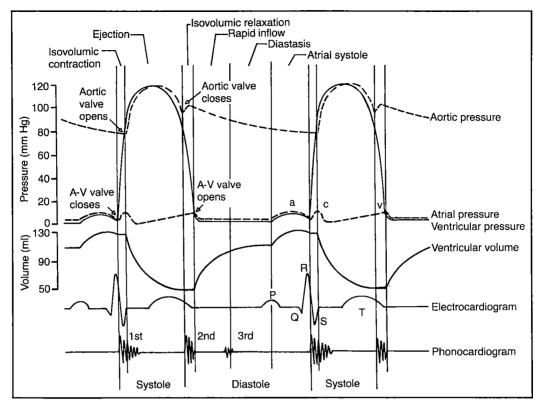

Figure 2-24.

The events of the cardiac cycle, showing changes in left atrial pressure, left ventricular pressure, aortic (systemic) pressure, ventricular volume, electrocardiogram, and phonocardiogram. (From Guyton AC. Textbook of Medical Physiology. 8th ed. Philadelphia, WB Saunders, 1991, p 102.)

ventricles—an atrial "kick." Then the ventricles provide the primary motive force to move blood through the vascular system.

The cardiac cycle may be divided further into two periods: **systole** and **diastole.** Systole is the period of ventricular contraction; diastole is the period of ventricular relaxation. Left-sided pressure and volume, ECG tracing, and phonocardiographic events associated with the cardiac cycle are illustrated in Figure 2-24. Closure of the tricuspid and mitral valves generates the first heart sound (S_1), signaling the onset of ventricular systole, and is shown on the phonocardiographic tracing just after the peak of the R wave on the ECG tracing. In early ventricular systole, the ventricular volume remains unchanged despite a rapid rise in ventricular pressure. This **isovolumic contraction** occurs until the aortic valve opens, at which time the **ventricular ejec-**

tion phase begins. The retrograde bulging of the mitral valve into the left atrium is responsible for the rise in atrial pressure seen during the isovolumic ventricular contraction, the *c wave.* Ventricular ejection continues until the aortic valve closes, terminating systole and generating the second heart sound. Immediately following aortic valve closure, a phase of **isovolumic relaxation** continues until the mitral valve opens when ventricular pressure falls below atrial pressure. The rise in atrial pressure indicated by the *v wave* of the atrial pressure tracing is probably brought about by the relative negative pressure resulting from ventricular relaxation. Once the mitral valve opens, ventricular volume begins rising as the ventricle passively fills during the **rapid-filling phase.** Immediately after the rapid-filling phase is the slow-filling phase, also called **diastasis,** which continues until atrial systole.

Atrial systole is indicated on the atrial pressure tracing as the *a wave.*

Preload, Afterload, and Contractility

The same physical principles and equations discussed with respect to the behavior of gases in the bronchi and lungs are applicable to a consideration of the behavior of blood in the cardiovascular system. Figure 2–25 graphically depicts the general relationships between pressure, vol-

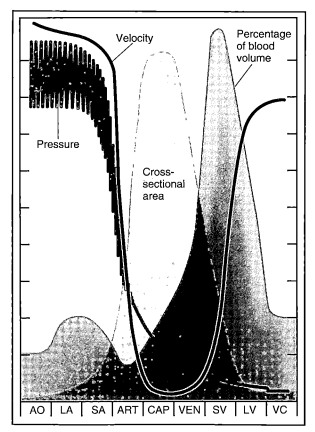

Figure 2–25.

The relationship among pressure, velocity of blood flow, cross-sectional area, and capacity of the blood vessels of the systemic circulation. Note the inverse relationship between velocity and cross-sectional area. AO, aorta; LA, large arteries; SA, small arteries; ART, arterioles; CAP, capillaries; VEN, venules; SV, small veins; LV, large veins; VC, vena cavae. (Redrawn from Berne RM, Levy MN. Cardiovascular Physiology. 6th ed. Chicago, Mosby–Year Book, 1992, p 3.)

ume, flow velocity, and cross-sectional area throughout the systemic circulation. Blood flow is generally expressed in units of ml · min⁻¹ or L · min⁻¹. The normal total blood flow in an adult male at rest is approximately 5.6 L · min⁻¹; in women, it is about 10% to 20% less. For general purposes, it may be easier to consider a non–gender-specific value of 5 L · min⁻¹ as a representative average value of the amount of blood ejected into the aorta each minute, called the **cardiac output.** The similar amount of blood flowing from the veins into the right atrium per minute is called the **venous return.** The amount of blood ejected from the ventricles with each systolic contraction is called the **stroke volume.**

Essentially, only three factors interact to influence the stroke volume of each ventricular systole:

- The amount of tension on the muscle before it contracts — the **preload**
- The load against which the muscle exerts its contraction — the **afterload**
- Other changes in stroke volume that are not attributable to either the preload or afterload — **contractility**

Preload is generally described in terms of the end-diastolic volume or end-diastolic pressure because they are the determinants of the tension on the ventricular walls (recall Laplace's law); up to a point, a larger end-diastolic tension tends to produce a larger stroke volume. Afterload is generally described in terms of end-systolic pressure generated during ejection because at a higher aortic or systolic blood pressure, the muscular walls of the ventricle have to develop more tension to eject the blood. Contractility is an ill-defined concept that represents muscular performance at any given preload and afterload.[30]

The left ventricular pressure-volume diagram in Figure 2–26 illustrates the idea of ventricular elastance. Since the ventricle is an elastic container, the pressure and the volume of blood in the ventricle determine its elastance. The diastolic curve is derived by incrementally filling the ventricle with blood and measuring the diastolic pressure immediately before ventricular contraction begins. The systolic curve is derived by preventing the ejection of blood from the ventricle

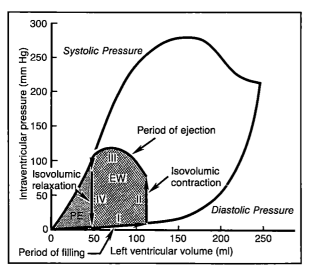

Figure 2-26.

The relationship of left ventricular systolic and diastolic pressure and volume curves. The diastolic pressure does not rise significantly and, in fact, is relatively independent of ventricular volumes below 150 ml. However, at volumes greater than 150 ml, the diastolic pressure rises rapidly and retards the flow of blood into the ventricle. The changes in intraventricular volume and pressure during a typical cardiac cycle are shown by the highlighted lines labeled I to IV. (From Guyton AC. Textbook of Medical Physiology. 8th ed. Philadelphia, WB Saunders, 1991, p 105.)

and measuring the maximal systolic pressure that is achieved at incremental volumes of filling.

As blood fills the ventricle during diastole, the resultant rise in ventricular pressure depends on the elastance of the ventricle. If, for some reason, the ventricular elastance becomes greater than normal, the end-diastolic volume is reduced unless the diastolic pressure increases concomitantly. From the diastolic pressure curve in Figure 2-26 it can be seen that diastolic volumes of up to about 150 milliliters result in minimal ventricular pressure changes, and thus blood can flow readily from the atrium into the ventricle. However, above 150 milliliters, the diastolic pressure increases rapidly. From the ventricular pressure curve it may be seen that the systolic pressure increases rapidly, with progressively increasing ventricular volumes up about 160 milliliters. Thereafter, the pressure drops off rapidly because the actin and myosin filaments are not optimally overlapped. Recall, that Laplace's law

tells us that more force is required to eject a given volume from the ventricle if it is enlarged from overfilling.

The inclusion of the normal left ventricular pressure-volume loop in Figure 2-26 shows that the elastance of the ventricle increases progressively from its minimum during diastole to its maximum at the end of systole. If elastance did not continue to increase after the opening of the aortic valve, the ventricular pressure would fall and the aortic valve would close. Thus, the larger the end-systolic elastance, the greater the stroke volume.

Figure 2-27 illustrates how changes in preload, afterload, and contractility affect stroke volume. Loop *n* shows normal ventricular pressure-volume loop for one contraction; the end-diastolic volume is 125 milliliters. An increase in venous return, causing an increase in end-diastolic volume for the next contraction to 150 milliliters, is shown by loop *p*. If the end-systolic pressure and contractility remain unchanged, the end-systolic volume for loops *n* and *p* is the same. Thus, the stroke volume increased from 75 milliliters to 100 milliliters, which mirrors the increase in venous return. In an oversimplified manner, this is an example of the Frank-Starling law, which says that if venous return increases, stroke volume increases by the same amount, so that the cardiac output equals the venous return. For many years, this self-regulating (not dependent on neural or hormonal influences) property of cardiac muscle was attributed to the amount of overlap between actin and myosin filaments. However, it is now known that two mechanisms are responsible. First, the sensitivity of the thin filaments for Ca^{++} is enhanced as the sarcomere lengthens. Therefore, more actin-myosin crossbridges can form at the same $[Ca^{++}]$ in the cytoplasm. Second, as sarcomere length is increased, more Ca^{++} enters the cytoplasm.

If, as in the case of hypertension, which increases afterload, the ventricle has to generate a higher end-systolic pressure, the stroke volume will be reduced. In Figure 2-27, loop *n* is a normal ventricular pressure-volume loop for one contraction, showing a normal end-systolic pressure of about 112 mm Hg (15 kPa). The effect of

Figure 2-27.

The effect of changes in preload, afterload, or contractility on the stroke volume of the left ventricle. Refer to text for details.

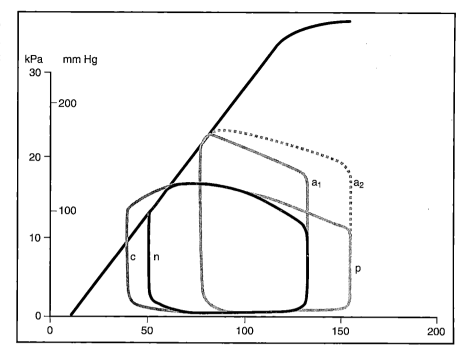

a sudden increase in systemic (aortic) blood pressure on the next contraction is indicated by loop a_1. Although the end-diastolic volumes of loops n and a_1 are the same, it takes a higher ventricular pressure of 150 mm Hg (20 kPa) in loop a_1 to push the aortic valve open because of the elevated aortic pressure. Because the contractility is the same, the maximal systolic elastance is also the same, so that loop a_1 intersects the end-systolic pressure-volume curve at a point above and to the right of loop n. Therefore, the end-systolic volume is increased to 75 milliliters instead of 50 milliliters, and the stroke volume is reduced from 75 milliliters to 50 milliliters. This effect is transient though, because if the venous return is unchanged, the subsequent diastole delivers another 75 milliliters of blood to the ventricle. The resultant new end-diastolic volume is 150 milliliters, which is 50 milliliters more than normal. The increased end-diastolic volume increases the ensuing stroke volume, as seen in loop a_2. The net result is an eventual return of stroke volume to a "normal" 75 milliliters, despite an increase in both the end-diastolic and end-systolic volumes. This is one of the reasons why hypertension causes problems: the ventricle

is working harder to pump a normal cardiac output, so little reserve capacity is left for situations in which an increased cardiac output might be necessary.

If contractility is increased, the stroke volume can increase even though end-diastolic volume and aortic pressure are unchanged. Loop c shows just such a case, in which stroke volume has increased to 85 milliliters. Clinically, however, it is more common for an increase in contractility to be the compensatory result of the body's effort to maintain a normal stroke volume in the face of an increased aortic pressure or a decreased end-diastolic volume. Anything that increases contractility is said to have a **positive inotropic** effect. However, the most common example of decreased contractility is a failing heart.

Cardiac Reflexes

Several of the rapid-acting nervous system mechanisms that have roles in arterial pressure control also influence the heart rate. The **baroreceptor** reflexes are probably the most readily recognized. These stretch receptors are located in the walls of almost all the large arteries, although they are particularly plentiful in the walls of the internal carotid arteries superior to the carotid bifurcation in an area called the *carotid sinuses* and in the walls of the arch of the aorta. The baroreceptors are stimulated only at pressures in excess of 60 mm Hg, peaking in activity at about 180 mm Hg.[7] The resultant reflex has two basic effects: (1) vasodilation, via inhibition of the vasomotor centers of the medulla; and (2) decreased heart rate and strength of contraction, via vagal stimulation. **Bainbridge's reflex** is an atrial stretch reflex that causes changes in heart rate; it is elicited when the right atrial pressure rises sufficiently to distend the right atrium. Bainbridge's reflex causes an increase in the heart rate if the heart is beating at normal rates, but it causes a decrease in the heart rate if the heart is beating at high rates. The **chemoreceptor reflex** manifests itself predominantly as an increase in the depth and rate of ventilation in response to a lack of oxygen, but it also influences heart rate. When ventilatory stimulation is mild, the heart rate usually decreases; when ventilatory stimulation is pronounced, the heart rate usually increases. Respiratory variation in heart rate is observable in most individuals; typically, the heart rate accelerates during inspiration and decelerates during expiration (sympathetic activity apparently increases on inhalation, whereas vagal activity increases on exhalation).

Resistance to Flow and Its Control

As shown in Figure 1–27, the arterioles have been labeled as resistance vessels and given the look of a spigot and faucet. The arterioles are portrayed this way because, just as the opening or closing of a spigot on a faucet controls flow, the changing of arteriolar resistance controls the flow of blood to each of the body's individual capillary beds. With respect to the flow of blood through the various blood vessels, the determinants of resistance are described by Poiseuille's law, which says that the resistance to flow of a fluid through a tube depends on the viscosity of the fluid, the length of the tube, and the fourth power of the radius of the tube:

$$R = \frac{8\eta \, l}{\pi r^4}$$

where R is the resistance to flow; η is the viscosity of the fluid, which in the case of blood is reflected by the fraction of the blood that is cells (normally 0.38 in females and 0.45 in males); l is the length of the vessel, which usually varies little over the short term; and r is the radius of the tube, the most important factor. So in very general terms $Q \propto r^4$; thus, a small change in the radius of the tube produces a large change in the flow through the tube. Because of the anatomic arrangement and distribution of the blood vessels, they may be thought of as exerting resistances to flow in both series and parallel. Note that the total resistance through the vessels arranged in series is the sum of the resistances through the individual vessels, but the total resistance through the vessels arranged in parallel is less than any of the individual resistances.

In addition to the Frank-Starling principle, three additional factors play a role in controlling the radii of arterioles:

● local metabolic needs
● locally released vasoactive substances
● the central nervous system

The best explanation of the mechanism for local regulation suggests that the degree of arteriolar smooth muscle contraction depends on the concentration of fuels (substrates) or metabolic wastes (metabolites) or both in the interstitial fluid immediately surrounding the arteriole. Basically, when fuels are in short supply or when wastes are accumulating, the arterioles are prompted to dilate, thus increasing blood flow to deliver more fuel and carry away accumulated wastes. Or when fuel is in abundant supply and waste concentration is low, blood flow is decreased, thereby obviating any excess cardiac output. The specific substrates and metabolites that link metabolism and smooth muscle tone are not known. Foremost among the potential candidates for the role is adenosine, a by-product of the breakdown of ATP that is able to pass readily into the extracellular fluid. Other candidates include carbon dioxide, hydrogen ions, and inorganic phosphates, each of which can dilate the arterioles. Another possibility is that oxygen causes arteriolar constriction, thus reducing blood flow when oxygen is abundant.

Other locally mediated control mechanisms that are not directly concerned with substrate supply or metabolite elimination are also active in the regulatory process of blood flow. For example, when antigens are detected by the immune system, mast cells in the connective tissue or basophils in the blood release histamine. Histamine first binds with receptors on the preganglionic sympathetic terminals, thus inhibiting the release of norepinephrine; it also binds with receptors inside the arterioles on their endothelial membranes. The endothelial cells then produce the substance endothelial-derived relaxing factor, which diffuses out of the arterioles to the smooth muscles and causes vasodilation.

Local metabolic control of arteriolar resistance only accounts for the needs of the cells in the immediate vicinity of the individual vascular bed that is affected, whereas the central nervous system takes into account how the flows to each of the many vascular beds combine to affect the entire body. Table 2–3 summarizes the cardiovascular effects of autonomic, sympathetic, and parasympathetic activity.

The sympathetic branch of the central nervous system exerts the most important influence on the arterioles. Although the density of the innervation varies from vascular bed to vascular bed, almost all arterioles are innervated by postganglionic sympathetic fibers. The neurotransmitter norepinephrine, released by these postganglionic neurons, binds with the alpha$_1$-adrenoceptors on the cell membranes of the arterial and arteriolar smooth muscle, resulting in muscular contraction and thus increased resistance. In a negative feedback loop that manifests itself when there is an overabundance of norepinephrine, alpha$_2$ receptors in the presynaptic cell membrane bind with some of the norepinephrine and exert an inhibitory effect on its further release. The arterioles of certain tissues are also innervated by postganglionic fibers of the parasympathetic branch of the nervous system, and to a much lesser extent, parasympathetic stimulation can also play a role

in the control of arteriolar resistance. By releasing acetylcholine, the postsynaptic parasympathetic neurons can reduce arteriolar resistance to flow by relaxing arteriolar smooth muscle. Additionally, acetylcholine may play an inhibitory role presynaptically by inhibiting the release of norepinephrine from postganglionic sympathetic neurons.

In addition to the direct neural release of vasoconstricting and vasorelaxing factors, hormonal release into the blood is another way in which the central nervous system can affect arteriolar resistance. For example, in response to low blood volume the posterior pituitary gland is stimulated to release vasopressin (a potent vasoconstrictor) into the blood. Likewise, as part of a general sympathetic response, the adrenal gland releases the **catecholamines** epinephrine and norepinephrine into the blood. Both catechols bind to alpha receptors on vascular smooth muscle, but epinephrine prefers to bind to beta$_2$ receptors in those vascular beds that have them. Thus, low concentrations of epinephrine circulating in the blood cause vasodilation because epinephrine binds to beta$_2$ receptors, but high concentrations cause overall vasoconstriction because epinephrine also binds to alpha receptors if there are not enough beta$_2$ receptors to accept it.

Clearly, the coordinated interaction between local and central nervous system mediation of arteriolar smooth muscle tone determines the final flow of blood into the vascular beds. Furthermore, this interplay yields different results in different tissues. Alpha and beta functions can be either excitatory or inhibitory. Neither is necessarily associated with excitation or inhibition, rather with the affinity of the receptor for a particular hormone in a given effector organ.

Once blood enters the capillaries, two mechanisms control the exchange of nutrients (e.g., oxygen, amino acids, glucose) from the blood for wastes (e.g., carbon dioxide, urea) from the cells: diffusion (the same mechanism that was discussed for the exchange of gases at the alveolar-capillary membrane) and filtration. Diffusion may be the principal mechanism, but filtration is important as a means of maintaining the fluid balance between the vascular and extravascular compartments.

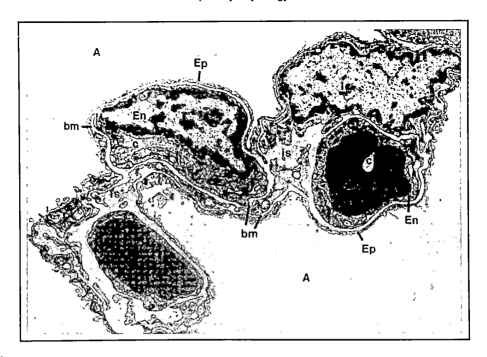

Figure 2-28.

A cross-sectional electron micrograph showing the alveolar-capillary membrane of the normal human parenchyma. Air in the alveolar lumina (A) is separated from the erythrocytes (Ec) in the capillaries (c) by epithelial cells (Ep), basement membranes (bm), endothelial cells (En), and the interstitial space (is). (From Dantzker DR. Cardiopulmonary Critical Care. 2nd ed. Philadelphia, WB Saunders, 1991, p. 6.)

Although diffusion across the capillary membrane is governed by the same factors that govern diffusion across the alveolar-capillary membrane (mentioned earlier), filtration is a bit more complicated. Filtration is the bulk flow of fluids through the tight junctions of the capillary walls (Fig. 2-28). Its success is dependent on how easily water can move through the tight junctions, which, in turn, is dependent on just how "tight" the tight junctions are and on the pressure gradient from inside the capillary to the interstitial fluid. The pressure gradient has two components:

- the fluid pressure gradient (hydrostatic pressure gradient), which is the difference between the fluid pressure inside the capillary (P_{cap}) and the interstitial fluid ($P_{interstit}$). The blood pressure in the capillary is the same as P_{cap} (P_{cap} = 30 mm Hg or 4 kPa at the arteriolar end; 15 mm Hg or 2 kPa at the venular end), and $P_{interstit}$ is considered to be 0 (possibly even negative).
- the osmotic pressure gradient, which depends

on the concentration of impermeable solutes in the fluid. These are mostly proteins (like albumin) that are much more abundant in the blood than in the interstitial fluid. Thus, the capillary osmotic pressure (Π_{cap}, about 25 mm Hg or ≈ 3 kPa) is much higher than the interstitial fluid osmotic pressure ($\Pi_{interstit}$, about 2 mm Hg or ≈ 0.26 kPa). Because the osmotic pressure gradient is the force tending to attract water, water is pulled toward the higher osmotic pressure.

The balance of these two forces (sometimes called **Starling's forces**) is described by the **Starling's hypothesis**:

$$\text{filtration or absorption} = k[(P_{cap} + \Pi_{interstit}) - (P_{interstit} + \Pi_{cap})]$$

where P_{cap} is the hydrostatic pressure in capillaries; $P_{interstit}$ is the hydrostatic pressure of interstitial fluid; Π_{cap} is the osmotic pressure of plasma protein (also called oncotic pressure); $\Pi_{interstit}$ is the osmotic pressure of the interstitial

Figure 2-29.

Pressure gradients across the wall of a typical capillary. The numbers at the arteriolar and venular ends of the capillary are the respective hydrostatic pressures. Filtration occurs at the arteriolar end of the capillaries because the arteriolar pressure exceeds the sum of the plasma colloid osmotic and the interstitial pressures (30 > 25 + 1). Absorption occurs because the sum of the interstitial and colloid osmotic pressures is greater than the venular pressure (0 + 25 > 15). The arrows indicate the approximate magnitudes of filtration (outgoing arrows) or absorption (ingoing arrows). (Adapted from Ganong WF. Review of Medical Physiology. 15th ed. East Norwalk, Conn, Appleton & Lange, 1991, p 546.)

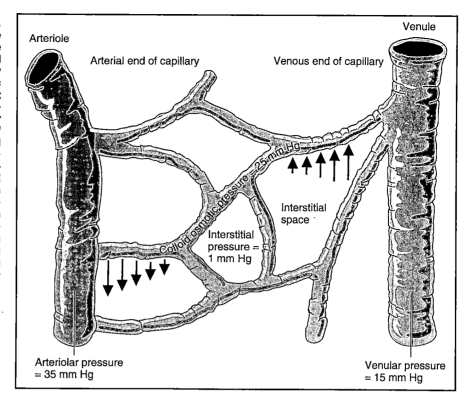

fluid; and k is the filtration constant for the capillary membrane. When the equation yields a positive number, filtration occurs; absorption occurs if the sum is negative.[18,23]

Because the capillary blood pressure decreases from one end of the capillary to the other (greater at the arteriolar end than at the venular end), the filtration rate also changes along the capillary. Normally, capillary blood pressure is greater than plasma osmotic pressure at the arteriolar end, whereas plasma osmotic pressure is greater than capillary blood pressure at the venular end. Figure 2-29 illustrates the pressure gradients across the wall of a muscular capillary.

Some organs have a higher filtration to reabsorption ratio than others. For example, more fluid is filtered out of the liver than is reabsorbed. In contrast, the capillaries of the lungs reabsorb any other fluid that enters the lungs in addition to fluids that are filtered. The balance of filtration and reabsorption is greatly influenced by arteriolar resistance. Because the capillaries are connected in series with the arterioles, an increase in arteriolar resistance leads to a de-

crease in capillary blood pressure. Lower capillary blood pressure leads to more reabsorption. For example, after a large blood loss, the baroreflex causes generalized vasoconstriction to maintain blood pressure. The resultant arteriolar constriction and the lowered total plasma volume lead to a lower capillary blood pressure, thus favoring reabsorption.

Edema, which results from fluids leaving the capillaries at a faster rate than they are reabsorbed, can be caused by anything that increases filtration relative to reabsorption or that decreases lymph drainage. For example, pregnancy causes an increase in extracellular fluid volume, which leads to an increase in venous pressure and yields an increase in capillary pressure, thereby increasing filtration pressure.

References

1. Ahlquist RP. Study of adrenotropic receptors. Am J Physiol 153:586–600, 1948.
2. Lands AM, Arnold A, McAuliff JP, et al. Differentiation of receptor systems activated by sympathomimetic amines. Nature (London) 214:597–598, 1967.

3. Gerber JG, Nies AS. Beta-adrenergic blocking drugs. Annu Rev Med 36:145–164, 1985.

4. Celli BR. Clinical and physiologic evaluation of respiratory muscle function. Clin Chest Med 10:199–214, 1989.

5. West JB. Respiratory Physiology—The Essentials. 4th ed. Baltimore, Williams & Wilkins, 1990.

6. Mines AH. Respiratory Physiology. 2nd ed. New York, Raven Press, 1986.

7. Guyton AC. Textbook of Medical Physiology. 5th ed. Philadelphia, WB Saunders, 1991.

8. Meyer D, Groebe K, Thews G. Theoretical analysis of factors influencing recovery of ventilation distributions from inert gas washout data. Adv Exp Med Biol 277:615–624, 1990.

9. Goerke J. Lung surfactant. Biochem Biophys Acta 344:241–261, 1974.

10. Comroe JH. Physiology of Respiration. Chicago, Year Book Medical Publishers, 1974.

11. Wasserman K, Hansen JE, Sue DY, Whipp BJ. Principles of Exercise Testing and Interpretation. Philadelphia, Lea & Febiger, 1987.

12. Shapiro BA, Harrison RA, Cane RD, Templin R. Clinical Application of Blood Gases. 4th ed. Chicago, Year Book Medical Publishers, 1989.

13. Samsel RW, Schumacker PT. Determination of the critical O_2 delivery from experimental data: Sensitivity to error. J Appl Physiol 64:2074–2082, 1988.

14. McGilvery RW. Biochemical Concepts. Philadelphia, WB Saunders, 1975.

15. Mitchell P. Chemiosmotic coupling in oxidative and photosynthetic phosphorylation. Biol Rev 41:455, 1965.

16. Chenevey B. Overview of fluids and electrolytes. Nursing Clin North Am 22:749–759, 1987.

17. Lindsey BG. Neural control of breathing. Recent advances and hypotheses. J Fla Med Assoc 78:241–243, 1991.

18. Ganong WF. Review of Medical Physiology. 15th ed. East Norwalk, Conn, Appleton & Lange, 1991.

19. Mitchell RA, Berger A. State of the art: Review of neural regulation of respiration. Am Rev Respir Dis 111:206–224, 1975.

20. von Euler C. Central pattern generation during breathing. Trends Neurosci 3:275–277, 1980.

21. McDonald DM, Mitchell RA. The innervation of glomus cells, ganglion cells, and blood vessels in the rat carotid body: A quantitative ultrastructural study. J Neurocytol 4:177–230, 1975.

22. Berger AJ, Hornbein TF. Control of respiration. In: Patton HD, Fuchs AF, Hille B, et al. (eds). Textbook of Physiology, 21st ed. Vol. 2. Philadelphia, WB Saunders, 1989.

23. Berne RM, Levy MN. Cardiovascular Physiology. 6th ed. St. Louis, Mosby–Year Book, 1992.

24. Goerke J, Mines AH. Cardiovascular Physiology. New York, Raven Press, 1988.

25. Sperelakis N. Regulation of calcium slow channels of cardiac muscle by cyclic nucleotides and phosphorylation. J Mol Cell Cardiol 2:75–105, 1988.

26. Civan MM, Bookman RJ. Transepithelial Na^+ transport and the intracellular fluids: A computer study. J Membr Biol 65:63–80, 1982.

27. Moore RL, Musch TI, Cheung JY. Modulation of cardiac contractility by myosin light chain phosphorylation. Med Sci Sports Exerc 23:1163–1169, 1991.

28. Bers DM. Ca regulation in cardiac muscle. Med Sci Sports Exerc 23:1157–1162, 1991.

29. Morgan JP, Perreault CL, Morgan KG. The cellular basis of contraction and relaxation in cardiac and vascular smooth muscle. Am Heart J 121:961–968, 1991.

30. Westerhof N. Physiological hypotheses—intramyocardial pressure. A new concept, suggestions for measurement. Basic Res Cardiol 85:105–119, 1990.

SECTION 2
PATHOPHYSIOLOGY

3 ISCHEMIC CARDIAC CONDITIONS

INTRODUCTION

Coronary heart disease (CHD), the clinical signs and symptoms caused by the myocardium's becoming ischemic, is the most prevalent disease in the United States.[1] The clinical presentation of the patient with CHD was first, and probably most colorfully, described by Heberden in his lecture on "Disorders of the Breast" in 1772.[2]

There is a disorder of the breast, marked with strong and peculiar symptoms considerable for the kind of danger belonging to it, and not extremely rare, of which I do not recollect any mention among medical authors. The seat of it, and sense of strangling and anxiety, with which it is attended, may make it not improperly be called angina pectoris. Those, who are afflicted with it, are seized while they are walking and most particularly when they walk soon after eating, with a painful and most disagreeable sensation in the breast, which seems as if it would take their life away, if it were to increase or to continue; the moment they stand still, all this uneasiness vanishes.

The prevalence of this disease and its surprising presence in seemingly healthy young men was not fully appreciated until 1953, when Enos and colleagues published the results of their autopsies performed on soldiers killed in the Korean conflict.[3] This study, originally performed to evaluate the cause of death from different ballistic injuries,[4] determined that 77.3% of 300 soldiers examined (mean age = 22.1 years) had detectable blockages in their coronary arteries. In 10 of these cases, complete obstruction of one or more coronary arteries was found.

The study by Enos and colleagues was followed by the now famous Framingham Heart Study.[5] In the course of the original Framingham study, 5209 men and women between the ages of 30 and 62 years who were free of clinically significant coronary disease at entry were followed for 20 years. During this period, these subjects were seen for biennial examinations, which consisted of questionnaires on activity and smoking history, blood chemistry studies, blood pressure measurement, and a resting 12-lead electrocardiogram. Although no one specific cause of **coronary artery disease (CAD)** could be identified in the Framingham cohort, several major and minor risk factors for its development were discovered and are discussed later in this chapter.

The most recent data available indicate that CHD continues to be the most prevalent and costly disease process in the industrialized world.[1] Deaths due to disease of the heart and blood vessels in the United States in 1987 were more than double those of the next leading cause (Fig. 3–1) and accounted for close to 50% of all

deaths that occurred in the United States that year.

It is encouraging to note that the total number of deaths from this process declined during the 1980s. Unfortunately, the decline was due not to a decrease in the incidence of CHD but to improvements in emergency medical care. The number of new **myocardial infarctions** reported in the United States each year has remained 1.5 million per year since 1984.

This chapter presents the microscopic anatomy and physiology of normal myocardial perfusion, followed by a description of the pathologic changes that occur in coronary arteries. The risk factors that have been shown to be related to the development of CHD are discussed, and the three major patterns of the clinical presentation of CHD—chronic stable angina, unstable angina, and sudden cardiac death—are described.

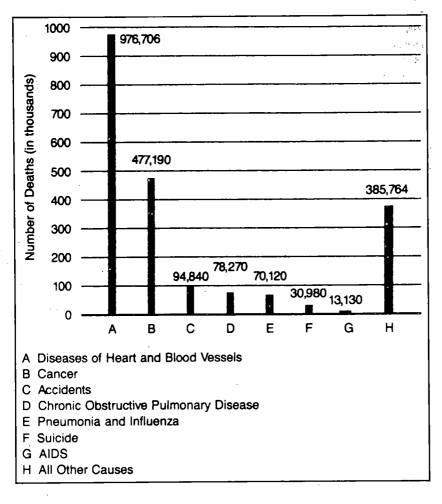

A Diseases of Heart and Blood Vessels
B Cancer
C Accidents
D Chronic Obstructive Pulmonary Disease
E Pneumonia and Influenza
F Suicide
G AIDS
H All Other Causes

Figure 3–1.
Leading causes of death in the United States, 1987 (estimated). *Sources:* National Center for Health Statistics, U.S. Public Health Service, Department of Health and Human Services, and the American Heart Association. (Reproduced with permission. *1991 Heart and Stroke Facts,* 1990. Copyright American Heart Association.)

ANATOMY OF THE CORONARY ARTERY

The microscopic anatomy of the coronary artery has been well known for several years. To fully understand what is known about **coronary atherosclerosis,** a basic understanding of the normal structures of arteries is necessary.[6]

Outer Layer

The outer layer of an artery (the **adventitia**), consists chiefly of collagenous fibers, mostly fibroblasts, and provides the basic support structure for the artery (Fig. 3–2). This portion of the artery also houses the vasa vasorum, which are the vessels that furnish the middle layer of the artery with its blood supply.

Middle Layer

The middle layer **(media)** of all arteries (of which the coronary arteries are considered medium sized) consists of multiple layers of smooth muscle cells separated from the inner and outer layers by a prominent elastic membrane, or lamina. Through alterations in vasomotor tone, as demands for changes in blood flow to the myocardium are perceived, this muscular layer is responsible for making adjustments to the luminal diameter. These smooth muscle cells are also capable of synthesizing collagen, elastin, and glycosaminoglycans, especially when they react to different physical and chemical stimuli.

Inner Layer

The inner layer **(intima)** consists of an endothelial layer, the basement membrane, and variable amounts of isolated smooth muscle cells as well as collagen and elastin fibers. The boundary of the intima and media is marked by the internal elastic lamina.

The two inner layers of the artery wall have received the most attention with regard to the development of the processes that lead to myocardial ischemia.

The arterial endothelium is selectively permeable to macromolecules of the size of a **low-density lipoprotein (LDL).** The concentration of LDL in the lymph of the arterial wall has been

Figure 3–2.

Structure of the normal arterial wall, consisting of the adventitia (outer), the media (middle), and the intima (inner) layers. (Reproduced with permission from Ross R, Glomset J. The pathogenesis of atherosclerosis. N Engl J Med 295:369, 1976.)

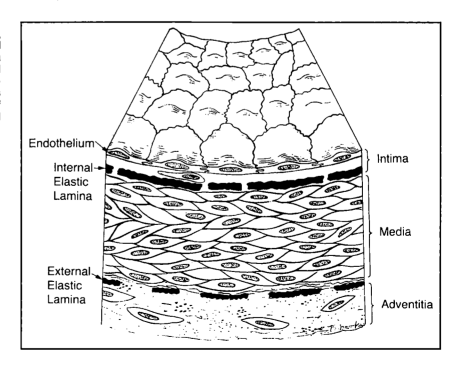

found to be approximately one tenth of that in the bloodstream.[7] Although many plasma proteins can enter the artery wall in this concentration, lipoproteins and fibrinogen are particularly likely to accumulate in the intima.[8]

PERFUSION

Before discussing the particulars of myocardial perfusion, it is important to review two basic rules of fluid dynamics. First, all fluids flow according to a pressure gradient, that is, from an area of higher pressure to an area of lower pressure. Second, all fluids follow the path of least resistance. If an obstruction is encountered, the fluid tends to follow another path, thereby decreasing the volume of fluid crossing the obstruction and the pressure driving that fluid farther down the path distal to the obstruction.

As with all muscle beds, myocardial perfusion occurs primarily during periods of muscle relaxation, in this case, during diastole.[9] In Figure 3-3, the relationship between mean aortic pressure and blood flow in the coronary arteries is shown. Blood flow increases in both the right and left coronary arteries at the onset of systole (first vertical dotted line). When the aortic valve is closed, aortic diastolic pressure is transmitted through the dilated Valsalva's sinuses to the openings of the coronary arteries themselves. The sinuses then act as miniature reservoirs, facilitating maintenance of relatively uniform coronary inflow through diastole. The pressure generated by the right ventricle during systole is in the range of 15 to 20 mm Hg, whereas the left ventricle produces pressures of 120 mm Hg or higher. Therefore, the occlusive pressure on the right coronary artery terminal vessels is less than that on the left during systole, so there is less difference in flow in the right coronary artery between systole and diastole.

The coronary arteries, like all arteries, become distended as blood is forced back into them by the contracting muscle. This pressure within the coronary artery is less than that in the aorta, so therefore, the coronary arteries themselves, like the Valsalva's sinuses, become reservoirs for the storage of blood and provide an initial "pressure

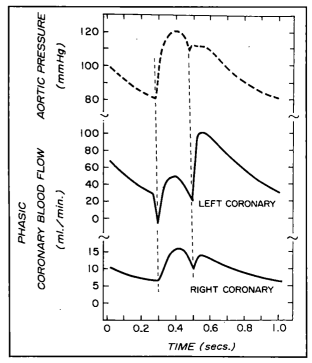

Figure 3-3.

The relationship between blood pressure in the aorta *(top)* and blood flow in the left *(middle)* and right *(bottom)* coronary arteries. The first vertical dotted line is the beginning of systole, and the second is the beginning of diastole. (Reproduced with permission from Boucek R, Morales A, Romanelli R, Judkins M. Coronary Artery Disease: Pathologic and Clinical Assessment. Baltimore, Williams & Wilkins, 1984, p 132.)

head" to drive blood into the myocardium as soon as the intramyocardial pressure drops following systole.

One especially important difference between the coronary vascular bed and most others is that anastomotic connections without intervening capillary beds (known as **collateral vessels**) are present (Fig. 3-4). In human hearts, the distribution and extent of collateral vessels are quite variable.[10] Under normal conditions, such vessels are generally less than 40 microns in diameter and appear to have little or no functional role. However, when myocardial perfusion is compromised by obstructions that affect major vessels, these collateral vessels enlarge over several weeks, and blood flow through them increases.[11] Given the time to make this adaptation, perfu-

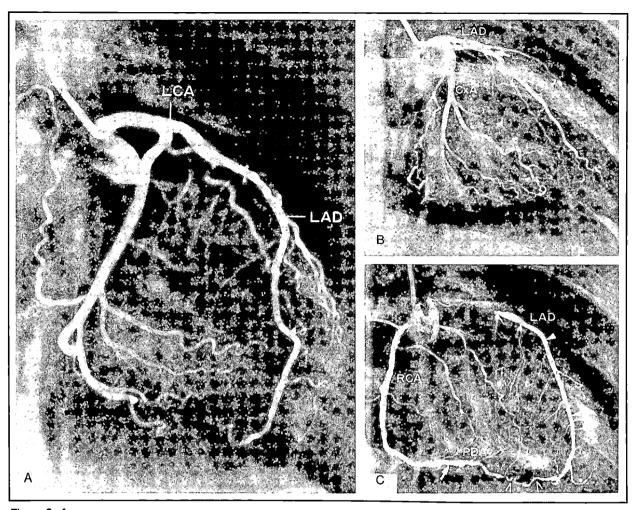

Figure 3–4.

A, Angiogram of a normal left coronary artery (LCA) as seen from the right anterior oblique view. *B*, Angiogram of a patient with a totally obstructed left anterior descending (LAD) coronary artery as seen from the right anterior oblique view. *C*, Angiogram of the right coronary artery (RCA) and its major branch, the posterior descending artery (PDA), of the patient in *B*. The LAD is seen because of collateral vessels connecting the LAD and the RCA system. (Reproduced with permission from Boucek R, Morales A, Romanelli R, Judkins M. Coronary Artery Disease: Pathologic and Clinical Assessment. Baltimore, Williams & Wilkins, 1984, pp 4, 9.)

sion via collateral vessels may equal or exceed perfusion via the obstructed vessel.

Major Determinants of Myocardial Blood Flow

● **Diastolic blood pressure (DBP)**—the primary driving force to move blood into the myocardial tissue.
● **Vasomotor tone (VMT)**—plays a major role in determining the volume of blood passed along to the tissue by regulating the caliber of the artery. This is usually uniform throughout the coronary vascular tree. It aids or opposes diastolic blood pressure.
● **Resistance to flow (R)**—most commonly caused by atherosclerosis. A significant increase in the size and number of collateral vessels decreases total resistance to flow by providing an alternative route for the blood to take around an obstruction.

- **Left ventricular end-diastolic pressure (LVEDP)**—pressure within the ventricle at end diastole causes an occlusive force on the capillary beds of the muscle closest to the pumping chamber, the endocardium.

The entire process can be considered in this relationship:

$$F = DBP \pm VMT - R - LVEDP$$

where F = flow of blood to the myocardium, DBP = diastolic blood pressure, VMT = vasomotor tone (additive if the vessel is in a dilated state and subtractive if constricted), R = the resistance to flow offered by an obstructive lesion, and LVEDP = left ventricular end-diastolic pressure.

ATHEROSCLEROSIS

The development of atherosclerosis is indeed a complex process dependent on the interaction of several risk factors and the sensitivity of the individual to these factors. Atherosclerotic plaques are composed of lipid and thrombus; the relative concentrations of each varies widely from individual to individual. In an effort to clarify this process, atherosclerosis is presented here as two processes—"atherosis" and "sclerosis"—that occur within the intima and endothelium of arterial walls. Undoubtedly, one of these components is more prominent than the other in each person who develops this disease. However, in very rare cases (homozygous familial hypercholesterolemia), atherosis is the only cause of the obstructive lesion.

Atherosis

The first detectable lesion of atherosclerosis is the often discussed fatty streak, which consists of lipid-laden macrophages and smooth muscle cells. Fatty streaks have been found in the arteries of patients as young as 10 years of age,[12] at the sites where major lesions appear later in life.

In animal studies, fatty streaks have been found in the lining of the aorta within 12 days of the initiation of a high-fat, high-cholesterol diet. Clusters of monocytes have been found in junctional areas, between endothelial cells, where they accumulate lipid and are known as **foam cells.**[13] The subendothelial accumulation of these macrophages constitutes the first stage of fatty streak development in primates; these streaks are similar to the fatty streaks observed in humans.

After several months, accumulations of lipid-laden macrophages grow so large that the endothelium is stretched and begins to separate over them. Such endothelial separation exposes the intima-based lesion and the underlying connective tissue to the circulation. Consequently, platelets aggregate and thrombus forms at these locations, a hallmark characteristic of the "sclerotic" phase of atherosclerosis.

Sclerosis

The sclerotic components of the lesions of atherosclerosis are those that reduce the blood vessel compliance. Atherosclerotic intimal lesions that produce symptoms or end-organ damage (ischemia or infarction in the organs fed by the vessel involved) invariably have a major fibrous component. Increased lesion collagen and destruction of medial elastin, in addition to changes in the composition of these fibrous proteins, are important mechanisms underlying sclerosis in atherosclerosis.[14]

Pure atherosis (lipid deposition alone), such as that in fatty streaks, does not produce end-organ damage (except with homozygous familial hypercholesterolemia) but may contribute to sclerosis. The exposure of subendothelial structures to the raw material of thrombus formation and the subsequent effect of such exposure on endogenous factors such as endothelium-derived relaxation factor (see later discussion) contribute to the process of sclerosis.

One of the long-standing theories of the development of the atherosclerotic lesion is that of encrustation, that is, the formation of organized thrombi over advanced plaques that had developed on the endothelial lining. This theory has never adequately accounted for the exact origin of the lesions but has always been considered an important part of the process because of the findings of extensive thrombus formation on microscopic examination of these plaques.

Ross[13] and Wissler[6] have described a "fibrous cap" that consists of intimal smooth muscle cells (that have for some reason proliferated) and connective tissue, mostly fibrin. Ross and Glomset[15] first described the "response to injury" hypothesis in an attempt to define the initial stages of development of the atherosclerotic plaque. In this report, the role of **platelet-derived growth factor (PDGF)** was shown to be a major factor in the development of the sclerotic component of arterial lesions.

Platelet-derived growth factor has been shown to contribute to these lesions in two ways. First, as the name implies, PDGF stimulates the replication of connective tissue cells in the areas in which it is released. Second, PDGF has been found to be a "chemoattractant." Released from tissue at the sites of endothelial injury, PDGF attracts smooth muscle cells so that they migrate from the media into the intima.[16]

The response to injury hypothesis does not identify which agent or process is responsible for initiating either the attachment of macrophages to the endothelium, triggering lipid deposition, or the adherence of platelets to this lining, since normal endothelium is known to secrete heparin and other platelet-inhibiting agents. However, recent investigation of vasospasm, an area thought to be a separate and distinct syndrome for myocardial ischemia, has provided some clues to the origin of these processes.

VASOSPASM

At the beginning of this century, Sir William Osler was the first to suggest that a basic abnormality existed in the smooth muscle of coronary arteries that were affected by atherosclerosis when he reported to the Royal College of Physicians: "We have, I think, evidence that sclerotic arteries are specially prone to spasm."[17] For the next 50 years, coronary vasospasm was considered only a minor factor in the myocardial blood flow equation.

In 1959, Prinzmetal and colleagues first identified the connection between vasospasm and what they called "variant angina."[18] This type of angina was different from "typical angina" as first described by Heberden in that it was associated with ST-segment elevation instead of depression, occurred at rest (typically in the early morning) instead of during a predictable level of activity, and was not associated with any preceding increase in myocardial oxygen demand. There was also a much stronger anatomic correlation between the electrocardiogram leads involved during these attacks and the site of subsequent myocardial infarctions in those patients who went on to have them when compared with the data for patients who experienced exertional angina. This syndrome, which became known as **Prinzmetal's angina,** was similar to typical angina in that it was promptly relieved with nitroglycerin and other vasodilators.

Subsequent investigators found that this syndrome was considerably more widespread than had been thought earlier, and this was in fact a "proved hypothesis" by 1976.[19] Maseri and coworkers further defined this syndrome with a report on 107 patients who experienced angina at rest and also underwent coronary angiography.[20] Of these, only nine (7%) had no visibly detectable atherosclerosis, whereas 93% had established disease.

It has long been known that hyperplasia of intimal smooth muscle cells is a hallmark of advanced atherosclerosis.[13,21] It is not unexpected, therefore, that coronary arteries so afflicted should be prone to spasm. What is less understood, just as it was with Ross's inability to specify the injury in his response to injury hypothesis, is what trigger sets these processes in motion.

Furchgott and Zawadzki[22] identified a substance secreted by the endothelium that causes the underlying smooth muscle cells to relax, hence the name **endothelial-derived relaxation factor (EDRF).** Furchgott[23] and others[24-28] have since demonstrated, both in the laboratory and in patients, that when the endothelium of the coronary artery is either removed experimentally or damaged (i.e., atherosclerosis), the intimal smooth muscle constricts instead of relaxing when stimulated by acetylcholine, a substance that causes normally functioning endothelium to release EDRF.

Work by Yasue and colleagues[29] has shown that this response is present not only in subjects with known atherosclerosis but also in subjects without detectable atherosclerosis. The investigators performed angiograms on 74 subjects who were divided into three groups: (1) 26 subjects between the ages of 9 and 29 years who had no detectable coronary disease, (2) 23 patients between the ages of 31 and 68 who had no detectable coronary atherosclerosis, and (3) 25 patients who had angiographically detectable atherosclerosis.

They found that there was a significant increase in the amount of coronary vasospasm in response to injection of acetylcholine in all subjects older than 30 years regardless of whether atherosclerosis was present. The only significant difference between the older than 30 and the younger than 30 groups who had no angiographic stenoses was the greater prevalence of risk factors for coronary disease in the older than 30 group.

The proof that the risk factors for CAD not only are what accelerate the disease process once it is established but in fact may themselves constitute the "injury" was provided by Vita and colleagues in 1990.[30] In their research on subjects with normal coronary arteries, documented by coronary angiography, they found that only those subjects who lacked the traditional risk factors for CAD had the normal vasodilatory response to acetylcholine. There was a highly significant correlation between the presence of certain risk factors (e.g., cholesterol level, male gender, family history, and age) and a vasoconstrictor response to acetylcholine, with the likelihood of response increasing when the number of risk factors increased in each subject. This means that the risk factors themselves probably are the triggers that set atherosclerosis in motion because their presence precedes the first detectable abnormalities in the coronary arteries and because no abnormalities were found in subjects who lacked them.

RISK FACTORS

The relationship among many genetic and behavioral factors and their contribution to the development of coronary atherosclerosis was first discussed by Heberden in the late eighteenth century. It was the Framingham study[5] that first tested these relationships in a long-term, large-scale epidemiologic trial. The following section of this chapter presents a brief discussion of each of the risk factors and some of what is known about how each factor contributes to the development of atherosclerosis. References are provided for a more in-depth study of these topics.

In any discussion of risk factors, the variability of the response of individuals to the same risk factor (host susceptibility) must be considered. The presence or absence of significant CAD cannot be determined by any simple arithmetic formula. Considerable evidence exists, however, to support the contention that the greater the number of risk factors present, the greater the likelihood that CAD is present as well.[30-32]

It is also important to remember the significance of the work of Enos and colleagues,[3] which is that CAD is present for many years before the individual becomes aware of it. Because of this, a distinction is made between CAD—the presence of an obstruction that does not limit flow significantly and thereby does not inhibit normal heart muscle function—and CHD—the presence of an obstruction that has caused permanent damage to the heart muscle fibers downstream.

Major Risk Factors

The three major risk factors for coronary atherosclerosis are cigarette smoking, hypertension, and elevated cholesterol. The relative risk, that is, the increase in risk above that experienced by the normal population of developing coronary atherosclerosis, for persons having any combination of the three major risk factors is depicted in Figure 3–5. Although all of the risk factors are discussed individually, it is critical to remember that only in the scientist's laboratory do these factors exist individually. As Figure 3–5 illustrates, each additional factor has not only an additive effect but in fact a multiplicative effect on the ability of the other factors to contribute to CAD and to subsequent CHD.

It is also important to note the wide distribu-

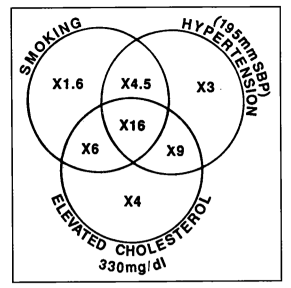

Figure 3-5.

The increase in risk of developing coronary heart disease for someone who has any combination of the three major risk factors compared with the risk for a nonsmoking, normotensive 45-year-old man with a cholesterol level of 185 mg/dL, based on the Framingham cohort. (Reproduced with permission from Kannel WB. Importance of hypertension as a major risk factor in cardiovascular disease in hypertension. In: Genest J, Koiw E, Kuchel O [eds]. Hypertension: Physiopathology and Treatment. New York, McGraw-Hill, 1977, pp 888-910.)

tion of these risk factors in the U.S. population. Figure 3-6 shows that the majority of U.S. workers have at least one major risk factor for CAD. The projected cost to American business in 1990 in the form of medical expenses and lost productivity of workers who have coronary disease was $127 billion, underscoring the impact of CAD on worker productivity.[33]

Cigarette Smoking

Cigarette smoking has been associated with increased risk of cardiovascular disease since 1958.[34] Although no one component of cigarette smoke has been identified as the causative agent for this association, a number of studies have shown how cigarette smoking has a deleterious effect on other known factors involved in the development of atherosclerosis.

As few as four cigarettes a day increases a smoker's risk of developing CAD and CHD above that of a nonsmoker or an exsmoker.[35] Factors that are known to be present in individuals who smoke and that have been identified as possible causes of this increased risk are a reduction in **high-density lipoprotein (HDL)** levels,

Figure 3-6.

Percentage of U.S. workers with major cardiovascular disease risk factors. *Sources:* For high blood pressure and high blood cholesterol: National Health and Nutrition Examination Survey, 1976-80 (NHANES II), National Center for Health Statistics; for smoking: National Health Interview Survey, 1985, National Center for Health Statistics. (Reproduced with permission from NHLBI Data Factsheet: Workplace Facts, July 1990.)

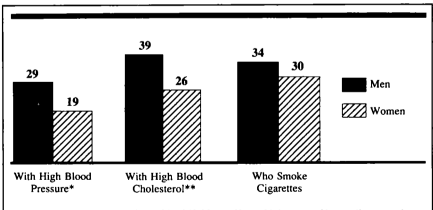

leukocytosis, elevated fibrinogen levels, and increased blood pressure and plasma catecholamine levels.[36,37] These alterations of risk factor profiles have also been observed in the preadolescent children of smoking parents, showing that cigarette smoking increases the risk of developing CHD in both the smoker and the nonsmoking family members.[38]

The power of smoking as an independent risk factor for developing atherosclerosis is illustrated by Kelly and associates, who evaluated 2955 patients admitted to the hospital for acute myocardial infarction.[39] Those patients who smoked were an average of 10 years younger than those who did not smoke and had a much lower prevalence of concomitant risk factors. This demonstrates that cigarette smoking can accelerate the atherosclerotic process in patients otherwise not at significant risk for it.

Hypertension

Hypertension, or high blood pressure, is known to be one of the most prevalent disease states in America, estimated to be present in 61 million people.[1] It has been found to be an independent risk factor for the development of CAD and peripheral and cerebral vascular disease. This finding applies individually to both systolic (>140 mm Hg) and diastolic hypertension (>90 mm Hg).[40]

In the 1960s and 1970s, large-scale studies, such as the Hypertension Detection and Follow-up Program,[41] were able to show impressive reductions in hypertension with concomitant reduction in cerebral vascular accident morbidity and mortality. No such improvements, however, were noted in CHD morbidity or mortality. These results have been reproduced in three separate large-scale clinical trials,[42-44] which has led some investigators to the hypothesis that high blood pressure and coronary vascular disease merely "co-exist" rather than have a causal relationship.[45]

Overwhelmingly, the epidemiologic evidence still points to hypertension as a significant risk factor for the development of CAD.[46] The theoretic basis for this finding is related to the sheer stresses exerted on the coronary endothelial lin-

ing during periods of high blood pressure.[47] This stress eventually leads to endothelial dysfunction, allowing platelet adhesion, release of PDGF, and subsequent onset of the proliferative process described earlier in this chapter.

The failure of medication trials to show success in reducing the incidence of CHD is thought to be due to the negation of any benefit derived from lowering of blood pressure by adverse effects on blood lipids (increased cholesterol, decreased HDL) caused by the drugs used.[48]

Elevated Cholesterol

From the publication of the results of the Framingham study to the present day, the relationship between abnormal levels of cholesterol and its related carrier substances, the lipoproteins, to the development of CHD has been well established.[5,49] Because these studies were epidemiologic in nature, they did not establish a strict cause and effect relationship between the abnormalities in blood lipids and the CAD that was significantly associated with them. Soon after the release of the Framingham study findings, several programs were instituted to screen and treat persons with high blood pressure, but there was no concerted effort to do the same for those with elevated cholesterol.

One of the frequently cited reasons for this was the difference between what is considered an "average" and a "desirable" cholesterol level.[50] Most laboratories identified normal ranges, with the statistical definition of normal being between the fifth and ninety-fifth percentile of the distribution curve. What this statistical definition failed to take into account was that more than 50% of the deaths in the United States at that time were from CHD. By virtue of its prevalence, CHD had become a "normal" disease in this and other industrialized countries.

Figure 3-7 shows the cholesterol levels of the participants at the time of entry in the Framingham study. As can be seen, when cholesterol level alone is analyzed, a significant overlap is present when comparing those who develop CHD with those who do not. Recently, the National Cholesterol Education Project identified a total cholesterol of less than 200 mg/dL as "de-

Figure 3-7.

Total cholesterol levels of individuals in the Framingham study who developed coronary heart disease (CHD) *(dashed line)* compared with those who did not *(solid line)*. (Reproduced with permission from Castelli WP, Anderson K. A population at risk: Prevalence of high cholesterol levels in hypertensive patients in the Framingham Study. Am J Med 80(suppl 2A):28, 1986.)

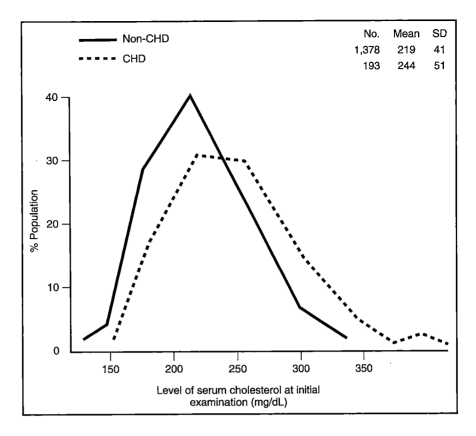

sirable" and more than 240 mg/dL as "high" (Table 3-1).[51]

In 1984, the Lipid Research Clinics Coronary Primary Prevention Trial (LRC-CPPT) established convincingly that elevated levels of cholesterol, especially LDL-transported cholesterol, contributed to the development of CHD.[52] Thirty-eight hundred subjects with elevated cholesterol levels were divided into a control group and an experimental group, which received the bile acid–binding resin cholestyramine. After a mean follow-up of 7.4 years, those subjects in the experimental group had experienced significantly fewer clinical episodes consistent with developing CHD, for example, heart attacks, angina, positive stress test results, and even coronary disease–related death.

In a companion article, the LRC-CPPT established a relationship between percentage of reduction in cholesterol level and reduction of risk of subsequently developing coronary disease for their subjects.[53] It was noted that for every 1% reduction in cholesterol level, there was a 2% reduction in risk of developing subsequent coronary-related events (Table 3-2).

Other studies have documented the importance of HDL as an independent predictor of risk

TABLE 3-1. National Cholesterol Education Program Recommendations for Blood Cholesterol Levels for Adults

Desirable blood cholesterol:
<200 mg/dL (<5.17 mmol/L)

Borderline high blood cholesterol:
200–239 mg/dL (5.17–6.18 mmol/L)

High blood cholesterol:
≥240 mg/dL (≥6.21 mmol/L)

(From National Cholesterol Education Program: Report of the expert panel on detection, evaluation and treatment of high blood cholesterol in adults. Bethesda, Md, US Department of Health and Human Services, Public Health Service, National Heart, Lung, and Blood Institute, NIH Pub. No. 88-2925, January 1988.)

TABLE 3-2. Percentage of Reduction of Risk of Developing Coronary Heart Disease Based on Cholesterol Reduction LRC-CPPT

Cholesterol Reduction	CHD Risk Reduction
4.4%	10.9%
11.5%	26.1%
19.0%	39.3%

(From Lipid Research Clinics Program. LRC-CPPT results II: Relationship of reduction in incidence of coronary heart disease to cholesterol lowering. JAMA 251:365–374, 1984.)

as well.[54,55] The exact mechanism by which increased levels of HDL provide protection from development of coronary disease is not known. Several theories have been proposed, but the one most often mentioned is the probability of HDL having a role in "reverse cholesterol transport," bringing free cholesterol from the tissues back to the liver for safe storage.[56] Analysis of the Framingham data revealed that the best predictor of risk for developing cholesterol-related blockages in an artery is the ratio of total cholesterol to HDL (CHOL/HDL). A level of greater than 4.5 increases an individual's risk of developing atherosclerosis.[57]

Elevated levels of triglycerides (>185 mg/dL) alone were found to be significant indicators for the development of coronary disease in women but not in men. They become a marker for the development of coronary atherosclerosis in men as well when they are associated with low levels of HDL (<35 mg/dL).[58]

Two important considerations regarding cholesterol and its role in the pathogenesis of atherosclerosis are amount of dietary fat intake and cell recognition and utilization of cholesterol. Intake of cholesterol in the diet is *not* the predominant factor in determining the level of cholesterol in the blood. The nutritionally dependent variable most related to increasing levels of blood cholesterol is the amount of saturated fat in the diet.[59] This hypothesis was first proposed by Keys and colleagues and again by Hegsted and associates,[60,61] both in 1965. It was recently revised by Connor and co-workers with the development of a cholesterol to saturated fat index

(CSI).[62] This CSI is a valuable tool that illustrates the variability between dietary and serum levels of cholesterol.

The formula for the determination of the CSI is shown in Figure 3–8. The formula demonstrates that the contribution of saturated fat in any particular food item can be as much as 20 times more atherogenic than its cholesterol content.

Probably the most important factor in the determination of an individual's blood cholesterol level is the ability of each cell to identify and then internalize cholesterol from the bloodstream. Brown and Goldstein received the Nobel Prize in 1985 for their work in identifying the functions of the LDL receptors located on all cells.[63] It is the function of these receptors to provide a binding site for LDL, which is the most abundant cholesterol carrier, to allow it to deliver the cholesterol to the cell. Remember that cholesterol is a major component of all cell membranes and therefore is vital to life. When a genetic defect causes someone to be born without properly functioning LDL receptors (homozygous familial hypercholesterolemia), a six- to tenfold increase occurs in the normal concentrations of plasma LDL from birth, and heart attacks in childhood are common.[64] As long as these cell surface receptors remain active, cholesterol is taken from the circulation and utilized by the cell. If they become inactive or "down regulated" or are exposed to more plasma cholesterol than they can handle, then more water-insoluble lipid in the circulation is available to interact with macrophages accumulating at the site of damaged coronary artery endothelium.

$$CSI = (1.01 \times gm\ sat.\ fat) + (0.05 \times mg\ chol.)$$

CSI - Cholesterol Saturated Fat Index
gm sat. fat - grams saturated fat
mg chol - milligrams cholesterol

Figure 3–8.

The cholesterol saturated fat index. (Reproduced with permission from Connor S et al. The cholesterol/saturated-fat index: An indication of the hypercholesterolaemic and atherogenic potential of food. Lancet 1229–1232, 1986.)

Minor Risk Factors

The minor or "contributing" risk factors are not independently significant in predicting the likelihood of an individual's developing CHD. As their name implies, however, they do play a role in its establishment and growth.

Diabetes

Nonenzymatic glycosylation, or the chemical attachment of glucose to proteins without the involvement of enzymes, is known to affect many of the substances involved in the evolution of CAD.[65] Proteins such as fibrinogen, collagen, and antithrombin III as well as both HDL and LDL have been shown to be adversely affected by this process. The attachment of glucose to these molecules renders them less sensitive to the enzymes and other substances with which they interact. For example, antithrombin III activity, which normally inhibits excessive blood coagulation, is decreased when it undergoes glycosylation, and fibrinogen is less likely to perform its function of degrading fibrin when so affected. In both these cases, thrombus formation is enhanced. This process may even be the principal cause of basement membrane thickening, long known to be a major tissue change associated with prolonged diabetes (see Chapter 7).

Sedentary Lifestyle

The role of exercise in the management of CHD has been discussed since Morris reported a decreased incidence of myocardial infarction in conductors, when compared with drivers, of British double-decker buses.[66] The Centers for Disease Control has reported that lack of adequate exercise is the most prevalent risk factor for coronary heart disease and that more than 90% of Americans do not perform the minimum amount of exercise that has been associated with a reduced risk for the development of atherosclerosis.[67]

Aerobic exercise is known to have a beneficial effect on many of the "building blocks" of CAD, for example, by increasing HDL, decreasing blood pressure (in selected populations), and helping to normalize blood glucose.[68-70] Some of the lesser-known benefits of long-term endurance training are an increase in fibrinolysis and red blood cell deformability as well as a decrease in platelet aggregability,[71-73] which may be beneficial in preventing initial or subsequent coronary ischemic events. It has been shown that exercise of adequate intensity, duration, and frequency is beneficial in preventing cardiovascular disease and increasing longevity in the normal population.[74,75]

Obesity

Several studies have identified obesity (weight >20% above ideal body weight) as a risk factor for CHD.[76] This relationship is known to apply for both men[77] and women.[78] It appears to be more significant if the excess body fat is concentrated in the abdomen ("central obesity") as opposed to being more evenly distributed throughout the body.[79]

It is difficult to prove that being overweight is an independent risk factor for CAD because it is associated with so many other risk factors, for example, hypertension, diabetes, and sedentary lifestyle.

Family History

Family history of CHD, defined as its presence in a parent or sibling, has been shown to be a minor risk factor for the development of CAD. This risk factor has been identified as "nonmodifiable."[1] With the exception of the familial hypercholesterolemias, no genetic link has been established for CHD. Like obesity, which has been shown to be at least 50% determined by lifestyle factors,[80] the atherogenic contribution of family history is not entirely genetic. Kannel has noted that "families share more than genes, and spouses as well as siblings share propensities to disease."[31]

In a 9-year study of 4000 people, Khaw and Barrett-Connor noted that modification of risk factors in subjects who have a strong family history of premature coronary disease provides a greater reduction in overall risk of developing subsequent disease than does the same modification in persons without this family history.[81] This finding suggests that some inherited aspects of coronary disease are in fact modifiable.

Age

Increased age (older than 65) is known to be a risk factor for CHD.[82] Whether older age is an independent pathologic process or simply a consequence of prolonged exposure to other risk factors is less clear. Studies of interventions on other risk factors have proved to be beneficial in older subsets of patients and have resulted in the reduction of clinical endpoints, for example, myocardial infarction and symptoms.[74,83] Also, both patients and subjects without known disease in the young-old and middle-old age groups (67–76) have responded to the same extent as young subjects to attempts at risk factor reduction.[84–86]

Although biochemical changes are known to occur as people age, for example, decreased nerve conduction velocity and decreased aerobic enzyme activity, the functional significance of these changes appears to be negligible if they are not complicated by preexisting disease.[87,88]

Gender

It is a common perception that premenopausal women are "immune" from CHD. Men are six times more likely than women to experience a myocardial infarction before age 55, and the overall onset of clinically significant coronary heart disease in women lags 10 years behind that in men.[89]

Although it is true that, in general, women experience less CHD morbidity and mortality than men, this disease still represents a significant health risk to women. Coronary heart disease is the second leading cause of death in all women younger than 45; it is the leading cause of death in black women younger than 45, an age when the majority are still premenopausal.[90] In terms of age group, the largest "gain" in either sex during which the greatest increase in CHD occurs is in women aged 55 to 64.[89]

Once a myocardial infarction occurs, women of all age groups have a higher mortality rate than men. Slightly more women have unrecognized or "silent" myocardial infarctions than men (34% vs. 27%), but interestingly, the initial clinical event in women is most often angina, whereas in men it is an acute myocardial infarction. Women who have diabetes are more susceptible to developing CHD than are men.[91]

Because the gap between CHD incidence in men and women closes between the fifth and sixth decades, it has been argued that menopause plays some nonspecific role in regulating this disease process. It has been found, however, that the risk of developing CHD is no different in women who had natural menopause, were premenopausal, or had "surgical" menopause and were undergoing estrogen replacement therapy. Estrogen is a factor, however, for it was noted that women who had surgical menopause but did not take estrogen replacement therapy did have a significant increase in the incidence of CHD.[92]

Stress

In 1910, Osler described a stereotypic "behavior pattern" for angina patients.[93] It is noteworthy that Osler commented to the Royal College of Physicians that little progress had been made in this area since Heberden's earlier publication. In 1974, Romeo and associates stated that "our present knowledge of the role played by psychological factors in the pathogenesis of coronary heart disease is not very different from that described by Osler!"[94,95]

Although the pathogenesis may not have been defined, in 1959, Friedman and Rosenman related the sense of time urgency and easily aroused hostility—what they termed *Type A* behavior—to a sevenfold increase in prevalence of CHD.[96] That this behavior is an independent risk factor for CHD was confirmed by the Review Panel on Coronary-Prone Behavior in 1981.[97]

The exact mechanism by which this predominantly psychologic trait increases the risk for the tissue changes of CHD is believed to be related to platelet activation. This contribution to the sclerotic component of CHD is known to be related to increases in levels of catecholamines and platelet-secreted proteins, which have been found in subjects undergoing emotional stress.[98] It is known also that alterations in this Type A behavior provide reduction in morbidity and mortality for the postmyocardial infarction patient.[99]

CLINICAL COURSE

The clinical presentation of the patient with CHD typically occurs in one of three ways:

- sudden cardiac death
- chronic stable angina
- unstable angina

Sudden Cardiac Death

In 20% to 25% of patients with CHD, **sudden cardiac death** (death within 1 hour of onset of symptoms) is the *initial* presenting syndrome![100] Ventricular fibrillation, leading to cessation of cardiac output, is the usual cause of death. For these patients, prompt delivery of bystander cardiopulmonary resuscitation and entry into the emergency medical system within 10 minutes is their only chance of survival.[101]

Angina

The majority of patients with CHD first seek medical attention because of those "peculiar symptoms" that Heberden described in 1772 as "angina" (old English for "strangling") pectoris.[2] This sensation, most commonly described as a substernal pressure, can occur anywhere from the epigastric area to the jaw and is described as squeezing, tightness, or crushing. It is now known to be caused by an imbalance in supply and demand of myocardial oxygen.

Chronic Stable Angina

Chronic stable angina, as its name implies, usually has a well-established level of onset. Pa-

tients are able to predict reliably those activities that provoke their discomfort; this condition is usually associated with a set level of myocardial oxygen demand. As mentioned earlier, myocardial oxygen demand is closely related to heart rate and systolic blood pressure. By multiplying these values, the so-called double product or rate-pressure product, an index that is useful in correlating functional activities with myocardial capabilities, can be obtained. Wall stress, the third determinant of the myocardial oxygen consumption rate (MV_{O_2}), can be accurately measured only with invasive monitoring and is therefore not usually available to the patient performing routine activities.

Patients with stable angina are usually able to bring their symptoms under control by reducing slightly the intensity of the exercise they are performing or by taking sublingual nitroglycerin. Patients have some variability in their tolerance for activity, that is, "good days and bad days," which is probably related to variations in coronary vascular tone, but overall, stable angina is a predictable syndrome.

Unstable Angina

The patient who presents with **unstable angina** or has been experiencing chronic stable angina that develops an unstable pattern (see later discussion) requires quick recognition and referral for treatment. The allied health professional is not responsible for making the diagnosis of unstable angina. However, he or she may be the person who first detects its presence while following a patient in a cardiac rehabilitation program. It is therefore important for such professionals to have a basic understanding of the mechanisms of unstable angina and how to detect it.

Patients who have unstable angina are known to have increased morbidity and mortality when compared with those who have stable angina, even though the absolute amount of coronary atherosclerosis in both groups is not significantly different.[102] Unstable angina can be defined as the presence of signs, symptoms, or both of an inadequate blood supply to the myocardium in the absence of the demands that usually provoke this imbalance. The major physiologic difference between unstable and chronic stable angina is the absence of the need for an increase in myocardial oxygen demand to provoke the syndrome. The notion that imbalances in myocardial blood flow could be related to a primary reduction in oxygen supply without an increase in demand was proved by Chierchia and colleagues.[103] They were able to show that a fall in cardiac vein oxygen saturation always preceded the electrocardiographic or hemodynamic indicators of ischemia in 137 patients who experienced angina while at rest.

Factors That Contribute to Unstable Angina. Several factors have been implicated as contributors to this syndrome. Circadian variations in

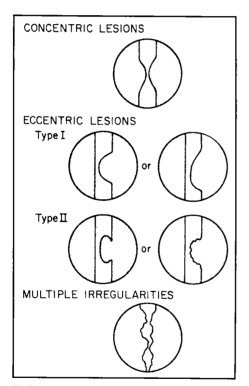

Figure 3–9.
Concentric lesions, usually smooth and symmetric, are more often seen in patients with chronic stable angina. Eccentric lesions, more often seen in patients with unstable angina, are asymmetric and either are smooth (type I) or have irregular borders (type II) or have multiple irregularities. (Reproduced with permission from the American College of Cardiology: Ambrose JA, Winters SL, Arora RR, et al. Coronary angiographic morphology in myocardial infarction. J Am Coll Cardiol 6:1234, 1985.)

catecholamine levels (e.g., epinephrine), which increase heart rate and blood pressure; increased plasma viscosity, known to occur in the first 4 hours of awakening; increases in platelet activation; and pathologic changes in the atherosclerotic plaques themselves have all been proposed as triggers of unstable angina.[104–106]

The atherosclerotic plaque is known to undergo physical changes when a patient is experiencing unstable angina. Ambrose and co-workers have described distinct differences in the morphology of atherosclerotic lesions of persons who are experiencing unstable angina compared with that of persons who have stable angina (Fig. 3–9).[107] More recent developments in fiberoptic technology have allowed direct visual inspection of coronary atherosclerotic lesions, thus permitting differentiation of plaques by their appearance. Sherman and associates were able not only to detect the presence of complex plaques and thrombus formation—the anatomic correlates for unstable angina—with greater accuracy using fiberoptic visualization, but also to identify specific "culprit" lesions by their appearance.[108]

The fact that the coronary plaque is a dynamic entity and not just a mound of debris is helpful in understanding how the stability of the disease can be altered so quickly. The clinical clues to the development of unstable angina that should alert the health professional to notify a patient's physician are

● angina at rest
● occurrence of the patient's typical angina at a significantly lower level of activity than usual
● deterioration of a previously stable pattern, for example, discomfort occurring several times a day compared with several times a week
● evidence of loss of previously present myocardial reserve, such as a drop in blood pressure or increase in heart rate with levels of activity previously well tolerated.

Unstable angina should be distinguished from Prinzmetal's or vasospastic angina. Both are most likely to occur in the first few hours of rising, but vasospastic discomfort is usually not as severe and is often relieved with minor activity, whereas unstable angina is not. Also patients with vasospastic angina are able to perform high levels of work later in the day without discomfort, but patients with unstable angina are unable to increase their cardiac output significantly without further provoking discomfort, even if their earlier pain has waned.

NATURAL HISTORY

Although many population and longitudinal studies have been carried out that document the relative importance of single factors or combinations of risk factors,[5,49,109] still little is known about the natural history of CHD as it applies to an individual patient. Knowledge of risk factors has allowed the establishment of a model from which relative risk can be approximated (Fig. 3–10), but such tools decrease in value for those who are at either end of the normal distribution of the population. The only "guarantee" that can be offered to the patient with known CHD is that if the factors that caused the disease to be present in the first place remain unchanged, it will progress.

There is some evidence that this progression is not inevitable. Blankenhorn and Kramsch have detailed the factors that are known to influence both the atherotic and sclerotic components of CHD.[14]

In regard to the sclerotic component of the disease, it appears that aspirin in small doses (e.g., 80 mg/day) successfully inhibits platelet

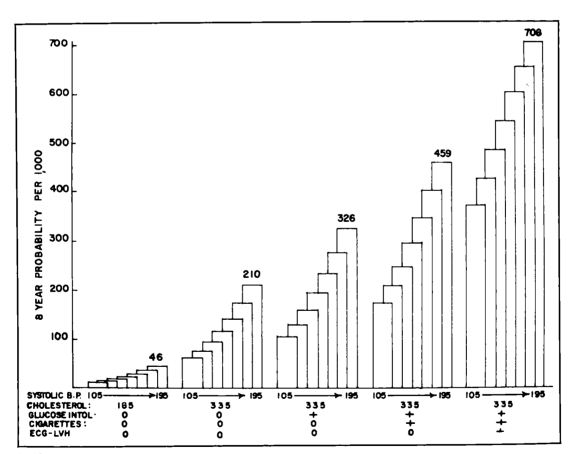

Figure 3–10.

The probability of the development of coronary heart disease in 40-year-old men, Framingham study, at 18-year follow-up. ECG-LVH, electrocardiographic evidence of left ventricular hypertrophy; B.P., blood pressure in mm Hg. (Reproduced with permission from Kannel WB: Importance of hypertension as a major risk factor in cardiovascular disease. In: Genest J, Koiw E, Kuchel O [eds]. Hypertension: Physiopathology and Treatment. New York, McGraw-Hill, 1977, pp 888–910.)

aggregation.[110] Strict control of diabetes also appears to decrease changes in endothelial and intimal elastin, which would lead to decreased vessel wall compliance.

Because cholesterol and related products comprise 60% of the advanced lesions of atherosclerosis, it is possible that strategies geared to alter this percentage would affect the progression of atherosclerotic plaques. Thus far, only two angiographic, controlled clinical trials in humans have addressed this issue.

The Cholesterol Lowering in Atherosclerosis Study achieved significant cholesterol reduction through the use of medications (colestipol and niacin).[111] All subjects in this study had undergone coronary artery bypass graft surgery, and lesions in both their graft and native coronaries were examined. There was significant coronary artery and graft lesion regression in 16.2% of the drug-treated group compared with 2.4% in the placebo-treated group over a 2-year period.

In the Lifestyle Heart Trial, a combination of strict diet, supervised exercise, and stress management constituted the experimental interventions.[112] This program provided detectable regression of stenoses in 82% of the intervention group, whereas 53% of the control group had detectable progression of lesions after only 1 year.

SUMMARY

- Coronary heart disease is the most common disease in the industrialized world.
- Its presence in a given individual is dependent on the presence of any of 10 risk factors for the disease and the susceptibility of the individual to those factors.
- The plaques that obstruct the coronary arteries are a combination of atheroma and thrombus, and they begin to form probably early in the second decade of life.
- Coronary artery disease remains undetected until it occludes approximately 70% of the original coronary lumen.
- The majority of the risk factors for CAD are modifiable.
- Through normalization of these risk factors, the progress of CAD can be arrested and in some cases, reversed.

CASE STUDIES

CASE 1

Mr. H is a 38-year-old white male who, at the age of 30, was experiencing angina with low levels of exertion and was found to have severe obstructions of his left anterior descending (LAD), first diagonal (D1), circumflex (CIRC), first obtuse marginal (OM1), and right coronary arteries (RCA). He underwent five-vessel coronary artery bypass grafting, which relieved his angina. He now has a 2-year history of chronic stable angina, which in the past month has become more frequent, occurring with minimal exertion and occasionally while at rest. Mr. H was admitted to the hospital.

He underwent a repeat cardiac catheterization, which revealed total obstructions of his native proximal LAD, mid-CIRC, and RCA. His venous bypass grafts to his LAD and D1 were also 100% occluded, whereas the grafts to his OM1 and distal RCA were patent.

He has a 20 pack/year (number of packs per day multiplied by the number of years smoked) history of smoking, which he stopped at the time of his bypass surgery. He has a 12-year history of hypertension, which is controlled by medication. He is 67 inches tall and weighs 270 pounds, which is 50 pounds more than he weighed at the time of his bypass surgery. His current blood lipids are cholesterol—188, triglycerides—147, HDL—27, and CHOL/HDL—6.96. He had been employed as an accountant but stated that he had to quit his job because he was experiencing frequent angina during stressful situations at work. He has never engaged in an organized exercise program.

Study Questions—Case 1

- What is this patient's admitting diagnosis?
- Why did this patient's angina return less than 5 years after bypass surgery?
- Which risk factors did Mr. H modify after his bypass surgery?
- Which risk factors did he not modify after his surgery?
- What lifestyle changes should this patient make to keep his remaining grafts patent?

CASE 2

Mr. S is a 65-year-old white male who first experienced chest pressure at rest on September 16. He was admitted to the hospital, and a myocardial infarction was ruled out. While awaiting a diagnostic study, he again had a sudden onset of severe substernal chest pressure, which was associated with ST-segment elevation in his anterior electrocardiogram leads. He was taken for cardiac catheterization, which revealed a complete obstruction of his proximal LAD and a 90% obstruction in his CIRC. His LAD blockage opened to 70% following streptokinase infusion. He went on to have percutaneous transluminal coronary angioplasty of these obstructions, which reduced them to 30%, and he was referred to cardiac rehabilitation.

At the time of admission, he was a 50 pack/year smoker, had poorly controlled hypertension, was 68 inches tall, and weighed 200 pounds. His blood lipids were cholesterol—181, triglycerides—139, HDL—34, and CHOL/HDL—5.32. He is retired and lives alone; he has never engaged in a regular exercise program.

Study Questions—Case 2

● Which of this patient's risk factors will respond favorably to diet and exercise?
● Which risk factors will not?
● What would be his clinical diagnosis during the first few days of his hospitalization?

CASE 3

Mr. C is a 56-year-old white male who has a known history of CHD, having had two myocardial infarctions and coronary artery bypass graft surgery in 1988. He was admitted to the hospital on April 13 with a 2-day history of palpitations associated with nausea and vomiting. He was found to be in sustained ventricular tachycardia, which converted to normal sinus rhythm spontaneously. His peak creatine phosphokinase level of 250 was 100% from skeletal muscle. His medical history included several admissions to the hospital between 1988 and 1992 for conges-tive heart failure, and during one of these, his left ventricular ejection fraction was noted to be 22%.

He had been a 75 pack/year smoker but had stopped smoking 15 years earlier. His blood pressure is well controlled at rest but following minimal activity is 230/90. Mr. C is diabetic and requires oral hyperglycemic agents; he is 6 feet tall and weighs 260 lbs. He admits to being "angry" when things do not go as he had planned and in fact has become dependent on diazepam, which he has been taking for 20 years to help with his "hyper" personality. His current blood lipids are cholesterol—208, triglycerides—240, HDL—29, CHOL/HDL—7.17, and glucose—145. He is limited by leg fatigue at a work load of less than 5 mets.

Study Questions—Case 3

● Is this patient's cholesterol level significantly elevated?
● Does this patient have a blood lipid "problem"? If so, what is it?
● What changes in this patient's medication program should be made before he begins cardiac rehabilitation?
● In view of this patient's ejection fraction, should he be considered a candidate for cardiac rehabilitation? Why or why not?

CASE 4

Mr. G is a 44-year-old white male who was in his usual state of health until December 19. On that date, he had a sudden onset of severe substernal chest pressure, which radiated to his left shoulder. He was admitted to the hospital and was diagnosed as having an acute anterior myocardial infarction. He was taken to the cardiac catheterization laboratory and underwent emergent percutaneous transluminal coronary angioplasty to his LAD, reducing his blockage from 100% to 30%. The remainder of his hospital stay was uncomplicated.

He has a 60 pack/year history of smoking and was smoking two packs per day at the time of admission to the hospital. Both his father and an older brother had had myocardial infarctions. He is 6 feet tall and weighs 242 pounds. His current blood lipids are cholesterol—247, triglycerides —165, HDL—38, CHOL/HDL—6.50, and glucose—100. His first marriage ended in divorce, and he reports that the onset of his chest discomfort at the time of his myocardial infarction occurred when he was arguing with his second wife about their mutually owned business. He states that because he works 60 to 70 hours per week, he has never participated in a regular exercise program.

Study Questions—Case 4

● What two major risk factors does this patient have for developing more atherosclerosis?
● What two lifestyle changes would increase this patient's HDL level?
● What *one* aspect of this patient's personality is likely to contribute to the progression of his CHD?

References

1. American Heart Association. 1990 Heart and Stroke Facts. Dallas, Tex, 1991.
2. Heberden W. An account of a disorder of the breast. Med Trans R Coll Physicians 2:59–67, 1786.
3. Enos W, Holmes R, Beyer J. Coronary disease among United States soldiers killed in action in Korea. JAMA 152:1090–1093, 1953.
4. Strong J. Coronary atherosclerosis in soldiers: A clue to the natural history of atherosclerosis in the young. JAMA 256:2863–2868, 1986.
5. Kannel W, Castelli W, Gordon T, McNamara P. Serum cholesterol, lipoproteins, and the risk of coronary heart disease: The Framingham Study. Ann Intern Med 24:1–12, 1971.
6. Wissler R. Principles of the pathogenesis of atherosclerosis. In: Braunwald E (ed). Heart Disease: A Textbook of Cardiovascular Medicine. 2nd ed. Philadelphia, WB Saunders, 1984.
7. Reichl D, Simons L, Myant N, et al. The lipids and lipoproteins of human peripheral lymph with observations on the transport of cholesterol from plasma and tissues into lymph. Clin Sci Mol Med 45:313, 1973.
8. Day C, Levy R. Control of the precipitation reaction between low density lipoproteins and polyions. Artery 1:150, 1975.
9. Gorlin R. Coronary anatomy. In: Gorlin R. Coronary Artery Disease. Philadelphia, WB Saunders, 1976, p 40.
10. Fulton W. The Coronary Arteries. Springfield, Ill, Charles C Thomas, 1965.
11. Schaper W. The physiology of the collateral circulation in the normal and hypoxic myocardium. Rev Physiol Biochem Pharmacol 63:102, 1971.
12. Stary HC. Evolution of atherosclerotic plaques in the coronary arteries of young adults. Atherosclerosis 3:471a, 1983 (abstract).
13. Ross R. The pathogenesis of atherosclerosis—An update. N Engl J Med 314:488–500, 1986.
14. Blankenhorn D, Kramsch D. Reversal of atherosis and sclerosis, the two components of atherosclerosis. Circulation 79:1–7, 1989.
15. Ross R, Glomset J. The pathogenesis of atherosclerosis. N Engl J Med 295:420–425, 1976.
16. Grotendorst G et al. Platelet-derived growth factor is a chemoattractant for vascular smooth muscle cells. J Cell Physiol 113:261–266, 1982.
17. Osler W. Second Lumleian lecture on angina pectoris. Lancet March 26, 1910:839–844.
18. Prinzmetal M, Ekemecki A, Kennamer R, et al. Angina pectoris. 1. A variant form of angina pectoris. Am J Med 27:375–388, 1959.
19. Meller J, Pichard A, Dack S. Coronary arterial spasm in Prinzmetal's angina: A proved hypothesis. Am J Cardiol 37:938–940, 1976.
20. Maseri A, Severi S, DeNes M, et al. "Variant" angina: One aspect of a continuous spectrum of vasospastic myocardial ischemia. Am J Cardiol 42:1019–1035, 1978.
21. Burke J, Ross R. Synthesis of connective tissue macromolecules by smooth muscle. Int Rev Connect Tis Res 8:119–157, 1979.
22. Furchgott R, Zawadzki J. The obligatory role of endothelial cells in relaxation of arterial smooth muscle by acetylcholine. Nature 288:373–376, 1980.
23. Furchgott R. Role of endothelium in responses of vascular smooth muscle. Circ Res 53:557–573, 1983.
24. Luscher T, Vanhoutte P. Endothelium-dependent contractions to acetylcholine in the aorta of the spontaneously hypertensive rat. Hypertension 8:344–348, 1986.
25. Freiman P, Mitchell G, Heistad D, et al. Atherosclerosis impairs endothelium-dependent vascular relaxation to acetylcholine and thrombin in primates. Circ Res 58:783–789, 1986.
26. Jayakody L et al. Endothelium-dependent relaxation in experimental atherosclerosis in the rabbit. Circ Res 60:251–264, 1987.
27. Forstermann U, Mugge A, Alheid V, et al. Selective attenuation of endothelium-mediated vasodilation in atherosclerotic human coronary arteries. Circ Res 62:185–190, 1988.
28. Ludmer P, Selwyn A, Shook T, et al. Parodoxical vasoconstriction induced by acetylcholine in atherosclerotic coronary arteries. N Engl J Med 315:1046–1051, 1986.
29. Yasue H, Matsuyama K, Matsuyama K, et al. Responses of angiographically normal human coronary arteries to intracoronary injection of acetylcholine by age and segment. Circulation 81:482–490, 1990.
30. Vita J, Treasure C, Nabel E, et al. Coronary vasomotor response to acetylcholine relates to risk factors for coronary disease. Circulation 81:491–497, 1990.
31. Kannell W. Some lessons in cardiovascular epidemiology from Framingham. Am J Cardiol 37:269–282, 1976.

32. Mancia G. Opening remarks: The need to manage risk factors of coronary heart disease. Am Heart J 115:240–241, 1988.

33. U.S. Department of Health and Human Services, Public Health Service, National Heart, Lung, and Blood Institute. Workplace facts. July 1990.

34. Hammond E, Horn D. Smoking and death rates—Report on 44 months of follow-up of 187,783 men. II. Death rates by cause. JAMA 166:1294–1308, 1958.

35. Wilhelmsen L. Coronary heart disease: Epidemiology of smoking and intervention studies of smoking. Am Heart J 115:242–249, 1988.

36. McGill H. The cardiovascular pathology of smoking. Am Heart J 115:250–257, 1988.

37. Trap-Jensen J. Effects of smoking on the heart and peripheral circulation. Am Heart J 115:263–267, 1988.

38. Moskowitz W, Mosteller M, Schieken R, et al. Lipoprotein and oxygen transport alterations in passive smoking in preadolescent children: The MCV twin study. Circulation 81:586–592, 1990.

39. Kelly T, Gilpin H, Ahnve S, et al. Smoking status at the time of acute myocardial infarction and subsequent prognosis. Am Heart J 110:535–541, 1985.

40. Rutan G, Kuller L, Neaton J, et al. Mortality associated with diastolic hypertension and isolated systolic hypertension among men screened for the Multiple Risk Factor Intervention Trial. Circulation 77:504–514, 1988.

41. Hypertension Detection and Follow-Up Program Cooperative Group. Five year findings of the Hypertension Detection and Follow-Up Program, I. Reduction in mortality of persons with high blood pressure, including mild hypertension. JAMA 242:2562–2571, 1979.

42. Medical Research Council Working Party. MRC trial of treatment of mild hypertension: Principal results. Br Med J 291:97–104, 1985.

43. Wilhelmsen L, Berglund G, Elmfeldt O, et al. Beta blockers versus diuretics in hypertensive men: Main results for the HAPPHY trial. J Hypertens 5:561–572, 1987.

44. The IPPPSH Collaborative Group. Cardiovascular risk and risk factors in a randomized trial of treatment based on the beta-blocker oxprenolol: The International Prospective Primary Prevention Study in Hypertension. J Hypertens 3:379–392, 1985.

45. Doyle A. Does hypertension predispose to coronary disease? Conflicting epidemiological and experimental evidence. Am J Hypertens 1:319–324, 1988.

46. Assmann G, Schulte H. The prospective Cardiovascular Munster Study: Prevalence and prognostic significance of hyperlipidemia in men with systemic hypertension. Am J Cardiol 59:9G–17G, 1987.

47. O'Rourke M. Arterial Function in Health and Disease. Edinburgh, Churchill Livingstone, 1982.

48. MacMahon S, MacDonald G. Antihypertensive treatment and plasma lipoprotein levels: The associations in data from a population study. Am J Med 80(suppl 2A):40–47, 1986.

49. Pekkanen J, Linn S, Heiss G, et al. Ten year mortality from cardiovascular disease in relation to cholesterol level among men with and without preexisting cardiovascular disease. N Engl J Med 322:1700–1707, 1990.

50. Steinberg D. The cholesterol controversy is over, why did it take so long? Circulation 80:1070–1078, 1989.

51. National Cholesterol Education Program. Report of the expert panel on detection, evaluation and treatment of high blood cholesterol in adults. Bethesda, Md, US Department of Health and Human Services, Public Health Service, National Heart, Lung, and Blood Institute, NIH Pub. No. 88-2925, January 1988.

52. Lipid Research Clinics Program. The lipid research clinics coronary primary prevention trial results. JAMA 251:351–364, 1984.

53. Lipid Research Clinics Program. LRC-CPPT results II: Relationship of reduction in incidence of coronary heart disease to cholesterol lowering. JAMA 251:365–374, 1984.

54. Gordon D, Probstfield J, Garrison B, et al. High density lipoprotein cholesterol and cardiovascular disease: Four prospective American studies. Circulation 79:8–15, 1989.

55. Miller M, Mead L, Kwiterovich P, Pearson T. Dyslipidemias with desirable plasma total cholesterol levels and angiographically demonstrated coronary artery disease. Am J Cardiol 65:1–5, 1990.

56. Gwynne J. High density lipoprotein cholesterol levels as a marker of reverse cholesterol transport. Am J Cardiol 64:10G–17G, 1989.

57. Castelli W, Anderson K. A population at risk: Prevalence of high cholesterol levels in hypertensive patients in the Framingham study. Am J Med 80(2A):23–32, 1986.

58. Castelli W. The triglyceride issue: A view from Framingham. Am Heart J 112:432–437, 1986.

59. Kris-Etherton P, Krummel D, Dreon D, et al. The effect of diet on plasma lipids, lipoproteins and coronary heart disease. J Am Diet Assoc 88:1373–1400, 1988.

60. Keys A, Anderson J, Grand F. Serum cholesterol response to changes in the diet. Metabolism 14:747–787, 1965.

61. Hegsted D, McGandy R, Meyers M, Stare F. Quantitative effects of dietary fat on serum cholesterol in man. Am J Clin Nutr 17:281–295, 1965.

62. Connor S, Artaud-Wild S, Gustafson J, et al. The cholesterol/saturated-fat index: An indication of the hypercholesterolaemic and atherogenic potential of food. Lancet May 31, 1986:1229–1232.

63. Brown M, Goldstein J. A receptor-mediated pathway for cholesterol homeostasis. Science 232:34–47, 1986.

64. Goldstein J, Brown M. In: Stanbury JB, Wyngaarden J, Frederickson D (eds). Metabolic Basis of Inherited Disease. New York, McGraw-Hill, 1983.

65. Brownlee M et al. Nonenzymatic glycosylation and the pathogenesis of diabetic complications. Ann Intern Med 101:527–537, 1984.

66. Morris J. Coronary heart disease and physical activity of work. Lancet 1053–1057, 1953.

67. Centers for Disease Control. Progress toward achieving the 1990 national objectives for physical fitness and exercise. MMWR 38:449–453, 1989.

68. Astrand PO. Exercise physiology and its role in disease prevention and in rehabilitation. Arch Phys Med Rehabil 68:305–309, 1987.

69. Duncan J, Farr J, Upton S, et al. The effects of aerobic exercise on plasma catecholamines and blood pressure in patients with mild essential hypertension. JAMA 254:2609–2613, 1985.

70. Horton ES. Role and management of exercise in diabetes mellitus. Diabetes Care 11:201–211, 1988.

71. Williams RS, Logue E, Lewis J, et al. Physical condi-

tioning augments the fibrinolytic response to venous occlusion in healthy adults. N Engl J Med 302:987–991, 1980.

72. Ernst E. Influence of regular physical activity on blood rheology. Eur Heart J 8:59G–62G, 1987.

73. Rauramaa R, Salonen J, Seppanen K, et al. Inhibition of platelet aggregability by moderate intensity physical exercise: A randomized clinical trial in overweight men. Circulation 74:939–944, 1986.

74. Paffenbarger R, Hyde R, Wing A, Hsieh C. Physical activity, all-cause mortality, and longevity of college alumni. N Engl J Med 314:605–613, 1986.

75. Blair S, Kohl H, Paffenbarger R, et al. Physical fitness and all-cause mortality: A prospective study of healthy men and women. JAMA 262:2395–2401, 1989.

76. Bray G. Overweight is risking fate: Definition, classification, prevalence and risk. Ann NY Acad Sci 499:14–28, 1987.

77. Phillips A, Shaper A. Relative weight and major ischaemic heart disease events in hypertensive men. Lancet 8645:1005–1008, 1989.

78. Manson J, Colditz G, Stampfer M, et al. A prospective study of obesity and risk of coronary heart disease in women. N Engl J Med 322:882–889, 1990.

79. Donahue R, Abbott R, Bloom E, et al. Central obesity and coronary heart disease in men. Lancet 8537:821–824, 1987.

80. Burns T, Moll P, Lauer R. The relation between ponderosity and coronary risk factors in children and their relatives: The muscatine ponderosity family study. Am J Epidemiol 129:973–987, 1989.

81. Khaw K, Barrett-Connor E. Family history of heart attack: A modifiable risk factor? Circulation 74:239–244, 1986.

82. Salter L, Green C, Wallace R, Rackley C. Coronary artery disease in the elderly. Am J Cardiol 63:245–248, 1989.

83. Hermanson B, Omenn G, Kronmal R, et al. Beneficial six-year outcome of smoking cessation in older men and women with coronary disease. N Engl J Med 319:1365–1369, 1988.

84. Haber P, Honiger B, Kliepers M, Niederberger M. Effects in elderly people 67–76 years of age of three-month endurance training on a bicycle ergometer. Eur Heart J 5:37E–39E, 1984.

85. Opasich C, Cobelli F, Assandri J, et al. Is old age a contraindication to cardiac rehabilitation after acute myocardial infarction? European Heart J 5:105E–107E, 1984.

86. Williams M, Maresh C, Aronow W, et al. The value of early out-patient cardiac exercise programmes for the elderly in comparison with other selected age groups. Eur Heart J 5:113E–115E, 1984.

87. Morley J, Reese S. Clinical implications of the aging heart. Am J Med 86:77–86, 1989.

88. Rodeheffer R, Gerstenblith G, Becker L, et al. Exercise cardiac output is maintained with advancing age in healthy human subjects: Cardiac dilatation and increased stroke volume compensate for a diminished heart rate. Circulation 69:203–213, 1984.

89. Lerner D, Kannel W. Patterns of coronary heart disease morbidity and mortality in the sexes: A 26 year follow up on the Framingham population. Am Heart J 111:383–390, 1986.

90. National Center for Health Statistics. Monthly vital statistics report. 32(4):October 1983.

91. Kannel W. Metabolic risk factors for coronary heart disease in women: Perspective from the Framingham study. Am Heart J 114:413–419, 1987.

92. Colditz G, Walter B, Willetts W, et al. Menopause and the risk of coronary heart disease in women. N Engl J Med 316:1105–1110, 1987.

93. Osler W. The Lumleian lectures on angina pectoris I. Lancet March 12, 1910:697–702.

94. Romeo M, Siltanen P, Theorell T, et al. Work behavior, time urgency and life dissatisfaction in subjects with myocardial infarction: A cross-cultural study. J Psychosom Res 18:1–8, 1974.

95. Morgan W, Raglin J. Psychological aspects of heart disease. In: Pollack M, Schmidt D (eds). Heart Disease and Rehabilitation. 2nd ed. New York, Wiley Medical Publications, 1986.

96. Friedman M, Rosenman RH. Association of specific overt behavior pattern with blood and cardiovascular findings. JAMA 169:1286–1296, 1959.

97. The review panel on coronary-prone behavior and coronary heart disease: A critical review. Circulation 63:1199–1215, 1981.

98. Levine S et al. Platelet activation and secretion associated with emotional stress. Circulation 72:1129–1134, 1985.

99. Friedman M, Thoresen C, Gill J, et al. Alteration of type A behavior and its effect on cardiac recurrences in post myocardial infarction patients: Summary results of the recurrent coronary prevention project. Am Heart J 112:653–665, 1986.

100. Myerburg R, Castellanos A. Cardiac arrest and sudden cardiac death. In: Braunwald E (ed). Heart Disease: A Textbook of Cardiovascular Medicine. 3rd ed. Philadelphia, WB Saunders, 1988, pp 742–777.

101. American Heart Association. Standards and guidelines for cardiopulmonary resuscitation (CPR) and emergency cardiac care (ECC). JAMA 255:2905–2914, 1986.

102. Moise A, Theroux P, Taeymans Y, et al. Unstable angina and progression of coronary atherosclerosis. N Engl J Med 309:685–689, 1983.

103. Chierchia S, Brunelli C, Simonetti I, et al. Sequence of events in angina at rest: Primary reduction in coronary flow. Circulation 61:759–768, 1980.

104. Muller J, Toffler G, Stone P. Circadian variation and triggers of onset of acute cardiovascular disease. Circulation 79:733–743, 1989.

105. Fitzgerald D, Roy L, Catella F, FitzGerald G. Platelet activation in unstable coronary disease. N Engl J Med 315:983–989, 1986.

106. Davies M, Thomas A. Plaque fissuring—The cause of acute myocardial infarction, sudden ischaemic death, and crescendo angina. Br Heart J 53:363–373, 1985.

107. Ambrose J, Winters S, Arora R, et al. Coronary angiographic morphology in myocardial infarction: A link between the pathogenesis of unstable angina and myocardial infarction. J Am Coll Cardiol 6:1233–1238, 1985.

108. Sherman CT, Litvack F, Grundfest W, et al. Coronary angioscopy in patients with unstable angina pectoris. N Engl J Med 315:913–919, 1986.

109. Reed D, Yano K, Kagan A. Lipids and lipoproteins as predictors of coronary heart disease, stroke, and cancer

in the Honolulu heart program. Am J Med 80:871–878, 1986.

110. Hennekens C, Buring J, Sandercook P, et al. Aspirin and other antiplatelet agents in the secondary and primary prevention of cardiovascular disease. Circulation 80:749–756, 1989.

111. Blankenhorn D, Nessim S, Johnson R, et al. Beneficial effects of combined colestipol-niacin therapy on coronary atherosclerosis and coronary venous bypass grafts. JAMA 257:3233–3240, 1987.

112. Ornish D, Brown S, Scherwitz L, et al. Can lifestyle changes reverse coronary heart disease? The lifestyle heart trial. Lancet 336:129–133, 1990.

4 CARDIAC MUSCLE DYSFUNCTION

INTRODUCTION

Cardiac muscle dysfunction (CMD) is a term that has gained popularity in describing an apparently common finding in patients with heart and lung disease.[1-3] This is probably because CMD effectively, yet very simply, describes the most common cause of congestive heart failure (CHF).[2] It is estimated that 2 million or more Americans suffer from CHF and that 400,000 new cases occur yearly, requiring 900,000 hospitalizations each year.[4] In addition, years of cardiovascular data compiled in Framingham, Massachusetts, show a 1% prevalence of CHF in those aged 50 to 59 years, which increases progressively with advancing age to approximately 10% in 80 to 89 year olds.[5] Therefore, individuals with a wide variety of heart and lung diseases very likely will develop CHF at some time during their lives,[3] which frequently manifests itself as **pulmonary congestion** or **pulmonary edema**.[1] This chapter describes the clinical manifestations resulting from CMD and demonstrates the interrelatedness of all bodily systems.

Many of the signs and symptoms of CHF are the result of a "sequence of events with a resultant increase in fluid in the interstitial spaces of the lungs, liver, subcutaneous tissues, and **serous cavities**."[6] The etiology of CHF is varied, but it is most commonly the result of CMD. Nevertheless, the interdependence and interrelationship between the cardiac and pulmonary systems are evident. In fact, Table 4–1 classifies the mechanisms responsible for pulmonary edema, of which increased pulmonary capillary pressure is the most common. Left ventricular failure is the most common cause of such increased pulmonary capillary pressure, which produces the congestion of CHF. Therefore, the term CMD accurately describes the primary cause of pulmonary edema as well as the underlying pathophysiology of CHF because CMD essentially *impairs* the heart's ability to *pump blood* or the left ventricle's ability to *accept blood*.[6] Subsequent sections in this chapter review the many interrelated pathophysiologies of CHF as well as the treatment and training of patients with CHF.

CAUSES AND TYPES OF CARDIAC MUSCLE DYSFUNCTION

The varied causes of CMD can be best classified according to the 10 most common primary pathologies.[6-8]

- Myocardial infarction or ischemia
- Cardiac arrhythmias
- Renal insufficiency
- **Cardiomyopathy**
- Heart valve abnormalities
- **Pericardial effusion or myocarditis**
- **Pulmonary embolism** or pulmonary hypertension
- Spinal cord injury
- Congenital abnormalities
- Aging

Of these, cardiomyopathy, congenital abnormalities, renal insufficiency, and aging are more commonly associated with *chronic* heart failure, whereas the others are associated with *acute* CHF. Acute and chronic heart failure can be more specifically described as forward or backward, right-sided or left-sided, low-output or high-output, or systolic or diastolic heart failure.[6]

TABLE 4–1. Mechanisms Responsible for Pulmonary Edema

Increased pulmonary capillary pressure
(e.g., left ventricular failure)

Decreased plasma oncotic pressure
(e.g., hypoalbuminemia secondary to multisystem dysfunction)

Increased negativity of interstitial pressure
(e.g., asthma)

Altered alveolar-capillary membrane permeability
(e.g., aspiration of acidic gastric contents or infectious pneumonia)

Lymphatic insufficiency
(e.g., after lung transplant)

Unknown or incompletely understood
(e.g., high altitude, after cardiopulmonary bypass)

Congestive Heart Failure

Right-sided or left-sided CHF simply describes which side of the heart is failing, as well as the side that is initially affected and behind which fluid tends to localize. For example, left-sided heart failure is frequently the result of left ventricular insult (e.g., myocardial infarction, hypertension, aortic valve disease), which causes fluid to accumulate behind the left ventricle. This, in turn, produces an accumulation of fluid in the lungs, liver, abdomen, and ankles (manifestations of right heart failure).[6] Thus, right-sided CHF may occur because of left-sided CHF or because of right ventricular failure (e.g., secondary to pulmonary hypertension, pulmonary embolus, right ventricular infarction). In either case, fluid backs up behind the right ventricle and produces the accumulation of fluid in the liver, abdomen, and ankles mentioned earlier.

Low-output CHF is the description most frequently associated with heart failure and is the result of a low cardiac output at rest or during exertion. **High-output CHF** usually results from a volume overload as in pregnancy, **thyrotoxicosis** (overactivity of the thyroid gland, such as in **Graves's disease**), and renal insufficiency.[6,9,10] Of particular importance is that although the term *high-output* implies a greater cardiac output, it is nonetheless lower than it was before CHF developed.

Systolic versus diastolic heart failure is perhaps the most informative and useful distinction in CHF because optimal cardiac performance is dependent on both proper systolic and diastolic functioning. The impaired contraction of the ventricles during systole that produces an inefficient expulsion of blood is termed systolic heart failure. Diastolic heart failure is associated with an inability of the ventricles to accept the blood ejected from the atria. Both types are very important in the overall scheme of CHF and often occur simultaneously, as in the patient who suffers a massive anterior myocardial infarction (loss of contracting myocardium producing systolic heart failure) with subsequent replacement of the infarcted area with nondistensible fibrous scar tissue (which does not readily or adequately

accept the blood ejected into the left ventricle from the left atria and produces diastolic heart failure).[1]

Hypertension and Coronary Artery Disease

Hypertension and coronary artery disease are the most common causes of CMD,[3] which occurs because of dysfunction of the left or right ventricle or both.[11-13] This is demonstrated in the example given earlier of a patient who, after suffering a massive anterior myocardial infarction, loses a significant amount of strategically located cardiac muscle, which subsequently decreases the performance of the left ventricle; this decrease produces a decreased **ejection fraction** and, in many instances, a decreased physical work capacity.

Cardiac Arrhythmias and Renal Insufficiency

Cardiac arrhythmias and renal insufficiency can also cause CMD for reasons similar to those given for myocardial infarction.[6] Extremely rapid or slow cardiac arrhythmias or volume overload impairs the functioning of the left or right ventricle, or both, and an overall CMD ensues. Correcting the arrhythmia or decreasing the volume overload can remedy this type of CMD quickly.[14,15]

Cardiomyopathy

Individuals with cardiomyopathy are often less fortunate because no apparent treatment can reverse the fatal progression of this disease at present (except for **palliative** treatment via cardiac transplantation). Cardiomyopathy is a disease in which the contraction and relaxation of myocardial muscle fibers are impaired.[16] This impaired contractility can result from either primary or secondary causes.[17] The *primary* causes are the result of pathologic processes in the heart muscle itself, which impair the heart's ability to contract. The *secondary* causes of cardiomyopathy are the result of a systemic disease process rather than of pathologic myocardial processes and can be classified according to the systemic disease that subsequently affects myocardial contraction. These include diseases that are

- inflammatory
- metabolic
- toxic
- infiltrative
- **fibroplastic**
- hematologic
- hypersensitive
- genetic
- the result of physical agents
- acquired (miscellaneous)
- idiopathic (unknown)[16]

Each secondary cause can be further subdivided, as in Table 4–2.

Cardiomyopathies are also classified from a *functional* standpoint, emphasizing three basic categories:

- dilated cardiomyopathy
- hypertrophic cardiomyopathy
- restrictive cardiomyopathy[16]

Dilated cardiomyopathy is characterized by ventricular dilation and cardiac muscle contractile dysfunction. **Hypertrophic cardiomyopathy** is distinguished by inappropriate and excessive left ventricular hypertrophy and normal or even enhanced cardiac muscle contractile function. **Restrictive cardiomyopathy** is identified by marked endocardial scarring of the ventricles, with resulting impaired diastolic filling. Patients often present with a combination of these functional classifications.[16]

Unfortunately, research suggests that cardiomyopathy is perhaps much more common than was originally believed. Myopathic change in cardiac and skeletal muscle has been associated with hypertension[3] and diabetes[18,19]; it has also been found in individuals with and without skeletal muscle disease[20,21] and in patients with CHF.[21,22] These findings have great implications for the health care providers of the 1990s and beyond, as the aged population increases and

TABLE 4–2. Secondary Causes of Cardiomyopathy
Inflammation
viral infarction
bacterial infarction
Metabolic
selenium deficiency
diabetes mellitus
Toxic
alcohol
bleomycin
Infiltrative
sarcoidosis
neoplastic
Fibroplastic
carcinoid fibrosis
endomyocardial fibrosis
Hematologic
sickle cell anemia
leukemia
Hypersensitivity
cardiac transplant rejection
methyldopa
Genetic
hypertrophic cardiomyopathy
Duchenne's muscular dystrophy
Miscellaneous acquired
postpartum cardiomyopathy
obesity
Idiopathic
idiopathic hypertrophic cardiomyopathy
Physical agents
heat stroke
hypothermia
radiation

(Adapted from Braunwald E. Heart Disease: A Textbook of Cardiovascular Medicine. 3rd ed. Philadelphia, WB Saunders, 1988, Table 42–1, p 1411.)

newer technologies are used to prolong and sustain life.

Heart Valve Abnormalities

Heart valve abnormalities can also cause CMD, as blocked valves **(valvular stenosis)** or incompetent valves **(valvular insufficiency** due to abnormal or poorly functioning valve leaflets), or both, cause heart muscle to contract more forcefully to expel the cardiac output. This subsequently produces myocardial hypertrophy, which can decrease ventricular distensibility and produce a mild diastolic dysfunction; if prolonged, this dysfunction can lead to more profound dia-stolic as well as systolic dysfunction.[23] Incompe-tent valves are frequently associated with myo-cardial dilation in addition to hypertrophy, because regurgitant blood fills the atria or ventri-cles forcefully.[23] Atrial dilation often accompanies mitral and tricuspid insufficiency, whereas ven-tricular dilation accompanies aortic or pulmonic insufficiency. Aortic insufficiency can dilate the left ventricle, while pulmonic insufficiency can dilate the right ventricle. Mitral insufficiency fre-quently dilates the left atrium, whereas tricuspid insufficiency dilates the right atrium. Such dila-tion can lengthen individual cardiac muscle fibers in the atria and ventricles to such a degree that myocardial contraction is impaired severely, but frequently the accompanying myocardial hy-pertrophy prevents such extreme dilation. How-ever, the abnormal hemodynamics from hyper-trophy and dilation often produce CMD.[23]

Acute heart valve dysfunction or rupture can cause rapid and life-threatening CMD because a ruptured valve impairs cardiac output and regur-gitant blood fills the heart's chambers rather than exiting the aorta.[7] If left untreated, valve rupture will ultimately produce pulmonary edema and eventually death.

Pericardial Effusion

Injury to the pericardium of the heart can cause acute *pericarditis* (inflammation of the pericardial sac surrounding the heart), which may progress to pericardial effusion, occasionally resulting in *cardiac compression* as fluid fills the pericardial sac.[16] Increased fluid accumulation within the pericardial space increases intraperi-cardial pressure and produces *cardiac tamponade.* Cardiac tamponade is characterized by elevated intracardiac pressures, progressively limited ven-tricular diastolic filling, and reduced stroke vol-ume.[16] Thus, the mechanism of CMD, which is primarily a diastolic dysfunction (limited ventric-ular diastolic filling because of cardiac compres-sion), produces a secondary systolic dysfunction. The same sequence of primary diastolic CMD producing secondary systolic CMD occurs in myocarditis.

Pulmonary Embolism

Cardiac muscle dysfunction from a pulmonary embolus is the result of elevated pulmonary ar-tery pressures, which dramatically increase right ventricular work. Right as well as left ventricular failure can occur because of decreased oxygen-ated coronary blood flow and decreased blood flow to the left ventricle.[24] A similar, but often less extreme, condition occurs in pulmonary hy-pertension.

Spinal Cord Injury

Spinal cord injury also can produce CMD be-cause of cervical spinal cord transection, which "causes an imbalance between parasympathetic and sympathetic control of the cardiovascular system."[25] Several studies have identified pul-monary edema as a frequently fatal complication of cervical spinal cord transection.[26-28]

Congenital Abnormalities and Aging

Although distinctly different processes, con-genital or acquired heart diseases and the aging process can produce a similar type of CMD, which is often initially well tolerated but as the dysfunction persists may become more sympto-matic and troublesome. The adaptability of in-fants and children to extreme conditions is evident in congenital heart disease, which fre-quently can be managed for many years with specific medications before surgical intervention is necessary.[29,30] The CMD associated with the aging process is initially well tolerated not be-cause of the aged individual's ability to adapt but because the degree of CMD is usually mild. Aging appears to decrease cardiac output by al-tered contraction and relaxation of cardiac mus-cle.[31,32] However, heart disease, hypertension, and other pathologic processes can increase CMD substantially and subsequently can impair functional abilities.[31,32]

CARDIAC MUSCLE DYSFUNCTION IN PHYSICAL THERAPY

Cardiac muscle dysfunction can produce observable and measurable signs and symptoms, such as a reduced physical work capacity, which, if thoroughly understood, could help physical therapists determine realistic and obtainable goals for their patients. The goal of the following sections is to assist the physical therapist in identifying the presence and severity of CMD.

Study of the demographics of CMD in physical therapy have revealed two very important findings.[33] The first is that physical therapists in all specialty areas, not just those in cardiopulmonary physical therapy, are treating a significant number of patients with CMD. The second and perhaps most important finding is that practicing clinicians may be unfamiliar with the specifics of CMD (its presence and effect on patient treatment).

The large number of patients with CMD whom we have been treating at St. Luke's Hospital in Cedar Rapids, Iowa, reflects what is occurring throughout the United States and abroad in industrialized countries. This increase in the number of patients is due to the increasing numbers of the aged population, improved technology, such as **tissue plasminogen activator** and **streptokinase** (anticlotting agents that frequently salvage oxygen-deprived myocardium during an acute myocardial infarction), **percutaneous transluminal coronary angioplasty**, and heart and heart-lung transplantation, and newer cardiovascular medications.[3,7] These improved and innovative technologies have decreased mortality from cardiovascular disease while increasing the morbidity rate in many of those who otherwise would have expired. It is our responsibility to help assess the functional status of these patients and to provide proper treatment to improve the quality of their lives and possibly to lessen the morbidity rate, or at least provide primary physicians with information to enhance medical therapy.

Characteristics of Congestive Heart Failure

Congestive heart failure is commonly associated with several characteristic signs and symptoms:

- Dyspnea
- Tachypnea
- Paroxysmal nocturnal dyspnea
- Orthopnea
- Peripheral edema
- Weight gain
- Hepatomegaly
- **Jugular venous distention**
- Rales
- Tubular breath sounds and consolidation
- Presence of an S_3 heart sound
- Sinus tachycardia
- Decreased exercise tolerance or physical work capacity

Only when CMD is so great that the heart's functional compensatory mechanisms are inadequate does CHF occur. Identification of several of the signs and symptoms listed earlier frequently suggests the presence of CHF, but radiologic and occasionally laboratory findings usually confirm the diagnosis and provide a baseline from which to evaluate therapy.[6]

Radiologic Findings in Congestive Heart Failure

Radiologic evidence of CHF is dependent on the size and shape of the cardiac silhouette (evaluating left ventricular end-diastolic volume) as well as the presence of interstitial, perivascular, and alveolar edema (evaluating fluid in the lungs).[6] Interstitial, perivascular, and alveolar edema are the radiologic hallmark of CHF and generally occur when pulmonary capillary pressures (which reflect the left ventricular end-diastolic pressure) exceed 20 to 25 mm Hg.[6] Pleural effusions (**parenchymal** fluid accumulations) and **atelectasis** (collapsed lung segments) may also be present.

Laboratory Findings in Congestive Heart Failure

Proteinuria; elevated urine specific gravity, **blood urea nitrogen (BUN)**, and **creatinine** levels; and decreased **erythrocyte sedimentation rates** (because of decreased fibrinogen concentrations resulting from impaired fibrinogen synthesis) are associated with CHF.[6] Frequently, but not consistently, Pa_{O_2} and oxygen saturation levels are reduced and Pa_{CO_2} levels elevated.[34] Liver enzymes (e.g., serum glutamic-oxaloacetic transaminase [SGOT], alkaline phosphatase) are often elevated, and **hyperbilirubinemia** commonly occurs, resulting in subsequent **jaundice.**[6] Serum electrolytes are generally normal, but individuals with chronic CHF may demonstrate **hyponatremia** during rigid sodium restriction and diuretic therapy, or **hypokalemia,** which also may be the result of diuretic therapy.[1] **Hyperkalemia** may occur for several reasons but most commonly is due to a marked reduction in the **glomerular filtration rate** (especially if individuals are receiving a potassium-retaining diuretic) or overzealous potassium supplementation (when a non–potassium-retaining diuretic is used).[6]

Symptoms of Congestive Heart Failure

Dyspnea

Dyspnea (breathlessness or air hunger) is probably the most common finding associated with CHF and is frequently the result of poor gas transport between the lungs and the cells of the body. The cause of poor transport at the lungs is often excessive blood and extracellular fluid in the alveoli, producing a shunt "characterized by a reduction of vital capacity as a consequence of the replacement of the air in the lungs with blood or interstitial fluid or both."[6] However, the cause of poor transport at the cellular level may be less apparent. A review of Wasserman and associates' "gas transport mechanisms" (Fig. 4–1) reveals the interrelationship

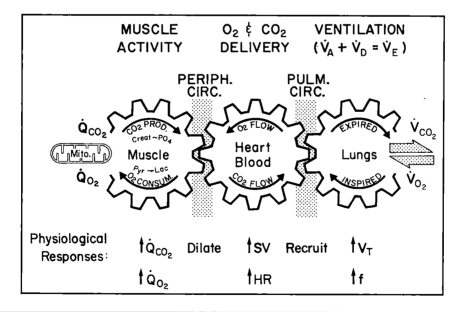

Figure 4–1.

Physiologic interdependence. The interdependence of the muscular, cardiopulmonary, and metabolic systems is evident as mitochondrial and metabolic activity are enhanced by the increased physiologic responses of the cardiopulmonary systems. (From Wasserman K, et al. Principles of Exercise Testing and Interpretation. Philadelphia, Lea & Febiger, 1987. Used with permission.)

of the lungs, heart, and muscle and shows that inadequate oxygen supply either at rest or during muscular activity undoubtedly increases the frequency of breathing (respiratory rate) or the amount of air exchanged (tidal volume) or both.[35] For this reason, subjects with CHF characteristically complain of easily provoked dyspnea or, in severe cases of CHF, dyspnea at rest.

Paroxysmal Nocturnal Dyspnea

Another common complaint of individuals suffering from CHF is **paroxysmal nocturnal dyspnea,** in which sudden, unexplained episodes of shortness of breath occur as patients with CHF assume a more supine position to sleep.[6] After a period of time in a supine position, excessive fluid fills the lungs. Earlier in the day, this fluid was shunted to the lower extremities because upright positions and activities permitted more effective minute ventilation ($\dot{V}$) and **perfusion** ($\dot{Q}$) of the lungs (correcting the $\dot{V}$-$\dot{Q}$ mismatch). During upright activity, the effects of gravity keep the lungs relatively fluid free, depending on the degree of CHF (which, if severe, would fill the lungs even in upright positions). Individuals suffering from paroxysmal nocturnal dyspnea frequently place the head of the bed on blocks or sleep with more than two pillows and often find it difficult to breathe with fewer than two pillows. Patients with marked CHF often assume a sitting position to sleep and are sometimes found sleeping in a recliner instead of a bed.

Orthopnea

The term **orthopnea** describes the development of dyspnea in the recumbent position.[6] Sleeping with two or more pillows puts the body in a more upright position and enables gravity to draw excess fluid from the lungs to the more distal parts of the body. The severity of CHF can sometimes be inferred from the number of pillows used to prevent orthopnea. Thus, the terms two-, three-, or four- or more pillow orthopnea indirectly allude to the severity of CHF (e.g., four-pillow orthopnea suggests more severe CHF than two-pillow orthopnea).

Signs Associated with Congestive Heart Failure

Breathing Patterns

A rapid respiratory rate at rest, characterized by quick and shallow breaths, is common in patients with CHF. Such **tachypnea** is apparently not due to hypoxemia (which may or may not be of sufficient magnitude) but rather to stimulation of interstitial **J-type receptors** (stretch receptors in the interstitium). The quick, shallow breathing of tachypnea may assist the pumping action of the lymphatic vessels, thus minimizing or delaying the increase in interstitial liquid.[34]

A clinical finding observed in many patients with CMD is extreme dyspnea after a change in position, most frequently from sitting to standing. This response appears to be occasionally but inconsistently associated with **orthostatic hypotension** and increased heart rate activity. The orthostatic hypotension and dyspnea (tachypnea) may be the result of (1) lower extremity muscle deconditioning, producing a pooling of blood in the lower extremities when standing, with a subsequent decrease in blood flow to the heart and lungs, which may result in marked dyspnea and increased heart rates; or (2) attenuation of the atrial **natriuretic** factor (release of a regulatory hormone from the atria because of elevated atrial pressure, which produces a brisk **diuresis** to reduce fluid volume), which may suggest advanced atrial distention and poor left ventricular function.[36] It appears that the more pronounced the dyspnea, the more severe the CMD, and vice versa. This pattern of breathing, therefore, is another clinical finding that can be timed (time for the dyspnea to subside) and occasionally measured (blood pressure and heart rate) to document progress or deterioration in patient status.

In addition, frequently associated with CHF is a breathing pattern characterized by waxing and waning depths of respiration with recurring periods of apnea. Although the Scottish physician John Cheyne and the Irish physician William Stokes first observed this breathing pattern in asthmatics and thus coined the term **Cheyne-Stokes respiration,** it has been observed in individuals who are suffering central nervous system damage (particularly those in comas) and in individuals with CMD.[6]

Rales (Crackles)

Carefully obtained subjective information can suggest a specific pathophysiology, but objective information obtained from physical examination frequently confirms one's suspicions. **Rales** are one such objective finding. Pulmonary rales, sometimes referred to as crackles, are abnormal breath sounds that, if associated with CHF, occur during inspiration and represent the movement of fluid in the alveoli and subsequent opening of alveoli that previously were closed because of excessive fluid.[6] A rather crude example of the dynamics (as well as the sound) responsible for rales is the sound heard when a sailboat sail suddenly fills with wind and becomes fully drawn. This is analogous to the opening of alveoli and airways that previously had no air; after the sound associated with such an opening is transmitted through the tissues overlying the lungs, the characteristic sound of rales is identical to that of hair near the ears being rubbed between two fingers. Rales are frequently heard at both lung bases in individuals with CHF but may extend upward depending on the patient's position, the severity of CHF, or both. Therefore, auscultation of all lobes should be performed in a systematic manner, allowing for bilateral comparison.

The importance of the presence and magnitude of rales was addressed in 1967 and provided data for the Killip and Kimball classification of patients with acute myocardial infarction.[37] Table 4–3 defines classes I through III, each of which is associated with an approximate mortality. Individuals with rales extending over more than 50% of the lung fields were observed to have a far poorer prognosis. Before continuing, the outline that follows should prove useful in planning a subjective and objective assessment of cardiopulmonary status.

Assessment of Cardiopulmonary Status

- notation of symptoms of CHF (dyspnea, paroxysmal nocturnal dyspnea, and orthopnea)
- evaluation of pulse and electrocardiogram to determine heart rate and rhythm
- evaluation of respiratory rate and breathing pattern
- auscultation of the heart and lungs with a stethoscope
- evaluation of radiographic findings to determine the existence and magnitude of pulmonary edema
- performance of laboratory blood studies to determine the Pa_{O_2} and Pa_{CO_2} levels
- evaluation of the oxygen saturation levels via oximetry
- palpation for **fremitus** and percussion of the lungs to determine the relative amount of air or solid material in the underlying lung
- performance of sit-to-stand test to evaluate heart rate and blood pressure (orthostatic hypotension) as well as dyspnea
- objective measurement of other characteristic signs produced by fluid overload, such as peripheral edema, weight gain, and jugular venous distention
- assessment of cardiopulmonary response to exercise (e.g., heart rate, blood pressure, electrocardiogram)

The methods to perform palpation and percussion are presented in Chapter 14, but a detailed description of auscultation of the heart follows because it is crucial to the assessment of patients with CMD.[38]

	Definition	Approximate Mortality (%)
Class I	Absence of rales and S₃ heart sound	8
Class II	Presence of S₃ heart sound or rales in 50% or less of the lung fields	30
Class III	Rales extending over more than 50% of the lung fields	44

TABLE 4–3. Killip Classification of Patients with Acute Myocardial Infarction and Approximate Mortality

Heart Sounds

Heart sounds can provide a great deal of information regarding cardiopulmonary status but unfortunately are forgotten in most physical therapy examinations. The normal heart sounds include a first heart sound (S_1), which represents closure of the mitral and tricuspid valves, and a second sound (S_2), which represents closure of the aortic and pulmonic valves. The most common abnormal heart sounds are the third (S_3) and fourth (S_4), which occur at specific times in the cardiac cycle as a result of abnormal cardiac mechanics. This can be best understood by viewing Figure 4–2, which displays graphically the normal and abnormal heart sounds and their respective locations in the cardiac cycle. Note that S_3 may be normal in children and young adults.[39] As displayed, S_4 is presystolic, and S_3 occurs during early diastole. Splitting of S_1 and S_2 is also occasionally heard and represents the closure of both the mitral and tricuspid valves in S_1 and the aortic and pulmonic valves in S_2.

Differentiating between a split S_1 and an S_4 or a split S_2 and an S_3 may cause confusion. However, a graphic and audible difference does exist (see Fig. 4–2). S_3 and S_4 are lower-frequency sounds and thus are heard best with light pressure while using the bell of the stethoscope (smaller-diameter, "bell-shaped" head of the stethoscope). If firm pressure is applied while listening with the bell of the stethoscope, higher-frequency sounds are more audible and lower-frequency sounds are difficult to hear. This is because as firm pressure is applied, the patient's skin tightly surrounds the edge of the bell and

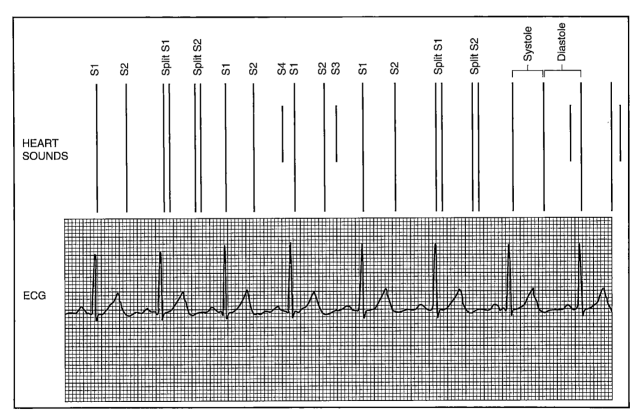

Figure 4–2.

The relationship of heart sounds to the electrocardiogram. The physiologic and mechanical events of myocardial activity are depicted. Assessment of the electrocardiogram and heart sounds provides important information about cardiac performance and patient status.

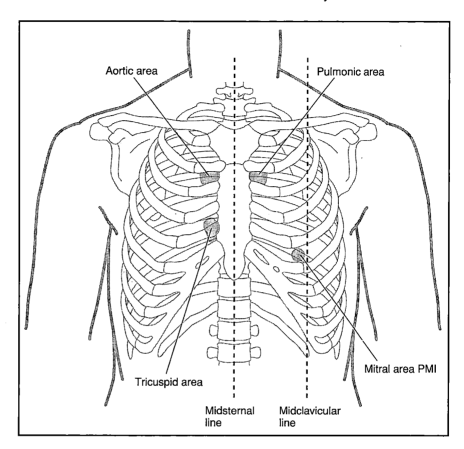

Figure 4-3.

Primary auscultatory areas. Auscultation of the heart is performed in a systematic fashion using both the bell and diaphragm of the stethoscope at the indicated sites.

constructs a rather primitive diaphragm (the flat, larger-diameter head of the stethoscope), which identifies the higher-frequency sounds. In this manner (alternating light and then firm pressure while listening with the bell of the stethoscope), S_4 and S_3 can be differentiated from a split S_1 and a split S_2, respectively. Therefore, light pressure identifies an extra sound, which if an S_4 or S_3 disappears with firm pressure and if a split S_1 or S_2, grows louder.

Different areas of auscultation also produce differences in the heart sounds. The four main areas are typically named for the area of the heart that is best heard in the chest wall area and include the aortic (base), pulmonic, apical, and tricuspid (Fig. 4-3). In general, the mitral (PMI) area yields the greatest amount of information because S_1 and S_2 are usually heard well here, and S_3 and S_4 are typically easier to identify in this area. However, auscultation of all areas should be performed in a systematic man-

ner to thoroughly evaluate the cardiopulmonary system.

The presence of an S_3 indicates a noncompliant left ventricle and occurs as blood passively fills a poorly relaxing left ventricle that appears to make contact with the chest wall during early systole.[39] The presence of an S_3 is considered the hallmark of CHF.[40] There are several reasons why the left ventricle may be noncompliant, of which fluid overload and myocardial scarring (via myocardial infarction or cardiomyopathy) appear to be the most common.[39]

The presence of an S_4 represents "vibrations of the ventricular wall during the rapid influx of blood during atrial contraction."[39] It is commonly heard in patients with hypertension, left ventricular hypertrophy, increased left ventricular end-diastolic pressure, pulmonary hypertension, and **pulmonic stenosis.**[39]

Auscultation of the heart may also reveal **adventitious** (additional) sounds, most frequently murmurs. They not only are common in patients with CMD but also appear to be of great clinical significance. Stevenson and co-workers demonstrated that the systolic murmur of secondary mitral regurgitation was an important marker in the treatment of a subgroup of patients with congestive cardiomyopathy.[41] The patients who benefited from afterload (the resistance to ventricular ejection or peripheral vascular resistance) reduction were those with a very large left ventricle (left ventricular end-diastolic dimension >60 cm) and a resultant **systolic murmur.**[41] This study demonstrated the importance of auscultation at rest and immediately after exercise to gain insight into the dynamics of myocardial activity.

In general, specific types of murmurs are associated with specific types of heart disease. Systolic murmurs occur during systole and are associated with mitral regurgitation, tricuspid regurgitation, aortic stenosis, pulmonic stenosis, and ventricular septal defects. Diastolic murmurs occur during diastole and are associated with aortic regurgitation, pulmonic regurgitation, tricuspid stenosis, and mitral stenosis. However, systolic and diastolic murmurs frequently occur together during each respective cycle of systole and diastole. Nevertheless, each murmur is associated with certain physical findings, which assist in the diagnosis of the specific disease process.

Peripheral Edema

Peripheral edema frequently accompanies CHF, but in some clinical situations it may be absent when, in fact, a patient has significant CHF.[6] In CHF, fluid is retained and not excreted because the **pressoreceptors** of the body sense a decreased volume of blood as a result of the heart's inability to pump an adequate amount of blood. The pressoreceptors subsequently relay a message to the kidneys to retain fluid so that a greater volume of blood can be ejected from the heart to the peripheral tissues.[42] Unfortunately, this compounds the problem and makes the heart work even harder, which further decreases its pumping ability. The retained fluid commonly accumulates bilaterally in the dependent extracellular spaces of the periphery.[6] Dependent spaces such as the ankles and pretibial areas tend to accumulate the majority of fluid and can be measured by applying firm pressure to the pretibial area for 10 to 20 seconds, then measuring the resultant indentation in the skin (pitting edema). This is frequently graded as mild, moderate, or severe or it is given a numerical value depending on the measured scale (Table 4–4). Peripheral edema can also accumulate in the sacral area (the shape of which resembles the popular fanny packs) or in the abdominal area (ascites).

Therefore, using the pitting edema scale to determine the severity and location of peripheral edema (pretibial or sacral, distal or proximal) and obtaining girth measurements of the lower extremities and the abdomen, important information regarding patient status can be obtained. However, it should be noted that peripheral edema is a sign that is associated with many other pathologies and does not by itself imply CHF.

Jugular Venous Distention

Jugular venous distention also results from fluid overload. As fluid is retained and the heart's ability to pump is further compromised, the retained fluid "backs up," not only into the lungs but also into the venous system, of which the jugular veins are the simplest to identify and evaluate. The external jugular vein lies medial to the external jugular artery, and with an individual in a 45-degree semirecumbent position, it can be readily measured for signs of distention. Although individuals with marked CHF may demonstrate jugular venous distention in all positions (supine, semisupine, and erect), typically jugular venous distention is measured when the head of the bed is elevated to 45 degrees.[38,39] The degree

TABLE 4–4. Pitting Edema Scale
1+ Barely perceptible depression (pit)
2+ Easily identified depression (EID) (skin rebounds to its original contour within 15 sec)
3+ EID (skin rebounds to its original contour within 15–30 sec)
4+ EID (rebound >30 sec)

of elevation should be noted as well as the magnitude of distention (mild, moderate, severe). More detailed measurements can be obtained by rotating the head slightly away from the vein being examined; at the point of elevation of the bed at which distention is first observed, pressure should be applied to the external jugular vein just above and parallel to the clavicle for approximately 10 to 20 seconds. This amount of time should allow the lower part of the vein to fill, and after quickly withdrawing the finger that was occluding the vein, the height of the distended fluid column within the vein should be measured. Normally, the level is less than 3 to 5 centimeters above the sternal angle of Louis. Measurements of the internal jugular vein may be more reliable than those of the external jugular vein. Nonetheless, the highest point of visible pulsation is determined as the trunk and head are elevated and the vertical distance between this level and the level of the sternal angle of Louis is recorded[38,39] (Fig. 4-4).

Evaluation of the jugular waveforms can also be performed in this position, but catheterization of the pulmonary artery for assessment of pulmonary arterial pressures provides the greatest amount of information. A tremendous amount of

information can be projected to a hemodynamic monitor, where the pulmonary artery pressure can be assessed and specific waveforms may be observed. The **a wave** of venous distention from right atrial systole occurring just before S_1 and the **v wave** frequently indicating a regurgitant tricuspid valve are two such examples and are displayed in Figure 4-5.[38,39] Although the assessment of hemodynamic function via pulmonary artery pressure monitoring is considered an advanced skill, it is relatively simple to interpret the typical intensive care unit monitor and thus obtain important hemodynamic information. Perhaps the most important aspect of such monitoring is identifying the pulmonary artery pressure, which is schematized in Figure 4-5. Pulmonary artery pressure greater than 25 mm Hg is the definition of pulmonary hypertension and appears to be associated with a variety of pathophysiologic phenomena (hypoxia, cardiac arrhythmias, and pulmonary abnormalities).

Pulsus alternans (mechanical alteration of the femoral or radial pulse characterized by a regular rhythm and alternating strong and weak pulses) can frequently identify severely depressed myocardial function and CHF in general. This is performed using light pressure at the radial pulse with the patient's breath held in *mid expiration* (to avoid the superimposition of respiratory variation on the amplitude of the pulse).[39] **Sphygmomanometry** can more readily recognize this phenomenon, which commonly demonstrates ≥20 mm Hg alternating systolic blood pressure. Characteristically, if pulsus alternans exists, a 20 mm Hg or greater decrease in systolic blood pressure occurs during breath holding because of increased resistance to left ventricular ejection. It should be noted that a difference exists between pulsus alternans and **pulsus paradoxus,** the latter of which is characterized by a marked reduction of both systolic blood pressure (≥20 mm Hg) and strength of the arterial pulse during *inspiration.* Pulsus paradoxus can also be detected by sphygmomanometry[39] and is occasionally seen in CHF. However, it is associated more frequently with cardiac tamponade and constrictive pericarditis primarily due to increased venous return and right heart volume, which bulges the interventricular septum into the left ventricle,

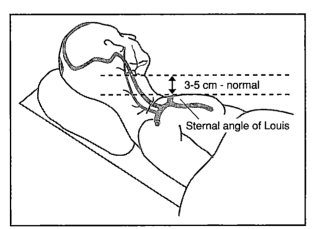

Figure 4-4.

Evaluation of venous pressure. Elevated venous pressure frequently represents right and left heart failure, which is characterized by pulmonary congestion and distention of the external jugular vein that is greater than 3 to 5 cm above the sternal angle of Louis.

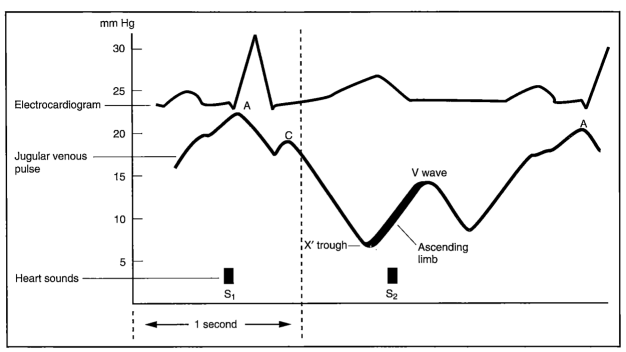

Figure 4-5.

The relationship of the jugular venous pulse to the electrocardiogram and heart sounds. The jugular venous pulse (and its various component wave patterns, C, V, and A wave) can be observed in the external jugular vein or via intensive care monitoring (which is often accompanied by an electrocardiogram). The physiologic and mechanical events producing the above wave patterns can be better analyzed by assessing the heart sounds and their respective location in the cardiac and venous pulse cycles.

thus decreasing the amount of blood present in the left ventricle and the amount of blood ejected from it (because of decreased left ventricular volume and opposition to stroke volume from the bulging septum).[39]

Weight Gain

As fluid is retained, total body fluid volume increases as does total body weight. Fluctuations of a few pounds from day to day are usually considered normal, but increases of several pounds per day (>3 lbs) are suggestive of CHF in a patient with CMD.[6] Body weight should always be measured from the same scale at approximately the same time of day with similar clothing before exercise is started.

Sinus Tachycardia

Sinus tachycardia or other tachyarrhythmias may occur in CHF as the pressoreceptors and

chemoreceptors of the body detect decreased fluid volume and decreased oxygen levels, respectively.[6] The body attempts (via increased heart rate) to increase the delivery of fluid and oxygen to the peripheral tissues where it is needed. Unfortunately, this attempt, much like the message to the kidneys to retain fluid, only compounds the problem and makes the heart work even harder, which further impairs its ability to pump.

Decreased Exercise Tolerance

Decreased exercise tolerance is ultimately the culmination of all of the preceding pathophysiologies that produce the characteristic signs and symptoms just discussed. It is apparent that as individuals at rest become short of breath, gain weight, and develop a faster resting heart rate, their ability to exercise is dramatically decreased. This has repeatedly been observed in patients with CHF and is the result of the interrelationships among the pathophysiologies briefly discussed.[6]

The methods of measuring exercise tolerance in patients with CHF have improved significantly in the past few years, but many investigators still utilize the criteria set forth by the New York Heart Association in 1964.[43] These criteria categorize patients into one of four classes, depending on the development of symptoms and the amount of effort required to provoke them. In short, patients in class I have no limitations in ordinary physical activity, whereas patients in class IV are unable to carry on any physical activity without discomfort. Patients in classes II and III are characterized by slight limitation and marked limitation in physical activities, respectively (Table 4–5).

A great deal of investigation has been done on measuring functional capacity in patients with CHF. Measurement of the **anaerobic threshold** (or ventilatory threshold) and the "slope of the rate of CO_2 output from aerobic metabolism plus the rate of CO_2 generated from buffering of lactic acid, as a function of the VO_2," as well as the change in oxygen consumption to change in work rate above the anaerobic threshold, appear to be useful and relatively reliable in determining exercise tolerance in patients with CHF.[44-48]

Unfortunately, most physical therapists do not have access to equipment (or training in its use) to measure respiratory gases. However, simple but thorough exercise assessments that evaluate symptoms, heart rate, blood pressure, heart rhythm via electrocardiogram, oxygen saturation via oximetry, and respiratory rate at specific workloads can provide important and useful information to compare patient response from day to day. Examples of such an assessment include treadmill ambulation, bicycle ergometry, hallway ambulation, or gentle calisthenic or strength training. Then, through this type of assessment, progress or deterioration can be documented and appropriate therapy implemented.

Several important responses observed during exercise testing in patients with CMD include (1) a more rapid heart rate response during submaximal workloads; (2) a lower oxygen consumption and oxygen pulse (an indirect measure of stroke volume obtained by dividing the heart rate into oxygen consumption) during submaximal and maximal work; (3) a flat, blunted, and occasionally hypoadaptive systolic blood pressure response to exercise; (4) a possible increase in diastolic blood pressure; (5) electrocardiographic signs of myocardial ischemia; (6) more easily provoked dyspnea and fatigue, often accompanied by angina; (7) lower maximal workloads when compared with those of subjects without heart disease; and (8) a chronotropic (increased heart rate response) and possibly an inotropic (increased force of myocardial contraction) *incompetence* (resulting in an inability to increase the heart rate or force of myocardial contraction) during exercise in patients with severe coronary artery disease and multisystem disease that may be partially due to an autonomic nervous system dysfunction.

The signs and symptoms associated with CHF can be ascribed, therefore, to some degree of failure of the several systems that were discussed earlier. However, further investigation of the problems in several of the systems that are affected by CHF is necessary to improve the assessment and treatment of patients, specifically, the pathophysiology occurring in the cardiovascular, pulmonary, renal, hepatic, neurohumoral, hematologic, musculoskeletal, nutritional, and pancreatic systems. This will provide a more

TABLE 4–5. New York Heart Association Functional Classification of Heart Disease

Class I	Patients with cardiac disease but without resulting limitations of physical activity. Ordinary physical activity does not cause undue fatigue, palpitation, dyspnea, or anginal pain.
Class II	Patients with cardiac disease that results in a slight limitation of physical activity. Patients are comfortable at rest, but ordinary physical activity results in fatigue, palpitations, dyspnea, or anginal pain.
Class III	Patients with cardiac disease that results in a marked limitation of physical activity. Patients are comfortable at rest, but less than ordinary activity causes fatigue, palpitations, dyspnea, or anginal pain.
Class IV	Patients with cardiac disease resulting in an inability to carry on any physical activity without discomfort. Fatigue, palpitations, dyspnea, or anginal pain may be present even at rest. If any physical activity is undertaken, symptoms increase.

complete understanding of CMD as well as the treatment and progression of patients with CMD, but first a brief review of the methods used to assess cardiac performance is presented.

Specific Assessment of Cardiac Performance

Cardiac performance is assessed in many ways, the most common of which are echocardiography (M-mode, two-dimensional, and *transesophageal*), thallium exercise testing (and most recently resting dipyridamole [Persantine] and adenosine thallium), radionuclide ventriculography (interventriculogram [IVG] and multigated angiogram [MUGA] studies), and cardiac catheterization[49] (Table 4–6). Cardiac catheterization is considered the gold standard with which other measurements are compared, but the other methods listed earlier provide considerable information regarding cardiovascular function and do so noninvasively. However, cardiac catheterization can provide important information about the coronary arteries as well as the pressures in the heart. The pressures obtained at the time of catheterization can help determine cardiac performance.[50–53]

Patient progress or deterioration in CMD is closely related to the preload and afterload status of the cardiovascular system. Preload is essentially the pressure (left ventricular end-diastolic pressure) in the left ventricle before ejection of the stroke volume. This is analogous to the preloading (or pulling backward on the rubber band) of a slingshot before releasing the rubber band to eject an object. Afterload is the resistance that the stroke volume ejected from the left ventricle encounters, that is, peripheral vascular resistance. Much of the treatment for CMD involves lowering both the preload and afterload of the cardiovascular system.

Specific Pathophysiologies Associated with Congestive Heart Failure

The pathophysiologies associated with CMD appear to be the result of eight independent, yet interrelated, systems and one process, which include the following:

- cardiovascular
- pulmonary
- renal
- hepatic
- neurohumoral
- hematologic
- musculoskeletal
- pancreatic
- biochemical

The remainder of this section describes and explains each of these systems as they relate to CHF in CMD. In addition, the specific pathophysiologies that produce CMD that are associated with spinal cord injury, congenital and acquired heart disease, and the aging process conclude this section.

CARDIOVASCULAR FUNCTION IN CONGESTIVE HEART FAILURE AND CARDIAC MUSCLE DYSFUNCTION

The cardiac pathologies that have the potential to produce CMD have been described as the result of "one or more of 12 mechanisms" that produce CHF primarily via pump failure or secondarily via mechanical complications. Although pump failure (of which myocardial infarction and ischemia are the most common) and mechanical complications can be divided into the

---

TABLE 4–6. Methods to Assess Cardiac Performance in Cardiac Muscle Dysfunction

Echocardiography
Impedance cardiography
Radionuclide ventriculography
  (multigated acquisition study—MUGA)
Thallium and technetium imaging
  (thallium testing/persantine thallium)
Cardiac catheterization
MUGA scan
Transesophageal echocardiography
Computed tomography (CT)
Magnetic resonance imaging (MRI)
Indirect assessment of cardiac performance
  (heart rate, blood pressure, rate-pressure product, tension/time index)

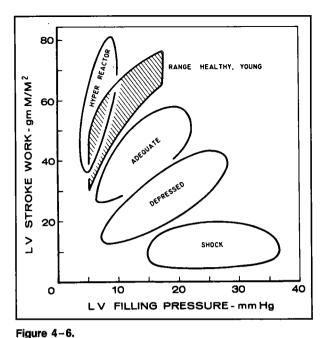

Figure 4-6.

Left ventricular (LV) function. Left ventricular performance is dependent on left ventricular filling (utilizing the Frank-Starling mechanism) and the resultant pressure, which, if extensive, dramatically decreases left ventricular work. (From Sodeman WA, Sodeman TM. Sodeman's Pathologic Physiology: Mechanisms of Disease. 7th ed. Philadelphia, WB Saunders, 1985, p 343.)

primary and secondary causes of CHF, the rationale for both to cause CHF can be understood best by describing the Frank-Starling mechanism. The Frank-Starling mechanism was one of the earliest efforts to better understand cardiac muscle relaxation and contraction or, in essence, "the relation between ventricular filling pressure (or end-diastolic volume) and ventricular mechanical activity,"[49] expressed as the volume output of the heart or the stroke volume (cardiac output divided by heart rate because CO = HR × SV).

In the early 1900s, Frank and Starling discovered that the stroke volume is dependent on both diastolic cardiac muscle fiber length and myocardial contractility (force of contraction and heart rate).[54] This relationship can be better understood by studying Figure 4-6, in which left ventricular stroke work is plotted against left ventricular filling pressure. The figure shows that an optimal range of left ventricular filling pressures exists that, when exceeded, decreases left ventricular stroke work considerably.[49,55] As the left ventricular filling pressure increases, so does the stretch on cardiac muscle fiber during diastole. Taken a step further, the left ventricular filling pressure is representative of the left ventricular end-diastolic volume, which determines the degree of stretch on the myocardium.[49,54] This is apparent in Figure 4-7, which *also* demonstrates that an optimal range of ventricular

Figure 4-7.

Determinants of myocardial stretch and ventricular performance. The Frank-Starling mechanism is based on adequate "stretch" of the myocardium that produces an increased end-diastolic volume (E.D.V.) and subsequently increases ventricular performance. The major influences that contribute to the stretching of the myocardium are depicted in the figure. (Reproduced with permission from Braunwald E, Ross J, Sonnenblick E, et al. Mechanisms of Contraction of the Normal and Failing Heart. 2nd ed. Boston, Little, Brown, 1976.)

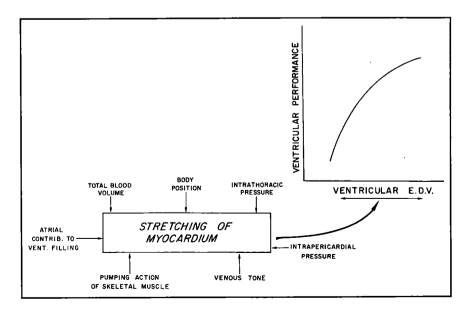

end-diastolic volume (or filling pressure) exists, which, if exceeded or insignificant, decreases ventricular performance. In addition, Figure 4–7 shows the major influences that determine the degree of myocardial stretch—atrial contribution to ventricular filling, total blood volume, body position, intrathoracic pressure, intrapericardial pressure, venous tone, and pumping action of skeletal muscle, all of which should be considered when evaluating and treating patients.[55]

The stroke volume was described earlier as the result of the degree of myocardial stretch (or as previously stated, the diastolic cardiac muscle fiber length) as well as that of myocardial contractility. Myocardial contractility is influenced by many variables; the major ones are illustrated in Figure 4–8. These include force-frequency relations, circulating **catecholamines,** sympathetic nerve impulses, intrinsic depression, loss of myocardium, pharmacologic depressants, **digitalis** or other **inotropic** agents, anoxia, **hypercapnia,** and acidosis.[55]

Despite these major influences, without adequate diastolic filling (and the "necessary degree of myocardial stretch"), stroke volume remains unchanged. The importance of diastolic filling of the ventricles is apparent in patients with **pericardial effusion** (i.e., cardiac tamponade) or **myocarditis,** who, because of cardiac compression or infectious agents, respectively, are unable to attain adequate diastolic filling, which results in a decreased stroke volume that can be hemodynamically significant, producing pulsus paradoxus as well as a **hypoadaptive** systolic blood pressure response to exercise.

The left ventricular filling pressure discussed earlier can be closely approximated by the pulmonary capillary wedge pressure, which is frequently monitored in patients in coronary care or intensive care units.[38] Left ventricular systolic performance appears to deteriorate when the pulmonary capillary wedge pressure is greater than 15 to 20 mm Hg. The effects of extremely elevated pressures in the left ventricle increase ventricular noncompliance and in the presence of cardiac arrhythmias can impair cardiac performance significantly. This condition is analogous to motor nerve lesions and the subsequent dysfunction of skeletal muscle. Central nervous system

activity is needed for proper function of skeletal muscle in much the same way as cardiac muscle function is dependent on proper intrinsic electrical activity (the heart rhythm resulting from the automaticity of cardiac cells).

Cardiac Arrhythmias

Ventricular function is intimately related to cardiac rhythm. Any abnormally fast, slow, or unsynchronized rhythm can impair ventricular and atrial function quickly and progress to CHF and even death.[56] Many patients with CMD have preexisting arrhythmias that must be controlled, typically with medication, but sometimes by other methods (e.g., ablation, automatic implantable cardiac defibrillator)[57] to prevent further deterioration of a muscle that is already compromised.

Left Ventricular Hypertrophy

The extremely elevated ventricular and occasionally elevated atrial pressures commonly seen in patients with CMD tend to produce a less effective pump as the myocardial contractile fibers become overstretched, thus increasing the work of each myocardial fiber in an attempt to maintain an adequate cardiac output.[51,58] Myocardial work continued in this manner eventually produces left ventricular hypertrophy as the contractile fibers adapt to the increased workload.[16,58] The primary problem with left ventricular hypertrophy is the increased energy expenditure (metabolic cost) required for myocardial contraction because of increased myocardial cell mass.[16,51,58] This scenario is typical of that commonly seen in cardiomyopathies.

Cardiomyopathies

As previously discussed, cardiomyopathies can be the result of either primary (due to pathologic heart muscle) or secondary (due to systemic diseases, which subsequently affect heart muscle) causes, which, when classified via heart function,

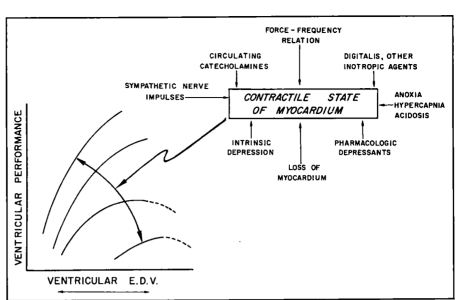

Figure 4-8.
Determinants of myocardial contraction and ventricular performance. The major "contractile" influences affecting ventricular performance are depicted in the figure, of which end-diastolic volume (E.D.V.) is a major factor. (Reproduced with permission from Braunwald E, Ross J, Sonnenblick E, et al. Mechanisms of Contraction of the Normal and Failing Heart. 2nd ed. Boston, Little, Brown, 1976.)

include dilated cardiomyopathies, hypertrophic cardiomyopathies, and restrictive cardiomyopathies.

Dilated Cardiomyopathies

Dilated cardiomyopathies "probably represent a final common pathway that is the end result of myocardial damage produced by a variety of toxic, metabolic, or infectious agents."[16] Possible causes of dilated cardiomyopathies include

- long-term alcohol abuse
- systemic hypertension
- a variety of infections
- cigarette smoking
- pregnancy
- carnitine deficiency[16]

These conditions may not be primarily responsible for dilated cardiomyopathy but may act to lower the threshold for its development.

Little is known regarding the further development of dilated cardiomyopathies, but the dilation that occurs in this type of cardiomyopathy, and that sets it apart from hypertrophic cardiomyopathy, appears to be due to myocardial mitochondrial dysfunction.[16] Dysfunction of myocardial mitochondria leads to a lack of energy necessary for proper cardiac function, which

produces a less effective pump.[16] Ineffective pumping increases both the left ventricular end-diastolic volume and pressure, which dilates the left ventricle (and frequently the other heart chambers). Because of inappropriate energy sources, the left ventricle is unable to contract properly or to relax individual muscle fibers in response to increased workload, therefore preventing myocardial hypertrophy but producing ineffective *systolic* (pumping) function.

Hypertrophic Cardiomyopathy

Hypertrophic cardiomyopathy should be thought of as the opposite of dilated cardiomyopathy, both functionally and etiologically. The hypertrophy associated with hypertrophic cardiomyopathy is inappropriate for the applied hemodynamic load and is associated with proper myocardial mitochondrial function. Furthermore, the dysfunction of hypertrophic cardiomyopathy is one of *diastolic* dysfunction, which impairs the filling of the ventricles during diastole.[16] This increases the left ventricular end-diastolic pressure and eventually increases left atrial, pulmonary artery, and pulmonary capillary pressures, all of which cause a hypercontractile left ventricle. The hypercontractile myocardial muscle fibers of hypertrophic cardiomyopathy are frequently disorganized and demonstrate a "quantitative relationship between the extent of cellular disarray and hypertrophic cardiomyopathy, since the disorganization of myocardial fibers is far greater in hypertrophic cardiomyopathy than in other disorders (coronary artery disease, congenital heart disease, and cor pulmonale)."[16]

Susceptibility to hypertrophic cardiomyopathy appears to be genetically transmitted as an *autosomal dominant trait*. It has been suggested that the apparent myocardial *isometric* contraction of hypertrophic cardiomyopathy is the result of malaligned myocardial muscle fibers[59] or an abnormal configuration of the interventricular septum response to a genetic influence.[60] Other causes of hypertrophic cardiomyopathy have been suggested, including abnormal sympathetic stimulation, subendocardial ischemia, and abnormal calcium ion dynamics.[16]

The characteristic findings of hypertrophic cardiomyopathy are rapid ventricular emptying and high ejection fraction, which are the opposite of those found in dilated cardiomyopathy but somewhat similar to those found in restrictive cardiomyopathy.[16]

Restrictive Cardiomyopathy

Restrictive cardiomyopathy is, like hypertrophic cardiomyopathy, a cardiomyopathy of *diastolic* dysfunction and frequently unimpaired contractile function. Little is known about restrictive cardiomyopathy, but certain pathologic processes, including myocardial fibrosis, hypertrophy, infiltration, or a defect in myocardial relaxation, may result in its development.[16]

The functional classification of cardiomyopathies just discussed as well as the cardiovascular pathophysiologies (i.e., left ventricular hypertrophy and cardiac arrhythmias) all tend to contribute to the progression of CMD, which is managed *initially* by several of the body's *compensatory mechanisms*, of which atrial natriuretic peptide is an important factor.

Atrial Natriuretic Peptide

The increased fluid volume that typically produces increased left ventricular end-diastolic volume "backs up" into the left atrium and likewise

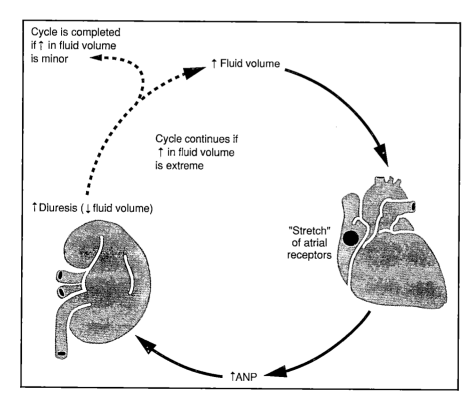

Cycle is completed if ↑ in fluid volume is minor

↑ Fluid volume

Cycle continues if ↑ in fluid volume is extreme

↑ Diuresis (↓ fluid volume)

"Stretch" of atrial receptors

↑ANP

Figure 4–9.

Atrial natriuretic peptide (ANP). Elevated vascular volume releases ANP, which increases the glomerular filtration rate (GFR) and facilitates natriuresis and diuresis.

produces elevated atrial pressure. The elevated atrial pressure produces significant cardiovascular change and stimulates the release of a specific regulatory hormone, atrial natriuretic peptide (ANP). Atrial natriuretic peptide is released from atrial myocyte granules when atrial pressure or volume exceeds an unknown value (Fig. 4–9).[42]

Once released, ANP binds to receptors in target tissues, such as the aorta, vascular smooth muscle, renal cortex and medulla, and adrenal zona glomerulosa.[42] It then produces a brisk **natriuresis** (excretion of sodium) and diuresis (excretion of water) as well as an increase in the excretion of most other electrolytes (chloride, potassium, calcium, magnesium, and phosphorus).[42] In addition, ANP suppresses secretion of renal renin and aldosterone and release of angiotensin-

stimulated aldosterone, which, in effect, attempts to maintain the blood pressure–electrolyte homeostasis.[61] Although ANP produces these effects to reduce fluid volume, they are only minor forces, which, unfortunately, are no match for the profound fluid retention produced by the kidneys.

RENAL FUNCTION IN CONGESTIVE HEART FAILURE AND CARDIAC MUSCLE DYSFUNCTION

The subtle, yet devastating, effects of the renal system in CHF can be appreciated best in Figure 4–10, which outlines the five major steps for the

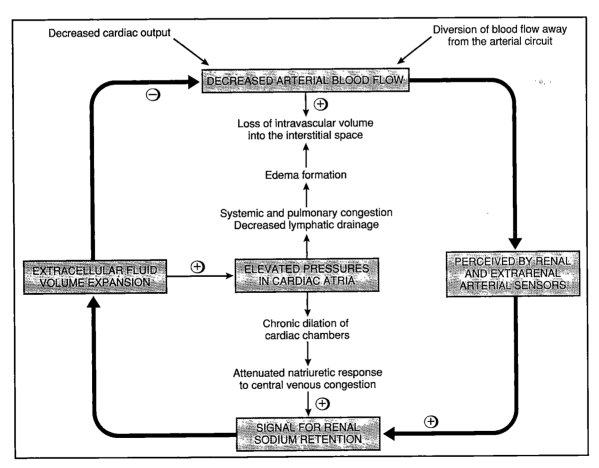

Figure 4–10.

Mechanisms of congestive heart failure. Cardiac muscle dysfunction decreases the cardiac output and resultant arterial blood flow, which initiates the cycle illustrated in the figure. (From Skorecki KL, Breuner BM. Body fluid homeostasis in congestive heart failure and cirrhosis with ascites. Am J Med 72:323, 1982.)

initiation and maintenance of renal sodium retention. As previously mentioned, sodium (and ultimately water) is retained in CHF because of inadequate cardiac output.[51,58] The arterial system of the body senses, via renal and extrarenal sensors, that the arterial blood flow is inadequate, often because of a poor cardiac output, and initiates a process to retain fluid (to increase arterial blood flow), which is identical to that initiated in **hypovolemic** states.[42] In effect, the kidneys in CHF act like those in an individual with a reduced volume of body fluid.

The subsequent retention of sodium and water are due to

- augmented alpha-adrenergic neural activity
- circulating catecholamines (e.g., epinephrine, norepinephrine)
- increased circulating and locally produced angiotensin II, which results in renal vasoconstriction, thus decreasing the glomerular filtration rate (GFR) as well as renal blood flow[42]

These effects increase the renal filtration fraction (the ratio of GFR to renal blood flow), which increases the protein concentration in the peritubular capillaries and decreases the postglomerular capillary hydrostatic pressure (increasing renal vascular resistance), thus decreasing the transcapillary hydraulic pressure gradient.[42] The resulting reduction in peritubular capillary hydrostatic pressure and elevation of peritubular oncotic pressure enhance the peritubular capillary uptake of proximal tubular fluid, thereby increasing the quantity of sodium reabsorbed in the proximal tubule.[62,63] The reabsorption process and a thorough overview of renal function in CHF are presented in Figure 4–11.

Laboratory findings suggestive of impaired renal function in CHF include increases in BUN or other nitrogenous bodies (**azotemia**), as well as in blood creatinine levels. This prerenal azotemia is the result of enhanced water reabsorption in the collecting duct, which becomes more pronounced with increased **antidiuretic hormone** levels and which augments the passive reabsorption of **urea** (the rate of which can be increased with an acute myocardial infarction and by the catabolic state of CHF).[42] Therefore, an increase

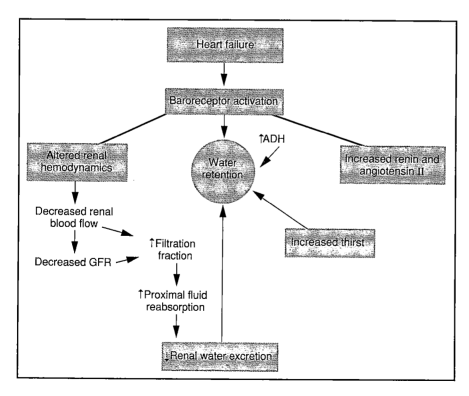

Figure 4–11.

Physiologic effects of myocardial failure. Heart failure produces a variety of altered responses that lead to retention of water and often congestive heart failure.

in urea production, a decrease in excretion of urine, and an increased BUN may occur even before a decrease in GFR. However, a decreased GFR is the primary reason for the increased BUN and serum creatinine levels commonly seen in patients with CHF.[42]

In summary, the viciousness of the renal sodium retention cycle is clearly seen in Figure 4–10, which demonstrates that if left untreated, the cycle will continue and ultimately lead to death. As previously noted, the extreme overload of fluid produced by the kidneys in CHF exceeds the volume that the left ventricle and eventually the left atrium can maintain, after which the fluid ultimately "backs up" into the lungs and produces CHF. The following section presents the pathophysiology observed when such a condition exists.

PULMONARY FUNCTION IN CONGESTIVE HEART FAILURE AND CARDIAC MUSCLE DYSFUNCTION

As previously mentioned, one of the characteristic signs of CHF is the presence of inspiratory rales during auscultation of the lungs. The following review of the pulmonary pathophysiology associated with CHF assists in the understanding of pulmonary edema in general and inspiratory rales in particular.

Pulmonary edema can be **cardiogenic** (hemodynamic) or noncardiogenic (caused by alterations in the pulmonary capillary membrane) in origin.[6] The differential diagnosis can be made by history, physical examination, and laboratory examination, as shown in Table 4–7. Despite the different origins of pulmonary edema, the "sequence of liquid accumulation"[34] is similar for both and appears to consist of three distinct stages.

Stage 1 of pulmonary edema is unfortunately difficult to detect or quantify because it seems to represent "increased lymph flow without net gain of interstitial liquid."[34] The edema associated with the increased lymph flow may actually improve gas exchange in the lung as more of

TABLE 4–7. Differentiation of Cardiogenic from Noncardiogenic Pulmonary Edema

Cardiac Pulmonary Edema	Noncardiac Pulmonary Edema
History	
Cardiac muscle dysfunction	Cardiac muscle dysfunction is uncommon
Clinical Examination	
Cool skin	Warm skin
S_3 gallop or cardiomegaly	Bounding pulses
Jugular venous distention	No S_3 gallop
Wet crackles	No jugular venous distention
	Dry crackles
Laboratory Tests	
Rapid or slow rhythm	ECG: Usually normal
CXR: Perihilar distribution	CXR: Peripheral distribution
Cardiac enzymes may be elevated	Cardiac enzymes usually normal
PCWP > 18 mm Hg	PCWP < 18 mm Hg

CXR, chest x-ray; PCWP, pulmonary capillary wedge pressure; ECG, electrocardiogram.

the small pulmonary vessels are distended. However, if lymph flow continues, pulmonary edema increases, and the airways and vessels become filled with increased liquid, particularly in the gravity-dependent portions of the lung.[34] This compromises the small airway lumina, resulting in a mismatch between ventilation and perfusion, which produces hypoxemia and wasted ventilation (stage 2).[34] As a result, the tachypnea of CHF often ensues.[34] In addition, the degree of *hypoxemia* appears to be correlated to the degree of *elevation* of the *pulmonary capillary wedge pressure.*[64]

As lymph flow continues, pulmonary edema increases, increasing the pulmonary capillary wedge pressure and eventually flooding the alveoli. This flooding represents stage 3 pulmonary edema, which significantly compromises gas exchange, producing severe hypoxemia and hypercapnia.[34] In addition, severe alveolar flooding can produce the following: (1) filling of the large airways with blood-tinged foam, which can be expectorated; (2) reductions in most lung volumes (e.g., vital capacity); (3) a right-to-left intrapulmonary shunt; and (4) hypercapnia with acute respiratory acidosis.[34]

Perhaps the most important principle regarding pulmonary edema is that of *"maintaining pulmonary capillary pressures at the lowest possible levels,"*[34] because it has been demonstrated that pulmonary edema can be decreased by more than 50% when pulmonary capillary wedge pressures are decreased from 12 to 6 mm Hg.

NEUROHUMORAL EFFECTS OF CONGESTIVE HEART FAILURE AND CARDIAC MUSCLE DYSFUNCTION

The neurohumoral system profoundly affects heart function in physiologic (fight-or-flight mechanism) and pathologic states (CMD). In general, the neural effects are much more rapid, whereas humoral effects are slower. This is because the information sent by the autonomic nervous system via efferent nerves travels faster than the information traveling through the vascular system.[65]

Normal Cardiac Neurohumoral Function

Neurohumoral signals to the heart are perceived, interpreted, and augmented by the transmembrane signal transduction systems in myocardial cells.[65] The primary signaling system in the heart appears to be the **receptor-G protein–adenylate cyclase** (RGC) complex as it regulates myocardial contractility. Figure 4–12 illustrates the complexity of this system, which consists of (1) membrane receptors; (2) guanine nucleotide-binding regulatory proteins (the G proteins, which transmit stimulatory or inhibitory signals); and (3) adenylate cyclase, which converts **adenosine triphosphate** (ATP) to **cyclic adenosine monophosphate** (cAMP). Adenylate cyclase is an effector enzyme activated by a receptor agonist, thus enhancing cAMP synthesis. The lower portion of Figure 4–12 shows that increased cAMP synthesis ultimately increases the force of myocardial contraction (the inotropic effect).[65]

The top portion of Figure 4–12 shows the receptor agonists responsible for the initial activation of the "receptor-G protein–adenylate cyclase complex." They include norepinephrine, epinephrine, histamine, vasoactive intestinal peptide, adenosine, and acetylcholine.

Although Figure 4–12 is more than complete, it does not reveal the degree of influence each receptor agonist has on cardiac function. In general, the most influential receptor agonists are the sympathetic neurotransmitters norepinephrine and epinephrine as they relay excitatory autonomic nervous system stimuli to both postsynaptic alpha- and beta-adrenergic receptors (primarily beta for norepinephrine) in the myocardium.[65] Inhibitory autonomic nervous system stimuli are transmitted by the parasympathetic nervous system via the vagus nerve and the neurotransmitter acetylcholine. The adrenergic receptors (alpha$_1$, alpha$_2$, beta$_1$, and beta$_2$) are discussed briefly later so that Figure 4–12 can be appreciated fully, as well as the neurohumoral changes that accompany CMD.

Alpha-Adrenergic Receptors

Stimulation of **alpha$_1$-adrenergic receptors** appears to activate the phosphoinositide transmembrane signaling system,[66,67] which increases **phosphodiesterase** and activates protein kinase, thus marginally increasing the inotropic effect.[68] Conversely, stimulation of **alpha$_2$-adrenergic receptors** activates the G-inhibitory protein and inhibits adenylate cyclase, which decreases the inotropic effect.[69]

Beta-Adrenergic Receptors

The importance of the beta-adrenergic pathway cannot be overemphasized because it has been proposed that the heart is a **beta-adrenergic** organ.[70] Two beta-adrenergic receptors have been identified, beta$_1$ and beta$_2$, which are "distinguished by their differing affinities for the agonists epinephrine and norepinephrine."[65] The beta$_2$-adrenergic receptor has a thirtyfold greater affinity for epinephrine than for norepinephrine.[71] In brief, beta$_2$ receptor stimulation promotes vasodilation of the capillary beds and

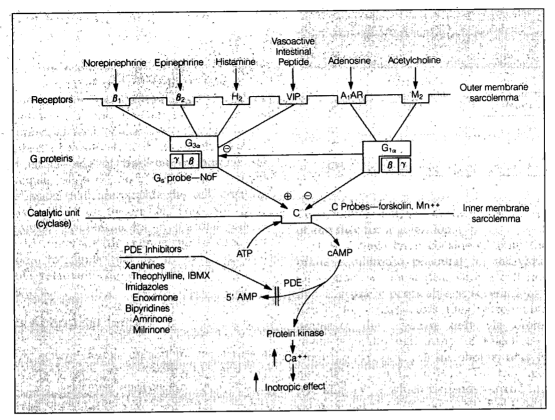

Figure 4-12.

Neural control of cardiopulmonary function. The receptor G protein–adenylate cyclase complex and other important receptors, all of which affect the inotropic state of the heart. G_s, G stimulatory protein; G_i, G inhibitory protein; PDE, phosphodiesterase; IBMX, isobutylmethylxanthine; ATP, adenosine triphosphate; cAMP, cyclic adenosine monophosphate. (From Feldman AM, Bristow MR. The β-adrenergic pathway in the failing human heart: Implications for inotropic therapy. Cardiology 77 [Suppl 1]:1–32, 1990. Reproduced by permission of Karger, Basel.)

muscle relaxation in the bronchial tracts, whereas beta$_1$-adrenergic receptor stimulation increases heart rate and myocardial force of contraction.[65]

Guanine Nucleotide-Binding Regulatory Proteins

As briefly discussed, the G proteins transmit stimulatory (G_s) or inhibitory (G_i) signals to the catalytic unit (inner membrane sarcolemma) of myocardial contractile tissue. The stimulatory and inhibiting signals are dependent on a very complex, and only partially understood, mechanism of receptor-mediated activation. Activation depends on several rate-limiting steps, mainly the dissociation of guanosine diphosphate (GDP) in exchange for guanosine triphosphate (GTP)

and the action of GTPase enzyme intrinsic to alpha-G_s.[65]

Catalytic Unit of Adenylate Cyclase

The activation of adenylate cyclase (and subsequent increase in myocardial force of contraction) is, unfortunately, poorly understood but has been observed to be decreased in patients with CHF. This is the result of "a paradoxical diminution in the function of the RGC complex,"[65] which alters the receptor-effector coupling and "limits the ability of both endogenous and exogenous adrenergic agonists to augment cardiac contractility."[65] The inability of **endogenous** (produced in the body) or **exogenous** (medications) adrenergic agonists to increase the force of myocardial contraction is frequently seen in patients with CHF, which may be a contributing factor in CMD.[65-76]

Neurohumoral Alterations in the Failing Human Heart

Abnormalities in Sympathetic Neural Function in Congestive Heart Failure

The sympathetic neural function of the heart is profoundly affected in CHF. The effects are due to abnormal RGC complex function primarily, despite increased concentrations of interstitial (in the interspaces of the myocardium), intrasynaptic, and systemic norepinephrine, which is less effective because of abnormal RGC complex function.[65]

The abnormal RGC complex function in CHF appears to be associated with the insensitivity of the failing heart to beta-adrenergic stimulation.[65] This insensitivity to beta-adrenergic stimulation is apparently the result of a decrease in $beta_1$-adrenergic receptor density[65] and is very important because the heart contains a ratio of 3.3 to 1.0 $beta_1$- to $beta_2$-adrenergic receptors.[65] In CHF, the ratio decreases to approximately 1.5 to 1.0, producing a 62% decrease in the $beta_1$-adrenergic receptors and no significant increase in $beta_2$ density.[72,73] Although the number of $beta_2$ receptors does not appear to change in CHF, the $beta_2$ receptor "is partially 'uncoupled' from the effector enzyme adenylate cyclase."[74,75] This uncoupling only mildly desensitizes the $beta_2$-adrenergic receptors, which *initially* are able to compensate for the decreased number of $beta_1$ receptors by providing substantial inotropic support.[65] However, the duration of inotropic support appears to be short lived, and myocardial failure becomes more pronounced.[65]

LIVER FUNCTION IN CONGESTIVE HEART FAILURE AND CARDIAC MUSCLE DYSFUNCTION

The fluid overload associated with CHF affects practically all organs and bodily systems, includ-ing liver function. Increased fluid volume eventually leads to hepatic venous congestion, which prevents adequate perfusion of oxygen to hepatic tissues. Subsequent hypoxemia from the hypoperfusion produces a **cardiac cirrhosis,** which is characterized histologically by central lobular necrosis, atrophy, extensive fibrosis, and occasionally sclerosis of the hepatic veins.[16]

Hepatomegaly, or liver enlargement, is frequently associated with CHF and can be identified readily as tenderness in the right upper quadrant of the abdomen. Patients with long-standing CHF, however, are generally not tender to palpation, although hepatomegaly is frequently present.

HEMATOLOGIC FUNCTION IN CONGESTIVE HEART FAILURE AND CARDIAC MUSCLE DYSFUNCTION

The normal morphology of the blood and blood-forming tissues is frequently disrupted in CHF. The most common abnormality is a secondary **polycythemia** (excess of red corpuscles in the blood), which is due to either a reduction in oxygen transport or an increase in **erythropoietin** production.[76] Erythropoietin is an alpha$_2$-globulin responsible for red blood cell production, and its important role is demonstrated in Figure 4–13. This figure shows that the hypoxia occasionally observed in patients with CHF may stimulate erythropoietin production, which increases not only red blood cell mass, but also blood volume in an already compromised cardiopulmonary system (partly because of fluid volume overload). This potentially vicious cycle can progress and further deteriorate cardiopulmonary function.

Clinically, **anemia,** which may be present in some patients with CHF, is a paradox, for when it is severe it can produce CHF independently, but when it precedes CHF, anemia may actually allow for a more efficient and effective cardiac function.[77] Improved cardiac output may occur because blood viscosity is reduced in patients with anemia, which subsequently decreases systemic vascular resistance. Anemia, therefore, acts as an afterload reducer and may promote an in-

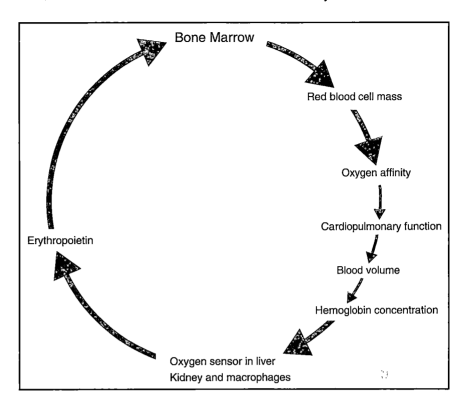

Figure 4-13.

Hematologic function. Hematologic function is occasionally disrupted in congestive heart failure and can further impair cardiopulmonary function and patient status.

creased cardiac output but at the cost of lower arterial oxygen and oxygen saturation levels as well as increased work for the heart.[77] A term that is frequently heard when such a condition (and others) exists is that there is "a shift in the oxyhemoglobin curve." The curve can be shifted to the right or left but normally follows a pattern depicted in Figure 2-10, which represents a specific percentage of oxygen saturation for a given concentration of arterial oxygen. Oxygen saturation remains relatively stable, with arterial oxygen concentrations greater than 60 mm Hg, but below this level the oxygen saturation drops dramatically. The chart that follows shows the oxygen saturation levels when arterial oxygen concentrations are less than 60 mm Hg.

Pa_{O_2}	40	50	60
O_2 sat	70	80	90

Various conditions move this normal curve to the right or left, which subsequently affects the respective oxygen saturation. For example, anemia shifts the curve to the right, representing a lower concentration of arterial oxygen, which moves the critical point of oxygen saturation to 70 mm Hg (therefore, to the right). This means that at levels of less than 70 mm Hg, the level of oxygen saturation decreases dramatically compared with the normal level of 60 mm Hg. Thus, patients with anemia have less reserve before their oxygen stores **desaturate.**[77]

The paradox thus unfolds, and patients with such a condition must be monitored carefully (especially if exercising). A blood transfusion may be given to improve oxygen transport to needed tissues, even though it may further increase the volume overload and potentially worsen the CHF. Therefore, breath sounds, heart rate, blood pressure, and symptoms must be monitored carefully during exercise in patients who have received a transfusion or who are anemic so that adverse reactions or medical emergencies can be prevented.

Also of concern for patients with advanced CMD (or CHF in general) is the state of **hemostasis** (the mechanical and biochemical aspects of platelet function and coagulation), which is frequently disrupted as a result of accompanying liver disease.[6] Normal platelet function is an interrelated process involving a reflex vasoconstriction, formation of platelet plugs, and aggregation of platelets to one another.[78] The aggregation of platelets is an energy-requiring process, which is stimulated by agonists and inhibited by antagonists. The most important stimulants appear to be adenosine diphosphate (ADP), epinephrine, thrombin, and collagen. Inhibition of platelet function to the point at which the platelet count drops below 150,000 per millimeter is termed **thrombocytopenia** and is due to hereditary factors or drugs or often is acquired from systemic disease.[78] Inherited thrombocytopenia is uncommon; however, thrombocytopenia due to drugs is much more common and frequently is an adverse reaction associated with use of aspirin, corticosteroids, antimicrobial agents (penicillins and cephalothins), phosphodiesterase inhibitors (dipyridamole), caffeine, sympathetic blocking agents (beta antagonists), and heparin.[78] Acquired disorders of platelet function are due to systemic disease states or complications arising from a disease. Renal failure frequently leads to **uremia,** which prolongs bleeding time and impairs platelet formation. This is usually corrected by renal **dialysis,** but patients with chronic CHF may demonstrate a mild-to-moderate level of platelet dysfunction.[78]

SKELETAL MUSCLE FUNCTION IN CONGESTIVE HEART FAILURE

Skeletal muscle activity in patients with CHF has been a topic of investigation for many years. Studies have identified a skeletal muscle **myopathy** in patients with CHF and in those with CHF and preexisting cardiomyopathy.[21,79] This section presents information regarding skeletal muscle function when CHF *alone* is present and when CHF is present as a result of a cardiomyopathy. It is essential that the material be presented in

this manner because skeletal muscle myopathies are common with cardiomyopathy.[21,79]

Skeletal Muscle Activity in Congestive Heart Failure without Cardiomyopathy

Unfortunately, the function of skeletal muscle in patients with CHF has been studied far less in patients without cardiomyopathy than in those with cardiomyopathy. However, two well-done studies have evaluated skeletal muscle activity in the presence of CHF without preexisting cardiomyopathy.[21,79] The first histopathologic study by Shafiq and colleagues examined skeletal muscle in patients with and without **idiopathic** cardiomyopathy.[79] Electromyographic, histochemical, and electron microscopic studies were performed on 15 subjects (four normal subjects, six with CHF and cardiomyopathy, and five with signs and symptoms of CHF but *without* cardiomyopathy). Results revealed no abnormalities in the normal subjects, a decrease in the average diameters of the type I and type II fibers in the patients with CHF but without cardiomyopathy, and in the patients with CHF and cardiomyopathy, three distinct skeletal muscle abnormalities (selective atrophy of type II fibers, pronounced nonselective myopathy, and hypotrophy of type I fibers).[79] Patients with diseases known to affect skeletal muscle (diabetes, collagen vascular disease, and alcoholism) were excluded from the study.

More recently, Lipkin and associates investigated the abnormalities of skeletal muscle in patients with chronic heart failure.[21] Three of the nine CHF subjects in this study had a dilated cardiomyopathy, five had coronary artery disease, and one had a previous aortic valve surgery for aortic regurgitation. Patients with myocardial ischemia, ventricular tachycardia during exercise testing, obstructive valvular heart disease, pulmonary disease, or peripheral vascular disease (history of intermittent claudication, thrombocytopenia, or patients on anticoagulation therapy) were excluded from this study because of potential effects on skeletal muscle. Participants underwent (1) a symptom-limited exercise test with respiratory gas analysis; (2) assessment of muscle strength (maximal voluntary isometric contractions of the quadriceps); and (3) analysis of quadriceps muscle **mitochondrial enzyme** activity, **histochemistry,** and fiber size. Mean maximal oxygen consumption was very low (11.7 ml $\cdot$ kg^{-1} $\cdot$ min^{-1}), and isometric maximal voluntary contraction of the quadriceps was only 55% (range 31% to 75%) of the predicted value for weight. Eight of the nine biopsies were abnormal, showing increased intracellular acid phosphatase activity (n = 6), increased intracellular lipid accumulation (n = 4), and atrophy of type I and type II muscle fibers (n = 4).[21] In conclusion, the results of a nuclear magnetic resonance spectroscopy study have shown that skeletal muscle fatigue in patients with CHF is associated with intracellular acidosis and **phosphocreatinine** depletion,[80] which if prolonged may predispose to myopathic processes.

Skeletal Muscle Activity in Congestive Heart Failure and Cardiomyopathy

Skeletal muscle activity is apparently impaired by chronic CHF as well as by cardiomyopathy. Skeletal muscle abnormalities due to dilated[81-83] and hypertrophic[84-88] cardiomyopathies have been reported previously and have consistently revealed type I and type II fiber atrophy.[81-88]

A detailed study of skeletal muscle abnormalities in patients with hypertrophic and dilated cardiomyopathy was performed by Caforio and co-workers.[20] In addition to investigating skeletal muscle activity, heart function was assessed 1 to 3 weeks before entry into the study by M-mode and two-dimensional echocardiography and right- and left-sided cardiac catheterization, including coronary arteriography and left ventriculography.

Eleven patients with dilated cardiomyopathy and eight patients with hypertrophic cardiomyopathy underwent neuromuscular and **electromyographic** analysis of the right biceps brachii during a maximal voluntary contraction. Six of the 19 patients underwent muscle biopsy of the right biceps brachii, and three underwent biopsy of the deltoid muscle with light and electron mi-

croscopy analysis. Patient functional status was determined by the New York Heart Association method, which classified six patients in class I, six in class II, and seven in class III. The ejection fraction range was from 20% to 62% with a mean of 41 $\pm$ 12%.[20]

Results of the neuromuscular assessment were relatively insignificant, except that (1) all symptomatic patients with dilated and one with hypertrophic cardiomyopathy demonstrated a slight **hyposthenia** in the girdles or proximal limbs, and (2) none of the patients had muscular hypotrophy. Electromyography studies revealed abnormalities typical of **myogenic** myopathy in nine patients (five dilated, four hypertrophic), but none of the patients showed signs of **neurogenic** alteration (i.e., a reduction of nerve conduction velocities or an increase in single motor unit potential duration).[20]

Muscle biopsies consistently detected pathologic changes (primarily mitochondrial abnormalities) in the type I (slow-twitch) fibers in all nine patients from whom a biopsy was obtained; eight of the biopsies demonstrated increases of atrophy factors. No alteration of type II fibers was observed in any patient.[20]

Although echocardiographic and hemodynamic indices of ventricular function were similar in patients with and without electromyographic abnormalities, patients in functional class III were slightly, but not statistically, more likely to have such abnormalities.[20]

Caforio and colleagues believe the findings from this study support the hypothesis that skeletal myopathic changes, which are occasionally observed in patients with cardiomyopathy, are of a primary nature rather than a secondary nature (due to congestive heart failure). It is likely that both chronic CHF and cardiomyopathy have profound effects on skeletal muscle activity, as is evident from what follows.

Loss of muscle strength will reduce exercise capacity. At workloads corresponding to 50 and 100% of maximal oxygen consumption in normal subjects, the proportion of maximal muscle force utilised during an isometric contraction is 30 and 50%, respectively. In the patients we have studied, isometric maximal muscle strength was reduced to nearly 50% of the value for control age, sex and weight matched subjects. Loss of muscle strength will result in each muscle fibre operating nearer to its maximal capacity for a given absolute power output. Consequently, the changes in skeletal muscle metabolism that are associated with fatigue might be expected to occur at lower absolute workloads and hence limit maximal exercise capacity in these patients.[21]

THE PANCREAS AND CARDIAC MUSCLE DYSFUNCTION

Severe CMD can potentially reduce blood flow to the pancreas "as a consequence of splanchnic visceral vasoconstriction, which accompanies severe left ventricular failure."[89] The reduction in blood flow to the pancreas impairs insulin secretion and glucose tolerance, which are further impaired by increased sympathetic nervous system activity and augmented circulatory catecholamines (inhibiting insulin secretion) that stimulate **glycogenolysis** and elevate blood sugar levels.[89]

Reduced secretion of insulin is of paramount importance because hypoxic and dysfunctional heart muscle depends a great deal on the energy from the metabolism of glucose, which is reduced significantly if insulin secretion is impaired.[89] Ultimately, there is further deterioration of left ventricular function, creating a vicious cycle.

Normally, when oxygen is available, the heart obtains 60% to 90% of its energy requirements from the oxidation of free fatty acids, which inhibits glucose uptake, glycolytic flux, and glycogenolysis.[90] The oxidation of free fatty acids increases the production of acetylcoenzyme-A (acetyl-CoA), which inhibits pyruvate dehydrogenase and limits carbohydrate metabolism.[90] However, as previously noted, myocardial ischemia (because of the limited supply of oxygen) inhibits the oxidation of free fatty acids and long-chain acyl–carnitine palmitoyl transferase enzyme activity, thus preventing the transport of cytosolic acylcoenzyme-A (acyl-CoA) to the mitochondria for oxidation. "Accordingly, intracellular concentrations of acyl-CoA increase and acetyl-CoA content declines."[91]

Increased levels of acyl-CoA produce several deleterious effects on proper cardiac function:

- increased synthesis of triglycerides, which accumulate in the myocardium
- inhibition of further formation of CoA esters of fatty acids, limiting oxidation of free fatty acids
- inhibition of adenine nucleotide translocase, which is important for myocardial energy metabolism as it transports ATP synthesized in the mitochondria to the cytosol[90]

This final inhibition of adenine nucleotide translocase may be a key factor contributing to myocardial dysfunction.[90]

In addition to the previously mentioned changes in metabolism, "the pancreas has also been viewed as the source of a myocardial depressant factor which has been shown to decrease contractility of an isolated papillary muscle preparation."[92,93]

NUTRITIONAL ASPECTS OF CARDIAC MUSCLE DYSFUNCTION AND CONGESTIVE HEART FAILURE

Nutritional concerns are very important when assessing and treating patients with CMD. Stomach and intestinal abnormalities are not uncommon in these patients, who frequently receive many medications with profound side effects.[94] In addition, the interrelated disease processes occurring in other organs because of CMD and CHF frequently produce **anorexia**, which leads ultimately to malnutrition.[94] The primary malnutrition is a **protein-calorie deficiency**, but vitamin deficiencies have also been observed (folic acid, thiamine, and hypocalcemia-accompanied vitamin D deficiency).[94] These deficient states may simply be the result of decreased intake, but "abnormal intestinal absorption and increased rates of excretion may also contribute."[94]

Protein-calorie deficiency is common in chronic CHF because of cellular hypoxia and hypermetabolism that frequently produces **cachexia** (malnutrition and wasting).[94] A catabolic state may also develop, yielding an excess of urea or other nitrogenous compounds in the blood (**azotemia**). This, as with most organ pathologies associated with CHF, causes a vicious cycle, which, because of gastrointestinal hypoxia and decreased appetite (anorexia) and protein intake, produces cardiac atrophy and more pronounced CMD.[94]

One particular area of concern is thiamine deficiency due to improper nutrition, which can affect this population dramatically. The force of myocardial contraction and cardiac performance in general appear to be dependent on the level of thiamine, and it has been suggested that *"the possibility of thiamine deficiency should be considered in many patients with heart failure of obscure origin."*[9] In addition, patients undergoing prolonged treatment with furosemide (Lasix) (the first drug of choice in the treatment of CHF) have demonstrated significant thiamine deficiency, which may improve with replacement.[95]

Skeletal muscle carnitine deficiency has also been observed in a small population of patients with hypertrophic cardiomyopathy. When carnitine was replenished, cardiac symptoms and echocardiographic parameters apparently improved.[96]

These examples demonstrate the interrelatedness of all bodily functions and the importance of a thorough and comprehensive assessment, which is of even greater significance when kidney and liver diseases (frequently accompanying CHF) further complicate a patient's status. Complications associated with renal disease that are specifically related to nutritional aspects of CMD include

- decreased production of erythropoietin (a hormone synthesized in the kidney that is an important precursor of red blood cell production in bone marrow), causing anemia and possibly less free fatty acid oxidation[97,98]
- decreased synthesis of **1,25-dihydroxycholecalciferol,** which may lead to decreased calcium absorption from the gastrointestinal tract,[99] as well as the development of **hyperparathyroidism**[100]
- impaired intermediary metabolism (impaired **gluconeogenesis** and lipid metabolism, as well as degradation of several peptides, proteins, and peptide hormones including insulin, **glucagon,** growth hormone, and **parathyroid hormone)**[101]

These renal abnormalities can, by themselves, impair liver function (primarily via protein deprivation), which "predisposes to chronic liver disease with a loss of hepatocytes and a decrease in portal venous blood flow."[102] Liver dysfunction further impairs the normal metabolism of many organic and inorganic nutrients, of which three intrahepatic intermediary amino acid metabolic pathways have been identified: the urea cycle, the **phenylalanine-hydroxylase pathway,** and the **transsulfuration pathway.**[102]

Although protein deprivation may be a predisposing factor to liver disease, Fischer and colleagues discovered that the aromatic amino acids phenylalanine and tyrosine and the sulfur-containing methionine are elevated, whereas the branched-chain amino acids are depressed in patients with cirrhosis of the liver and **hepatic encephalopathy.**[103,104] This finding led to the current practice of administering enteral and parenteral products with reduced aromatic amino acids and increased branched-chain amino acids, which many patients with end-stage CHF frequently receive, to patients with liver disease.[102] Thus, the complexity of liver disease alone, not to mention a superimposed CHF and its many complications, makes the patient with CHF a complex challenge.

SPINAL CORD INJURY

Transection of the cervical spinal cord prevents sympathetic nervous system information from reaching the cardiovascular system (heart, lung, arterial and venous systems), thus *preventing* the sympathetic-driven changes necessary to maintain cardiac performance (i.e., increased heart rate and force of myocardial contraction, constriction of venous capacitance vessels or arterial constriction). Lacking these cardiovascular adaptations, patients with spinal cord injuries (who frequently are volume-depleted because of fluid loss from multiple injuries) may develop a specific type of CMD that produces pulmonary edema.[25]

In view of the possibility of volume depletion, it has been recommended that cardiac filling pressures be monitored, that "cardiac preload be increased by giving fluids,"[25] and that construction of a ventricular function curve may be useful in guiding therapy and treatment for patients with spinal cord injuries.[25] It appears, then, that a slightly elevated pulmonary capillary wedge pressure (not exceeding 18 mm Hg) may facilitate optimal cardiac performance in these patients.

CONGENITAL AND ACQUIRED HEART DISEASE

Congenital heart disease is the result of "altered embryonic development of a normal structure or failure of such a structure to progress beyond an early stage of embryonic or fetal development."[29] Approximately 0.8% of live births are complicated by cardiovascular malformations[105] such as **ventricular septal defect, atrial septal defect, patent ductus arteriosus, coarctation of the aorta,** and **tetralogy of Fallot.** The two most common cardiac anomalies are the "congenital nonstenotic bicuspid aortic valve and the leaflet abnormality associated with mitral valve prolapse."[29]

Heart disease can also be *acquired* in infancy and childhood. Such disease processes include

- rheumatic heart disease
- connective tissue disorders
- **mucopolysaccharidoses**
- **hyperlipidemia**
- nonrheumatic inflammatory diseases (infective myocarditis, infective pericarditis, and **post-pericardiotomy syndrome**)
- primary **(endocardial fibroelastosis)** and secondary cardiomyopathies (due to glycogen storage disease, neonatal **thyrotoxicosis,** infantile **beriberi,** protein-calorie malnutrition, tropical endomyocardial fibrosis, **anthracycline toxicity, Kawasaki's disease,** and diabetes in mothers)[29]

Although the disease processes are different in acquired and congenital heart disease, the resultant pathophysiologic processes are not unlike those seen in adults with CMD because it is dysfunctional cardiac muscle that eventually produces the clinical signs and symptoms.[29] The primary manifestations are

- congestive heart failure
- cyanosis
- hepatomegaly
- acid-base imbalances
- impaired growth
- pulmonary hypertension
- chest pain
- syncope
- arrhythmias

AGING AND CARDIAC MUSCLE DYSFUNCTION

The aging process involves several interrelated pathophysiologic processes, all of which have the potential to impair physical performance, including cardiac function. Although several earlier studies have revealed a reduced cardiac output in the elderly (at rest and with exercise),[106–108] a study that excluded subjects with ischemic heart disease demonstrated no "age effect" on cardiac performance.[109] In this study, the heart rates of the elderly were lower at most workloads, but increased stroke volume apparently compensated for the decreased heart rates and thus maintained cardiac output (cardiac output = heart rate × stroke volume).[109]

However, other age-associated changes such as increased systolic arterial pressure and decreased aortic distensibility probably contribute to the mild-to-moderate left ventricular hypertrophy commonly found in the elderly.[110] This hypertrophy preserves left ventricular systolic function but impairs left ventricular diastolic function. Diastolic dysfunction delays left ventricular filling, which is more profound in the presence of hypertension, coronary artery disease, and higher heart rates.[111] Additionally, increased norepinephrine levels (probably because of decreased catecholamine sensitivity) and decreased baroreceptor sensitivity and plasma renin concentrations have been reported in elderly subjects.[31]

These pathophysiologic processes, as well as other confounding variables such as coronary artery disease, exposure to environmental toxins (cigarette smoking, radiation), malnutrition, and other lifestyle habits, must be considered to accurately document the effects of aging on cardiac and exercise performance. Nonetheless, the consensus regarding the cardiovascular aging process is as follows:

- After neonatal development, the number of myocardial cells in the heart does not increase.
- There is moderate hypertrophy of left ventricular myocardium, probably in response to increased arterial vascular stiffness and dropout of myocytes.
- When myocardial hypertrophy occurs, it is out of proportion to capillary and vascular growth.
- The ability of the myocardium to generate tension is well maintained as a result of prolonged duration of contraction and greater stiffness despite a modest decrease in the velocity of shortening of cardiac muscle.
- There is a selective decrease in beta-adrenoceptor–mediated inotropic, chronotropic, and vasodilating cardiovascular responses with aging.
- Increased pericardial and myocardial stiffness and delayed relaxation during aging may limit left ventricular filling during stress.[32]

The primary cause of the changes associated with aging has been attributed to one or a combination of three theories: the genome, the physiologic, and the organ theories.[32] The genome theories are based on the programming of genes for aging, death, or both, whereas the physiologic theories (cross-linkage theory) are dependent on specific pathophysiologic processes. The organ theories (primarily immunologic and neuroendocrine) may be the most encompassing because immunologic and neurohormonal dysfunction is hypothesized to produce both general and specific aging effects.[32]

Muscular Changes Associated with Aging

The specific changes in skeletal and cardiac muscle are discussed in the following section, and a brief review of the effects of exercise training on cardiac and skeletal muscle in the

TABLE 4-8. Effects of Aging

Aging	Effect
Decreased elasticity in vascular system	Increased systolic and possibly diastolic blood pressure
Left ventricular hypertrophy	Decreased ventricular compliance (filling)
Decreased adrenergic responsiveness	Decreased heart rate with exercise and decreased Vo_{2max}
Decreased lean body mass	Decreased muscle strength and Vo_{2max}

elderly is presented. Table 4-8 provides a good overview of the effects of aging.

Cardiac Muscle

Animal studies have revealed that the contraction and relaxation times of cardiac muscle are prolonged in aged rats.[112-115] This prolongation "can be attributed to alterations in mechanisms that govern excitation-contraction coupling in the heart,"[32] primarily the increase and decrease of **cytosolic** calcium in the myofilaments. The rate that the sarcoplasmic reticulum pumps calcium is reduced in hearts of older animals and "appears to be a major contributor to the prolonged transient and prolonged time course of cardiac muscle relaxation."[32] The diminished ability of the sarcoplasmic reticulum to pump calcium may also be responsible for the following changes observed in elderly animals:

- prolonged time to peak force and half relaxation time of peak stiffness[116-118]
- lower muscular twitch force at higher stimulation rates[119]

In addition, the rate of ATP hydrolysis and myosin ATPase activity declines progressively with age, and in conjunction with the previously mentioned changes contributes to the reduction in the velocity of shortening as well as the prolonged contraction and relaxation times of cardiac muscle.[32]

In summary, in healthy elderly individuals, exercise cardiac output is, for the most part, maintained by the Frank-Starling mechanism (increasing end-diastolic volume) to increase stroke volume because of lower heart rates in the elderly. Aged subjects with hypertension are unable to fully utilize the beneficial effects of the Frank-Starling mechanism because of a hypertrophied and noncompliant myocardium and most likely will be unable to maintain exercise cardiac output, as demonstrated in Figure 4–14.[31] Finally, the lower exercise heart rates seen in the elderly are probably mediated by an age-associated decreased responsiveness to beta-adrenergic stimulation.[120]

Skeletal Muscle

Many of the same changes observed in cardiac muscle also occur in the skeletal muscles of elderly persons. However, skeletal muscle change may be more profound than cardiac muscle change in view of the following observations in the elderly: skeletal muscle atrophy,[121] slowed muscle contraction and reduced capacity for twitch potentiation,[122] decreased insulin sensitivity and skeletal muscle enzyme activity,[123] decreased skeletal muscle mitochondrial respiratory chain function,[124] impaired cardiopulmonary (primarily vascular and neurohumoral) receptor reflex activity,[125] increased defects and pseudotu-

mors of the diaphragm,[126] and greater percentage of type I (slow oxidative) fibers.[127–128] The last finding is important and may be one reason that older athletes (masters) are able to perform as well as younger athletes, despite having a lower $\dot{V}O_{2max}$.[128] Although this finding is somewhat paradoxical, it exemplifies the importance and benefits of exercise training in the elderly, who seem to gain increased endurance and functional capacity (via a greater capillary-to-fiber ratio and improved oxidative skeletal muscle enzyme activity)[128] as well as enhanced psychosocial function.[129] Therefore, exercise training appears to decrease the magnitude of impairment seen in elderly individuals.

Exercise Training in the Elderly

The study of cardiac performance in elderly rats performing long-term exercise has revealed

- a diminution or elimination of the age-associated increase in duration of myocardial contraction and dynamic stiffness
- a modest augmentation of cytochrome-C oxidase activity in heart muscle

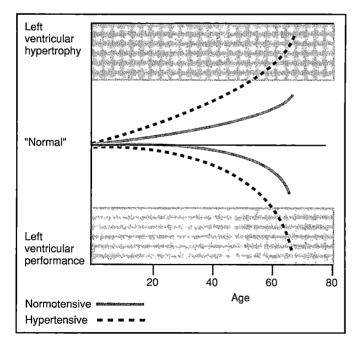

Figure 4–14.

The effects of aging and hypertension on cardiovascular performance. Aging is accompanied by an increase in left ventricular mass and a subsequent decrease in left ventricular performance (possibly owing to less distensible myocardium). These changes are partly responsible for the increased incidence of congestive heart failure in the elderly.

- a diminution or elimination in the progressive decline of myocardial calcium-activated acto-myosin ATPase activity[32]

Studies that evaluate changes in cardiac performance of elderly humans during long-term exercise training have been scarce or poorly conducted. However, exercise training adaptations in the elderly have been suggested to include increased joint stability and mobility (via increased muscle and tendon strength), improved neuromuscular coordination, increased flexibility and muscular strength, and the previously mentioned increase in endurance and physical work capacity.[120] In addition, several beneficial effects of exercise training may occur, such as the modification of coronary risk factors (obesity, hypertension, hyperglycemia, and hyperlipidemia), retardation of mineral loss from bone, enhanced self-confidence and a sense of well-being, and possibly improved cognitive function.[120]

"Exercise of almost any kind, suitable in degree and duration . . . can and does play a useful role in the maintenance of both physical and mental health of the aging individual . . . ,"[129] despite the reduction in cardiovascular performance.

TREATMENT OF CARDIAC MUSCLE DYSFUNCTION AND ASSOCIATED PATHOPHYSIOLOGIES

The treatment of CMD, in general, is directed at the underlying cause or causes. Therefore, the following treatments are presented in view of the primary pathology producing CMD, that is, cardiac arrhythmias, heart valve abnormalities (stenosis, insufficiency, or rupture), pericardial effusion and myocarditis, pulmonary embolus, renal insufficiency, myocardial infarction, and cardiomyopathy. More specific treatments of CMD and CHF are discussed in the section entitled, Specific Treatment for Congestive Heart Failure. This is followed by a review of the specific treatment effects of exercise training in patients with CMD. Finally, six case studies of patients treated at our facilities are presented that should provide an overview of the treatments and pathophysiologies associated with CMD.

Cardiac Arrhythmias

Cardiac arrhythmias that produce CMD are the result of prolonged very slow or very fast heart rates and frequently are due to a **sick sinus node syndrome** or heart blocks (producing very slow heart rates), prolonged supraventricular tachycardia (i.e., rapid atrial fibrillation or flutter), or ventricular tachycardia (the last two of which produce very fast heart rates).[56,57]

Very slow heart rates or heart blocks are often an adverse reaction or side effect of a specific medication, but when medications are withheld and slow rates or a heart block persists, the implantation of a permanent pacemaker is generally performed.[56] This type of CMD is readily amenable to treatment and quite reversible.

Cardiac muscle dysfunction due to very rapid heart rates is also reversible. Rapid atrial fibrillation or flutter can produce CMD and is often easily treated by the administration of verapamil or digoxin[56] (see Chapter 12). If these drugs fail, electrical cardioversion is usually performed, after which rapid heart rates frequently become much more normal as the cyclic "circus movement" propagating the rapid rhythm is disrupted and the sinoatrial node is allowed to resume control of the heart's rhythm.[56] Ventricular tachycardia and fibrillation are life-threatening cardiac arrhythmias, which, if prolonged, rapid, or both, can also produce CMD and death. The treatment of ventricular tachycardia and fibrillation is dependent on the clinical status of the patient and follows the guidelines set forth by the American Heart Association.[56] The use of automatic implantable cardiac defibrillators (AICDs) has been a treatment of choice for patients with recurrent ventricular tachycardia and fibrillation that is unresponsive to antiarrhythmic medications.[57]

Heart Valve Abnormalities

Heart valve abnormalities that cause CMD appear to be reversible to a point. If the abnormality persists for too long, cardiac function appears to be permanently impaired.[23] Acute problems such as heart valve rupture can affect proper cardiac muscle function profoundly and are fatal if not surgically repaired within a relatively short period of time. The most common valvular surgeries are valvular replacement, **valvuloplasty** (pressurized reduction of atherosclerotic plaque, similar to angioplasty of the coronary arteries), **valvulotomy** (incision), and **commissurotomy** (incision to separate adherent, thickened leaflets).[23]

Other heart valve conditions can be classified as chronic conditions. These include the stenotic and regurgitant abnormalities of the aortic, pulmonic, mitral, or tricuspid valves. Prolonged valvular stenosis or regurgitation affects cardiac function and can eventually lead to CMD, but cardiac function is less likely to return to normal after valvuloplasty or surgical repair or replacement of a chronic valvular condition.[23]

Pericardial Effusion (Cardiac Tamponade) and Myocarditis

The prompt treatment of pericarditis with nonsteroidal anti-inflammatory agents (aspirin or indomethacin) or corticosteroids (usually prednisone) frequently prevents pericardial effusion. Treatment of the causative inflammatory process in myocarditis (most commonly viral) should prevent the diastolic and systolic CMD of pericardial effusion and myocarditis.[16] However, patients who do not respond to this therapy must undergo more extensive treatment, including drainage of fluid from the pericardium (**pericardiocentesis**) for pericardial effusion; immunosuppressive, antibiotic, and possibly antiviral agents for myocarditis; and aggressive CHF management (digitalization, diuresis, and afterload or preload reduction) for both pericardial effusion and myocarditis.[16]

Pulmonary Embolus

An acute pulmonary embolus is also a potentially life-threatening condition. As previously mentioned, the primary CMD resulting from a pulmonary embolus is due to a very high pulmonary artery pressure (because of damaged lung tissue and less area for proper pulmonary perfusion), which increases the work of the right ventricle and eventually produces right-sided heart failure. Left-sided heart failure may accompany right-sided failure because of decreased blood volume and coronary perfusion to the left ventricle, impairing the pumping ability of the heart.[24]

The treatment of a pulmonary embolus consists of the following treatment:

- a thrombolytic agent (typically heparin) to decrease the blood clot
- a sedative to decrease the patient's anxiety and pain
- oxygen to improve the Pa_{O_2} and decrease the pulmonary artery pressure
- occasionally an **embolectomy**[24]

Cardiac muscle dysfunction due to a pulmonary embolus occasionally can be reversed (especially if treatment is initiated immediately), but quite frequently some degree of CMD ensues because of infarcted lung tissue, which increases the work of the right ventricle.[24] When such a condition exists, the pulmonary artery pressure rises and may produce pulmonary hypertension. Pulmonary hypertension can produce CMD often by increasing right ventricular work, resulting in right ventricular hypertrophy (and inefficient right ventricular performance). This may reduce the right ventricular stroke volume, thereby decreasing the left ventricular stroke volume and cardiac output.

Renal Insufficiency

As previously discussed, acute or chronic renal insufficiency tends to produce a fluid overload, which frequently progresses to CMD and CHF that can often be reversed if it is the only underlying pathophysiologic process. However, other pathophysiologic processes may produce the fluid overload that caused CMD.[42] Therefore, CMD is seldom reversed by the correction of fluid volume alone. Nevertheless, the primary treatment is to decrease the reabsorption of fluid from the kidneys so that more fluid is eliminated (in essence, diuresed).[42] The diuretic most commonly used is furosemide (Lasix), which can be given intravenously or orally. The dosage is dependent on the degree of fluid overload and the desired diuretic effect; furosemide is commonly given orally at a dosage of 20 to 80 milligrams every 6 to 8 hours.[42] Patients receiving a diuretic such as Lasix in the acute care setting are carefully monitored (hourly measurement of input and output) and frequently undergo titrated doses to achieve the desired effects. There is a certain degree of guesswork associated with the assessment and treatment of fluid overload. However, it appears that **bioimpedance analysis,** a method frequently used to evaluate percentage body fat and lean body mass, may also be of assistance in assessing fluid volume (total body water).[130] The measurement of total body water may prove to be invaluable in the treatment of patients receiving diuretics so that less guesswork and more objective information can direct the proper dosage of diuretics.

In addition to and as a result of the administration of a diuretic, electrolyte levels are carefully monitored, ensuring that potassium and sodium levels are within the normal range to prevent further retention of fluid from high levels of potassium and sodium or the detrimental effects of low levels (cardiac arrhythmias, muscle weakness, etc.).

Severe renal insufficiency, demonstrating advanced azotemia, is best treated by **peritoneal hemodialysis,** which is designed to

- remove solutes
- alter the electrolyte concentration of the extracellular fluid
- remove as much as 1 liter of extracellular fluid per hour[42]

Myocardial Ischemia and Infarction

The specific treatment of acute myocardial infarction depends on many factors, primarily the presence or absence of CHF, ventricular arrhythmias, recurrent angina, and persistent hypotension.[89] The primary treatments are

- oxygen
- nitroglycerin
- analgesia
- electrical defibrillation
- atropine
- lidocaine
- pacemaker
- thrombolytic agents
- beta blocker
- calcium-channel blocker
- anticoagulant and platelet-inhibitory agents
- percutaneous transluminal coronary angioplasty
- intra-aortic balloon counterpulsation and other circulatory assist devices
- surgical intervention[131]

These therapies are considered most crucial in the treatment of acute myocardial infarction, and a variety of patient variables dictate which of the above treatments should be used. A detailed review of the early management of patients with acute myocardial infarction with an emphasis on patient identification, stratification, and treatment progression has previously been published and provides detailed information regarding the treatment of myocardial infarction.[131]

Postperfusion (postpump) syndrome is a complication associated with cardiopulmonary bypass surgery and essentially represents "organ and subsystem dysfunction."[132] Not only is CMD common after bypass surgery,[133] but abnormal bleeding, inflammatory reactions, renal dysfunction, hemodynamic and metabolic problems (from peripheral and possibly central vasoconstriction), breakdown of red blood cells, and possibly increased susceptibility to infection have all been reported as "damaging effects of cardiopulmonary bypass."[132] The following quote indicates the importance of investigating for the presence of any of the previously mentioned complications because "the fact that most patients convalesce normally after cardiopulmonary bypass attests only to patients' abilities to compensate for these damaging effects and not to their absence."[132]

In conclusion, several important risk factors have been recognized to be associated with the postpump syndrome, including

- duration of cardiopulmonary bypass (if greater than 90 to 120 minutes for young infants or 150 minutes for adults)
- patient age
- presence of preoperative cyanosis
- perfusion flow rate
- composition of the **perfusate**
- oxygenating surface
- patient temperature during perfusion[132]

Coronary angioplasty has also been associated with a certain degree of myocardial damage or "stunning," the clinical significance of which is still under investigation.[134,135]

Cardiomyopathy

The specific treatment of cardiomyopathy is dependent on the underlying cause but in general includes "physical, dietary, pharmacological, mechanical, and surgical intervention."[16] One pharmacologic intervention worth mentioning is beta-adrenergic blockade, which appears to improve symptoms and survival via "(1) negative chronotropic effect with reduced myocardial oxygen demand, (2) reduced myocardial damage due to catecholamines, (3) improved diastolic relaxation, (4) inhibition of sympathetically mediated vasoconstriction, and (5) increase in myocardial beta-adrenoceptor density."[16] These factors are important because they are the basic mechanisms supporting the use of beta blockers for dilated, restrictive, and hypertrophic cardiomyopathies as well as CHF in general, since "treatment is on the same basis as that for heart failure."[16]

Specific Treatments for Congestive Heart Failure

The basic treatment for CHF involves controlling the mechanisms responsible for its existence (i.e., the heart's ability to pump, the heart's workload, and the amount of sodium and water retention).[136] These are outlined in Table 4-9.

TABLE 4-9. Control of Congestive Heart Failure

Correct the underlying cause of heart failure
(causes 1-9 in Table 4-2)

Improve cardiac muscle performance
(e.g., use of digitalis, other agents, pacemaker)

Reduce the workload of the heart
(e.g., physical and emotional rest, treatment of obesity, vasodilator therapy, assisted circulation)

Control excessive salt and water retention
(e.g., low-sodium diet, diuretics, dialysis)

The specific treatments for CHF include the restriction of sodium intake, use of medications (diuretics, digitalis and other positive inotropic agents, dopamine, dobutamine, amrinone, vasodilator therapy, venodilators, angiotensin-converting enzyme inhibitors, and beta-adrenergic blockers), and other special measures. These treatments are outlined in Table 4-10.

Medications

Diuretics. Diuretics "remain the cornerstone" of treatment for CHF.[136] As outlined in Table 4-10, moderate diuretics and loop diuretics are commonly used to reduce the fluid overload of CHF by increasing urine flow.[136] Most of these diuretics act directly on kidney function by inhibiting solute (substances dissolved in a solution) and water reabsorption. As previously discussed, furosemide is the most commonly used diuretic, and its principle site of action is the thick ascending limb of Henle's loop, where it inhibits the cotransport of sodium, potassium, and chloride.[136]

Digoxin and Other Positive Inotropic Agents. Digoxin (digitalis) is one of medicine's oldest drugs, and most of the digitalis drugs in use today are steroid glycosides derived from the leaves of the flowering plant foxglove, or *Digitalis purpurea*. Despite its long history, there is still controversy over its use in patients with CHF and normal sinus rhythm.[137-139] However, several studies have demonstrated favorable hemodynamic and clinical responses in selected

TABLE 4–10. Outline of Treatment of Chronic Congestive Heart Failure

Proper Prescription of Physical Activity

Decrease or discontinue exhaustive activities

Decrease or discontinue full-time work or equivalent activity, introducing rest periods during the day

Gradual progressive exercise training that fluctuates frequently from day to day

Exercise intensity determined by level of dyspnea or adverse physiologic effort (i.e., angina or decrease in systolic blood pressure)

Restriction of Sodium Intake

Institute a low-sodium diet

Digitalis, Glycoside, and other Inotropic Agents

Dopamine

Dobutamine

Amrinone

Diuretics

Moderate diuretics (thiazide)

Loop diuretic (furosemide)

Loop diuretic plus distal tubular (potassium-sparing) diuretic

Loop diuretic plus thiazide and distal tubular diuretic

Vasodilators or Venodilators

Captopril, enalapril, or combination of hydralazine plus isosorbide dinitrate

Intensification of oral vasodilator regimen

Intravenous nitroprusside

Angiotensin Converting Enzyme

Captopril—may prevent cardiac dilation

Enalapril maleate

Lisinopril

Beta Blockers

Metoprolol

Bucindolol

Xamoterol

Special Measures

Dialysis and ultrafiltration

Assisted circulation (intra-aortic balloon, left ventricular assist device, artificial heart)

Cardiac transplantation

---

patients.[140–144] The most significant clinical observations tend to be related to the positive inotropic (increased force of contraction) effect evidenced by increased left ventricular ejection fraction.[145] In addition, the electrophysiologic effects of digoxin on the heart help control rapid supraventricular arrhythmias (primarily atrial fibrillation or flutter) by increasing the parasympathetic tone in the sinus and atrioventricular nodes, thereby slowing conduction.[145]

Dopamine. Dopamine hydrochloride is a chemical precursor of norepinephrine, which stimulates dopaminergic, beta$_2$-adrenergic, and alpha-adrenergic receptors as well as the release of norepinephrine. This results in increased cardiac output and, at doses greater than 10 μg/kg/min, markedly increased systemic vascular resistance and preload.[56] For this reason, the primary indication for dopamine is hemodynamically significant hypotension in the absence of hypovolemia.[56] Dopamine is also useful for patients with refractory CHF, in which case it is carefully titrated until urine flow or hemodynamic parameters improve. In such patients, the hemodynamic and renal effects of dopamine can be profound, and frequently it is infused together with nitroprusside or nitroglycerin to counteract the vasoconstricting action. In addition, dopamine is frequently administered (as are dobutamine and amrinone) during and after cardiac surgery to improve low cardiac output states.[56]

Dobutamine. Dobutamine is a **sympathomimetic** amine that stimulates beta$_1$- and alpha-adrenergic receptors in the myocardium, thus providing potent inotropic effects.[146] Like dopamine, dobutamine increases cardiac output, but the peripheral resistance decreases; with the use of dopamine, there is a potentially significant increase in peripheral resistance. For this reason, "dobutamine and moderate volume loading are the treatment of choice in patients with hemodynamically significant right ventricular infarction."[56]

Amrinone. Amrinone is a phosphodiesterase inhibitor that produces rapid inotropic and vasodilatory effects but unfortunately can exacerbate myocardial ischemia if coronary occlusion exists.[147] Amrinone can also cause thrombocytopenia in 2% to 3% of patients as well as a variety of other side effects (e.g., gastrointestinal dysfunction, myalgia, fever, hepatic dysfunction, cardiac arrhythmias). Despite these adverse effects, amrinone is recommended and has proved to be therapeutic for patients with severe CHF that is refractory to diuretics, vasodilators, and other inotropic agents.[148]

Several other phosphodiesterase inhibitors (milrinone, pimobendan, and enoximone) appear to be promising for patients in the previously mentioned category.[149,150] In particular, an increase in exercise tolerance has been observed with the use of milrinone.[149]

Vasodilators and Venodilators. Vasodilators are given to patients with CHF or CMD to relax smooth muscle in peripheral arterioles, which produces peripheral vasodilation that decreases the afterload, lessens the work of the heart, and potentially decreases the degree of CMD.[145] Two important studies have demonstrated a 38%[151] and 31%[152] improvement in survival rates in patients with classes II to III CHF and class IV CHF, respectively, utilizing hydralazine and isosorbide dinitrate. Isosorbide dinitrate not only dilates peripheral arterioles, but also relaxes smooth muscle in the peripheral vessels and thus produces a venodilation that redistributes "blood volume away from the heart and thereby lowers right and left ventricular filling pressures."[145] This action reduces the preload and afterload, which is of major importance for patients with moderate to severe CMD. The clinical management of patients with CHF and CMD frequently combines vasodilators, venodilators, and angiotensin converting enzyme inhibitors.

Angiotensin Converting Enzyme Inhibitors. The combined use of **angiotensin converting enzyme** inhibitors, vasodilators, and venodilators has been demonstrated to be very effective in reducing symptoms and improving exercise tolerance.[153] The primary mechanism of action of these inhibitors is probably via the reduction of **angiotensin II,** a hormone that causes vasoconstriction,[145] but other less well-defined actions may be responsible for the therapeutic effects of angiotensin converting enzyme inhibitors in patients with CHF. Other poorly understood mechanisms of such inhibitors include "nonspecific vasodilation with unloading of the ventricle, inhibition of excessive sympathetic drive and perhaps modulation of tissue receptor systems."[145]

A great deal of interest has focused on the "prevention" hypothesis regarding the use of angiotensin converting enzyme inhibitors and the prevention of progressive CMD (dilation and CHF).[154-157] Notably, captopril may prevent such progressive cardiac dilation.[154,155]

Beta-Adrenergic Antagonists and Partial Agonists. Perhaps one of the most confusing groups of medications used in treating CHF and CMD is the beta-adrenergic blockers. One of the many uses of beta blockers is to lower blood pressure, primarily via a reduction in cardiac output.[145] This reduction in cardiac output is the result of a decrease in heart rate and stroke volume, which causes an increase in end-diastolic volume and end-diastolic pressure (primarily because of a slower heart rate, which allows more time for the ventricles to fill before the next myocardial contraction) but somewhat paradoxically reduces the myocardial oxygen requirement.[158] This paradoxical reduction in oxygen requirement is probably the result of a decrease in sympathetic nervous system stimulation because of beta blocker therapy. Sympathetic (catecholamine-driven) increases in heart rate, force of myocardial contraction, velocity, and extent of myocardial contraction, as well as systolic blood pressure, are prevented by beta blockade.[158,159]

Although the mechanisms of action of beta blocker therapy may appear to be helpful to patients in CHF, the use of these medications is still considered experimental because of a lack of large multicenter controlled studies[145] and because the use of beta blockers may "exacerbate CHF by removing sympathetic support from a diseased myocardium."[160] Several uncontrolled observational studies have suggested that small doses of metoprolol (Lopressor) may be efficacious for some patients with CHF and idiopathic dilated cardiomyopathy.[151-165] These studies have hypothesized that the excessive sympathetic nervous system activity common in CHF further depresses myocardial performance, and that "down-regulation of myocardial beta-adrenergic receptors occurs in heart failure."[145] One placebo-controlled trial did confirm the above hypothesis, but other studies utilizing beta blockers with intrinsic sympathomimetic activity (e.g., oxyprenolol and pindolol), which provide a slight stimulation of the blocked receptor that preserves adequate beta-adrenergic sympathetic tone and maintains cardiac output) have failed to demonstrate clinical benefit in patients with CHF.[166-168] However, beta blockers with peripheral dilating activity (bucindolol) as well as partial beta agonists (drugs with both beta-adrenergic agonist and beta-blocking activity, i.e., xamoterol) may be much more effective in CHF and CMD.[169-172] Partial beta agonists may possibly protect "the heart from down-regulation of beta receptors during the progressive rise in sympathetic activity that presumably occurs in advanced heart failure."[145]

Special Measures for the Treatment of Congestive Heart Failure and Cardiac Muscle Dysfunction

Patients who respond unfavorably to the aforementioned methods of treatment for CHF and CMD and who demonstrate signs and symptoms of severe CHF are frequently managed using several rather extreme methods. As noted in Table 4-10, there are three "special measures" categories for treating CHF and CMD: dialysis and ultrafiltration, assisted circulation, and cardiac transplantation.

Dialysis and Ultrafiltration. The mechanical removal of fluid from the pleural and abdominal cavities of patients with CHF is usually unnecessary, but patients unresponsive to diuretic therapy because of severe CHF or insensitivity to diuretics may be in need of peritoneal dialysis or **extracorporeal ultrafiltration.**[136] The mechanical removal of fluid in patients with acute respiratory distress because of large pleural effusions or diaphragms elevated by ascites (both of which compress the lungs) frequently brings rapid relief of dyspnea. However, mechanical removal of fluid (primarily peritoneal dialysis) may be associated with risk of **pneumothorax,** infection, **peritonitis, hypernatremia, hyperglycemia, hyperosmolality,** and cardiac arrhythmias.[136,173] Cardiovascular collapse may also occur if too much fluid is removed or if removal takes place too rapidly. It is recommended that no more than 200 milliliters of fluid per hour be removed and no greater than 1500 milliliters of pleural fluid be removed during dialysis.[136,173]

For these reasons as well as for simplicity, cost effectiveness, and long-lasting effects, ultrafiltration has recently been the treatment of choice for patients in need of mechanical fluid removal.[173] Extracorporeal ultrafiltration is a relatively new technique, which removes plasma water and sodium via an ultrafiltrate (a blend of water, elec-trolytes, and other small molecules with concentrations identical to plasma) from the blood by convective transport through a highly permeable membrane.[173] Ultrafiltration can be performed vein-to-vein using an extracorporeal pump or with an arteriovenous approach.[173]

Although hemodynamic side effects (hypotension, organ malperfusion, and hemolysis) are also possible with ultrafiltration, proper monitoring of the rate of blood flow through the filter (rates <150 ml/min or <500 ml/hr are tolerated without side effects) as well as right atrial pressure (ultrafiltration should be discontinued when the pressure falls to 2-3 mm Hg)[174] and hematocrit levels (should not exceed 50%) should, for the most part, prevent them.[173]

Assisted Circulation. Several methods of treatment exist that assist the circulation of blood throughout the body. Perhaps the most widely used is intra-aortic balloon counterpulsation via the intra-aortic balloon pump. The intra-aortic balloon pump catheter is positioned in the thoracic aorta just distal to the left subclavian artery via the right or left femoral artery (Fig. 4-15). Inflation of the balloon occurs at the beginning of ventricular diastole, immediately after closure of the aortic valve. This increases intra-aortic pressure as well as diastolic pressure in general and forces blood in the aortic arch to flow in a retrograde direction into the coronary arteries. This mechanism of action is referred to as *diastolic* augmentation and profoundly improves oxygen delivery to the myocardium.[89] In addition to this physiologic assist (greater availability of oxygen for myocardial energy production) to improve cardiac performance, hemodynamic assistance is also obtained as the balloon deflates just before systole, which decreases left ventricular afterload by forcing blood to move from an area of higher pressure to one of lower pressure to fill the space previously occupied by the balloon.[89] Consequently, the intra-aortic balloon pump causes "a 10 to 20% increase in cardiac output as well as a reduction in systolic and increase in diastolic arterial pressure with little change in mean pressure, a diminution of heart rate, and an increase in urine output."[89] In addition, intra-aortic balloon counterpulsation produces a reduction in myocardial oxygen consumption "and

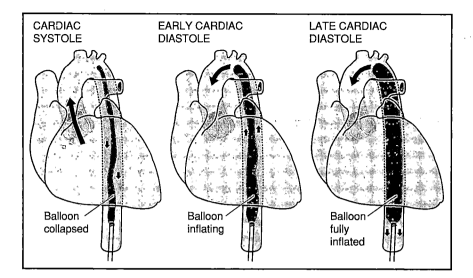

CARDIAC SYSTOLE

EARLY CARDIAC DIASTOLE

LATE CARDIAC DIASTOLE

Balloon collapsed

Balloon inflating

Balloon fully inflated

Figure 4–15.

The intra-aortic balloon pump. Inflation and deflation of the intra-aortic balloon pump improve diastolic and systolic heart function, respectively.

decreased myocardial ischemia and anaerobic metabolism,"[89] all of which are very important in the management of CHF and CMD.

The intra-aortic balloon pump is occasionally used in conjunction with a slightly different (in the pulmonary artery vs. the thoracic aorta) but similar treatment called **pulmonary artery balloon counterpulsation (PABC),** which is helpful in treating right ventricular and biventricular failure unresponsive to inotropic drugs and the intra-aortic balloon pump alone.[89]

Temporary Left Ventricular Assist Devices

Patients awaiting heart transplantation, or those in whom ventricular function is expected to return, occasionally benefit from prosthetic devices that consist of a flexible polyurethane blood sac and diaphragm placed within a rigid case outside of the body (Fig. 4–16). Pulses of compressed carbon dioxide from a pneumatic drive line are delivered between the rigid case and the diaphragm and provide the force necessary to eject blood that has traveled to the prosthetic device via a cannula inserted into the left ventricle through a Dacron graft into the ascend-

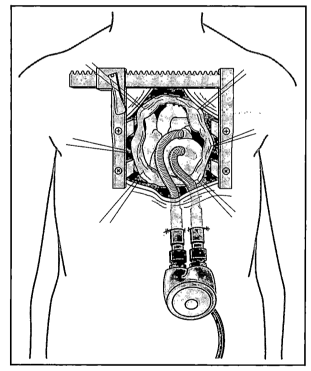

Figure 4–16.

Left ventricular assist device. The left ventricular assist device provides myocardial assistance until heart transplantation or corrective measures are taken.

ing aorta and finally to the periphery. This device can handle "almost the total left heart output,"[136] which provides rest or assistance to impaired myocardium.

A fully implanted left ventricular assist device, similar to the previously discussed prosthetic device, that requires no external machinery has been developed.[176] This device, manufactured by the Novacor Corporation, "has an internal computer that serves as a miniaturized controller, with electrical power supplied by a wire buried beneath the skin around the waist"[176] and is activated by inducing a gentle current through the skin. This allows the patient mobility and almost totally eliminates the risk of infection, which is common with the pneumatic-driven devices.

Surgical Treatments Utilized in Congestive Heart Failure and Cardiac Muscle Dysfunction

Reparative, reconstructive, excisional, and ablative surgeries are sometimes performed in the treatment of CHF and CMD. Reparative procedures correct cardiac malfunctions such as ventricular septal defect, atrial septal defect, and mitral stenosis, and frequently improve cardiac hemodynamics, resulting in improved cardiac performance. Coronary artery bypass graft surgery is probably the most common reconstructive surgery because myocardial ischemia and infarction are the primary causes of CMD and CHF.[175] Its effects are often profound, improving cardiac muscle function and eliminating CHF. Reconstruction of incompetent heart valves is also common.[132] Excisional procedures, in patients with atrial **myxomas** (tumors) and large left ventricles, are employed less often. The excision of a tumor or **aneurysm** is occasionally performed, and the excised area is replaced with Dacron patches.[132] Ablative procedures are also used less frequently, but for patients with persistent and symptomatic **Wolff-Parkinson-White** syndrome or intractable ventricular tachycardia, ablation (via laser or cryotherapy, etc.) of the reentry pathways appears to be very therapeutic.[132] The surgical implantation of automatic implantable defibrillators has become increasingly common and also appears to be of great therapeutic value

for those with ventricular tachycardia that is unresponsive to medications and ablative procedures.[132]

Left Ventricular Muscle Flaps. Although somewhat unusual, the use of muscle flaps (cardiomyoplasty), usually dissected from the latissimus or trapezius muscle, may be an alternative treatment for a limited number of patients with severe CMD and CHF.[176] The muscle flap is wrapped around the left ventricle and attached to a pacemaker, which stimulates the flap to contract, thus contracting the left ventricle. Many years of animal research have provided procedural treatment protocols and have resulted in the use of muscle flap techniques in approximately 12 human subjects who apparently "carry on a reasonably normal life with adequate exercise tolerance."[176]

The major problem with the use of muscle flaps is muscle fatigue, because skeletal muscle, unlike cardiac muscle, does not have the ability to contract continuously. However, it has been demonstrated that skeletal muscle, after careful training and conditioning, "could adapt itself and assume the functions of the cardiac muscle."[176] This is an area in which physical therapy has the potential to make significant contributions, but further investigation is needed.

Cardiac Transplantation. Cardiac transplantation is the last treatment effort for a patient with CHF and CMD because "potential recipients of cardiac transplants must have end-stage heart disease with severe heart failure and a life expectancy of less than one year."[136] Heart transplantation can be **heterologous** (or xenograft—from a nonhuman primate) or more commonly **homologous** (or allograft—from another human).[136] **Orthotopic** homologous cardiac transplantation is performed by removing the recipient's heart, leaving the posterior walls of the atria with their venous connections in place on which the donor's atria are sutured. In heterotopic homologous cardiac transplantation, the recipient's heart is left intact and the donor heart is placed in parallel, with anastomoses between the two right atria, pulmonary arteries, left atria, and aorta. Heterotopic heart transplantation may be preferable to orthotopic transplantation because if the donor heart is rejected (a primary

TABLE 4-11. Relative Contraindications to Exercise Training

Resting HR > 130 bpm, < 40 bpm

Resting SBP > 180 mm Hg
   DBP > 100 mm Hg

Any recent ECG change

Electrolyte abnormalities (e.g., hypokalemia or hyperkalemia)

Easily provoked angina or nocturnal angina

Extreme dyspnea (resting respiratory rate > 35 breaths/min)

Profound fatigue

Mental confusion

Hemoglobin < 8 gm/100 ml, hematocrit < 26%

Frequent arrhythmias (premature ventricular contractions, rapid atrial fibrillation)

Acute ventricular aneurysm

Moderate-to-severe valvular heart disease (e.g., aortic stenosis and/or insufficiency, and mitral stenosis and/or insufficiency)

Acute systemic illness or fever > 100°F

Profound and debilitating musculoskeletal, neuromuscular, or rheumatoid disorders

Pulmonary artery pressure > 35 mm Hg

HR, heart rate; SBP, systolic blood pressure; DBP, diastolic blood pressure; ECG, electrocardiogram; bpm, beats per minute.

complicating factor, as are infection and nephrotoxicity secondary to vigorous immunosuppression), the presence of the patient's own heart may improve the likelihood of survival.[136] However, orthotopic heart transplantation is most commonly performed.

A more complete description of cardiac transplantation is provided in Chapter 10, but in summary, "in the absence of rejection, the transplanted heart, which is denervated and lacks autonomic neural control, exhibits normal contractility and contractile reserve . . . ," and "as a consequence of this near-normal circulatory response, the transplanted heart permits excellent functional and social and vocational rehabilitation in 90 percent of long-term survivors."[136]

Proper Levels of Physical Activity

Historically, physical activity was restricted in persons with CHF.[136] Patients were commonly confined to their home and often to a bed or chair. Patients with severe CHF are often unable to do little more than sit in a bed or chair, but the use of properly prescribed exercise training may have a profound impact on their quality of life (Tables 4-11 to 4-13).

EXERCISE TRAINING IN PERSONS WITH CONGESTIVE HEART FAILURE

Historical Perspective

Until recently, the diagnosis of CHF was typically a contraindication for participation in a car-

TABLE 4-12. Absolute Contraindications to Exercise Training

Resting systolic BP > 200 mm Hg
   diastolic BP > 110 mm Hg

Profound orthostatic hypotension: drop in systolic BP > 20 mm Hg with symptoms

Rapid and prolonged atrial or ventricular arrhythmias (e.g., paroxysmal atrial tachycardia, ventricular tachycardia)

Third-degree heart block

Symptomatic and hemodynamically significant (hypoadaptive systolic BP response to exercise) pericarditis, pericardial effusion, or myocarditis

Acute pulmonary embolism (< 2 days after the event)

Acute thrombophlebitis

Acute hypoglycemia or other metabolic disorder

Digoxin toxicity

Pa_{O_2} < 60

O_2 saturation < 86%

Pending laboratory tests (e.g., myocardial enzymes, hemoglobin, and hematocrit)

Acute MI (< 2 days after an MI)

New ECG signs and symptoms of myocardial ischemia

Any profound symptom (e.g., nausea, dyspnea, lightheadedness)

Suspected or known dissecting aneurysm

Significant emotional distress

Profound CHF with complaints of dyspnea and a resting respiratory rate > 45 breaths/min, as well as other signs or symptoms (Table 4-4)

BP, blood pressure; ECG, electrocardiogram; CHF, congestive heart failure; MI, myocardial infarction.

TABLE 4–13. Measurement of Dyspnea

Magnitude of Effort	Change in Magnitude of Effort
—— Grade 4: *Extraordinary.* Becomes short of breath only with the greatest imaginable effort. No shortness of breath with ordinary effort.	—— −3: *Major Deterioration.* Severe decrease in effort from baseline to avoid shortness of breath. Activities now take 50–100% longer to complete than required at baseline.
—— Grade 3: *Major.* Becomes short of breath with effort distinctly submaximal, but of major proportion. Tasks performed without pause unless the task requires extraordinary effort that may be performed with pauses.	—— −2: *Moderate Deterioration.* Some decrease in effort to avoid shortness of breath, although not as great as in preceding category. There is greater pausing with some activities.
—— Grade 2: *Moderate.* Becomes short of breath with moderate effort. Tasks performed with occasional pauses and requiring longer to complete than the average person might require.	—— −1: *Minor Deterioration.* Does not require more pauses to avoid shortness of breath, but does things with distinctly less effort than previously to avoid breathlessness.
—— Grade 1: *Light.* Becomes short of breath with little effort. Tasks performed with little effort or more difficult tasks performed with frequent pauses and requiring 50–100% longer to complete than the average person might require.	—— 0: *No Change.* No change in effort to avoid shortness of breath.
	—— +1: *Minor Improvement.* Able to do things with distinctly greater effort without shortness of breath. For example, may be able to carry out tasks somewhat more rapidly than previously.
—— Grade 0: *No effort.* Becomes short of breath at rest, while sitting, or lying down.	—— +2: *Moderate Improvement.* Able to do things with fewer pauses and distinctly greater effort without shortness of breath. Improvement is greater than in preceding category, but not of major proportion.
	—— +3: *Major Improvement.* Able to do things with much greater effort than previously with few, if any, pauses. For example, activities may be performed 50–100% more rapidly than at baseline.

(Adapted from Mahler DA, et al: The measurement of dyspnea. Chest 85:6, 1984.)

diac rehabilitation program or, more specifically, for exercise training.[177] In the 1970s and early 1980s, it was not uncommon to exclude patients with heart failure from cardiac rehabilitation, including the acute phase (phase I cardiac rehabilitation).[178] However, several investigations that included patients with CHF discovered that these patients demonstrated marked improvements in exercise tolerance when properly managed.[179–181] One of the earliest studies evaluating the effects of exercise on CHF was designed to evaluate the effects of isosorbide dinitrate on exercise capacity in CHF.[179] The findings suggested that peripheral training effects may occur in patients with CHF who are undergoing exercise training.

Approximately 1 year before the previously mentioned study, a team of physicians and physical therapists studied patients who did not demonstrate signs of significant CHF, but who

had impaired left ventricular function (left ventricular ejection fraction ≤40%).[180] The subjects were able to increase their exercise duration (mean increase of 6.4 to 7.4 min; p = 0.03) without significant change in heart rate or blood pressure at maximal exertion after a 12- to 42-month exercise training program.[180] In addition, resting heart rates were decreased (71 to 63 bpm; p = 0.01) as well as heart rates during standardized submaximal work (117 to 109 bpm; p = 0.05). Finally, cardiac catheterization revealed no change in resting left ventricular ejection fraction, left ventricular end-diastolic pressure, or left ventricular end-diastolic volume, all of which further suggested the importance of peripheral adaptation in skeletal muscle.[180]

These concepts were further evaluated by researchers at Duke University[182] and others[183–188] who investigated the peripheral adaptations to exercise training in patients with CHF. Important findings have included

- the apparent ability of some patients to maintain normal exercise capacity despite a markedly abnormal ejection fraction, suggesting a poor relationship between left ventricular performance (assessed via ejection fraction) and exercise capacity (assessed via Vo_{2max})[182]
- the role of increased pulmonary capillary wedge pressure during exercise in some patients with ventricular dysfunction, producing pulmonary vascular congestion and exercise intolerance because of marked dyspnea[175]
- the prevalence and limitations of anaerobic metabolism during exercise in patients with CHF[187]
- the strong relationship between the dysfunctional heart's chronotropic response and the a-vO_2 difference at maximal exercise to an individual's exercise capacity, again suggesting the importance of peripheral skeletal muscle adaptation.[188]

To further evaluate these findings, Conn and associates investigated the effects of exercise training in 10 patients with severely impaired ventricular function (left ventricular ejection fraction <27%), of whom six had clinical CHF.[181] Exercise training was performed for 4 to 37 months (mean of 13 months), during which no adverse effects occurred and all patients demonstrated a reduction in heart rate during standardized submaximal exercise. In addition, six of the patients demonstrated improved work performance (assessed via treadmill exercise testing), with significant change in group mean MET levels (7.0–8.5; p = 0.05) and **oxygen pulse** (12.8–15.7 ml/beat; p = 0.01).[181]

All of these studies have provided important clinical information about the treatment of patients with CMD and CHF, and much of it has been presented in an informative chapter entitled, "Exercise Training of Patients with Ventricular Dysfunction and Heart Failure."[175] Although somewhat conservative in approach, this 1985 publication appears to have provided the groundwork for more recent recommendations for exercise training in patients with CMD and CHF.[189-190] Since 1985, a number of paramount studies have been performed, of which

the most notable are presented in the following pages.

Current Perspectives

Much of the investigation into the issue of CHF and exercise has focused on one of the earlier findings regarding exercise tolerance and anaerobic metabolism. Many patients with CHF apparently have a lower **anaerobic threshold** than normal individuals, and the resultant anaerobic metabolism becomes the limiting factor (because of lactate acidosis) in exercise performance. The lower anaerobic threshold may be due in part to reduced blood flow to exercising muscles in patients with CHF and is probably the reason that these patients were observed to have a 40% lower exercise capacity than a group of control subjects.[191]

In view of these findings, it seems likely that exercise training should improve the **oxidative capacity** of skeletal muscle, which would reduce lactate production and thereby increase exercise capacity. Three studies have demonstrated such benefits from exercise training in patients with mild-to-moderate CHF (many of whom had cardiomyopathy).[192-194] Perhaps the most detailed study was performed by Sullivan and colleagues, who evaluated the effects of exercise training in patients with chronic heart failure due to left ventricular dysfunction (ejection fraction of 24% ± 10%).[192] Twelve patients with stable symptoms underwent a 4- to 6-month training program of stationary bicycling, walking, jogging, and stair climbing 4 hours per week at approximately 75% of maximal oxygen consumption (Vo_2). After the training period, central hemodynamic and peripheral metabolic adaptations to heart failure were improved, including an increased exercise tolerance and increased Vo_{2max}.[192]

Similar results were also observed in a study of a larger number of subjects (n = 41) with moderately impaired left ventricular function,[193] as well as in a study that utilized **arm ergometry** exercise training alone.[194] Apparently arm ergometry was chosen because of greater exercise demand (heart rate, rate-pressure product, minute ventilation, and oxygen consumption) compared with that observed during legwork. Exercise training on an arm ergometer was performed two times per week for 30 minutes. Each session was performed at an intensity of 90% of maximal work capacity. The results of this study of 11 patients with a mean left ventricular ejection fraction of 30.1 ± 9.5% showed an increased work capacity, peak heart rate, peak rate-pressure product, and left ventricular ejection fraction.[194] An important observation in all of these studies was that no complications occurred during the exercise training programs and no further deterioration of ventricular function occurred.

Another study by Coats and associates evaluated the effects of physical training in 11 patients with chronic heart failure due to ischemic heart disease.[195] The subjects had very low ejection fractions (mean of 19%) and underwent 8 weeks of home-based exercise training (5 days per week for 20 minutes at 70% to 80% of maximum heart rate) and 8 weeks of activity restriction in this physician-blind, random-order, crossover trial. Exercise training increased exercise duration (14.2–16.8 min) and peak oxygen consumption (14.3–16.7 ml/min/kg) and reduced heart rates at submaximal workloads, rate-pressure products, and patient-rated symptom scores.[195] No complications occurred during the home exercise training program, but patients were reassessed every week during the training period. Even though the patients were provided sophisticated pulse-rate monitors and thorough exercise instructions, the absence of complications and the noted improvements in patients with markedly reduced left ventricular ejection fractions are two very important findings. The improvements noted in this study with very low ejection fractions reinforce the earlier findings of Port and co-workers,[182] suggesting a weak relationship between left ventricular ejection fraction alone and exercise performance. More appropriate predictors of exercise performance may be related to left and right ventricular diastolic function, other hemodynamic variables (e.g., pulmonary capillary wedge pressure and left ventricular end-diastolic pressure), or myocardial ischemia.[175,196] These predictors may prove to be

useful in the future but will require more thorough investigation and analysis.

Two other studies have demonstrated the importance of a thorough assessment and reassessment as well as an understanding of each patient's disease process to identify specific criteria necessary to promote training effects.[196,197] Arvan demonstrated that to obtain training effects (for a 12-week training period), patients with left ventricular dysfunction must not exhibit electrocardiographic signs of myocardial ischemia.[196] This finding is not surprising because an individual with left ventricular dysfunction and myocardial ischemia has a poor prognosis from the start.[198] Despite the inability of this group to attain a training effect, routine cardiopulmonary exercise assessments of patients with left ventricular dysfunction *can* better direct medical therapy and reduce risk factors and *possibly* promote training effects if the exercise training program is performed for an appropriate period of time. As in the study by Coats and colleagues, no complications were reported, but 20 patients were excluded for various reasons (e.g., symptomatic CHF, arrhythmias, severe hypertension). The exclusion of these 20 patients suggests that some patients with left ventricular dysfunction may be inappropriate for exercise training but appropriate for exercise assessments to evaluate symptoms, rhythm, and blood pressure response to varying levels of exertion.

A study by Jugdutt and associates identified patients with left ventricular dysfunction who would benefit least from exercise training.[197] If left ventricular dysfunction was below a specific echocardiographic index of contractility and exercise training was performed, left ventricular function actually deteriorated, decreasing the ejection fraction and functional capacity.[197] These results suggest that initial and follow-up echocardiograms as well as thorough cardiopulmonary exercise assessments must be performed to evaluate patient progression or deterioration.

In summary, based on clinical experience[199] and that of others,[192–197] exercise assessments and exercise training in patients with poor left ventricular dysfunction can be (1) done safely if patients are thoroughly assessed,[200] (2) quite beneficial (e.g., improve exercise tolerance and awareness of physical capabilities), and (3) invaluable to the primary physician by providing important information that *completes* the physician's assessment and better directs medical therapy. These concepts are evident in the following quotation:

Exercise training appears to be a therapeutic modality that should be considered for patients with ventricular dysfunction related to coronary artery disease. When patients are carefully selected and when exercise training sessions are conducted under close supervision, life-threatening complications of exercise training are infrequent, and favorable physiologic adaptations, most prominently an increase in functional work capacity, occur in most patients. Although only limited data are available, increased levels of physical activity do not appear to have adverse effects on subsequent cardiac mortality or on ventricular function in patients with ventricular dysfunction. In addition, these patients may derive psychologic benefits from participation in exercise training, and the close medical surveillance available in the content of a supervised exercise program may facilitate better clinical decisions concerning pharmacologic therapy, interpretation of symptoms, or the necessity for and timing of operative procedures.[175]

The end result of such exercise assessments and exercise training is an improved quality of life for this rather unfortunate population of patients.

Guidelines for Exercise Training in Congestive Heart Failure and Cardiac Muscle Dysfunction

The aforementioned studies and a number of others evaluating the effects of exercise training in patients with CHF have demonstrated improvements in exercise tolerance, cardiopulmonary function, and patient symptoms. However, the exercise training was performed in different manners with varying modes, intensities, durations, and frequencies of exercise (Table 4-14). What, therefore, is the optimal method of training patients with CHF and CMD? Rather than arbitrarily choosing a specific intensity, duration, frequency, or even mode of exercise, it is imperative that the patient be screened for cardiovascular and orthopedic complications (not to mention the complications associated with the interrelated pathophysiologies previously discussed) as well as personal desires and goals. In

addition, because the status of patients with CHF and CMD can change daily, exercise prescriptions must also change to more appropriately meet the demands of each patient's bodily functions (see Table 4-13). Although these guidelines seem vague, the ever-changing status of patients with CHF and CMD prevents general exercise training guidelines, but Tables 4-11 and 4-12 should be helpful. In addition, the use of heart rate monitoring to determine exercise intensity may be less reliable for patients with CHF, who often suffer from some degree of renal dysfunction. Reduction in maximal heart rate "may be as much as 20-40 beats per minute"[201] lower in such patients and frequently is accompanied by a blunted systolic blood pressure response, despite elevated plasma norepinephrine levels.[202] These results may be due to autonomic dysfunction, which is known to exist in this population of patients.[203] However, specific exercise training guidelines can be obtained for each *individual* patient with CHF or CMD by performing a simple exercise assessment. Although heart rate monitoring may be less reliable, it still appears to be a common method for exercise prescription, as is evident in the following statement by Williams:

For patients who can exercise to fatigue without adverse hemodynamic effects or symptoms, we calculate the training range as 60 to 80 percent of the increment between the resting heart rate and the maximal heart rate attained, adding back to the resting heart rate. For patients who develop angina, a fall in left ventricular ejection fraction, an elevation of pulmonary capillary wedge pressure, or a fall in systemic arterial pressure during exertion, we attempt to quantitate the heart rate at which such adverse effects first occur and prescribe the upper limit of subsequent exercise at a level 10 bpm below the heart rate at which such evidence for hemodynamic compromise occurs."[175]

In addition, the level of dyspnea appears to correlate well with the training heart rate ranges mentioned by Williams and frequently results in mild-to-moderate dyspnea, which enables patients to carry on a conversation with another comfortably. However, many patients with CMD and CHF are prescribed beta blockers, which often results in little or no change in resting and exercise heart rates. Therefore, the basic guideline of increasing the respiratory rate to a level

TABLE 4–14. Review of Exercise Training Studies of Patients with Cardiac Muscle Dysfunction or Congestive Heart Failure *

		Exercise Training				Training Period	Training Effect
Author	N	Type	Duration	Frequency	Intensity		
Williams, et al.	121	?	?	?	?	2–57 mo	Positive
Cody, et al.	32	?	?	4×/week	?	12 mo	Positive
Jensen, et al.	19	IT, W, J	30–50 min	3×/week	65–86% $\dot{V}O_{2max}$	6 mo	Positive
Verani, et al.	16	W, J, B	60 min	3×/week	80% HR max	3 mo	15 of 16 Positive
Letac, et al.	15	W, R, B, RW, G	60–75 min	3×/week	80% HR max	2 mo	Positive
Sklar, et al.	21	?	?	?	?	3 mo	Positive
Lee, et al.	18	W, J, B	20–45 min	2–6×/week	85% HR max	12–42 mo	Positive
Conn, et al.	10	B, W/J	35–45 min	3–5×/week	70–80% $\dot{V}O_{2max}$	4–37 mo	Positive
Sullivan, et al.	16	W, J, B, SC	60 min	3–5×/week	75% $\dot{V}O_{2max}$	4–6 mo	Positive
Hoffman	41	?	?	3–7×/week	70–85% HR max	4 mo	Positive
Kellerman, et al.	11	AE	?	2×/week	90% subj max wrk cap	36 mo	Positive
Kellerman, et al.	11	C	?	2×/week	2.2–7.5 kcal/min	12 mo	Positive
Coats, et al.	11	B	20 min	5×/week	80% HR max	2 mo	Positive
Arvan,	65	B, W, AE	30–45 min	3×/week	75–85% $\dot{V}O_{2max}$	3 mo	Positive†
Jugdutt, et al.	22	C, SR	11 min	7×/week	?	3 mo	Positive§

* Thirty patients entered the study, but only 16 completed the entire training program. No information on the other 14 patients was provided.
† Except in patients with left ventricular dysfunction and myocardial ischemia (Group II).
‡ Twenty patients were excluded from the initial study group for various reasons (symptomatic CHF, dysrhythmias, severe hypertension).
§ Positive in both groups, but Group II demonstrated a worsening in left ventricular function.
‖ Nine patients who did not complete exercise training were excluded from analysis (secondary to MI, CVA, CABG, and other surgical procedures).

IT, Interval training; W, walking; J, jogging; B, bicycling; R, running; SR, stationary running; RW, rowing; G, gynmastics; W/J, walking/jogging; SC, stair climbing; AE, arm ergometry; C, calisthenics; EF, ejection fraction; LVEDP, left ventricular end-diastolic pressure; PA, pulmonary artery; MI, myocardial infarction; CVA, cardiovascular accident; CABG, coronary artery bypass graft; CHF, congestive heart failure.

Mean EF (%)		Mean LVEDP (mm Hg)		PA Pressure		Complications	
Before Training	After Training	Before Training	After Training	Before Training	After Training	Morbidity	Mortality
8–26 (n = 14)	?	?	?	?	?	?	?
30–49 (n = 23)	?						
51–86 (n = 84)	?						
18	?	?	?	?	?	4 of 32	0
57 ± 13	55 ± 13	?	?	?	?	0	0
52 ± 4	57 ± 4	?	?	?	?	?*	?*
45 ± 12.6	44 ± 13	13.1 ± 8.5	13.7 ± 5.6	?	?	0	0
47	49	?	?	?	?	?	?
35 ± .04	35 ± .06	14.8 ± 3.9	14.9 ± 6.5	24.6 ± 3.3	22.4 ± 3.3	0	0
20	?	?	?	?	?	0	0
24 ± 10	Unchanged	?	?	−14	Unchanged	1 of 16	0
?	?	?	?	?	?	0	0
30 ± 9.52	?	?	?	?	?	0	0
25.5 ± 6.8	?	?	?	?	?	0	0
19	?	?	?	?	?	0	0
I: 55 ± 9	I: 55 ± 7	?	?	?	?	?‡	0‡
II: 29 ± 7	II: 27 ± 7						
I: 59 ± 4	I: 58 ± 7						
II: 43 ± 7	II: 30 ± 5	?	?	?	?	7 of 22	0‖

that allows one to converse comfortably may be an effective method to prescribe exercise training since (1) it has been previously evaluated following a format similar to that in Table 4–13, and (2) it has proved beneficial in treating patients with CHF as well as other patient populations (primarily those with morbid obesity and coronary artery disease).[175] This principle is useful not only for exercise training intensity but also for determining patient appropriateness for entry into a cardiac rehabilitation program.[175] Determining the suitability of patients with CMD for exercise training in cardiac rehabilitation programs appears to depend on "the patient performing any level of exertion, however low, for several minutes without subjective *dyspnea* or *excessive fatigue* and without adverse *hemodynamic effects, arrhythmias,* or *evidence of myocardial ischemia.*"[175] In addition, the key signs and symptoms previously discussed in the section on the assessment of cardiopulmonary status should be employed to prescribe and check the progress of exercise training programs for patients with CMD. The Borg scale of perceived exertion can also be used in a similar manner, with patients instructed to train at a level observed during the exercise assessment to be safe and of adequate training stimulus (Table 4–15).

With this in mind, and to finally summarize, "it is important to emphasize that exercise training of patients with severe ventricular dysfunction does not necessarily involve levels of effort that normal individuals would regard as strenuous. For a person with congestive heart failure whose activities have been limited to sitting in a chair and walking to the bathroom, walking continuously for 15 minutes at 1.5 to 2.0 mph may represent a level of exertion sufficient to induce favorable physiologic adaptations and therefore constitute physical conditioning."[175]

CONCLUSION

Physical therapists have much to offer patients with CMD, and a more sincere effort in understanding and treating these patients undoubtedly will improve their quality of life. The value of the ejection fraction may be overemphasized; the left ventricular end-diastolic volume and pressure as well as clinical signs and symptoms of myocardial ischemia appear to be better predictors of exercise performance and patient prognosis.

The material presented in this chapter clearly demonstrates the widespread occurrence of CMD and its potential implications for physical therapy treatment. Cardiac muscle dysfunction and CHF are disease processes that physical therapists undoubtedly will encounter and be challenged by, as was demonstrated in the study of Cardiac Muscle Dysfunction in Physical Therapy.[35]

CASE STUDIES

CASE 1

This 85-year-old woman with a past medical history of coronary artery bypass graft surgery in 1982 to the right coronary artery and left anterior diagonal, cholecystectomy, hiatal hernia, gastritis, and peptic ulcer disease, was admitted 8/9/90 with angina (a myocardial infarction was ruled out). The patient underwent cardiac catheterization on 8/16/90, which revealed 99% occlusion of

TABLE 4–15. Borg Scale for Ratings of Perceived Exertion			
Original Scale		**Modified Scale**	
		0	Nothing at all
		0.5	Very, very slight
6			
7	Very, very light	1	Very slight
8			
9	Very light	2	Slight
10			
11	Fairly light	3	Moderate
12			
13	Somewhat hard	4	Somewhat severe
14			
15	Hard	5	Severe
16		6	
17	Very hard		
18		7	Very severe
19	Very, very hard		
20		8	
		9	Very, very severe (almost maximal)
		10	Maximal

(From Borg GV. Psychophysical basis of perceived exertion. Med Sci Sports Exerc 14[5]:377–381, 1982. © American College of Sports Medicine.)

the right coronary artery graft, 85% occlusion of the left anterior diagonal graft, 95% stenosis of the circumflex artery, moderate mitral regurgitation, dilated left atrium, inferior hypokinesis, and ejection fraction of approximately 30%. Echocardiographic study revealed severe left ventricular hypertrophy with a small left ventricular chamber size, inferior hypokinesis, calcified mitral valve with moderate mitral regurgitation, abnormal left ventricular compliance (left ventricular stiffness), and a dilated left atrium.

The referral for cardiac rehabilitation was written on 8/11/90, at which time the patient was assessed and complained of left scapular pain that increased with deep breathing (different from previous angina and altered with breathing pattern). Physical examination revealed normal sinus rhythm and slightly decreased breath sounds in the left lower lobe. The patient ambulated approximately 250 feet with an adaptive heart rate and blood pressure response, without angina. The patient continued with twice-daily cardiac rehabilitation, increasing the distance ambulated to 800 feet, and underwent a thallium treadmill stress test on 8/13/90. The patient completed 2 minutes 25 seconds of the modified Bruce protocol (attaining a maximal heart rate of 104 bpm, 67% of the age-predicted maximal heart rate), which was terminated because of leg fatigue. The patient experienced no angina and demonstrated no electrocardiographic (ECG) changes consistent with myocardial ischemia. The thallium scan demonstrated moderately severe stress-induced ischemic change in the inferior and septal areas.

Cardiac rehabilitation was performed 8/14/90 through 8/16/90, during which the patient walked 5 to 10 minutes (500–1000 feet) with adaptive heart rate and blood pressure responses to exercise, without angina. On 8/17/90, while resting in bed, the patient developed severe angina and dyspnea, which required morphine sulfate, nitroglycerin, and heparin, suggesting impending graft occlusion. In view of these findings, coronary artery bypass graft surgery was repeated on 8/20/90, after which the patient developed numerous complications, requiring intra-aortic balloon pump assistance from which weaning was difficult. In addition, the patient experienced a postoperative anterolateral myocardial infarction as a result of a third-degree heart block that decreased the blood supply to the myocardium, respiratory failure that required full ventilatory support, congestive heart failure, and severe abdominal distention.

The patient's status further deteriorated as she became anemic and was unable to maintain adequate nutritional requirements. However, a radiograph on 8/24/90 revealed no evidence of CHF, and ventilatory measurements demonstrated improved pulmonary function. In addition, hemoglobin and hematocrit levels were slightly increased (10.7 and 29.4, respectively). The patient was extubated on 8/25/90 and began ambulation with nursing on 8/26/90, during which she complained of severe abdominal pain and a feeling of increased abdominal swelling. Because of persistent abdominal pain and distention, an exploratory laparotomy was performed on 8/28/90, resulting in resection of the small bowel.

The patient remained on bedrest for 3 days, after which she began ambulating with nursing. On 9/4/90, the patient ambulated 50 feet with physical therapy, during which she complained of severe dyspnea and mild-to-moderate abdominal discomfort. For this reason, physical therapy discontinued ambulation but continued chest physical therapy and bedside exercise to the upper and lower extremities. However, nursing continued to ambulate the patient approximately four times per day despite her complaints of severe shortness of breath and abdominal discomfort. On 9/6/90 immediately after walking, she developed severe abdominal discomfort associated with nausea and vomiting. Nonetheless, that evening, the patient was ambulated 200 feet, walking approximately 15 minutes, at which time she complained of severe abdominal pain; her respiratory rate was noted to be in the high 50s. On 9/7/90, the patient was again walked approximately 75 feet with a walker and maximal assist of three, at which time she became unresponsive. Physician examination at this time revealed severe tachypnea and abdominal distention. On 9/10/90, the patient's status further deteriorated with effusion and atelectasis of the left lung base, ischemic bowel, possible abdominal infection, anemia, and azotemia. She expired on 9/11/90.

Discussion

This case study is an example of an 85-year-old patient who underwent bypass surgery after (1) she remained asymptomatic during prolonged cardiac rehabilitation exercise assessments with adaptive heart rate and blood pressure responses, but somewhat paradoxically developed angina at rest, (2) a thallium treadmill stress test demonstrated moderately severe ischemic change, and (3) a cardiac catheterization revealed occluded grafts to the right coronary artery and left anterior diagonal and high-grade occlusion of the circumflex artery, inferior hypokinesis, and depressed ejection fraction (approximately 30%).

Unfortunately, after bypass surgery was performed, the patient developed numerous complications caused primarily by pump failure and improper exercise training that was not appropriately adjusted to the patient's needs. At no time should a patient be ambulated with moderate-to-severe pain (whatever the location or cause), as it most likely represents a pathologic process (in this case, ischemia of the small intestine). In addition, inappropriate responses to exercise training, such as a rapid heart rate or respiratory rate with minimal exercise, must be reassessed and treated before subsequent exercise is performed, or at least changes must be made in the type of exercise performed. Sitting lower extremity exercise was much more appropriate for this patient, who demonstrated many interrelated pathophysiologic processes that were exacerbated by improper exercise training and ultimately led to her death.

CASE 2

This 64-year-old man was admitted 11/5/90 after returning home from a 5-hour appointment at the university hospital heart transplant clinic. On his return from the clinic, the patient became increasingly short of breath and fatigued and complained of moderate-to-severe chest pain. He reported to the emergency department, where he was diagnosed with moderate to severe CHF and unstable angina, neither of which was present earlier that day during examination at the heart transplant clinic.

The patient's past history included hyperlipidemia; previous coronary artery bypass graft surgeries in 1979 and 1984; multiple percutaneous transluminal coronary angioplasties (a total of 15), including dilation of the vein grafts; ischemic cardiomyopathy; mitral regurgitation; peripheral vascular disease; left carotid endarterectomy; and recent anterior myocardial infarction (9/18/90), at which time the following treatments were provided:

10/15/90   Cardiac rehabilitation initiated (approximately 1 month was required to stabilize the patient), at which time patient ambulated 50 feet with an adaptive heart rate response but demonstrated a decrease in systolic blood pressure in response to exercise and complaints of lightheadedness.

10/16/90   Patient seen twice a day, ambulating 100 to 200 feet with moderate dyspnea and a flat heart rate and systolic blood pressure response.

10/18/90   Patient ambulated 500 feet twice a day, at which time he complained of mild nausea but demonstrated a blunted heart rate and systolic blood pressure response.

10/22/90   Patient ambulated 800 feet but complained of mild+ angina. Nitroglycerin patch increased from 5 to 10 mg/cm.

10/23/90   Patient ambulated 700 feet with adaptive heart rate and systolic blood pressure responses to exercise, without angina.

10/27/90   Patient ambulated 800 feet with adaptive heart rate and systolic blood pressure response, without angina. Patient discharged home with a home exercise program consisting of activities of daily living and home ambulation of 5 to 6 minutes, equivalent to approximately 600 to 800 feet.

Because of the patient's past hospitalization and previous history of diffuse coronary artery disease and ischemic cardiomyopathy with recurrent angina and CHF, he was considered a candidate for cardiac transplantation. However, the 5-hour interview process was apparently more than the patient could tolerate and caused the emergency department admission of 11/5/90. At this time, the patient's hemoglobin was 9.9, hematocrit 25%, BUN 35, and creatinine 1.5. Chest radiograph showed moderately severe CHF, and physical examination revealed jugulovenous distention of 8 centimeters, with distended and rigid abdomen as well as tenderness over his liver. Auscultation identified moderate-to-severe rales throughout most lobes bilaterally and distant heart sounds with a soft S_3. The patient was transferred on 11/8/90 to university hospital for heart transplantation.

11/9–15/90	Preoperative assessments and preparation for heart transplantation while awaiting a donor heart. Cardiac rehabilitation treatments were provided twice a day, consisting of baseline measurements of endurance, muscle strength, and pulmonary function during morning sessions and educational and stress reduction classes during afternoon sessions.
11/16/90	Orthotopic heart transplantation performed.
11/18/90	Patient extubated and physical therapy initiated, consisting of gentle passive range of motion to upper and lower extremities.
11/19/90	Passive range of motion repetitions increased and patient encouraged to perform independent lower extremity movements (5–10 reps) every hour awake.
11/20/90	Sitting active assist range of motion exercises to the upper and lower extremities and standing pregait activities (weight shifting and plantar flexion).
11/21/90	Ambulation in room (starting with several steps and progressing to 12 feet) and upper extremity wand exercises.

11/22/90	Twice a day ambulation in room, 20 to 30 feet, and 2 minutes of stationary bicycle ergometry.
11/23/90	Patient transferred out of isolation, and ambulation in hallway begun (50 feet).
11/28/90	Ambulation in hallway of 500 feet, and bicycle ergometry for 5 minutes twice a day.
12/2/90	Bicycle ergometry for 10 minutes and independent hallway ambulation.
12/4/90	Bicycle ergometry for 15 minutes. Patient discharged home with instructions to begin phase II cardiac rehabilitation in 3 days.

CASE 3

This 69-year-old man had undergone a mitral valve replacement with a porcine Carpentier-Edwards valve in 1983 due to myomatous degeneration. The artificial valve later failed, producing recurrent episodes of CHF and requiring numerous hospitalizations. Cardiac assessment via transesophageal echocardiography revealed moderately severe left ventricular hypertrophy and thickened porcine mitral valve leaflets with "some" prolapse, causing moderate to severe mitral regurgitation with an eccentric jet into the left atrium. Cardiac catheterization showed normal coronary arteries, slightly impaired left ventricular function (ejection fraction of approximately 50%), elevated left ventricular end-diastolic pressure (28 mm Hg), and significant prosthetic mitral insufficiency without stenosis. Soon after a second mitral valve replacement was performed on 5/16/90, he developed adult respiratory distress syndrome (requiring a ventilator and tracheostomy); staphylococcal septicemia; a cerebrovascular accident causing left hemiparesis; and a reduced cardiac output that required an intra-aortic balloon pump, which maintained adequate perfusion except to the distal extremities (right great toe, left second toe, and right index finger). The patient's past medical history otherwise included a bleeding ulcer and left forearm trauma in 1949 that caused a left median nerve injury.

The patient finally recovered and began inpatient cardiac rehabilitation in addition to rehabilitation for his neurologic dysfunction. During inpatient cardiac rehabilitation, the patient progressed slowly at first, performing fewer than 10 repetitions of lower and upper extremity exercises in bed, but soon increased his strength and began to perform the exercises while sitting. He then began ambulating and by week 2 was walking 200 feet without assistive device but with moderate dyspnea. The patient was then discharged from the hospital and referred to outpatient neurologic rehabilitation, at which time the neurologic physical therapist referred the patient to cardiopulmonary physical therapy services because of marked dyspnea during gait training. The patient was evaluated by cardiopulmonary physical therapy services and was observed to be in moderate CHF, which quickly resolved after the primary physician was contacted and the patient's dosage of Lasix was slightly increased. The patient was then followed by outpatient cardiac rehabilitation, where he slowly progressed to a rather independent and active lifestyle. The following data were obtained during exercise assessments and training sessions, which were initially performed three times per week and gradually decreased to once per week after significant improvement was made.

9/26/90

S: Patient reports mild-to-moderate dyspnea during activities of daily living, and community outings have been easier since using the wheelchair, which he frequently pushes (for increased stability) and occasionally sits in (for rest periods).

O: Weight 167.5 (up 1.5 lb since 9/24/90). Meds: potassium 2 qd, Lanoxin 1 qd, Lasix 40 mg bid.
RHR: 80   PHR: 110 (bike); 112 (arms and ambulation)
RBP: 94/70   PBP: 110/70 (bike); 120/70 (arms and ambulation)
Appearance: No peripheral edema or jugular venous distention.

Auscultation: No S_3 or S_4 at rest. Mild-to-moderate rales bilateral lower lobes (left greater than right). Intermittent S_3 during exercise.
Respiratory rate: Resting 34 breaths per minute, exercise 40–46 breaths per minute.
Vital capacity: 420 liters (350 L after exercise).
Bicycle ergometry: 0 watts, 40 rpm × 20 minutes = 20 minutes total.
Arm ergometry: 0 watts × 32 revolutions, brief rest, 0 watts × 78 revolutions.
Ambulation: 1.0–1.2 mph, 0% grade, ×2 minutes without complaint but with ventricular tachycardia versus aberrantly conducted supraventricular beats, because of which ambulation was terminated.

A: Occasional to frequent premature ventricular contractions (couplets and triplets) with one 10- to 12-beat salvo of ventricular tachycardia versus aberrantly conducted beats (Fig. 4–17). Exercise terminated at this point.

P: Case discussed with primary physicians; therapists instructed to continue exercise and to monitor rhythm and symptoms. Information regarding physician discussion and signs and symptoms of ventricular tachycardia relayed to patient and wife.

11/3/90

S: Patient reports slightly increased dyspnea with exercise. No other complaints. Activity is status quo.

O: Weight 172.8. Meds: Unchanged.
RHR: 70   PHR: 110 (bike); 100 (arms); 110 (ambulation).
RBP: 120/70 supine, 90/70 sit, 100/70 stand.
PBP: 120/70 (bike); 124/70 (arms); 110/70 (ambulation).
Appearance: No peripheral edema or jugular venous distention.
Auscultation: Moderate rales lower lobes and middle lobes bilaterally.
Respiratory rate: 28 to 30 breaths per minute.
Vital capacity: 500 liters (400 L after exercise).
Resting oxygen saturation: 94   *Exercise oxygen saturation:* 92–96

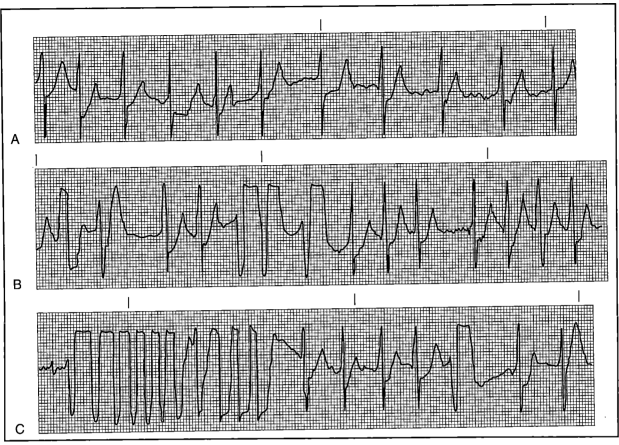

Figure 4-17.

Electrocardiogram obtained during an exercise assessment. The single-lead electrocardiograms obtained during an exercise assessment show controlled atrial fibrillation (A), atrial fibrillation with frequent premature ventricular contractions or aberrantly conducted beats (B), and ventricular tachycardia (C).

Fitron bicycle ergometry: 90 rpm setting (40 rpm) × 10 min, 80 rpm setting (40 rpm) × 5 min = 15 min total.

Arm ergometry: 0 watts (500 revolutions) in 15 minutes.

Treadmill ambulation: 1.0–1.2 mph, 0% × 2 min; 1.2–1.4 mph, 0% × 2 min; 1.6–1.8 mph × 3 min = 7 total minutes. Moderate fatigue and dyspnea.

ECG: Less ectopy.

A: Patient progressing but still demonstrating chronic rales on auscultation of lungs before exercise.

P: Discuss with primary physicians.

Discussion

This case history demonstrates the interrelatedness of all bodily systems and the use of specialized physical therapy services (neurologic and cardiopulmonary) to facilitate the patient's recovery. In addition, it supports the concept of exercise training in patients with chronic CHF who, although demonstrating only mild left ventricular systolic dysfunction, continue to exhibit signs and symptoms of mild-to-moderate CHF. This was undoubtedly the result of left ventricular diastolic dysfunction as evidenced by the elevated left ventricular end-diastolic pressure and the moderately severe left ventricular hypertrophy.

The patient maintained his increased level of exercise tolerance as the sessions were decreased from three times to once per week. However, shortly thereafter, he reported blood in his stool, which was evaluated by his primary physician, who scheduled a lower gastrointestinal tract test the following week. Unfortunately, the patient died suddenly while sleeping before the test could be performed. Five days earlier during his exercise assessment and training session he demonstrated no signs or symptoms suggestive of cardiac, respiratory, hematologic, or intestinal abnormality. It seems likely because of the "sudden" death that the patient died as a result of a fatal arrhythmia.

CASE 4

This 56-year-old man was admitted on 2/22/89 after a cardiac arrest associated with a large anterolateral myocardial infarction that was complicated by recurrent ventricular tachycardia and CHF. Cardiac rehabilitation was initiated on day 3 of hospitalization, during which increased ventricular ectopy and mild angina with minimal activity prompted an increased dosage of antiarrhythmic (quinidine) and antianginal (nitrates) medications. Chest radiograph revealed only slightly less CHF. Subsequent cardiac catheterization on day 5 revealed 100% occlusion of the left anterior descending artery, 60% occlusion of the right coronary artery, and a large dyskinetic anterolateral wall of the left ventricle with an ejection fraction of 25%.

The patient was treated medically with antiarrhythmics, nitrates, diuretics, and low-dose beta blockers, which significantly decreased the ventricular ectopy and CHF and eliminated the angina during days 6 to 10 after the myocardial infarction. The CHF resolved, and a low-level exercise test performed on day 11 revealed rare to occasional premature ventricular contractions without ventricular tachycardia, fair exercise tolerance (9 min of the Sheffield protocol, representing 3 min of the Bruce protocol) to a prede-

termined end point (heart rate of 130 bpm), and hypoadaptive systolic blood pressure response at maximal exercise (from 150/70 to 120/70).

The patient was enrolled in phase II cardiac rehabilitation and participated without angina or significant arrhythmia and with great interest. His primary mode of home exercise training was bicycling for 15 to 30 minutes daily, which he seldom missed, in addition to the three times a week cardiac rehabilitation schedule. The patient's cardiopulmonary responses to exercise improved, and he began demonstrating signs and symptoms of exercise conditioning, including lower resting heart rates, adaptive blood pressures, and significantly lower exercise heart rates during increased workloads, which were tolerated with less dyspnea and fatigue. After 2 months of home exercise training and cardiac rehabilitation, the patient began bicycling with the SCOR Cardiac Cycling Club during Saturday bicycle rides. He began riding on a tandem bicycle with a physical therapist who continuously monitored the patient's symptoms and heart rate (via a Polar Vantage Heart Rate Monitor) and occasional blood pressures during the 5- to 10-mile rides. On several of the weekend bicycle rides the patient wore a 24-hour Holter monitor, which revealed a well-controlled heart rhythm without significant arrhythmias.

After 1 month of bicycling on a tandem and completing a distance of 20 miles without complaint or complication, it was decided by the primary cardiologist and physical therapist that the patient was safe for independent bicycling, which he performed once a week with the cycling club as well as 4 to 5 days per week as home exercise training. This training routine continued for 4 months, during which no complications occurred. The patient lost approximately 50 pounds and was comfortably bicycling 20 to 50 miles, 4 to 5 days per week. His goal was to participate in an annual 100-mile bicycle ride that was scheduled 2 months later. The patient began increasing his bicycling distance (increased duration versus increased intensity) to an average of 30 to 70 miles, 3 to 4 days per week, and did so comfortably without complication. He began the 100-mile event at 6:00 AM and completed the ride 11 hours later. During the ride, the patient's heart rate and symptoms were monitored intermittently, and he took rests as needed.

He continued to ride an average of 20 miles per day, 3 to 4 times per week, after the 100-mile event, even to the day of his death when he suffered a cardiac arrest several hours after a bicycle ride that coincidentally was approximately 1 year after the 100-mile ride. He considered the 100-mile ride one of his greatest accomplishments.

Discussion

This case history demonstrates (1) that proper exercise progression is essential to cardiac rehabilitation; (2) the importance of exercise training in patients with left ventricular dysfunction; (3) the importance of encouraging exercise that is interesting to the patient, allows goals to be set (100-mile bicycle ride), and provides rewards (camaraderie, increased self-esteem); and (4) the enigma and reality of heart disease in a patient who had progressed so far and done so well, yet still suffered from atherosclerotic heart disease and increased likelihood of death secondary to an impaired left ventricular function and a history of cardiac arrest and CHF.

CASE 5

This 86-year-old man was admitted on 11/25/90 with an acute anterolateral myocardial infarction complicated by rapid atrial fibrillation, occasional short runs of ventricular tachycardia, and mild renal failure. His past medical history included a myocardial infarction in 1980 and a transient ischemic attack several years ago. Chest radiograph on admission revealed mild cardiomegaly and moderate increase in pulmonary vasculature, resulting in a diagnosis of moderate CHF. An echocardiogram performed on 11/26/90 revealed right ventricular and right atrial hypertrophy as well as left ventricular hypertrophy, septal and anterior wall hypokinesis, moderate mitral regurgitation with a dilated left atrium, and mild aortic regurgitation.

The patient's CHF, renal failure, and cardiac arrhythmias were further evaluated and treated, and on 12/3/90 cardiac rehabilitation was initiated. The patient's initial treatment consisted of passive and active upper and lower extremity active range of motion in bed while semisupine and then sitting, which was followed by ambulation (with moderate assist of two) of 3 to 4 steps (from bed to commode) with an adaptive heart rate response and blunted systolic blood pressure response to exercise without significant arrhythmia. The afternoon treatment on 12/3/90 consisted of sitting upper and lower extremity active range of motion exercise, followed by 5 feet of ambulation, requiring minimal assist of two, during which the heart rate and rhythm were adaptive but the systolic blood pressure decreased from 124/62 standing to 86/52 during ambulation, at which time the patient complained of dizziness.

On 12/4/90, the patient ambulated 45 feet in 2½ minutes with minimal assist of two, during which he was asymptomatic, and demonstrated an adaptive heart rate response (60–84 bpm) without arrhythmia. Again he experienced a hypoadaptive systolic blood pressure response but of a lesser magnitude (126/74 to 116/64 mm Hg). The same distance was ambulated in the afternoon with a similar response to exercise. On the morning of 12/5/90, the patient ambulated 90 feet in 2½ minutes with an adaptive heart rate response (60–102 bpm) and rhythm but with a 30 mm Hg hypoadaptive systolic blood pressure response and complaints of mild dizziness. That afternoon, the patient ambulated approximately 35 feet, at which time he became very dyspneic and diaphoretic and collapsed to the floor. Electrocardiographic monitoring revealed a very slow normal sinus rhythm of 30 beats per minute and a blood pressure of 60/30. The patient's legs were elevated and atropine was administered. He was further stabilized and the following day underwent cardiac catheterization, which revealed a 90% blockage of the left main coronary artery as well as two 90% occlusions of the left anterior descending, a 50% blockage of the circumflex, and an 80% occlusion in the right coronary artery. In addition, the patient demonstrated significant mitral regurgitation and a mildly enlarged left ventricle with anteroapical akinesis, an elevated left ventricular end-diastolic pressure, and an ejection fraction of 27%.

Discussion

This case history demonstrates the interrelatedness of all the bodily systems (mild renal failure resulting from CHF that was due to the poorly contracting *hypokinetic* septal and anterior walls of the left ventricle from a myocardial infarction) as well as the effects of myocardial ischemia on cardiac performance. As the patient's exercise was increased, his heart was required to perform more work than it was able to do because the severe 90% blockage in the left main coronary artery decreased the blood flow to the heart. As a result, the myocardium received less blood and became ischemic, and its ability to pump (an ischemic CMD) decreased, which is why the systolic blood pressure repeatedly decreased with progressive exercise.

CASE 6

A 29-year-old male with a history of congenital aortic stenosis secondary to a bicuspid valve underwent a valvulotomy (excision of diseased valve) at age 10 because of persistent CHF but recently developed progressive dyspnea and exertional angina. The patient had been evaluated annually since age 10 via echocardiography and exercise interventriculograms. The last evaluation was made approximately 1 year ago, and the patient demonstrated fairly good exercise tolerance without complaint and without a significantly abnormal interventriculogram. However, recently he has developed paroxysmal nocturnal dyspnea and orthopnea and has exhibited a gradual increase in exertional symptoms.

The patient was admitted on 11/26/90 for evaluation of these conditions, and the results of his hospitalization follow.

11/26/90   Physical examination:
Appearance: Mildly apprehensive and dyspneic with a respiratory rate of 32 breaths per minute.
Pulmonary: Few crackles (rales) in both bases.
Cardiac: Precordial thrill; PMI displaced laterally, diffuse and sustained; S_3 with a grade IV/VI holosystolic murmur and III/VI decrescendo diastolic murmur.
Laboratory findings: Prothrombin time 11.8 seconds with a 12-second control.

11/27/90   Two-dimensional echocardiography revealed good left ventricular function but moderate-to-severe aortic stenosis with moderate dilation of the left ventricle.

11/28/90   Cardiac catheterization revealed mild left ventricular hypertrophy with moderate dilation, normal coronary arteries, and moderately severe aortic stenosis with a gradient of 86%.

11/29/90   Aortic valve replacement was performed without complication using a St. Jude prosthetic aortic valve.

12/1/90   Cardiac rehabilitation was initiated, and a chart review revealed a hemoglobin level of 11.1 (reference 14–17.7 g/100 ml) and a hematocrit level of 24.3 (reference 40–52 vol%). White blood cell count and bands were elevated, and temperature was 99.5 degrees F. Radiographic findings revealed clear lungs.

S: The patient complained of moderate fatigue.

O: *Auscultation:* Lungs clear with prosthetic valve sounds; possible distant S_3, no S_4 or murmur heard.
Heart rate: 110 (rest), 120 (exercise).
Blood pressure: 104/70 (rest), 110/70 (exercise).
Ambulation: 300 feet in approximately two minutes.

Electrocardiogram: Sinus tachycardia.

A: The patient tolerated exercise well, considering low hemoglobin and hematocrit levels, infection, and complaints of fatigue before exercising. Heart rate, blood pressure, and rhythm responses were adaptive.

P: Continue twice daily cardiac rehabilitation.

12/3/90   The patient ambulated 800 feet in 6 minutes without complaint and with adaptive heart rate, blood pressure, and rhythm responses to exercise.

12/5/90   Hemoglobin level 13.2, hematocrit level 28.6, white blood cell count and bands decreased to within normal limits, temperature 98.4 degrees F, and radiograph again reveals clear lungs.

Treatment: The patient ambulated on a treadmill at 1 to 1.4 miles per hour, 0% grade, for 5 minutes without complication or arrhythmia but with complaints of moderate fatigue.

12/6/90   The patient ambulated on a treadmill at 1.4 miles per hour, 0% grade, for 6 minutes, and ascended and descended 20 steps with a blunted heart rate and systolic blood pressure response and complaints of moderate fatigue.

Heart rate: 120 (rest), 120 (exercise).

Blood pressure: 100/70 (rest), 100/70 (exercise).

Patient discharged home and instructed to return for occasional cardiopulmonary exercise assessments.

Discussion

This patient was evaluated annually to determine cardiac performance because of a congenital valvular abnormality. These annual assessments were unchanged from previous examinations, but apparently cardiac function rapidly deteriorated within a relatively short period of time and produced signs and symptoms of CHF. This case also presents important hematologic information, such as the role of anticoagulation in patients with valvular abnormalities (prothrombin time at admit was near control) as well as the common reduction of hemoglobin and hematocrit levels in surgically treated patients. This reduction, as well as the increased temperature from infection, produced elevated heart rates and symptoms of fatigue. Although the patient progressed very well during his hospitalization, his limited exercise tolerance (5–6 min of ambulation at 1–1.5 mph, 0% grade) was probably due to his low hemoglobin and hematocrit levels (anemia), which decreased the oxygen-carrying capacity of his blood and produced higher resting and exercise heart rates, thus lowering his threshold for fatigue.

SUMMARY

● The term *cardiac muscle dysfunction* accurately describes the primary cause of pulmonary edema as well as the underlying pathophysiology, which essentially impairs the heart's ability to pump blood or the left ventricle's ability to accept blood.

● Causes of CMD include (1) myocardial infarction or ischemia, (2) cardiomyopathy, (3) cardiac arrhythmias, (4) heart valve abnormalities, (5) pericardial effusion or myocarditis, (6) pulmonary embolus, (7) renal insufficiency, (8) spinal cord injury, (9) congenital abnormalities, and (10) aging.

● Cardiomyopathy, congenital abnormalities, renal insufficiency, and aging are associated more commonly with chronic heart failure, whereas the others tend to cause acute CHF.

● Right-sided or left-sided CHF simply describes which side of the heart is failing, as well as the side initially affected behind which fluid tends to localize.

● Low-output CHF is the description associated with heart failure and is the result of a low cardiac output at rest or during exertion.

● High-output failure usually results from a volume overload.

- The impaired contraction of the ventricles during systole that produces an inefficient expulsion of blood is termed *systolic heart failure*.
- Diastolic heart failure is associated with an inability of the ventricles to accept the blood ejected from the atria.
- Hypertension and coronary artery disease are the most common causes of CMD.
- Cardiac arrhythmias and renal insufficiency can also cause CMD for reasons similar to those of myocardial infarction.
- Cardiomyopathies are classified from a functional standpoint, emphasizing three categories: dilated, hypertrophic, and restrictive.
- Heart valve abnormalities can also cause CMD as blocked or incompetent valves, or both, cause heart muscle to contract more forcefully to expel the cardiac output.
- Injury to the pericardium can cause acute pericarditis, which may progress to pericardial effusion.
- CMD from a pulmonary embolus is the result of elevated pulmonary artery pressures, which dramatically increase right ventricular work.
- Spinal cord injury can also produce CMD because of cervical spinal cord transection, which causes an imbalance between sympathetic and parasympathetic control of the cardiovascular system.
- Congestive heart failure is commonly associated with several characteristic signs and symptoms, including dyspnea, tachypnea, paroxysmal nocturnal dyspnea, orthopnea, hepatomegaly, peripheral edema, weight gain, jugular venous distention, rales, tubular breath sound and consolidation, presence of an S_3 heart sound, sinus tachycardia, and decreased exercise tolerance.
- Proteinuria; elevated urine specific gravity, blood urea nitrogen and creatine levels; and decreased erythrocyte sedimentation rates are associated with CHF.
- Dyspnea is probably the most common finding associated with CHF.
- A rapid respiratory rate at rest, characterized by quick and shallow breaths, is common in patients with CHF.
- The presence of an S_3 indicates a noncompliant left ventricle and occurs as blood passively fills a poorly relaxing left ventricle.
- The retention of sodium and water is due to (1) augmented alpha-adrenergic neural activity; (2) circulating catecholamines; and (3) increased circulating and locally produced angiotensin II, which result in renal vasoconstriction.
- Laboratory findings suggestive of impaired renal function in CHF include increases of BUN as well as blood creatinine levels.
- Pulmonary edema can be cardiogenic or noncardiogenic in origin.
- The most common hematologic abnormality is a secondary polycythemia, which is due to either a reduction in oxygen transport or an increase in erythropoietin production.
- Skeletal muscle abnormalities due to dilated and hypertrophic cardiomyopathies have been reported previously and consistently reveal type I and type II fiber atrophy.
- Severe CMD has the potential to reduce blood flow to the pancreas, which impairs insulin secretion and glucose tolerance.
- The primary malnutrition in CHF is a protein-calorie deficiency, but vitamin deficiencies have also been observed.
- The specific treatments for CHF include restriction of sodium intake, use of medications, and other special measures.
- Many patients with CHF apparently have lower anaerobic thresholds, and the resultant anaerobic metabolism (due to acidosis) becomes the limiting factor in exercise performance.

References

1. The European "Corwin" Study Group. Xamoterol in mild to moderate heart failure: A subgroup analysis of patients with cardiomegaly but no concomitant angina pectoris. Br J Clin Pharmacol 28:67S, 1989.
2. Kannel WB. Epidemiological aspects of heart failure. Cardiol Clin 7:1, 1989.
3. Kannel WB, Belanger AJ. Epidemiology of heart failure. Am Heart J 121:951, 1991.
4. Yancy CW, Firth BG. Congestive heart failure. Dis Mon 34:467, 1988.
5. McKee PA, Castelli WP, McNamara PM, et al. The natural history of congestive heart failure: The Framingham Study. N Engl J Med 26:1441, 1971.
6. Braunwald E. Clinical manifestations of heart failure. In: Braunwald E (ed). Heart Disease: A Textbook of Cardiovascular Medicine. Vol. 1. Philadelphia, WB Saunders, 1988, chap 16.
7. Cheng TO. Cardiac failure in coronary heart disease. Am Heart J 120:396, 1990.
8. Hildner FJ. Pulmonary edema associated with low left ventricular filling pressures. Am J Cardiol 44:1410, 1979.

9. Grossman W, Braunwald E. High-cardiac output states. In: Braunwald E (ed). Heart Disease: A Textbook of Cardiovascular Medicine. Vol. 1. Philadelphia, WB Saunders, 1988, chap 25.

10. Perloff JK. Pregnancy and cardiovascular disease. In: Braunwald E (ed). Heart Disease: A Textbook of Cardiovascular Medicine. Vol. 2. Philadelphia, WB Saunders, 1988, chap. 60.

11. Goldberger JJ, Peled HB, Stroh JA, et al. Prognostic factors in acute pulmonary edema. Arch Intern Med 146:489, 1986.

12. Baigrie RS, Haq A, Morgan CD, et al. The spectrum of right ventricular involvement in inferior wall myocardial infarction. J Am Coll Cardiol 6:1396, 1983.

13. Cintron GB, Hernandez E, Linares E, Aranda JM. Bedside recognition, incidence and clinical course of right ventricular infarction. Am J Cardiol 47:224, 1981.

14. Rabbani LE, Wang PJ, Couper GL, Friedman PL. Time course of improvement in ventricular function after ablation of incessant automatic atrial tachycardia. Am Heart J 121:816, 1991.

15. Holt W, Auffermann W, Wu ST, et al. Mechanism for depressed cardiac function in left ventricular volume overload. Am Heart J 121:531, 1991.

16. Wynne J, Braunwald E. The cardiomyopathies and myocarditides. In: Braunwald E (ed). Heart Disease: A Textbook of Cardiovascular Medicine. Vol. 2. Philadelphia, WB Saunders, 1988, chap 42.

17. Abelmann WH. Classification and natural history of primary myocardial disease. Prog Cardiovasc Dis 27:73, 1984.

18. Zarich SW, Nesto RW. Diabetic cardiomyopathy. Am Heart J 118:1000, 1989.

19. Jermendy G, Khoor S, Koltai MZ, Pogatsa G. Left ventricular diastolic dysfunction in type 1 (insulin-dependent) diabetic patients during dynamic exercise. Cardiology 77:9, 1990.

20. Caforio ALP, Rossi B, Risaliti R, et al. Type 1 fiber abnormalities in skeletal muscle of patients with hypertrophic and dilated cardiomyopathy: Evidence of subclinical myogenic myopathy. J Am Coll Cardiol 14:1464, 1989.

21. Lipkin DP, Jones DA, Round JM, Poole-Wilson PA. Abnormalities of skeletal muscle in patients with chronic heart failure. Int J Cardiol 18:187, 1988.

22. Poole-Wilson PA. The origin of symptoms in patients with chronic heart failure. Eur Heart J 9(suppl H):49, 1988.

23. Braunwald E. Valvular heart disease. In: Braunwald E (ed). Heart Disease: A Textbook of Cardiovascular Medicine. Vol. 2. Philadelphia, WB Saunders, 1988, chap 33.

24. Goldhaber SZ, Braunwald E. Pulmonary embolism. In: Braunwald E (ed). Heart Disease: A Textbook of Cardiovascular Medicine. Vol. 2. Philadelphia, WB Saunders, 1988, chap 47.

25. MacKenzie CF, Shin B, Krishnaprasad D, et al. Assessment of cardiac and respiratory function during surgery on patients with acute quadriplegia. J Neurosurg 62:843, 1985.

26. Woolman L. The disturbance of circulation in traumatic paraplegia in acute and late stages. A pathological study. Paraplegia 2:213, 1965.

27. Meyer GA, Berman IR, Doty DB, et al. Hemodynamic

28. Bellamy R, Pitts FW, Stauffer ES. Respiratory complications in traumatic quadriplegia. Analysis of 20 years' experience. J Neurosurg 39:596, 1973.

29. Friedman WF. Congenital heart disease in infancy and childhood. In: Braunwald E (ed). Heart Disease: A Textbook of Cardiovascular Medicine. Vol. 1. Philadelphia, WB Saunders, 1988, chap 30.

30. Borow KM, Braunwald E. Congenital heart disease in the adult. In: Braunwald E (ed). Heart Disease: A Textbook of Cardiovascular Medicine. Vol. 1. Philadelphia, WB Saunders, 1988, chap 31.

31. Moser M. Physiological differences in the elderly. Are they clinically important? Eur Heart J 9(suppl D):55, 1988.

32. Weisfeldt ML, Lakatta EG, Gerstenblith G. Aging and cardiac disease. In: Braunwald E (ed). Heart Disease: A Textbook of Cardiovascular Medicine. Vol. 2. Philadelphia, WB Saunders, 1988, chap 50.

33. Cahalin LP, Wadsworth JB, Fisher DS. Cardiac muscle dysfunction in physical therapy. Cardiopulmonary Phys Ther J 2:15, 1991.

34. Ingram RH Jr, Braunwald E. Pulmonary edema: Cardiogenic and noncardiogenic. In Braunwald E (ed). Heart Disease: A Textbook of Cardiovascular Medicine. Vol. 1. Philadelphia, WB Saunders, 1988, chap 18.

35. Wasserman K, Hansen JE, Sue DY, Whipp BJ. Principles of Exercise Testing and Interpretation. Philadelphia, Lea & Febiger, 1987.

36. Moe GW, Canepa-Anson R, Howard RJ, Armstrong PW. Response of atrial natriuretic factor to postural change in patients with heart failure versus subjects with normal hemodynamics. J Am Coll Cardiol 16:599, 1990.

37. Killip T, Kimball JT. Treatment of myocardial infarction in a coronary care unit. A two-year experience with 250 patients. Am J Cardiol 20:457, 1967.

38. Andreoli KG, Fowkes VH, Zipes DP, Wallace AG. Comprehensive Cardiac Care. 4th ed. St. Louis, CV Mosby, 1979.

39. Braunwald E. The physical examination. In: Braunwald E (ed). Heart Disease: A Textbook of Cardiovascular Medicine. Vol. 1. Philadelphia, WB Saunders, 1988, chap 2.

40. Chezner MA. Cardiac auscultation: Heart sounds. Cardiology in Practice Sept/Oct:141, 1984.

41. Stevenson LW, Brunken RC, Belil D, et al. Afterload reduction with vasodilators and diuretics decreases mitral regurgitation during upright exercise in advanced heart failure. J Am Coll Cardiol 15:174, 1990.

42. Pastan SO, Braunwald E. Renal disorders and heart disease. In: Braunwald E (ed). Heart Disease: A Textbook of Cardiovascular Medicine. Vol. 2. Philadelphia, WB Saunders, 1988, chap 59.

43. Criteria Committee, New York Heart Association, Inc. Diseases of the Heart and Blood Vessels. Nomenclature and Criteria for Diagnosis. 6th ed. Boston, Little, Brown, 1964.

44. Sullivan MJ, Cobb FR. The anaerobic threshold in chronic heart failure. Relation to blood lactate, ventilatory basis, reproducibility, and response to exercise training. Circulation 81(suppl II):47, 1990.

45. Tavazzi L, Gattone M, Corra U, De Vito F. The anaer-

obic index: Uses and limitations in the assessment of heart failure. Cardiology 76:357, 1989.

46. Wasserman K, Beaver WL, Whipp BJ. Gas exchange theory and the lactic acidosis (anaerobic) threshold. Circulation 81(suppl II):14, 1990.

47. Koike A, Itoh H, Taniguchi K, Marumo F. Relationship of anaerobic threshold (AT) to AVO_2/WR in patients with heart disease. Circulation 78(suppl II):624, 1988 (abstract).

48. Wenger NK. Left ventricular dysfunction, exercise capacity and activity recommendations. Eur Heart J 9(suppl F):63, 1988.

49. Braunwald E. Assessment of cardiac function. In: Braunwald E (ed). Heart Disease: A Textbook of Cardiovascular Medicine. Vol. 1. Philadelphia, WB Saunders, 1988, chap 15.

50. Gurry MK, Freedson PS, Kline G, et al. A comparative analysis of an automated noninvasive estimate of cardiac output with Direct Fick and thermodilution techniques. J Cardiopulmonary Rehabil 9:122, 1989.

51. Auchincloss JH, Gilbert R, Morales R, Peppi D. Reduction of trial and error in the equilibrium rebreathing cardiac output method. J Cardiopulmonary Rehabil 9:87, 1989.

52. Davis CC, Jones NL, Sealey BJ. Measurements of cardiac output method in seriously ill patients using a CO_2 rebreathing method. Chest 73:167, 1978.

53. Franciosa JA. Evaluation of the CO_2 rebreathing cardiac output method in seriously ill patients. Circulation 55:449, 1977.

54. Parmley WW. Hemodynamic monitoring in acute ischemic disease. In: Fishman AP (ed). Heart Failure. New York, McGraw-Hill, 1978, p 114.

55. Braunwald E, Sonnenblick EH, Ross J Jr. Mechanisms of cardiac contraction and relaxation. In: Braunwald E (ed). Heart Disease: A Textbook of Cardiovascular Medicine. Vol. 1. Philadelphia, WB Saunders, 1988, chap 13.

56. American Heart Association. Textbook of Advanced Cardiac Life Support. Dallas, American Heart Association, 1987.

57. Cruz FES, Cheriex EC, Smeets JL, et al. Reversibility of tachycardia-induced cardiomyopathy after cure of incessant supraventricular tachycardia. J Am Coll Cardiol 16:739, 1990.

58. Braunwald E. Pathophysiology of heart failure. In: Braunwald E (ed). Heart Disease: A Textbook of Cardiovascular Medicine. Vol. 1. Philadelphia, WB Saunders, 1988, chap 14.

59. Perloff JK. Pathogenesis of hypertrophic cardiomyopathy: Hypothesis and speculation. Am Heart J 101:219, 1981.

60. Silverman KJ, Hutchins GM, Weiss JL, Moore GW. Catenoidal shape of the interventricular septum in idiopathic hypertrophic subaortic stenosis: Two dimensional echocardiographic confirmation. Am J Cardiol 49:27, 1982.

61. Laragh JH. Atrial natriuretic hormone, the renin-aldosterone axis, and blood pressure-electrolyte homeostasis. N Engl J Med 313:1330, 1985.

62. Skorecki KL, Brenner BM. Body fluid homeostasis in congestive heart failure and cirrhosis with ascites. Am J Med 72:323, 1982.

63. Hostetter TH, Pfeffer JM, Pfeffer MA, et al. Cardio-renal hemodynamics and sodium excretion in rats with myocardial infarction. Am J Physiol 245:H98, 1983.

64. Fillmore SJ, Giumaraes AC, Scheidt AC, Killip T. Blood gas changes and pulmonary hemodynamics following acute myocardial infarction. Circulation 45:583, 1972.

65. Feldman AM, Bristow MR. The beta-adrenergic pathway in the failing human heart: Implications for inotropic therapy. Cardiology 77(suppl I):1, 1990.

66. Lefkowitz RJ, Caron MG. Adrenergic receptors: Models for the study of receptors coupled to guanine nucleotide regulatory proteins. J Biol Chem 263:4993, 1988.

67. Exton JH. Molecular mechanisms involved in alpha-adrenergic responses. Mol Cell Endocrinol 23:233, 1981.

68. Scholz A, Schaefer B, Schmitz W, et al. Alpha$_1$-mediated positive inotropic effect and inositol triphosphate increase in mammalian heart. J Pharmacol Exp Ther 245:327, 1988.

69. Gilman AG. G proteins: Transducers of receptor-generated signals. Ann Rev Biochem 56:615, 1987.

70. Bristow MR. The beta-adrenergic receptor. Configuration, regulation, mechanism of action. Postgrad Med Feb 29:19, 1988.

71. Bristow MR, Minobe W, Rasmussen R, et al. Alpha$_1$-adrenergic receptors in the non-failing and failing human heart. J Pharmacol Exp Ther 247:1039, 1989.

72. Bristow MR, Ginsburg R, Umans V, et al. Beta$_1$- and beta$_2$-adrenergic receptor subpopulations in nonfailing and failing human ventricular myocardium: Coupling of both receptor subtypes to muscle contraction and selective beta$_1$-receptor down-regulation in heart failure. Circ Res 59:297, 1986.

73. Fowler MB, Laser JA, Hopkins GL, et al. Assessment of the beta-adrenergic receptor pathway in the intact failing human heart: Progressive receptor down-regulation and subsensitivity to agonist response. Circulation 74:1290, 1986.

74. Bristow MR, Hershberger RE, Port D, et al. Beta$_1$ and beta$_2$ adrenergic receptor mediated adenylate cyclase stimulation in non-failing and failing human ventricular myocardium. Mol Pharmacol 35:295, 1989.

75. Feldman MA, Copelas L, Gwathney JK, et al. Deficient production of cyclic AMP: Pharmacologic evidence of an important cause of contractile dysfunction in patients with end-stage heart failure. Circulation 75:331, 1987.

76. Feldman AM, Cates AE, Bristow MR, et al. Altered expression of alpha-subunits of G proteins in failing human hearts. J Mol Cell Cardiol 21:359, 1989.

77. Rosenthal DS, Braunwald E. Hematological-oncological disorders and heart disease. In: Braunwald E (ed). Heart Disease: A Textbook of Cardiovascular Medicine. Vol. 2. Philadelphia, WB Saunders, 1988, chap 55.

78. Jandl JH. Blood: Textbook of Hematology. Boston, Little, Brown, 1987.

79. Shafiq SA, Sande MA, Carruthers RR, et al. Skeletal muscle in idiopathic cardiomyopathy. J Neurol Sci 15:303, 1972.

80. Wilson JR, Fink L, Maris J, et al. Evaluation of energy metabolism in skeletal muscle of patients with heart failure with gated phosphorus-31 nuclear magnetic resonance. Circulation 71:57, 1985.

81. Isaacs H, Muncke G. Idiopathic cardiomyopathy and skeletal muscle abnormality. Am Heart J 90:767, 1975.

82. Dunnigan A, Pierpont ME, Smith SA, et al. Cardiac and skeletal myopathy associated with cardiac dysrhythmias. Am J Cardiol 53:731, 1984.

83. Dunnigan A, Staley NA, Smith SA, et al. Cardiac and skeletal muscle abnormalities in cardiomyopathy: Comparison of patients with ventricular tachycardia or congestive heart failure. J Am Coll Cardiol 10:608, 1987.

84. Smith ER, Heffernan LP, Sangalang VE, et al. Voluntary muscle involvement in hypertrophic cardiomyopathy: A study of 11 patients. Ann Intern Med 85:566, 1976.

85. Hootsmans WJM, Meerschwam IS. Electromyography in patients with hypertrophic obstructive cardiomyopathy. Neurology 21:810, 1971.

86. Meerschwam IS, Hootsmans WJM. An electromyographic study in hypertrophic obstructive cardiomyopathy. In: Wolsterholme GEW, O'Connor M, London J, Churchill A (eds). Hypertrophic Obstructive Cardiomyopathy. Ciba Foundation Study Group No. 37. New York, Wiley, 1971.

87. Przybosewki JZ, Hoffman HD, Graff AS, et al. A study of family with inherited disease of cardiac and skeletal muscle. Part 1: Clinical electrocardiographic, echocardiographic, hemodynamic, electrophysiological and electron microscopic studies. S Afr Med J 59:363, 1981.

88. Lochner A, Hewlett RH, O'Kennedy A, et al. A study of a family with inherited disease of cardiac and skeletal muscle. Part 2: Skeletal muscle morphology and mitochondrial oxidative phosphorilation. S Afr Med J 59:453, 1981.

89. Pasternak RC, Braunwald E, Sobel BE. Acute myocardial infarction. In: Braunwald E (ed). Heart Disease: A Textbook of Cardiovascular Medicine. Vol. 2. Philadelphia, WB Saunders, 1988, chap 38.

90. Braunwald E, Sobel BE. Coronary blood flow and myocardial ischemia. In: Braunwald E (ed). Heart Disease: A Textbook of Cardiovascular Medicine. Vol. 2. Philadelphia, WB Saunders, 1988, chap 37.

91. Neely JR, Rovetto MJ, Whitmer JT, Morgan HE. Effects of ischemia on ventricular function and metabolism in the isolated working rat heart. Am J Physiol 225:651, 1973.

92. Lefer AM. Vascular mediators in ischemia and shock. In: Cowley RA, Trump BF (eds). Pathophysiology of Shock, Anoxia, and Ischemia. Baltimore, Williams & Wilkins, 1982.

93. Lefer AM. Pharmacologic and surgical modulation of myocardial depressant factor formation and action during shock. Prog Clin Biol Res 111:111, 1983.

94. Williams GH, Braunwald E. Endocrine and nutritional disorders and heart disease. In: Braunwald E (ed). Heart Disease: A Textbook of Cardiovascular Medicine. Vol. 2. Philadelphia, WB Saunders, 1988, chap 58.

95. Yui Y, Fujiwara H, Mitsui H, et al. Furosemide-induced thiamine deficiency. Jpn Circ J 42:744, 1978.

96. Bautista J, Rafel E, Martinez A, et al. Familial hypertrophic cardiomyopathy and muscle carnitine deficiency. Muscle Nerve 13:192, 1990.

97. Eschbach JW, Adamson JW. Anemia of end-stage renal disease (ESRD). Kidney Int 28:1, 1985.

98. Eschbacch JW, Egrie JC, Downing MR, et al. Correction of the anemia of end-stage renal disease with recombinant human erythropoietin: Results of a combined phase I and II clinical trial. N Engl J Med 316:73–78, 1987.

99. Wilson L, Felsenfeld A, Drezner MK, Llach F. Altered divalent ion metabolism in early renal failure: Role of 1,25(OH)$_2$D. Kidney Int 27:565, 1985.

100. Madsen S, Olgaard K, Ladefoged J. Suppressive effect of 1,25-dihydroxyvitamin D$_3$ on circulating parathyroid hormone in renal failure. J Clin Endocrinol Metab 53:823, 1981.

101. Klahr S. Nonexcretory functions of the kidney. In: Klahr S (ed). The Kidney and Body Fluids in Health and Disease. New York, Plenum Medical Publishing, 1983.

102. Rudman D, Feller AG. Liver disease. In: Brown ML (ed). Present Knowledge in Nutrition. Washington, DC, International Life Sciences Institute-Nutrition Foundation, 1990, chap 46.

103. Fischer JE, Baldessarini R. False neurotransmitters and hepatic failure. Lancet 2:75, 1971.

104. Fischer JE, Funovics JM, Aguirre A, et al. The role of plasma amino acids in hepatic encephalopathy. Surgery 78:276, 1975.

105. Mitchell SC, Korones SB, Berendes HW. Congenital heart disease in 56,109 births. Incidence and natural history. Circulation 43:323, 1971.

106. Brandfonbrener M, Landowne M, Shock NW. Changes in cardiac output with age. Circulation 12:557, 1955.

107. Strandell T. Circulatory studies on healthy old men. Acta Med Scand 175:1, 1964.

108. Conway J, Wheeler R, Sannerstedt R. Sympathetic nervous activity during exercise in relation to age. Cardiovasc Res 5:577, 1971.

109. Rodeheffer RJ, Gerstenblith G, Becker LC, et al. Exercise cardiac output is maintained with advancing age in healthy human subjects: Cardiac dilatation and increased stroke volume compensate for a diminished heart rate. Circulation 69:203, 1984.

110. Sjorgen AL. Left ventricular wall thickness determined by ultrasound in 100 subjects without heart disease. Chest 60:341, 1971.

111. Gerstenblith G, Fleg JL, Becker LC, et al. Maximum left ventricular filling rate in healthy individuals measured by gated blood pool scans: Effect of age. Circulation 68:III–101, 1983.

112. Capasso JM, Malhotra A, Remily R, et al. Effects of age on mechanical and electrical performance of rat myocardium. Am J Physiol 245:H72, 1983.

113. Lakatta EG, Yin FCP. Myocardial aging: Functional alterations and related cellular mechanisms. Am J Physiol 242:H927, 1982.

114. Bhatnagar GM, Walford GD, Beard ES, et al. ATPase activity and force production in myofibrils and twitch characteristics in intact muscle from neonatal, adult, and senescent rat myocardium. J Mol Cell Cardiol 16:203, 1984.

115. Wei JY, Spurgeon HA, Lakatta EG. Excitation-contraction in rat myocardium: Alterations with adult aging. Am J Physiol 246:H784, 1984.

116. Spurgeon HA, Steinbach MF, Lakatta EG. Chronic exercise prevents characteristic age-related changes in rat cardiac contraction. Am J Physiol 244:H513, 1983.

117. Spurgeon HA, Thorne PR, Yin FCP, et al. Increased dynamic stiffness of trabeculae carneae from senescent rats. Am J Physiol 232:H373, 1977.

118. Yin FCP, Spurgeon HA, Weisfeldt ML, Lakatta EG. Mechanical properties of myocardium from hypertrophied rat hearts. A comparison between hypertrophy induced by senescence and by aortic banding. Circ Res 46:292, 1980.
119. Orchard CH, Lakatta EG. Intracellular calcium transients and developed tensions in rat heart muscle. A mechanism for the negative interval-strength relationship. J Gen Physiol 86:627, 1985.
120. Wenger NK. Exercise for the elderly: Highlights of preventive and therapeutic aspects. J Cardiopulmonary Rehabil 9:9, 1989.
121. Oertel G. Morphometric analysis of normal skeletal muscles in infancy, childhood and adolescence. An autopsy study. J Neurol Sci 88:303, 1988.
122. Petrella RJ, Cunningham DA, Vandervoort AA, Paterson DH. Comparison of twitch potentiation in the gastrocnemius of young and elderly men. Eur J Appl Physiol 58:395, 1989.
123. Kruszynska YT, Petranyi G, Alberti G. Decreased insulin sensitivity and muscle enzyme activity in elderly subjects. Eur J Clin Invest 18:493, 1988.
124. Cardellach F, Galofre J, Cusso R, Urbano-Marquez A. Decline in skeletal muscle mitrochondrial respiration chain function with ageing. Lancet 2:44, 1989 (letter).
125. Cleroux J, Giannattasio C, Grassi G, et al. Effects of ageing on the cardiopulmonary receptor reflex in normotensive humans. J Hypertens 6(suppl):S141, 1988.
126. Caskey CI, Zerhouni EA, Fishman EK, Rahmouni AD. Aging of the diaphragm: A CT study. Radiology 171:385, 1989.
127. Melichna J, Zauner CW, Havlickova L, et al. Morphologic differences in skeletal muscle with age in normally active human males and their well-trained counterparts. Hum Biol 62:205, 1990.
128. Coggan AR, Spina RJ, Rogers MA, et al. Histochemical and enzymatic characteristics of skeletal muscle in master athletes. J Appl Physiol 68:1894, 1990.
129. White PD. Exercise for the elderly. JAMA 165:70, 1957.
130. Subramanyan R, Manchanda SC, Nyboer J, Bhatia ML. Total body water in congestive heart failure. A pre and post treatment study. J Assoc Physicians India 28:257, 1980.
131. American College of Cardiology/American Heart Association Task Force. Guidelines for the early management of patients with acute myocardial infarction. J Am Coll Cardiol 16:249, 1990.
132. Kirklin JW, Blackstone EH, Kirklin JK. Cardiac surgery. In: Braunwald E (ed). Heart Disease: A Textbook of Cardiovascular Medicine. Vol. 2. Philadelphia, WB Saunders, 1988, p 1663.
133. Breisblatt WM, Stein KL, Wolfe CJ, et al. Acute myocardial dysfunction and recovery: A common occurrence after coronary bypass surgery. J Am Coll Cardiol 15:1261, 1990.
134. Klein LW, Kramer BL, Howard E, Lesch M. Incidence and clinical significance of transient creatine kinase elevations and the diagnosis of non-Q wave myocardial infarction associated with coronary angioplasty. J Am Coll Cardiol 17:621, 1991.
135. Fischell TA, Derby G, Tse TM, Stadius ML. Coronary artery vasoconstriction routinely occurs after percutaneous transluminal coronary angioplasty. A quantitative arteriographic analysis. Circulation 78:1323, 1988.
136. Smith TW, Braunwald E, Kelly RA. The management of heart failure. In: Braunwald E (ed). Heart Disease: A Textbook of Cardiovascular Medicine. Vol. 1. Philadelphia, WB Saunders, 1988, chap 17.
137. Parmley WW. Should digoxin be the drug of first choice after diuretics in chronic congestive heart failure? J Am Coll Cardiol 12:265, 1988.
138. Pitt B. Antagonists viewpoint. J Am Coll Cardiol 12:271, 1988.
139. Mulrow CD, Feussner JR, Velez R. Reevaluation of digitalis efficacy. Ann Intern Med 101:113, 1984.
140. Arnold SB, Byrd RC, Meister W, et al. Long-term digitalis therapy improves left ventricular function in heart failure. N Engl J Med 303:1443, 1980.
141. Lee DC-S, Johnson RA, Bingham JB, et al. Heart failure in outpatients. A randomized trial of digoxin versus placebo. N Engl J Med 306:699, 1982.
142. Gheorghiade M, St Clair J, St Clair C, Beller GA. Hemodynamic effects of intravenous digoxin in patients with severe heart failure initially treated with diuretics and vasodilators. J Am Coll Cardiol 9:849, 1987.
143. Guyatt GH, Sullivan MJJ, Fallen EL, et al. A controlled trial of digoxin in congestive heart failure. Am J Cardiol 61:371, 1988.
144. The Captopril-Digoxin Multicenter Research Group. Comparative effects of therapy with captopril and digoxin in patients with mild to moderate heart failure. JAMA 259:539, 1988.
145. Francis GS. Which drug for what patients with heart failure, and when? Cardiology 76:374, 1989.
146. Leier CV. Acute inotropic support. In: Leier CV (ed). Cardiotonic Drugs: A Clinical Survey. New York, Marcel Dekker, 1986.
147. Rude RE, Kloner RA, Maroko PR, et al. Effects of amrinone on experimental acute myocardial ischemic injury. Cardiovasc Res 14:419, 1980.
148. Taylor SH, Verma SP, Hussain M, et al. Intravenous amrinone in left ventricular failure complicated by acute myocardial infarction. Am J Cardiol 56:29B, 1985.
149. DiBianco R, Shabetai R, Kostuk W, et al. Oral milrinone and digoxin in heart failure: Results of a placebo-controlled, prospective trial of each agent and the combination (abstract). Circulation 76(suppl IV):IV-256, 1978.
150. Ruegg J. Effects of new inotropic agents on calcium ion sensitivity of contractile proteins. Circulation 73(suppl III):78, 1986.
151. Cohn JN, Archibald DG, Ziesche S, et al. Effect of vasodilator therapy on mortality in chronic congestive heart failure. Results of a Veterans Administration cooperative study. N Engl J Med 314:1547, 1986.
152. The CONSENSUS Trial Study Group. Effects of enalapril on mortality in severe congestive heart failure. Results of the cooperative north Scandinavian enalapril survival study (CONSENSUS). N Engl J Med 316:1429, 1987.
153. Massie BM, Packer M, Hanlon JT, Combs DT. Combined captopril and hydralazine for refractory heart failure: A feasible and efficacious regimen. J Am Coll Cardiol 2:338, 1983.
154. Sharpe N, Smith H, Murphy J, Hannon S. Treatment of patients with symptomless left ventricular dysfunction after myocardial infarction. Lancet 1:255, 1988.
155. Pfeffer MA, Lamas GA, Vaughan DA, et al. Effect of

captopril on progressive ventricular dilatation after anterior myocardial infarction. N Engl J Med 319:80, 1988.

156. Pfeffer JM, Pfeffer MA, Braunwald E. Hemodynamic benefits and prolonged survival with long-term captopril therapy in rats with myocardial infarction and heart failure. Circulation 75(suppl I):I149, 1987.

157. Pfeffer MA, Pfeffer JM. Ventricular enlargement and reduced survival after myocardial infarction. Circulation 75(suppl IV):IV-93, 1987.

158. Rutherford JD, Braunwald E, Cohn PF. Chronic ischemic heart disease. In: Braunwald E (ed). Heart Disease: A Textbook of Cardiovascular Medicine. Vol. 2. Philadelphia, WB Saunders, 1988, chap 39.

159. Cahalin LP. Cardiovascular medications. In: Malone T (ed). Physical and Occupational Therapy: Drug Implications for Practice. Philadelphia, JB Lippincott, 1989, chap 3.

160. Goldberg AN. The effects of pharmacological agents on human performance. In: Naughton JP, Hellerstein HK (eds). Exercise Testing and Exercise Training in Coronary Heart Disease. New York, Academic Press, 1973, chap 9.

161. Waagstein F, Hjalmarson A, Varauskas E, Wallentin I. Effect of chronic beta-adrenergic receptor blockade in congestive cardiomyopathy. Br Heart J 37:1022, 1975.

162. Swedberg K, Waagstein F, Hjalmarson A, Wallentin I. Prolongation of survival in congestive cardiomyopathy by beta-receptor blockade. Lancet 1:1374, 1979.

163. Swedberg K, Hjalmarson A, Waagstein F, Wallentin I. Adverse effects of beta blockade withdrawal in patients with congestive cardiomyopathy. Br Heart J 44:134, 1980.

164. Swedberg K, Hjalmarson A, Waagstein F, Wallentin I. Beneficial effects of long-term beta blockade in congestive cardiomyopathy. Br Heart J 44:117, 1980.

165. Engelmeier RS, O'Connell JB, Walsh R, et al. Improvement in symptoms and exercise tolerance by metoprolol in patients with dilated cardiomyopathy: A double-blind, randomized, placebo-controlled trial. Circulation 72:536, 1985.

166. Taylor SH, Silke B. Haemodynamic effects of beta-blockade in ischaemic heart failure. Lancet 2:835, 1981.

167. Binkley PF, Lew RF, Lima JJ, et al. Hemodynamic-inotropic response to beta-blocker with intrinsic sympathomimetic activity in patients with congestive cardiomyopathy. Circulation 74:1390, 1986.

168. Majid PA, Niznick J, Nishizaki S, et al. Acute hemodynamic and neurohumoral effects of pindolol: A beta adrenoceptor antagonist with high intrinsic sympathomimetic activity in patients with dilated cardiomyopathy. J Cardiovasc Pharmacol 10:309, 1987.

169. Gilbert EM, Anderson JL, Deitchman D, et al. Chronic beta blockade with bucindolol improves resting cardiac function in dilated cardiomyopathy. Circulation 76(suppl IV):IV-358, 1987 (abstract).

170. Pouleur H, Van Mechelen H, Balasim H, et al. Comparisons of the inotropic effects of the beta$_1$ adrenoceptor partial agonists SL 75,177.10 and ICI 118,587 with digoxin in the intact canine heart. J Cardiovasc Pharmacol 6:720, 1984.

171. Rousseau MF, Pouleur H, Vincent MF. Effects of a cardioselective beta$_1$-partial agonist (Corwin) on left ventricular function and myocardial metabolism in patients with a previous myocardial infarction. Am J Cardiol 51:1267, 1983.

172. Kullmer T, Kindermann W, Urhausen A, Hess H. Influence of xamoterol, a partial beta$_1$-selective agonist, on physical performance capacity and cardiocirculatory, metabolic and hormonal parameters. Eur J Clin Pharmacol 34:255, 1988.

173. L'Abbate A, Emdin M, Piacenti M, et al. Ultrafiltration: A rational treatment for heart failure. Cardiology 76:384, 1989.

174. Rimondini A, Cipolla CM, Della Bella P, et al. Hemofiltration as short-term treatment for refractory congestive heart failure. Am J Med 83:43, 1987.

175. Williams RS. Exercise training of patients with ventricular dysfunction and heart failure. In: Wenger NK (ed). Exercise and the Heart. 2nd ed. Philadelphia, FA Davis, 1985.

176. Cardiac Alert 11. April 1990, p 6.

177. Brock L. Early reconditioning for post-myocardial infarction patients: Spalding Rehabilitation Center. In: Naughton JP, Hellerstein HK (eds). Exercise Testing and Exercise Training in Coronary Heart Disease. New York, Academic Press, 1973, chap 22B.

178. Wenger NK. Early ambulation after myocardial infarction: Grady Memorial Hospital-Emory University School of Medicine. In: Naughton JP, Hellerstein HK (eds). Exercise Testing and Exercise Training in Coronary Heart Disease. New York, Academic Press, 1973, chap 22C.

179. Franciosa JA, Goldsmith SR, Cohn JN. Contrasting immediate and long-term effects of isosorbide dinitrate on exercise capacity in congestive heart failure. Am J Med 69:59, 1980.

180. Lee AP, Ice R, Blessey R, et al. Long-term effects of physical training on coronary patients with impaired ventricular function. Circulation 60:1519, 1979.

181. Conn EH, Williams RS, Wallace AG. Exercise responses before and after physical conditioning in patients with severely depressed left ventricular function. Am J Cardiol 49:296, 1982.

182. Port S, McEwan P, Cobb FR, et al. Influence of resting left ventricular response to exercise in patients with coronary artery disease. Circulation 63:856, 1981.

183. Litchfield RL, Kerber BE, Benge JW, et al. Normal exercise capacity in patients with severe left ventricular dysfunction: Compensatory mechanisms. Circulation 66:129, 1982.

184. Franciosa JA, Park M, Levine B. Lack of correlation between exercise capacity and indices of resting left ventricular performance in heart failure. Am J Cardiol 47:33, 1981.

185. Letac B, Cribier A, Desplanches JF. A study of left ventricular function in coronary patients before and after physical training. Circulation 56:375, 1977.

186. Williams RS, Conn EH, Wallace AG. Enhanced exercise performance following physical training in coronary patients stratified by left ventricular ejection fraction. Circulation 64:IV-186, 1981.

187. Wilson JR, Ferraro N. Exercise intolerance in patients with chronic left heart failure: Relation to oxygen transport and ventilatory abnormalities. Am J Cardiol 51:1358, 1983.

188. Higgenbotham MB, Morris KG, Conn EH, et al. Determinants of variable exercise performance among pa-

tients with severe left ventricular dysfunction. Am J Cardiol 51:52, 1983.

189. Greenland P, Chu JS. Efficacy of cardiac rehabilitation services with emphasis on patients after myocardial infarction. Ann Intern Med 109:650, 1988.

190. Greenland P, Chu JS. Cardiac rehabilitation services. Ann Intern Med 109:671, 1988.

191. Roubin GS, Anderson SD, Shen WF, et al. Hemodynamic and metabolic basis of impaired exercise tolerance in patients with severe left ventricular dysfunction. J Am Coll Cardiol 15:986, 1990.

192. Sullivan MJ, Higginbotham MB, Cobb FR. Exercise training in patients with severe left ventricular dysfunction: Hemodynamic and metabolic effects. Circulation 78:506, 1988.

193. Hoffman A. The effects of training on the physical working capacity of MI patients with left ventricular dysfunction. Eur Heart J 8 (suppl G):43, 1987.

194. Kellermann JJ, Shemesh J, Fisman E, et al. Arm exercise training in the rehabilitation of patients with impaired ventricular function and heart failure. Cardiology 77:130, 1990.

195. Coats AJS, Adamopoulos S, Meyer TE, et al. Effects of physical training in chronic heart failure. Lancet 335:63, 1990.

196. Arvan S. Exercise performance of the high risk acute myocardial infarction patients after cardiac rehabilitation. Am J Cardiol 62:197, 1988.

197. Jugdutt BI, Bogdon L, Michorowski BL, Kappagoda CT. Exercise training after anterior Q wave myocardial infarction: Importance of regional left ventricular function and topography. J Am Coll Cardiol 12:362, 1988.

198. Epstein SE, Palmeri ST, Patterson RE, et al. Evaluation of patients after acute myocardial infarction: Indications for cardiac catheterization and surgical intervention. N Engl J Med 307:1487, 1982.

199. Cahalin LP, Ice RG, Irwin S. Program planning and implementation. In: Irwin S, Tecklin JS (eds). Cardiopulmonary Physical Therapy. 2nd ed. St. Louis, CV Mosby, 1989, chap 9.

200. Blessey RL, Irwin S. Patient evaluation. In: Irwin S, Tecklin JS (eds). Cardiopulmonary Physical Therapy. St. Louis, CV Mosby, 1985.

201. Hagberg JM. Patients with end-stage renal disease. In: Franklin BA, Gordon S, Timmis GC (eds). Exercise in Modern Medicine. Baltimore, Williams & Wilkins, 1989, chap 7.

202. Kettner A, Goldberg AP, Hagberg JM, et al. Cardiovascular and metabolic responses to submaximal exercise in hemodialysis patients. Kidney Int 26:66, 1984.

203. Tyler HR. Neurological aspects of dialysis patients. In: Drukker W, Parsons FM, Maher JF (eds). Replacement of Renal Function by Dialysis. The Hague: Martinus Nijhoff Medical Division, 1978, p 601.

5 RESTRICTIVE LUNG DYSFUNCTION

189

INTRODUCTION

Pulmonary pathology can be organized and discussed in a number of ways. Within this text pulmonary function abnormalities have been divided into two main categories: obstructive dysfunction and restrictive dysfunction. If the flow of air is impeded, the defect is obstructive. If the volume of air or gas is reduced, the defect is **restrictive.** Although this organization of pulmonary pathology may in some ways clarify the discussion, it must be remembered that a number of diseases and conditions result in both obstructive and restrictive lung impairment. This chapter discusses those pathologies and interventions that result in restrictive lung dysfunction.

ETIOLOGY

Restrictive lung dysfunction (RLD) is an abnormal reduction in pulmonary ventilation. Lung expansion is diminished. The volume of air or gas moving in and out of the lungs is decreased.[1]

Restrictive lung dysfunction is not a disease. In fact, this dysfunction may result from many different diseases arising from the pulmonary system or almost any other system in the body. It can also result from trauma or therapeutic interventions, such as radiation therapy or the use of certain drugs.

PATHOGENESIS

Three major aspects of pulmonary ventilation must be considered to understand the pathophysiology of RLD. They are compliance of both the lung and the chest wall, lung volumes and capacities, and the work of breathing (Fig. 5-1).

Compliance

Pulmonary compliance encompasses both lung and chest wall compliance. It is the physiologic link that establishes a relationship between the pressure exerted by the chest wall or the lungs and the volume of air that can be contained within the lungs.[1] With RLD chest wall or lung compliance, or both, is decreased.

As discussed in Chapter 2, a decrease in compliance of the lungs indicates that they are becoming stiffer and thus more difficult to expand. It takes a greater **transpulmonary pressure** to expand the lung to a given volume in a person with decreased lung compliance.[2] If the amount of pressure used to move air into the lungs is constant, the volume of air would be decreased in the person with decreased lung compliance. The pressure-volume or compliance curve is shifted to the right (Fig. 5-2 and discussion of compliance in Chapter 2, Fig. 2-8). A chest wall low in compliance limits thoracic expansion and therefore lung inflation even if the lung has normal compliance.

Because pulmonary compliance is decreased in RLD, resistance to lung expansion is increased. In other words, decreased pulmonary compliance requires an increase in pressure just to maintain adequate lung expansion and ventilation. This means the patient has to work harder just to move air into the lungs.

Lung Volumes

Restrictive lung dysfunction eventually causes all the lung volumes and capacities to become decreased. Because the distensibility of the lung is decreased, the **inspiratory reserve volume (IRV)** is diminished. **Tidal volume (VT)** is the volume of air or gas normally moved in and out of the lungs at rest. Although the body tries to preserve the tidal volume in RLD, the compliance gradually decreases and the work of breathing increases; thus the tidal volume decreases. The **expiratory reserve volume (ERV)** is the volume of air or gas that can be exhaled following a normal exhalation. No matter the etiology, RLD effects a reduction in the ERV; this reduction is particularly pronounced if a decrease in lung compliance is the principal etiologic factor. However, the **residual volume (RV)** is invariably decreased whether the RLD results from a decrease in lung or chest wall compliance. However, the amount of the decrease may be less than seen in the IRV or the ERV.

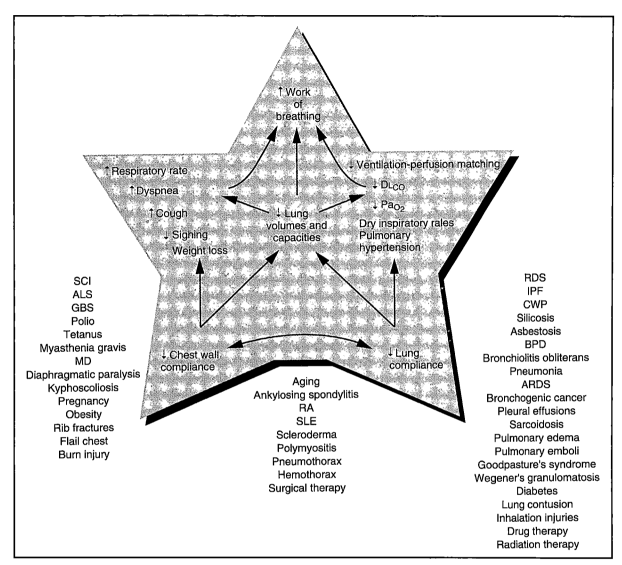

Figure 5-1

Interactive star diagram in restrictive lung dysfunction. SCI, spinal cord injury; ALS, amyotrophic lateral sclerosis; GBS, Guillain Barré syndrome; MD, muscular dystrophy; RA, rheumatoid arthritis; SLE, systemic lupus erythematosus; RDS, respiratory distress syndrome; IPF, idiopathic pulmonary fibrosis; CWP, coal workers' pneumoconiosis; BPD, bronchopulmonary dysplasia; ARDS, adult respiratory distress syndrome; DL_{CO}, diffusing capacity of the lungs for carbon monoxide; Pa_{O_2}, arterial partial pressure of oxygen.

Because all lung volumes are decreased with RLD, all lung capacities are also decreased. **Total lung capacity (TLC)** and **vital capacity (VC)** are the two most common **spirometric measurements** used in the identification of RLD (Fig. 5-3). Decreases in TLC and **functional residual capacity (FRC)** are a direct result of a decrease in

lung compliance. At TLC the force of the inspiratory muscles is balanced by the inward elastic recoil of the lung. Because the recoil pressure is increased if lung compliance is decreased, this balance occurs at a lower volume, and thus the TLC is diminished. At FRC the outward recoil of the chest wall is balanced by the inward elastic

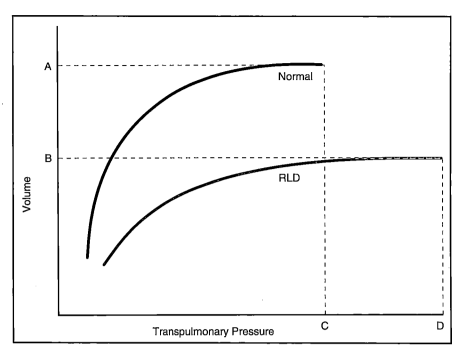

Figure 5–2

Compliance curve. Diagram shows how the lung compliance curve is shifted down and to the right in restrictive lung dysfunction (RLD). Total lung capacity (TLC) (B) in RLD is less than normal TLC (A). The amount of transpulmonary pressure needed to achieve TLC (D) in RLD is greater than the transpulmonary pressure needed to achieve a normal TLC (C). (Reproduced with permission from Weinberger SE. Principles of Pulmonary Medicine. Philadelphia, WB Saunders, p 120.)

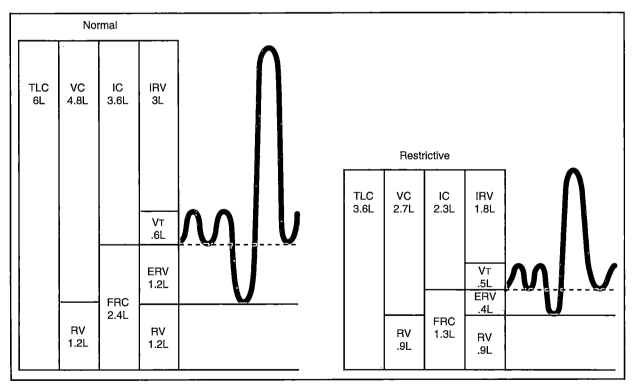

Figure 5–3

Lung volumes and capacities. Comparison between normal and restrictive lung dysfunction. TLC, total lung capacity; VC, vital capacity; RV, residual volume; IC, inspiratory capacity; FRC, functional residual capacity; IRV, inspiratory reserve volume; VT, tidal volume; ERV, expiratory reserve volume.

recoil of the lung. Becuase this elastic recoil is increased, the balance is achieved at a lower lung volume and so the FRC is decreased (Fig. 5−4).[2]

Work of Breathing

With RLD the work of breathing is increased. The respiratory system normally finely tunes the respiratory rate and the V_T to minimize the mechanical work of breathing. As previously mentioned, a greater transpulmonary pressure is required to achieve a normal V_T. The result is that the patient's work of breathing is increased and a new equilibrium, with a decreased V_T and an increased respiratory rate, is sought in an effort to reduce energy expenditure. However, if the respiratory rate is too high, energy is wasted in overcoming airway resistance and in ventilating the anatomic dead space. Furthermore, if the tidal volume is larger than required, energy is wasted overcoming the natural recoil of the lung and in expanding the chest wall. Anything that increases airway resistance, increases flow rates, or decreases lung or chest wall compliance increases the work of breathing. In RLD both lung and chest wall compliance and lung volumes may decrease. These changes can significantly change the work of breathing.[3] To overcome the decrease in pulmonary compliance, the respiratory rate is usually increased; the normal inspiratory muscles, especially the diaphragm (see Fig. 1−7), work harder; and the accessory muscles of respiration, the scaleni and the sternocleidomastoid (see Fig. 1−7), are recruited to assist in expanding the thorax.[4] These additional efforts require additional oxygen (O_2) expenditure. In

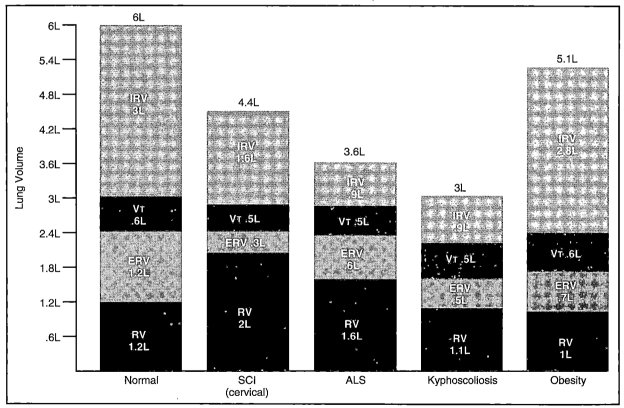

Figure 5−4

Examples of lung volumes in different restrictive impairments. IRV, inspiratory reserve volume; VT, tidal volume; ERV, expiratory reserve volume; RV, residual volume; SCI, spinal cord injury; ALS, amyotrophic lateral sclerosis.

normal persons at rest, the body uses less than 5% of the oxygen consumption per minute ($\dot{V}o_2$) or 3 to 14 ml $O_2 \cdot min^{-1}$ to support the work of breathing.[3,5] With RLD the percentage of $\dot{V}o_2$ needed to support the work of breathing can reach and exceed 25%.[3,5] This change is usually very insidious as the RLD progresses and is countered by the concurrent decrease in activity seen in these patients. Although the respiratory muscle pump is very resistant to fatigue, these patients can experience respiratory muscle fatigue, overuse, and failure as RLD progresses.

CLINICAL MANIFESTATIONS

Signs

Six classic signs often indicate and are always consistent with RLD. The first is **tachypnea** or an increased respiratory rate. Because the inspiratory muscles have to work so hard to overcome the decreased pulmonary compliance, an involuntary adjustment is made to increase the respiratory rate and decrease the volumes so that the minute ventilation is maintained. Early in the course of RLD there may be *overcompensation*, with the respiratory rate increasing to the point that minute ventilation is increased and **alveolar hyperventilation** occurs, resulting in greater exhalation of carbon dioxide (CO_2).

Ventilation-perfusion mismatching, an invariable finding in RLD, leads to the second classic sign: **hypoxemia.** This mismatching may be due to changes in the collagenous framework of the lung, scarring of capillary channels, distortion or narrowing of the small airways, compression from tumors within the lung or bony abnormalities of the chest wall, or a variety of other causes. Even if patients are not hypoxemic at rest, they may quickly become hypoxemic with exercise.

The third classic sign of RLD is decreased breath sounds with dry inspiratory **rales** (velcro crackles), which is thought to be caused by **atelectatic** alveoli opening at end-inspiration and is most often heard at the bases of the lungs.

The fourth and fifth classic signs are apparent from pulmonary function testing. The decrease in lung volumes and capacities, determined by spirometry, comprises the fourth classic sign of RLD. The fifth classic sign is the decreased **diffusing capacity (DL_{CO}).** This arises as a consequence of a widening of the interstitial spaces due to scar tissue, fibrosis of the capillaries, and ventilation-perfusion abnormalities. In RLD the DL_{CO} has been measured at less than 50% of predicted.[6]

The sixth classic sign usually apparent with RLD is **cor pulmonale.** This right-sided heart failure is due to hypoxemia, fibrosis, and compression of the pulmonary capillaries, which leads to pulmonary hypertension. The rise in pressure in the pulmonary circulation increases the work of the right ventricle. Because the pulmonary capillary bed is fibrotic it is also less able to distend to handle the ordinary increase in cardiac output expected with exercise. Therefore, during exercise hypoxemia may occur earlier or be more pronounced. Other signs include a decrease in chest wall expansion and possible **cyanosis** or **clubbing** (Table 5-1).

Symptoms

Three hallmark symptoms are usually experienced with RLD. The first is dyspnea or shortness of breath. This symptom typically manifests itself with exercise, but as RLD progresses, dyspnea at rest may also be experienced. The second symptom and the one that usually brings the patient into the physician's office is an irritating, dry, and nonproductive cough. The third hallmark symptom of RLD is the wasted, emaciated appearance these patients present as the disease progresses. With the work of breathing increased

TABLE 5-1. Signs and Symptoms of Restrictive Lung Dysfunction

Signs	Symptoms
Tachypnea	Dyspnea
Hypoxemia	Cough
Decreased lung volumes	Weight loss
Decreased diffusing capacity	Muscle wasting
Decreased breath sounds	
Altered chest radiograph (often reticulonodular pattern)	
Pulmonary hypertension	

as much as twelvefold over normal, these individuals are using caloric requirements similar to those necessary for running a marathon 24 hours a day.[3] Additionally, because breathing is such hard work and eating makes breathing more difficult, these patients usually are not eager to eat and often report a decrease in appetite. Because their energy expenditure is up and their caloric intake is down, they are very often in a continual weight loss cycle, which becomes more severe as the RLD progresses.

TREATMENT

Treatment interventions for RLD are discussed briefly for each disease and traumatic or therapeutic entity that can result in its appearance. Generally, however, if the etiologic factors that are causing RLD are permanent **(spinal cord injury)** or progressive **(idiopathic pulmonary fibrosis)**, the treatment consists primarily of supportive measures. Supportive interventions include supplemental oxygen to support the arterial partial pressure of oxygen (Pa_{O_2}), antibiotic therapy to fight secondary pulmonary infection, measures to promote adequate ventilation and prevent the accumulation of pulmonary secretions, and good nutritional support. However, if the changes that are causing the RLD are acute and reversible **(pneumothorax)** or chronic but reversible **(Guillain-Barré syndrome)**, the treatment consists of specific corrective interventions (e.g., chest tube placement) as well as supportive measures (e.g., temporary mechanical ventilation) to assist the patient to maintain adequate ventilation until the patient is again able to be independent in this activity.

MATURATIONAL CAUSES OF RESTRICTIVE LUNG DYSFUNCTION

Abnormalities in Fetal Lung Development

- **Agenesis** is the total absence of the bronchus and the lung **parenchyma.** Unilateral agenesis is rare.[7]

- **Aplasia** is the development of a rudimentary bronchus without the development of the normal lung parenchyma. This condition is also rare.[7]
- **Hypoplasia** is the development of a functioning although not always normal bronchus with the development of reduced amounts of lung parenchyma. This developmental abnormality is much more common and may affect one lung or one lobe of a lung. It is often present in infants born with a large diaphragmatic hernia and displaced abdominal organs.[7]

Clinical Manifestations

Depending on the amount of lung parenchyma lost, these infants can be asymptomatic or can exhibit severe pulmonary insufficiency. The pulmonary impairment is restrictive in that the volumes are decreased even though the lung compliance may be normal.

Respiratory Distress Syndrome

Respiratory distress syndrome (RDS), also known as **hyaline membrane disease,** is a disorder of prematurity or lack of complete lung maturation in the human fetus. It usually takes 36 weeks of normal gestation to achieve lung maturity in the fetus. Infants born with a gestational age less than 36 weeks often exhibit respiratory distress and may develop the full complement of signs and symptoms associated with RDS.[8]

Etiology

Insufficient maturation of the lungs is the cause of RDS, and it is usually linked directly to the gestational age of the fetus at birth. The incidence of RDS in infants with a gestational age of 26 to 28 weeks at birth is approximately 75%.[8] In contrast, the incidence of RDS in infants with a gestational age of 36 weeks at birth is less than 5%.[8] Other factors that seem to contribute to the development of RDS are gender, race, and diabetes in the mother. Premature male infants are more at risk to develop RDS than premature female infants. White premature infants have a greater incidence of RDS than black premature infants. Fetal lung maturation is delayed in pregnant women with diabetes, so infants born of diabetic mothers are at increased risk of developing RDS. Worldwide 1% of infants are affected by RDS. In the United States 4000 infants die of RDS annually.[8]

Pathophysiology

RDS is caused primarily by abnormalities in the **surfactant** system and inadequate surfactant production. Structural abnormalities, such as alveolar septal thickening, within the immature lung may also contribute to the pathophysiology of this syndrome. The surfactant dysfunction causes the overall retractive forces of the lung to be greater than normal, which decreases lung compliance; increases the work of breathing; and leads to progressive diffuse **microatelectasis**, alveolar collapse, increased ventilation-perfusion mismatching, and impaired gas exchange. In addition, alveolar epithelial and endothelial permeability are abnormal in the immature lung. Therefore, when these premature infants are mechanically ventilated without sufficient normal surfactant, the bronchiolar epithelium is disrupted. This leads to pulmonary edema and the generation of hyaline membranes. Further, because the proximal and distal airways in the infant are very compliant and the alveoli may be less compliant owing to atelectasis and the formation of **hyaline membrane,** the mechanical ventilator pressures used can disrupt, dilate, and deform the airways. Mechanical ventilator pressures can also cause air leaks, **tension pneumothorax,** and extensive pulmonary interstitial emphysema.

Another cause of decreased gas exchange is the often severe pulmonary hypertension evident in infants with RDS. These infants have hypoxemia and are acidotic, both of which cause vasoconstriction. This response is exaggerated in the infant and causes severe pulmonary hypertension, increased ventilation-perfusion mismatching, and decreased gas exchange. Restrictive lung dysfunction may be complicated further by persistent *patency of the ductus arteriosus,* resulting in a left-to-right shunt within the infant's heart. The patent ductus arteriosus increases pulmonary pressures and blood flow and could allow plasma proteins to leak into the alveolar space, causing pulmonary edema and further interfering with surfactant function.

Complications common in infants with RDS include intracranial hemorrhage, sepsis, pneumonia, pneumothorax, pulmonary hemorrhage, and pulmonary interstitial emphysema. This syndrome can also result in the development of **bronchopulmonary dysplasia.** Recovery in RDS is usually preceded by an abrupt unexplained diuresis.[8]

Clinical Manifestations

Signs
Pulmonary Function Tests. Infants with RDS have an increased respiratory rate and decreased lung volumes, particularly FRC and VC.

Chest Radiograph. The lung parenchyma of infants with RDS has a fine **reticulogranular pattern.** If the RDS is severe, air bronchograms are prominent, and the **cardiothymic silhouette** becomes indistinct owing to severe diffuse microatelectasis.

Arterial Blood Gases. There is a marked decrease in the Pa_{O_2}. The arterial partial pressure of carbon dioxide (Pa_{CO_2}) is increased, and the pH is decreased or acidotic. Ventilation-perfusion mismatching is prominent. Dead space ventilation is increased, whereas alveolar ventilation is decreased.

Breath Sounds. An *expiratory grunt* is the most common abnormal breath sound associated with RDS. The diffuse atelectasis may also cause rales and decreased breath sounds.

Cardiovascular Findings. Infants may experience **bradycardia.** There may also be cerebral, pulmonary, or intraventricular hemorrhage as a result of the exaggerated changes in vascular pressures due to the hypoxemia and **acidemia.**

Symptoms. The infant's respiratory pattern is usually rapid and very labored, with significant intercostal and substernal retractions. Nasal flaring and grunting are common. Infants with RDS often are cyanotic, and their crying is decreased in volume and strength.

Treatment

Treatment of this syndrome is unusual in that the syndrome sometimes can be prevented by treating the mother before the premature birth of an infant at high risk for RDS. Administration of corticosteroids to the mother before delivery can stimulate surfactant synthesis, induce changes in the elastic properties of the fetal lung, stimulate alveolarization, and decrease the permeability of the airway and alveoli epithelium. These changes would decrease the incidence or severity of RDS.

Once the infants are delivered, however, treatment is supportive as the lung continues to mature. The infants are placed in a neutral thermal environment. Their nutritional status is maintained via supplemental glucose or **hyperalimentation.** Electrolyte and fluid balance are also closely monitored and managed. Supplemental oxygen is supplied via a hood. If the infant is unable to maintain sufficient tissue oxygenation, mechanical ventilation is initiated. **Continuous positive airway pressure (CPAP)** is used to maintain an adequate Pa_{O_2} and decrease the inspired oxygen concentration in an effort to decrease the risk of oxygen toxicity. Surfactant replacement therapy is employed to increase lung compliance. Infants with RDS are monitored closely for any complications. Infants who respond to treatment and require limited mechanical ventilation or none at all may recover and have normal pulmonary function. Infants who require prolonged mechanical ventilation or respond less well to treatment may develop bronchopulmonary dysplasia (BPD).[8]

Normal Aging

Maturation of the various body systems is a natural process that takes place throughout a lifetime. Normal aging usually refers to physiologic changes that occur with regularity in the majority of the population and can therefore be predicted. Physiologic changes that commonly are considered part of the aging process can begin as early as 20 years of age.[9]

Etiology

The normal aging process in the pulmonary system is very slow and insidious, and because we have great ventilatory reserves the changes are often not felt functionally until the sixth or seventh decade of life.[10] Universally, the normal aging process in the lungs is complicated by the fact that throughout life the lungs have had to cope with the external environment. Environmental factors that affect the aging process include general pollution, noxious gases, specific occupational exposures, inhaled drug use, and of course cigarette smoking.[9]

Physiology

The compliance of the pulmonary system starts to decrease at about age 20 and decreases approximately 20% over the next 40 years.[9] Maximum voluntary ventilation decreases by 30% between the ages of 30 and 70.[9] Vital capacity also drops by about 25% between 30 and 70 years of age.[10] However, as stated previously, although some changes start as early as the second and third decades of life, functional status often is not affected until the sixth and seventh decades.

The control of ventilation undergoes significant change. The peripheral chemoreceptors are not as responsive to hypoxia, and the central receptors are not as responsive to acute **hypercapnia.** These changes mean that the ventilatory response mediated by the central nervous system is significantly depressed.[3,8] The normal Pa_{O_2} in a 70 year old is 75, a measurement that is not interpreted as hypoxia by the central nervous system.[9]

The thorax undergoes a number of changes, including decalcification of the ribs, calcification of the costal cartilages, arthritic changes in the joints of the ribs and vertebrae, dorsal thoracic kyphosis, and increased anteroposterior diameter of the chest (barrel chest). The effects of these changes combine to decrease the compliance of the chest wall and increase the work of breathing. Oxygen consumption in the respiratory muscles is increased, causing an increase in the minute ventilation. The strength and endurance of the inspiratory muscles gradually diminishes. This results in a decreased maximal ventilatory effort.[3] The forced expiratory volume in 1 second (FEV_1) is reduced by about 40 milliliters per year.[9]

The lung tissue itself shows enlargement of the air spaces owing to enlargement of the alveolar ducts and terminal bronchioles. The alveolar surface area and the alveolar parenchymal volume are decreased. The alveolar walls become thinner, and the capillary bed incurs considerable loss, with an increase in ventilation-perfusion mismatching. Distribution of inspired air and pulmonary blood flow becomes less homogeneous with age. Diffusing capacity is therefore reduced, and physiologic dead space is increased.[9]

The static elastic recoil of the alveolar tissue decreases, which means that alveolar compliance is increased and the lungs do not empty well. The lung compliance curve is shifted to the left in the elderly. Thus, although TLC may not change with age, RV increases and dynamic volumes therefore decrease[9,10] (Fig. 5–5).

Closing volumes are increased, which results in early closure of the small airways, particularly in the dependent lung regions. By approximately age 55 small airways are closed at or above FRC in the supine position. In the upright position, with the attendant increase in FRC, this change occurs at approximately age 70.[9]

Of course, normal concomitant aging changes take place in the cardiovascular system, including a decrease in maximum heart rate and cardiac output. These changes combine with the decreased oxygen exchange capability of the lungs and result in a decrease in the maximum oxygen uptake with exercise and therefore a decrease in the anaerobic threshold. After 50 years of age, the maximum oxygen uptake usually declines at a rate of $0.45 \text{ ml} \cdot \text{kg} \cdot \text{min}^{-1}$ for each year.[3,8]

Ventilation during sleep is altered in the el-

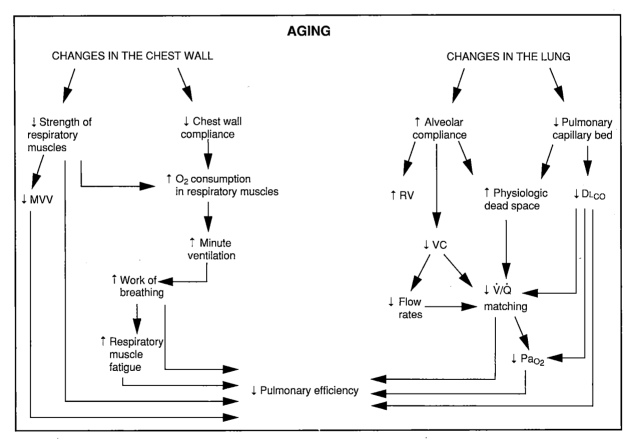

Figure 5–5

Respiratory changes with aging. MVV, maximum voluntary ventilation; O_2, oxygen; RV, residual volume; VC, vital capacity; V/Q, ventilation-perfusion; Pa_{O_2}, arterial partial pressure of oxygen; DL_{CO}, diffusing capacity of the lungs for carbon monoxide.

derly. **Electroencephalographic (EEG)** studies have shown that total nocturnal sleep time is shorter with more frequent and longer nocturnal awakenings in the elderly. The pattern of ventilation during sleep is irregular more often in the elderly than in young adults. Repetitive periodic apneas occur in 35% to 40% of the elderly, predominantly in males during sleep stages 1 and 2.[8]

Clinical Manifestations

Signs
Pulmonary Function Tests. Total lung capacity and airway resistance are usually unchanged. The RV is increased, and the VC is decreased by approximately 25% by age 70.[10] Flow rates are decreased. **Maximum voluntary ventilation (MVV)** is decreased by about 30%[9]; DL_{CO} is also decreased.

Chest Radiograph. The chest film can show a variety of changes in the bony thorax (e.g., decalcification of ribs, barrel chest, kyphosis) and in the lung parenchyma (e.g., larger air spaces, altered vascular markings).

Arterial Blood Gases. The Pa_{O_2} normally is decreased to about 75 mm Hg at age 70.[9] Usually the Pa_{CO_2} is normal or slightly elevated.

Breath Sounds. Auscultation often reveals slightly diminished breath sounds.

Cardiovascular Findings. With increased age maximum heart rate, stroke volume, and cardiac output usually decrease. Often systolic blood pressure increases.

Symptoms. The pulmonary reserve is so great that individuals usually do not consciously note any changes until the seventh or eighth decade. But even before changes in the pulmonary system are recognized, an individual has often made changes in activity patterns and recreational pursuits because of normal aging processes taking place in other body systems.

Treatment

Aging is normal—no treatment is required. The elderly should be encouraged to remain active and fit. Although even with regular activity about 0.45 ml · kg^{-1} · min^{-1} of oxygen consumption is lost each year, the fit elderly person

has a greater maximum oxygen consumption than the sedentary person. In fact, a sedentary elderly person beginning regular exercise can improve maximum oxygen consumption by 5% to 25% and can regain the exercise capability that was present as much as 5 to 10 years earlier.[9]

PULMONARY CAUSES OF RESTRICTIVE LUNG DYSFUNCTION

Idiopathic Pulmonary Fibrosis

Idiopathic pulmonary fibrosis (IPF) is an inflammatory process involving all of the components of the alveolar wall that progresses to gross distortion of lung architecture. The components of the alveolar wall include the epithelial cells, the endothelial cells, the cellular and noncellular components of the interstitium, and the capillary network. These components are supported by the connective tissue framework made up of collagen and elastic fibers and containing a milieu of ground substance. Other synonyms used for IPF are **cryptogenic fibrosing alveolitis, interstitial pneumonitis,** and **Hamman-Rich syndrome.**[11,12]

Etiology

By definition, IPF is of unknown origin. It may be due to viral, genetic, or immune-mediated disorders. It seems to begin with an inflammation, but then the response to the inflammation continues to generate the abnormalities seen in IPF.

Pathophysiology

The lung involvement in IPF often shows patchy focal lesions scattered throughout both lungs. These lesions first show inflammatory changes and then scar and become fibrotic, distorting the alveolar septa and the capillary network. The alveolar spaces become irregular in size and shape. There can be significant progressive destruction of the capillary bed. These changes combine to cause decreased lung compliance; decreased lung volumes; increased ventilation-perfusion mismatching; decreased surface area for gas exchange; decreased diffusing capacity; increased pulmonary arterial pressure, which increases the work of the right ventricle; increased work of breathing; increased caloric requirements; and decreased functional capacity.[11]

The two major pathologic components of IPF are (1) an inflammatory process in the alveolar wall (sometimes called an *alveolitis*), and (2) a scarring or fibrotic process that is thought to be secondary to the active inflammation. Both of these pathologic processes occur simultaneously within the lung.[11]

Clinical Manifestations

Signs

Pulmonary Function Tests. Patients with IPF typically show decreases in TLC, VC, FRC, and RV. These patients have normal flow rate values or slightly decreased flow rates owing to the decrease in lung volumes. The $D_{L_{CO}}$ is also decreased. As the disease progresses, the V_T is decreased and the respiratory rate increased.

Chest Radiograph. The chest films usually show a diffuse **reticulonodular pattern** throughout both lungs (Fig. 5–6). Some patients have a predominance of abnormal markings in the upper or lower lung fields. Interestingly, some IPF patients with symptoms of the disease have normal chest radiographs.

Arterial Blood Gases. The Pa_{O_2} is often decreased, but the Pa_{CO_2} is usually within normal limits. Patients are hypoxemic first with exercise; as the disease progresses, they are hypoxemic at rest.

Breath Sounds. Auscultation reveals bibasilar end-inspiratory dry rales and possibly decreased breath sounds.

Cardiovascular Findings. As the pulmonary capillary bed is destroyed, pulmonary hypertension develops. This change from a low-pressure system to a high-pressure system puts a strain on the right ventricle and can cause cor pulmonale.

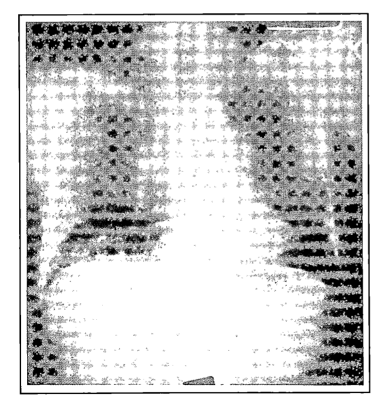

Figure 5–6

Chest radiograph of a patient with idiopathic pulmonary fibrosis, showing a diffuse reticulonodular pattern and elevated diaphragms. (Reproduced with permission from Mitchell RS. Synopsis of Clinical Pulmonary Disease. 2nd ed. St. Louis, CV Mosby, p 244.)

Late in the course of IPF, patients may be cyanotic, and 40% to 75% of IPF patients have clubbing of the digits.[11]

Symptoms. Patients with IPF usually complain of an insidious onset of dyspnea on exertion, which progresses until the patient may feel short of breath even at rest. Often patients also complain of a repetitive, nonproductive cough. Patients also usually report weight loss and decrease in appetite as well as complain of fatigue. Another symptom of IPF reported by some patients is sleep disturbances with a loss of rapid eye movement sleep.[11]

Treatment

Corticosteroids are frequently used in the treatment of IPF. The active alveolitis seems to have some positive response to these drugs. The progressive fibrosis is nonreversible, and corticosteroids have no effect on lung tissue that is already fibrotic. The remaining treatment measures are supportive. They consist of maintaining adequate oxygenation, ventilation, and nutrition.

Coal Workers' Pneumoconiosis

Coal workers' pneumoconiosis (CWP) is an interstitial lung disease, an occupational **pneumoconiosis,** caused by the inhalation of coal dust. This disease is most commonly divided into simple CWP and complicated CWP.[13]

Etiology

Coal workers' pneumoconiosis is caused by repeated inhalation of coal dust over a long period of time; usually 10 to 12 years of underground work exposure is necessary for the development of simple CWP.[14] Complicated CWP, sometimes called *progressive massive fibrosis,* usually occurs only after even longer exposure to coal dust. Anthracite coal is more hazardous than bituminous in the development of this disease.[15]

Coal workers' pneumoconiosis is not the most common respiratory disease found in this occupational group. Chronic bronchitis is even more common, usually occurs earlier, and often coexists with CWP in coal miners.

Pathophysiology

The pathologic hallmark of CWP is the coal macule, which is a focal collection of coal dust with little tissue reaction either in terms of cellular infiltration or fibrosis. These coal macules are often located at the division of respiratory bronchioles and are often associated with focal emphysema.[14] Lymph nodes are enlarged and homogeneously pigmented and are firm but not fibrotic. The pleural surface appears black owing to the deposits of coal dust. Simple CWP is a benign disease if complications do not develop. Less than 5% of cases progress to complicated CWP.[16]

The mechanism for the progression of simple CWP to complicated CWP is unknown. It has been suggested that simple CWP may progress when it is combined with infection, or silicosis, or tuberculosis, or altered immunologic mechanisms. Complicated CWP results in large confluent zones of dense fibrosis that are usually present in apical segments in one or both lungs. These zones are made up of dense, acellular, collagenous, black-pigmented tissue. The normal lung parenchyma can be completely replaced, and the blood vessels in the area then show an obliterative arteritis. These fibrous zones can completely replace the entire upper lobe.[14]

Common complications associated with complicated CWP include emphysema, chronic bronchitis, tuberculosis, cor pulmonale, and pulmonary **thromboembolism.**

Clinical Manifestations

Signs
Pulmonary Function Tests. In simple CWP, spirometric tests may be normal or may show a slight decrease in VC with a small increase in RV. There may also be a small reduction in DL_{CO}. In complicated CWP, a marked reduction occurs in TLC, VC, and FRC. Lung compliance is decreased. The diffusing capacity is also decreased. Respiratory rate is often increased.

Chest Radiograph. The chest radiograph in simple CWP shows small, discrete densities more nodular than linear. They may appear throughout both lung fields but usually are predominantly in the upper regions. In complicated CWP, the chest radiograph shows **coalescent opacities** of black fibrous tissue, usually in the posterior segments of the upper lobes or the superior segments of the lower lobes. Cavities also may be evident that are due to superimposed tuberculosis or are secondary to ischemic necrosis.

Arterial Blood Gases. The Pa_{O_2} is decreased.

Breath Sounds. With simple CWP, breath sounds may be slightly diminished, with rhonchi heard owing to the concomitant chronic bronchitis. In complicated CWP, breath sounds vary: they are markedly decreased over areas of fibrotic tissue; abnormal bronchial breath sounds are present over compressed or atelectatic lung areas; and rhonchi and rales are heard with chronic bronchitis and excess secretions.

Cardiovascular Findings. In complicated CWP, fibrotic pulmonary hypertension and cor pulmonale are common when significant portions of the lungs and pulmonary capillary beds are involved.

Symptoms. The major symptoms include severe dyspnea and cough, usually with the appearance of moderate to copious amounts of black sputum. Patients are often barrel chested and wasted in appearance. Progressive weight loss is common.

Treatment

Complicated CWP with pulmonary fibrosis is nonreversible; there is no cure for it. Supportive treatment includes cessation of exposure to coal dust, good nutrition, interventions to ensure adequate oxygenation and ventilation, and progressive exercise training to maximize the remaining lung function.

Silicosis

Silicosis, one of the occupational pneumoconioses, is a fibrotic lung disease caused by the inhalation of the inorganic dust known as free or **crystalline silicon dioxide.**[13]

Etiology

The disease is caused by the repeated inhalation of free or crystalline silicon dioxide, which is very common and widely distributed in the earth's crust in a variety of forms including quartz, flint, cristobalite, and tridymite.[14] Industries in which silicon dioxide exposure can occur include mining, tunneling through rock, quarrying, grinding and polishing rock, sandblasting, ship building, and foundry work.[16]

Pathophysiology

Inhaled silica causes macrophages to enter the area to ingest these particles. But the macrophages are destroyed by the cytotoxic effects of the silica. This process releases lysosomal enzymes that then induce progressive formation of collagen, which eventually becomes fibrotic. Another characteristic of silicosis is the formation of acellular nodules composed of connective tissue called *silicotic nodules.* Initially these nodules are small and discrete, but as the disease progresses they become larger and coalesce. Silicosis normally affects the upper lobes of the lung more than the lower lobes. Silicosis also seems to predispose the patient to secondary infections by mycobacteria including *Mycobacterium tuberculosis.* Complicated silicosis follows a steadily deteriorating course that leads to respiratory failure (Fig. 5–7).[2,16]

Clinical Manifestations

Signs

Pulmonary Function Tests. As would be expected, TLC and VC are decreased. Pulmonary compliance is decreased, and FEV_1 is diminished.

Chest Radiograph. The chest films may show small rounded opacities or nodules (simple silicosis), which can become larger over time and coalesce (complicated silicosis). The pathologic findings are seen more in the upper lung fields. The hilar lymph nodes may be enlarged and calcified.

Figure 5-7

Lungs with widespread silicosis showing scarring and honeycombing. (Reproduced with permission from Fishman AP. Pulmonary Diseases and Disorders. 2nd ed. New York, McGraw-Hill, p 2238.)

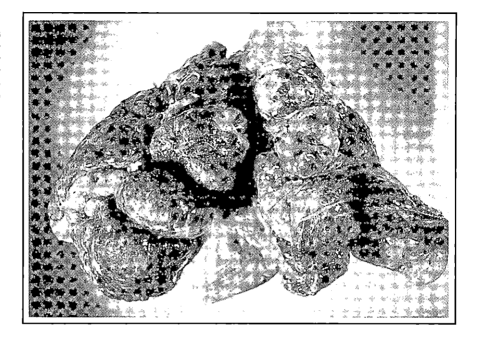

Arterial Blood Gases. The Pa_{O_2} is decreased with exercise.

Breath Sounds. Breath sounds are decreased, particularly over the upper lobes. Rhonchi may or may not be present.

Cardiovascular Findings. There are no specific findings.

Symptoms. The major symptom is shortness of breath. Cough is also very common, and it may be productive or nonproductive.

Treatment

There is no treatment except to avoid further exposure to silica. Supportive therapy is used to counteract the patient's symptoms and includes measures to provide adequate oxygenation, ventilation, and nutrition.

Asbestosis

Asbestosis is a diffuse interstitial pulmonary fibrotic disease caused by asbestos exposure.[15]

Occupational asbestos exposure is also associated with an increased incidence of primary cancer of the larynx, oropharynx, esophagus, stomach, and colon.[14]

Etiology

The term *asbestos* is used generically to name a specific group of naturally occurring fibrous silicates. There are four types of commercially significant asbestos. *Chrysolite* accounts for more than 70% of the asbestos used in the United States and is primarily mined in Canada and the Commonwealth of Independent States. *Crocidolite* and *amosite* are mined primarily in South Africa. *Anthophyllite* comes from Finland.[15]

Asbestos is valued because of its resistance to fire; it has been used widely since the 1930s. Those at most risk for asbestosis are asbestos miners and millers, construction workers, shipbuilders, insulation workers, pipefitters, steamfitters, sheet metal workers, welders, workers who remove old asbestos insulation, workers employed in building renovation or demolition, and auto mechanics who work on brake linings.

Pathophysiology

How asbestos causes a fibrotic reaction is not understood. There seems to be a considerable latency period after an initial exposure, which can extend to 15 to 20 years. It is hypothesized that the asbestos fiber causes an alveolitis in the area of the respiratory bronchioles, which then progresses to peribronchiolar fibrosis owing to the release of chemical mediators. Plaques, which are localized fibrous thickenings of the parietal pleura, are common and are usually seen posteriorly, laterally, or on the pleural surface of the diaphragm. Pleural effusions may also occur with asbestosis. Also "asbestos bodies" or ferruginous bodies appear in the lungs and sputum of these patients. These rod-shaped bodies with clubbed ends seem to be an asbestos fiber coated by macrophages with an iron-protein complex.[2,7,14,15]

Studies have shown conclusively that cigarette smoking has a multiplicative effect in the development of primary lung cancer in persons who have been exposed to asbestos. In addition several studies have shown a dose-response relationship between the amount of cigarette smoking and the degree of fibrotic response to inhaled asbestos.[14] Complications of asbestosis include **bronchiectasis,** pleural **mesothelioma,** and **bronchogenic carcinoma.**[7]

Clinical Manifestations

Signs

Pulmonary Function Tests. Lung compliance and therefore lung volumes are decreased. Specifically the TLC and the VC are decreased with a lesser decrease usually seen in the RV. The FEV_1, which is a measure of flow rate, is often decreased also. The DL_{CO} is decreased.

Chest Radiograph. The chest films show irregular or linear opacities distributed throughout the lung fields that are more prominent in the lower zones. Often a loss of distinct heart and diaphragmatic borders occurs owing to pleural involvement. These usually clear borders take on a "shaggy" appearance. There also may be radiographic evidence of diaphragmatic or pericardial calcification. Late in the course of the disease, the chest radiograph may show cyst formation, and the lungs may take on a honeycomb appearance.

Arterial Blood Gases. The Pa_{O_2} is decreased with exercise and, as the disease progresses, may be decreased at rest. Hypercapnia is not a usual manifestation of asbestosis, so the Pa_{CO_2} is commonly within normal limits.

Breath Sounds. Auscultation usually reveals bibasilar rales with decreased breath sounds due to the pleural thickening. Percussion is often dull at the bases.

Cardiovascular Findings. As the pulmonary capillary bed is destroyed, pulmonary hypertension develops and increases the work of the right ventricle. This can progress to cor pulmonale and cyanosis. Clubbing is more common in asbestosis than in silicosis or coal workers' pneumoconiosis.

Symptoms. The major patient complaints with asbestosis are dyspnea on exertion that progresses to shortness of breath even at rest, recurrent pulmonary infections, and chronic cough with or without sputum production. In addition, patients often report weight loss with decreased appetite and exercise tolerance.

Treatment

There is no curative treatment for asbestosis, and the disease progresses even though exposure to asbestos has ceased. Symptomatic support includes cessation of smoking, good nutrition, exercise conditioning to maximize lung function, and prompt treatment of recurrent pulmonary infections.

Bronchopulmonary Dysplasia

Bronchopulmonary dysplasia is a chronic pulmonary syndrome in neonates that occurs in some survivors of RDS who have been ventilated mechanically and have received high concentrations of oxygen over a prolonged period of time. Other names used for this syndrome are **pulmonary fibroplasia** and **ventilator lung.**[7,8]

Etiology

The incidence of BPD following RDS varies from 2% to 68% in different studies.[8] The incidence increases in neonates who had low birth weights (<1000 g); required mechanical ventilation, particularly using continuous positive pressure; received inspired oxygen concentrations ($F_{I_{O_2}}$) at 60% or higher; or received supplemental oxygen for more than 50 hours.[7,8] In fact, BPD almost invariably develops in neonates who received oxygen at an $F_{I_{O_2}}$ of 60% or higher for 123 hours or more.[7] See Chapter 6 for more details on BPD.

Bronchiolitis Obliterans

Bronchiolitis obliterans is a fibrotic lung disease that affects the smaller airways. It can produce restrictive and obstructive lung dysfunction. This syndrome has been known and discussed under a variety of names including bronchiolitis, bronchiolitis obliterans with organizing pneumonia (BOOP), bronchiolitis fibrosa obliterans, follicular bronchiolitis, and bronchiolitis obliterans with diffuse interstitial pneumonia.[11]

Etiology

Bronchiolitis obliterans was first recognized in children, usually those under the age of 2 years. Pediatric bronchiolitis obliterans is commonly caused by a viral infection, most commonly by the *respiratory syncytial virus, parainfluenza virus, influenza virus,* or *adenovirus.*[15] An adult form of the disease has now been recognized that can occur in persons from 20 to 80 years of age and has a wider variety of causes. In the adult, bronchiolitis obliterans may be caused by toxic fume inhalation (nitrogen dioxide) or by viral, bacterial, or mycobacterial infectious agents, particularly *Mycoplasma pneumoniae.* It may be associated with connective tissue diseases, such as rheumatoid arthritis; related to organ transplantation and graft versus host reactions; or allied with other diseases, such as idiopathic pulmonary fibrosis. It also may be idiopathic, with no known cause.[11]

Pathophysiology

Bronchiolitis obliterans is characterized by necrosis of the respiratory epithelium in the af-
fected bronchioles. This necrosis allows fluid and debris to enter the bronchioles and alveoli, causing alveolar pulmonary edema and partial or complete obstruction of these small airways. With complete obstruction, the trapped air is absorbed gradually, and the alveoli then collapse, causing areas of atelectasis. When the destruction of the respiratory epithelium is severe or widespread, it may be followed by a significant inflammatory response. This causes fibrotic changes in the adjacent peribronchial space, the alveolar walls, and the air spaces. The fibrotic changes are patchy and usually occur primarily within the bronchial tree and alveoli rather than in the interstitial lung tissue, as happens in IPF. All these changes combine to increase ventilation-perfusion mismatching; decrease lung compliance; impair gas transport; and, in some patients, cause demonstrable airway obstruction.[11]

Clinical Manifestations

Signs
Pulmonary Function Tests. The $D_{L_{CO}}$ is usually reduced. Lung volumes may be normal or decreased. Respiratory rate is increased. Flow rates are more frequently within normal limits but may be decreased.

Chest Radiograph. The chest radiographic findings are variable depending on the causative factor and the extent of involvement. In pediatric bronchiolitis obliterans, the chest radiograph may show hyperinflation with increased bronchial markings or subsegmental consolidation and collapse. Some children have patchy alveolar infiltrates, and others have a diffuse nodular or reticulonodular pattern consistent with interstitial inflammation and scarring. In adults the chest radiograph may first show pulmonary edema; bilateral patchy alveolar infiltrates may also be seen. Later in the clinical course, a nodular pattern consistent with fibrotic changes within the bronchial tree and alveoli may be seen.

Arterial Blood Gases. Hypoxemia is present in almost all patients; the Pa_{O_2} is therefore reduced. Carbon dioxide may be retained, resulting in respiratory acidosis, or the Pa_{CO_2} may be within normal limits.

Breath Sounds. Rales and often expiratory wheezing are heard on auscultation. Areas of decreased breath sounds are also common.

Cardiovascular Findings. Tachycardia is common.

Symptoms. Patients are often **dyspneic,** with an increased respiratory rate and a hacking, nonproductive cough. In infants chest wall retractions are often evident. Patients may be **cyanotic.** If the cause of the bronchiolitis obliterans is infectious, fever and malaise are common.

Treatment

In children treatment is supportive, usually consisting of hydration and supplemental oxygen. If the child is unable to clear secretions, postural drainage and suctioning are employed. Mechanical ventilation is rarely needed. If respiratory syncytial virus is the causative pathogen, then the antiviral agent *ribavirin* may be administered via aerosol.[15] Corticosteroids, antibiotics, and bronchodilators are not recommended in the treatment of pediatric bronchiolitis obliterans. In adults supplemental oxygen and proper fluid balance are also very important. Corticosteroids have proved very effective in treating adult bronchiolitis obliterans that is idiopathic, caused by toxic fume inhalation, or associated with connective tissue disease.

Pneumonia

Pneumonia is an inflammatory process of the lung parenchyma. This inflammation usually begins with an infection in the lower respiratory tract that may be caused by various microbes, including bacteria, mycoplasmas, viruses, protozoa, or a **psittacosis** agent. There are two categories of pneumonias: community-acquired pneumonias and hospital-acquired or **nosocomial** pneumonias.[10,17]

Etiology

Community-acquired pneumonias can be traced to the causative agent in approximately 50% of cases.[15] Although bacteria account for the majority of these pneumonias, viruses cause about one third of the pneumonias in this category.[15] More than 1 million cases of bacterial pneumonia occur each year in the United States. Approximately 50,000 people die of this disease, making it the fifth most common cause of death in the nation.[2] The most common agent causing bacterial pneumonia is *Streptococcus pneumoniae,* commonly called *pneumococcus.* Other bacterial agents that cause community-acquired pneumonias are *Legionella pneumophila, Haemophilus influenzae,* enteric gram-negative bacteria, *Staphylococcus aureus,* and anaerobic bacteria often found in the oropharynx. The mycoplasma agent *M. pneumoniae,* the psittacosis agent *Chlamydia psittaci,* and the protozoan *Pneumocystis carinii,* can also cause community-acquired pneumonias. The viruses that are most commonly involved in community-acquired pneumonias are adenovirus, influenza virus, herpes group viruses (including cytomegalovirus), parainfluenza virus, and respiratory syncytial virus. Although there are many infectious agents in the environment, few pneumonias develop because of the efficient defense mechanisms in the lung. Those who develop community-acquired pneumonias usually have been infected with an exceedingly virulent organism or a particularly large **inoculum** or have impaired or damaged lung defense mechanisms.[15]

Hospital-acquired or nosocomial pneumonias are defined as infections in the lower respiratory tract with an onset of 72 hours or more after hospitalization; they are characterized by the development of a new or progressive lung infiltrate.[15] Nosocomial pneumonias account for 10% of all nosocomial infections.[8] These opportunistic infections prey on the sickest patients in the hospital. The rate of nosocomial infections in the United States is 5.7 per 100 admissions or more than 2 million per year.[8] The most commonly identified causative agent of nosocomial pneumonias is a gram-negative bacillus, *Pseudomonas aeruginosa.*[15] Other microbes also capable of causing hospital-acquired pneumonias are *S. aureus, Klebsiella pneumoniae,* and *P. carinii.* The patients most likely to develop a nosocomial pneumonia have one or more of the following risk factors: nasogastric tube placement; intubation; **dysphagia;** tracheostomy; mechanical ventilation; thoracoabdominal surgery; lung injury; diabetes; chronic cardiopulmonary disease; intra-abdominal infection; **uremia; shock;** history of smoking; advanced age; poor nutritional status; or certain therapeutic interventions, such as the administration of broad spectrum antibiotics, corticosteroids, antacids, or high oxygen concentrations.

Pathophysiology

Bacteria and other microbes commonly enter the lower respiratory tract. It has been estimated that during sleep 45% of healthy people aspirate oropharyngeal secretions into the lower respiratory tract.[8] However, microbial entrance into the lower respiratory tree usually does not lead to pneumonia because of the elaborate defense mechanisms within the pulmonary system. The mechanical defenses include cough, bronchoconstriction, angulation of the airways favoring impaction and subsequent transport upward, and action of the mucociliary escalator. The immune defenses include bronchus-associated lymphoid tissue, phagocytosis by polymorphonuclear cells and macrophages, immunoglobulins A and 'G, complement, surfactant, and cell-mediated immunity by T lymphocytes.[15]

The most common routes for infection leading to pneumonia are inhalation and aspiration (Table 5–2). When the causative agent is bacterial, the first response to infection is an outpouring of edema fluid. This is followed rapidly by the appearance of polymorphonuclear leukocytes that are involved in active **phagocytosis** of the bacteria, and then fibrin is deposited in the inflamed area. Usually by day 5, specific antibodies are in the area fighting the bacterial infection. Clinically, bacterial pneumonia usually has an abrupt onset and is characterized by lobar **consolidation,** high fever, chills, dyspnea, tachypnea, productive cough, pleuritic pain, and leukocytosis.[1,14,15] When the causative agent is viral, the virus first localizes in respiratory epithelial cells and causes destruction of the cilia and mucosal surface, leading to the loss of mucociliary function. This impairment may then predispose the patient to bacterial pneumonia. If viral infection reaches the level of the alveoli, there may be edema, hemorrhage, hyaline membrane formation, and possibly the development of adult respiratory distress syndrome. Primary viral pneumonia is a serious disease with diffuse infiltrates, extensive parenchymal injury, and severe hypoxemia. Clinically, viral pneumonia usually has an insidious onset and is characterized by patchy diffuse bronchopulmonary infiltrates, moderate fever, dyspnea, tachypnea, nonproductive cough, **myalgia,** and a normal white blood cell count.[15] Usually it is impossible to identify the specific pathogen by clinical signs and symptoms or chest radiographic findings. Specific laboratory test results and other data are needed.

Clinical Manifestations

Signs
Pulmonary Function Tests. Pneumonias from any cause result in decreased lung volumes, decreased lung compliance, decreased gas exchange, increased respiratory rate, increased inspiratory pressure, and increased work of breathing. These changes are due to fluid-filled alveoli; increased ventilation-perfusion mismatching; decreased oxygen uptake; possible pulmonary capillary leakage; and pneumonia resolution, including fibrosis and scarring. For these reasons, pneumonias are usually classified as primarily restrictive in the lung dysfunction they cause.

Chest Radiograph. Bacterial pneumonia usually shows a lobar consolidation on radiographic examination. This may involve more than one lobe in one lung or may involve lobes in both lungs with confluent shadows that usually terminate at pleural surfaces. Viral pneumonia presents a different radiographic picture, which is usually of a bilateral bronchopneumonia. It appears on a chest radiograph as diffuse scattered fluffy shadows, indicating patchy alveolar infiltrates, and follows the distribution of the central conducting airways. When cavities are seen in addition to the other chest radiographic findings, the pneumonia is described as a necrotizing pneumonia.

Arterial Blood Gases. Patients with penumonia are usually hypoxemic, having a decreased Pa_{O_2}. Because most patients with pneumonia are dyspneic and tachypneic, they are

TABLE 5–2. Pneumonia Transmission and Treatment

Pneumonia Type	Transmission Route	Susceptible Populations	Preferred Drug
Bacterial			
Streptococcus pneumoniae	Droplet inhalation, direct contact with infected respiratory secretions, indirect contact with articles soiled by infected respiratory secretions	Infants, elderly; patients having congestive heart failure, COPD, splenectomy, alcoholism, multiple myeloma, or a predisposing viral infection	Penicillin G Erythromycin
Legionella pneumophila	Inhalation of an aerosolized infected water source (drinking water, air conditioning, shower heads, lakes)	Elderly; patients having diabetes, COPD, AIDS, renal transplantation, malignancy, and alcoholism; smokers	Erythromycin
Haemophilus influenzae	Droplet inhalation, direct contact with infected respiratory secretions, indirect contact with articles soiled by infected respiratory secretions	Elderly; patients having chronic bronchitis, AIDS, alcoholism, splenectomy, chronic debilitation, or a predisposing viral infection	Ampicillin
Klebsiella pneumoniae	Droplet inhalation, direct contact with infected respiratory secretions, indirect contact with articles soiled by infected respiratory secretions	Elderly in nursing homes; patients having COPD, alcoholism, diabetes, malignancy, chronic renal failure, and chronic debilitation	Aminoglycosides Cephalosporin
Pseudomonas aeruginosa	Droplet inhalation, direct contact with infected respiratory secretions, indirect contact with articles soiled by infected respiratory secretions, hematogenously, wound infection	Patients having cystic fibrosis, ARDS, or neutropenia; patients on mechanical ventilation	Antipseudomonal penicillin Cephalosporin Aminoglycosides
Staphylococcus aureus	Droplet inhalation, direct contact with infected respiratory secretions, indirect contact with articles soiled by infected respiratory secretions, hematogenously, aspiration	Patients having cystic fibrosis, drug addictions, splenectomy, or a predisposing viral infection	Antistaphylococcol penicillin Cephalosporin Vancomycin
Mycoplasma			
Mycoplasma pneumoniae	Droplet inhalation, direct contact with infected respiratory secretions, indirect contact with articles soiled by infected respiratory secretions	School children; college students; patients with AIDS	Erythromycin Tetracycline
Viral			
Respiratory syncytial virus	Droplet inhalation, direct contact with infected respiratory secretions, indirect contact with articles soiled by infected respiratory secretions	Infants 2–5 months of age and school-aged children	Ribavirin
Adenovirus	Droplet inhalation, direct contact with infected respiratory secretions or infected feces, indirect contact with articles soiled by infected respiratory secretions or feces	Children 6 months to 5 years and military recruits	None
Cytomegalovirus	Contact with infected body fluids including tears, saliva, blood, breast milk, urine, semen; can be infected in utero and by infected transplanted organs	Fetuses; patients having malignancy, AIDS, major organ transplantation, or chronic debilitation	Acyclovir analogue DHPG
Influenza virus	Droplet inhalation, direct contact with infected respiratory secretions, indirect contact with articles soiled by infected respiratory secretions	Women in the third trimester of pregnancy; elderly; patients having malignancy, heart disease, COPD, diabetes, chronic renal failure, neuromuscular disorders, or chronic debilitation	Amantadine
Protozoan			
Pneumocystis carinii	Unknown, probably droplet inhalation	Premature infants, patients with AIDS, or chronic debilitation	Trimethoprim-sulfamethoxazole
Psittacosis			
Chlamydia psittaci	Inhalation of infected droplets, droplet nuclei, or dust from the desiccated dropping of infected birds (parrots, parakeets, turkeys, pigeons, chickens)	Persons with pet birds and workers on poultry farms and in poultry processing plants	Tetracycline Chloramphenicol

COPD, chronic obstructive pulmonary disease; AIDS, acquired immunodeficiency syndrome; ARDS, adult respiratory distress syndrome.

blowing off an excess of carbon dioxide and so the Pa_{CO_2} may be decreased.

Breath Sounds. Auscultation findings vary depending on the amount of consolidation and the course of the particular pneumonia. Breath sounds could include any of the following: bubbling rales, rhonchi, bronchial breath sounds, decreased or absent breath sounds, a pleural friction rub, egophony, and **whispered pectoriloquy.** There is a dullness to **mediate percussion.**

Cardiovascular Findings. Patients usually have some tachycardia, particularly with high fever. Arrhythmias are uncommon.

Symptoms. Generally the symptoms of bacterial pneumonia include high fever, chills, dyspnea, tachypnea, productive cough, and pleuritic pain. A viral pneumonia produces symptoms of moderate fever, dyspnea, tachypnea, nonproductive cough, and myalgias.

Treatment

Drug therapy is the primary focus in the treatment of pneumonia, particularly antibiotics for treating bacterial pneumonia. Antibiotic therapy should be pathogen specific if the pathogen can be determined; if not, an empiric regimen of multiple antibiotics may be needed. Oxygen and temporary mechanical ventilation may be necessary in patients with refractory hypoxemia ($Pa_{O_2} < 60$ mm Hg). Other supportive therapy includes postural drainage, percussion, vibration, and assisted coughing techniques for patients who are producing more than 30 milliliters per day of mucus or have an impaired cough mechanism.[15] Adequate hydration and nutrition are also important. Nosocomial pneumonias can also be prevented by rigorous environmental controls in hospitals. Such controls include strict guideline adherence for the prevention of contamination of ventilators and other respiratory equipment, careful aseptic patient care practices, and surveillance of infections and antibiotic susceptibility patterns in high-risk areas.

Specific Pneumonias

Bacterial Pneumonias
Streptococcus Pneumoniae

S. pneumoniae is more common in the elderly, in alcoholics, and in those with **asplenia,** multi-ple myeloma, congestive heart failure, or chronic obstructive lung disease. Seventy percent of patients report a preceding viral illness.[15] This type of pneumonia occurs more frequently during the winter and early spring. Specific signs and symptoms include rusty colored sputum, hemoptysis, bronchial breath sounds, egophony, increased tactile fremitus, pleural effusion in 25% of patients, and slight liver dysfunction.[15] Complications can include **lung abscess,** atelectasis, delayed resolution in the elderly, pericarditis, **endocarditis, meningitis,** jaundice, and arthritis.[14] *S. pneumoniae* is treated with penicillin G or erythromycin. There is also a pneumococcal vaccine; this injection provides lifetime protection against 23 **serotypes** of the pneumococcus that account for 85% of all cases of pneumococcal pneumonia.[15]

Legionella pneumophila

L. pneumophila can occur in epidemic proportions because the organism is water borne and can emanate from air conditioning equipment, drinking water, lakes, river banks, water faucets, and shower heads. *L. pneumophila* accounts for 7% to 15% of all community-acquired pneumonias.[15] It is found more commonly in patients who have undergone renal transplantation or are on dialysis; in persons who have a malignancy, a chronic obstructive pulmonary disease (COPD), a smoking history, or an age older than 50 years; and in persons who are alcoholics or diabetics. Signs and symptoms in addition to those characteristic of bacterial pneumonias include headache, myalgias, preceding diarrhea, mental confusion, **hyponatremia,** bradycardia, and liver function abnormalities. Half the patients have productive coughs with **purulent** sputum, and half have nonproductive coughs. The chest radiograph may show **lobar** consolidation or unilateral or bilateral bronchopneumonia; rounded densities with **cavitation** may also be seen. Fifteen percent of these patients have pleural effusions. The antibiotic of choice is erythromycin. Rifampin may also be used in addition to erythromycin.[15]

Haemophilus influenzae

H. influenzae causes pneumonia particularly in children who have had their spleen removed, in patients with COPD, in alcoholics, in patients with **hypogammaglobulinemia,** and in the elderly. In addition to the expected signs and symptoms of bacterial pneumonia, *H. influenzae* often causes a sore throat. The chest radiograph may show focal lobar, lobular, multilobar, or patchy bronchopneumonia or segmental pneumonia that usually involves the lower lobes. Complications can include empyema, lung abscess, epiglottitis, otitis media, pericarditis, meningitis, and arthritis. The preferred antibiotic is ampicillin; however, 20% of patients have been shown to be resistant to ampicillin. In these cases cephalosporins, trimethoprim-sulfamethoxazole, and chloramphenicol are used.[14,15]

Klebsiella pneumoniae

K. pneumoniae may cause either a community-acquired pneumonia or a nosocomial pneumonia. The community-acquired *Klebsiella* pneumonia is seen most commonly in men over the age of 40 who are alcoholic or diabetic or who have underlying pulmonary disease. These patients may show purulent blood-streaked sputum, hemoptysis, cyanosis, and hypotension. Chest radiographic findings most frequently show right-sided involvement of the posterior segment of the upper lobe or the lower lobe segments. There may be outward bulging of a lobar fissure due to edema, and 25% to 50% of these patients have lung abscesses.[14] Complications include empyema, lung abscess, pneumothorax, chronic pneumonia, pericarditis, meningitis, and anemia. Treatment includes a two-drug therapy: an aminoglycoside and a cephalosporin. Oxygen is also used to maintain an oxygen saturation level of 80% to 85%. The mortality rate for this gram-negative pneumonia is 20%.[14]

Nosocomial *Klebsiella* pneumonia is a **fulminant** infection that causes severe lung damage and has a 50% mortality rate.[15] It affects debilitated patients in hospitals and nursing homes, middle-aged or older, who suffer from concomitant alcoholism, diabetes, malignancy, or chronic renal or cardiopulmonary disease. Their sputum is thick, purulent, and bloody or is thin and has a "currant jelly" texture. Tachycardia is common. The chest radiograph can show lobar consolidation, usually in the upper lobes, with lung abscesses, cavities, scarring, and fibrosis. A bronchopneumonia appearance may also occur. Complications are the same as those in community-

acquired *Klebsiella* pneumonia. Drug therapy includes the use of aminoglycosides, cephalosporin, and antipseudomonal penicillin.[14,15]

Pseudomonas aeruginosa

P. aeruginosa is a gram-negative bacillus and is the most common cause of nosocomial pneumonias. It causes 15% of all hospital-acquired pneumonias and affects 40% of all mechanically ventilated patients.[15] Those at most risk for this infection are patients with cystic fibrosis, bronchiectasis, **tracheostomy,** or **neutropenia** or those who are on mechanical ventilation or corticosteroid therapy. This necrotizing pneumonia causes alveolar septal necrosis, microabscesses, and vascular thrombosis and has a mortality rate of 70% in postoperative patients.[15] Signs and symptoms include confusion, bradycardia, and hemorrhagic pleural effusion. The chest radiograph shows bilateral patchy alveolar infiltrates, usually in the lower lobes with nodular infiltrates and cavitation. Treatment always involves two drugs. Antipseudomonal penicillin or cephalosporin is used with an aminoglycoside or with the monobactam aztreonam.[15]

Staphylococcus aureus

S. aureus causes approximately 5% of community-acquired pneumonias and can also cause nosocomial pneumonia.[15] This type of pneumonia is usually seen in infants and children under the age of 2 years, in patients with cystic fibrosis or COPD, or in patients who are recovering from influenza. Signs and symptoms include a more insidious onset, with cough, fever, and dyspnea, but usually an absence of chills and pleuritic pain. Other manifestations commonly seen in children are cyanosis, labored breathing, grunting, flaring of the nostrils, and chest wall retractions. The chest radiograph shows a diffuse bronchopneumonia, with bilateral infiltrates, cavitary lung abscesses, **pneumatoceles,** and pleural effusions. Complications include pneumothorax, lung abscess, endocarditis, and meningitis. Treatment is with antistaphylococcal penicillin, cephalosporin, and vancomycin.[14,15]

Mycoplasma Pneumonias

Mycoplasma are the smallest free-living organisms that have yet been identified. This class of organisms is intermediate between bacteria and viruses. Unlike bacteria they have no rigid cell wall, and unlike viruses they do not require the intracellular machinery of a host cell to replicate.

Mycoplasma pneumoniae

M. pneumoniae is seen in all age groups but is more common in persons under 20 years of age. Mycoplasma pneumonias account for 20% of all community-acquired pneumonias.[15] This infection is common year round, but usually the incidence increases in the fall and winter. Mycoplasma pneumonia has also been termed *walking pneumonia* because the respiratory symptoms are often not severe enough for people to seek medical attention. The course of the disease is approximately 4 weeks, and it is very infectious; whole families may become ill once a child brings it into the home. The signs and symptoms often include many extrapulmonary manifestations that are not common in bacterial or viral pneumonias. Patients may have fever, shaking chills, dry cough, headache, **malaise,** sore throat, ear ache, arthralgias, immune dysfunction with an **autoantibody response, meningoencephalitis,** meningitis, **transverse myelitis,** cranial nerve palsies, myocarditis, pericarditis, gastroenteritis, pancreatitis, glomerulonephritis, hepatitis, and generalized lymphadenopathy. The chest radiograph shows interstitial infiltrates, usually unilateral in the lower lobe; 20% of patients have a pleural effusion. Treatment is with erythromycin or tetracycline.[15]

Viral Pneumonias

Cytomegalovirus, varicella zoster, and **herpes simplex** cause viral pneumonias most commonly in immunocompromised hosts, such as patients who have had major organ transplants or who have acquired immunodeficiency syndrome (AIDS) or malignancy. The respiratory syncytial virus and the parainfluenza virus cause viral pneumonias in children. The adenovirus is a source of viral pneumonias in children and in military recruits. Viral pneumonias in the debilitated elderly are most commonly caused by the influenza virus. Persons at most risk for a viral pneumonia are those who have an underlying cardiopulmonary disease or who are immunosuppressed or pregnant. Complications of viral pneumonias include secondary bacterial infections, bronchial hyperreactivity and possibly asthma, chronic air flow obstruction, **tracheitis,** bronchitis, **bronchiolitis,** and **acellular hyaline membrane** formation.

Some antiviral agents are now available. **Acyclovir** is used against herpes simplex and varicella zoster. **Amantadine** is the drug of choice for influenza A. **Ribavirin** is used in children to treat the respiratory syncytial virus. Cytomegalovirus is treated with acyclovir analogue dehydroxyphenylglycol (DHPG). No drug therapy is available for all the varieties of viral agents, so treatment is often limited to supportive measures.[14,15]

Protozoan Pneumonias
Pneumocystis carinii

P. carinii is a parasitic protozoa that causes the pneumonia most commonly associated with AIDS. Patients with AIDS have impairment of T cell function as well as humoral immune dysfunction and thus are susceptible to infection from bacteria, viruses, fungi, and parasites. *P. carinii* pneumonia damages the parenchymal cells within the lung and alters the alveolar-capillary permeability. This type of pneumonia usually has a subacute course of fever, dyspnea, cough, chest pain, malaise, fatigue, weight loss, and *night sweats*. The chest radiograph most commonly shows bilateral diffuse interstitial or alveolar infiltrates, and a solitary pulmonary nodule may be seen. Treatment is with trimethoprim-sulfamethoxazole. If this drug is not tolerated, then pentamidine is prescribed.[10,15]

Psittacosis Pneumonias

C. psittaci causes approximately 12% of the community-acquired pneumonias in the student population and about 6% of the community-acquired pneumonias in the elderly.[15] The onset is usually insidious, with a dry cough, headache, and splenomegaly. Complications include laryngitis, pharyngitis, encephalitis, **hemolytic** anemia, bradycardia, hepatitis, renal failure, and **macular** rash. Treatment is with tetracycline or chloramphenicol.

Adult Respiratory Distress Syndrome

Adult respiratory distress syndrome (ARDS) is a clinical syndrome caused by acute lung injury and characterized by severe hypoxemia and increased permeability of the alveolar capillary membrane. It also has been known as noncardiogenic pulmonary edema, shock lung, increased permeability pulmonary edema, and post-traumatic pulmonary insufficiency.[2,8,15,17,18]

Etiology

Adult respiratory distress syndrome can result from a variety of causes. Some of the primary causes of ARDS include

- trauma—fat emboli, lung contusion, heart-lung transplantation
- aspiration—drowning, gastric contents
- drug associated—heroin, barbiturates, narcotics
- inhaled toxins—smoke, high oxygen concentrations
- shock—any cause
- massive blood transfusion—sepsis
- metabolic—acute pancreatitis, uremia
- primary pneumonias—viral, bacterial, *P. carinii*
- other—increased intracranial pressure, postcardiopulmonary bypass, amniotic fluid embolism, ascent to high altitudes[2,8,15,17,18]

Approximately 150,000 cases of ARDS are diagnosed annually in the United States.[15]

Pathophysiology

The primary pathologic change is an increase in the permeability of the microvascular pulmonary membrane. The specific cause of this change is unknown. It seems that a variety of mechanisms can be involved, depending on the specific associated etiology. Therefore, the exact mechanisms that damage the pulmonary capillary endothelial cells and the alveolar epithelial cells are still under investigation. The current theories under investigation involve the role of the neutrophils, the complement pathway, the superoxide radicals, the proteolytic enzymes, and the coagulation system.[2] When the permeability of the microvascular membrane increases, excess fluid and plasma proteins are allowed to move out of the vascular channel. This fluid leaks into the interstitial tissue and then crosses the usually tight alveolar epithelium to fill the alveoli. The change from an air-filled to a fluid-filled organ decreases markedly the compliance of the lung and all lung volumes and capacities; the work of breathing is increased. Pulmonary vascular resistance is increased; an intrapulmonary right-to-left shunt takes place; ventilation-perfusion mismatching is increased; and gas exchange is drastically reduced. In addition, surfactant production is decreased. The significant atelectasis due to edema in the interstitial spaces leads to increased pressure on the adjacent bronchioles and alveoli.[6,15]

Following this acute phase, ARDS may resolve completely so that the patient regains normal lung function after a period of a few months. However, some patients enter a **subacute** phase following ARDS. During this phase, alveolar fibrosis and capillary obliteration develop within the lung, which leads to chronic significant restrictive dysfunction. It is not clear why ARDS in some patients resolves completely whereas in others significant permanent lung damage occurs. It is known that the longer the patient is on mechanical ventilation and high concentrations of oxygen, the poorer is the long-term prognosis.[15]

Clinical Manifestations

Signs
Pulmonary Function Tests. The FRC, VC, and V_T are all decreased. Owing to the decreased lung compliance, the work of breathing is increased and the respiratory rate is high. Flow rates may be normal or somewhat decreased. The DL_{CO} is usually decreased.

Chest Radiograph. Symmetric, bilateral, diffuse, fluffy infiltrates are found on the chest radiograph. These may coalesce into a diffuse haze, which essentially whites out the lung. Other findings may be present that are consistent with concomitant COPD, atelectasis, or pneumonia.

Arterial Blood Gases. The Pa_{O_2} by definition is less than 60 mm Hg in ARDS.[8] The Pa_{CO_2} is usually decreased also because of the markedly impaired gas exchange; however, if the patient has a chronic carbon dioxide–retention problem, the Pa_{CO_2} may be elevated.

Breath Sounds. Decreased breath sounds are heard over the fluid-filled areas of lung, and wet rales are a common finding. Wheezing and rhonchi may be heard also, depending on the precipitating cause of ARDS.

Cardiovascular Findings. Tachycardia is common with ARDS. Arrhythmias may occur also, owing to the decreased oxygenation of the myocardium and the stress placed on the heart.

Symptoms. These patients appear acutely ill. They are dyspneic even at rest, and their breathing pattern is fast and labored. They often are cyanotic. Other symptoms include headache, impaired mental status, restlessness, and increased anxiety.

Treatment

The treatment of ARDS can be divided into four areas, each with a distinct goal. The first area is treatment of the precipitating cause of the ARDS. Because of the wide variety of causes for ARDS, there is a wide variety in the treatment protocols used to address the underlying cause. The second area of treatment is aimed at supporting adequate gas exchange and tissue oxygenation until the ARDS resolves. Maintaining an adequate airway and oxygenation is usually accomplished by intubating and mechanically ventilating the patient. Most often the patient is placed on a volume-cycled ventilator with supplemental oxygen. **Positive end-expiratory pressure (PEEP)** of approximately 5 to 15 cm H_2O is often utilized.[15] The PEEP helps inflate poorly ventilated alveoli; improves gas exchange; and permits the inspired oxygen concentration to be lowered, decreasing the risk of oxygen toxicity. The third area of treatment is supportive, managing the patient's nutritional status and fluid balance. Fluid and electrolyte balance is very important in these patients. Management may mean monitoring input and output and using diuretics. Or because ARDS can be associated with multiorgan failure, it may mean the use of highly technical interventions such as **continuous arteriovenous hemofiltration (CAVH)** or dialysis in patients with chronic renal insuffi-

ciency.[8] The final focus of treatment is to prevent and treat complications of the patient's condition and intensive care measures. Complications common in patients with ARDS are nosocomial infections, pulmonary barotrauma due to the use of PEEP, and coagulation disturbances. The prognosis in ARDS is always guarded; mortality can be as high as 50% to 70%, especially if this syndrome is associated with failure in other organ systems or is complicated by serious or repeated infections.[8,15]

Bronchogenic Carcinoma

Bronchogenic carcinoma is a malignant growth of abnormal epithelial cells arising in a bronchus.[15] This growth or tumor may spread by infiltrating surrounding tissues or by metastasizing to other body organs, or both. The World Health Organization has established a standard classification system that organizes bronchogenic carcinoma into four major types. They are squamous cell carcinoma, small cell carcinoma, adenocarcinoma, and large cell carcinoma.[15]

Etiology

The causes of lung cancer are many. However, it has now been well established through numerous studies that the primary causative factor is tobacco use. The average cigarette smoker has 10 times the risk of developing lung cancer as the nonsmoker. The heavy cigarette smoker may have up to 25 times the risk of developing lung cancer as the nonsmoker.[15] Occupational agents have also been implicated in the development of bronchogenic carcinoma. The known carcinogens present in the workplace include radioactive material, asbestos, chromates, nickel, mustard gas, isopropyl oil, hydrocarbons, arsenic, hematite, vinyl chloride, and bischloromethyl ether.[15] Increased exposure to significant air pollution also seems to increase the incidence of lung cancer, although this relationship is very difficult to quantify. Finally, in some individuals and families, a genetic predisposition for the development of lung cancer seems to be present.

Currently lung cancer accounts for 16% of all malignant tumors and 28% of all cancer deaths in the United States.[15] It is now the leading cause of death from cancer in both men and women (surpassing breast cancer). In 1990 approximately 142,000 Americans died of lung cancer, 92,000 men and 50,000 women. In the same year almost 157,000 new cases of lung cancer were diagnosed.[15] Because the 5-year survival rates have not changed significantly in the past 2 decades, the vast majority of these people will be dead well before 1995. The majority of these people could have been spared this diagnosis, with its pain, health care costs, morbidity, and unrelenting mortality, if they had given up smoking.

Pathophysiology

Each of the four major types of bronchogenic carcinoma is discussed separately.

Squamous cell carcinoma accounts for 30% to 32% of all lung cancer. It arises from the bronchial mucosa after repeated inflammation or irritation caused by cancer stimuli. It is therefore the type of lung cancer most closely associated with cigarette smoking. Squamous cell carcinoma often arises in the segmental or subsegmental bronchi but can also cause a hilar tumor. It is considered a centrally located tumor and occurs in the peripheral lung only about 30% of the time. Squamous cell tumors are bulky. They cause obstructive dysfunction because they extend into the bronchial lumen, which can prevent airflow and lead to atelectasis and pneumonia. They cause restrictive dysfunction because the tumor can compress the surrounding lung tissue; cause atelectasis and pneumonia, both of which decrease the ventilation-perfusion matching; and impair gas exchange. These tumors often cavitate but do not **metastasize** early. When squamous cell cancer does metastasize, it most often involves the liver, adrenal gland, central nervous system, and pancreas.[15]

Small cell carcinoma, also called *oat cell carcinoma*, accounts for 20% to 25% of all lung cancer.[2] It may arise in any part of the bronchial tree; however, 75% of the time it presents as a centrally located proximal lesion.[15] It often has hilar or mediastinal lymph node involvement. This tumor usually does not extend into the bronchial lumen but spreads through the submucosa and can cause obstructive and restrictive dysfunction through compression of the surrounding lung tissue. This type of lung cancer rapidly involves the vascular channels, lymph nodes, and soft tissue. It is known to metastasize widely and early and in most patients has metastasized by the time the diagnosis is made. This tumor rarely cavitates but commonly produces hormones that can lead to a wide variety of symptoms in many different body systems not involved in direct metastasis.

A number of body organs, however, are involved in direct metastasis. Seventy-five percent of small cell carcinoma metastasizes to the central nervous system, 65% to the liver, 58% to the adrenal gland, 30% to the pancreas, 28% to bone, 20% to the genitourinary system, 10% to the thyroid, and 10% to the spleen.[15] The metastases to the central nervous system and the bone often produce clinical symptoms such as hemiplegia, epilepsy, personality changes, confusion, speech deficits, headache, bone pain, and pathologic fractures. Metastases to the liver and the adrenal glands are often clinically silent.[8] Other clinical symptoms caused by tumor hormone production that are of particular interest to the physical therapist include abnormalities in the neurologic or muscular systems. These complications of small cell carcinoma can include progressive dementia, ataxia, vertigo, sensory neuropathy with numbness and loss of reflexes, motor neuropathy with progressive muscle weakness and wasting, atrophic paresis of the proximal limb girdle musculature, marked fatigability, osteoarthropathy, arthralgia, and peripheral edema.[15]

Adenocarcinoma includes acinar adenocarcinoma, papillary adenocarcinoma, and bronchioalveolar carcinoma and accounts for 33% to 35% of all lung cancer.[2] The majority of these tumors are located in the periphery of the lung and may not be spatially related to the bronchial tree. These tumors may arise as a solitary nodule and may involve the pleura, causing a carcinogenic pleural effusion. Adenocarcinomas metastasize widely and often involve the central nervous system, which produces neurologic symptoms already listed under small cell carcinoma. Approximately half of these tumors involve the hilar and mediastinal lymph nodes.[15]

Large cell carcinoma includes all tumors not categorized in the first three groups and accounts for 15% to 18% of all lung cancer.[2] These tumors are most frequently subpleural in location. Peripheral tumors are often large, lobulated, and bulky, causing compression of the normal lung tissue. They are usually sharply defined lesions, which may be necrotic or cavitate. This type of tumor spreads locally by invasion and also metastasizes widely, with more than 50% metastasizing to the brain.[15]

Prognosis for lung cancer is usually discussed in terms of 5-year survival rates according to the stage of the disease. The assigned stage number is determined by the International Cancer Staging System and is determined by the degree of lung involvement, the location of the lesion, and the metastatic spread of the disease. The 5-year survival rate for stage I is 50%, for stage II is 30%, for stage IIIa is 17%, for stage IIIb is less than 5%, and for stage IV is 0%.[15]

Clinical Manifestations

Signs
Pulmonary Function Tests. There are no characteristic pulmonary function abnormalities associated with bronchogenic carcinoma. Some obstructive or restrictive dysfunction may be reflected in the pulmonary function test values, depending on the location and size of the lesion.

Chest Radiograph. Squamous cell carcinoma appears most often as a hilar or perihilar cavitary lesion with bronchial obstruction and atelectasis or postobstructive consolidation.[8,15] Small cell carcinoma usually appears as a central mass, often with bulky hilar and mediastinal adenopathy.[8] Adenocarcinoma is usually seen as a peripheral tumor, often with pleural involvement and pleural effusions.[15] Large cell carcinoma is seen on a chest radiograph as a sharply defined, large, often lobulated mass in the periphery of the lung; the lesion may cavitate.[15] The chest radiograph may also show elevated diaphragms

if the tumor compresses the phrenic nerve and causes paralysis of the diaphragm.

Arterial Blood Gases. Hypoxemia and hypocapnia are common as the lung cancer progresses.

Breath Sounds. Wheezing and **stridor** may be heard if the tumor is obstructing the bronchial lumen. Patients may also have breath sounds consistent with atelectasis or postobstructive pneumonia if the tumor causes these complications.

Cardiovascular Findings. Superior vena cava syndrome may be present if the tumor compresses the superior vena cava. This compression would result in neck enlargement, neck vein distention, and edema in one or both arms. Anemia is common. Recurrent or migratory **thrombophlebitis** may occur. Cardiac arrhythmias and **tamponade** may also be complications of lung cancer.

Symptoms. The symptoms and physical findings with lung cancer can be extremely variable because they result from (1) the location and growth of the primary tumor with compression of the surrounding tissue, (2) regional extension into the mediastinum, (3) metastases to other body organs, and (4) tumor-produced hormones that can affect a number of body systems.[8] The pulmonary symptoms most common to lung cancer are a cough—productive or nonproductive—and chest pain—dull or acute. Central lesions more often cause the dull, vague, persistent but poorly localized type of chest pain.[8] Peripheral lesions usually cause a more localized, sharp, pleuritic-type chest pain.[8] If the patient's cough is productive, blood streaking of the sputum is common, but massive hemoptysis is rare. Clubbing of the digits is a common finding. Some patients develop dyspnea. Most patients have experienced an unexplained weight loss.

Treatment

The three most widely accepted forms of therapy remain surgery, radiation, and chemotherapy. Newer treatment interventions being applied to patients with lung cancer include immunotherapy, laser, brachytherapy, and nutritional therapy. Unfortunately, none of these newer treatment options has affected the overall survival rate of lung cancer patients. Surgical removal of the tumor remains the treatment of choice for all non–small cell lung carcinoma when the location of the tumor makes resection possible.[15] The more defined and smaller the lesion, the better the surgical success rate. Radiation has been used to treat all types of lung cancer. However, small cell lung carcinoma is the most radiosensitive, followed by squamous cell carcinoma and adenocarcinoma. Large cell carcinoma is the least responsive to radiation.[15] The response to radiation therapy depends on the size of the tumor and the intrathoracic spread of the cancer. Chemotherapy does not significantly benefit non–small cell lung carcinoma. The response rates are low, and the toxicity rates for the drugs used are high. Chemotherapy is the treatment of choice for small cell lung carcinoma.[15] Because small cell carcinoma metastasizes so early, surgery has little to offer patients with this type of cancer. Chemotherapy and radiation in combination with chemotherapy are often used to treat small cell carcinoma. See Chapter 7 for the effects of chemotherapy and radiation on the cardiopulmonary system.

Pleural Effusions

Pleural effusion is the accumulation of fluid within the pleural space. The fluid is a **transudate** if it has a low-protein content and accumulates owing to changes in the hydrostatic pressure within the pleural capillaries. The fluid is an **exudate** if it has a high-protein content and accumulates because of changes in the permeability of the pleural surfaces.[16]

Etiology

Numerous disease entities can cause pleural effusions. Transudative pleural effusions can be caused by congestive heart failure, left ventricular failure, **cirrhosis,** nephrotic syndrome, pericardial disease, myxedema, pulmonary emboli, or peritoneal dialysis. Exudative pleural effusions can be caused by bacterial or viral pneumonias,

parasitic or fungal infections, tuberculosis, mesotheliomas, bronchogenic carcinoma, **systemic lupus erythematosus (SLE), rheumatoid arthritis (RA),** acute **pancreatitis,** esophageal perforations, intra-abdominal abscess, asbestos exposure, uremia, sarcoidosis, or drug hypersensitivity.[14,16]

Pathophysiology

The capillaries in the parietal pleura receive blood via the high-pressure systemic arterial circulation. The capillaries in the visceral pleura receive blood via the low-pressure pulmonary circulation. Because of this pressure gradient, fluid is constantly moving from the parietal pleural capillaries into the pleural space and is then reabsorbed into the visceral pleural capillaries. Approximately 5 to 10 liters of fluid pass through the pleural space each day using this route.[2] Additionally, each day up to one half a liter of fluid and solutes can be moved out of the pleural space via the pleural lymphatics.[2,15] Normally pleural fluid formation and pleural fluid resorption are balanced, so fluid does not accumulate in the pleural space. When this balance is disrupted by any cause and a significant amount of fluid is allowed to accumulate in the pleural space, a restrictive pulmonary impairment results.[2] The excess pleural fluid within the thorax does not allow the lungs to expand fully.

Transudative pleural effusions are associated with an elevation in the hydrostatic pressure in the pleural capillaries. This is most commonly due to left-sided heart failure, right-sided heart failure, or both. Because of the increase in the hydrostatic pressure, more fluid is moved out of the pleural capillaries and less fluid is reabsorbed. There is therefore excess fluid in the pleural space, causing a bilateral pleural effusion. Congestive heart failure is the single most common cause of transudative pleural effusions.[2]

Exudative pleural effusions are associated with an increase in the permeability of the pleural surfaces that allows protein and excess fluid to move into the pleural space. Therefore, in exudative pleural effusions the pleurae are in some way involved in the pathologic process. Most commonly, the pleurae may be involved in an inflammatory process or with neoplastic disease. Inflammatory processes such as pneumonia, tuberculosis, or pulmonary emboli with infarction can begin in the lung but extend into the visceral pleura, causing disruption of the normal pleural permeability. Cancer can also cause disruption of the normal pleural permeability, either by direct extension of a lung tumor to the pleural surface or by hematogenous dissemination of tumor cells to the pleural surface from a distant source. Tumor cells are also spread via the lymphatic system and therefore can alter the normal lymphatic clearance of the pleural space or be brought into the pleural space by the pleural lymphatics.[2]

Clinical Manifestations

Signs
Pulmonary Function Tests. The larger the pleural effusion, the more compromised the lung volumes. Flow rates and DL_{CO} are unaffected by the pleural effusion. Pulmonary function tests may show a variety of abnormalities, depending on the underlying cause of the pleural effusion.

Chest Radiograph. Smaller pleural effusions are usually seen by noting a blunting of the costophrenic angle. Larger effusions cause a homogeneous opacity of fluid density, which may spread over the entire lung but is usually more pronounced at the bases when the patient is upright. The underlying cause of the pleural effusion if located within the thorax may also be evident on the chest radiograph.

Arterial Blood Gases. The Pa_{O_2} and the Pa_{CO_2} usually remain within normal limits. Even if the pleural effusion is large and is compressing a significant amount of lung tissue, ventilation-perfusion matching is maintained. This is accomplished by reflex vasoconstriction in the hypoventilated areas of the lung.

Breath Sounds. Bronchial breath sounds and egophony are usually present just above a pleural effusion. Directly over the pleural effusion, breath sounds are decreased. A pleural friction rub may also be heard if the pleural surfaces are inflamed.

Cardiovascular Findings. There are none specific to the pleural effusion. However, there may be abnormal cardiovascular findings if the pleural effusion is due to cardiovascular disease.

Symptoms. Patients may exhibit no symptoms. If the pleural effusion is large, the patient may be short of breath. If there is inflammation of the parietal pleura, the patient may have **pleuritic** chest pain. Some patients report a dry, nonproductive cough, which may result from irritation of the pleural surfaces.

Treatment

The underlying cause of the pleural effusion must be identified and treated. This procedure in many cases causes the pleural effusion to resolve. **Thoracentesis** can also be performed, using a large-bore needle to remove excess pleural fluid. However, this procedure does not seem to benefit patients significantly and is being used less frequently. Another treatment option that is used if a large infected pleural effusion (empyema) is present is the placement of a pleural space chest tube for drainage of this fluid.

Sarcoidosis

Sarcoidosis is an enigmatic multisystem disease that is characterized by the presence of **noncaseating** epitheloid granulomas in many organs. Clinically the lung is the most involved organ.[11,12]

Etiology

The etiology of this disease is unknown. It most commonly affects young adults, with 70% of the cases diagnosed in persons 20 to 40 years of age. It is more common in women than in men. The incidence is increased tenfold in black Americans when compared with whites. It is rare in native American Indians.[16]

Pathophysiology

This disease presents with three distinctive features within the lung: **alveolitis,** formation of well-defined round or oval granulomas, and pulmonary fibrosis.[11] The alveolitis usually appears earliest and is an infiltration of the alveolar walls by inflammatory cells, especially macrophages and T lymphocytes. The core of the sarcoid granuloma contains epitheloid cells and multinucleated giant cells; there is rarely any necrosis in the core. The core is surrounded by monocytes, macrophages, lymphocytes, and fibroblasts. These granulomas may resolve without scarring, but many go on to become obliterative fibrosis, which is characterized by the accumulation of fibroblasts and collagen around the granuloma. Diffuse fibrosis of the alveolar walls is not typical in this disease, although it can occur late in the disease progression. Approximately 25% of patients with pulmonary sarcoidosis experience a permanent decrease in lung function, which over time proves fatal in 5% to 10% of patients.[11] This loss of lung function is due to restrictive lung impairment primarily, but this disease also has an obstructive component. Prognosis seems to be better if the onset of pulmonary symptoms is acute. If the onset is insidious, with progressive dyspnea, then the prognosis is worse.

Sarcoidosis is a multisystem disease, and although the pulmonary system is the most commonly involved, other systems are affected also. Twenty to thirty percent of patients have ocular involvement, which can lead to blindness.[11] The most common ocular presentation is granulomatous uveitis, which causes redness and watering of the eyes, cloudy vision, and photophobia.[19] Five percent of patients have neurologic involvement, which can include encephalopathy, granulomatous meningitis, or involvement of the cranial nerves.[11] Other organs and systems that can be involved are the skin, heart, liver, spleen, kidney, muscles, joints, and immune system.[2,7,11,12,16,19]

The progression of this disease is extremely variable. The disease can be active and resolve spontaneously, both clinically and radiographically. The disease can be inactive and stable for long periods of time with no change in clinical symptoms. The disease also can be persistent and active, with progressive loss of lung function leading to a fatal outcome.[11]

Clinical Manifestations

Signs
Pulmonary Function Tests. The TLC and all lung volumes including RV are decreased. Lung compliance is decreased. The $D_{L_{CO}}$ is decreased primarily because of the increase in the ventilation-perfusion mismatching. Late in the disease there may be superimposed obstructive deficits, which result in decreased flow rates.

Chest Radiograph. Bilateral hilar **lymphadenopathy** is commonly seen on the chest radiograph. The lung parenchyma shows diffuse infiltrates with an interstitial reticulonodular pattern.

Arterial Blood Gases. Blood gas values may remain within normal limits. Late in the disease as pulmonary involvement progresses, the Pa_{O_2} falls.

Breath Sounds. Patient's respiratory rate is increased, and chest expansion is decreased. Auscultation commonly reveals bibasilar rales, decreased breath sounds in the apices due to bullae, and sometimes wheezes from bronchial obstruction.

Cardiovascular Findings. Because of the pulmonary involvement, approximately 15% of patients develop pulmonary hypertension, but this complication rarely progresses to cor pulmonale.[11] Direct effects on the heart in sarcoidosis include dysrhythmias, congestive heart failure, and papillary muscle dysfunction.

Symptoms. Approximately one third of patients with sarcoidosis experience dyspnea during the course of the disease.[16] Cough with or without sputum production is common also, and some patients complain of a vague retrosternal discomfort or fullness. Other constitutional symptoms include fever, fatigue, weight loss, and erythema nodosum.

Treatment

Treatment of this disease is difficult because it is known that some cases resolve spontaneously and others can go into long periods of remission. In treating the three pulmonary manifestations of this disease, corticosteroids are used early to suppress the alveolitis and granuloma formation.

Established granulomas with pulmonary fibrosis are relatively fixed lesions and do not respond to therapy.

CARDIOVASCULAR CAUSES OF RESTRICTIVE LUNG DYSFUNCTION

Pulmonary Edema

Pulmonary edema is an increase in the amount of fluid within the lung. Usually the pulmonary interstitium is affected first and then the alveolar spaces.[13,15]

Etiology

Pulmonary edema has two primary causes. One is an increase in the pulmonary capillary hydrostatic pressure secondary to left ventricular failure. This is called cardiogenic pulmonary edema and is discussed in this section. Pulmonary edema can also be caused by increased alveolar capillary membrane permeability secondary to various causes. This type of pulmonary edema is also named ARDS and was discussed under the section on Pulmonary Causes of RLD. Cardiogenic pulmonary edema is also known as high-pressure pulmonary edema, hydrostatic pulmonary edema, and hemodynamic pulmonary edema.[8,15]

Pathophysiology

As the left ventricle fails, its ability to contract and pump blood into the systemic circulation efficiently is diminished. This results in an increase in left atrial pressure, which is transmitted back to the pulmonary circulation. Because of this impedance to blood flow, the pressure in the microcirculation of the lung is increased, which increases the *transvascular* flow of fluid into the interstitium of the lung. The interstitial space can accommodate a small amount of excess fluid, approximately 500 milliliters.[15] The lymphatic drainage can be enhanced to move some excess

fluid out of the thorax. However, when the left atrial pressure rises above 30 mm Hg, these protective mechanisms are overcome.[15] The interstitial edema fluid disrupts the tight alveolar epithelium, floods the alveolar spaces, and moves through the visceral pleura, causing pleural effusions. The pulmonary edema fluid in cardiogenic pulmonary edema is characterized by low-protein concentrations. This finding is in contrast to that in ARDS in which the pulmonary edema fluid has elevated protein concentrations. With fluid in the alveoli and the interstitium, lung compliance is decreased; ventilation-perfusion mismatching is increased; gas exchange is disrupted; the work of breathing is increased; and there is restrictive lung dysfunction.[8,13,15]

Clinical Manifestations

Signs
Pulmonary Function Tests. Respiratory rate is increased and lung volumes are decreased. Flow rates are usually normal. The DL_{CO} is normal or decreased.

Chest Radiograph. Increased vascular markings in the hilar region are characteristic of cardiogenic pulmonary edema. **Kerley B lines** are present because of prominent thickened interlobular septa. Interstitial and alveolar infiltrates can be diffuse, and pleural effusions are common.

Arterial Blood Gases. The Pa_{O_2} is decreased owing to the increased ventilation-perfusion mismatching. The Pa_{CO_2} is usually decreased with the pH increased, denoting a respiratory alkalosis. Later in the clinical course, there may be carbon dioxide retention.

Breath Sounds. Wet rales with decreased breath sounds are the most common auscultatory finding. Some patients may develop marked bronchospasm and wheezing.

Cardiovascular Findings. Many patients with pulmonary edema may have a history of significant cardiac problems, including myocardial infarction. These patients commonly have arrhythmias.

Symptoms. Patients with pulmonary edema appear in respiratory distress and may report a sense of suffocation. They are short of breath, cyanotic, and their respiratory pattern is usually fast and labored. The patient's cough is productive of pink frothy sputum. **Pallor, diaphoresis,** and restlessness are also common symptoms.

Treatment

Treatment is aimed at decreasing the cardiac preload and maintaining oxygenation of the tissues. To decrease cardiac preload, venous return to the heart is decreased, which decreases the left ventricular filling pressure. Venodilators and diuretics are used to decrease the venous return. Other drugs may be given to improve cardiac contractility. To maintain oxygenation, supplemental oxygen is provided. Intubation with mechanical ventilation may also be necessary.

Pulmonary Emboli

Pulmonary emboli are a complication of venous thrombosis, in which blood clots or thrombi travel from a systemic vein through the right side of the heart and into the pulmonary circulation, where they lodge in branches of the pulmonary artery.[2,12]

Etiology

Pulmonary embolism is the most common acute pulmonary problem among hospitalized patients in the United States. Each year 500,000 to 1 million Americans have a pulmonary embolic event.[15] Many of these events may go unnoticed because they are clinically silent. However, approximately 10% of pulmonary embolisms result in the patient's death.[15] Thus, between 50,000 and 100,000 Americans die annually because of a pulmonary embolism, making it the third most common cause of death in the United States.[15] About one third of the deaths occur within 1 hour of the acute event. And more than half of these fatalities occur in patients in whom the diagnosis was not clinically suspect.[15]

In more than 95% of the cases, the thrombi that caused the pulmonary emboli were formed in the lower extremities.[2] In the remaining 5% of the cases, the thrombi may be formed in the pelvis, the arms, or the right side of the heart. Numerous risk factors increase the likelihood of thrombus formation in the lower extremities. These risk factors include immobilization owing to bed rest, long periods of travel, or fracture stabilization. Increased age, congestive heart failure, obesity, cancer, chronic deep venous insufficiency, trauma, cerebral vascular accident, oral contraceptives, pregnancy and the postpartum period, sickle-cell anemia, and thrombocytosis are also risk factors for pulmonary embolism. The highest risk group for thrombophlebitis is orthopedic patients. Some studies have shown that more than half of the patients with hip fractures have thrombus formation in the legs.[2,15]

Pathophysiology

The pathophysiologic changes that occur following pulmonary embolism affect the pulmonary system and the cardiovascular system. The occlusion of one or more pulmonary arterial branches causes edema and hemorrhage into the surrounding lung parenchyma. This is known as *congestive atelectasis*. The lack of blood flow causes coagulative necrosis of the alveolar walls; the alveoli fill with erythrocytes, and there is an inflammatory response. Another change within the pulmonary system is the increase in the alveolar dead space because a portion of the lung is being ventilated but no longer perfused. Pneumoconstriction of the affected area occurs, with the marked decrease in alveolar carbon dioxide owing to the lack of gas exchange and the patient's respiratory pattern of hyperventilation. In addition, the alveolar surfactant decreases over a period of approximately 24 hours, which results in alveolar collapse and regional atelectasis. These changes combine to cause an acute increase in the ventilation-perfusion mismatching, a decrease in lung compliance, and impaired gas exchange. If the oxygen supply is completely cut off to a portion of lung, then frank necrosis and infarction of lung tissue results. This happens in less than 10% of all pulmonary embolisms because lung tissue has three sources of oxygen: the pulmonary vascular system, the bronchial vascular system, and the alveolar gas.[15] However, infarction of lung tissue is followed by contraction of the affected tissue and scar formation.

The first cardiovascular change that occurs because of a pulmonary embolism is an increase in the pulmonary arterial resistance due to a decrease in the cross-sectional area of the pulmonary arterial bed. If this cross-sectional area is decreased by more than 50%, then the pressure needed to maintain pulmonary blood flow rises and pulmonary hypertension results.[15] This also increases the work of the right ventricle and can lead to right ventricular failure. If the pulmonary embolus is massive, right ventricular failure and cardiac arrest can occur within minutes.[2,13,15]

Clinical Manifestations

Signs

Pulmonary Function Tests. Lung volumes are decreased owing to the decrease in lung compliance and the congestive atelectasis. Expiratory flow rates also may be decreased owing to bronchoconstriction. Respiratory rate is increased, often markedly. These changes are transient and can resolve completely with resolution of the pulmonary embolism. If lung infarction occurs, then lung volumes remain decreased in proportion to the amount of lung tissue infarcted.

Chest Radiograph. A chest radiograph may appear normal. If changes take place, they usually occur in the lower lobes, where the blood supply is best. The chest radiograph may show a transient cone-shaped infiltrate fanning out and extending to the visceral pleura or a rounded nodular lesion. One of the pulmonary arteries may appear larger and the other smaller than normal. There may be evidence of a small pleural effusion. With unilateral pulmonary embolism and pneumoconstriction, one of the hemidiaphragms may appear elevated. These changes resolve with lysis or fragmentation of the pulmonary embolism. The only permanent change seen on chest radiograph is the scar formation secondary to lung infarction.

Arterial Blood Gases. Commonly the Pa_{O_2} is decreased, and the patient is hypoxic, although if the pulmonary embolism is small, the Pa_{O_2} may

be normal. The Pa_{CO_2} is decreased, and the patient's pH is elevated, denoting a respiratory alkalosis.

Breath Sounds. Breath sounds are decreased in the area of pneumoconstriction; there may be some wheezing. Sometimes fine rales due to the surfactant loss and resultant atelectasis also are evident.

Cardiovascular Findings. Tachycardia is almost always present. Electrocardiographic (ECG) changes are common but are usually minor and nonspecific. Arrhythmias may develop, particularly when hypoxemia develops. If the pulmonary embolism is massive, right ventricular failure and cardiac arrest can occur.

Symptoms. The acute onset of dyspnea is the most common symptom; more than 90% of patients who have a pulmonary embolism complain of shortness of breath.[15] This is the only symptom for the majority of patients. The severity of the dyspnea is directly related to the amount of pulmonary vasculature involved in the embolic event. Rapid shallow breathing and tachycardia are commonly present. Apprehension and cough may be present in some patients. Syncope may be evident with a massive pulmonary embolism. Pleuritic chest pain and hemoptysis may occur with pulmonary infarction but usually do not develop for some hours following the vascular occlusion. Patients may run a low-grade fever following a pulmonary embolism.

Treatment

Treatment begins with prevention of deep-vein thrombosis. This can be accomplished by decreasing the risk factors when possible and by heparin therapy. With repeated thrombus formation and embolic events, surgical placement of a transvenous device (e.g., Greenfield filter) to prevent migration of thrombi may be utilized.

Heparin therapy is most commonly used to treat pulmonary embolism. To maintain adequate tissue oxygenation, mechanical ventilation with supplemental oxygen may be required. In addition, if the patient is hypotensive or in shock, fluid therapy and vasopressors may be needed. Mild sedation and analgesia may be used to decrease anxiety and pain. Thromboembolic lysing agents (e.g., streptokinase) can be used to lyse the emboli, but this therapeutic intervention is no more effective than heparin therapy in terms of the patients' morbidity or mortality. Pulmonary **embolectomy** is being performed less frequently owing to the increased mortality when results are compared with those for conventional medical treatment. However, this emergent surgical intervention may be indicated in patients who have large emboli and cannot receive heparin therapy or have overt right ventricular heart failure leading to cardiac arrest. The ultimate prognosis following pulmonary embolism is extremely variable. In patients who experience no shock and are treated medically, the mortality rate is 8%. Patients who have pulmonary embolism and a simultaneous cardiac arrest have a 45% mortality rate. Patients who have a pulmonary embolism with extreme increases in right ventricular pressures have a 90% mortality rate.[15]

NEUROMUSCULAR CAUSES OF RESTRICTIVE LUNG DYSFUNCTION

Spinal Cord Injury

Spinal cord injury is damage to or interruption of the neurologic pathways contained within the spinal cord.[13,20]

Etiology

A spinal cord injury can result from an acute traumatic event, often a motor vehicle accident or a diving accident, or from a pathologic process that invades the spinal cord and damages it or in some way interrupts the neurologic transmissions.

Pathophysiology

For this discussion, spinal cord injuries include cervical injuries only. A spinal cord injury in the cervical region produces paralysis or paresis in the arms, legs, and trunk, therefore resulting in **tetraplegia.** With this type of injury, the expiratory muscles are paralyzed or very weak, leading to an inability to cough. This ineffective cough

may cause an increase in the incidence of pulmonary infections. The external intercostals are inactive, and the patient may have a functional, weak, or absent diaphragm, depending on the level of the injury (Table 5–3).[8,20] Weakness in the inspiratory muscles results in alveolar hypoventilation, hypoxemia, and hypercapnia. Because the alveoli are not well ventilated, the patient is prone to atelectasis, particularly in the dependent lung regions, which could lead to recurrent pulmonary infections. With parts of the lung underventilated, the ventilation-perfusion matching is impaired and the diffusing capacity reduced. A cervical injury also results in the loss of the sigh reflex, which increases the incidence of atelectasis and contributes to alveolar collapse. If the patient retains use of the diaphragm, breathing dynamics are altered markedly, resulting in **paradoxical** breathing. In paradoxical breathing the diaphragm descends on inspiration, causing the abdomen to rise and the paralyzed thoracic wall to be pulled inward. The diaphragm relaxes on exhalation, causing the abdomen to fall and the chest wall to move outward. Immediately after a cervical injury, the VC and the maximum voluntary ventilation are markedly reduced.

Approximately 6 months after injury, the VC has improved significantly if the patient has an intact diaphragm. And although it may not be normal, the VC may have doubled since the acute postinjury period. Paradoxical breathing is also diminished or eliminated because of the developing *spasticity* in the thorax and abdomen.[8,10,20]

TABLE 5–3. Innervation Levels of the Respiratory Muscles

Muscles	Level
Inspiratory	
Diaphragm	C3, C4, C5 (phrenic nerve)
External intercostals	T1–T12
Sternocleidomastoids	Cranial nerve XI (spinal accessory nerve)
Scalenes	C1, C2
Expiratory	
Internal intercostals	T1–T12
Abdominals	T7–L1

Over time pulmonary compliance is decreased owing to the shallow breathing and atelectasis within the lung and the paralysis and lack of mobility in the chest wall. This increases the work of breathing and can lead to diaphragmatic fatigue. All these pathophysiologic alterations lead to RLD and a chronic state of hypoxemia. The patient may therefore need mechanical ventilation part time or full time or an enriched $F_{I_{O_2}}$ (Fig. 5–8).[2,8,14]

Clinical Manifestations

Signs

Pulmonary Function Tests. The TLC, VC, and inspiratory capacity (IC) are decreased. The ERV is eliminated if there are no active expiratory muscles and the RV equals the FRC. The RV is increased. Flow rates are decreased. Peak inspiratory and expiratory pressures are decreased. The respiratory rate is routinely increased and the tidal volume diminished.[20]

Chest Radiograph. The chest radiograph may be within normal limits or may show evidence of pulmonary infections and infiltrates. Over time the ribs take on a more horizontal configuration.

Arterial Blood Gases. Hypoxemia is normal in high cervical lesions of the spinal cord. The more profound the respiratory muscle weakness, the more significant the level of hypercapnia.

Breath Sounds. Usually auscultation reveals diminished breath sounds, with abnormal or adventitious breath sounds being consistent with current pulmonary infections or infiltrates.

Cardiovascular Findings. Patients with spinal cord injuries above the T7 level may have epi-

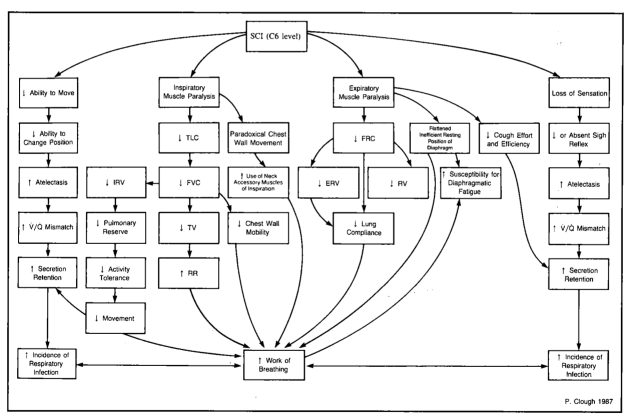

Figure 5–8

Pulmonary compromise in cervical spinal cord injury (SCI). TLC, total lung capacity; FVC, forced vital capacity; IRV, inspiratory reserve volume; Tv, tidal volume; RR, respiratory rate; FRC, functional residual capacity; ERV, expiratory reserve volume; RV, residual volume; V, ventilation; Q, perfusion; ($\downarrow$), decreased; ($\uparrow$), increased. (Reproduced with permission from Peat M [ed]. Current Physical Therapy. Philadelphia, BC Decker, 1988, p 34.)

sodes of **autonomic dysreflexia (hyperreflexia).** This may result in vasoconstriction below the level of the injury, which causes hypertension. The central nervous system above the level of the injury may then try to compensate in an effort to decrease the blood pressure, causing vasodilation and bradycardia.

Symptoms. Patients with acute cervical spinal cord injuries often complain of fatigue. This fatigue is due to the inefficiency of the breathing pattern and the effort that must be made by the remaining respiratory muscles. Patients also report shortness of breath, inability to cough, inadequate voice volume, and morning headaches, this last complaint being a significant symptom of hypoxia during sleep. Patients may also be restless or irritable, both of which can be caused by hypercapnia.

Treatment

Patients with spinal cord injuries must be taught ways to strengthen and increase the endurance of any remaining ventilatory muscles via use of an inspiratory muscle trainer, resistance exercises to the diaphragm, or an incentive spirometer. Patients must learn how to perform active and passive chest wall stretching, using rolling, positioning, side leaning, and air shift maneuvers. Patients, family members, or caregivers need to know how to assist the patient in clearing excess secretions with postural drainage, percussion, assisted coughing, and possibly suctioning. Learning how to perform glossopharyngeal breathing or how to operate a portable ventilator may also be necessary for selected patients.[20]

Amyotrophic Lateral Sclerosis

Amyotrophic lateral sclerosis (ALS) is a progressive degenerative disease of the nervous system that involves both upper and lower motor neurons, causing both flaccid and spastic paralysis.[1,2]

Etiology

The cause of the disease is unknown. It occurs worldwide, and onset is usually after the age of 40. Males are affected 1.7 times as often as females.[13]

Pathophysiology

The anterior horn cells of the cervical, lower thoracic, and lumbosacral spinal segments usually are the most involved, which means that the respiratory muscles may be affected severely. Muscles innervated by the cranial nerves as well as the spinal nerves frequently are involved, causing problems with dysarthria and dysphagia. Muscle weakness and wasting are profound. Following the onset of neurologic symptoms, the average life expectancy is 3.6 years.[18] Death is often the result of acute respiratory failure.[14]

Clinical Manifestations

Signs
Pulmonary Function Tests. The TLC, IC, VC, and ERV are all decreased, and RV is usually increased, resulting in an FRC that may be within normal limits. The patient's respiratory rate usually increases as the weakness of ventilatory muscles progresses and V_T is diminished. The maximum voluntary ventilation is severely reduced. Because of the profound weakness, the maximum inspiratory and expiratory pressures are also reduced.

Chest Radiograph. This parameter may be within normal limits or may show retained secretions and infiltrates that the patient is not able to clear.

Arterial Blood Gases. Owing to the compromised ventilatory pump, the Pa_{O_2} is decreased, and these patients experience marked hypoxemia. The Pa_{CO_2} is elevated because of the alveolar hypoventilation.

Breath Sounds. Auscultation usually reveals very decreased breath sounds, often with rales and rhonchi due to pulmonary infiltrates or infections.

Cardiovascular Findings. There are no specific clinical cardiovascular manifestations.

Symptoms. Patients often first notice a weakness or wasting in the muscles of the hands, although presentation of the disease can begin in the lower extremities or the trunk. This weakness may be accompanied by pain. Weakness is followed by atrophy of the muscles and muscular **fasciculations** ("snakelike movements").[1] Patients retain normal sensation and may complain of cramping of the muscles. Patients fatigue easily, lack endurance for activities, and become dyspneic with even mild exertion.

Treatment

There is no treatment for this disease except supportive therapy to make the patient more comfortable. Physical exertion is not recommended because it tires the patient so rapidly. However, the patient should be encouraged to get out of bed and be as mobile as possible.

Poliomyelitis

Poliomyelitis (polio) is a viral disease that attacks the motor nerve cells of the spinal cord and brain stem and can result in muscular paralysis.[2]

Etiology

Polio is caused by an acute viral infection, which can reach epidemic proportions in at-risk populations. It is reported most commonly in children. This infection can now be prevented by vaccine.

Pathophysiology

The virus is **neurotropic** and has a predilection for the motor cells of the anterior horn and the brain stem. The lesions are patchy and asymmetric, and microscopically healthy and diseased cells can be seen side by side. This results in a patchy flaccid paralysis or paresis of the lower motor neuron type. Both the diaphragm and intercostal muscles may be affected, resulting in a respiratory muscle weakness that can progress to respiratory failure. There are two stages. The preparalytic stage is characterized by fever, headache, malaise, and symptoms in the gastrointestinal and upper respiratory tracts. For some patients this stage is followed by the paralytic stage, which includes tremulousness of the limbs, tenderness in the muscles, and swollen painful

joints, as well as flaccid paralysis of from one to two muscles to all four limbs and the trunk.[1,2,14]

Clinical Manifestations
(Polio with Respiratory Involvement)

Signs
Pulmonary Function Tests. The paralysis of the diaphragm, intercostals, or both results in RLD, with the lung volumes being decreased. Respiratory rate is increased and V_T diminished. The maximum inspiratory and expiratory pressures are decreased. The DL_{CO} is decreased owing to the increase in ventilation-perfusion mismatching and alveolar hypoventilation.

Chest Radiograph. Films may show atelectasis or infiltrates. If the diaphragm is paralyzed, it appears elevated. Over time, if trunk musculature is paralyzed or paretic, a kyphoscoliosis may develop that would be evident on chest radiograph.

Arterial Blood Gases. The Pa_{O_2} is decreased, and the Pa_{CO_2} is elevated owing to alveolar hypoventilation and increased ventilation-perfusion mismatching.

Breath Sounds. Breath sounds are usually diminished. **Rhonchi** may be present, particularly in bulbar polio, which affects the brain stem and can result in the loss of the swallowing reflexes, thus leading to aspiration problems.

Cardiovascular Findings. There may be some transient rise in the systolic or diastolic pressures. Occasionally ECG changes may be found.

Symptoms. Patients are short of breath and anxious. Cough effort may be weak and ineffective in clearing secretions. Patients may experience any of the clinical symptoms described in the pathophysiology section.

Treatment

There is no specific treatment for poliomyelitis. Prevention through the use of oral or parenteral vaccine is very effective. Supportive therapy consisting of rest during the acute phase, with proper positioning, pain relief, good nutrition, and ventilatory support, as needed, is appropriate. Later, active range of motion exercises, strengthening exercises, bracing, and other equipment evaluation are required for patients with paralysis.

Guillain-Barré Syndrome

Guillain-Barré syndrome is a demyelinating disease of the motor neurons of the peripheral nerves.[14]

Etiology

This *idiopathic polyneuritis* is a disorder that seems to be linked to the immune system. The history of most patients with Guillain-Barré syndrome includes a viral illness followed by the ascending paralysis of this syndrome. However, the specific cause of the syndrome remains unknown.[2]

Pathophysiology

Guillain-Barré syndrome is characterized by a rapid bilateral ascending flaccid motor paralysis. The loss of muscular strength is usually fully realized within 30 days, often within 10 to 15 days, and may leave the patient so involved that mechanical ventilation is required. Approximately 10% to 20% of all patients with Guillain-Barré syndrome develop acute respiratory failure and must be placed on a ventilator.[8] The duration of mechanical ventilation is variable but is usually between 2 weeks and 2 months.[1,2,8,14]

Clinical Manifestations

Signs

Pulmonary Function Tests. Because of the profound muscular weakness seen in this syndrome, all the dynamic lung volumes are decreased. This includes the TLC, VC, IRV, ERV, and VT. The RV is usually within normal limits. Peak inspiratory and expiratory pressures are decreased. Respiratory rate is usually increased in an effort to maintain minute ventilation with a decreased VT. The $D_{L_{CO}}$ may also be decreased because of the increase in ventilation-perfusion mismatching and alveolar hypoventilation.

Chest Radiograph. Findings on chest films may vary widely during the course of the disease. They may include atelectasis, infiltrates, pneumonia, or neurogenic pulmonary edema.

Arterial Blood Gases. Owing to the weakness of the ventilatory pump, both hypoxia and hypercapnia are common.

Breath Sounds. Auscultation reveals diminished breath sounds that are usually most decreased at the bases. Adventitious breath sounds may also be heard during periods of pneumonia or with pulmonary infiltrates.

Cardiovascular Findings. Autonomic abnormalities can occur in Guillain-Barré syndrome, including cardiac dysrhythmias, hypertension, or postural hypotension.

Symptoms. Patients usually complain of weakness of both legs. Muscles may feel tender, and often paresthesias of the fingers and toes occur. Other sensory loss is slight.[1] When the respiratory muscles become involved, patients often report feeling dyspneic, anxious, and suffocated. Cough effort is often ineffective in clearing secretions. Patients report decreased endurance for activities and increased fatigue.

Treatment

Patients are supported throughout the syndrome's progression. Heat may be used to decrease muscular pain. Passive range of motion is begun immediately. Active exercises, including breathing exercises to assist the patient in weaning from the ventilator, should be begun as soon as the patient's condition has stabilized. Although exercise is important, patients with Guillain-Barré syndrome fatigue easily and should not be overly stressed. This polyneuropathy usually leads to complete recovery with minimal permanent sequelae. Recurrence of Guillain-Barré syndrome in the same patient is possible; in fact, patients with this syndrome are at slightly higher risk than the general public. However, even a second bout of the syndrome usually resolves.[2,13]

Myasthenia Gravis

Myasthenia gravis is a chronic neuromuscular disease characterized by progressive muscular weakness on exertion.[1]

Etiology

Myasthenia gravis is caused by an autoimmune attack on the acetylcholine receptors at the postsynaptic neuromuscular junction. What causes the production of this antibody is unknown. This disease predominantly affects women, and its onset is usually between 20 to 40 years of age.[13]

Pathophysiology

The antibody IgG binds to the acetylcholine receptor sites, which impairs the normal transmission of impulses from the nerves to the muscles. The muscles most characteristically involved are those innervated by the cranial nerves. This causes **ptosis, diplopia, dysarthria,** dysphagia, and proximal limb weakness. The signs and symptoms of this disease may fluctuate over a period of hours or days. Severe generalized quadriparesis may develop. Approximately 10% of patients develop respiratory muscle involvement that can be life threatening.[13,21]

Clinical Manifestations

Signs
Pulmonary Function Tests. With ventilatory pump failure, all the dynamic lung volumes and capacities are decreased. The peak inspiratory and expiratory pressures are decreased. As expected in a patient with RLD, the respiratory rate is increased and the VT decreased. The $D_{L_{CO}}$ is diminished owing to alveolar hypoventilation and ventilation-perfusion mismatching.

Chest Radiograph. The chest radiograph may be consistent with atelectasis or pneumonia.

Arterial Blood Gases. The patient's Pa_{O_2} is decreased, and the Pa_{CO_2} is increased because of alveolar hypoventilation and increased ventilation-perfusion mismatching.

Breath Sounds. Decreased breath sounds are common. If the patient retains secretions and cannot clear them, adventitious sounds also are heard.

Cardiovascular Findings. There are no specific clinical cardiovascular manifestations.

Symptoms. Patients with myasthenia gravis complain of weakness and fatigue of voluntary muscles, particularly those innervated by the cranial nerves. They may not be able to focus their eyes properly or to swallow. Patients are often short of breath, and their cough is weak and ineffective.

Treatment

Treatment of the disease's symptoms is with an **anticholinesterase** (pyridostigmine or neostigmine) and **plasmapheresis.** Corticosteroids, immunosuppressive drugs, and thymectomy are used in an effort to alter the disease's progression by interfering with the autoimmune abnormality.[13,14]

Tetanus

Tetanus is a disease of the neuromuscular system caused by the neurotoxin *Clostridium tetani.*[1] This anaerobic bacillus is found in the soil and the excreta of humans and animals and usually enters via a contaminated wound. The **neurotoxin** binds to the **ganglioside** membranes of the nerve synapses and blocks release of the inhibitory transmitter. This action causes severe muscle spasticity with superimposed tonic convulsions. This muscle rigidity can become so severe that the chest wall is immobilized, resulting in **asphyxia** and death. Tetanus can produce the most severe example of decreased chest wall compliance, leading to a restrictive impairment incompatible with life. The best treatment for tetanus is prevention via immunization. Prompt and careful wound débridement is also important. Once a patient has developed the disease, the tetanus antitoxin can be used to neutralize nonfixed toxin in the system. Once fixed or bound, the toxin cannot be neutralized. Supportive therapy is primarily focused on maintaining an airway and ensuring adequate ventilation.[1,13]

Pseudohypertrophic (Duchenne's) Muscular Dystrophy

Pseudohypertrophic muscular dystrophy is a genetically determined, progressive degenerative myopathy.[13,21]

Etiology

Pseudohypertrophic muscular dystrophy is a sex-linked (X chromosome) recessive disorder that occurs only in boys and is transmitted by female carriers. It is the most common of the *muscular dystrophies,* with a prevalence rate of 4 per 100,000 in the United States.[13,21]

Pathophysiology

Pseudohypertrophic muscular dystrophy typically appears when boys who have this recessive gene are 3 to 7 years of age.[13] Muscle biopsy at this time shows both muscle fiber hypertrophy and necrosis with regeneration. There is also excessive infiltration of the muscle with fibrous tissue and fat. Muscle innervation is not normal in this disease, but the abnormality is due to loss of motor end plates when muscle fibers degenerate and not to neurogenic disease. The pelvic girdle is affected first, and then the shoulder girdle muscles become involved. Although the calf often shows **pseudohypertrophy,** the quadriceps usually appear atrophied. The progression of the disease is steady, and most patients are confined to wheelchairs by 10 to 12 years of age. Involvement of the diaphragm occurs late in the course of this disease. However, respiratory failure and infection are the causes of death in 75% of these patients, which occurs usually by age 20.[8,13,21]

Clinical Manifestations

Signs

Pulmonary Function Tests. All lung volumes are decreased except the RV, which is usually increased. The TLC and VC are decreased. Because the patient is so weak, the respiratory pattern becomes inefficient with the VT decreased and the respiratory rate increased. Maximum inspiratory and expiratory pressures are also decreased.[2] The maximum voluntary ventilation is markedly decreased, often by one third of the predicted normal.[14] Chest wall compliance is decreased, and because of the microatelectasis that develops, lung compliance is also decreased. Gas diffusion is decreased owing to the increased ventilation-perfusion mismatching.

Chest Radiograph. Chest films may show atelectasis, pulmonary infection with infiltrates, or both.

Arterial Blood Gases. The Pa_{CO_2} is increased owing to alveolar hypoventilation and ventilation-perfusion mismatching. The Pa_{O_2} is often decreased, with the patient becoming hypoxic.

Breath Sounds. Breath sounds are often diminished; when a pulmonary infection and infiltrates are present, rales, rhonchi, and bronchovesicular breath sounds may be heard.

Cardiovascular Findings. The cardiac muscle is often involved, and fibrosis of the myocardium can be extensive. This change may cause abnormalities in the ECG, indicating a conduction block.

Symptoms. The usual presenting symptoms are a waddling gait, toe walking, lordosis, frequent falls, difficulty standing up from the floor, and difficulty in climbing stairs, all of which are caused by proximal pelvic girdle muscle weakness. With respiratory muscle involvement, patients first feel dyspnea on exertion and so will decrease their activity level. The dyspnea may worsen so the patient becomes dyspneic at rest and feels anxious and suffocated. Cough is weak and often ineffective in clearing secretions.

Treatment

There is no curative treatment. Supportive treatment is aimed at preserving the patient's mobility as long as possible and making the patient comfortable.

Other Muscular Dystrophies

Facioscapulohumeral Muscular Dystrophy

Facioscapulohumeral muscular dystrophy is an *autosomal dominant* disorder characterized by weakness of the facial and shoulder girdle muscles. Respiratory involvement or failure is uncommon in this type of muscular dystrophy.[8,13]

Limb-Girdle Muscular Dystrophy

Limb-girdle muscular dystrophy is a disorder in which adults exhibit weakness of the pelvic and shoulder girdle musculature. There can be severe involvement of the diaphragm early in the course of this disease.[8,13]

Myotonic Muscular Dystrophy

Myotonic muscular dystrophy is an autosomal dominant disorder that combines myotonia with progressive peripheral muscle weakness. Respiratory involvement and failure are common as this disease progresses.[8,13]

MUSCULOSKELETAL CAUSES OF RESTRICTIVE LUNG DYSFUNCTION

Diaphragmatic Paralysis or Paresis

Diaphragmatic paralysis or **paresis** is the loss or impairment of motor function of the diaphragm because of a lesion in the neurologic or muscular system. The paralysis or paresis may be temporary or permanent.[14,15]

Etiology

Unilateral paralysis or paresis of the diaphragm is most commonly caused by invasion of the phrenic nerve by bronchogenic carcinoma.[15] Another very common cause is open heart surgery. An estimated 20% of patients who undergo cardiac surgery suffer injury to the phrenic nerve owing to either cold or stretching of the nerve.[15] In hemiplegic patients it is not uncommon to find paralysis of the corresponding **hemidiaphragm.** The left hemidiaphragm is involved in left hemiplegia more frequently than the right hemidiaphragm is involved in right hemiplegia.[14] Other causes of unilateral diaphragmatic dysfunction include poliomyelitis; Huntington's chorea; herpes zoster; or peripheral neuritis associated with measles, tetanus, typhoid, or diphtheria. Bilateral paralysis or paresis of the diaphragm may result from high spinal cord injury, thoracic trauma, Guillain-Barré syndrome, multiple sclerosis, muscular dystrophy, or anterior horn cell disease.[14,15]

Pathophysiology

Normally as the crural portion of the diaphragm contracts, the pleural space pressure decreases; the central tendon moves caudally; the lungs inflate; and the abdominal pressure increases, which moves the abdominal wall outward. Contraction of the costal portion of the diaphragm accomplishes these same effects and in addition causes the anterior lower ribs to expand and move in a *cephalad* direction.[8] In diaphragmatic paralysis or significant weakness, the negative pleural space pressure moves the diaphragm in a cephalad direction so that the diaphragm's resting position is elevated. During inspiration, as the pleural space pressure becomes more negative, the paralyzed diaphragm is pulled farther upward and the anterior lower ribs are pulled inward rather than being expanded.[15] These changes in ventilatory mechanics cause alveolar hypoventilation with secondary changes that are seen in the lung parenchyma. The decreased inspiratory capacity leads to microatelectasis, ventilation-perfusion mismatching, alveolar collapse, and hypoxemia. The atelectasis leads to a decrease in lung compliance and an increase in the work of breathing. These pathologic changes are heightened in the supine position. The rib cage is less compliant in the supine position, and the rib cage musculature is less active. Therefore, in the supine position, diaphragmatic dysfunction produces a more significant decrease in alveolar ventilation than that produced in the upright position. The changes in the ventilatory mechanics and within the lung parenchyma combine to increase the risk of pulmonary infection or pneumonia in patients with diaphragmatic dysfunction.[8,14,15]

Clinical Manifestations

Signs
Pulmonary Function Tests. All lung capacities and all dynamic lung volumes are decreased in

proportion to the degree of diaphragmatic dysfunction. With unilateral paralysis, the TLC and VC are decreased approximately 25%.[15] With full diaphragmatic paralysis, the VC may fall below the predicted V_T, which would necessitate mechanical ventilation for the patient. Lung volumes may be further decreased when these patients change positions; the VC is decreased 30% by moving a patient with diaphragmatic paralysis from the sitting to the supine position.[14] Flow rates are also decreased in proportion to the decrease in lung volumes. The degree of weakness of the diaphragm is best measured by transdiaphragmatic pressure. The normal transdiaphragmatic pressure is higher than 98 cm H_2O.[14] When the transdiaphragmatic pressure is lower than 20 cm H_2O, the patient exhibits significant respiratory distress.[14] The maximum transdiaphragmatic pressure is decreased 50%, and the maximum inspiratory pressure is decreased 40% with unilateral paralysis.[15] The reduction is even more profound with bilateral involvement.

Chest Radiograph. An elevated hemidiaphragm is the classic radiographic finding. The diaphragm may show decreased, absent, or paradoxical movement on inspiration. Areas of atelectasis, especially at the bases, or pneumonia may also be evident.

Arterial Blood Gases. The Pa_{O_2} is decreased with diaphragmatic dysfunction, and the decrease is more pronounced when the patient is in the supine position. The Pa_{CO_2} usually remains within normal limits with unilateral involvement. With bilateral involvement, hypercapnia results when the patient is not able to maintain an adequate V_T and minute ventilation.

Breath Sounds. Breath sounds are usually decreased on the side of the paralysis or paresis, particularly at the base.

Cardiovascular Findings. Severe hypoxemia can cause pulmonary hypertension, which can progress to cor pulmonale.

Symptoms. The patient's most common complaint is dyspnea, which is worse in the supine position. Therefore, patients often report **orthopnea** and use two or three pillows because they are uncomfortable and short of breath when lying flat. Patients also report difficult or labored inspiration, daytime somnolence, and morning headache.

Treatment

Patients with unilateral diaphragmatic involvement usually do not require treatment because of the large pulmonary reserve and the other respiratory muscles that are still functional. With bilateral involvement, either full-time or part-time mechanical ventilation is often required. Diaphragmatic pacing via an intact phrenic nerve is also a possibility for some of these patients; however, the success rate with this treatment intervention is estimated at only 50%.[14]

Kyphoscoliosis

Kyphoscoliosis is a combination of excessive anteroposterior and lateral curvature of the thoracic spine[2,8] (Fig. 5–9). This bony abnormality occurs in 3% of the population. However, lung dysfunction occurs in only 3% of the population with kyphoscoliosis.[15]

Etiology

The cause of kyphoscoliosis is unknown or idiopathic in 85% of the cases. Idiopathic kyphoscoliosis is usually divided into three groups by age at onset: infantile, juvenile, and adolescent (10–14 years of age), with most cases appearing in the adolescent group. There is a 4 to 1 ratio of females to males in this group. The other 15% of the cases are due to known congenital causes (e.g., hemivertebrae) or develop in response to a neuromuscular disease (e.g., poliomyelitis, syringomyelia, muscular dystrophy).[15]

Pathophysiology

In addition to the excessive anteroposterior and lateral curvature, the lateral displacement causes two additional structural changes. A second lateral curve develops to counterbalance the primary curve. In addition, the spine rotates on its longitudinal axis so that the ribs on the side

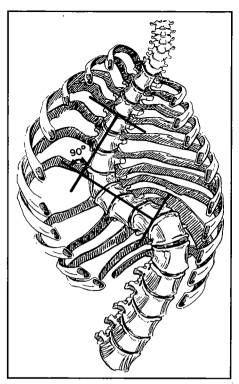

Figure 5-9

Kyphoscoliosis, showing the primary and secondary curves. The angle of curvature (90°) is determined by the intersection of two lines drawn through the upper and lower limbs of the primary curve. (Reproduced with permission from Fishman AP. Pulmonary Diseases and Disorders. 2nd ed. New York, McGraw-Hill, p 2300.)

of the convexity are displaced posteriorly and splayed, creating a *gibbous* hump, whereas the ribs on the side of the concavity are compressed. Significant spinal curvature must be present before pulmonary symptoms develop. Usually angles less than 70 degrees do not produce pulmonary symptoms. Angles between 70 degrees and 120 degrees cause some respiratory dysfunction, and respiratory symptoms may increase with age as the angle increases and as the changes associated with aging affect the lung. Angles greater than 120 degrees are commonly associated with severe RLD and respiratory failure.[8] These skeletal abnormalities decrease the chest wall compliance, which may be as low as 25% of predicted.[8] Lung compliance is also decreased and dead space increased. The distribu-

tion of ventilation is disturbed, with more air going to the apices. Ventilation-perfusion matching is markedly impaired. These changes lead to a state of alveolar hypoventilation and a profound increase in the work of breathing—as high as 500% over normal.[8] The hypoventilation causes pulmonary hypertension, which over time causes structural changes in the vessels and thickening of the pulmonary arteriolar walls, leading to cor pulmonale. Although the respiratory muscles need to work harder to overcome the decreased pulmonary compliance, they are impaired because of the mechanical disadvantages from the thoracoabdominal deformity. When the VC is decreased to less than 40% of the predicted value, cardiorespiratory failure is likely to occur.[14] This usually occurs in the fourth or fifth decade of life. Sixty percent of deaths are due to respiratory failure or cor pulmonale.[14]

Clinical Manifestations

Signs
Pulmonary Function Tests. All the dynamic lung volumes and lung capacities are decreased in proportion to the degree of deformity. The RV may be normal. Flow rates are decreased in proportion to the decrease in the VC. Because so much energy is needed to move the chest wall, even V_T is decreased, and so to try to maintain minute ventilation the respiratory rate is increased. The DL_{CO} is usually within normal limits unless the angle is 120 degrees or more, in which case it is decreased.

Chest Radiograph. The thoracic film appears grossly abnormal because of the severe deformity of the ribs and spine. The geography of the underlying lungs also is disrupted. It is not uncommon to see some lung tissue compressed with increased vascular markings, whereas other lung tissue is distended and may be emphysematous.

Arterial Blood Gases. If the angle is great enough, there is a decrease in the Pa_{O_2} and an increase in the Pa_{CO_2} owing to the chronic alveolar hypoventilation. The long-term elevation of the Pa_{CO_2} may blunt the responsiveness of the central chemoreceptors to acute changes in the Pa_{CO_2} that can put the patient at risk.

Breath Sounds. Breath sounds are usually decreased over the compressed lung.

Cardiovascular Findings. The hypoventilation causes pulmonary hypertension to develop. The arteriolar walls thicken, and cor pulmonale is common. Another complication of the chronic hypoxemia is that **polycythemia** may develop.[2]

Symptoms. Patients have dyspnea on exertion, and their exercise tolerance decreases as the pulmonary restrictive impairment increases. The structural abnormality may overstretch the muscles, make them subject to spasm or overuse, or cause them to be underused and atrophied. Patients appear wasted owing to the very high caloric expenditure necessary to maintain ventilation.

Treatment

Kyphoscoliosis is treated conservatively with orthotic devices and an exercise program. Surgical intervention includes placement of Harrington's distraction strut bars. Serious pulmonary involvement, including recurrent episodes of respiratory failure, seems to benefit from long-term nocturnal mechanical ventilation either through a chest cuirass or a positive-pressure ventilator.[14,15]

Ankylosing Spondylitis

Ankylosing spondylitis is a chronic inflammatory disease of the spine characterized by immobility of the sacroiliac and vertebral joints and by **ossification** of the paravertebral ligaments.[1,10]

Etiology

Ankylosing spondylitis is an inherited arthritic condition that ultimately immobilizes the spine and results in a fixed thoracic cage.[15]

Pathophysiology

The pulmonary impairment caused by this disease results from the markedly decreased compliance of the chest wall. With thoracic expansion so markedly decreased, ventilation becomes dependent almost entirely on diaphragmatic movement. Displacement of the abdomen during inspiration may be increased to compensate for the lack of rib expansion. Because the diaphragm is the major muscle of inspiration, the restrictive impairment involving the chest wall may result in only minimal respiratory symptoms.[8,15] However, approximately 6% of patients with ankylosing spondylitis develop specific fibrosing lesions in the upper lobes as part of this disease process.[7] Why these lesions occur in some patients is unknown, but the immune system may be involved.[16] The pulmonary lesions may be unilateral or bilateral; they begin as small irregular opacities in the upper lobes. These lesions then increase in size, coalesce, and contract the lung parenchyma. Cavitation is frequent. The lung architecture becomes distorted, which can lead to bronchiectasis and repeated pulmonary infections and an obstructive pulmonary deficit superimposed on the RLD.[7,16]

Clinical Manifestations

Signs. The VC and IC are decreased. However, unlike many other RLD entities, the RV and the FRC are increased.[8] If upper lobe fibrosis is present, it is apparent on chest radiograph. Breath sounds are usually normal unless the upper lobes are involved, and then rhonchi consistent with bronchiectasis can be heard.

Symptoms. The major symptom is **dyspnea** on exertion owing to the restrictive lung impairment. With involvement of the upper lobes, symptoms may include a productive cough, progressive dyspnea, fever, and possible **hemoptysis.**

Treatment

There is no curative treatment for ankylosing spondylitis. It is important to maintain good body alignment and as much thoracic mobility as possible. If there is direct lung involvement, then treatment of repeated pulmonary infections is required.

Pectus Excavatum

Pectus excavatum (funnel chest) is a congenital abnormality characterized by sternal depression and decreased anteroposterior diameter. The lower portion of the sternum is displaced posteriorly, and the anterior ribs are bowed markedly. Pulmonary function values are normal or near normal, and respiratory symptoms are uncommon. If the deformity is very severe, the patient may have decreased TLC, VC, and maximum voluntary ventilation and may complain of dyspnea on exertion, precordial pain, palpitation, and dizziness. Usually no treatment is indicated because the deformity is only cosmetic with no functional deficits.[1,14,15]

Pectus Carinatum

Pectus carinatum (pigeon breast) is a structural abnormality characterized by the sternum protruding anteriorly. Fifty percent of patients with atrial or **ventricular septal defects** have pectus carinatum. It also has been associated with severe prolonged childhood asthma. There is no pulmonary compromise associated with this structural abnormality, and no treatment is indicated.[15]

CONNECTIVE TISSUE CAUSES OF RESTRICTIVE LUNG DYSFUNCTION

Rheumatoid Arthritis

Rheumatoid arthritis is a chronic process characterized by inflammation of the peripheral joints that results in progressive destruction of articular and periarticular structures.[1,13]

Etiology

The etiology is unknown. There is a high prevalence of RA in the United States; 4 to 6 million adults have been diagnosed with this chronic condition.[11] One third of these patients, almost 2 million people, have some pulmonary involvement as part of their disease, although it remains unclear why one or more pulmonary lesions may develop in a given patient.[16] Lung involvement with RA usually occurs between 50

to 60 years of age and is very rare in children who have RA.[11] Another distinction is that although RA is more prevalent in women, pulmonary involvement, particularly pulmonary fibrosis, is more common in men.[16]

Pathophysiology

Pulmonary involvement in RA was first recognized and reported by Ellman and Ball in 1948.[19] Rheumatoid arthritis can affect the lungs in six different ways: pleural involvement, **pneumonitis,** interstitial fibrosis, development of pulmonary nodules, pulmonary **vasculitis,** and obliterative bronchiolitis. These different pulmonary manifestations of RA may occur individually or in combination within the lungs.[19] Pleural involvement may include pleuritis, pleural friction rub, repeated small exudative pleural effusions, and pleural thickening and fibrosis.[11,16,17] These pulmonary abnormalities can result in pain and some RLD. Pneumonitis causes an inflammatory reaction in the lung, including patchy infiltrates, which can resolve spontaneously or can progress to fibrotic changes. The cause of interstitial fibrosis in the patient with RA is unknown but seems to correlate with increased manifestations of **autoimmunity.**[19] Patients with a high titer of rheumatoid factor are more likely to develop interstitial fibrosis.[11]

There seems to be a temporal relationship between joint involvement and development of fibrosing alveolitis, with the joint involvement usually coming first.[11] Interstitial fibrosis can be diffuse but predominates in the lower lobes. Rheumatoid (necrobiotic) nodules usually occur subpleurally in the upper lung fields or in the interlobular septa. They may be single, multiple, unilateral, or bilateral. Spontaneous resolution of these nodules can occur. Cavitation is common.[14,19] If a patient with RA is exposed to coal dust, pulmonary nodules known as *Caplan's syndrome* can develop. These multiple peripheral pulmonary nodules have a pigmented ring of coal dust surrounding the lesion. Rheumatoid nodules and Caplan's syndrome rarely produce significant RLD.[16,19]

Pulmonary vasculitis often occurs adjacent to pulmonary nodules. There is intimal fibrosis in the pulmonary arterioles.[7,19] Obliterative bronchiolitis is rare; however, the onset is usually acute and progresses within 2 years to a fatal outcome. The bronchioles become inflamed and edematous and are then replaced with granulation tissue. The bronchial lumen is severely narrowed or obliterated.[7,14]

In addition to lung involvement with RA, chest wall compliance may be decreased significantly owing to increased rigidity of the thorax because of RA, decreased inspiratory muscle power because of rheumatoid myopathy, or decreased mobility because of pain caused by **pleurisy.** Therefore the RLD that can result in RA patients may be due to a decrease both in lung and in chest wall compliance.[11]

Clinical Manifestations

Signs
Pulmonary Function Tests. With interstitial fibrosis the VC and the volumes that make up this lung capacity decrease. The DL_{CO} also decreases, especially if there is evidence of pulmonary vasculitis. Lung compliance is reduced.

Chest Radiograph. Early pulmonary involvement may show patchy alveolar infiltrates and increased **reticulation** in the lower lobes. Later as interstitial fibrosis develops, a dense reticular or reticulonodular pattern with honeycombing appears.

Arterial Blood Gases. As lung involvement becomes significant, the typical restrictive lung impairment values of a decreased Pa_{O_2} with a normal Pa_{CO_2} emerge.

Breath Sounds. Bibasilar rales are common. With fibrosis, decreased breath sounds may also occur.

Cardiovascular Findings. With pulmonary vasculitis, pulmonary hypertension occurs if enough of the pulmonary vessels are involved.

Symptoms. The common articular symptoms are warm, swollen, painful joints, with progressive destruction of the joint surfaces and impairment of the joint mechanics. The major pulmonary symptoms are progressive dyspnea with a nonproductive cough. Other symptoms can include pleuritic pain, fever, clubbing, cyanosis;

hemoptysis can occur with cavitation of pulmonary nodules.[11,14,17]

Treatment

Corticosteroids and immunosuppressant drugs are commonly used to treat pulmonary involvement in RA.[14,19]

Systemic Lupus Erythematosus

Systemic lupus erythematosus is a chronic inflammatory connective tissue disorder.[1,13,14]

Etiology

The etiology is unknown, although the immune system seems to be involved.[1,14] Ninety percent of cases occur in women, and SLE is more common in black women.[8] It usually occurs between the ages of 15 and 45, most frequently in the second and third decades of life.[8] It is interesting that certain drugs (procainamide hydrochloride, phenytoin, hydralazine hydrochloride, penicillamine, isoniazid) can evoke a clinical syndrome indistinguishable from spontaneous SLE.[11]

Pathophysiology

This disorder involves the autoimmune system and is characterized by a variety of reactive **antigen-antibody reactions.**[1] Systemic lupus erythematosus can involve the skin, joints, kidneys, lung, nervous tissue, and heart. In 50% to 70% of the cases it does involve the lungs or pleura; this incidence of pulmonary involvement is higher than that of any other connective tissue disorder.[17] The most common lung involvement is pleurisy, often with the development of small bilateral exudative pleural effusions that may be recurrent, may be associated with **pericarditis,** and may lead to fibrinous pleuritis.[8,17] Acute lupus pneumonitis is another manifestation of lung involvement. It usually causes hypoxemia, severe shortness of breath, cyanosis, tachypnea, and tachycardia.[8,14,17] There may be an accompanying pleuritis with or without pleural effusion. Acute lupus pneumonitis may resolve or may lead to chronic interstitial pneumonitis and fibrosis. Alveolar hemorrhage is a rare but life-threatening pulmonary manifestation of SLE. It can occur suddenly with no prior hemoptysis and can carry a mortality as high as 70%.[8] The reasons some patients develop recurrent pulmonary hemorrhages or have a massive intra-alveolar hemorrhage are not known. Recurrent hemorrhages can lead to interstitial fibrosis.

It has been found that diaphragmatic weakness is relatively common in SLE patients. It is now appreciated that the "shrinkage" of the lower lobes, elevated diaphragms, and bibasilar atelectasis can be attributed largely to diaphragmatic weakness. The diaphragm may show muscle atrophy and fibrosis with minimal inflammation.[8] Other ventilatory muscles may also be weak, even with no noticeable weakness in the muscles of the extremities. This muscle involvement may cause a marked restrictive ventilatory impairment. Nephritis occurs in more than 50% of patients and is the major cause of mortality in SLE.[8]

Clinical Manifestations

Signs
Pulmonary Function Tests. With interstitial fibrosis or fibrosing alveolitis, lung volumes are decreased due to the decrease in lung compliance. Lung volumes could also be decreased owing to respiratory muscle weakness or recurrent alveolar hemorrhage. Diffusing capacity is decreased due to the increased ventilation-perfusion mismatching.

Chest Radiograph. The chest radiograph can show atelectatic pneumonitis with alveolar consolidation, particularly at the bases of the lungs; elevated hemidiaphragms; the reticulonodular pattern of interstitial infiltrates; pleural effusions; or **cardiomegaly** from a pericardial effusion.

Arterial Blood Gases. The Pa_{O_2} is decreased with significant restrictive impairment, and the Pa_{CO_2} is usually within normal limits.

Breath Sounds. On auscultation bibasilar rales may be heard or a pleural friction rub, or both.

Cardiovascular Findings. Pericarditis is often present; pericardial effusions and pulmonary hypertension can also occur.

Symptoms. Approximately 90% of SLE patients report articular symptoms, including arthralgias and polyarthritis.[14] Pulmonary symptoms reported depend on the type of pulmonary involvement but may include dyspnea, cough without or with only scant sputum production, hemoptysis, fever, pleuritic pain, cyanosis, and clubbing. Other symptoms may include skin lesions, photosensitivity, fatigue, weight loss, **Raynaud's phenomenon,** oral or nasal septal ulcerations, and neurologic disturbances.

Treatment

Corticosteroids cause rapid improvement of acute lupus pneumonitis and, together with plasmapheresis, are also used to treat alveolar hemorrhage.[8,17] Fibrotic changes in the lungs are irreversible, so only supportive therapy is indicated.

Scleroderma

Scleroderma (progressive systemic sclerosis) is a progressive fibrosing disorder that causes degenerative changes in the skin, small blood vessels, esophagus, intestinal tract, lung, heart, kidney, and articular structures.[1,14]

Etiology

The etiology is unknown, and the pattern of involvement, progression, and severity of the disease varies widely. It is four times more common in women than in men and is rare in children. The majority of patients are diagnosed between 30 and 50 years of age.[17]

Pathophysiology

Within the lung, scleroderma appears as progressive diffuse interstitial fibrosis, in which collagen replaces the normal connective tissue framework of the lung. There is fibrotic replacement of the connective tissue within the alveolar walls. The pulmonary arterioles undergo obliterative changes; however, necrotizing vasculitis is rare.[14] These changes may be accompanied by parenchymal cystic sclerosis, thus increasing the restrictive impairment in the lung. At autopsy 75% to 80% of scleroderma victims show evidence of interstitial pulmonary fibrosis.[16] Pleuritis and pleural effusions are unusual, unlike in the other collagen diseases that have pulmonary involvement.[16] Carcinoma of the lung also has been reported in association with scleroderma.[14]

Esophageal dysfunction is the most frequent visceral disturbance and occurs in most patients.[17] The disease is often slowly progressive. However, if cardiac, pulmonary, or renal involvement is early, the prognosis is poor. Death is usually due to cardiac or renal failure.[16]

Clinical Manifestations

Signs
Pulmonary Function Tests. The TLC, VC, and all lung volumes are decreased. Lung compliance is reduced owing to the interstitial fibrosis, and chest wall compliance also may be reduced because of the scleroderma. These changes can increase markedly the work of breathing and usually result in an increased respiratory rate in an effort to maintain minute ventilation. The $D_{L_{CO}}$ is impaired early in this disease.

Chest Radiograph. The chest films early in the course of the disease show pulmonary infiltrates. Later the chest radiograph may show an interstitial reticular pattern with honeycombing, particularly at the bases of the lungs; pleural thickening; or aspiration pneumonia, which is common because of the decreased esophageal motility. Pericardial effusions and right heart enlargement may also be seen.

Arterial Blood Gases. Because of the RLD, the Pa_{O_2} is decreased, whereas the Pa_{CO_2} is usually within normal limits.

Breath Sounds. Bibasilar rales are the most common finding. Breath sounds may be diminished, and rhonchi can be present if the patient has pulmonary infiltrates or an aspiration pneumonia.

Cardiovascular Findings. Pulmonary hypertension is common and can progress to cor pulmonale. Other common cardiac findings are pericarditis with pericardial effusions, arrhythmias, and conduction disturbances.

Symptoms. The most prominent symptom is exertional dyspnea, and this occurs in approximately 40% of all scleroderma patients. It is even more common in patients with Raynaud's phenomenon.[16] A nonproductive cough and clubbing of the digits are also common.

Treatment

There is no effective treatment for sclerodermatous pleuropulmonary disease. The interstitial fibrosis is progressive and nonreversible. There is also no drug therapy that has been shown to be effective in altering the course of scleroderma. A number of agents are used to treat specific symptoms in affected organs.[17]

Polymyositis

Polymyositis is a systemic connective tissue disease characterized by symmetric proximal muscle weakness and pain.[13,14,17]

Etiology

The etiology is unknown but may involve an autoimmune reaction. The disease can occur throughout life but most commonly appears before age 15 or between 40 and 60 years of age. The disease is twice as common in women.[13,17]

Pathophysiology

Approximately 5% of patients exhibit involvement of the lung parenchyma.[17] Changes can include interstitial pneumonitis and fibrosis, bronchiolitis obliterans, **aspiration pneumonia,** or diffuse pulmonary infiltrates. The pleura is usually not involved. In addition to these changes, which result in a restrictive pulmonary impairment, the respiratory muscles may be weak, which increases the restrictive dysfunction. Striated muscle involvement includes inflammation, degeneration, atrophy, and necrosis. This results in profound weakness of the limb girdle muscles, the respiratory muscles, the laryngeal muscles, and the pharyngeal muscles. When the disease occurs in children, diffuse soft tissue calcification may occur also, which could decrease chest wall compliance further. Dysphagia and aspiration problems are common. Although characteristics of the disease are similar in children and adults, the onset is often more acute in children and more insidious in adults. The disease may enter long periods of remission. However, it seems to be more severe and unrelenting in patients with pulmonary or cardiac involvement.[14,16,17]

Clinical Manifestations

Signs. With chest wall and lung parenchymal involvement, the lung volumes are decreased and the $D_{L_{CO}}$ is also reduced. The chest radiograph shows small irregular shadows in the lower zones. Because of weakness in the ventilatory pump, alveolar hypoventilation occurs, which leads to a decrease in the Pa_{O_2}. Auscultation reveals bibasilar rales.

Symptoms. Patients experience progressive shortness of breath with a nonproductive cough. Neck flexors may become extremely weak so that the patient has difficulty lifting or supporting the head. Weakness of the laryngeal and pharyngeal muscles can cause dysphonia and dysphagia. As the respiratory muscles become weak, breathing becomes labored. There may also be muscle pain and tenderness and polyarthralgia. Raynaud's phenomenon is present in 9% of these patients.[14]

Treatment

Pulmonary involvement is treated with corticosteroids with good results if started early during the inflammatory phase.[14]

Dermatomyositis

Dermatomyositis is a systemic connective tissue disease characterized primarily by inflammatory and degenerative changes in the skin. The pulmonary involvement that occurs with this disease mirrors the involvement that occurs with polymyositis described earlier. The incidence of

lung involvement in dermatomyositis patients is also 5%.[10,16]

IMMUNOLOGIC CAUSES OF RESTRICTIVE LUNG DYSFUNCTION

Goodpasture's Syndrome

Goodpasture's syndrome is a disease of the immune complex that is characterized by interstitial or intra-alveolar hemorrhage, glomerulonephritis, and **anemia.**[16]

Etiology

This rather rare disease is most often brought on by the presence of *antiglomerular basement membrane (anti-GBM) antibodies* that react with the vascular basement membranes of the alveolus and the glomerulus, causing pulmonary hemorrhage and glomerulonephritis. How these antibodies come to be formed is still unknown. **Prodromal** viral infections or exposure to chemical substances such as hydrocarbon solvents may be involved. Why these anti-GBM antibodies cannot be demonstrated in all patients with Goodpasture's syndrome is another mystery. This syndrome is approximately four times more prevalent in men than in women. The onset of the disease occurs between the ages of 17 and 27 in 75% of the cases.[15]

Pathophysiology

Whatever the cause of these autoantibodies, it has been shown that when they are present in the circulating blood, they crossreact with the basement membrane of the alveolar wall and deposit along the glomerular basement membrane. This results in the release of **cytotoxic** substances that damage the pulmonary and glomerular capillaries. Blood leaks from the damaged pulmonary capillaries into the interstitium and the alveolar spaces, which over time can lead to significant and widespread pulmonary fibrosis. The pulmonary hemorrhages are episodic and seem to be precipitated by nonimmunologic factors such as fluid overload, smoking, toxic exposure, or infection. Within the kidney, the damaged glomerular capillaries lead to a rapidly progressive, often necrotizing type of glomerulonephritis and renal failure.[8,15,16]

Clinical Manifestations

Signs

Pulmonary Function Tests. Lung volumes are decreased in proportion to the amount of pulmonary fibrosis present. The area of the lung involved and affected by the fibrosis is variable.

Chest Radiograph. The chest radiograph shows the distribution, volume, and temporal sequence of repeated pulmonary hemorrhages. Confluent densities are visible shortly after a hemorrhage into the interstitial tissue or the alveolar spaces. These diffuse, fluffy infiltrates may clear completely during remission of the disease. However, with repeated episodes of pulmonary hemorrhage, accentuated interstitial pulmonary markings persist and become visible on the radiograph. When pulmonary fibrosis develops, permanent reticulonodular infiltrates can be seen. It is also possible to see fluffy alveolar densities superimposed on a reticulonodular pattern when there is a new pulmonary hemorrhage in an already damaged and fibrotic area of lung.[15]

Arterial Blood Gases. Hypoxemia is common owing to the increase in ventilation-perfusion mismatching. Pa_{CO_2} may also be decreased.

Breath Sounds. Auscultatory findings vary. With active pulmonary hemorrhage, breath sounds are decreased, and rales or rhonchi may be heard. Over areas of permanent pulmonary fibrosis, the most common findings are decreased breath sounds and dry inspiratory rales.

Cardiovascular Findings. Usually the ECG is normal.

Symptoms. The most characteristic symptom is hemoptysis, which can vary from blood-tinged sputum to massive amounts of frank red blood. Hemoptysis is most often the initial symptom; it occurs at some time during the course of the disease in virtually every case. Other pulmonary symptoms include dyspnea and substernal chest pain. Patients may also experience weakness, hematuria, and fever, and 5% of these patients report arthralgias or arthritis.[8]

Treatment

Treatment usually combines plasmapheresis and immunosuppressive therapy to lower the levels of anti-GBM antibodies circulating in the blood. Cyclophosphamide with prednisone are the drugs of choice. Methylprednisolone may be used to treat pulmonary hemorrhage. Dialysis is used to counteract renal failure. The overall prognosis for Goodpasture's syndrome is poor. Approximately 50% of the patients die within 1 year of diagnosis. One half of the deaths are due to pulmonary hemorrhage and the other half to renal failure.[8,15,16]

Wegener's Granulomatosis

Wegener's granulomatosis is a multisystem disease characterized by granulomatous vasculitis of the upper and lower respiratory tracts, glomerulonephritis, and widespread small vessel vasculitis.[15]

Etiology

The etiology is unknown. Some studies seem to indicate that the disease may be due to a hypersensitivity reaction to an undetermined antigen. During the active disease process, circulating immune complexes have been identified. Immune reactants and complexlike deposits have also been identified in renal biopsies of patients with Wegener's granulomatosis. Although histologically the immune system and hypersensitivity reactions seem to be involved, the disease appears clinically as an infectious process due to some unknown pathogen. This disease can occur at any age, but the average age at onset is 40 years. The disease is twice as common in males as in females.[15]

Pathophysiology

The disease often seems to start in the upper respiratory tract with necrotizing granulomas and ulceration in the nasopharynx and paranasal areas. Inflammation with perivascular exudative infiltration and fibrin deposition in the pulmonary arteries and veins causes focal destruction. Multiple nodular cavitary infiltrates develop in one or both lungs. These lesions often consist of a necrotic core surrounded by granulation tissue. Early in the disease, the kidney shows acute focal or segmental glomerulitis with hematuria. As the disease progresses, necrotizing glomerulonephritis leading to kidney failure often occurs.[12,15]

Clinical Manifestations

Signs
Pulmonary Function Tests. Lung volumes are decreased if the lung parenchyma is significantly involved. There may also be an obstructive component to this disease if granulomatous lesions invade and block bronchial airways. Gas diffusion can also be impaired if the pulmonary capillary bed has been extensively destroyed.

Chest Radiograph. The pulmonary infiltrates seen on radiograph may be of any size or shape and seem to have no predilection for location within the lung. These nodular infiltrates may appear in any lobe—bilaterally or unilaterally—and may appear hazy or with sharply defined borders. Cavitation of these lesions is common.[12,15]

Arterial Blood Gases. A decrease in the Pa_{O_2} is evident as more of the lung tissue and the pulmonary capillary bed are unable to participate in gas exchange.

Breath Sounds. Auscultatory findings are variable, depending on the size and location of the pulmonary lesions.

Cardiovascular Findings. These findings are variable, depending on the severity of the disseminated small vessel vasculitis. Myocardial infarction can result from the vasculitis.

Symptoms. The initial symptoms often involve the upper respiratory tract and include severe **rhinorrhea;** paranasal sinusitis; nasal mucosal ulcerations; and otitis media, often with hearing loss. With pulmonary involvement, the usual symptoms include dyspnea, cough, hemoptysis, vague chest pain, or pleuritic chest pain. Other more generalized symptoms commonly noted in this disease are fever, fatigue, malaise, anorexia, weight loss, and migratory arthralgias.

Treatment

The treatment of choice is with cyclophosphamide. This drug can produce long-term remission in most patients. Without drug therapy, this disease progresses rapidly and is fatal. The mean duration between diagnosis and death is 5 months when not treated.[15] Death is most often due to renal disease progressing to kidney failure. Kidney transplantation has been used successfully in cases of renal failure.

REPRODUCTIVE CAUSES OF RESTRICTIVE LUNG DYSFUNCTION

Pregnancy

During the third trimester of pregnancy, ventilation to the dependent regions of the lungs is impaired by the growth and position of the developing fetus. This restrictive change in ventilation is due to a decrease in chest wall compliance caused primarily by the decreased downward excursion of the diaphragm. The decreased ventilation in the bases of the lungs results in early small airway closure and increased ventilation-perfusion mismatching. The voluntary lung volumes are decreased, particularly the ERV. Respiratory rate is increased. The work of breathing is increased, and the woman may feel she is unable to take a deep breath, particularly in the supine position. To counteract some of these changes and to keep the Pa_{O_2} within the normal range, the body increases the progesterone level during this trimester. The increased level of progesterone increases the woman's ventilatory drive and ensures that she and the fetus do not become hypoxemic.[10]

NUTRITIONAL AND METABOLIC CAUSES OF RESTRICTIVE LUNG DYSFUNCTION

Obesity

Obesity is defined as an increase in weight of 20% or more over the ideal body weight.[13]

Etiology

Obesity is the result of an imbalance between the calories ingested and the calories expended. This imbalance may be due to overeating, inadequate exercise, a pathologic process that alters metabolism, or a psychological need or coping mechanism.

Pathophysiology

The increase in body weight represents a significant increase in body mass, and this extra tissue requires additional oxygen from the lungs and produces additional carbon dioxide, which must be eliminated by the lungs. The excess soft tissue on the chest wall decreases the compliance of the thorax and therefore increases the work of breathing. The excess soft tissue in the abdominal wall exerts pressure on the abdominal contents, forcing the diaphragm up to a higher resting position. This shift results in decreased lung expansion and early closure of the small airways and alveoli, especially at the bases or the dependent regions of the lung. These areas are hypoventilated relative to their perfusion, which can markedly increase the ventilation-perfusion mismatching and result in hypoxemia.[2,8]

Clinical Manifestations

Signs

Pulmonary Function Tests. The ERV is especially decreased, but all lung capacities and volumes are slightly diminished. The V_T may be smaller, so to maintain minute ventilation the respiratory rate is increased. In the supine position, the lung volumes are even further reduced, which can lead to alveolar hypoventilation during sleep.

Chest Radiograph. The chest film shows an increase in the adipose tissue overlying the ribs. Compression of the lung tissue in the dependent lung regions may also be evident.

Arterial Blood Gases. In very obese patients, alveolar hypoventilation, increased ventilation-perfusion mismatching, oxygenation demands of the extra adipose tissue, increased work and oxygen uptake in the inspiratory muscles, and inef-

ficient breathing patterns all combine to cause hypoxemia. The Pa_{O_2} is therefore decreased, and in some patients the Pa_{CO_2} is continually elevated, which blunts the response to acute changes in the Pa_{CO_2}.

Breath Sounds. Breath sounds are diminished, particularly at the bases of the lungs.

Cardiovascular Findings. The circulatory response to obesity is an increase in the cardiac output and the circulating blood volume. This response creates more work for the heart, and both systemic and pulmonary hypertension are not uncommon, with both the right and left ventricles being stressed. Alveolar hypoventilation leads to further pulmonary hypertension. Over time, cardiac arrhythmias and congestive heart failure can result.

Symptoms. The primary symptom is dyspnea on exertion, which can become more limiting as the obesity increases. **Sleep apnea** can also occur owing to the extra soft tissue in the neck that surrounds the upper airways, causing airway obstruction during sleep.[2]

Treatment

It is becoming better recognized that obesity is a very complex disorder. It involves virtually all the body's systems via the patient's metabolism, the psychological and mental processes within the patient, and the patient's behaviors and habits. Treatment consisting of dieting and will power is usually not effective over an extended period of time. Patients who have been markedly obese over a long period usually can demonstrate expertise in dieting and remarkably significant will power. It is not unusual for these patients to have lost three or four times their body weight over their lifetime, only to regain the lost weight and more. Current treatment strategies for the obese patient combine interventions. Weight loss programs now often include extensive medical evaluation and a variety of therapeutic interventions, including diet, increased activity, behavior modification, psychological support, nutritional counseling, and family involvement. A great deal is still to be learned and understood about the body's metabolism; how food is broken down, stored, and eliminated; and how obesity can be reversed so that recurrence is not the norm. See Chapter 7 for more details on obesity.

Diabetes Mellitus

Diabetes mellitus is a syndrome that results from abnormal carbohydrate metabolism and is characterized by inadequate insulin secretion and hyperglycemia.[13]

Etiology

Diabetes mellitus has no distinct etiology but seems to result from a variable interaction of hereditary and environmental factors.[13]

Pathophysiology

The most common pathologic changes seen in diabetes mellitus result from hyperglycemia, large vessel disease, microvascular disease (particularly involving the retina and kidney), and neuropathy.[13] Recently, the effects of this metabolic disorder on the lungs have been reported, and although the incidence of pulmonary involvement does not seem to be high, it can be significant in some patients. Hyperglycemic patients have an increased incidence of pulmonary infections and tuberculosis, which is manifest more frequently in the lower lobes.[14] Diffuse alveolar hemorrhage has also been reported in diabetics and may be due to inflammation and necrosis of the pulmonary capillary endothelium. This could then be followed by fibrotic changes.[11] In a study of more than 31,000 patients with diabetes mellitus, pulmonary fibrosis was found in 0.8% of the diabetic population, which is a moderately greater incidence than that reported for the general population.[14] Juvenile diabetics have shown a decrease in elastic recoil of the lungs and in lung compliance, causing a decrease in TLC.[14,19] These abnormalities in ventilatory mechanics are thought to be due to changes in the elastin and collagen within the lung. Another mechanism that can cause a restrictive impairment in the lung is *diabetic keto-acidosis*, which can produce a noncardiogenic pulmonary edema. The physiologic cause for this change is unclear but may be due to an alteration in the pulmonary capillary permeability.[14] See Chapter 7 for more details on diabetes.

TRAUMATIC CAUSES OF RESTRICTIVE LUNG DYSFUNCTION

Crush Injuries

Crush injuries to the thorax are usually caused by blunt trauma that results in pathologic damage, particularly rib fractures, flail chest, or lung contusion.[1]

Etiology

The leading cause of blunt trauma to the thorax is motor vehicle accidents. The second most common cause of thoracic crush injuries is falls, which usually occur in the home.[15]

Pathophysiology

Rib Fractures. Rib fractures most commonly involve the fifth through the ninth ribs because they are anchored anteriorly and posteriorly and are less protected than ribs 1 through 4 from the kinetic energy of a traumatic blow.[15] Even nondisplaced rib fractures can be very painful, and it is the pain on any movement of the chest wall that causes the restrictive impairment. Patients with rib fractures breathe very shallowly in an effort to keep the thoracic wall still. The muscular splinting around the fracture site also decreases chest wall excursion and lung expansion. In addition, fractured ribs may be accompanied by a **hemothorax**, which can progress to a large sanguinous effusion and empyema. This fluid in the pleural space compresses the underlying lung parenchyma and can cause fibrosis and scarring of the pleura, leading to permanent restrictive dysfunction.[8] More frequently, the pain of the rib fractures decreases significantly during the first 2 weeks after the injury, and normal lung function is restored, although coughing may cause pain for up to 6 months. Patients who have multiple rib fractures, are older than 50 years, or have underlying pulmonary or cardiovascular disease are at greater risk of developing a pneumonia following rib fracture.[4,15]

Flail Chest. Flail chest refers to a free-floating segment of ribs due to multiple rib fractures both anteriorly and posteriorly that leave this part of the thoracic wall disconnected to the rest of the thoracic cage.[15] This segment can usually be identified by its paradoxical movement during the respiratory cycle. It moves inward during inspiration, drawn by the increase in the negative pleural space pressure. It moves outward during expiration, as the pleural space pressure approaches atmospheric pressure. Both the pain and the paradoxical movement of a part of the thoracic cage during the respiratory cycle contribute to the restrictive dysfunction. Lung volumes are decreased, and the distribution of ventilation is altered, causing an increase in ventilation-perfusion mismatching. The force of the blunt trauma that causes a flail chest is usually greater than that causing a simple rib fracture. Because the force is greater, flail chest is often associated with lung contusion.[4,15]

Lung Contusion. Lung contusion occurs when the lung strikes directly against the chest wall. The local pulmonary microvasculature is damaged, causing red blood cells and plasma to move into the alveoli.[15] This immediately decreases the compliance of the lung, changes the distribution of inspired gases, and increases ventilation-perfusion mismatching. Although the injury due to the lung contusion may resolve in approximately 3 days, patients are at high risk for serious pulmonary complications. Approximately 50% to 70% develop a pneumonia in the contused segment, 35% develop an empyema, and some patients develop ARDS, with complete "white out" of the injured lung on chest radiograph.[4,15]

Clinical Manifestations

Signs
Pulmonary Function Tests. The crush injuries increase the respiratory rate and decrease Vt, FRC, VC, and TLC.

Chest Radiograph. The chest radiograph may appear normal if the rib fractures are not dis-placed. Displaced rib fractures and flail chest are easily recognized on the posteroanterior (PA) view of the chest film. A lung contusion on chest radiograph shows as focal infiltrates occurring in nonsegmental and nonlobar distribution. These infiltrates usually clear within 3 days. More diffuse infiltrates that remain more than 3 days following injury may denote a pneumonia or the development of ARDS.

Arterial Blood Gases. The Pa_{O_2} is decreased in proportion to the amount of chest wall damage and lung contusion.

Breath Sounds. Breath sounds are diminished owing to the decrease in lung volumes and possible fluid in the pleural space. Rales may also be heard over areas of atelectasis.

Cardiovascular Findings. Because the heart may be directly involved in the precipitating trauma, changes in the cardiovascular system are variable.

Symptoms. With rib fracture and flail chest, the primary symptom is chest wall pain and tenderness to palpation. Pain is exacerbated with movement of the chest wall, particularly coughing and sneezing. Patients splint the chest wall to decrease movement during the respiratory cycle. Respiratory rate is increased, and with larger injuries patients may appear in some respiratory distress.

Treatment

Rib Fractures. Pain control is the primary treatment and can be accomplished by oral analgesics, intercostal nerve block, or epidural anesthesia depending on the extent of the injury.[15] The goal is to allow the patient to reestablish a normal breathing pattern. In patients at high risk for developing pneumonia, hospital admission may be indicated for close observation and for aggressive pulmonary hygiene in addition to pain relief.

Flail Chest. Flail chest may have to be managed by mechanical ventilation when the patient's respiratory rate exceeds 40 beats per minute, the VC progressively decreases to less than 10 to 15 milliliters per kilogram of body weight, the arterial oxygenation falls to less than 60 mm Hg with an $F_{I_{O_2}}$ of 50%, hypercapnia develops with the Pa_{CO_2} higher than 50 mm Hg, or other injuries sustained in the trauma necessitate its use.[15] Mechanical ventilatory support may be needed for 2 to 4 weeks. With severe chest wall injuries or marked displacement of the fracture fragments, surgical stabilization may be required. Surgery usually shortens the time the patient needs to be on mechanical ventilation, decreases the pain, and increases anatomic alignment during the healing process.[15] With less severe injuries, the flail chest may be able to be treated with excellent pain control and aggressive breathing exercises, use of an **incentive spirometer,** positioning, and coughing.

Lung Contusion. Treatment is supportive and preventive. Mechanical ventilation and supplemental oxygen may be required. Fluid monitoring to ensure against volume overload, which could lead to pulmonary edema, is important. Although corticosteroids have been used, there is no conclusive proof that they improve the patient's morbidity or mortality. Deep breathing exercises, positioning, and coughing are also used to assist in clearing infiltrates and to decrease the incidence of pneumonia.[15]

Penetrating Wounds

Penetrating wounds to the thorax are usually caused by gunshot or stabbing and result in pathologic damage, particularly pneumothorax, hemothorax, pulmonary laceration, tracheal or bronchial disruption, diaphragmatic injury, esophageal perforation, or cardiac laceration. Only the first three are discussed within the scope of this chapter.[1,4]

Etiology

The leading cause of penetrating wounds to the thorax is gunshot wounds and stab wounds. Penetrating wounds to the chest are usually more specific and defined and are less likely to have the multisystem involvement more commonly seen with thoracic crush injuries.[4,15]

Pathophysiology

Pneumothorax. Traumatic pneumothorax is defined as the entry of free air into the pleural space (Fig. 5–10). This often occurs after a penetrating wound to the thorax. A traumatic pneumothorax can be further classified as an open pneumothorax or a **tension pneumothorax.**[1]

An open pneumothorax means the air in the pleural space communicates freely with the outside environment. When air can move freely through the chest wall, into and out of the pleural space, the patient is unable to maintain a negative pleural space pressure. Because an effective negative pleural space pressure cannot be maintained in both the affected and unaffected hemithorax, the patient's ability to move air into

Figure 5–10

Diagram of the pleural space. (Reproduced with permission from Weinberger SE. Principles of Pulmonary Medicine. Philadelphia, WB Saunders, p 178.)

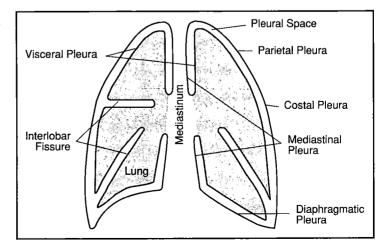

the lungs is severely diminished. Lung volumes are decreased; lung compliance is decreased; ventilation-perfusion mismatching is increased; and gas exchange is impaired.[1]

A tension pneumothorax means air can enter the pleural space but cannot escape into the external environment. This is an acute life-threatening situation.[16] As air continues to enter and become trapped in the pleural space the intrapleural pressure rapidly increases. This causes the lung on the involved side to collapse. The mediastinal structures are pushed away from the affected side. The increased thoracic pressure causes a decrease in venous return; cardiac output falls; and systemic hypotension and shock are the result. Lung volumes are signficantly reduced; lung compliance is decreased; and the alveolar-capillary surface area available for gas exchange is cut by more than 50%.[1,4,15]

Hemothorax. Hemothorax is the presence of blood in the pleural space. It can occur with both penetrating wounds and crush injuries to the thorax. Approximately 70% of patients with chest trauma develop a hemothorax. Collection of blood in the pleural space causes compression of the underlying lung tissue and prevents lung expansion. This process usually affects the lower lobes because the blood in the pleural space is pulled by gravity to the most dependent area. Compression of the lung tissue causes an increase in ventilation-perfusion mismatching, decreases lung compliance, and promotes atelectasis. Occasionally trauma to the thorax results in a massive hemothorax, which almost always means that the heart or great vessels were injured directly. Hemothorax can have serious sequelae if all the blood is not evacuated from the pleural space. The residual blood becomes organized into nonelastic fibrous tissue, which can form a restrictive pleural rind. This condition is known as *fibrothorax* and can limit lung expansion markedly, causing a restrictive lung dysfunction and predisposing the patient to atelectasis and pneumonic complications. In addition, approximately 5% of patients wtih hemothorax develop an infection within the pleural space called an empyema, which can lead to further scarring of the pleural surfaces.[1,4,15]

Pulmonary Laceration. A laceration directly into the lung parenchyma is usually caused by a penetrating wound. It results in air and blood escaping from the lung into the pleural space and often into the environment. Therefore, a pulmonary laceration most commonly appears as a combination pneumothorax and hemothorax. The hemothorax is usually not massive because the lung is perfused at low pressures, so the bleeding is not profuse. The restrictive impairments caused by pneumothorax and hemothorax described earlier are present, and in addition the damaged lung tissue is not participating in gas exchange.[15]

Clinical Manifestations

Signs
Pulmonary Function Tests. Respiratory rate is increased. Lung volumes are decreased; this is most marked in a tension pneumothorax. Lung volume changes are usually transient in pneumothorax and hemothorax and can return to normal. If a fibrothorax or empyema develops, lung volumes remain diminished owing to the decrease in chest wall and lung compliance.

Chest Radiograph. In pneumothorax lung collapse can readily be seen on the chest radiograph. In tension pneumothorax, the diaphragm may be flattened, the mediastinal structures shifted, the trachea deviated, and the neck veins distended, in addition to lung collapse. Hemothorax, unless massive, may be more difficult to visualize on the chest radiograph. It may appear as a subtle uniform increase in the density over the affected hemithorax. Upright and decubitus films are very helpful in determining the presence of a hemothorax because the blood shifts within the pleural space with the change in position.[4,15]

Arterial Blood Gases. Hypoxemia results from all penetrating wound injuries. The degree of hypoxemia depends on the extent of the injury and the subsequent restrictive lung dysfunction. **Hypercapnia** is also common.

Breath Sounds. With a pneumothorax, the patient has markedly decreased or absent breath sounds over the affected hemithorax. Breath sounds are also decreased in hemothorax, fibrothorax, and empyema.

Cardiovascular Findings. Tachycardia is common in pneumothorax and decreased cardiac output, and systemic hypotension is present with a tension pneumothorax. Other cardiovascular changes are variable, depending on the involvement of the heart or great vessels in the thoracic trauma.

Symptoms. Shortness of breath is severe in pneumothorax and can also be present in hemothorax, fibrothorax, and empyema. Patients may appear in respiratory distress with an increased respiratory rate, intercostal retractions, cyanosis, and increased anxiety and agitation. Pain at the site of the chest wound is to be expected. Patients may also appear pale, cyanotic, or unconscious owing to loss of blood, systemic hypotension, hypoxemia, and shock.

Treatment

Pneumothorax. The definitive treatment of an open pneumothorax is the application of an airtight, sterile dressing over the sucking chest wound and the placement of a chest tube into the pleural space of the affected hemithorax. The chest tube is connected to suction so that the air and any fluid or blood within the pleural space can be evacuated. These measures will re-expand the collapsed lung. Mechanical ventilation and supplemental oxygen may be required until the patient can maintain tissue oxygenation independently.[15]

A tension pneumothorax is treated as an emergency by inserting a needle into the pleural space to allow air to escape. This is immediately followed by placement of a chest tube connected to suction so that air can be continuously evacuated from the pleural space along with any blood or fluid.[4,15]

Hemothorax. The definitive treatment for hemothorax is to evacuate the blood from the pleural space by placement of a dependent chest tube. This chest tube is connected to suction. Autotransfusion devices are becoming more common so that the patient's own blood can be returned to the cardiovascular system to replace lost blood volume. If the wound involves the lung parenchyma, the bleeding in most patients stops because of clotting and internal repair mechanisms. Only 4% of these patients require thoracotomy and surgical intervention to control the bleeding.[15] If the wound involves the heart or great vessels, then emergency surgery may be required to stop massive bleeding; this surgery takes precedence over all other treatment other than respiratory and cardiac resuscitation. Following placement of the chest tube, the patient should be monitored carefully by chest radiograph to be sure all the blood is evacuated from the pleural space. An additional chest tube may be required to accomplish this goal. If a fibrothorax does develop and impairs lung expansion, a surgical procedure known as a *decortication* may be required. A decortication removes the restrictive pleural rind, which is usually done through a minithoracotomy.[15,16] An empyema may also develop if the hemothorax is not completely resolved. The empyema would be treated with placement of a chest tube and antibiotics.[15]

Thermal Trauma

Thermal trauma involving the pulmonary system is usually due to inhalation injuries, direct burn injuries to the thorax, or a combination of both.[10]

Etiology

Thermal trauma is usually caused by exposure to fire and smoke, particularly in an enclosed space. The effects of this exposure are dependent on what is burning, the intensity or the temperatures generated by the fire, the length of the exposure, and the amount of body surface involved.[22]

Pathophysiology

Smoke inhalation causes pulmonary dysfunction in three different ways. First is a direct injury from inhaling hot, dry air containing heated particulate matter. This injury is localized in the upper airway because most of the heat is dissipated in the nasopharynx. Nasal hairs may be scorched. There is usually edema of the laryngeal and tracheal mucosa with **laryngospasm** and **bronchospasm** almost always present. Mucus production is increased, and commonly there is damage to the mucociliary clearance mechanism. This can lead to bronchopneumonia.[10,22]

The second cause of pulmonary dysfunction is the inhalation of carbon monoxide, a gas present in smoke. Carbon monoxide is a colorless, odorless, tasteless, nonirritating gas. Exposure to carbon monoxide can be life threatening; many suicides are committed by overexposure to carbon monoxide. This gas has more than 200 times the affinity for hemoglobin when compared with oxygen.[10] This means that when carbon monoxide is taken into the lungs it diffuses quickly into the pulmonary capillaries, enters the red blood cells, and binds with hemoglobin to form **carboxyhemoglobin.** This abnormal process decreases the available hemoglobin binding sites for oxygen and significantly decreases the oxygen-carrying capacity of the blood.

The third cause of pulmonary dysfunction is the inhalation of noxious and toxic gases, the effects from which are dependent on the materials being burned. The specific pulmonary abnormalities depend on the specific gas inhaled and the length of time exposed to the gas. However, exposure to noxious gases often results in surfactant inactivation and chemical pneumonitis.[10,18,22]

Direct burn injuries to the thorax cause pulmonary dysfunction in five ways.

- The pain of the burn decreases chest wall mobility.
- If the depth of the burn is third degree, involving chest wall musculature, then the effectiveness of the respiratory pump is diminished.
- Major burns involving 25% of the body surface area or more result in a massive shift of fluid from the intravascular to the interstitial spaces, causing pulmonary edema and possibly acute pulmonary insufficiency.
- With circumferential burns of the thorax, **eschar** formation may severely restrict chest wall expansion.
- Because these patients may have to be on bedrest for protracted periods of time, the pulmonary system is at risk for atelectasis and bronchopneumonia.[10,22]

Clinical Manifestations

Signs

Pulmonary Function Tests. Constriction of the airways and edema of the airway mucosa cause marked obstructive lung dysfunction. Flow rates are decreased. Lung volumes are decreased both by decreased lung compliance due to surfactant inactivation, pulmonary edema, and atelectasis and by decreased chest wall compliance due to the direct burn injury and pain. Gas diffusion is decreased. Respiratory rate is increased in an effort to maintain minute ventilation.

Chest Radiograph. The chest radiograph often shows diffuse interstitial and intra-alveolar infiltrates owing to the shift of body fluid. Superimposed on these findings may be areas of bronchopneumonia or atelectasis.

Arterial Blood Gases. Hypoxemia is common owing to the increased ventilation-perfusion mismatching and hypoventilation. If the patient was exposed to carbon monoxide for a period of time, the Pa_{O_2} may be so low that it becomes incompatible with life.

Breath Sounds. Auscultation usually reveals decreased breath sounds; wheezing, wet rales, and rhonchi are common.

Cardiovascular Findings. Tachycardia is common. Significant thermal trauma can cause shock, cardiac arrhythmias, hypertension, hypotension, or myocardial infarction.[22]

Symptoms. Patients with thermal trauma appear dyspneic and have a repetitive, hacking, productive cough. Sputum may be **carbonaceous.**[22] Respiratory rate is increased. Stridor and wheezing may be heard. Patients are usually very anxious and may be cyanotic.

Treatment

Treatment of the seriously burned patient is usually divided into emergency, acute, and rehabilitative care and involves monitoring and providing support and care for every body system. Treatment of the pulmonary system includes humidification, supplemental oxygen, bronchodilators, appropriate positioning, and pulmonary hygiene techniques. Intubation, ventilatory support, and suctioning may be necessary in some patients.[22]

THERAPEUTIC CAUSES OF RESTRICTIVE LUNG DYSFUNCTION

Surgical Therapy

Surgery can be defined as a planned entry into the human body by a trained practitioner under well-controlled conditions.[1]

Etiology

The pulmonary dysfunction that results from surgical therapy is due to three primary factors: (1) the anesthetic agent, (2) the surgical incision or procedure itself, and (3) the pain caused by the incision or procedure.[1,15]

Pathophysiology

The anesthetic agent causes a decrease in the pulmonary arterial vasoconstrictive response to hypoxia. This increases ventilation-perfusion mismatching and decreases pulmonary gas exchange. Anesthesia also depresses the respiratory control centers so that ventilatory response to hypercapnia and hypoxia is decreased. Placement of an endotracheal tube increases airway resistance. During surgery the shape and configuration of the thorax change. The anteroposterior diameter decreases, and the lateral diameter increases. The vertical diameter of the thorax also decreases, with the diaphragm moving in a cephalad direction. These changes in configuration result in decreased thoracic volumes; the FRC is decreased by approximately 20%.[15]

If the site of surgery is in the upper abdomen or the thorax, the surgical incision causes a significant, although temporary, restrictive impairment. Following upper abdominal surgery, the VC is decreased by 55% and the FRC by 30%.[15]

These decreases in lung volumes reach their greatest values 24 to 48 hours following surgery. Lung volumes then return to relatively normal values in 5 days, although full recovery may take 2 weeks.[15] Postoperative lung volume changes after upper abdominal surgery resemble changes seen in patients with unilateral diaphragmatic paralysis. In fact, diaphragmatic dysfunction has been demonstrated in some abdominal surgery patients. Diaphragmatic dysfunction also can occur following thoracic surgery, particularly if the phrenic nerve experiences hypothermic damage because of external cardiac cooling. Some studies have shown that a transverse abdominal incision results in better postoperative lung volumes and fewer postoperative pulmonary complications than the vertical midline abdominal incision. This is not a universal finding.[15] However, it is well accepted that the median sternotomy incision is better tolerated and results in fewer pulmonary complications than the posterolateral thorocotomy.[15]

The surgical procedure itself can result in a permanent restrictive impairment when lung tissue is excised. Because pulmonary reserves are significant, a *pneumonectomy* or possibly a *lobectomy* has to be performed before any measurable restrictive dysfunction results. *Thoracoplasty* is another surgical procedure that results in restrictive dysfunction. This procedure removes portions of several ribs so that the soft tissue of the chest wall can be used to collapse underlying lung parenchyma. Thoracoplasty was used to treat tuberculosis and was designed to close cavities caused by tuberculosis in the upper lobes. Currently this procedure is rarely performed, although it has been used to treat *bronchopulmonary fistulas.*[1]

Surgical incisions invariably cause pain, particularly abdominal incisions and posterolateral thoracotomies. Because of the pain, the tone in the muscles of the thorax and the abdominal wall increases, thereby decreasing the chest wall compliance. This change contributes to decreased lung volumes and increased work of breathing during the postoperative period. The phenomenon of increased muscle tone in and around the incision is known as *muscular splinting of the incision.*

Clinical Manifestations

Signs

Pulmonary Function Tests. All lung volumes are decreased; the VC is decreased by 55% and the FRC by 30% following upper abdominal surgery.[15] Flow rates are usually within normal limits but may be slightly decreased. Gas exchange is decreased temporarily because of the increase in ventilation-perfusion mismatching.

Chest Radiograph. Postoperative films often show atelectasis, which can occur at rates up to 80% following abdominal or thoracic surgery.[15] The chest radiograph may also show pneumonia, often involving the lower lobes, or pulmonary embolism.

Arterial Blood Gases. Hypoxia is common during the postoperative period, especially in obese or elderly patients who have cardiac or pulmonary insufficiency or in those who undergo thoracic or upper abdominal surgery. The Pa_{CO_2} may be increased, normal, or decreased, depending on the patient's breathing pattern, functioning lung tissue, and degree of pain.

Breath Sounds. The most common finding following surgery is decreased breath sounds. Rales or rhonchi also may be noted if the patient has atelectasis or pneumonia.

Cardiovascular Findings. Possible cardiovascular complications following pulmonary surgery include arrhythmias, myocardial infarction, and cardiac arrest. If a significant portion of the lung is removed, pulmonary hypertension can result.[8]

Symptoms. After surgery, patients commonly have an altered breathing pattern characterized by an increase in respiratory rate and a decrease in Vт. The cough reflex is suppressed because of the anesthesia, and voluntary coughing is difficult because of the pain. Cough is often productive of blood-streaked sputum if the patient has been intubated.

Treatment

The pulmonary status of surgical patients should be evaluated before surgery. Many patients require preoperative treatment, including deep breathing and coughing exercises and practice with an incentive spirometer. In addition, patients should abstain from smoking a minimum of 6 weeks before surgery. To prevent aspiration pneumonia, patients usually fast for 12 hours or longer before surgery. Drugs such as cimetidine or ranitidine can be used preoperatively to increase gastric pH and decrease gastric volume.[23] Postoperatively, hypoxia can be treated with inflation-hold breathing techniques, positive end-expiratory pressure, **continuous positive airway pressure (CPAP),** and occasionally with increased oxygen concentrations. Common techniques used to treat postoperative atelectasis include deep breathing exercises, early mobilization of the patient out of bed, incentive spirometry, and CPAP. Nosocomial pneumonias following surgery are not uncommon and are treated with an appropriate antibiotic and possibly with postural drainage, percussion, and vibration if the patient's secretion clearance mechanisms are impaired. Postoperative pulmonary embolism is usually treated with low-dose heparin. Prevention of venous thromboembolism should include simple leg exercises (ankle dorsi and plantar flexion) and elastic support hose when the patient is confined to bed.

Drug Therapy

More than 100 drugs are capable of causing RLD. Approximatley 80 of these drugs adversely affect the lung parenchyma directly, causing drug-induced interstitial lung disease.[11] Other drugs affect the ventilatory pump, ventilatory drive, or chest wall compliance.[1] Most drug-induced interstitial lung disease is reversible if it is recognized early and the drug is discontinued. Drug-induced RLD contributes to the morbidity of an estimated several hundred thousand patients in the United States annually. Approximately 50% of patients treated with chemotherapeutic drugs develop some degree of interstitial pneumonitis.[11] Some patients who take chemotherapeutic drugs demonstrate pathologic alterations with no radiologic, symptomatic, or physiologic abnormalities. Therefore, probably less than 5% of all adverse drug-induced interstitial lung disease is reported or recognized.[11]

It is very difficult to predict which drugs may affect a particular person's lung adversely. The basic reason for this difficulty is insufficient knowledge. First, knowledge of the metabolites of different drugs and their effects on the lung is lacking. Second, some patients seem to have a genetic predisposition to react adversely to certain drugs but this is not well understood. Third, many patients are on multiple drugs, and the interaction of the various metabolites has not been well studied.[11]

Drug-induced interstitial lung disease probably results from a combination of mechanisms including

● toxic effects of the drug or its metabolites
● an indirect inflammatory reaction
● some immunologic processes[11]

Drugs capable of causing drug-induced interstitial lung disease are discussed by drug category.

Oxygen

High concentrations of oxygen for more than 24 hours can produce interstitial lung disease. The lung damage occurs in two phases. First is the *exudative phase*, which begins after using high oxygen concentrations for 24 to 72 hours. During this phase, perivascular, interstitial, and alveolar edema and alveolar hemorrhage and atelectasis occur. The second or *proliferative phase* is marked by **hyperplasia** and deposition of collagen and elastin in the interstitium, and is irreversible. Oxygen toxicity can result in significant RLD. Treatment is primarily preventive. Oxygen toxicity can be minimized by keeping the $F_{I_{O_2}}$ under 40% and the Pa_{O_2} under 120 mm Hg.[11]

Antibiotics

Some antibiotics used to fight infections can be neurotoxic. Drugs such as polymyxin, gentamicin, and kanamycin, when given intravenously, can cause neuromuscular blockade. This neuromuscular blockade can result in respiratory muscle paralysis, failure of the ventilatory pump, and such significant restrictive lung impairment that assisted ventilatory support may be necessary.

The significance of the respiratory impairment is even greater when these drugs are used with anesthetic agents or muscle relaxants.[23]

Nitrofurantoin. This drug is used to fight specific urinary tract infections. It can cause acute or chronic interstitial pneumonitis and is one of the most commonly reported drugs that causes drug-induced pulmonary disease. There seems to be no relation between the acute and chronic reactions. The acute pneumonitis is characterized by fever, dyspnea, cough, and rales; approximately 35% of patients experience pleuritic pain. The acute pneumonitis is completely reversible if the drug is discontinued. Chronic pneumonitis mimics IPF and usually begins 6 to 12 months after initiation of the drug. Patients complain of dyspnea and a mild, nonproductive cough. There can be diffuse fibrosis with lower zone predominance. Treatment includes discontinuation of the drug, lung biopsy, and possibly corticosteroids. Therapeutic results are inconsistent.[11,23]

Sulfasalazine. This drug is used to treat inflammatory bowel disease (chronic ulcerative colitis). Patients who develop lung complications complain of dyspnea and cough approximately 1 to 8 months after the initiation of the drug. Approximately half the patients also complain of fever. This can develop into interstitial pulmonary fibrosis. Treatment is to discontinue the drug. Pulmonary involvement and symptoms are reversible in most patients. One fatality was recorded as caused by sulfasalazine-induced diffuse pulmonary fibrosis.[11]

Anti-inflammatory Drugs

Gold. Gold is used in the treatment of rheumatoid arthritis, but in some patients it causes diffuse interstitial pneumonitis and fibrosis. These patients develop dyspnea and a nonproductive cough approximately 6 weeks to many months after initiation of gold therapy. Treatment is the discontinuation of the drug, which allows the reaction to regress spontaneously. Some patients with respiratory distress are given corticosteroids to speed this process.[7,11]

Penicillamine. This drug is used to treat **Wilson's disease, cystinuria,** and patients with severe rheumatoid arthritis who have failed to respond to conventional therapy. However, it can cause bronchiolitis obliterans, which contributes to both obstructive and restrictive lung dysfunction; Goodpasture's syndrome; or penicillamine-induced SLE. The drug is discontinued in patients who develop any of these pulmonary complications. Patients who have developed Goodpasture's syndrome are also treated with hemodialysis, immunosuppression, and plasmapheresis. Patients who have penicillamine-induced SLE may also receive corticosteroids to accelerate the resolution of this pulmonary complication.[11,23]

Cardiovascular Drugs

Amiodarone. This antiarrhythmic drug is given for ventricular dysrhythmias that are refractory to other antiarrhythmic drugs. The pulmonary complications seem to be dose related and rarely occur if the dose is under 400 milligrams per day. The incidence of pulmonary complications is approximately 6%, and the pulmonary complications may be fatal in a small number of patients. Patients with pulmonary involvement experience an insidious onset of dyspnea and a nonproductive cough with occasional fever and chills. Rales are heard on auscultation, and the chest radiograph shows asymmetric lesions in the lung, which appear mostly in the upper lung fields. Treatment is to discontinue the drug; corticosteroids may help in reversing the interstitial pneumonitis.[11]

Hexamethonium. Hexamethonium compounds are used to treat hypertension. In the lungs this group of drugs can cause exudation of fluid that contains fibrin into the alveolar spaces. Exudation usually begins centrally and spreads outward from the hilar regions. This process can lead to intra-alveolar fibrosis, significant RLD, and death.[7]

Chemotherapeutic Drugs

These cytotoxic drugs used in cancer chemotherapy are a major cause of morbidity and mortality in the immunocompromised individual. It has been reported that the majority of these drugs can cause pulmonary fibrosis.[7] They are also responsible for causing pulmonary infiltrates, secondary neoplasms, and **non-Hodgkin's lymphoma,** all of which compromise lung function. The precise mechanism that incites the inflammatory and fibrotic response in the lung is unknown.

Dyspnea appears gradually, usually within a few weeks of the drug therapy, followed by fever and a nonproductive cough. With some drugs, symptoms may be delayed for months or years (e.g., cyclophosphamide). Early chest radiographs show asymmetric parenchymal changes in one lobe or lung; eventually these changes progress and become diffuse and uniform in distribution. Pulmonary function tests show a classic restrictive impairment. The $D_{L_{CO}}$ usually falls before the patient experiences the onset of any overt symptoms (except with methotrexate). Rales are heard on auscultation. Treatment is the discontinuation of the drug and the use of corticosteroids.[11]

Bleomycin. Bleomycin is an antibiotic used as an antineoplastic agent against squamous cell carcinomas, seminomas, and lymphomas. Ten percent of patients on this drug develop parenchymal lung disease, which proves to be fatal in 1% of the patients. The risk of lung involvement increases with higher dosages of bleomycin, if it is used with previous or concomitant thoracic radiation or if it is prescribed with current or subsequent use of high oxygen concentrations.[11,23]

Mitomycin C. Mitomycin C is an antibiotic used in conjunction with other chemotherapeutic drugs, particularly for adenocarcinoma of the stomach or pancreas. Approximately 3% to 12% of patients on this drug develop pulmonary complications. Frequency of lung involvement increases if this drug is used with other drugs, particularly fluorouracil or the Vinca alkaloids.[11,23]

Busulfan. Busulfan is an alkylating agent used to treat myeloid leukemia. Patients usually have to take the drug over a period of 6 to 8 months for any pulmonary complications to occur. Clinical symptoms appear insidiously, often after the drug has been discontinued.[11,23]

Cyclophosphamide. Cyclophosphamide is an alkylating agent used in the treatment of malignant **lymphomas,** multiple myeloma, and leukemias. Diffuse interstitial fibrosis can occur a few months to a few years after use of this drug. There seems to be no age or dose correlation with the development of pulmonary complications. The drug-induced pulmonary disease can range from one with a very long-term course to one with a rapid downhill course resulting in death.[11,23]

Chlorambucil. Chlorambucil is an alkylating agent used to treat chronic lymphatic malignancies. If pulmonary complications develop, it is usually 1 to 12 months before symptoms appear.[11]

Melphalan. Melphalan is an alkylating agent used in the treatment of multiple myeloma that can cause significant RLD.[11]

Azathioprine. Azathioprine is an antimetabolite used for treating neoplastic disease, Wegener's granulomatosis, connective tissue diseases, and organ transplants. This drug rarely causes interstitial lung disease; however six cases have been reported in the literature.[11]

Cytarabine. Cytarabine is an antimetabolite used primarily to induce a remission in acute leukemia. Unlike the other drugs under discussion, cytarabine causes minimal parenchymal abnormalities. However, it can cause a noncardiac pulmonary edema, which results in RLD and has been fatal in all recognized cases.[11]

Methotrexate. Methotrexate is an antimetabolite taken for acute lymphatic leukemia in children. The complication of interstitial lung disease is not dose or age related. Symptoms begin a few days to a few weeks after drug initiation, and approximately one third of patients who develop interstitial pneumonitis have poorly formed granulomas. Treatment is the discontinuation of the drug; in almost all patients the lung involvement is spontaneously resolved. Corticosteroids are sometimes used.[11]

Nitrosoureas. Nitrosourea drugs (BCNU [carmustine], CCNU [lomustine], methyl-CCNU [semustine]) are used against a variety of neoplasms. Anywhere from 1% to 50% of patients on these drugs develop interstitial lung disease. Patients have a higher risk of developing pulmonary complications when higher dosages are prescribed or when these drugs are prescribed along with other agents, particularly cyclophosphamide.[11]

Poisons

Paraquat. Paraquat is used as a weed killer. If it is ingested, it causes acute pulmonary fibrosis. There are usually no symptoms for 24 hours after ingestion, and then the person experiences progessive respiratory distress leading to death in 1 to 38 days.[7]

Other drugs can cause RLD via a variety of pathophysiologic mechanisms other than that of producing alveolar pneumonitis and fibrosis. A few of these drug categories or specific drugs are discussed.

Anesthetics

Anesthetic agents such as halothane (Fluothane), methoxyflurane (Penthrane), or thiopental sodium (Pentothal) are used to provide anesthesia during surgical procedures. These agents also inhibit the respiratory centers in the medulla and therefore depress ventilation so that lung volumes are significantly reduced. Assisted mechanical ventilation is usually required with the use of these drugs. The effects of these drugs and the effects of the assisted mechanical ventilation usually result in significant but brief RLD.[1,23]

Muscle Relaxants

Muscle relaxants such as pancuronium bromide (Pavulon), dantrolene sodium (Dantrium), diazepam (Valium), and cyclobenzaprine hydrochloride (Flexeril) are used to enhance surgical relaxation, overcome muscle spasm, and control shivering (with systemic hypothermia). However, because these drugs act on skeletal muscle, they also decrease thoracic expansion, decrease chest wall compliance, and decrease pulmonary ventilation. As soon as the drug effects have worn off, the transient RLD also disappears.[1,23]

Drug-Induced Systemic Lupus Erythematosus

Nearly 50 drugs have been reported to induce SLE, but only 5 regularly induce antinuclear antibodies and therefore symptomatic SLE. They are procainamide hydrochloride, isoniazid, hydralazine hydrochloride, hydantoins, and penicillamine. Patients who take one of these drugs for months or years may develop clinical SLE, and of these, 50% develop pleuropulmonary involvement, including interstitial lung disease. In the majority of patients, these changes are reversible by discontinuing the drug. Use of corticosteroids may accelerate the resolution.[11]

Illicit Drugs

Heroin. An overdose of methadone hydrochloride, propoxyphene hydrochloride, or heroin can lead to a noncardiac pulmonary edema with interstitial pneumonitis. This reaction can begin within minutes of an intravenous injection or within an hour of oral ingestion. Respiration is depressed; lung compliance is decreased; hypoxemia and hypercapnia result. Treatment includes mechanically assisted ventilation and usually antibiotics to deal with the invariable aspiration pneumonia.[11]

Talc. Talc (magnesium silicate) is used as a filler in oral medications such as amphetamines, tripelennamine hydrochloride, methadone hydrochloride, meperidine, and propoxyphene hydrochloride (Darvon). When addicts inject these drugs intravenously, talc granulomatosis results. Talc granulomatosis is characterized by granulomas in the arterioles and the pulmonary interstitium. The clinical picture includes dyspnea, pulmonary hypertension, and restrictive lung impairment with a decreased $D_{L_{CO}}$. Treatment is abstinence from further intravenous talc exposure. Use of corticosteroids has afforded variable results.[11]

Radiation Therapy

Radiation Pneumonitis or Fibrosis

Radiation pneumonitis or fibrosis is a primary complication of irradiation to the thorax. It usually occurs 1 to 3 months after this treatment intervention.[15]

Etiology. Irradiation of the thorax is a treatment option for lymphoma **(Hodgkin's disease)**, breast cancer, lung cancer, and esophageal cancer. Not all patients who receive irradiation to the thorax develop radiation pneumonitis or fibrosis. This serious pulmonary complication of irradiation seems to depend on the rate of delivery of the irradiation, the volume of lung being irradiated, the total dose, the quality of the radiation, and the concomitant chemotherapy.[2,8,11] Time-dose relationships are extremely important in predicting the occurrence of radiation pneumonitis or fibrosis. The number of fractions into which a dose is divided seems to be the most important factor.[8] Also important is the total dose and the span of time over which the radiation is delivered. Approximately, 20% to 70% of patients undergoing irradiation of the thorax show radiologic changes in the lung.[2] However, only 5% to 15% of patients who receive radiation to the thorax actually develop signs and symptoms of pulmonary injury.[2]

Currently one group of patients seems to be at higher risk for developing radiation pneumonitis or fibrosis. Bone marrow transplant patients receive whole lung irradiation; they are also on cytotoxic chemotherapeutic agents that can intensify the pneumonitis; and these patients often have a graft versus host reaction that can add to radiation damage.[8]

Pathophysiology. The pathogenesis of radiation pneumonitis or fibrosis is uncertain. The pulmonary tissues that are most sensitive to radiation are the capillary endothelial cells, the type I alveolar epithelial cells, and the type II pneumocytes.[11] This pulmonary injury usually is divided into three phases. The acute or early phase is marked by an increased capillary permeability with fragmentation of the connective tissue. This phase leads to engorgement and thrombosis of capillaries and arterioles, alveolar edema, and cellular infiltration. The subacute or intermediate phase is characterized by infiltration of alveolar walls with cells and fibroblasts and obstruction of the capillaries by platelets, collagen, and fibrin. The chronic or late phase shows alveolar fibrosis, capillary sclerosis, obliteration of the alveoli, and increased deposition of collagen and basement membrane material.[8,11] It seems that the earlier the onset, the more serious and protracted the complications.[16] Usually one third to one half of the volume of one lung must be irradiated for pneumonitis to develop and show any clinical symptoms.[8] Some patients have a complete resolution of the pneumonitis, but many show a gradual evolution to permanent fibrosis. Occasionally pleural effusion, spontaneous pneumothorax, or **tracheoesophageal fistula** may further complicate the clinical picture. With whole-lung irradiation, the involved fibrotic lung may contract to a remarkable degree, even causing shifts in the mediastinal structures, overexpansion of the other lung, and death.

Clinical Manifestations

Signs

Pulmonary Function Tests. Both lung volumes and flow rates are decreased, with the maximum impairment occurring at approximately 4 to 6 months after irradiation.[2,11,15] With regional irradiation, the VC and ERV are the primary volumes decreased. As more lung is irradiated, all lung volumes, the TLC, VC, IC, and RV are all decreased. The DL_{CO} is decreased because of the increased ventilation-perfusion mismatching and the decreased capillary-alveolar surface area. The respiratory rate is increased and tidal volume decreased in an effort to decrease the work of breathing. Lung compliance is decreased. The compliance of the chest wall is usually not affected.

Chest Radiograph. The chest radiograph shows sharply demarcated alveolar or interstitial parenchymal infiltrates limited to the radiation port.[15] Lungs may have a ground-glass or soft appearance, and the lung markings may appear hazy or indistinct. This can progress to a reticulonodular pattern that conforms in shape and location to the region of lung irradiated. Mediastinum and heart borders may become indistinct. Irradiated regions of lung may also adopt a bronchiectatic, cystic, or honeycomb appearance.[14] Some patients do develop additional changes outside the field of irradiation.

Arterial Blood Gases. Because of the increased respiratory rate, the Pa_{CO_2} may be decreased. Hypoxemia is a common finding with respiratory distress evident even on mild exertion.

Breath Sounds. During the early phase, some rales and rhonchi may be heard. Breath sounds are normally diminished over the involved area and this can progress to essentially absent breath sounds. Pleural rubs can occasionally be heard.

Cardiovascular Findings. With the obliteration of the capillary beds, pulmonary hypertension develops, which puts an added burden on the right ventricle and can lead to cor pulmonale. Thrombolytic occurrences are common. Tachycardia is extremely common in these patients.

Symptoms

The primary symptom is shortness of breath on exertion progressing to dyspnea with even minimal effort. Patients often have a repetitive, irritating cough, which may be nonproductive or may produce a white or pink sputum. Heart rate is increased. Exercise tolerance is invariably decreased. Cyanosis and clubbing of the digits may also develop. Patients may run a low-grade fever or have temperature spikes. Some patients may complain of pleuritic pain or sharp chest wall pain, which is usually due to fractured ribs caused by coughing.[11,14]

Treatment. Corticosteroids are used during the acute phase and may produce dramatic results. They offer no help in the later phases and should not be used prophylactically because terminating corticosteroid therapy may actually precipitate radiation pneumonitis. Pneumonectomy has been reported to treat severe unilateral radiation fibrosis. Otherwise treatment is supportive and consists of oxygen therapy, cough suppression medications, and antibiotics to treat any superimposed infection.[2,8,14]

Prevention is the ultimate treatment, and the occurrence of radiation injury to the lung is decreasing with the refinement of radiotherapy techniques, particularly the careful tailoring of radiation fields.[7,8]

SUMMARY

● Restrictive lung dysfunction is not a disease; it is an abnormal reduction in pulmonary ventilation.

- Restrictive lung dysfunction can be caused by a variety of disease processes occurring in different body systems, trauma, or therapeutic measures.
- In RLD one or more of the following is abnormal; lung compliance, chest wall compliance, lung volumes, or the work of breathing.
- The classic signs of RLD include tachypnea, hypoxemia, decreased breath sounds, dry inspiratory rales, decreased lung volumes, decreased diffusing capacity, and cor pulmonale.
- The hallmark symptoms of RLD include shortness of breath, cough, and a wasted emaciated appearance.
- Treatment interventions for RLD vary and are dependent on the cause of the restrictive impairment. Sometimes corrective measures are possible. However, once the lung has undergone fibrotic changes, the pathologic alterations are irreversible and only supportive interventions are used.
- Idiopathic pulmonary fibrosis is the pulmonary disease entity most commonly associated with RLD.
- Pneumonia is an inflammatory process within the lung which can be caused by bacteria, mycoplasmas, viruses, protozoa, or psittacosis agents.
- There are four major types of lung cancer: squamous cell carcinoma, small cell carcinoma, adenocarcinoma, and large cell carcinoma. All types can cause a restrictive impairment within the lung. This restrictive impairment may be due to direct pressure from the tumor, may result from susceptibility to other disease processes in the weakened cancer patient, may be related to changes that occur as the tumor metastasizes to other body systems, or may be produced by hormones arising from the tumor, which can cause a variety of symptoms in different body systems.
- Cigarette smoking has been linked to a variety of pathologic conditions, including bronchogenic carcinoma, cancer of the mouth and larynx, esophageal cancer, kidney and urinary bladder cancer, pancreatic cancer, chronic bronchitis, emphysema, increased incidence of respiratory infection, increased frequency and severity of asthmatic attacks, coronary artery disease, myocardial infarction, peripheral vascular disease, hypertension, stroke, low birth weights in infants, increased incidence of still-

births, impotence, burn injuries, and reduced exercise capacity.
- Neuromuscular causes of RLD include spinal cord injury, ALS, polio, Guillain-Barré syndrome, muscular dystrophy, and myasthenia gravis, and any of these disease entities can cause such a significant decrease in alveolar ventilation that a mechanical ventilator is required to maintain life.
- Crush injuries and penetrating wounds to the thorax can cause significant RLD but are almost always reversible with corrective interventions.
- More than 100 drugs have the side effect of causing restrictive lung impairment, including oxygen and the majority of drugs used in the treatment of cancer.
- Radiation fibrosis of the lung is a complication of radiation therapy and is dependent on the number of fractions into which the radiation dose is divided, the total dose of radiation, the volume of lung being irradiated, and the quality of the radiation.

References

1. Hercules PR, Lekwart FJ, Fenton MV. Pulmonary Restriction and Obstruction. Chicago, Year Book Medical Publishers, 1979.
2. Weinberger SE. Principles of Pulmonary Medicine. Philadelphia, WB Saunders, 1986.
3. Whipp BJ, Wasserman K. Exercise Pulmonary Physiology and Pathophysiology. New York, Marcel Dekker, 1991.
4. Divertie MB. The CIBA Collection of Medical Illustrations. Vol. 7: Respiratory System. 2nd ed. Summit, NJ, CIBA Pharmaceutical Company, 1980.
5. Basmajian JV. Therapeutic Exercise. 3rd ed. Baltimore, Williams & Wilkins, 1978.
6. Klusek-Hamilton H. Respiratory Disorders. Springhouse, Pa, Springhouse, 1984.
7. Dunhill MS. Pulmonary Pathology. 2nd ed. New York, Churchill Livingston, 1987.
8. Fishman AP. Pulmonary Diseases and Disorders. 2nd ed. New York, McGraw-Hill, 1988.
9. Fishman AP. Update: Pulmonary Diseases and Disorders. New York, McGraw-Hill, 1982.
10. Scully RM, Barnes MR. Physical Therapy. Philadelphia, JB Lippincott, 1989.
11. Schwarz MI, King TE Jr. Interstitial Lung Disease. Philadelphia, BC Decker, 1988.
12. Glauser FL. Signs and Symptoms in Pulmonary Medicine. Philadelphia, JB Lippincott, 1983.
13. Berkow R, Fletcher AJ. The Merck Manual of Diagnosis and Therapy. 15th ed. Rahway, NJ, Merck Sharp and Dohme Research Laboratories, 1987.

14. Baum GL, Wolinsky E. Textbook of Pulmonary Diseases. 3rd ed. Boston, Little, Brown, 1983.
15. George RB, Light RW, Matthay MA, Matthay RA. Chest Medicine: Essentials of Pulmonary and Critical Care Medicine. 2nd ed. Baltimore, Williams & Wilkins, 1990.
16. Hinshaw HC, Murray JF. Diseases of the Chest. 4th ed. Philadelphia, WB Saunders, 1980.
17. Mitchell RS. Synopsis of Clinical Pulmonary Disease. 2nd ed. St. Louis, CV Mosby, 1978.
18. Boyda EK. Respiratory Problems. Oradell, NJ, Medical Economics Company, 1985.
19. Cannon GW, Zimmerman GA. The Lung in Rheumatic Diseases. New York, Marcel Dekker, 1990.
20. Peat M. Current Physical Therapy. Philadelphia, BC Decker, 1988.
21. Adams JH, Corsellis JAN, Duchen LW. Greenfield's Neuropathology. 4th ed. New York, John Wiley & Sons, 1984.
22. Mc Donald K, Wisniewski JM. Basic Burn Seminar Notebook (unpublished). Ann Arbor, Physical Therapy Division, University of Michigan Medical Center, 1988.
23. Angel JE. Physician's Desk Reference. 37th ed. Oradell, NJ, Medical Economics Company, 1983.

6 CHRONIC OBSTRUCTIVE PULMONARY DISEASES

INTRODUCTION

UNIQUE FEATURES OF OBSTRUCTIVE LUNG CONDITIONS

KEY CONCEPTS

PEDIATRIC OBSTRUCTIVE LUNG CONDITIONS

Bronchopulmonary Dysplasia

PEDIATRIC, ADOLESCENT, AND ADULT OBSTRUCTIVE LUNG CONDITIONS

Cystic Fibrosis
Asthma
Bronchiectasis

ADULT OBSTRUCTIVE LUNG CONDITIONS

Chronic Bronchitis
Emphysema

CASE STUDIES

SUMMARY

INTRODUCTION

Chronic obstructive pulmonary diseases (COPD) are diseases of the respiratory tract that produce an obstruction to airflow and that ultimately can affect both the mechanical function and gas exchanging capability of the lungs.

Certain physical symptoms are characteristic of obstructive lung conditions. These include chronic cough, expectoration of mucus, wheezing, and dyspnea on exertion. Obstructive lung conditions are diagnosed by changes in the results of pulmonary function tests. Important markers for COPD are a decrease in expiratory flow rates and an increase in residual volume (RV) (see Chapter 10).

In terms of pathologic changes, other similarities are also notable, including

- increased mucus production (or impairment of mucus clearance)
- inflammation of the mucosal lining of the bronchi and bronchioles

- mucosal thickening
- spasm of the bronchial smooth muscle

All of these changes decrease the size of the bronchial lumen and increase the resistance to airflow. In addition, the loss of normal elastic recoil of lung tissue and the tendency for bronchial walls to collapse and thereby to trap air contribute to decreased airflow. Over time the entire lung may become hyperinflated.

Obstructive pulmonary conditions affect the efficiency and function of the lung in many ways. Respiratory muscles must work harder to overcome the resistance to airflow and to enlarge a thorax that already may be in an inflated position. Alveolar ventilation (gas exchange at the alveolar level) is reduced. Capillary bed surface area and alveolar wall surface area may be reduced owing to destructive changes that occur in the structure of lung tissue. This reduction results in ventilation-perfusion mismatching and decreased gas exchange (see Chapters 2 and 10).

Ultimately, oxygen delivery to the tissues is

reduced, and carbon dioxide clearance is inadequate; decreases in Pa_{O_2} and increases in Pa_{CO_2} are noted. If **hypoxemia** (decreased Pa_{O_2}) is chronic, the patient may develop **pulmonary arterial hypertension** owing to vasoconstriction of the pulmonary artery in response to the hypoxia. **Polycythemia** (increased red blood cell count), also secondary to chronic hypoxemia, increases the **viscosity** of the blood and further increases pulmonary vascular resistance. Increased pressure in the pulmonary artery can also take place if the pulmonary capillary bed suffers a gradual loss of capillaries and area.

Cor pulmonale (right ventricular hypertrophy or dilation resulting from diseases that affect the function or structure of the lung) may ultimately develop from the resistance encountered as the right ventricle attempts to pump blood through the narrowed pulmonary artery. The development of cor pulmonale with **respiratory failure** ($Pa_{O_2} < 60$ mm Hg and $Pa_{CO_2} > 55$ mm Hg) is frequently the cause of death in individuals with obstructive lung conditions.

Physical therapists encounter COPDs as primary or secondary diagnoses in many of the patient populations they treat. An understanding of the diseases, their responsiveness to treatment, and their general course of progression enhances our ability to provide appropriate cardiopulmonary care and complete physical therapy programs for these individuals.

UNIQUE FEATURES OF OBSTRUCTIVE LUNG CONDITIONS

Despite many similarities, important differences in etiology, pathology, and pathophysiology should be recognized in the diseases grouped under the heading of obstructive lung conditions. The dominant cause of obstruction is one important factor. The reversibility of the obstructing lesion is another important variable. In addition, the differing locations of the major sites of obstruction should be understood. By appreciating these differences, we can become more effective in designing a pulmonary care program that considers the characteristics of each disease as well as those of each patient.

Pulmonary obstructive conditions to be covered include

- **Bronchopulmonary dysplasia**
- **Cystic fibrosis**
- **Asthma**
- **Bronchiectasis**
- Chronic bronchitis
- Emphysema

Obstructive conditions may occur independently, or, frequently, they may coexist. For ease of understanding, they are presented individually, but three combinations that often develop are asthmatic bronchitis, chronic bronchitis with emphysema, and cystic fibrosis with bronchiectasis.

Over time, some obstructive conditions may result in **fibrosis** and decreased **compliance** of the lung, so that some elements of restrictive lung disease may be evident as well (see Chapter 5).

KEY CONCEPTS

Chronic airflow obstruction is defined as permanent diminution of airflow, usually assessed by testing forced expiratory airflow. There are many tests of forced expiratory airflow of which FEV_1 is just one of many.[1] Airflow limitation can result from two basic causes. Airflow is determined both by the pressure applied and by the resistance encountered. In the lung, pressure applied during expiratory airflow is due to the normal elastic recoil of lung tissue after it has been released from the stretched position it assumes during inspiration. Resistance encountered to airflow results from narrowing of the airways. Narrowing may be caused by inflammation, airway thickening, increased mucus, or constriction of the bronchial walls **(bronchospasm)** (Fig. 6–1).

For purposes of classifying the location of obstructive diseases, the anatomic generations of the airways are divided into

- bronchi or airways with cartilage in their walls (usually > 2 mm in diameter)
- **bronchioles** or airways without cartilage in their walls (usually < 2 mm in diameter)
- lung **parenchyma,** or alveolar units, the gas exchanging part of the lung.

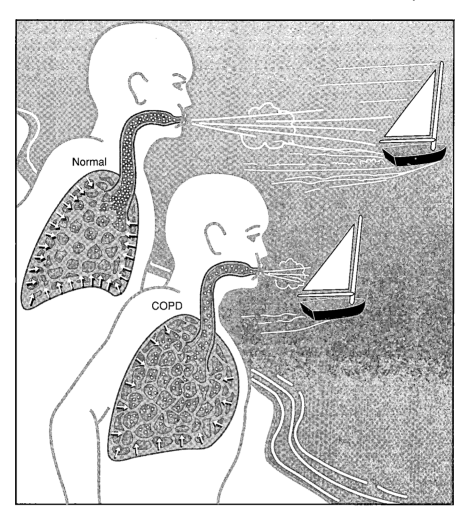

Figure 6-1.

The loss of elastic recoil in lung tissue and the increased airway resistance decrease the expiratory airflow in a patient with chronic obstructive pulmonary disease as compared with the expiratory airflow in a normal subject.

Abnormalities in both the airways and the parenchyma may be present in some conditions, whereas in others one area of abnormal function may dominate.

PEDIATRIC OBSTRUCTIVE LUNG CONDITIONS

In the pediatric population, four chronic obstructive pulmonary conditions are seen:

● Bronchopulmonary dysplasia
● Cystic fibrosis
● Asthma
● Bronchiectasis

Bronchopulmonary Dysplasia

Bronchopulmonary dysplasia (BPD) is a chronic lung disease of infancy characterized by respiratory distress and oxygen dependency lasting beyond 1 month of age that follows the use of oxygen and ventilatory support to treat neonatal respiratory distress.[2] Bronchopulmonary dysplasia most commonly and more easily develops in premature infants being treated for **respiratory distress syndrome,** but it also may develop in full-term infants following **meconium aspiration,** neonatal pneumonia, **persistent fetal circulation,** or surgery when long-term ventilatory support and oxygen exposure are required.[3]

Prevalence

Bronchopulmonary dysplasia occurs in 10% to 20% of infants who require prolonged assisted ventilation and exposure to high oxygen concentrations to survive respiratory distress syndrome.[4] However, cases of BPD have been reported in infants who received only a high FI_{O_2} (fraction of inspired oxygen concentration) without mechanical ventilation and in infants mechanically ventilated with a low FI_{O_2}.[5] The exact mechanism for development of BPD is unknown.

Pathology

The typical pathologic progression of BPD has four distinct phases, classified by age of occurrence (days of life).[6]

Stage I. Stage I (days 1–3 of life) is associated with the presence of **hyaline membrane disease,** a restrictive lung condition caused by a deficiency of pulmonary **surfactant** in immature lungs. Inadequate production of surfactant causes high **surface tension** in the alveoli and leads to the development of severe **atelectasis.** Histologic examination of autopsy results from infants has revealed complete collapse of many alveoli. In patent airways, hyaline membranes containing some **fibrin** were usually present, along with capillary congestion and edema in the **interalveolar septa** and **lymphatic spaces.**[7]

Stage II. Stage II (days 4–10 of life) is classified as the regeneration phase. Repair and regeneration are the most important features during this period. The medium-sized and small bronchi as well as the terminal airways become lined with **granulation** tissue. In 50% of cases, an **obliterating bronchitis** is seen, as proliferating fibroblasts combine with cellular debris and exudates, blocking the lumina of many bronchi and terminal airways.[7] Epithelial regeneration is also sometimes excessive and reduces the lumina of some small bronchi.

Stage III. Stage III (10–20 days of life) is considered the transition stage to the chronic condition of BPD. Hyaline membranes disappear, and mucus production increases.[6] The autopsy results of infants dying at this stage show that the lungs are divided into differing regions, some with

emphysematous changes (distended terminal airways and open alveoli separated by thin septa) and some with restrictive changes (contracted airways, fibrous septa, and residual collapse).[7]

Stage IV. Stage IV (first month to 2–3 years) is defined as the chronic phase of BPD. A continuation of alternating emphysematous (with bullae formation) and atelectatic areas are present. Hypertrophy of smooth muscle and **subepithelial fibrosis** are seen in medium-sized and small bronchi. Pulmonary arterial walls are thicker, and **right ventricular hypertrophy** is also seen. The ductus arteriosus is usually patent.

Because pathologic changes caused by BPD have been documented in the autopsy results of very severe cases, milder pathologic changes may actually be present in survivors of BPD.[5]

Pathogenesis

Barotrauma (injury caused by pressure) resulting from high airway pressures utilized during ventilator management of respiratory distress syndrome plays an important role in the development of BPD.[4] Infants who are **intubated** (insertion of an endotracheal tube, necessary for mechanical ventilation) are almost five times more likely to develop BPD than infants who have only face masks or nasal prongs to provide positive airway pressure or oxygen.[8]

The use of high oxygen concentrations for prolonged periods has also been implicated in the development of BPD. The precise concentration of oxygen that is toxic depends on many factors, including maturation, nutritional status, and length of oxygen exposure. **Oxygen toxicity** increases capillary permeability, impairs **mucociliary transport,** and causes an influx of leukocytes containing proteolytic enzymes (enzymes that digest proteins in the lung's elastic fiber network).[4]

The presence of **pulmonary interstitial edema** or extra-alveolar air due to alveolar rupture from positive pressure ventilation may contribute to the development of BPD.[9] Other factors that may contribute include nutritional deficits, infectious complications, and a **patent ductus arteriosus** that increases pulmonary blood flow and interstitial fluid and further impairs pulmonary function.[4] Table 6–1 identifies contributing factors in the development of BPD.

Clinical Features

Infants with mild BPD may only have transient **tachypnea** (rapid respiratory rate) and **cyanosis** with feeding or crying. Infants with severe BPD show typical signs of acute hypoxemic respiratory distress, including tachypnea; cyanosis on room air; suprasternal, intercostal, and subcostal retractions; nasal flaring; and grunting. Infants with severe BPD may also develop pulmonary hypertension and right heart failure. These infants have an increased incidence and increased severity of lower respiratory tract infections, such as **bronchiolitis** or pneumonia, and may require hospitalization for treatment. Many of their respiratory symptoms diminish with time, most likely owing to growth of parenchyma and airways.[5] Oxygen dependency and ventilator support via **tracheostomy** in some cases, however, may be necessary for 1 to 2 years.

Pathophysiology

Young children are difficult to study by pulmonary function test, but use of the **partial expiratory flow volume (PEFV)** has revealed low forced expiratory rates.[10] Generally decreased lung compliance and functional residual capacity (FRC) have been reported in the early stages of BPD. An increased work of breathing has also

been reported. In later tests, lung compliance continues to improve but remains below normal up to 3 years of age.[5]

Pulmonary function test results of older children with BPD have demonstrated a wide variety of responses, ranging from evidence of normality to evidence of airway obstruction and bronchial narrowing.[11]

In terms of arterial blood gases, persistent ventilation-perfusion mismatching results in hypoxemia and the need for long-term oxygen therapy and possibly ventilator support. Some infants may have long-term carbon dioxide retention.

Radiographic Findings. Initially a *ground glass appearance* is seen on the radiograph (indicating hyaline membrane disease). This progresses to a radiograph demonstrating both atelectatic and cystic areas. Chronically, radiographs show atelectatic and fibrotic changes with some element of hyperinflation.

Medical Treatment

Medical treatment for BPD consists of the use of bronchodilators, diuretics, potassium supplements, corticosteroids, and nutritional support and in some cases prolonged oxygen support. Prompt management of lower respiratory tract infections with the appropriate antibiotic therapy is essential.

Surfactant replacement for treatment of respiratory distress syndrome is being studied in hopes of removing the need for the long-term ventilatory support that leads to the lung injury of BPD.[4]

Prognosis

The outcome for children with BPD depends on the severity of the initial disease. A small but significant number of infants die within the first year of life. In survivors, the lung grows and repairs itself, and pulmonary function may gradually improve. However, respiratory tract infections and recurrent bouts of wheezing and **pulmonary insufficiency** may develop during the first 2 years of life.[12] Infants with BPD appear to be at greater risk for growth retardation and de-

TABLE 6–1. Contributing Factors to the Development of Bronchopulmonary Dysplasia
Immature lungs
Barotrauma (excessive positive-pressure ventilation)
Oxygen toxicity
Endotracheal intubation
Pulmonary interstitial edema
Infection
Congestive heart failure

velopmental delay than infants with respiratory distress syndrome.[13]

Graded exercise stress tests and pulmonary function tests demonstrate that abnormalities persist at 10 years of age. Children with BPD continue to show evidence of airway obstruction, hyperinflation, and **airway reactivity** (bronchospasm).[14] The oldest survivors of BPD are in their early twenties, and as they mature their lung function will continue to be studied. The possibility that they may be more susceptible to progressive obstructive pulmonary disease as adults has been raised by Northway, who originally described BPD in 1967.

PEDIATRIC, ADOLESCENT, AND ADULT OBSTRUCTIVE LUNG CONDITIONS

Cystic Fibrosis

Cystic fibrosis (CF) is a multisystem disorder involving the **exocrine glands.** Pulmonary and pancreatic problems are the most prominent clinical features, but the extent and type of involvement of different organ systems may vary in each individual.

Genetics

Cystic fibrosis is a recessively inherited genetic disorder. The incidence of the disease in whites is approximately 1 in 2500 live births, and 4% to 5% of white Americans are *heterozygous* carriers of the CF gene.[15] Although skilled medical care has resulted in increased years of survival, CF is invariably fatal. The disease is rare in orientals and blacks.

The role of genetic counseling is very important in families who have had a child, or first cousin, diagnosed with CF. The genetic defect has been localized to the long arm of chromosome 7.[15] As more is learned about the gene responsible for CF, the likelihood increases that DNA testing eventually can be used to identify carriers and those affected by CF.

At this time the diagnosis of CF is based on demonstrating an abnormally high level of chloride in the sweat of an individual who has a characteristic history and symptoms of CF. Two positive sweat tests using the **quantitative pilocarpine iontophoresis** method (sweat chloride > 60 mEq/L); clinical symptoms of chronic pulmonary disease, pancreatic insufficiency, or both; and a family history are necessary to make the diagnosis with confidence. The diagnosis of CF may be difficult to make in adolescents or young adults because of the subtle and variable manifestations of the disease.[16]

Pathogenesis

Although the CF gene has been localized, the basic defect causing the disease has not been identified. However, it appears that a block in the chloride permeability at the epithelial surface is a common factor in all tissues affected by CF.[15] Abnormality in ion transport explains the increased sweat chloride concentration found in the perspiration of children with CF. To explain the physiologic changes in pancreatic and lung function, however, other yet undiscovered mechanisms may also come into play.[15]

Every exocrine gland (a gland that does not secrete its product directly into the bloodstream) can be affected, although they may be affected to different degrees in individuals. Progressive obstruction of the exocrine ducts by viscous secretions seems to play a primary role in the pathogenesis of almost all manifestations of the disease. In 10% to 20% of all CF patients, the first manifestation is **meconium ileus,** or obstruction of the intestines by thick viscous meconium stool. Chronic pulmonary disease, pancreatic insufficiency, and **focal biliary cirrhosis** progress gradually throughout the course of the disease.

Pathology and Pathophysiology

Respiratory Tract. At birth the lungs of CF patients are both morphologically and functionally normal. However, soon after birth, thick secretions plug the airways and bacterial infection occurs in the lung. Once established, the infection is difficult to eradicate despite aggressive antibiotic therapy.[15] It is unclear how the infection occurs initially, but first *Staphylococcus aureus* is found in the sputum of CF patients. Later in the disease, most patients become colonized with *Pseudomonas aeruginosa*. Less commonly found organisms include *Escherichia coli, Klebsiella,* and *Haemophilus influenzae.*[16] In later stages of CF, *Pseudomonas* is usually the predominant organism. Intensive antibiotic therapy may be partially to blame for the persistence of these pathogens, but alterations in the immune system of CF patients cannot be excluded.[15]

The lung disease of CF appears to begin in the small airways with inflammation and destruction of the airway walls. Alveolar units are usually spared, but damage spreads centrally to the larger airways, and ultimately all conducting airways are inflamed. Persistent infiltration with neutrophils is the hallmark of the inflammatory process in CF.[15] There is *hyperplasia* of mucus-secreting cells, and thick secretions plug the airways. In the lungs of CF patients, the combination of hypersecretion of viscid mucus and chronic bacterial infection combine to produce an obstructive pulmonary disease that progresses eventually to severe diffuse bronchiectasis.

Repeated episodes of infection have a cumulative effect and gradually impair pulmonary function. Pulmonary function tests may be useful in tracing the natural history of the disease and also in evaluating the effectiveness of various therapeutic interventions.[16] Initially these tests reflect small airway dysfunction with reduced midexpiratory flow and increased RV (increased air trapping).[15] Later frank obstruction to airflow occurs; the FEV_1 falls; and the ratio of RV to total lung capacity (TLC) increases markedly.[15] Mild bronchoconstriction may be seen owing to slight increases in muscle tone in the airways.

Hemodynamic Changes. Early in the disease, ventilation-perfusion abnormalities widen the alveolar-arterial difference in Po_2 and increase the ratio of dead space to tidal volume.[16] As the disease progresses, the imbalance between ventilation and perfusion increases, and arterial hypoxemia follows. Generally pulmonary hypertension develops; cor pulmonale and right

ventricular failure may follow. Late in the disease, **hypercapnia** (increased CO_2) and **respiratory acidosis** (decreased pH) are prominent features as respiratory failure develops.[16] Figure 6–2 is a diagram of the pathogenesis and progression of pulmonary disease in CF.

Clinical Features of Respiratory Involvement

In patients who have pulmonary involvement, increased *sputum* production and chronic cough are evident, with symptoms becoming more pronounced when a viral respiratory infection is superimposed on airways colonized with *Pseudomonas.* An increased respiratory rate and increased work of breathing may be seen with acute illness. Diffuse coarse rales, rhonchi, or wheezing may be evident, along with fever and **leukocytosis** (elevated white blood cell count). **Digital clubbing** (broadening and thickening of ends of fingers and nails seen in chronic pulmonary disease) may occur early in the course of CF.

Radiographic Findings. Radiographic findings become more abnormal as CF progresses (Fig. 6–3). Hyperinflation is frequently seen in children and may be the only abnormality initially.[15] In adults, hyperinflation is accompanied by **peribronchial** thickening due to inflammation. In advanced disease, ring shadows and **cystic lesions** may occur with areas of bronchiectasis and atelectasis also evident. The upper lobes are usually more involved than the lower lobes, and the right side is more involved than the left.[17] The pulmonary and bronchial arteries often begin to enlarge in the middle stages of disease, but the **cardiac silhouette** remains within normal limits until the disease is far advanced.

Other Organ Involvement

Upper Airway. Sinusitis and nasal **polyps** are common in CF. Approximately 50% of adult CF patients have nasal polyps at some point.[14]

Pancreas. The pancreas is involved in 80% to 90% of CF patients. Infants with pancreatic insufficiency demonstrate failure to thrive owing to

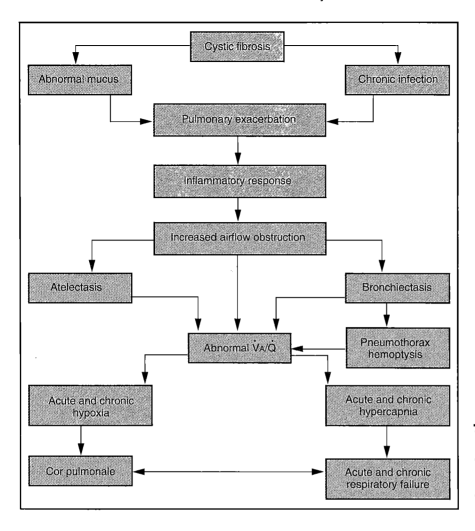

Figure 6-2.

The pathogenesis and progression of pulmonary disease in cystic fibrosis. (Redrawn with permission from Fishman A. Pulmonary Diseases and Disorders. Vol. 2. 2nd ed. New York, McGraw-Hill, 1988.)

malabsorption, and older children may have **steatorrhea** (excessive fat in the feces). Pancreatic function becomes progressively more abnormal as the ducts become more obstructed by thick viscous secretions. Pancreatic enzymes that are trapped in the ducts lead to autodestruction of the pancreas. Both cystic and fibrotic changes are seen, and in advanced stages, fibrosis of the pancreas affects the **islets of Langerhans** and causes diabetes.

Liver and Biliary Tract. The liver and gallbladder are also affected by obstruction of their ducts with abnormally viscid secretions. Biliary cirrhosis may be present in infancy, and in some patients it may progress to diffuse cirrhosis and portal hypertension. **Obstructive jaundice** may

also be present. **Microgallbladder** is seen in 20% to 30% of CF patients. Because of malabsorption of bile salts, gallstones are present in 13% of adults with CF.[14]

Gastrointestinal Tract. In the intestinal tract, goblet cells and hyperplasia of the mucous glands are evident. Abnormalities in intestinal mucins contribute to malabsorption of specific nutrients. Malabsorption can generally be corrected by administering pancreatic enzymes. Also water content in the intestinal tract is reduced, probably owing to abnormalities in ion transport.[15] This reduction in liquid leaves the intestinal contents in a semisolid or solid state, in contrast to their normal, more liquid state, which can result in **fecal impaction.** Fecal impaction

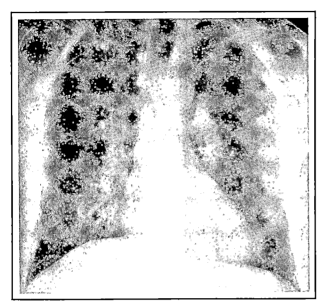

Figure 6-3.

Chest radiograph of a patient with cystic fibrosis. Coarse reticulation is seen throughout the lungs with cyst formation secondary to bronchiectasis more pronounced in the upper lobes. (Courtesy of Dr. Dorothy McCauley, New York University Medical Center.)

can also lead to **volvulus** (intestinal obstruction due to twisting of the bowel into a loop) or **intussusception** of the bowel (infolding of one segment of the intestine into an adjacent part).

Reproductive Organs. Female CF patients appear to be less fertile than other women. They demonstrate increased viscosity of cervical mucus, which fails to thin at midcycle, making sperm penetration more difficult. However, pregnancy is possible and has been carried to term in hundreds of cases.[15] In males affected with CF, the vas deferens is partially or completely obstructed, and approximately 98% of CF males are aspermatic.[16]

Laboratory Findings

A sputum culture demonstrating *P. aeruginosa* and *S. aureus*, either alone or in combination, is most common. **Sputum** cultures and sensitivities guide antibiotic therapy during treatment of exacerbations of the disease. Once present, these organisms, especially *Pseudomonas*, are rarely eradicated from the sputum.

Laboratory evaluation of malabsorption due to pancreatic insufficiency requires stool collection for 72 hours to test for residual fat content while ingestion of 100 grams of fat per day is maintained. A coefficient of malabsorption of greater than 7% is considered abnormal; patients with CF often have coefficients of malabsorption of 20% to 30%.

Medical Treatment

Comprehensive and intensive medical treatment of CF patients has led to a dramatic increase in the median age of survival (age 25).[15] Individual programs must be tailored to improve or maintain function of the organs involved.

Management of Pulmonary Disease. The goals of treatment of the pulmonary disease are to prevent and treat the complications of obstruction and infection in the airways. This is done by practicing bronchial hygiene, including postural drainage with percussion and vibration, to prevent plugging of the airways (see Chapter 15) and antibiotic therapy when appropriate. Administration of aerosol, mucolytic, or bronchodilator therapies may precede the bronchial hygiene therapy.

Antibiotics. Antibiotics have been the key factor responsible for the increased survival of CF patients during the past few decades. When signs of pulmonary infection are evident, the appropriate antibiotic, determined by culture and sensitivity testing, is given, and bronchial hygiene therapy is increased.

Signs of Pulmonary Infection

Increased cough
Increased sputum production
Fever
Increased respiratory rate
Increased white blood cell count
New findings on auscultation or on the radiograph
Decreases in the pulmonary function test values

Antibiotics currently used to treat staphylococcal infections include dicloxacillin, cephalexin, the newer cephalosporins, and chloramphenicol.[16] Early in the pulmonary disease, *Pseudomonas* organisms may respond to tetracycline. If the *Pseudomonas* organisms are resistant to oral antibiotics, the patient must be admitted for a 2-week course of intravenous antibiotics. Usually a combination of two antibiotics are used intravenously, an aminoglycoside and a semisynthetic penicillin. The most commonly used combinations are gentamicin and carbenicillin or tobramycin and ticarcillin.[16] The combination of antibiotics is believed to work synergistically on *Pseudomonas*, and the organism is less likely to become resistant to either antibiotic.

Larger doses and more frequent administration of the aminoglycoside are prescribed to achieve higher levels of the antibiotic in the airways and the secretions. Serum concentrations of the antibiotics, renal function, and hearing are monitored to avoid toxic reactions.[16] When antibiotic therapy is required for longer than 2 weeks, use of a heparin lock or inhaled antibiotics may allow the patient to return home.

Mucolytics and Bronchodilators. Mist tents, historically used with CF patients, have been found not to be helpful in thinning secretions. However, intermittent **aerosols** are used to deliver **mucolytics** and bronchodilators. These medications should be delivered before performing **postural drainage.**

Nutrition. Management of pancreatic insufficiency is partially accomplished by ingestion of pancreatic enzyme replacements, which should be taken along with any food that contains protein, fat, or complex carbohydrates. The dose of enzymes is adjusted to attempt to maintain an adequate weight gain or an ideal weight and a relatively normal bowel pattern with a decrease in cramping and flatulence. Enzyme replacement cannot totally correct pancreatic insufficiency, so patients also require increased caloric intake. This is accomplished through the use of nutritional supplements taken orally or via nasogastric feeding. Multivitamin preparations and increased salt intake are also recommended for individuals with CF.[16]

Complications and Prognosis

The general course of CF is characterized by a gradual decrease in pulmonary function over the life span, with abrupt declines in pulmonary function when infections are present. Malnutrition may be present with severe pulmonary impairment. Certain complications, however, may occur suddenly and be life threatening. Complications include electrolyte depletion, usually seen in hot weather, or intestinal obstruction due to an impacted fecal mass.

Pneumothorax, caused by rupture of bronchiectatic cysts or subpleural blebs, is a serious complication in CF. About 20% of patients do not survive the hospitalization during which their pneumothorax is treated.[17] Because the recurrence rate is about 50% following pneumothorax, and collapse of a lung could be fatal in CF patients, surgical treatment of pneumothorax is usually recommended.[15] **Pleurectomy, pleural abrasion,** and **oversewing** of the tear is usually effective. Atelectasis of a segment or lobe may occur, which if untreated may lead to the development of bronchiectasis in that segment. **Hemoptysis** (coughing up blood) may occur, ranging from streaking of blood in the sputum to larger quantities. When 30 to 60 milliliters of fresh blood is expectorated, the patient is usually hospitalized. Massive hemoptysis is uncommon in CF.[15]

With progression of the disease and during acute infections, increased hypoxia can lead to pulmonary arterial hypertension and cor pulmonale. During acute infections, oxygen and diuretics may be used to treat right heart failure. When the patient is considered to be in respiratory failure, management becomes very difficult. If the respiratory failure is due to an acute problem such as viral infection or **status asthmaticus** and prior PFTs were relatively good, mechanical ventilation is more likely to be successful. Mechanical ventilation is usually of no help when respiratory failure is due to a progressive pulmonary insufficiency despite adequate medical management.[16]

Prognosis

As mentioned earlier, the comprehensive medical treatment now available to manage patients with CF has improved median survival to 25 years of age. Thirty years ago, median survival was only a few years of age. However, most experts believe the median survival rate is now plateauing. Also because CF is such a complex clinical disorder, the variability in outcomes is wide. Some severely affected children still die at a young age, despite skillful medical management, whereas others who are more mildly affected may live into their thirties and forties. Because more than 98% of CF patients die of respiratory failure or pulmonary complications, the possibility of using heart-lung or single-lung transplantation to prolong their lives is being explored.

Asthma

Asthma is a disease of the airways characterized by increased responsiveness of the tracheobronchial tree to a variety of stimuli. Widespread narrowing of the airways occurs when the individual comes in contact with these stimuli. Clinical manifestations of asthma include cough, dyspnea, wheezing, and an inability to expel air completely. Generally asthma is episodic in nature, with acute episodes being separated by symptom-free time periods.

Prevalence

Asthma affects both children and adults. It is estimated that approximately 4% of the population in the United States has the disorder. Fifty percent of individuals with asthma develop the disease before age 10, and another 30% develop it before age 40.[18] Asthma that begins in childhood and is triggered by allergens is called **extrinsic asthma.** Many children outgrow this type of asthma. Asthma that begins after age 35 is called **intrinsic asthma** and is more severe in nature.

Pathology

Airways are dynamic structures that dilate when large amounts of air need to be moved, as during exercise, and constrict when the airways need to be protected, as during exposure to irritant gases. The ability of the airways to alter their diameter in response to both internal and external stimuli is called airway reactivity. In asthmatic individuals, airway reactivity is increased, and they develop more intense bronchoconstriction than do nonasthmatic individuals when exposed to a specific stimulus. Certain biologic functions vary during a 24-hour period, and airway reactivity appears to follow this pattern. Some asthmatics experience increased respiratory symptoms during the night and early morning. Nocturnal asthma may occur in as many as 70% to 80% of patients with asthma.[18]

Pathogenesis

Seven major types of stimuli induce acute episodes of asthma:

- Allergens
- Exercise
- Infections
- Occupational stress
- Environmental stress
- Pharmacologic stress
- Emotional stress[18]

An allergic component can be found in 35% to 55% of asthma patients. Most allergens that provoke asthma are airborne.

Initially allergens must be abundant to produce an asthmatic response, but once sensitization has occurred, only minute quantities of the substance are necessary to provoke bronchospasm. Allergens cause constriction of bronchial smooth muscle, increased secretion of mucus by bronchial glands, reduced ciliary activity, and vasodilation of blood vessels[18] (Fig. 6–4).

In a sensitized individual, inhalation of an allergen causes airflow limitation within minutes; the allergen's effect decreases in the next 30 to 60 minutes. In some individuals, the initial reaction is followed by a second wave of obstruction or what is sometimes called a *late reaction,* which may be more severe than the first and less responsive to treatment.[18]

Asthma that is exacerbated by physical exertion is identified as *exercise-induced asthma.* Attacks are characterized by cough, wheezing, and dyspnea, which resolve relatively quickly and spontaneously. The use of bronchodilators before exercise may often control attacks. The environment in which the exercise is performed may influence the development of asthma. The inha-

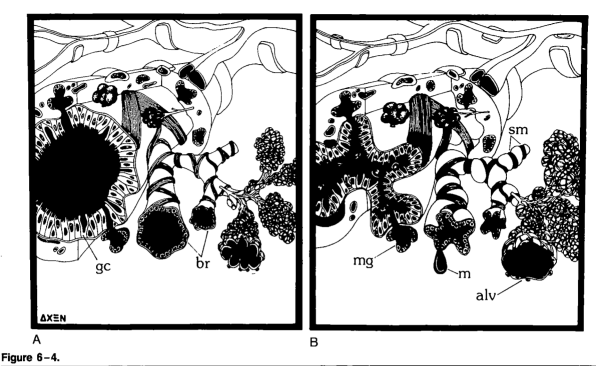

A   B

Figure 6-4.

Comparison of normal *(A)* and asthmatic *(B)* airways and their surrounding tissue; gc, goblet cell; br, bronchi; mg, mucous gland; m, mucus; sm, smooth muscle; alv, alveoli. (From Des Jardins T. Clinical Manifestations of Respiratory Disease. Chicago, Year Book Medical Publishers, 1984. Redrawn by Kenneth Axen.)

lation of cold air during exercise may precipitate an attack. Activities such as ice skating or skiing may be difficult for affected individuals. Both the lack of water content in the inspired air and the high levels of ventilation during exercise have been implicated in triggering asthmatic attacks.

Viral respiratory tract infections may also precipitate attacks. In children younger than 2 years of age, **respiratory syncytial virus** plays a major role, and with increasing age **rhinoviruses** (colds) become more important, along with influenza and *Mycoplasma* infections.[18] Bacterial infections are less likely to be a cause of asthma attacks.

Certain occupations may be associated with the development of asthma. Workers in the cotton industry (those involved in the carding and spinning processes) have a higher than average incidence of asthma. Bakers exposed to cereals and flours and animal handlers also show an increased incidence of asthma. The many substances implicated in occupational asthma include metal salts; wood and vegetable dusts; pharmaceutic agents; industrial chemicals and plastics; biologic enzymes (used in detergents); and animal, bird, fish, or insect proteins.[18]

Weather changes such as increased cold or dampness may worsen asthmatic symptoms. High levels of air pollution may also trigger asthma attacks, especially when there are stagnant air masses associated with heavy pollution.

Pharmacologic agents most frequently linked with acute episodes of asthma include aspirin, drug additives such as tartrazine (yellow dye no. 5), and food preservatives such as sulfites.[18] Asthma can also be aggravated by nonselective beta-blocking drugs such as propanolol.

Emotional or psychological factors can interact with an individual's predisposition to asthma attacks. Emotions can ease or worsen the severity of the attack in approximately half of the cases.[18] However, it is unusual for psychological factors to be the cause of an attack.

Clinical Features

Asthma is generally episodic in nature. It is a chronic disease in which acute episodes of bronchial narrowing are interspersed with symptom-free periods. Clinical signs include intermittent wheezing and dyspnea, usually accompanied by cough. Episodes may last for a few minutes or may persist for hours or days. Young children with severe asthma or late-onset asthmatics may wheeze continuously, with variation only in severity of the wheezing.

During an attack, the patient may be in respiratory distress, using primarily the accessory muscles of respiration. The chest is often hyperinflated and hyperresonant to percussion. Auscultation reveals a prolonged expiratory phase, and diffuse wheezing may be heard on both inspiration and expiration.

Patients with a severe persistent attack of asthma that is refractory to bronchodilation medication are said to have status asthmaticus. These patients are usually in severe respiratory distress and have cyanosis (bluish discoloration of skin and mucous membranes due to lack of oxygen in the blood). They may become physically exhausted by the increased work of breathing and from sleep deprivation.[19] Auscultation during an acute attack may reveal very little air movement, with wheezing faintly heard or even absent. This is an ominous sign during a severe attack.[19] Signs of acute respiratory failure such as carbon dioxide retention, alterations in level of consciousness, and signs of cardiac failure may be evident. Patients in this type of respiratory distress require immediate attention and may require mechanical ventilation.

In asthmatics who experience only intermittent attacks, there may be no clinical signs of airway disease between attacks.

Chest Radiograph. Between attacks and during mild asthma attacks the radiograph is often entirely normal. In severe attacks, however, a radiograph may look similar to that of a patient with emphysema, and marked hyperinflation may be seen. The diaphragms may be low and flattened; the ribs are horizontal with wide interspaces and sparse vascular markings, giving a dark appearance to the lung parenchyma (Fig. 6–5).

Pathophysiology

Obstruction to airflow, either episodic or continual with varying severity, is the predominant feature seen in the pulmonary function tests of asthmatic patients. The FEV_1 and the FEV_1 to FVC (forced vital capacity) ratio are reduced during an attack. When the FEV_1 to FVC ratio is less than 75%, obstruction to airflow is present.[19] **Maximal expiratory flow-volume (MEFV)** relationships may also be abnormal. The MEFV curve measures airflow at all lung volumes throughout the FVC maneuver, and even in asymptomatic asthma patients airflow may be reduced at lung volumes between 50% of **vital capacity (VC)** and RV.[19] This probably represents the presence of residual abnormalities in the peripheral airways. Other tests of peripheral airway function such as closing volume may also reveal abnormalities.

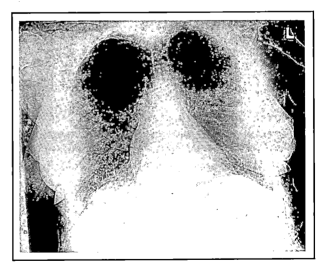

Figure 6–5.

Chest radiograph of a patient during an acute attack of asthma. Note the low flattened diaphragms and horizontal ribs, indicating hyperinflation of the lungs. (Courtesy of Dr. Dorothy McCauley, New York University Medical Center.)

In performing pulmonary function tests on patients suspected of having asthma, it is very important to repeat each test after the administration (usually by aerosol) of bronchodilators. An improvement of 15% or more in the FEV_1 is considered to indicate reversibility of obstruction to airflow. Normal individuals improve 10% or less in FEV_1 measurement when their resting bronchial tone is reduced by bronchodilators.

Asthmatics often have a reduced VC and an increased FRC and RV. These signs of hyperinflation usually improve with treatment of the airways obstruction. Work of breathing may be increased when hyperinflation is present, as inspiratory muscles are at a mechanical disadvantage.

In an asthma attack, the severity of airways obstruction may be nonuniform in the lungs so that distribution of ventilation is uneven. Initially perfusion is diverted away from underventilated areas, but if obstruction becomes more widespread and severe, ventilation-perfusion mismatching worsens and arterial hypoxemia occurs. Early in the attack, minute ventilation is increased to maintain alveolar ventilation, and initially, Pa_{CO_2} is decreased (30–35 mm Hg). In severe attacks of obstruction, alveolar ventilation decreases and hypercapnia ($Pa_{CO_2} > 45$ mm Hg) results.

Laboratory

A complete blood count with an absolute eosinophil count is usually ordered. Finding eosinophilia helps to identify an allergic cause of the asthma and is useful in predicting response to corticosteroids. In patients younger than 35 years of age, allergy testing (skin patch tests) may be done. Sputum should be examined for bacteria during a severe attack. If food substances are suspected allergens, the diet may need to be evaluated.

Medical Treatment

The goals of medical treatment are to relieve bronchospasm, mobilize secretions, and maintain alveolar ventilation. Drugs may be used for short-term control or long-term control with sta-bilization of the airway. Five categories of drugs that are used in the treatment and prevention of asthma are **sympathomimetics,** theophylline and its derivatives, anticholinergics, cromolyn, and corticosteroids (see Chapter 13).

Controlling exposure to environmental stimuli, such as smog, dust, and other irritants, may be critical in the control of asthma. Physical conditioning is believed to be beneficial in improving exercise tolerance.

Prognosis

Despite great advances in pharmacologic management, asthma-related deaths appear to be increasing. Possible explanations for this finding include complacency or lack of understanding of the disease. Overreliance on self-administered medications may be contributory also. An important goal for health care professionals working with asthmatics is to educate them and encourage them to enter the health care system earlier when experiencing symptoms of an asthma attack that is not resolving.

Bronchiectasis

Bronchiectasis is a permanent, abnormal dilation and distortion of one or more bronchi that is caused by destruction of the elastic and muscular components of the bronchial walls.

Clinical Features

Common clinical features include

- cough
- **copious mucopurulent** sputum and **fetid breath** (having a disagreeable odor)
- recurrent pulmonary infections
- recurrent hemoptysis

Prevalence

The incidence of bronchiectasis is decreasing. It was common and often fatal in the preantibiotic era and is still common in developing countries. The decrease in bronchiectasis is felt to be due to greater availability of antibiotics for the treatment of respiratory tract infections and widespread use of immunization in childhood against **pertussis** (whooping cough) and measles.

Pathology

The abnormal permanent bronchial dilation involves mainly the medium-sized bronchi but extends to the more distal bronchi and bronchioles as well. Dilation of the bronchi may reach as much as four times the normal diameter. Bronchiectatic areas are often filled with purulent secretions, and the mucosal surface is swollen, inflamed, and often ulcerated. Bronchial mucous glands are dilated. Infection denudes the epithelial lining and elastic tissue; smooth muscle and surrounding cartilage are destroyed.[20] In chronic bronchiectasis, marked fibrosis occurs in and around bronchial walls, replacing muscle, mucous glands, and cartilage.

Bronchiectasis is bilateral in 30% of cases. The lower lobes are most frequently involved, with the left lower lobe involved more than three times as often as the right lower lobe. This may be because of better drainage of the wider and straighter right mainstem bronchus. Also the left mainstem bronchus is slightly compressed as the left pulmonary artery crosses it. The left lower lobe posterior basal segment is the most frequently involved.[20]

The classification of bronchiectasis developed through a correlation between the findings of **bronchography** and the pathologic changes, both gross and microscopic, found in resected bronchiectatic lobes. Since the development of the computed tomography (CT) scan, bronchography (the instillation of a radiopaque dye into the tracheobronchial tree) is no longer used extensively in the diagnosis of bronchiectasis.

Types of Bronchiectasis

Cylindric Bronchiectasis. In **cylindric bronchiectasis,** the bronchi are tubular; the walls of the bronchi are straight and their diameter is only slightly increased. The involved bronchi come to an abrupt squared end rather than gradually tapering as do normal bronchi. The numbers of subdivisions of the bronchi appear normal by microscopic examination.

Varicose Bronchiectasis. In **varicose bronchiectasis,** the bronchi are generally dilated and irregular in form and size. As they extend peripherally, the bronchi terminate in a bulbous end pouch rather than tapering gradually. Irregular bulging contours are characteristic of varicose bronchiectasis. The average number of bronchial divisions is reduced to about one half of those in a normal lung on microscopic examination. In many areas the bronchial lumen is obliterated by fibrous tissue.

Saccular Bronchiectasis. In **saccular bronchiectasis,** bronchi are very dilated and ballooning in shape, especially as they progress to the periphery. The number of bronchial subdivisions is markedly reduced to one fourth or one fifth of the number normally found on microscopic examination.

Different classifications of bronchiectasis may coexist in the same lung, and no cause and effect relationship exists between etiology and type of bronchiectasis that develops. In general, with proper medical care bronchiectasis does not progress.

Pathogenesis. The cause of bronchiectasis is, most commonly, a **necrotizing** infection or a series of multiple infections involving the tracheobronchial walls and adjacent lung parenchyma. So-called congenital bronchiectasis is a rarer cause and is due to a variety of abnormalities in tracheobronchial structure, defects in ciliary structure or function, or alterations in the upper airway. These anatomic defects cause respiratory tract dysfunction that predisposes the child to developing bronchiectasis in early childhood. The bronchiectasis is usually not present at birth.

Before the 1950s, when extensive immunization against pertussis and measles began, pulmonary infections that developed during these childhood diseases were associated with bronchiectasis.[20] The association of measles with bronchiectasis is less prominent now in the United States, but in developing countries bronchiectasis may develop after the measles. Secondary necrotizing bacterial pneumonias that develop after pertussis can also lead to the development of bronchiectasis. Dried retained mucus and debris associated with pertussis may cause resorptive atelectasis (collapse of alveolar units caused by proximal plugging and reabsorption of distal air) and contribute to the development of bronchiectasis.

The bacterial pneumonias that predispose an individual to the development of bronchiectasis are usually necrotizing processes. These bacteria include *S. aureus, Klebsiella pneumoniae,* and *P. aeruginosa.* Tuberculosis has also been associated with subsequent bronchiectasis.

Other Causes of Bronchiectasis

Bronchial Obstruction. Bronchiectasis may develop years after an unrecognized foreign body aspiration. This type of bronchiectasis is usually localized rather than diffuse. Foreign bodies associated with aspiration include peanuts; chicken bones; or, in the pediatric population, grass aspiration (flowering head of the grass).[20] Obstructive emphysema, atelectasis, and infection usually develop behind the obstruction, setting the stage for the development of bronchiectasis.

Mucoid Impaction. Bronchiectasis may be associated with diffuse obstructive airways diseases such as asthma or chronic bronchitis. Hypersecretion of mucus may be present with these diseases, and continuing infection, mucoid impaction, blockage of peripheral bronchi, and bronchial inflammation can gradually progress to bronchiectasis.

Hereditary Conditions Associated with Bronchiectasis

Immotile Cilia Syndrome. Immotile cilia syndrome is a genetic disorder in which cilia are immotile or defective owing to a molecular lesion. Symptoms of immotile cilia syndrome include sinusitis, otitis, chronic rhinitis, chronic or recurrent bronchitis, bronchiectasis, and male sterility. Cilia from these patients lack structural components called dynein arms, which are important in mucus propulsion. Consequently, in affected individuals tracheobronchial or nasal mucociliary transport is totally or nearly totally absent. The frequency of bronchiectasis associated with immotile cilia syndrome is approximately 30%. The term *ciliary dyskinesia syndrome* is used to describe those individuals whose cilia are anatomically abnormal but do display some movement, although the movement is not entirely normal.

Kartagener's Syndrome. Kartagener's syndrome is a triad of bronchiectasis, sinusitis, and situs inversus (lateral transposition of the thoracic contents; heart is located on the right). Kartagener's syndrome occurs in approximately 50% of patients with ciliary dyskinesia syndrome.

Cystic Fibrosis. Cystic fibrosis is a predisposing factor in at least half of the cases of bronchiectasis seen in persons up to the age of 20 years. Bronchiectasis is found on examination of essentially all autopsied CF victims older than 6 months of age.[20]

Clinical Features

Cough is almost always present in individuals with bronchiectasis. **Purulent** (consisting of or containing pus) sputum, which separates into three layers on standing, is characteristic of the disease: an upper layer of white or slightly greenish brown frothy secretions, a middle thin mucoid layer, and a bottom layer of thick greenish plugs. Sputum production is present in 90% of patients, and it is often greatest in the morning, after accumulating during sleep in the recumbent position. During episodes of infection, sputum increases in volume and purulence. In rare cases, sputum production is not a prominent feature, and these cases are referred to as *dry bronchiectasis.*

Patients with bronchiectasis have a tendency to develop hemoptysis. Before the widespread use of antibiotics, 40% to 70% of bronchiectatic patients developed hemoptysis.[20] Hemoptysis varies in quantity from light blood streaking to massive life-threatening bleeding.

Sinusitis is frequently associated with bronchiectasis, especially in the predisposing syndromes, such as CF and immotile cilia syndrome.

Most patients with bronchiectasis have abnormalities on auscultation of the thorax. Moist rales, or crackles, are present over the involved lobes. Rhonchi are evident during periods of mucus retention, and dullness to percussion and decreased breath sounds may be present when mucus plugging occurs. Bronchovesicular or **bronchial breath sounds** may be noted during pneumonia. Observations of clubbing of the fingers and cyanosis were more frequent in the preantibiotic era. By the 1960s, clubbing was observed in only 7% of cases.[20] Cor pulmonale occurred formerly in 10% to 22% of cases. Now it is a less common complication.

Radiographic Findings. Radiographic findings may be unremarkable, especially early in the disease. Later in the disease, line shadows following a bronchovascular distribution may be evident. These are caused by thickened bronchial walls, peribronchial fibrosis, and adjacent alveolar collapse.[20] If mucus plugging is significant, atelectasis or collapse of whole lobes behind the obstruction may be visible on a radiograph. With advanced saccular bronchiectasis, large cystic areas with and without fluid levels may be seen.

Patchy areas of bronchopulmonary pneumonia may occur in patients with bronchiectasis.

Bronchography was done more frequently in the past to assist in diagnosis (Fig. 6–6). Currently it is done only when surgical resection of a localized bronchiectatic area is being considered. Adverse reactions to this procedure include possible allergic reactions to the dye and impairment of ventilation. Computed chest tomography (CT scan) is more frequently used for diagnostic purposes today.

Computed Tomography Scan. Cystic bronchiectasis is most easily diagnosed by a CT scan, but cylindric and varicose types may be diagnosed as well as long as pneumonia and other causes of consolidation are eliminated. Pneumonia may look similar to bronchiectasis on a CT scan. Findings on a CT scan include dilated bronchi extending peripherally and thickened

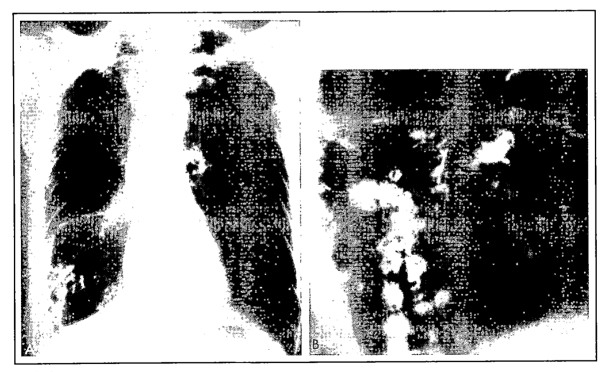

Figure 6–6.

Saccular bronchiectasis. Chest roentgenogram *(A)* of a 42-year-old man with severe chronic cough and sputum production showing increased markings extending into the right lower lobe and cystic lesions. Detail of bronchogram *(B)* confirms the presence of saccular bronchiectasis. (From Hinshaw HC, Murray JF. Diseases of the Chest. 4th ed. Philadelphia, WB Saunders, 1980, p. 597.)

bronchial walls. Air-fluid levels may be present, and in cystic bronchiectasis clusters of cysts may be seen[20] (Fig. 6–7).

Pathophysiology

Pulmonary Function Tests. Test results in bronchiectasis depend on the extent of disease present and the coexistence of other lung diseases such as chronic bronchitis or emphysema. Patients with mild or localized bronchiectasis and no other associated diseases may have relatively normal pulmonary function test results. However, in patients with diffuse involvement, results show a pattern of airway obstruction. A reduced FVC, FEV_1, FEV_1/FVC, and a reduced forced expiratory flow of 25% to 75% (FEF_{25-75}) are seen as well as increased RV. In patients with associated atelectasis and fibrosis, test results show a more mixed obstructive-restrictive pattern or a largely restrictive pattern with decreased VC and decreased FRC.

Arterial Blood Gases. With extensive bronchiectasis, arterial hypoxemia may develop due to ventilation-perfusion mismatching. Carbon dioxide retention occurs only in patients with bronchiectasis associated with severe chronic bronchitis and advanced emphysema.

Hemodynamic Changes. Extensive systemic to pulmonary anastomoses occur at the precapillary level in the granulation tissue surrounding bronchiectatic segments. These anastomoses can lead to bronchial artery enlargement and left to right shunts (recirculation of oxygenated blood). In patients with severe bronchiectasis and accompanying chronic bronchitis and emphysema, hypoxia, pulmonary hypertension, and cor pulmonale may develop. The development of pulmonary hypertension and cor pulmonale is uncommon in patients with bronchiectasis alone.[20]

Laboratory Findings

Bacteria commonly found in the sputum of bronchiectatic patients include *H. influenzae* and streptococcus pneumonia. Anaerobic bacteria may also play an important role in some cases of bronchiectasis. A gram-stained smear of sputum shows numerous polymorphonuclear leukocytes and mixed bacterial flora, often including fusiform bacteria as well as a variety of gram-negative and gram-positive cocci. Leukocytosis is variable and may be associated with infections and active **suppuration. Anemia** in long-standing disease is sometimes seen.[20]

Medical Treatment

The goals of treatment are to prevent the progression and to alleviate the symptoms of the disease. Control of infection and supportive measures to provide good pulmonary hygiene,

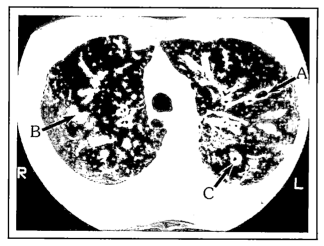

Figure 6–7.

Computed tomography (CT) scan showing bronchiectasis. A, dilated, irregularly shaped, air-filled bronchus; B, mucoid impaction of a bronchus; C, signet ring configuration common in bronchiectasis—a dilated bronchus with its accompanying pulmonary artery, resembling a signet ring. (CT scan courtesy of Dr. Dorothy McCauley, New York University Medical Center.)

including postural drainage with percussion, vibration, and shaking, are indicated. Hydration is very important to assist in thinning secretions. Eight to ten glasses of water are recommended daily. Control of bronchospasm may also be necessary.

Immunization against influenza and pneumonia is recommended for this population. Antibiotic therapy should be initiated promptly for acute infections and febrile exacerbations of bronchiectasis. The choice of antibiotic should be guided by sputum culture and sensitivity testing, which determines the most effective antibiotic for eradicating the organism. Bronchoscopy may be necessary for removal of foreign bodies if they are the cause of the bronchiectasis.

Surgical resection of a bronchiectatic segment is recommended only when symptoms of the disease are severe and interfere with the progress of a normal life. The disease must be fairly well localized. Surgery is also recommended when major hemorrhage from an eroded bronchial artery in a bronchiectatic segment cannot be controlled by bronchial arteriography and embolization.[20]

Complications and Prognosis

The complications of bronchiectasis include

- chronic bronchial infections and episodes of **bronchopneumonia**
- hemoptysis with possible pulmonary hemorrhage
- obliteration of peripheral airways, with associated bronchitis and emphysema
- chronic respiratory insufficiency
- cor pulmonale

The greatest disability results from a combination of bronchiectasis and emphysema that produces chronic respiratory failure.[20]

Despite the use of antibiotics, the bronchiectasis could become more severe over time, in already involved segments, but its spread to previously normal areas is rare, except when a diffuse underlying process is present, such as CF or immotile cilia syndrome.[20]

In the era before antibiotics and widespread childhood immunization, bronchiectasis was considered a highly lethal disease.[21] Today mortality has improved greatly. Aside from individuals with CF and bronchiectasis, many patients with bronchiectasis live into their seventies and eighties if they receive proper treatment.

ADULT OBSTRUCTIVE LUNG CONDITIONS

The prevalence of COPD is continuing to increase in the adult population. In 1990, COPD was predicted to affect as many as 30 million Americans, and it ranks as the fifth most common cause of death in the United States.[22] Although presented here separately, chronic bronchitis and emphysema are often considered together under the term COPD, because most patients have a combination of chronic bronchitis (airway disease) and emphysema (alveolar disease). The manifestation of each component may vary greatly from patient to patient. Both diseases are attributed to cigarette smoking.

Chronic Bronchitis

Chronic bronchitis is generally defined as hypersecretion of mucus sufficient to produce a productive cough on most days for 3 months during 2 consecutive years. Hypersecretion of mucus usually begins in the large airways and is not associated with airway obstruction (simple bronchitis). Later, hypersecretion progresses to the smaller airways, where the airway obstruction begins initially (chronic bronchitis).

Pathology

In chronic bronchitis, there is hypertrophy of the submucosal glands in the large and small bronchi and in the trachea. The ratio of gland thickness to wall thickness (Reid Index) is used as an indicator of mucous gland hypertrophy. In normal individuals this value is less than 3 to 10. In chronic bronchitis the ratio may increase to as high as 8 to 10.[23] In addition to mucous gland hypertrophy in the bronchi, there is an increase in surface epithelial secretory cells, or goblet cells, peripherally in the bronchioli, where usually they are sparse. Denudation of ciliated epithelium and **squamous metaplasia** are also seen. The degree to which the bronchioli, or small airways, are involved is the most important in determining disability.[23] When obstruction of the bronchioli occurs, a **bronchogram** demonstrates impairment of lung function. Peripheral filling is severely impaired, with the appearance of irregularities in the lumina of the airways and the presence of intraluminal mucus. Walls of the small airways are thickened owing to edema or inflammatory cell infiltration. The walls are also thickened by the hypertrophy of muscular and connective tissues and the increase in the height of the epithelium (Fig. 6–8). Some of these changes may also be associated with infection. Deterioration of pulmonary function, however, is usually gradual and is related more to hypersecretion and the presence of mucus within the airway lumina than to infection.[23]

Pathogenesis

Chronic bronchitis is a response to chronic irritation. Cigarette smoking is the most consistently important causal factor in the development of chronic bronchitis. A persistent productive cough is highly correlated with cigarette smoking, and its severity increases with the number of cigarettes smoked. Pipe and cigar smokers have fewer symptoms than cigarette smokers.[23] Chronic bronchitis is higher in inhalers than in noninhalers and in those who extinguish and relight their cigarettes.[23] It is likely that the response of airway epithelium, which is to secrete more mucus, is a nonspecific response to an irritant. The accumulation of mucus in the airways results both from epithelial hypersecretion and from defective mucociliary function.[24] Both components of mucociliary interaction are found to be impaired in smokers and in patients with chronic bronchitis.[24]

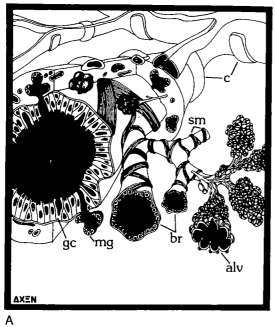
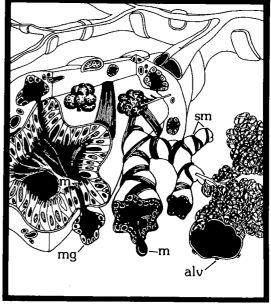

A   B

Figure 6–8.

Comparison of normal airway *(A)* and chronic bronchitic airway *(B)*; gc, goblet cell; c, cartilage; br, bronchi; mg, mucus gland; m, mucus; sm, smooth muscle; alv, alveoli. (From Des Jardins T. Clinical Manifestations of Respiratory Disease. Chicago, Year Book Medical Publishers, 1984. Redrawn by Kenneth Axen.)

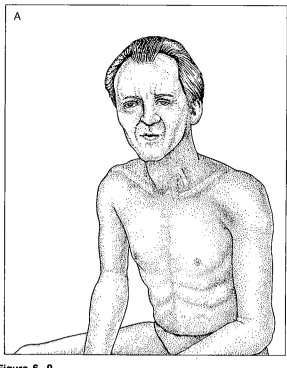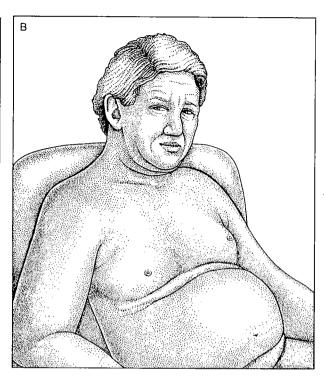

Figure 6-9.

Comparison of appearance of individuals with Type A dominant *(left)* and Type B dominant *(right)* chronic obstructive pulmonary disease. (From Goodman CC, Snyder TEK. Differential Diagnosis in Physical Therapy. Philadelphia, WB Saunders, 1990, pp 89, 90.)

Other factors that may contribute to a lesser extent to the development of chronic bronchitis include

● air pollution
● second-hand smoke
● occupational exposure to metal dusts, such as gold, coal, flurospar, and asbestos
● occupational exposure to vegetable dusts, such as cotton, flax, or hemp[23]

Exposure to gases and fumes has been less well studied but may also contribute in some individuals. Heredity may also play an important role, as relatives of bronchitic patients have a higher incidence of bronchitis than the relatives of control subjects. Also bronchitics have a higher incidence of childhood respiratory infections, such as pneumonia, **pleurisy,** and acute bronchitis, than people without bronchitis.[23]

Clinical Features

The clinical presentation of chronic bronchitis is dominated by a chronic productive cough with morning expectoration and clearing of secretions accumulated during the night. Sputum is usually clear and mucoid but can become purulent during the presence of infection. Recurrent chest infections are a common feature. Bronchitic patients have a tendency to be overweight with a cyanotic cast to their lips and nailbeds. The bronchitic patient is sometimes referred to as a blue bloater or a Type B COPD patient (Fig. 6-9). These patients frequently have edema of the lower extremities because of right heart failure.

Adventitious breath sounds, such as **rhonchi** and wheezes, are frequently heard during auscultation of the chest. The expiratory phase of breathing may become prolonged as obstruction to expiration becomes more severe.

Radiographic Findings

The radiograph may be normal or may show only mild increase in peripheral markings in a bronchitic patient. Severity of disease and functional impairment cannot be estimated by the radiograph. The main use of the radiograph in this population is to help identify other possible causes of their symptoms, such as pneumonia or tumors (Fig. 6–10).

Pathophysiology

The initial lesion in the development of chronic bronchitis may be respiratory bronchiolitis, with inflammatory and obliterative changes that have been initiated by inhaled irritants (cig-

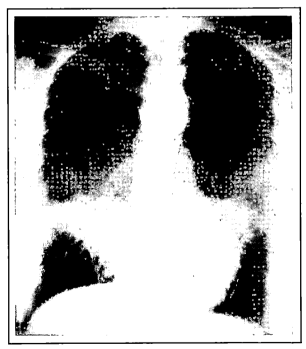

Figure 6–10.

Chest radiograph showing pneumonia in a patient with bronchitis. Patchy bilateral pneumonic infiltrates affect both the right middle lobe and the lingula. (Courtesy of Dr. Dorothy McCauley, New York University Medical Center.)

arette smoke) evident in the bronchioles. Early in the course of bronchitis, signs of *small airway disease* are evident. In addition to bronchiolitis and hypersecretion, other abnormalities may be seen in the small airways, such as fibrosis, ulceration, metaplasia, and increased smooth muscle mass.[23] At this point, conventional tests of airflow (FEV_1, FEV_1/FVC, maximum voluntary ventilation [MVV]) may still be normal, but special tests, such as closing volume or maximal expiratory flow-volume curves (see Chapter 10), can reveal obstruction in peripheral airways.[23] Edema of the airway, intraluminal mucus, loss of elastic recoil in surrounding structures, bronchospasm, or alterations in surface tension all may contribute to the obstruction, so the cause of the functional change cannot be identified clearly. Small airway disease may not be detectable clinically, but the abnormalities are sufficient to disturb alveolar ventilation–blood flow relationships and alveolar-capillary gas exchange.[23] Pulmonary function tests and arterial blood gases may revert to normal if a person stops smoking while manifesting small airway disease.[25]

Pulmonary Function Tests. To establish the diagnosis of true chronic bronchitis, an FEV_1 of less than 65% of predicted (age, height, and sex adjusted) is considered diagnostic for chronic airflow obstruction. Also an FEV_1 to FVC ratio of less than 70% is considered diagnostic. Residual volume is increased, but VC and dynamic lung compliance are decreased.[25]

Laboratory Findings

Initially arterial blood gases reveal a Pa_{O_2} at the lower limits of normal. As the disease progresses and ventilation-perfusion mismatching increases, the Pa_{O_2} falls further and may become markedly reduced (Pa_{O_2} of 40–50 mmHg); the Pa_{CO_2} may increase to 60 to 70 mm Hg or higher.

Polycythemia (increased red blood cell volume) is a commonly seen adaptation to chronic **hypoxia**. The body attempts to increase the blood's oxygen-carrying capacity by increasing the red blood cell volume. **Hematocrit** (red blood cell volume) levels may increase to 55% to 60% (normal hematocrit value is 42%–45%). An increased hematocrit level increases blood viscosity, which increases cardiac work and decreases cardiac output.[25]

Medical Treatment

Smoking cessation is very important in the management of chronic bronchitis. Several improvements in symptoms of the disease have been noted when smoking is discontinued: (1) a decrease or resolution of signs of mucous hypersecretion, (2) a reversal of small airways dysfunction, and (3) a slowing of the average rate of annual decline of FEV_1.[26]

Other approaches to treatment include attempts to prevent and to manage aggressively respiratory tract infections, which cause acute exacerbations of chronic bronchitis. Influenza and pneumonia vaccines are recommended.

An increased incidence of H. influenzae and Streptococcus pneumoniae bacteria have been noted in the secretions of the lower respiratory tract of patients with severe chronic bronchitis. Viruses and Mycoplasma pneumoniae have also been implicated as causes of acute exacerbations of chronic bronchitis.[26]

Antibiotics commonly used to manage acute exacerbations include tetracycline and erythromycin. H. influenzae is sensitive to tetracycline, and both S. pneumoniae and M. pneumoniae are affected by tetracycline and erythromycin. Ampicillin is also sometimes prescribed. Antiviral agents are not available for treatment.

Treatment of respiratory tract infections reduces time lost from work but does little to influence the natural history of chronic bronchitis.[27] Bronchodilators are indicated if bronchospasm is evident.

The use of low-flow oxygen (1–3 L/min) may help reduce pulmonary hypertension and polycythemia and therefore improve right heart function.

Complications and Prognosis

Polycythemia, pulmonary embolism, pulmonary hypertension, respiratory failure, and cor pulmonale are the most frequent complications of chronic bronchitis. Cor pulmonale develops earlier and more frequently in COPD patients with chronic bronchitis. The predominately bron-chitic patient generally has a poorer prognosis for longevity than the patient with emphysema because the former has ventilation-perfusion abnormalities that lead to respiratory failure and cor pulmonale.

Emphysema

Emphysema, an alveolar or parenchymal disease, is an abnormal and a permanent enlargement of the air spaces distal to the terminal nonrespiratory bronchioles, accompanied by destructive changes of the alveolar walls. Disturbances in lung function result from these anatomic changes, including loss of elastic recoil, excessive collapse of airways on exhalation, and chronic airflow obstruction[23] (Fig. 6–11). The diagnosis of emphysema is based on pulmonary function test findings; clinical findings, such as distant breath sounds; findings on physical examination; history; and CT scan.

Pathology

Several different types of emphysema are recognized anatomically according to the distribution of enlarged air spaces within the acinus.

Panacinar (Panlobular) Emphysema. In **panacinar emphysema,** all alveoli within the acinus are affected to the same degree; a nearly uniform destruction of most of the structures within a lobule is seen. The distinction between alveolar ducts and alveoli is lost. This type is seen in emphysema associated with **alpha$_1$-antitrypsin deficiency** and unilateral **hyperlucent lung syndrome.** The distribution is equally likely in lower as in upper lobes.

Centriacinar (Centrilobular) Emphysema. In **centriacinar emphysema,** alveoli arising from the respiratory bronchiole or the proximal portion of the acinus are most affected. Alveolar ducts and alveolar sacs remain normal. Individuals with centrilobular emphysema may have no respiratory disability. Centriacinar emphysema is commonly found in the upper lobes.

Paraseptal Emphysema. In **paraseptal emphysema,** the enlarged air spaces are located at the periphery of the acinus, just under the pleura

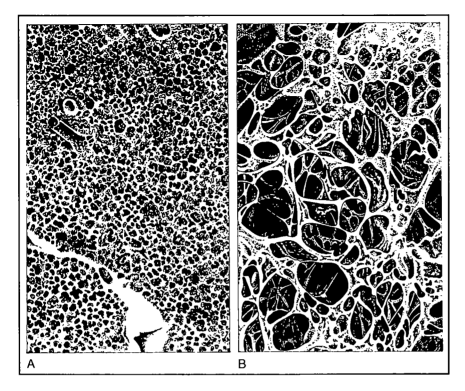

Figure 6-11.

Comparison of the appearance of normal lung tissue *(A)* with the pathologic changes observable in lung tissue damaged by emphysema *(B)*. (From Des Jardins T. Clinical Manifestations of Respiratory Disease. Chicago, Year Book Medical Publishers, 1984. Redrawn by Kenneth Axen.)

or along connective tissue septa. The enlargement is in the alveolar sacs and associated alveoli. These thin-walled, inflated areas located at the pleural surface may become bullae (subpleural air sacs of alveolar origin greater than 1 cm in diameter) and rupture, causing a spontaneous pneumothorax.

Irregular Emphysema. Irregular emphysema forms in the vicinity of scars and is related to the effects of scarring and contraction. This type is the most common and is of little clinical significance.

Pathogenesis

Cigarette smoking is the most important etiologic factor in the development of both emphysema and chronic bronchitis. Many studies suggest a rough dose-response relationship between smoking and development of emphysema. Emphysema is rare in those who have never smoked.[28] Other factors that are associated with the development of emphysema are environmental air pollution and hereditary deficiency of alpha$_1$-antitrypsin.

Emphysema is thought to result from disruption of the elastic fiber network of the lung because of an imbalance between **elastases** (proteolytic enzymes that digest elastin) and their inhibitors.[28] The degradation of **elastin** (one component of the lung's elastic fiber network) is most important in the pathogenesis of emphysema.

Smoking produces low-level, chronic inflammation in the lungs. Increased numbers of phagocytic cells, neutrophils, and alveolar macrophages can be recovered from the lungs of smokers by bronchoalveolar lavage. Neutrophils are located mainly in alveolar walls, whereas alveolar macrophages are found in the respiratory bronchioles.[28] These cells are produced in response to the particulate matter in tobacco smoke. Both neutrophils and macrophages may release proteolytic enzymes into the lungs and be involved in the breakdown of elastin in the lungs of smokers.[28]

Smoking may also predispose an individual to emphysema through inactivation of intrapulmonary elastase inhibitors, so that elastase is unchecked in its destruction of elastin. This hypothesis has been proved in animal models but not yet in humans.[28] In addition, biosynthetic repair of pulmonary elastic tissue is reduced by smoking.[28]

A rare cause of emphysema is the inherited deficiency of alpha$_1$-antitrypsin, a protein that functions as a *protease* (general term for a proteolytic enzyme) inhibitor. It occurs in 1 of 6000 people in the United States, but it is more common in Sweden, where it was first detected. The concentration of alpha$_1$-antitrypsin in the plasma of individuals who inherit this condition is only approximately 15% of normal.[28]

The primary role of alpha$_1$-antitrypsin appears to be the inhibition of neutrophil elastase, because it associates with neutrophil elastase faster than with trypsin.[28] Neutrophil elastase is released during phagocytosis and helps to dispose of microorganisms, such as bacteria, by digesting them. Neutrophil elastase is active against elastin and other components of the lung's fibroelastic network, such as fibronectin and basement membrane collagen.

This unrestrained activity of elastase in the lungs, due to a deficiency of alpha$_1$-antitrypsin, is expected to result in the development of emphysema. Eighty to ninety percent of individuals with alpha$_1$-antitrypsin deficiency develop COPD, and their rate of deterioration of lung function (measured by annual decline in FEV$_1$) is nearly twice the average rate of decline for COPD patients without the deficiency.[28] When individuals with alpha$_1$-antitrypsin deficiency also smoke, symptoms appear very early, with shortness of breath evident often at age 40; nonsmokers with the condition usually become symptomatic around age 55. Panacinar emphysema, worst at the basal segments of the lung, is most often seen. Liver disease is also associated with this condition. Children are at risk for the development of **hepatitis** and **cirrhosis**. Adults have an increased incidence of chronic liver disease and **hepatoma**.[28]

Clinical Features

Patients with emphysema usually present clinically with shortness of breath and scant sputum production. They may demonstrate a barrel-shaped configuration of the chest wall, with an increased subcostal angle[29] and horizontal rather than downsloping ribs, owing to hyperinflation of the lungs. Accessory muscles of respiration may be hypertrophied, with supraclavicular retraction evident. Pursed-lip breathing may be utilized even at rest, and postures in which the upper extremities are stabilized (hand on hips in standing or forearms on knees in sitting) are commonly used for more effective utilization of the accessory muscles of breathing. Shoulders are frequently rounded because of shortening of the pectoral muscles. The respiratory rate may be rapid with a shallow depth of respiration.

The typical type A COPD patient, one with a predominately emphysematous component, is sometimes called a "pink puffer" (see Fig. 6–9). The emphysematous patient tends to be thin, sometimes **cachectic** in body build, with rosy skin tones. Distant breath sounds are frequent because of hyperinflation of the lungs; adventitious sounds are less common than in the type B patient.

Radiographic Findings

A radiograph is not considered diagnostic for emphysema. In the early stages of disease and even in some patients with advanced disease, the radiograph may be relatively normal. Centrilobular emphysema is hardest to see on a radiograph, whereas panacinar emphysema is more readily identified. When findings characteristic of emphysema are found on a chest film, the disease is very advanced. Signs of lung hyperinflation include increase in anteroposterior diameter; kyphosis; increased retrosternal air; horizontal ribs; and low, flattened diaphragms. The cardiac silhouette may be narrow and elongated because of both low diaphragms and compression from the hyperinflation of the lungs. At times bullae may also be seen. Bullae are caused by destruction of air spaces distal to the terminal bronchioles (Fig. 6–12).

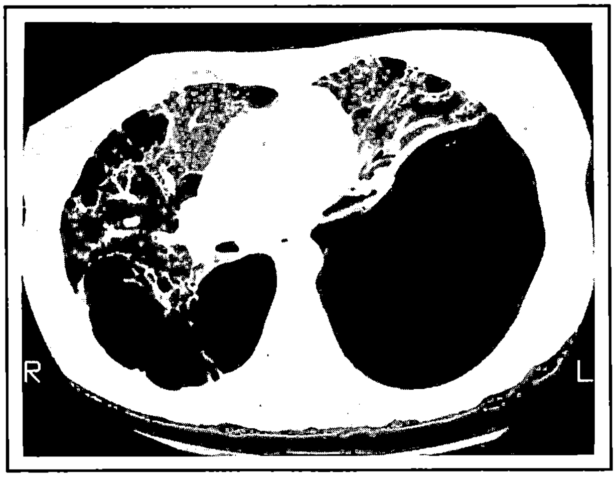

Figure 6-12.
Computed tomography scan of bullous emphysema. (Courtesy of Dr. Dorothy McCauley, New York University Medical Center.)

Pathophysiology

The enlargement of the terminal air spaces in the lungs and the destruction of alveolar walls seen in pure emphysema cause characteristic changes in the pulmonary function test results. In emphysema a low diffusing capacity for carbon monoxide is noted (using either the single-breath test or a rebreathing maneuver). However, in unaffected areas of the lung the relationship between bloodflow and ventilation is relatively well preserved so that overall Pa_{O_2} is only slightly to moderately reduced. Normally Pa_{CO_2} is slightly elevated only during acute respiratory infections.

Owing to loss of elastic recoil, some obstruction to airflow may be seen by a decrease in the FEV_1 or the FEV_1 to FVC ratio, although values are not as decreased as when chronic bronchitis is also present. Airway resistance in emphysema may be normal or slightly increased. The FRC, TLC, and RV are all markedly increased in emphysema patients.

Laboratory Findings

The hematocrit value and the pulmonary artery pressure are usually normal.

Medical Treatment

Cessation of smoking and prevention of respiratory infections are essential in the medical management of emphysema. Prophylactic immunizations against influenza and pneumonia are recommended. When emphysema coexists with bronchitis, some of the treatment methods outlined previously may be indicated.

Complications and Prognosis

Emphysema, in the absence of airway obstruction, can span 20 to 40 years of life, producing only undue breathlessness on exertion. In general, the prognosis for the patient with emphysema is much better than that for the patient with chronic bronchitis because of the preservation of ventilation and blood-flow relationships in emphysema. The emphysematous patient develops cor pulmonale only when hypoxemia is severe enough to produce pulmonary arterial hypertension.

CASE STUDIES

CASE 1 – Diagnosis: Asthma

M.A. is a 31-year-old man who was diagnosed with asthma at age 7.

Past Medical History: Wheezing intermittently over last 24 years. Symptoms of shortness of breath precipitated by exercise; change in temperature; and exposure to smoke, perfume, and animals. History of allergies to dogs, cats, and dust. Hospitalized once (6/87) for episode of severe bronchospasm. Pneumonia 4 times in 1988; collapsed left lower lobe 8/88.

Past Surgical History: none

Smoking History: negative

Medications: Ventolin inhaler TID (three times daily)
Intal inhaler TID
Theophylline 200 mg BID (two times daily)

**Pulmonary
Function Test
Results**

SPIROMETRY	PRED	Pre-RX ACTUAL	% PRED	Post-RX (Bronchodilator) ACTUAL	% PRED
$FEV_{0.5}$ Liters	3.10	2.33	75	2.68	86
FEV_1 Liters	4.37	3.33	76	3.77	86
$FEF_{25-75\%}$ L/sec	4.50	2.07	46	2.50	56

CASE 2 – Diagnosis: Bronchiectasis

R.A. is a 60-year-old woman diagnosed with bronchiectasis 9/87 following referral to a pulmonary specialist for unresolved right middle lobe and right lower lobe pneumonia.

Past Medical History: 10-year history of frequent sore throats, right nasal sinus infection, and postnasal drip. Productive of moderate amounts of yellow sputum with occasional small plugs; productive 8 to 10 times daily for past 10 years. Occasional hemoptysis. Recurrent pneumonias: first in 1984, followed by pneumonia several times per year; 1987—pneumonia 4 times. Has experienced shortness of breath during episodes of pneumonia, as well as pleuritic pain and darker colored sputum.

Past Surgical History: Hysterectomy for fibroids

Smoking History: negative

Medications: none

Diagnostic Testing: Blood gas and pulmonary function test results are within normal limits.

Sputum culture (9/87): Numerous gram-negative rods; many white blood cells. Final report: *Pseudomonas aeruginosa*, moderately sensitive to tetracycline, fully sensitive to trimethoprim sulfamethoxazole (Bactrim). CT scan (9/87): Inflammatory change within both the right middle lobe and lingula, with a suggestion of increased thickening in the region of the minor fissure and a small atelectatic area within the right middle lobe.

SUMMARY

- Changes seen in pulmonary function test results in obstructive pulmonary diseases are decreases in expiratory flow rates and increases in RV.

- Decreased airflow noted in COPD during expiration may be caused by loss of elastic recoil in lung tissue or resistance encountered in the airways.
- Resistance encountered in the airways in COPD may be caused by inflammation, airway thickening, mucus, or bronchospasm.
- Bronchopulmonary dysplasia is a lung disease of infancy characterized by respiratory distress and oxygen dependency lasting beyond 1 month of age following the use of oxygen and ventilatory support to treat neonatal respiratory distress.
- Cystic fibrosis is a genetic disorder resulting in abnormal function of the exocrine glands. Pulmonary and pancreatic problems are the most common clinical features.
- Asthma is a disease of the airways characterized by increased responsiveness of the tracheobronchial tree to various stimuli. Widespread narrowing of the airways occurs when these stimuli are encountered. Asthma is episodic in nature with relatively normal lung function between attacks.
- Bronchiectasis is a permanent abnormal dilation and distortion of one or more bronchi. Large amounts of mucopurulent sputum are usually produced, and recurrent pulmonary infections and hemoptysis are common.
- Chronic bronchitis (airway disease) is defined as hypersecretion of mucus sufficient to produce a productive cough on most days for 3 months during 2 consecutive years.
- Emphysema (alveolar disease) is an abnormal and permanent enlargement of the air spaces distal to the terminal nonrespiratory bronchioles accompanied by destruction of alveolar walls.
- Pulmonary diseases frequently coexist. Three common combinations are asthmatic bronchi-

tis, chronic bronchitis with emphysema, and cystic fibrosis with bronchiectasis.

● Common signs of obstructive pulmonary disease include chronic cough, expectoration of mucus, wheezing, and dyspnea on exertion.

● Clinical signs of infection in pulmonary disease include increased cough, increased sputum production, fever, increased respiratory rate, and change in auscultatory findings.

References

1. Thurlbeck WM. Pathology of chronic airflow obstruction. Chest 97 (Suppl): 6s–10s, 1990.
2. O'Brodovich HM, Mellins RB. Bronchopulmonary dysplasia. Unresolved neonatal lung injury. Am Rev Respir Dis 132:694–709, 1985.
3. Wedig KE, Bruce MC, Martin RJ, Fanaroff AA. Bronchopulmonary dysplasia. In: Nussbaum E, Galant S (eds). Pediatric Respiratory Disorders: Clinical Approaches. Orlando, Fla, Grune & Stratton, 1984, pp. 83–90.
4. Martin RJ, Davis PB. Relationship of neonatal and childhood lung disease to adult COPD. In: Cherniack NS (ed). Chronic Obstructive Pulmonary Disease. Philadelphia, WB Saunders, 1991, pp 286–293.
5. Katz R, McWilliams B. Bronchopulmonary dysplasia in the pediatric intensive care unit. Crit Care Clin 4:755–787, 1988.
6. Voyles JB. Bronchopulmonary dysplasia. Am J Nurs 81(3):510–514, 1981.
7. Taghizadeh A, Reynolds EOR. Pathogenesis of bronchopulmonary dysplasia following hyaline membrane disease. Am J Pathol 82:241–256, 1976.
8. Heimler R, Hoffman RG, Starshak RJ, et al. Chronic lung disease in premature infants: A retrospective evaluation of underlying factors. Crit Care Med 16:1213–1217, 1988.
9. Watts JL, Ariagno RI, Brady JP. Chronic pulmonary disease in neonates after artificial ventilation: Distribution of ventilation and pulmonary interstitial emphysema. Pediatrics 60:273, 1977.
10. Tepper RS, Morgan WJ, Cota K, Taussig LM. Expiratory flow limitation in infants with bronchopulmonary dysplasia. J Pediatr 109:1040–1046, 1986.
11. Smyth JA, Tabachnik E, Duncan WJ, et al. Pulmonary function and bronchial hyperactivity in long-term survivors of bronchopulmonary dysplasia. Pediatrics 68:336–340, 1981.
12. Phelan PD, Landau LI, Olinsky A. Neonatal respiratory disorders. In: Phelan PD, Landau LI, Olinsky A (eds). Respiratory Illness in Children. 3rd ed. Melbourne, Blackwell Scientific Publications, 1990, pp 17–21.
13. Meisels J, Plunkett JW, Roloff DW, et al. Growth and development of pre-term infants with respiratory distress syndrome and bronchopulmonary dysplasia. Pediatrics 77:345–352, 1986.
14. Bader D, Ramos AD, Lew CD, et al. Childhood sequelae of infant lung disease. Exercise and pulmonary function abnormalities after bronchopulmonary dysplasia. J Pediatr 110:693–699, 1987.
15. Davis PB. Cystic Fibrosis: A major cause of obstructive airways disease in the young. In: Cherniack NS (ed). Chronic Obstructive Pulmonary Disease. Philadelphia, WB Saunders, 1991, pp 297–307.
16. Scanlin TF. Cystic fibrosis. In: Fishman AP (ed). Pulmonary Diseases and Disorders. Vol. 2. 2nd ed. New York, McGraw-Hill, 1988, pp 1273–1294.
17. Davis PB, di Sant'Agnese PA. Diagnosis and treatment of cystic fibrosis: An update. Chest 85:802–809, 1984.
18. McFadden ER Jr. Asthma: General features, pathogenesis, and pathophysiology. In: Fishman AP (ed). Pulmonary Diseases and Disorders. Vol. 2. 2nd ed. McGraw-Hill, 1988, pp 1295–1310.
19. Costello JF. Asthma. In: Hinshaw HC, Murray JF (eds). Diseases of the Chest. 4th ed. Philadelphia, WB Saunders, 1980, pp 525–559.
20. Swartz MN. Bronchiectasis. In: Fishman AP (ed). Pulmonary Diseases and Disorders. Vol. 2. 2nd ed. New York, McGraw-Hill, 1988, pp 1553–1581.
21. Davis AL, Salzman SH. Bronchiectasis. In: Cherniack NS (ed). Chronic Obstructive Pulmonary Disease. Philadelphia, WB Saunders, 1991, pp 316–338.
22. Petty TL. Chronic obstructive pulmonary disease—Can we do better? Chest 97 (Suppl): 2s–5s, 1990.
23. Reid LM. Chronic obstructive pulmonary diseases. In: Fishman AP (ed). Pulmonary Diseases and Disorders. Vol. 2. 2nd ed. New York, McGraw-Hill, 1988, pp 1247–1272.
24. Wanner A. The role of mucus in chronic obstructive pulmonary disease. Chest 97 (Suppl): 11s–15s, 1990.
25. Hinshaw HC, Murray JF. Chronic bronchitis and emphysema. In: Diseases of the Chest. 4th ed. Philadelphia, WB Saunders, 1980, pp 560–590.
26. Tager IB. Chronic bronchitis. In: Fishman AP (ed). Pulmonary Diseases and Disorders. Vol. 2. 2nd ed. New York, McGraw-Hill, 1988, pp 1543–1551.
27. Higgins ITT. Epidemiology of bronchitis and emphysema. In: Fishman AP (ed). Pulmonary Diseases and Disorders. Vol. 2. 2nd ed. New York, McGraw-Hill, 1988, pp 1237–1246.
28. Senior RM, Kuhn C III. The pathogenesis of emphysema. In: Fishman AP (ed). Pulmonary Diseases and Disorders. Vol. 2. 2nd ed. New York, McGraw-Hill, 1988, pp 1209–1218.
29. Zadai CC. Rehabilitation of the patient with chronic obstructive pulmonary disease. In: Irwin S, Tecklin JS (eds). Cardiopulmonary Physical Therapy. St. Louis, CV Mosby, 1985, pp 367–381.

7 CARDIOPULMONARY IMPLICATIONS OF SPECIFIC DISEASES

INTRODUCTION

Many diseases of body systems other than the heart and lungs also affect cardiopulmonary function. Some, like **hypertension** or neuromuscular diseases, have obvious associations with cardiopulmonary dysfunction, but others, such as rheumatoid arthritis and other collagen vascular diseases, are not routinely associated with cardiac and pulmonary manifestations. This chapter presents the cardiopulmonary effects of a number of specific diseases and medical problems as well as their clinical implications for physical

therapy intervention. The medical information presented is merely a synopsis of current knowledge and therefore is meant only to introduce the reader to this area. The amount of detail provided is generally proportional to the frequency with which clinicians are likely to encounter each diagnosis. The goal is to make the reader aware of the potential for cardiopulmonary dysfunction in patients with the described diseases and to suggest modifications of treatment procedures that might be indicated. Further reading is indicated if the physical therapist has a patient with one of these diseases.

285

HYPERTENSION

Hypertension is defined by the American Heart Association as arterial pressure exceeding 140/90 mm Hg; according to the World Health Organization, it is 160/95 or greater, with values between 140/90 and 160/95 being considered borderline hypertension. *Labile* hypertension refers to a condition in which the blood pressure fluctuates between hypertensive and normal values. Usually individuals with hypertension have elevated levels of both **systolic blood pressure (SBP)** and **diastolic blood pressure (DBP);** however, isolated systolic hypertension occurs when SBP exceeds 160 mm Hg but DBP remains within the normal range. Approximately 90% of individuals with hypertension have no discernible cause for their disease and are said to have **essential (primary) hypertension.**[1] The remainder have **secondary hypertension** resulting from another identifiable medical problem, such as renovascular or endocrine disease.

The consequences of hypertension are related directly to the level of blood pressure, even within the accepted normal range. Actuarial data reveal that persons with DBPs of 88 to 92 mm Hg have 32% to 36% greater mortality over 20 years of follow-up than those with DBPs of less than 80 mm Hg.[2] Higher SBP levels at any given level of DBP have also been associated with increased morbidity in both men and women.[3,4,5] The most common complications of hypertension include cerebral vascular accidents, congestive heart failure, **atherosclerotic heart disease,** renal failure, **dissecting aneurysm, peripheral vascular disease,** and **retinopathy.**

Despite much research, the etiology of essential hypertension continues to be unknown. Both genetic and environmental factors, such as excess dietary sodium, stress, obesity, and excess alcohol consumption, have been implicated. Regardless of the underlying cause or causes, the result is failure of one or more of the control mechanisms that are responsible for lowering blood pressure when it becomes elevated.

The major determinants of arterial blood pressure are **cardiac output** and **total peripheral resistance.** If either one or both of these factors becomes elevated, blood pressure rises. However, both cardiac output and total peripheral resistance are determined by a number of other factors (Fig. 7–1). Cardiac output results from the product of heart rate and stroke volume; yet each of these has several determinants, as discussed in Chapter 2. Similarly, total peripheral resistance is affected by several variables, including the caliber of the arteriolar bed, the viscosity of the blood, and the elasticity of the arterial walls.

Thus, the abnormal functioning of many physiologic pathways can result in high blood pressure, and many of these pathways share a number of common features, as shown in Figure 7–1. Furthermore, it is probable that the mechanisms that are responsible for initiating hypertension differ from those that serve to maintain it. For example, many individuals with labile or early mild hypertension have a central redistribution of blood volume and increased cardiac output that probably is related to enhanced activity of the sympathetic nervous system with increased heart rate and more rapid left ventricular ejection.[6,7] Initially, this group appears to have normal peripheral resistance, though their ability to lower forearm vascular resistance during circumstances in which enhanced blood flow is required is impaired. Later, when hypertension becomes established, these individuals display the classical hemodynamic findings of elevated total peripheral resistance and normal or decreased cardiac output.[7]

Hypertensive Heart Disease

Regardless of its cause and pathophysiologic mechanisms, hypertension produces a pressure overload on the left ventricle (LV). To compensate for the increased stress placed on the heart, left ventricular hypertrophy develops.[8] Initially, normal systolic LV function is maintained by the hypertrophied LV. However, evidence of diastolic dysfunction with impairment of LV relaxation appears early in the course of essential hypertension.[9,10] The combination of left ventricular hypertrophy and diastolic dysfunction leads to reduced LV compliance (i.e., a stiffer LV), which

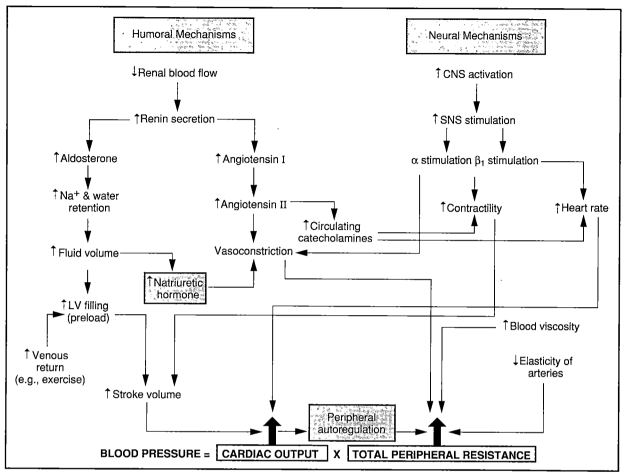

Figure 7-1.

Factors contributing to elevated blood pressure. Because blood pressure is a product of cardiac output and peripheral resistance, any influence that increases either of these factors results in a rise in blood pressure. The enclosed boxes identify some of the proposed mechanisms involved in the pathogenesis of essential hypertension. Note the number of interrelationships among the different mechanisms. CNS, central nervous system; SNS, sympathetic nervous system; LV, left ventricle; ↑, increased; ↓, decreased.

creates a greater load on the left atrium with resultant left atrial enlargement. If adequate filling volume is not achieved because of either atrial arrhythmias or insufficient filling time (i.e., tachycardia), stroke volume diminishes. Thus, symptoms of inadequate cardiac output, such as pulmonary congestion, can result from diastolic dysfunction rather than from impaired systolic function. However, as hypertension becomes more severe or prolonged or both, systolic dysfunction may develop, appearing as subnormal LV functional reserve initially during exercise and later at rest.[11]

Although normal cardiac output may be maintained for some time, at the expense of pulmonary congestion, the ultimate consequence of progressive left ventricular hypertrophy is the development of left ventricular failure, as shown in Figure 7-2. A number of factors, such as further elevation of blood pressure, increased venous return, or impairment of cardiac function, may precipitate decompensation and overt LV failure. Other cardiac manifestations commonly seen in patients with hypertension are myocardial ischemia or infarction, or both, which can result from the increased myocardial oxygen de-

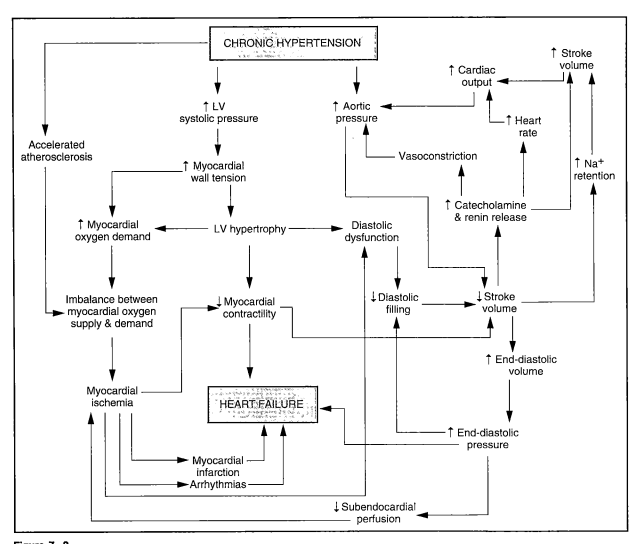

Figure 7-2.

Some of the mechanisms and interrelationships in hypertension that may lead to the development of left ventricle (LV) failure. Vicious cycles tend to aggravate the problem; ↑, increased; ↓, decreased.

mand of the hypertrophied LV as well as from the diminished blood supply, as hypertension is a major risk factor for the development of atherosclerotic heart disease (see Chapter 3). This interaction makes it difficult to differentiate between the effects of atherosclerotic heart disease and **hypertensive heart disease.**

Treatment of Hypertension

Pharmacologic therapy is the most commonly prescribed intervention in the management of hypertension. However, a number of nonpharmacologic interventions also can lower blood pressure: weight reduction, sodium restriction and other dietary manipulations, regular aerobic exercise, and relaxation training.[12] Although these interventions may not eliminate the need for antihypertensive medications in most patients, they often permit a lower dosage of medication to be used, thus reducing the potential for adverse side effects.

The medications used to treat hypertension fall into the following major categories:

- Diuretics
- **Beta-adrenergic blockers**
- Alpha-adrenergic blockers
- Vasodilators
- Centrally acting adrenergic antagonists
- Calcium channel blockers
- **Angiotensin converting enzyme inhibitors**

A summary of their antihypertensive effects and exercise interactions is provided in Table 7–1.[13–16]

Many of these drugs have other cardiovascular effects and side effects and may be used to treat other clinical problems. For more complete information on these drugs refer to Chapter 12.

Hypertension and Exercise

The normal blood pressure response to dynamic exercise is a rise in SBP that is propor-

TABLE 7–1. The Antihypertensive Effects and Exercise Interactions of the Different Classes of Medications Used to Treat Hypertension			
Medications	**Antihypertensive Action**	**Effects on Exercise**	**Side Effects re Exercise**
Beta blockers	↓ HR and contractility ↓ Renin secretion	↓ HR, ↓ SBP ↓ Ischemic ST-T changes ↓ Angina ↑ Ex. capacity in pts with angina ↓ Or ↔ ex. capacity if no angina ⊕ Training responses ? ↓ Arrhythmias May be ↑ BP during isometric ex.	Bronchospasm May mask S&S of hypoglycemia in DM ↑ Claudication Muscle fatigue and cramps ↑ K+ Beta-blocker withdrawal

Diuretics
    thiazides,
        loop diuretics
	↓ Peripheral resistance
	↓ Plasma volume
		Moderate ↓ BP response
		↔ HR
		↔ Ex. capacity
			Hypokalemia → ST depression, ↑ ventricular ectopy, muscle fatigue and cramps, weakness
			Excessive diuresis → ↑ ex.-induced tachycardia, ↑ postural hypotension

K+-sparing diuretics	Same	Same	↑ Serum K+ leads to ↑arrhythmias
Alpha-adrenergic blockers alpha₁	↓ Peripheral resistance	↓ SBP and DBP ↔ HR ↔ Ex. capacity	Orthostatic hypotension Post-ex. hypotension
alpha₂	Same + ↓ Cardiac output	Same	Same + Reflex tachycardia
Centrally acting alpha- adrenergic agonists	↓ Central and/or peripheral outflow of catecholamines → ↓ plasma norepinephrine	↓ Plasma norepinephrine ↓ Or ↔ HR, ↓ BP ↔ Ex. capacity ↓ Or ↔ BP response to isometric ex.	Rebound HTN on withdrawal of drug Post-ex. hypotension, dizziness, syncope
Ca++ channel blockers	Vasodilation	↓ BP ↓ HR (✗ nifedipine ↑ HR) ↓ Ischemic ST-T changes ↑ Ex. tolerance in pts with angina ↔ Ex. tolerance if no angina	Orthostatic hypotension
ACE inhibitors	Inhibits formation of angiotension II → ↓ Vasoconstriction	↓ BP ↔ Exercise tolerance	

HR, heart rate; BP, blood pressure; SBP, systolic blood pressure; DBP, diastolic blood pressure; ex., exercise; pts, patients; S&S, signs and symptoms; DM, diabetes mellitus; ST-T, ST segment; ACE, angiotensin converting enzyme; HTN, hypertension.

↑, increased; ↓, decreased; ↔, little or no change; →, results in; +, in addition; ⊕, positive.

tional to the workload (approximately 7–10 mm Hg per MET) and little or no change in DBP (±10 mm Hg).[17] However, once activity reaches an intensity that is predominantly anaerobic, the **pressor** response becomes more marked. Isometric exercise or exercise involving a small muscle mass (e.g., one arm) typically elicits minimal incremental changes in SBP and greater increases in DBP.[18]

Some individuals have normal or borderline blood pressure values at rest but develop excessive increases in SBP, DBP, or both during activity. This is particularly true for emergency response team members, such as police officers and firefighters, who produce large bursts of sympathetic nervous system activity in response to an alarm. After a period of time, this physiologic response may become generalized to any stressful situation, including physical exertion, and hypertensive blood pressure responses, especially the DBP response, are frequently observed during exercise.

Persons with moderate hypertension exhibit exaggerated blood pressure responses to isometric exercise and often to isotonic exercise compared with those of normotensive individuals because of a lack of change in total peripheral resistance during dynamic exercise.[19-21] In addition, their ability to increase cardiac output appropriately with greater demands may be impaired.[22] Individuals with more severe hypertension may display further impairment of cardiac output during exercise and more marked increases in total peripheral resistance.[23] The net effect of these two opposing factors on blood pressure determines whether SBP increases dramatically or appears as a more normal response; DBP responses are usually hypertensive.

Treatment of hypertension with medication may modify the physiologic responses to exercise. Antihypertensive medications lower resting blood pressure, but many do not maintain the same degree of effectiveness during exertion, especially with isometric activities.[20,24] Thus, patients on antihypertensive medications may have acceptable blood pressure levels at rest but may display exaggerated responses to exercise. Furthermore, some of these drugs have side effects that are affected by or have an effect on exercise,

as shown in Table 7–1. Of particular concern is the **hypokalemia** that can be induced by diuretic therapy using the thiazides and loop diuretics. When combined with the systemic demands of exercise, hypokalemia can precipitate dangerous arrhythmias, skeletal muscle fatigue and cramps, weakness, and occasionally **rhabdomyolysis** (destruction of skeletal muscle), secondary **aldosteronism**, and **hyperuricemia**. However, the potassium-sparing diuretics and beta blockers are associated with a greater risk of **hyperkalemia**, which can also cause arrhythmias.

A great deal of research has been directed at assessing the efficacy of exercise training for the treatment of hypertension. Although the data are not consistent, the consensus is that reductions of 10 to 20 mm Hg in both SBP and DBP can be achieved through exercise training, an amount that is significant enough to allow some patients to avoid or to discontinue drug treatment and many others to reduce their drug dosages.[12,19,21,25-28]

Implications for Physical Therapy Intervention

According to recent estimates, approximately 59 million Americans (about one in three adults) have high blood pressure, almost half of whom do not even know they have it.[29] Therefore, the percentage of patients referred to physical therapy who may have recognized or unrecognized hypertension is significant. Patients with any of the following diagnoses are particularly likely to have hypertension:

- Stroke
- Diabetes
- Coronary artery disease
- **Aortic aneurysm**
- Peripheral vascular disease
- Obesity
- Renal failure
- Alcoholism

In addition, patients with chronic pain syndromes may be at higher risk for hypertension, possibly because they tend to be inactive, obese, financially stressed, or a combination of these. Finally, patients in high-stress occupations, such as air traffic control, firefighting, and middle- and upper-level managing, have a higher incidence of hypertension.

With the growing trend toward independent practice, physical therapy may represent the route of entry into the medical care system for a number of adults. This fact combined with the prevalence of hypertension in the United States supports the need for inclusion of blood pressure monitoring during the physical therapy evaluation of all adults older than 35 years. In addition to the valuable information this might provide for both client and physician, the positive professional image created by such an arrangement could improve acceptance by the medical community of the position of physical therapists as independent health care providers.

Because blood pressure values can be normal or borderline at rest but excessively elevated during exertion, it is important to monitor blood pressure during exercise. The techniques for proper monitoring of blood pressure are described in Chapter 14, but a few points that are particularly relevant to the detection and monitoring of hypertension deserve emphasis here. First, proper cuff size is essential to accuracy. A cuff that is too narrow produces a reading that is falsely elevated, and one that is too wide yields a reading that is erroneously low. Second, because there may be an **"auscultatory gap"** of up to 40 mm Hg after the first audible sounds, it is especially important to palpate for the disappearance of the radial pulse as the cuff is inflated and then continue inflation for another 30 mm Hg; otherwise the SBP may be significantly underestimated. Third, the arm should be relaxed and supported at the level of the heart. If the arm is lower than the heart or if the arm muscles are not relaxed, the blood pressure readings, both systolic and diastolic, will be erroneously high. Finally, when the arms are so large or misshapen that a conventional cuff does not fit properly, measurements are not accurate; as an alternative, a standard blood pressure cuff can be placed on the forearm, and auscultation or palpation can be performed over the radial artery at the wrist.[30]

If the resting blood pressure is excessively high (SBP >200 mm Hg or DBP >105–110 mm Hg), physician clearance should be obtained before continuing with physical therapy evaluation or treatment. Furthermore, any evidence of target organ damage secondary to hypertension, such as retinopathy, renal disease, or left ventricular hypertrophy, necessitates that blood pressure be controlled both at rest and during exercise before physical therapy intervention. Exercise should be terminated if blood pressure becomes excessively high (SBP >250 or DBP >110).[31] If left ventricular hypertrophy has developed, the risk of myocardial ischemia during exercise is enhanced, and **angina** may ensue. Furthermore, if LV function is impaired, **LV end-diastolic pressure,** and therefore intrapulmonary pressures, will rise during exercise, and shortness of breath can occur.

As mentioned previously, the diastolic dysfunction that commonly occurs in hypertension may result in impaired LV filling, which becomes more clinically significant with advancing age and at elevated heart rates. Therefore, many elderly patients with hypertension may develop symptoms of inadequate cardiac output because of poor filling of their stiff hearts rather than because of systolic dysfunction. Atrial arrhythmias also reduce LV filling. Therefore, patients tolerate exercise better if their atrial arrhythmias are controlled and if exercise intensity and heart rate (HR) responses are appropriately modulated.

Physical therapists must also consider the side effects of antihypertensive medications when designing and implementing treatment programs. Many of the medications used to treat hypertension can result in hypotension, especially when combined with treatments that result in vasodilation. Of particular concern are heat treatments, such as the whirlpool or Hubbard tank. In addition, moderate to vigorous exercise of large muscle groups can produce significant vasodilation and can result in hypotension, particularly following exercise when venous return diminishes as exercise is abruptly ceased. Likewise, stationary standing, as in performing many activities of daily living, can produce hypotension. Also orthostatic hypotension is a common side effect, necessitating caution in making sudden changes of position.

Avoidance of breath holding and **Valsalva's maneuver,** which frequently occur during isokinetic exercise and stabilization activities, especially the all-fours position, is particularly important in patients with hypertension. The abrupt increase in blood pressure that is associated with Valsalva's maneuver may be dangerous in these patients.

In addition, exercise training should be prescribed as part of a comprehensive physical therapy treatment program to improve both functional capacity and hypertensive control. Aerobic exercise training can produce significant decreases (~10–20 mm Hg) in both systolic and diastolic resting blood pressure. In addition, the rise in SBP that occurs during exercise is attenuated. Exercise training should consist of aerobic activities, such as brisk walking, jogging, swimming and cycling, performed at least 4 days per week for 30 to 45 minutes. As with other populations, typical training intensities of 70% to 85% of maximum HR may be used, but some evidence suggests that lower intensity training may elicit greater reductions in blood pressure than higher intensity training.[26,32] When lower training intensities are used, the duration, frequency, or both, of exercise should probably be increased to achieve maximum benefit so that exercise is performed for 45 to 60 minutes 5 to 7 times a week. However, it is important to emphasize, when patients do not have time for a full exercise session, that any amount of exercise is better than none. In designing an exercise prescription for clients with hypertension, the standard HR formulas can be utilized when the HR response to exercise is not altered by medications (e.g., beta blockers).[33] Alternatively, a rating of perceived exertion (RPE) scale[34] can be used with patients—especially with those who take medications that affect HR—as an indicator of exercise intensity. Also the results of an exercise stress test, if available, can be very helpful if the patient was evaluated on current medications.

DIABETES MELLITUS

Diabetes mellitus (DM) is a chronic metabolic disorder characterized by **hyperglycemia** and caused by inadequate insulin production, ineffective insulin action, or both. Abnormalities in the metabolism of glucose, fats, and proteins result. In addition, the vascular and neuropathic components to DM result in abnormalities in both large vessels (macroangiopathy) and small vessels (microangiopathy) and in the peripheral and **autonomic nervous systems.**

The two types of DM differ in etiology, clinical presentation, and pathophysiology.[35,36]

- insulin-dependent DM (IDDM)
- non–insulin-dependent DM (NIDDM)

Additionally, a number of disorders are associated with secondary DM, such as pancreatic diseases (e.g., **hemochromatosis, pancreatitis,** cystic fibrosis), hormonal syndromes (e.g., **acromegaly, Cushing's syndrome, pheochromocytoma**), and drug-induced DM (e.g., phenytoin [Dilantin], glucocorticoids, estrogens).

Insulin-dependent diabetes mellitus, also called type I DM, usually develops before early adulthood as a result of pancreatic beta cell destruction. Although the exact cause of IDDM is unknown, three factors have been implicated: viral infections, immunologic processes, and genetics.[37] The result is little or no **endogenous** insulin production. Patients with IDDM develop extreme hyperglycemia, **ketosis,** and their associated symptoms, making survival dependent on exogenous insulin therapy.

Non–insulin-dependent diabetes mellitus, also called type II DM, usually appears later in life (rarely before the age of 40) and is associated with obesity (70%–90% of patients), lack of exercise, and familial tendency. Although endogenous insulin production is relatively preserved and may even be excessive in NIDDM, the great majority of patients are insulin resistant at the cellular level owing to receptor or postreceptor defects. Hyperglycemia results from an increased rate of hepatic glucose production as a consequence of hepatic insulin resistance. Ketosis is extremely rare in this group because of the presence of at least some effective insulin.

Insulin and Glucose Physiology

The major actions of insulin are the inhibition of glucose production by the liver and the promotion of glucose transport across the cell membrane and its subsequent metabolism within the cell. Insulin also plays a role in the synthesis of glycogen, fat, and protein. Insulin deficiency results in an inability to utilize glucose as fuel, an increased **lipolysis** of triglycerides (stored fat), and an increased level of **free fatty acids (FFAs)** in the blood. When the FFAs are metabolized in the liver, **ketone** bodies are formed and **ketoacidosis** may develop.

A number of anti-insulin or counterregulatory hormones also participate in the regulation of glucose metabolism: **glucagon, growth hormone, cortisol,** and **catecholamines.** Of these, glucagon plays the most important role in terms of DM, in which its levels are absolutely or relatively increased. Glucagon release is stimulated by hypoglycemia, amino acids, neural influences, and stress. In the liver, it promotes the conversion of glycogen to glucose **(glycogenolysis),** the formation of glucose or glycogen from proteins and fats **(gluconeogenesis),** and the production of ketone bodies **(ketogenesis).**

Normally, physical activity induces a reduction in insulin secretion and an enhanced secretion of the counterregulatory hormones, which result in the stimulation of hepatic glucose production and the enhanced mobilization of muscle glycogen and FFAs. Reduced insulin secretion is compensated for by a heightened sensitivity and responsiveness of the peripheral tissues to insulin. Hepatic glucose production intensifies according to glucose requirements so that blood glucose levels remain nearly constant despite large increases in glucose uptake. In DM, particularly in IDDM, the metabolic responses to exercise are altered, as is discussed later.

Treatment of Diabetes Mellitus

The major goal of treatment for DM is to control hyperglycemia. Achieving good control of blood glucose levels prevents acute metabolic derangements and minimizes the morbidity and mortality associated with the disease.[38-41] Treatment is individualized and varies according to the type of DM; it may include

- education
- diet
- insulin
- oral hypoglycemic agents
- exercise[42]

For patients with IDDM, insulin therapy is necessary and can be provided in a variety of forms. The most common form of therapy is daily injection of insulin preparations (Table 7–2). Usually some combination of short-, intermediate-, and long-acting insulin is prescribed to attempt to mimic a normal physiologic insulin profile with maintenance of basal levels between meals and at night and sharp peaks at mealtimes (Figs. 7–3 and 7–4). When compared with the normal insulin profile, the profile for patients using insulin injections often oscillates between states of insulin excess and insulin deficiency.

Intensive insulin therapy can be undertaken, using multiple daily injections or **continuous subcutaneous insulin infusion,** which involves the use of an open loop pump to provide a constant basal level of insulin along with **preprandial** boluses to achieve more normal glycemic control. Both of these forms of treatment require frequent self-monitoring of blood glucose levels (at least before each meal and at bedtime) so that the dosage of insulin can be adjusted according to pattern of need, size of impending meal, and anticipated exercise or activity level. Finally, implantable insulin pumps have become available, but their size and limited programmability make them impractical at this time.

TABLE 7–2. Insulin Preparations — Basic Types and Their Properties				
Class	Type	Onset	Peak Effect (hr)	Duration (hr)
Rapid acting	Regular, crystalline (CZI)	30–60 min	2–4	6–8
	Semilente	60–90 min	2–6	6–8
Intermediate acting	Neutral protamine (NPH), isophane	60–90 min	6–12	18–24
	Lente	60–90 min	6–12	18–24
Long acting	Protamine zinc (PZI)	4–8 hr	14–24	36
	Ultralente	4–8 hr	18–24	36

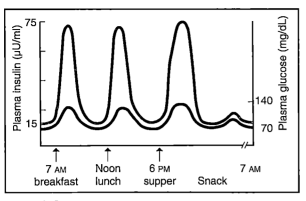

Figure 7–3.

Normal insulin-glucose interrelationships throughout the day. Red line, plasma insulin level; black line, plasma glucose level. (Reproduced with permission from Kozak GP. Clinical Diabetes Mellitus. Philadelphia, WB Saunders, 1982, p 77.)

The primary problem associated with insulin therapy is the risk of hypoglycemia. Because insulin therapy does not produce a normal physiologic insulin profile, the level of available insulin can exceed the individual's need at times. The risk of hypoglycemia increases when a meal is delayed or skipped or during strenuous or unexpected physical activity. In addition, unexpected episodes of hypoglycemia may occur because of variability in insulin activity due to the presence of insulin antibodies, which can cause insulin binding and resistance as well as allergic reactions.[43]

The treatment of NIDDM consists of

● diet
● exercise
● oral hypoglycemic agents
● insulin (sometimes)

The cornerstones of treatment are diet and exercise, especially for the control of obesity. Oral hypoglycemic agents are reserved for patients who have failed to control their hyperglycemia through diet and exercise (Table 7–3). Some individuals who are unable to achieve adequate glycemic control with diet, exercise, and oral hypoglycemic agents benefit from treatment with insulin; usually only one or two doses of intermediate-acting insulin are required each day. Insulin may also be necessary during acute ill-

ness or stress situations, such as infection, myocardial infarction, trauma, and anesthesia.

The measurement of **glycosylated hemoglobin (Hb A$_{1c}$)** is often used as an indicator of the degree of glycemic control achieved by a diabetic during the preceding 60-day period. In hyperglycemia, hemoglobin molecules become glycosylated (bound with glucose), which is a relatively

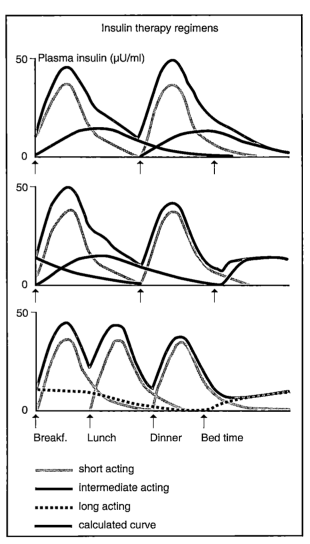

Figure 7–4.

Some common insulin therapy regimens and the insulin levels they produce. The calculated curve is the sum of the plasma insulin levels derived from the combined insulin dosages. (Reproduced with permission from Krall LP [ed]. World Book of Diabetes in Practice. Vol. 3. Amsterdam, Elsevier Science Publishers BV, 1988, p 157.)

TABLE 7–3. Oral Hypoglycemic Agents and Their Properties

Generic Name	Trade Name	Serum Half-life (hr)*	Duration of Action (hr)	Usual Daily Dose (mg)	Dosage Range (mg)
Tolbutamide	Orinase, Oramide	4–8	6–12	2000	500–3000
Chlorpropamide	Diabinese	36	24–72	250–500	100–750
Acetohexamide	Dymelor	6–8	12–24	500–1000	250–1500
Tolazamide	Ronase, Tolinase	5–7	10–24	250–500	100–1000
Glyburide	Micronase, DiaBeta	5–10	10–30	2.5–10.0	2.5–30.0
Glipizide	Glucotrol	2–4	10–30	15–25	5–40

*Half-life for parent drug plus active metabolite

irreversible process. Therefore, the level of Hb A_{1c} within the red blood cells reflects the average level of glucose that the cell has been exposed to during its life cycle (~120 days). Normal Hb A_{1c} levels are 3% to 6%, whereas diabetics usually have values of 6% to 22%.[44]

Diabetes and Exercise

Because of altered glucose and fat metabolism, individuals with DM, especially with IDDM, have a metabolic response to exercise that is different from that of nondiabetics. A number of important variables affect the metabolic responses to exercise in patients with IDDM:

- The type of insulin used
- The injection site
- The time between insulin injection and onset of exercise
- The time between the exercise and the last meal

Furthermore, the metabolic responses to exercise are influenced by the level of insulin at the onset of exercise.[45,46] Commonly, there is an excess of insulin, which inhibits hepatic glucose production and thus promotes the development of hypoglycemia. Factors associated with exercise-induced hypoglycemia include inadequate food intake preceding exercise, rapid absorption of depot insulin from an injection site near exercising muscle, and exercising at the time of peak insulin effect. However, when an insulin deficiency with marked hyperglycemia (>300 mg/dL) exists at the onset of exercise, glucose uptake by the exercising muscles is impaired, and addi-

tional glucose produced by the liver exceeds peripheral utilization, resulting in even more marked hyperglycemia. In addition, the excessive mobilization of FFAs may lead to accelerated ketogenesis and ketoacidosis, which can cause coma and death.

Because patients with IDDM often have excessively high glucose levels following meals, and because exercise enhances glucose utilization by peripheral tissues, scheduling exercise to occur after meals seems practical. Although this timing works well for some patients, research has revealed that the glycemic responses to postprandial exercise are quite variable[47]; therefore, appropriate self-monitoring of blood glucose levels is indicated. Also, delayed hypoglycemia may develop up to 24 hours after the completion of exercise.

Treatment with continuous subcutaneous insulin infusion appears to provide much more normal metabolic responses to exercise than standard insulin therapy. With a constant infusion of basal insulin, patients maintain steady state plasma glucose levels throughout exercise because muscle glucose uptake and hepatic glucose production are appropriate. Thus, patients are even able to exercise before breakfast with minimal risk of hypoglycemia.[48] The major disadvantages of continuous subcutaneous insulin infusion are the size of the currently available devices and the vulnerability of the subcutaneous infusion site to trauma or disruption. To overcome these problems, some patients remove the pumps before certain activities, such as contact or water sports. However, pump discontinuation for more than 2 hours can result in the relatively rapid development of insulin deficiency with hyperglycemia and ketosis.

Exercise plays a central role in the management of patients with NIDDM because of its beneficial effects on glycemic control and weight loss. Research has documented a significant decrease in plasma glucose levels in patients with NIDDM following 45 minutes of moderate exercise, which may last as long as 12 to 16 hours after the exercise.[49-51] For patients taking oral hypoglycemic drugs, therefore, there may be a tendency toward hypoglycemia during or following prolonged exercise.

A limited number of studies have evaluated the effect of exercise training on the long-term metabolic control in both IDDM and NIDDM. Researchers have documented increased insulin sensitivity and favorable alterations in lipoprotein concentrations with exercise training in both types of DM.[52-58] Although improved glucose tolerance has been demonstrated in patients with NIDDM following exercise training,[52,53,56,57] the magnitude of improvement has been small and often only temporary. In patients with IDDM, improved blood glucose control as measured by glycosylated hemoglobin has not been demonstrated.[59-62] However, the benefits of improved fitness level and modification of cardiovascular risk factors are sufficient reasons to encourage exercise training in patients with DM.

Cardiovascular and Pulmonary Complications of Diabetes

The organs most affected by DM are the eyes, the kidneys, the heart, and the peripheral nerves. Complications develop in these organs as a result of microangiopathy with thickening, damage, or both to the capillary basement membrane (e.g., retinopathy, nephropathy); macroangiopathy by atherosclerosis (e.g., coronary artery, cerebrovascular, and peripheral vascular disease), which tends to occur at an earlier age and with greater severity; and neuropathies involving the peripheral and autonomic nerves.[35,44] The combination of a peripheral neuropathy and an arterial insufficiency leads to the frequent complications of tissue necrosis and infection and sometimes to lower extremity amputation. Because of the prevalence of microangiopathy combined with macroangiopathy, vascular disease may be diffuse and not amenable to surgical intervention, such as coronary artery bypass grafting. However, there is strong evidence that good glycemic control can delay and possibly prevent the onset of retinopathy, nephropathy, and neuropathy.[38-41]

Cardiovascular disease is the major cause of death in patients with both types of DM.[63-66] Cardiovascular abnormalities that are more prevalent in diabetics in the United States include

- atherosclerotic heart disease
- hypertension
- defects in impulse conduction through the heart
- congestive heart failure
- autonomic neuropathy
- cerebrovascular disease
- peripheral vascular disease

Coronary artery disease, which probably results from both macroangiopathy and microangiopathy, is often diffuse and may appear as angina pectoris, myocardial infarction, sudden death, and occasionally as unexplained left ventricular failure. Symptoms associated with myocardial ischemia and infarction are frequently atypical in DM: both may appear "silently," that is, with little or no discomfort; or angina may appear as fatigue or shortness of breath in the absence of pulmonary disease, which comes on abruptly with exertion and resolves immediately with rest. Mortality associated with acute myocardial infarction is approximately two to three times (males versus females, respectively) that of nondiabetics.[63,67] The majority of deaths result from pump failure or arrhythmias and conduction disturbances and frequently occur up to 1 to 2 months after an acute myocardial infarction.[68] Diabetics appear to have twice the risk of ventricular fibrillation, which often appears after transfer from the cardiac care unit and is nearly always fatal.[67,69]

Hypertension is approximately twice as prevalent in diabetics as in nondiabetics.[44] This is particularly significant because hypertension accelerates both the microvascular and macrovascular complications of DM. Aggressive treatment of even borderline hypertension is indicated. However, effective treatment can be difficult to achieve in diabetics because many antihypertensive medications worsen glucose tolerance, increased lipids, or other severe side effects.

The incidence of congestive heart failure is markedly increased in the diabetic population. It most commonly results from atherosclerotic heart disease and hypertensive heart disease. In addition, congestive heart failure can occur in some diabetics who have myocardial dysfunction without significant coronary disease or hypertension. This **diabetic cardiomyopathy** may be due to either microvascular disease or accumulation of glycoprotein deposits, lipids, or collagen in the myocardial cells.[70,71]

Autonomic defects are also very common in long-standing diabetics but are often asymptomatic; when symptoms are noted, they are usually those associated with **postural hypotension.** The presence of autonomic neuropathy can be determined by observing HR responses to Valsalva's maneuver, deep breathing, and standing and the blood pressure responses to standing and sustained handgrip: HR response to stimuli, such as Valsalva's maneuver, standing up, and deep breathing is minimal; blood pressure falls during standing; and HR and blood pressure responses to exercise are blunted. The diagnosis of autonomic neuropathy carries a poor prognosis, with a 50% mortality rate within 2.5 years in patients with symptoms and abnormal function tests.[71]

Other cardiac abnormalities are also observed in patients with DM. Besides the relatively fixed HR described previously, autonomic dysfunction produces elevated resting HRs in most diabetics and sometimes actual resting tachycardia. In addition, the incidence of sinus node dysfunction and atrioventricular conduction abnormalities in diabetics is higher.

Many pulmonary disorders are associated with DM. Diabetics have a higher incidence of pulmonary infections than nondiabetics, and those with autonomic neuropathy have more sleep-related breathing problems. Pulmonary function testing often shows mild abnormalities in lung elastic recoil, diffusion capacity, and pulmonary

capillary blood volume, which are directly related to the duration of DM.[72] Also, diabetic ketoacidosis is related to a number of pulmonary problems, including hyperventilation, **pneumomediastinum,** and mucous plugging of the major airways.

Implications for Physical Therapy Intervention

The abnormal metabolic responses of diabetics to exercise and the frequency of cardiovascular complications necessitate caution in providing physical therapy to the diabetic population. Several factors should be considered:

- The necessity of pretreatment medical screening
- The importance of HR, blood pressure, and blood glucose monitoring
- The potential for exercise-induced hypoglycemia
- Attention to the timing of exercise
- The intensity, mode, and duration of exercise

Because of the increased incidence of asymptomatic myocardial ischemia and infarction, all patients should have a thorough medical evaluation, including graded exercise testing whenever possible, before starting any kind of exercise program. However, this evaluation is infrequently done in the acute care setting, especially when the admitting diagnosis is not cardiac in nature. In any event, HR and blood pressure monitoring should be included in all physical therapy evaluations and may be indicated during treatment sessions. Patients with DM who do not have autonomic dysfunction frequently have hypertensive responses to exercise as well as postexercise hypotension, which emphasizes the need for blood pressure monitoring. Diabetics, especially those with IDDM, tend to have blunted HR responses to activity and engage anaerobic metabolism at lower HRs[73]; therefore, exercise HRs should not exceed 50% to 60% of predicted maximum unless the patient has a good level of physical fitness. Use of the RPE scale can be very helpful for monitoring exercise intensity in diabetics, although HRs should still be checked periodically. Strenuous exercise should be avoided until reasonable diabetic control is achieved. Also, therapists should be watchful for any signs of exercise intolerance, as described in Chapter 14.

Exercise produces heightened sensitivity to insulin and so increases the risk of hypoglycemia, which may occur up to 24 hours after exercise. Therefore, patients require either a lower dose of insulin or an increased carbohydrate intake before, during, or after exercise. Clinicians should definitely be aware of the signs and symptoms of hypoglycemia, as described in Table 7–4. Carbohydrate snacks, such as fruit juice or soft drinks, should be readily available, with 5 to 10 grams provided for each 30 to 45 minutes of prolonged exercise, depending on its intensity. To minimize the risk of hypoglycemia, patients should

- avoid exercising at the time of peak insulin effect or eat a carbohydrate snack 30 minutes before exercise
- start with a moderate workload and increase intensity gradually
- choose a consistent pattern of exercise (time, duration, and intensity)
- choose exercise that can be quantified easily if possible (which can be difficult in many physical therapy programs)
- avoid tissue near the exercising muscles as the injection site for insulin

TABLE 7–4. Signs and Symptoms of Hypoglycemia

Adrenergic*	Neuroglucopenic†
Weakness	Headache
Sweating	Hypothermia
Tachycardia	Visual disturbances
Palpitations	Mental dullness
Tremor	Confusion
Nervousness	Amnesia
Irritability	Seizures
Tingling of mouth and fingers	Coma
Hunger	
Nausea‡	
Vomiting‡	

*Caused by increased activity of the autonomic nervous system
†Caused by decreased activity of the central nervous system
‡Unusual

Self-monitoring of blood glucose just before exercise is extremely helpful in predicting a patient's metabolic response to treatment and, when starting an exercise program, should be performed at frequent intervals following exercise so the patient's need for alterations in diet, insulin dosage, or both can be determined. Diabetics should avoid vigorous or prolonged exercise if blood glucose values are 250 to 300 milligrams per deciliter and should not exercise at all if blood glucose exceeds 300 milligrams per deciliter or if there is any ketosis.[74,75]

Because of the prevalence of autonomic dysfunction in diabetics and its associated risk for **silent ischemia** and decreased exercise tolerance, autonomic function testing may be included in the physical therapy evaluation by measuring the blood pressure response to standing. A fall in SBP of more than 30 mm Hg or in DBP of more than 20 mm Hg may be indicative of autonomic dysfunction.[76] A more reliable evaluation can be performed by measuring the beat-to-beat variation in HR during standing and deep breathing.[77] For the standing test, an electrocardiogram (ECG) is recorded in the supine position and then as the individual stands up quickly. Using the shortest R–R interval, which usually occurs around beat 15 after starting to stand, and the longest R–R interval, which occurs about the time of beat 30, the so-called 30 to 15 ratio can be calculated. If it is 1.0 or less, autonomic dysfunction is likely. To observe the response to deep breathing, an ECG strip is obtained at rest (sitting) and then during 1 minute of deep breathing at a rate of six breaths per minute; the longest and shortest R–R intervals during each breathing cycle are used to calculate the maximum and minimum HRs, and the difference between these two values is used to determine autonomic function. Differences of less than 15 to 20 beats per minute (older-younger individuals, respectively) indicate abnormal autonomic function.

A few other factors should be emphasized:

- Adequate fluid replacement, both during and after exercise, is very important for diabetics to avoid dehydration and maintain proper osmotic levels.

- Good footwear and careful foot hygiene with daily inspection are essential.
- Diabetics should *never* exercise alone.
- Diabetics should be alerted to the possibility of delayed exercise-induced hypoglycemia, which may occur up to 24 hours after exercise.

RENAL FAILURE

The kidneys are a complex organ whose major functions include

- the control of extracellular fluid volume
- the regulation of serum **osmolality**
- the maintenance of electrolyte and acid-base balances
- the secretion of hormones such as **renin** and **erythropoietin**

Thus, when renal function becomes impaired, the resultant metabolic disturbances affect virtually every other body system. Yet **renal failure** is usually an insidious process that often appears with symptoms of only vague general **malaise** and ill health until late in its progression. Only when renal failure becomes marked, with the accumulation of water, crystalloid solutes, and waste products, are the symptoms of **uremia** manifested. The **uremic syndrome** consists of the following derangements:

- Altered electrolyte homeostasis and acid-base imbalance
- Gastrointestinal distress
- Severe anemia
- Multiple other abnormalities involving the skin and the respiratory, cardiovascular, neurologic, musculoskeletal, endocrine, genitourinary, and immune systems

Chronic renal failure results in a number of major complications:

- Hypertension
- Pericarditis with pericardial effusion and sometimes **cardiac tamponade**
- Accelerated atherosclerosis
- Anemia
- Bleeding disorders
- Renal **osteodystrophy** (bone changes resembling osteomalacia and rickets occurring in patients with chronic renal failure)

- Proximal **myopathy** (wasting and weakness of the proximal skeletal muscles)
- Peripheral neuropathy
- **Peptic ulcer**
- **Immunosuppression** leading to **intercurrent** infections[78]

Although most of these complications are reversible with frequent **dialysis,** patients maintained on dialysis may develop other problems, as described later.

Cardiovascular complications cause nearly 50% of deaths in patients with **end-stage renal disease,** regardless of the type of treatment used.[79,80] The majority of these deaths are due to myocardial infarction, heart failure, and cerebrovascular accidents. Hypertension is both a cause and a consequence of renal disease and greatly aggravates renal dysfunction in chronic renal failure. Accelerated atherosclerosis is related to both hypertension and the **hyperlipidemia** associated with chronic renal failure. Heart failure in chronic renal failure results from fluid overload, hypertension, and atherosclerotic heart disease.

Treatment of Chronic Renal Failure

The treatment methods for managing chronic renal failure include conservative management of symptoms, dialysis, and transplantation. Because the clearance of toxic metabolic waste products and other substances by the kidneys remains superior to that achieved by dialysis until renal function deteriorates to 10% to 20% of normal, the conservative management of chronic renal failure is usually employed for as long as possible. The primary goals are to reduce the rate of progressive deterioration in renal function and to minimize the complications of chronic renal failure. The most common interventions include control of

- diet
- fluid balance
- blood pressure
- mineral metabolism
- symptoms of uremia[78]

When the symptoms or complications of chronic renal failure become troublesome despite the application of conservative therapies, dialysis is indicated. Dialysis is a process that replaces the filtration and excretory functions of the kidney by employing a semipermeable membrane and a rinsing solution **(dialysate)** to filter out toxic waste substances from the blood. In addition, dialysis allows for control of fluid and **electrolyte** balances. Several modes of dialysis are currently available, with hemodialysis and **continuous ambulatory peritoneal dialysis (CAPD)** being the most common. The major complications of chronic dialysis are

- renal osteodystrophy
- anemia
- vascular access infections and thromboses
- **pericarditis**
- **ascites**

Although many patients do well for more than 10 years on dialysis, success is limited by the inadequate clearance of waste products and other substances and the marked impairment of the regulatory and endocrine functions normally provided by the kidneys. Therefore, transplantation is the treatment of choice, particularly for younger patients. It offers the best opportunity for normalization of renal function and lifestyle, but its application is dependent on organ availability and on immunologic matching of donor kidneys, whether from living relatives or from cadavers. Furthermore, transplantation can be complicated by early and late immunologic, surgical, and medical events as well as problematic side effects of immunosuppressive medications.

Exercise and Chronic Renal Failure

Most patients with chronic renal failure are extremely sedentary and tolerate exercise poorly. Only 23% to 60% of patients (depending on presence or absence of DM, respectively) are able to do more than self-care,[81] and their mean exercise capacity is only 4 to 6 METs, or approximately 50% of that of normal sedentary values.[82-86] Factors that may contribute to their poor tolerance include

- anemia
- abnormal peripheral metabolism

- abnormal control of metabolic or systemic function during exercise
- ventricular dysfunction
- physical deconditioning

Heart rate responses are also altered in patients with chronic renal failure.[82-87] Patients do not reach their age-predicted maximal HRs on exercise stress testing. In addition, patients on hemodialysis compared with normal individuals exhibit blunted HR responses at any given relative workload despite higher levels of **norepinephrine,** which suggests diminished **adrenergic** sensitivity.[88]

A number of studies have evaluated the responses to exercise training in selected patients with end-stage renal disease who are receiving hemodialysis (e.g., patients without unstable angina pectoris; cardiac arrhythmias; hemodynamically significant valvular heart disease; clinically significant or symptomatic cerebrovascular, peripheral vascular, or coronary atherosclerosis; congestive heart failure; poorly controlled hypertension; electrolyte imbalance; severe retinal disease; IDDM; **hypothyroidism;** or orthopedic or musculoskeletal limitations).[82-86,89,90] Researchers have found that exercise training sessions can be scheduled safely and successfully during dialysis,[84,91] just before[82] or just after[90] dialysis, as well as on "off-dialysis" days.[85,86,89] Most studies have documented the ability to increase **maximal oxygen consumption ($\dot{V}O_{2max}$)** an average of 22% to 24% over a period of 10 weeks to 12 months of exercise training.[92] Other reported benefits of exercise training include

- improved lipid profiles
- enhanced blood pressure control with decreased dosage or discontinuation of medications
- normalization of insulin sensitivity and glucose metabolism
- increased red blood cell mass
- increased muscle strength
- improvements in mood, level of depression, and psychosocial functioning[93]

Thus, some of the complications experienced by hemodialysis patients may be caused by their sedentary lifestyle, rather than by their end-stage renal disease.

The major difficulty in implementing an exercise program for this patient population is that the majority of patients cannot or will not participate in the program. Compliance is improved if the sessions are scheduled on the days of dialysis and is highest when they are held during dialysis. In addition, subjective reports from patients who participated in their exercise program during dialysis indicated that they found it enjoyable, were more active at home and had better endurance, experienced less muscle cramping while on dialysis, and had fewer hypotensive responses to hemodialysis.[84]

Exercise training for selected patients after **renal transplantation** also has been shown to be feasible and beneficial. One study reported a 90% increase in estimated aerobic capacity by 8 weeks after surgery and an additional 12% a mean of 2.2 years after completion of the supervised program.[94] However, another study documented the same degree of improvement a mean of 3.25 years after transplantation in a group of patients who did not receive exercise training.[92] Despite this lack of consensus, exercise training offers additional benefits in this population

- Modification of coronary risk factors
- Prevention of **corticosteroid-related myopathy**
- Stress reduction

Implications for Physical Therapy Intervention

As discussed, patients with chronic renal failure are often very debilitated and have poor tolerance for activity. However, exercise training has been shown to offer a number of benefits for selected patients. Yet, the patients referred to physical therapy often have a number of the complex medical problems that excluded patients from previous research studies; for instance, a patient receiving neurologic rehabilitation for a stroke may also have diabetes, hypertension, peripheral vascular disease, and renal failure.

If safe treatment is to be offered, cardiovascular monitoring is essential, and appropriate adjustments should be made to accommodate potential complications, including volume overload and electrolyte imbalances (particularly hyperkalemia) that may develop from one day to the next. Ideally, patients should be on a stable regimen of dialysis, diet, and medications; however, this is not always possible in the acute care setting, in which case additional caution must be exercised. Blood pressure monitoring is also important for patients who have undergone renal transplantation owing to the prevalence of hypertensive exercise responses resulting from **cyclosporine** therapy.[95]

Exercise training programs for patients with chronic renal failure should be low intensity initially, with 5-minute exercise intervals alternating with brief (1 – 2 min) rests. The exercise intervals should increase gradually, and the number of rests should decrease, with an eventual goal being 30 to 45 minutes of continuous exercise. Aerobic activities, especially those that are non–weight bearing, are recommended. Intensity is best monitored using a rating of perceived exertion scale[34] because the intensing levels at most calculated HRs are not tolerated by most patients; a rating of perceived exertion range of 12 to 13 or "somewhat hard" has been shown to be more consistent than HR levels during dialysis.[85] Although benefits are observed using three sessions per week, five sessions per week have also been suggested.[75]

PERIPHERAL VASCULAR DISEASE

Peripheral vascular disease, or more specifically **atherosclerotic occlusive disease,** involves obstruction of the large or medium-sized arteries that supply blood to one or more of the extremities (usually lower) by atheromatous plaques. Atherosclerotic occlusive disease results from the same atherosclerotic process described in Chapter 3 and produces symptoms when the atheroma becomes so enlarged that it interferes with blood flow to the distal tissues; when it ruptures and extrudes its contents into the bloodstream or obstructs the arterial lumen; or when it encroaches on the media, causing weakness of that layer and aneurysmal dilation of the arterial wall. The hemodynamic significance of the disease is dependent on the location and number of lesions in an artery, the rapidity with which the atherosclerotic process progresses, and the presence and extent of any collateral arterial system.

When blood flow is not adequate to meet the demand of the peripheral tissues (e.g., during activity), the patient experiences symptoms of ischemia, such as **intermittent claudication** of a lower extremity. As the disease progresses, the patient experiences more severe symptoms, such as pain at rest and skin changes. Complete obstruction to flow causes tissue **necrosis** and possibly loss of the limb.

Because atherosclerosis is a generalized disorder, most individuals with peripheral vascular insufficiency also have involvement of the coronary arteries, the carotids, or the aorta. Individuals with lower extremity atherosclerotic occlusive disease should be assumed to have arteriosclerotic heart disease, which is their main cause of mortality.[96]

Exercise and Peripheral Vascular Disease

Individuals with atherosclerotic occlusive disease are unable to produce the normal increases in peripheral blood flow essential for increasing the oxygen supply to exercising muscles. If the oxygen supply is inadequate to meet the increasing demand of the exercising muscles, ischemia develops and leads to the production of lactic acid and other waste products. When excessive lactic acid accumulates in the muscle, pain is experienced; when it reaches the central circulation, respiration is further stimulated, and patients may experience shortness of breath.

Patients with **intermittent claudication** have moderate to severe impairment in walking ability. Their peak exercise capacity during graded treadmill exercise is severely limited, allowing for only very light to light activities.[97-99] Therefore, the energy requirements of many leisure and work-related activities exceed their capacity. Metabolic measurements during exercise testing reveal that maximal oxygen consumption and **anaerobic threshold** are reduced in patients with atherosclerotic occlusive disease.[97,98] Yet even though the anaerobic threshold may be so low that it cannot be detected, evidence of systemic lactic acidosis may be minimal because of the reduced muscle perfusion.

Several studies have documented the efficacy of exercise training in the management of patients with atherosclerotic occlusive disease.[96,100-107] Increases in pain-free and maximal walking tolerance on level ground and during constant-load treadmill exercise, in peak exercise capacity achieved during exercise testing, and in peak oxygen consumption have been reported. One study even concluded that greater symptomatic relief and functional improvement in patients with mild to moderate claudication not requiring immediate therapeutic intervention is achieved through supervised exercise therapy rather than through **percutaneous transluminal coronary angioplasty**.[101] In addition, some studies have shown benefit for patients with pain while at rest.[105,108] Several mechanisms have been postulated to account for these improvements: increased walking efficiency, increased peripheral blood flow through changes in the collateral circulation, reduced blood viscosity, regression of atherosclerotic disease, raising of the pain threshold, and improvements in skeletal muscle metabolism. The most likely of these appear to be enhanced biomechanical efficiency of walking and improved skeletal muscle metabolism.[101,103,107]

Implications for Physical Therapy Intervention

Because of the high prevalence of atherosclerotic heart disease in patients with peripheral vascular disease, all patients should be assumed to have atherosclerotic heart disease and therefore should receive HR and blood pressure monitoring during physical therapy evaluation and initial treatment. This is especially true when working with patients who have undergone amputation, because amputation implies severe disease. Notably, patients with atherosclerotic occlusive disease may exhibit precipitous rises in blood pressure during exercise owing to their atherosclerosis and diminished vascular bed.

It is very useful to use a subjective gradation of pain for expressing claudication discomfort, as described in Table 7-5.[31] It is generally believed that patients should not exercise at levels beyond

TABLE 7–5. Subjective Gradation of Claudication Discomfort

I	Initial discomfort (established, but minimal)
II	Moderate discomfort but attention can be diverted
III	Intense pain (attention cannot be diverted)
IV	Excruciating and unbearable pain

grades I to II pain, because more stressful exercise elicits anaerobic energy mechanisms that may exacerbate the claudication pain. Lower intensities are recommended, because they maximize the potential length of the exercise bouts.

Exercise training should consist of daily aerobic activities at least 5 days per week and preferably with two exercise periods per day. Again, exercise training will be performed at intervals, alternating brief exercise periods with frequent rests and gradually increasing exercise periods according to the patient's tolerance. Popular modes of exercise include recreational walking, treadmill walking, stationary cycling, swimming, or pool exercise programs. The goal should be to achieve a duration of at least 20 to 30 minutes, allowing intermittent rest periods whenever necessary to relieve pain.

OBESITY

Obesity can be defined as an increased accumulation of **adipose** tissue so that body mass index (body weight in kilograms divided by height in meters squared) is higher than 30 kg/m^2; body fat is greater than 25% for males or 30% for females; or body weight is more than 20% above the upper limit for height.[109] Approximately 26% of Americans are obese, a third of whom are extremely so.[110] There are two types of obesity, which vary according to the age of onset: juvenile-onset obesity is characterized by an increased number, or **hyperplasia,** of **adipocytes;** adult-onset obesity is usually associated with increased size, or hypertrophy, of the existing adiposites.

Obesity is the result of a positive energy balance due to an imbalance between energy intake and energy expenditure. Genetic, hormonal, and metabolic factors appear to play a role in the etiology of obesity. In fact, probably multiple factors, both physiologic and psychological, which vary among individuals, interact to induce obesity. Although it is generally assumed that overeating is a primary cause of obesity, research indicates that obese individuals of all ages may consume the same number or fewer calories than their lean counterparts.[111–117] Researchers are now discovering that there are other factors that shift the balance between energy intake and expenditure and thus promote either body fat deposition or metabolism. For instance, diet composition appears to be just as important as caloric content in the promotion or reduction of obesity. Evidence suggests that dietary fat and refined sugar intake may promote obesity,[117–119] whereas complex carbohydrates and dietary fiber may assist in body fat reduction, despite the same total caloric intake.[120–122] In addition, it is now recognized that severe calorie-restricted dieting elicits an energy conservation process and a reduction in metabolic rate, which persists after the dieting period ends and facilitates rapid weight regain.[121,123,124] Frequently this cycle is repeated a number of times, with the dieter experiencing progressive difficulty in losing weight and enhanced ability to regain any lost weight.

Obesity represents a major health problem in this country because of its association with increased prevalences of hypertension, cardiovascular disease, osteoarthritis, gastrointestinal problems, endometrial and breast cancers, glucose intolerance, type II DM, **obesity hypoventilation syndrome, sleep apnea,** and pulmonary hypertension.[109,125] In addition, it is associated with increased mortality rates, usually as a result of atherosclerotic heart disease, stroke, diabetes, digestive diseases, or cancer.[126,127]

The increased prevalence of atherosclerotic heart disease in obese individuals is probably related to its association with hypertension, hyperlipidemia, and glucose intolerance rather than with a direct role in the pathogenesis of atherosclerosis. However, a cardiomyopathy of obesity, which consists of a syndrome of chronic circulatory congestion associated with diastolic and sometimes systolic left ventricular dysfunction in the absence of hypertension or other cardiovascular disease, has been identified in morbidly obese individuals.[128] Blood volume, stroke volume, cardiac output, left ventricular end-diastolic volume, and end-diastolic filling pressure are increased with obesity, especially during exertion.[129] These result in left ventricular hypertrophy and dilation as well as left atrial hypertrophy due to the augmented pulmonary blood volume and flow. If hypertension is also present, left ventricular hypertrophy will be more marked, and congestive heart failure may develop. In addition, approximately 75% of very obese individuals have pulmonary hypertension at rest or during exercise, along with elevated systemic pressures in the majority of cases.[130]

The most specific pulmonary problems found in obesity are sleep apnea and obesity hypoventilation syndrome.[72] Sleep apnea tends to occur in moderately to extremely obese males, aged 40 to 60, and consists of **hypersomnolence** during the day and sleep apnea at night. During the apneic periods, significant increases in systemic and pulmonary arterial pressures occur and frequently cardiac arrhythmias, including sinus arrest, asystole up to 6 seconds, heart block, and ventricular tachycardia. The obesity hypoventilation syndrome occurs in approximately 5% of extremely obese individuals and includes hypoventilation, cyanosis, and somnolence. The results of these symptoms are chronic hypoxemia, hypercapnia, respiratory acidosis, and polycythemia. Chronic hypoxemia and hypercapnia stimulate pulmonary vasoconstriction, leading to a worsening of pulmonary hypertension. **Biventricular hypertrophy** with pulmonary and systemic congestion are characteristic of this syndrome.

Exercise and Obesity

In obesity the resting metabolic rate and therefore the cardiac output and minute ventilation relative to lean body mass are increased because of the greater body mass that must be provided with oxygen. During exercise the increase in oxygen consumption is even more marked because of the additional energy required to move the larger body segments. However, the hypoxemia

that may exist at rest as a result of peripheral atelectasis caused by chest wall obesity usually disappears during exercise, presumably because of deeper breathing. In obesity, the maximal oxygen consumption and anaerobic threshold are low when related to actual body weight but are normal when expressed as a ratio to height or lean body weight.

Because obesity is the result of a positive energy balance, it seems only logical that successful treatment of obesity would consist of reversing this energy balance through decreasing caloric intake, increasing energy expenditure, or a combination of both. Unfortunately, studies evaluating the efficacy of exercise, either as a single modality or combined with diet restriction, are very discouraging because of the rather low amount of weight loss and the high dropout rates.[131-135] Yet the reported findings have shown a great deal of variability. Some reports have documented that the percentage of body fat decreases more with less loss of lean body weight when exercise is added to dieting,[131,136-138] but others have not found this to be the case.[139,140] It has also been suggested that individuals with **hyperplastic** (increased number of fat cells) obesity may be more resistant to attempted dietary restriction than those with hypertrophic (enlarged fat cells but normal number) obesity,[136] but again not all data concur.[132] The disparity in published results may be due to a variety of factors: the type of obesity; the physiologic causes or sustaining factors involved in an individual's obesity; the age, sex, and body build of the subjects; the variations in frequency, intensity, and duration of exercise; the length of the training period (long term versus short term); the type of diet; and the motivation of the subjects.

Maintenance of any weight loss is a major problem for most people, but those who continue with their exercise program have been more successful.[141] In addition, exercise has other demonstrable benefits for the obese, even if their weight loss is not achieved. Physical training in obese individuals is associated with an improvement in glucose tolerance and a marked reduction in the insulin response to a **glucose tolerance test**.[142,143] Also, the lipid profiles of obese subjects, particularly males, may shift favorably as a result of exercise training.[131,134,143] As it does with other populations, exercise training in the obese improves exercise tolerance and increases efficiency so that daily activities can be performed more easily.[131,133,138,139,143] This is particularly important because obese individuals use more energy with exaggerated cardiovascular and respiratory stress to perform any form of physical work.

Implications for Physical Therapy Intervention

When prescribing exercise for obese individuals, a number of specific factors should be considered to maximize both safety and effectiveness. First, because of the increased prevalence of hypertension and atherosclerotic heart disease in obesity, monitoring of the physiologic responses to exercise is indicated during physical therapy evaluation and initial treatment. A tendency toward exercise-induced syncope due to fluid imbalance that results from calorie-restricted diets and is exacerbated by exercise-induced fluid loss further emphasizes the need for blood pressure monitoring. Second, an endurance training program should be prescribed for all patients to increase energy expenditure, lower cardiovascular risk factors, and improve functional efficiency. Intensity should be lower than the anaerobic threshold, or around 50% to 60% of functional capacity, to utilize predominantly FFAs as fuel. Duration and frequency should be prescribed so that a total of 1750 to 2000 calories are expended per week in a fairly even distribution. The goal is to perform 45 to 60 minutes of low- to moderate-intensity aerobic activity at least 3 to 5 days per week. Finally, non–weight-bearing exercise programs, such as cycling, swimming, or water aerobics, decrease the stress on joints that are often affected by osteoarthritis.

In addition, obese individuals should be encouraged to increase their general level of activity during daily routines. This can be accomplished by walking whenever possible, including for 2- to 5-minute periods every hour at work or at home or during lunchtime, and taking the stairs instead of the elevator for fewer than two to four flights.

OTHER SPECIFIC DISEASES AND DISORDERS

A wide variety of other specific diseases may be associated with cardiopulmonary complications. The presence of cardiac or pulmonary complications, or both, may affect patient tolerance of physical therapy intervention. Tables 7–6 to 7–9 summarize the cardiac and pulmonary manifestations of a number of specific diseases and disorders.

Collagen Vascular Diseases

The collagen vascular diseases are a diverse group of systemic diseases that are characterized by diffuse and variable abnormalities of the vasculature and inflammatory lesions involving the joints, muscles, and connective tissues, including the pericardium and pleura. Involvement of the kidneys, brain, and heart cause the most serious morbidity and mortality. Pericarditis and **cardiomyopathy** can occur in most of these conditions, but some have very characteristic cardiovascular lesions associated with them as well. As shown in Table 7–6, the following specific collagen vascular diseases may have major cardiopulmonary involvement:

- **Systemic lupus erythematosus (SLE)**
- **Polyarteritis nodosa**
- **Rheumatoid arthritis**
- **Ankylosing spondylitis**
- **Progressive systemic sclerosis**

In addition, other collagen vascular diseases, such as **polymyositis,** dermatomyositis, and Reiter's disease, are occasionally associated with cardiovascular or pulmonary dysfunction but are not presented here.

Systemic Lupus Erythematosus

Systemic lupus erythematosus is a multisystem autoimmune disease with diffuse and widespread

TABLE 7–6. Most Common Cardiac and Pulmonary Manifestations of the Collagen Vascular and Connective Tissue Diseases

| Disease | Cardiac Manifestations | | | | | | Pulmonary Manifestations | | | | |
	P	M	E/V	CA	ECG	Other	Pl.	I	Pn.	Vasc.	Mm.
Systemic lupus erythematosus	++	+/−	++	+	+/−	HTN, CHF	++	+	+	+/−	+
Polyarteritis nodosa	+	++	−	++	+	HTN, CHF	−	−	−	+/−	−
Rheumatoid arthritis	++	+	+	+	+	Rare intrapulm. nodules	++	+	+	+/−	−
Ankylosing spondylitis	−	+/−	++	−	+	Ankylosis of thorax	−	+/−	+	−	−
Progressive systemic sclerosis	+	++	−	++	+	HTN, CHF, pulm. HTN	++	+	+	++	−
Marfan's syndrome	−	−	++	+	−	Aortic dissection	−	−	−	−	−
Osteogenesis imperfecta	−	−	++	−	+	AR, MVP, MR	−	−	−	−	−

P, pericardial; M, myocardial; E/V, endocardial/valvular; CA, coronary arteries; ECG, ECG changes, arrhythmias, and conduction disturbances; Pl., pleural; I, interstitial; Pn., pneumonitis; Vasc., vascular; Mm., respiratory muscle weakness; HTN, hypertension; CHF, congestive heart failure; pulm., pulmonary; AR, aortic regurgitation; MVP, mitral valve prolapse; MR, mitral regurgitation.

+, convincing association; ++, very common; +/−, possible association; −, no association reported for specific disease or disorder.

vasculitis involving the skin, joints, brain, kidney, heart, and virtually all serous membranes. Clinical evidence of cardiac involvement is present in 18% to 56% of patients.[144] In addition, there is an increased incidence of coronary atherosclerosis, which is probably related to treatment with corticosteroids.[145] Systemic lupus erythematosus may cause a **pancarditis** (inflammation of all the structures of the heart) with abnormalities of the pericardium, endocardium, myocardium, and coronary arteries. Acute pericarditis is the most common lesion and is usually asymptomatic and without consequence; on rare occasions, however, constrictive pericarditis or **pericardial tamponade** may develop. Evidence of endocarditis with lesions on all four valves, particularly the aortic and mitral valves, can be identified in up to 40% to 50% of victims at

TABLE 7–7. Cardiac and Pulmonary Manifestations of a Number of Neurologic and Neuromuscular Diseases

| Disease/Disorder | Cardiac Manifestations | | Other | Pulmonary Manifestations | | |
	Myocardial	CA		Mm.	Obst.	Rest.
Hemiplegia	+/−	++	HTN, CAD if vascular pathology	+	−	+
Paraplegia	−	−	Depends on level of lesion	++	−	++
Parkinson's disease	−	−	Dyskinetic respiration	+	−	+
Amyotrophic lateral sclerosis	−	−	Respiratory failure	++	−	++
Landry-Guillain-Barré syndrome	−	−	Respiratory failure	++	−	++
Myasthenia gravis	+	−	Arrhythmias, rare CHF Respiratory failure	+	−	++
Progressive muscular dystrophy	++	−	Arrhythmias Pulmonary infections	++	−	++
X-linked muscular dystrophy	+	−	Sinus arrest, atrial paralysis AV blocks	+/−	−	+/−
Limb-girdle syndromes	+	−	Abnl ECG	+/−	−	+/−
Myotonic dystrophy	−	−	Heart blocks, v-tach	++	−	+
Friedreich's ataxia	++	+	Arrhythmias, CHF Scoliosis, chest deformity	+/−	−	+/−

CA, coronary arteries; Mm., respiratory muscle weakness; Obst., obstructive lung disease; Rest., restrictive lung disease; HTN, hypertension; CAD, coronary artery disease; CHF, congestive heart failure; AV, atrioventricular; abnl, abnormal; ECG, electrocardiogram; v-tach, ventricular tachycardia.

+, convincing association; ++, very common; +/−, possible association, −, no association reported for specific disease or disorder.

TABLE 7–8. Cardiac and Pulmonary Dysfunction Associated with Cancer Treatment

Treatment	Cardiac Problems				Comments	Pulmonary Problems		
	Ar/ECG	P	Isch.	CM		Pneum.	Fib.	Other
Radiation therapy to chest	+	++	+	+	Varies with prescription techniques	+	+	—
Chemotherapy Agents:								
Amsacrine (AMSA)	+	—	+/−	+		—	—	—
Azathioprine	+/−	—	—	—	Atrial fibrillation	—	—	—
Bleomycin	—	+/−	—	—	Dose dependent, O_2 sensitive	+	+	+
Busulfan	—	—	—	—	Poor prognosis	+	+	+
Carmustine (BCNU)	—	—	—	—		+	+	—
Chlorambucil	—	—	—	—	50% mortality	+/−	+/−	—
Chlorozotocin (DCNU)	—	—	—	—		+	+	—
Cyclophosphamide	—	+	—	+	Acute pericarditis-myocarditis	+	+	+
Cytosine arabinoside/cytarabine	—	+/−	—	—	Unexplained pulmonary edema	—	—	+
Dactinomycin	—	—	—	—		+	—	—
Daunorubicin (Daunomycin)	+	+	+	+	Dose dependent	—	—	—
Doxorubicin (Adriamycin)	+	+	+	+	Dose dependent	—	—	—
Etoposide	—	—	+/−	—		—	—	—
Fluorouracil (5-FU)	—	—	+	—		—	—	—
Interleukin-2	—	—	+	—		—	—	—
Lomustine (CCNU)	—	—	—	—		+	+	—
Mechlorethamine	+/−	—	—	—	PACs and tachycardia	—	—	—
Melphalan	—	—	—	—		+/−	+/−	—
Mercaptopurine	—	—	—	—	Very rare	—	—	+/−
Methotrexate	+/−	—	—	—	? Hypersensitivity	+	+/−	+
Mitomycin	—	—	—	—	Almost 50% mortality	+	+	+
Procarbazine	—	—	—	—	Allergic interstitial infiltrates	+	+/−	+
Semustine (methyl-CCNU)	—	—	—	—		+	+	—
Vinblastine/vincristine/vindesine	—	—	+	—	Accelerated CAD, coronary spasm	+	+	+

ar/ECG, arrhythmias/ECG changes; P, pericardial; Isch., myocardial ischemia or infarction; CM, chronic cardiomyopathy; Pneum., pneumonitis; Fib., fibrosis; CAD, coronary artery disease; PAC, premature atrial complex.
+, convincing association; ++, very common; +/−, possible association; −, no reported association.

TABLE 7–9. Cardiac and Pulmonary Manifestations of Some Other Specific Diseases

Disease	Cardiac Manifestations			Other	Pulmonary Manifestations			
	P	M	CA		Pl.	I	Pn.	Vasc.
Sickle cell disease	—	++	+	Cardiomegaly, ↓ exercise capacity	—	—	++	+
Bone marrow transplantation	—	+/−	—	Pulmonary edema, COPD, graft-versus-host disease	—	++	++	+
AIDS	+	—	—	Metastasis of Kaposi's sarcoma to heart and lungs, non-Hodgkin's lymphoma, opportunistic infections	—	+	+	—
Hepatic disease	—	+	—	Alcoholic cardiomyopathy, HTN, arrhythmias, chest pain, ascites → ↓ vital capacity pulmonary shunting and HTN	+	—	—	—
Anorexia nervosa	—	++	—	Arrhythmias, sudden death	—	—	—	—
Bulimia	—	+/−	—	Arrhythmias Aspiration pneumonia	—	—	—	—

P, pericardial; M, myocardial; E/V, endocardial/valvular; CA, coronary arteries; Pl., pleural; I, interstitial; Pn., pneumonitis; Vasc., vascular; AIDS, acquired immunodeficiency syndrome; COPD, chronic obstructive pulmonary disease; HTN, hypertension.
+, convincing association; ++, very common; +/−, possible association; −, no association reported for specific disease or disorder; →, resulting in; ↓, decreased.

autopsy, but it is usually asymptomatic.[145-148] **Myocarditis** is an uncommon manifestation of SLE. Occasionally widespread vasculitis may affect the smaller coronary arteries, resulting in myocardial necrosis and fibrosis, cardiomyopathy, and sometimes rhythm and conduction disturbances. Hypertension is common in patients with SLE and is the major cause of cardiac enlargement and heart failure.

Pulmonary involvement, which occurs in at least 50% of patients with SLE, most commonly affects the pleura.[72,149,150] Pleuritic chest pain is more common than chest radiograph evidence of pleural effusions might indicate, though massive effusions can occur. Acute **pneumonitis** develops in some patients; it is often infectious but can also result from the disease directly (acute lupus pneumonitis) or from **alveolar hemorrhage,** which can be fatal. **Chronic interstitial lung disease** is occasionally seen and is characterized by dyspnea on exertion and bibasilar rales. Approximately 50% of patients with SLE have decreased diffusion capacity and changes consistent with restrictive lung disease, which are probably related to respiratory muscle weakness and sometimes to interstitial lung disease.[151] Diaphragmatic weakness has been recognized as being relatively common in SLE and is manifested as dyspnea, especially when the patient is recumbent.[151] Patients can have mild to severe hypoxemia. Finally, pulmonary hypertension occurs in a small number of patients.

Polyarteritis Nodosa

Polyarteritis nodosa is a systemic disease characterized by segmental necrotizing inflammation of the medium- to small-sized arteries with resultant dysfunction of multiple organ systems, including the skin, kidneys, gastrointestinal tract, spleen and lymph nodes, central nervous and musculoskeletal systems, and heart. Approximately 78% of patients exhibit signs of cardiovascular involvement, particularly hypertension and congestive heart failure.[152] Polyarteritis of the coronary arteries and their branches occurs in approximately 70% of patients and can lead to myocardial infarction, which is often undiagnosed but found at autopsy.[153] Chest pain, heart

murmurs, pericardial friction rubs, cardiac enlargement, and ECG abnormalities are fairly common. Heart failure caused by a combination of infarction and renal failure is a frequent cause of death in patients with polyarteritis nodosa.[148,152] Clinical manifestations of pulmonary disease do not occur unless **allergic angiitis** or **granulomatosis** is present. Then there may be intractable asthma and transient or progressive episodes of pneumonia. Pulmonary lesions account for approximately 50% of the mortality in patients with allergic angiitis and granulomatosis.[153]

Rheumatoid Arthritis

Rheumatoid arthritis is a chronic inflammatory disease that predominantly involves the joints but may affect other systems, particularly when the disease is severe and long-standing. Although evidence of cardiovascular involvement, especially of the pericardium, is commonly seen during echocardiography and at autopsy, it is seldom a clinical problem.[152,154] However, occasionally, patients go on to develop constrictive pericarditis or tamponade. Other lesions that are sometimes seen in rheumatoid arthritis include myocardial inflammation, diffuse myocarditis with cell necrosis (which can cause heart failure and death), arteritis of the coronary arteries with resultant heart failure and arrhythmias, and granulomatous lesions involving the myocardium and mitral valve. Pulmonary involvement with rheumatoid arthritis tends to be asymptomatic but occasionally causes major problems.[72,155] Rheumatoid pleural disease is frequently found at autopsy.[151] In rare cases, intrapulmonary nodules are present, which may become infected; cause bronchial obstruction; cavitate; or rupture into the pleural space, causing a pneumothorax. Sometimes there is diffuse interstitial fibrosis with pneumonitis, which can progress to bronchiectasis, chronic cough, and progressive dyspnea, and, infrequently, respiratory insufficiency and right-sided heart failure. In addition, reports have appeared of other pulmonary problems in patients with rheumatoid arthritis, including a therapeutic drug-related pulmonary dysfunction, an unexplained pulmonary vasculopathy, and, rarely, a rapidly progressive obliterative bronchiolitis.

Ankylosing Spondylitis

Ankylosing spondylitis is a form of arthritis involving mainly the spine and sacroiliac joints resulting in chronic back pain, deforming dorsal kyphosis, and possibly fusion of the costovertebral and sacroiliac joints. Cardiac involvement takes the form of a sclerosing inflammatory lesion involving the aortic root area, both immediately above and below the level of the aortic valve, resulting in aortic insufficiency in up to 10% of patients with long-standing disease.[147,148] If the inflammatory process extends below the aortic valve to the mitral valve, mitral insufficiency can develop, or if it extends into the top of the ventricular septum, conduction disturbances through His's bundle and its branches may result. Patients with severe disease also may have chronic infiltrative and fibrotic changes in the upper lung fields that mimic tuberculosis. Ankylosis of the costovertebral joints results in a stiff thorax, which is revealed as restrictive changes during pulmonary function testing. Small airway disease may also be present in some patients. In addition, ankylosing hyperostosis of the cervical spine can cause dysphagia, foreign-body sensation, and aspiration.[72]

Progressive Systemic Sclerosis

Progressive systemic sclerosis, or scleroderma, is an uncommon disease characterized by slowly progressive fibrosis and diffuse vascular lesions of the skin and subcutaneous tissues and often the visceral organs, including the gastrointestinal tract, especially the esophagus, heart, lungs, and kidneys. Cardiovascular disease, which is found in more than 90% of patients with diffuse progressive systemic sclerosis, results either from primary involvement of the heart by the disease or secondary involvement of the kidneys or lungs.[156,157] Cardiomyopathy due to myocardial necrosis and fibrosis, which may result from a **Raynaud's phenomenon** of the coronary arteries, is found in 50% of cases at autopsy.[148,152] There may also be congestive heart failure, heart block due to fibrosis of conducting tissue, and asymptomatic pericarditis. Hypertension secondary to renal involvement is common. The primary cause of mortality in progressive systemic sclerosis is the combined effect of multiple pulmonary abnormalities.[157] Pulmonary hypertension, which occurs in 33% to 60% of patients, can develop suddenly as a result of a Raynaud's phenomenon of the pulmonary arteries, creating a medical emergency, or can be chronic because of obliterative vascular disease of the pulmonary arteries and arterioles.[156] Pleural effusions, which are usually asymptomatic, may appear, as well as pleurisy, interstitial lung disease with fibrosis, and ultimately restrictive pulmonary disease. More than 50% of asymptomatic patients have abnormal pulmonary function test results.[157] However, a sedentary lifestyle due to restrictions on skin and joint movement often masks the symptoms of shortness of breath or dyspnea on exertion until late in the disease process.

Connective Tissue Diseases

Abnormalities of connective tissue of the great arteries, cardiac valves, skeletal system, and skin are characteristic of a number of diseases, including **Marfan's syndrome, Ehlers-Danlos syndrome, osteogenesis imperfecta,** and **homocystinuria.** These diseases may cause minimal cardiovascular dysfunction, such as mitral valve prolapse or mild aortic root dilation, or severe problems, such as severe aortic or mitral insufficiency or aortic dissection and aneurysm. These manifestations probably reflect the response of abnormal connective tissue to prolonged hemodynamic stresses. Pulmonary problems may also develop in these patients.

Neuromuscular Diseases and Neurologic Disorders

A number of disorders that affect the neurologic or neuromuscular systems are associated with cardiac and pulmonary dysfunction (see Table 7–7). The incidence and severity of dysfunction in all of the disorders vary widely. Cardiac abnormalities include cardiomyopathy and disorders of impulse formation and conduction. Abnormalities of pulmonary function are usually related to respiratory muscle weakness that causes hypoventilation and weakness of cough, **bulbar** muscle weakness that results in aspiration pneumonia, or cardiomyopathy that leads to pulmonary edema. Respiratory muscle fatigue is probably the final event responsible for respiratory failure in the neuromuscular disorders; accordingly, nocturnal mechanical ventilation in the form of cuirass ventilators is being used in the homes of some patients with good results.[158]

Hemiplegia. Hemiplegia can result from a number of events:

- Cerebrovascular accidents due to thrombosis, embolism, or hemorrhage
- Surgical excision of a brain tumor
- Trauma

Regardless of cause, weakness or spastic paralysis of the affected side of the body can include the diaphragm and intercostal muscles. Left diaphragmatic dysfunction is more common than right diaphragmatic dysfunction. Pulmonary function testing reveals decreased volumes and flows to approximately 60% to 70% of predicted normal[159]; obviously, these abnormalities take on additional clinical significance in the presence of preexisting pulmonary disease. Respiratory failure can develop in patients whose vital capacity decreases to 25% of predicted normal, and mechanical ventilation will be required. The usual lack of clinical symptoms in hemiplegic patients is probably owing to their low level of physical exertion; however, more strenuous exertion or physical therapy activities may elicit dyspnea, especially when the patient is lying flat. Only hemiplegia due to vascular pathologies is clearly associated with cardiovascular abnormalities. Hypertension and atherosclerotic heart disease are common, though frequently not diagnosed. The majority of deaths following transient ischemic attacks, stroke, and **carotid endarterectomy** are due to cardiac disease; yet only 25% to 48% of patients presenting with cerebrovascular disease have a history of coronary artery disease.[160] One angiographic study designed to define the frequency of asymptomatic coronary artery disease in patients with cerebrovascular disease found

that 40% had severe coronary artery disease (defined by >70% stenosis of at least one coronary artery), 46% had mild to moderate disease, and only 27% had normal coronary arteries.[161] Needless to say, these data have direct implications for physical therapy evaluation and treatment of patients with strokes (see final discussion).

Spinal Cord Injury. Pulmonary dysfunction is common in patients with spinal cord injury, with the degree of dysfunction being related to the level of injury.[162] Lesions above C4 result in diaphragm as well as intercostal muscle paralysis and frequently necessitate permanent ventilator assistance. Lesions below this level have corresponding intercostal muscle involvement, and therefore some restrictive changes are observed on pulmonary function testing. A reasonable discussion of this topic is beyond the scope of this chapter but can be found elsewhere.[163] Interruption of autonomic nervous system signals in patients with spinal cord injuries at or above the T6 level can lead to serious disturbances of blood pressure. Orthostatic hypotension is common in the early phase of recovery but usually resolves over time. **Autonomic dysreflexia (hyperreflexia)** can produce elevated blood pressures when noxious visceral or cutaneous stimuli are sensed below the level of the lesion. In addition, autonomic denervation also interferes with temperature regulation so that body temperature tends to fluctuate according to the ambient temperature, especially in persons who have high lesions; therefore, hypothermia and hyperthermia can develop.

Parkinson's Disease. Parkinson's disease is a common dyskinetic disorder of the extrapyramidal system, which is characterized by resting muscle tremors, rigidity, slowness and poverty of motion, postural instability, and masklike facial expression. Although rarely recognized clinically, impaired ventilatory function occurs in nearly 87% of patients and tends to be proportional to the severity of the skeletal muscle disease.[164] Erratic, or chaotic, breathing due to the rigidity and weakness of the respiratory muscles is common but may be responsive to treatments that ameliorate other symptoms of the disease.[165] In addition, an obstructive pulmonary disease associated with Parkinson's disease may appear, which may be related to increased parasympathetic tone and infections.[166] No specific cardiac complications are associated with Parkinson's disease; however, patients often have the cardiovascular problems that are common in their same-aged peers (e.g., hypertension, arteriosclerotic heart disease).

Amyotrophic Lateral Sclerosis. Amyotrophic lateral sclerosis (ALS) is the most common motor neuron disease in the United States and is characterized by progressive neurologic deterioration without remission owing to anterior horn cell loss. The average life expectancy after the onset of symptoms is 3.6 years.[167] Irreversible hypoventilation leading to mechanical ventilator dependence and fatal respiratory failure is common in the later stages of the disease. Also, bulbar paralysis occurs in 25% of patients, which contributes to the frequent complication of **aspiration pneumonia.** Furthermore, repetitive episodes of aspiration and airway obstruction may be responsible for the increased incidence of obstructive lung disease in patients with amyotrophic lateral sclerosis.[159]

Landry-Guillain-Barré Syndrome. Landry-Guillain-Barré syndrome, or acute polyneuritis, is a **demyelinating** disease of motor neurons, manifested by symmetric ascending paralysis, which is usually temporary. Nearly 50% of patients develop complications due to respiratory muscle paralysis, including paralysis of the diaphragm.[159] Approximately 25% to 30% of patients require mechanical ventilatory support during the most severe phase of their disease.[168] The majority of deaths result from cardiopulmonary complications.[159]

Myasthenia Gravis. Myasthenia gravis is an acquired autoimmune disorder associated with **acetylcholine** receptor deficiency at the motor end plates that affects either the external ocular muscles selectively or the general voluntary muscle system. Abnormal fatigability is characteristic of the disease, though symptoms may fluctuate from hour to hour, day to day, or over longer periods. Cardiac involvement may occur in some patients, especially with thymoma, and may be due to myocardial necrosis with acute and chronic inflammatory infiltrates, concurrent coronary artery disease, or intercurrent respiratory problems.[169] Tachycardia and other arrhythmias;

dyspnea; and, rarely, heart failure may occur. Notably, drugs used to treat cardiovascular problems, such as quinidine, procainamide, lidocaine, and morphine, may adversely affect myasthenia gravis. Respiratory muscle weakness and respiratory failure are not uncommon and may necessitate prolonged ventilatory assistance. The risk of respiratory failure may be increased by surgery, infectious disease, and administration of corticosteroids or **antimicrobial** drugs.[159]

Progressive (Duchenne's) Muscular Dystrophy. Progressive (Duchenne's) muscular dystrophy is a lethal, X-linked recessive disorder of childhood. The disease is present at birth and usually becomes symptomatic during early childhood; the child is unable to walk by the age of 10 and usually dies by the age of 20. Up to 90% of patients develop typical ECG changes associated with scarring of the posterobasal portion of the left ventricle.[170,171] Arrhythmias and conduction disturbances also occur frequently, probably owing to multifocal dystrophic involvement of the conduction system. Involvement of the posteromedial papillary muscle sometimes causes mitral valve prolapse and mitral regurgitation. Clinically significant cardiomyopathy is uncommon, although approximately 10% of patient mortality is related to cardiac dysfunction.[172] The most common cause of death is respiratory failure, which is usually related to pulmonary infection. Chronic alveolar hypoventilation and poor cough due to weakness of the respiratory muscles is common by the age of 10 years.

Other Types of Muscular Dystrophy. Other types of muscular dystrophy are also associated with cardiac dysfunction. Cardiomyopathy may occur in **fascioscapulohumeral muscular dystrophy** and the **limb-girdle muscular dystrophy syndromes,** but ventricular dysfunction is usually mild to moderate and heart failure is unusual. There may be gallop sounds, cardiac enlargement, and ECG abnormalities. Atrial abnormalities are present in all patients with X-linked scapuloperoneal myopathy (Emery-Dreifuss dystrophy) and result in sinus arrest, atrial arrhythmias, varying atrioventricular block, and permanent atrial paralysis with junctional bradycardia. Because sudden death is common in young adults afflicted with the disease, permanent pacing is recommended for ventricular rates below 50, regardless of atrial activity. Fascioscapulohumeral dystrophy and the scapuloperoneal syndromes have also been associated with atrial paralysis. **Myotonic muscular dystrophy** is associated with cardiac involvement, especially with ECG abnormalities and arrhythmias, in at least two thirds of patients; high-grade heart block or ventricular tachycardia may cause sudden death.[173,174] Occasionally, acute left ventricular failure or congestive heart failure occur. Pulmonary problems related to the muscular dystrophies can result from either respiratory muscle weakness, which causes alveolar hypoventilation, hypercapnia, hypoxia, and increasing somnolence in severe cases, or pharyngeal muscle weakness, which may lead to aspiration pneumonia. In addition, chronic hypoxia can result in pulmonary hypertension and sometimes right ventricular failure.

Friedreich's Ataxia. Friedreich's ataxia is a hereditary disease characterized by progressive spinocerebellar degeneration that begins during adolescence. Cardiovascular involvement, including cardiomyopathy and ECG abnormalities, occurs in 50% to 100% of patients and often appears as the initial manifestation of the disease, though most patients are asymptomatic, except for dyspnea, which could be explained on the basis of their neurologic disability.[175,176] When other symptoms are noted, they usually consist of **palpitation** and angina. Arrhythmias are common, especially **atrial fibrillation** and **paroxysmal supraventricular tachycardia.** Cardiomyopathy with cardiac hypertrophy and dilation and interstitial fibrosis may result from a variety of abnormalities, including myocardial degeneration, **scoliosis** or other chest deformity causing cor pulmonale, or a distinctive coronary arteriopathy. Death is usually caused by congestive heart failure or intercurrent infections and commonly occurs within 20 years after the onset of symptoms.[148]

Cardiopulmonary Toxicity Resulting from Cancer Treatment

The development of aggressive treatment for a number of cancers has yielded increasing survival rates and periods but has also been associated with increasing frequency of cardiac and pulmonary toxicity. There may be a synergistic effect of irradiation and some of the chemotherapeutic agents, and some of the drugs when used in combination, which increases their degree of cardiac or pulmonary toxicity, or both. This effect has been documented in both early and late toxicity.[177-179]

Therapeutic radiation to the chest (e.g., for treatment of **Hodgkin's disease, non-Hodgkin's lymphoma,** lung and breast cancer) necessarily exposes the heart and lungs to varying degrees and dosages of radiation, depending on the extent of disease. The pericardium is the most commonly affected structure; pericarditis can occasionally be severe and can require **pericardiocentesis** or pericardiectomy for relief of tamponade or constrictive pericarditis, respectively. Other cardiac manifestations of radiation toxicity include

- acute myocardial infarction due to radiation-induced coronary artery disease
- restrictive cardiomyopathy and ECG changes, including varying degrees of heart block, due to endocardial fibrosis
- mitral regurgitation resulting from papillary muscle dysfunction
- aortic regurgitation as a consequence of endocardial valvular thickening

Fortunately, more refined treatment techniques have resulted in dramatic decreases in the incidence of these sequelae to less than 2.5%.[180]

Chest irradiation can also produce lung injury. Acute radiation pneumonitis occurs in approximately 3% to 5% of patients who receive irradiation to the chest but in almost 20% of patients who have Hodgkin's disease with massive mediastinal involvement (>one third chest diameter).[180] It usually develops 2 to 3 months following completion of treatment, requires no treatment, and resolves within days to months; however, some patients (<5%) develop severe pneumonitis that requires hospitalization and aggressive supportive care.[181] Although frequently asymptomatic, most patients then develop gradual progressive fibrosis, which is characterized primarily as a restrictive lung disease. In cases of persistent fibrosis of a large volume of lung tissue, late radiation fibrosis can be severe, with cor pulmonale and respiratory failure. The major variables associated with radiation injury to the lungs are total radiation dose (>4000 rads), dose rate (rads/min) and **fractionation** (rads/treatment), and volume of lung within the high-dose region. Patients undergoing total body irradiation in preparation for bone marrow transplantation or as systemic adjuvant treatment for pediatric and adolescent tumors such as **neuroblastoma, rhabdomyosarcoma,** and **Ewing's sarcoma** are also high-risk groups.

The treatment of cancer using chemotherapeutic agents is also associated with both cardiac and pulmonary toxicity. **Cardiotoxicity** most frequently results from the use of the **anthracycline** antibiotics doxorubicin (Adriamycin) and daunorubicin (Cerubidine) and can be acute or chronic. Arrhythmias and conduction disturbances are the most common manifestations of acute toxicity; more rarely, left ventricular dysfunction and possibly congestive heart failure can occur owing to cardiomyopathies, a pericarditis-myocarditis syndrome, sudden death, and myocardial ischemia and infarction. Late cardiotoxicity appears as a chronic cardiomyopathy in 50% to 60% of patients treated with doxorubicin,[178] although it is clinically apparent in only 1% to 2% of patients.[182] The risk factors associated with the development of a cardiomyopathy include increasing cumulative doses (especially >550 mg/m²) and previous mediastinal radiation. The prognosis with clinically apparent doxorubicin cardiomyopathy is poor, with mortality as high as 48%, especially in patients who present in the first month after therapy.[183] A number of other chemotherapeutic agents have also been associated with cardiotoxicity,[178] as shown in Table 7–8. Amsacrine, azathioprine, methotrexate, and mechlorethamine have been associated with arrhythmias. Cyclophosphamide (Cytoxan) in high doses has been reported to cause an acute lethal pericarditis-myocarditis in rare cases and occasionally a cardiomyopathy. Finally, 5-fluorouracil (5-FU), the Vinca alkaloids vinblastine and vincristine, and high-dose interleukin-2 therapy have been linked to myocardial ischemia and infarction in a small percentage of patients.

The lungs are a common site of chemotherapy-related toxicity, which is being recognized more frequently and is associated with an increasing number of drugs (see Table 7–8). Interstitial pneumonitis is the most frequently encountered manifestation of pulmonary toxicity, which appears clinically as dyspnea with or without a nonproductive cough and fever. Of all the chemotherapy drugs, bleomycin is the most likely to cause interstitial pneumonitis, which is related to total dose (especially if >450–500 mg/m² but can occur with <100 mg/m²).[177,181] Other drugs that can cause interstitial pneumonitis include busulfan, cyclophosphamide, chlorambucil, carmustine (BCNU), mitomycin, methotrexate, and procarbazine. The most common abnormalities seen on pulmonary function testing are

- decreased diffusion capacity for carbon monoxide
- decreased volumes, indicative of restrictive lung disease

Arterial hypoxemia may also occur, especially with exercise. Some drugs are associated with other forms of pulmonary toxicity; the most notable is cytosine arabinoside, which causes unexplained **pulmonary edema** in up to 38% of patients.[184]

Hematologic Disorders

Anemia

Anemia, or a reduced circulating red blood cell mass relative to the sex and age of an individual, results from excessive destruction of red blood cells, loss by hemorrhage, impaired red blood cell production, or a combination of these factors. The signs and symptoms associated with anemia depend on the cause of the anemia, its extent, the rapidity of onset, and the presence of any other problems that compromise the individual's health. Anemia commonly produces fatigue, headache, and exertional dyspnea. In addition, patients with coronary disease may have increased episodes of angina with even mild anemia. Compensatory mechanisms are available to preserve tissue oxygenation:

- Reduced hemoglobin-oxygen affinity
- Increased cardiac output
- Reduced peripheral vascular resistance and blood viscosity
- Decreased circulatory time
- Increased oxygen extraction
- Redistribution of blood flow

Elevated cardiac output appears to be due primarily to the reduction in left ventricular afterload and the increased stroke volume, rather than to an increase in HR, at least until the anemia is marked. Congestive heart failure can develop in severe anemia even in the absence of cardiac disease, but usually it occurs as a result of the increased workload imposed on an unhealthy heart.[185]

Sickle Cell Disease

Sickle cell disease is a genetic disorder found most commonly in blacks and is characterized by structurally abnormal hemoglobin; the red blood cell is "sickle" shaped, less pliable, and "sticky." These alterations result in hemolytic anemia due to the trapping and destruction of the abnormal red blood cells in the spleen and in tissue ischemia and infarction (painful crises) due to occlusion of the small capillaries and venules, particularly in the spleen, central nervous system, bones, liver, kidney, and lungs. Cardiopulmonary problems are common in sickle cell disease, as shown in Table 7–9, because both the cardiac output and oxygen extraction by the tissues are increased, and the reduced oxygen content of the red blood cells leads to further sickling. Cardiomegaly is a frequent finding and is usually associated with exertional dyspnea and systolic murmurs. Exercise capacity is reduced primarily because of the diminished oxygen-carrying capacity of the blood and may be associated with an exercise-induced drop in cardiac output or myocardial ischemia.[186] Specific cardiac manifestations may include biventricular hypertrophy and dilation; arteritis with proliferation and thrombosis; and myocardial degeneration, necrosis, and fibrosis.[148] Congestive heart failure is a late occurrence. The major pulmonary manifesta-

tions of sickle cell disease are **pneumococcal pneumonia,** which is a major cause of morbidity and mortality in children; pulmonary vascular occlusion; **capillary stasis;** thrombus formation; and infarction. Rarely, cor pulmonale may develop because of pulmonary infarction. Most patients have abnormal pulmonary function test results, with decreased diffusion capacity, reduced vital capacity, arterial oxygen desaturation (which further predisposes to sickling and its consequences), and a widened alveolar-arterial oxygen tension difference.[72]

Bone Marrow Transplantation

Bone marrow transplantation (BMT) may be used in the treatment of **aplastic anemia,** acute and chronic leukemias, malignant lymphomas, breast cancer, myeloma, immunodeficiency states, and some genetic hemoglobinopathies and metabolic disorders. Bone marrow transplantation can be achieved by transplanting normal bone marrow from an identical twin or a genetically different donor into an individual whose own diseased marrow has been ablated by chemotherapy, total body irradiation, or both (syngeneic or allogeneic bone marrow transplantation, respectively) or by reinfusing an individual's own bone marrow that was obtained during a period of complete remission or was treated in vitro to remove any contaminating cells (an autologous bone marrow transplant). Pulmonary complications are a major cause of morbidity and mortality following BMT and may occur early or late (see Table 7–9). Pulmonary edema is common during the first 2 to 4 weeks after BMT and may result from fluid overload, myocardial injury, cyclosporine toxicity, and transfusion reactions. The most dangerous complication of BMT is interstitial pneumonitis, which occurs in 10 to 80%[80] of transplant recipients and has a mortality rate of 40% to 75%.[72] It is most commonly due to active **cytomegalovirus** infection or is idiopathic, in which no specific cause can be identified but may be related to the combined effects of the chemotherapy and total body irradiation that were prescribed as treatment for the primary disease or for the conditioning program immediately preceding BMT. Graft-versus-host disease is also associated with pulmonary problems, aside from the increased incidence of infectious pneumonitis: lymphocytic bronchitis, obstructive small airways disease, chronic sinopulmonary infections, and chronic aspiration. Other less common pulmonary complications associated with BMT include alveolar hemorrhage, leukemic recurrence, **pleural effusion** associated with hepatic veno-occlusive disease, and pulmonary vascular abnormalities.

The incidence of cardiac toxicity after BMT has been reported as 5% to 43%.[187] Although cardiac involvement is generally not considered a major clinical problem following BMT, it is occasionally serious and even fatal. The most frequent manifestations of cardiac toxicity related to BMT are arrhythmias, usually bradycardias or tachyarrhythmias; ST–T changes; and decreased QRS voltage. Heart failure occurs in 5% to 30% of patients following BMT, and pericarditis affects 7% to 23% of patients; either one of these by itself or the two occurring together may be fatal in up to 30% of patients.[188] Because of reports of congestive heart failure, which is often progressive and fatal, developing 4 to 20 years after treatment with the anthracycline antibiotics, which include many BMT recipients,[189] there is concern that an increasing number of patients, especially those who were treated during childhood, might show evidence of late cardiac toxicity after BMT.

Acquired Immunodeficiency Syndrome

Acquired immunodeficiency syndrome (AIDS) is a syndrome characterized by severe **immunodeficiency** that is caused by infection of CD4(T4) lymphocytes with the human immunodeficiency virus (HIV). Pulmonary involvement is the major cause of morbidity and mortality in patients with AIDS (see Table 7–9).[72,155,190] **Opportunistic** pulmonary infections with *Pneumocystis carinii*, tuberculosis, cytomegalovirus, *Mycobacterium avium-intracellulare*, or a number of other pathogens are very common. Other pulmonary abnormalities include diffuse interstitial pneumonitis, either idiopathic or lymphocytic; the AIDS-related pulmonary malignancies **Kaposi's sarcoma** and non-Hodgkin's lymphoma; and adult respiratory distress syndrome. Notably, multiple pulmonary problems exist simultaneously in almost 20% of patients.[190]

Cardiac complications can also develop in patients with AIDS, though their prevalence has not yet been documented. The most frequent cardiac manifestation of AIDS is the metastasis of Kaposi's sarcoma to the heart.[191] Other more rare complications include involvement of the pericardium by tuberculosis and progressive cardiomyopathy due to opportunistic viral infections.[192]

Hepatic Diseases

Several diseases of the liver, including **cirrhosis** and **hepatitis,** produce or are associated with multiple cardiac and pulmonary problems, as shown in Table 7–9. Approximately 15% to 45% of patients with cirrhosis, the most prevalent type of chronic liver disease in the United States, exhibit pulmonary abnormalities, especially arterial hypoxemia, hyperventilation, and pleural effusions.[72] The presence of ascites further compromises pulmonary function because of diaphragmatic elevation and reduced lung volumes. Additionally, patients may develop intrapulmonary and **portopulmonary shunting,** ventilation-perfusion mismatching, and pulmonary hypertension. The cardiovascular system can also be affected by long-term alcohol consumption in a variety of ways, including hypertension, cardiac arrhythmias, chest pain, and heart failure. The major cardiac abnormality specific to hepatic disease is **alcoholic cardiomyopathy,** which is responsible for up to one third of the cases of congestive cardiomyopathy (see Chapter 4).[148] In addition, up to 50% of asymptomatic alcoholics demonstrate subclinical abnormalities, including left ventricular hypertrophy, left ventricular dilation, and diminished contractility.[193]

Eating Disorders

The two most common eating disorders are **anorexia nervosa** and **bulimia nervosa.** Both disorders occur predominantly in young, previously healthy females and have specific behavioral and psychological features as well as physiologic abnormalities, including those involving the heart and lungs, as summarized in Table 7–9.

Anorexia Nervosa

Anorexia nervosa is characterized behaviorally by severe self-induced weight loss (at least 15% below ideal body weight) through extreme restriction of food intake and sometimes ritualized exercise. The major psychological manifestations are a distorted body image and an unreasonable concern about being "too fat" as well as denial of hunger, fatigue, and emaciation. A number of medical problems besides the characteristic **amenorrhea** have been reported in anorexia nervosa:

- Salivary gland enlargement
- Pancreatitis
- Pancreatic insufficiency
- Liver dysfunction
- Thiamine deficiency
- **Coagulopathies**
- Electrolyte imbalance
- Decreased gastric emptying and intestinal mobility
- **Hypophosphatemia**
- Bilateral peroneal nerve palsies
- Hypoglycemia
- Osteoporosis
- **Hypothalamic dysfunction**
- Cardiac abnormalities

In addition to the considerable medical morbidity caused by anorexia nervosa, mortality is significant, with rates of approximately 6% over a 5-year period and 15% to 20% at 15 years.[194] Cardiac complications account for most of the deaths. Nutritional depletion results in decreased myocardial muscle mass, diminished glycogen stores, and evidence of myofibrillar destruction.[195] Both systolic and diastolic ventricular dysfunction may occur. **Mitral valve prolapse** is a frequent finding. Clinically, bradycardia, relative hypotension, and abnormal exercise performance with reduced exercise tolerance (approximately 50% of predicted normal) and

blunted heart rate and blood pressure responses are common.[196,197] Multiple ECG abnormalities have been documented; some of them, including hypokalemic-induced arrhythmias, may be responsible for episodes of sudden death. Also, there have been reports of congestive heart failure, especially during refeeding.

Bulimia Nervosa

Bulimia nervosa is a much more common disorder, which is characterized behaviorally by binge eating counterposed with dieting, purging, or both by self-induced vomiting, laxative abuse, or diuretic abuse. Psychologically, the patient is aware that the eating pattern is abnormal, fears that eating cannot be controlled, and feels depressed after binge eating. Because severe weight loss is not a problem for the majority of patients, many of the physiologic abnormalities evident in anorexia nervosa do not occur in most bulimic patients. However major complications are associated with bulimia, including

- tooth decay
- aspiration pneumonia
- esophageal or gastric rupture
- pneumomediastinum
- pancreatitis
- neurologic abnormalities

The most significant cardiac disorders consist of cardiac arrhythmias (due to hypokalemia from vomiting and laxative abuse), which can be fatal, and occasionally ipecac-induced cardiomyopathy.[196]

Clinical Implications for Physical Therapy

The most obvious implication of all the information presented in this chapter is that many patients with many different primary diagnoses can have cardiopulmonary dysfunction. Yet the symptoms of dysfunction are often nonspecific, such as shortness of breath, lightheadedness, and fatigue; or there may be no symptoms at all (e.g., hypertension). Therefore, the only way to determine if a patient is responding to exercise appropriately is to evaluate the physiologic responses. This is achieved by monitoring HR, blood pressure, and other signs and symptoms during every physical therapy evaluation. Only in this way can physical therapists design treatment programs that are both safe and effective.

Another important implication is that physical therapists must address the needs of the whole patient, not just those of the primary diagnosis, if our goal is truly to promote "optimal human health and function." Endurance training should be a component of the physical therapy program for every patient who is not already performing regular aerobic exercise, except for those who are acutely ill or have debilitating neuromuscular diseases that are adversely affected by exercise. Endurance exercise facilitates the other components of almost every physical therapy program and offers a number of additional health benefits, as discussed throughout this chapter.

Many specific guidelines have been presented in the sections on the most commonly encountered diagnoses seen by physical therapists, but many of them can also be applied to patients with the diagnoses presented in this last section. To summarize and reduce to the basics for practical application, the following recommendations are offered.

Guidelines for Physical Therapy Intervention

1. Heart rate, blood pressure, and signs and symptoms should be monitored during every physical therapy evaluation.

2. If the patient's responses are normal, it is safe to proceed with typical treatment planning (including, of course, endurance training).

3. If the responses are abnormal, caution is indicated (they may be so abnormal that consultation with a physician is warranted, or they may signal that the patient's tolerance is compromised and that the patient requires frequent rests during more strenuous activities and careful attention to maintain coordinated breathing during exertion).

4. Patients with moderate to severe cardiopulmonary dysfunction usually display symptoms of dyspnea, fatigue, and possibly lightheadedness or dizziness during activity, which should be associated with the physiologic responses detected during monitoring and

then used during future treatment sessions as indicators of patient tolerance.

5. A few patients will require continued monitoring of HR, blood pressure, or both during treatment sessions.

6. Some patients may benefit more from two shorter treatment sessions per day rather than one intense or prolonged session.

Guidelines for Endurance Training

1. Patients should start slowly and increase their activity gradually.

2. The mode of training can consist of any form of aerobic exercise, including walking, jogging, cycling, swimming, cross-country skiing, and aerobics classes, and can vary during the week.

3. Intensity may be most easily monitored by using a rating of perceived exertion scale; a good starting place is "somewhat hard" (13 on the 6–20 Borg scale[34]).

4. Duration starts with the length of time a patient can exercise until fatigue begins to occur and increases approximately 1 minute per day.

5. Short rest periods (1–2 min) can be alternated with exercise intervals if a patient has very limited endurance.

6. Patients benefit most from twice-daily exercise periods until the duration increases to at least 20 minutes of continuous peak activity.

7. Once a patient can perform the peak aerobic portion of his or her program for at least 30 minutes, the frequency can be decreased to 3 to 5 days per week, depending on the intensity and goals of the patient (e.g., for control of hypertension or reduction of body weight, longer durations are more successful).

8. Any amount of activity is better than no activity; if a patient has a hectic day and cannot complete the entire workout, a partial workout is preferable to skipping the whole thing.

9. Patients should be encouraged to increase the activity level of their daily routines, such as by parking farther away from their place of work or shopping and taking the stairs instead of the elevator for 1 to 2 flights.

10. Exercise time, distance, or both can be recorded on a calendar to keep track of progress and provide motivation.

11. And finally, exercise should be *fun!* Encourage patients to identify activities they enjoy or to create a social aspect into their program (e.g., involving family or friends) so it does not become a chore.

SUMMARY

- The major determinants of arterial blood pressure are cardiac output and total peripheral resistance, each of which is affected by a number of other factors.
- Hypertension produces a pressure overload on the left ventricle, resulting in left ventricular hypertrophy and diastolic dysfunction, which reduces left ventricular compliance.
- The ultimate consequence of progressive left ventricular hypertrophy is the development of congestive heart failure.
- Persons with hypertension may exhibit exaggerated blood pressure responses to exercise even though their resting blood pressure may be normal.
- Reductions of 10 to 20 mm Hg in both systolic and diastolic blood pressure may be achieved through aerobic exercise training.
- Avoidance of breath holding and Valsalva's maneuver is particularly important in patients with hypertension.
- Diabetes mellitus is frequently complicated by vascular and neuropathic abnormalities, including microangiopathy (i.e., retinopathy), macroangiopathy (e.g., coronary, cerebral, and peripheral vascular disease), and peripheral and autonomic neuropathies.
- Cardiovascular disease is extremely common in diabetics, especially hypertension, coronary ischemia and infarction (which may be silent), and congestive heart failure.
- Although exercise training offers many benefits for patients with DM, including increased insulin sensitivity and improved lipoprotein concentrations, physical therapists and patients must use caution in order to avoid abnormal heart rate and blood pressure responses, as well as hypoglycemia.
- End-stage renal disease is often associated with cardiovascular complications, which cause nearly 50% of deaths in these patients.
- Exercise tolerance is extremely poor in patients with chronic renal failure. Their heart rate and blood pressure responses are often abnormal.
- Exercise training offers a number of benefits for patients with chronic renal failure, such as improved functional capacity, modification of coronary risk factors, prevention of corticosteroid-related myopathy, and stress reduction.
- In peripheral vascular disease, blood flow becomes progressively impeded, resulting in poor exercise tolerance and symptoms of ischemia, such as intermittent claudication, which can be ameliorated through exercise training.
- Obesity carries an increased risk of atherosclerotic heart disease owing to its association with hypertension, hyperlipidemia, glucose intolerance, and lack of regular physical activity.
- A number of other medical diagnoses also may be complicated by cardiac or pulmonary problems, or both, including collagen vascular, connective tissue, neuromuscular and neurologic, hematologic, hepatic, and eating disorders or diseases.
- Treatment of cancer with radiotherapy, chemotherapy, or both may produce cardiopulmonary toxicity.
- The only way to determine whether a patient has any cardiopulmonary dysfunction is to monitor physiologic responses (e.g., heart rate, blood pressure, signs and symptoms) during physical therapy interventions.

References

1. Kaplan NM. Clinical Hypertension. 4th ed. Baltimore, Williams & Wilkins, 1986.
2. Blood Pressure Study 1979. Chicago, Society of Actuaries & Association of Life Insurance Medical Directors of America, 1980.
3. Kannel WB, Doyle JT, Ostfeld AM, et al. Original resources for primary prevention of atherosclerotic diseases. Circulation 70:157A–205A, 1984.
4. Kannel WB. Some lessons in cardiovascular epidemiology from Framingham. Am J Cardiol 37:269–282, 1979.
5. Rutan GH, Kuller LH, Neaton JD, et al. Mortality associated with diastolic hypertension and isolated systolic hypertension among men screened for the Multiple Risk Factor Intervention Trial. Circulation 77:504–514, 1988.
6. Cohn JN, Limas CJ, Guiha NH. Hypertension and the heart. Arch Int Med 133:969–979, 1974.
7. Frohlich ED. The heart in hypertension. In: Genest J, Koiw E, Kuchel O (eds). Hypertension—Physiopathology and Treatment. New York, McGraw-Hill, 1983.
8. Strauer BE. Left ventricular wall stress and hypertrophy. In: Messerli FH (ed). The Heart and Hypertension. New York, Yorke Medical Books, 1987.
9. Smith V-E, Katz AM. Left ventricular relaxation in hypertension. In: Messerli FH (ed). The Heart and Hypertension. New York, Yorke Medical Books, 1987.
10. Wikstrand J. Diastolic function of the hypertrophied left ventricle. In: Messerli FH (ed). The Heart and Hypertension. New York, Yorke Medical Books, 1987.
11. Borer JS, Jason M, Devereaux RB, et al. Systolic function of the hypertrophied left ventricle at rest and dur-

ing exercise: Hypertension and aortic stenosis. Am J Med 75(suppl):34–39, 1983.

12. Kaplan NM. Nonpharmacological control of high blood pressure. Am J Hypertens 2:55S–59S, 1989.

13. Kendrick ZV, Cristal N, Lowenthal DT. Cardiovascular drugs and exercise interactions. Cardiol Clin 5(2):227–244, 1987.

14. Lowenthal DT, Wheat M, Kuffler LA. Coordinating drug use and exercise in elderly hypertensives. Geriatrics 43(6):69–80, 1988.

15. McAllister RG Jr. Effect of adrenergic receptor blockade on the responses to isometric handgrip: Studies in normal and hypertensive subjects. J Cardiovasc Pharmacol 1:253–263, 1979.

16. Sannerstedt R, Julius S. Systemic hemodynamics in borderline arterial hypertension: Responses to static exercise before and under the influence of propranolol. Cardiovasc Res 6:398–403, 1972.

17. American Heart Association (The Committee on Exercise). Exercise Testing and Training of Individuals with Heart Disease or at High Risk for Its Development: A Handbook for Physicians. Dallas, Tex, American Heart Association, 1975.

18. Blomqvist CG, Lewis SF, Taylor WF, Graham RM. Similarity of the hemodynamic responses to static and dynamic exercise of small muscle groups. Circ Res (suppl I) 48:I87–I90, 1981.

19. Cahalin L. The effects of aerobic exercise upon hypertension. Cardiopulmonary Record 3(2):1–3, 1989.

20. Nyberg G. Blood pressure and heart rate response to isometric exercise and mental arithmetic in normotensive hypertensive subjects. Clin Sci Mol Med 51:681s–685s, 1976.

21. Ressl J, Chrastek J, Jandova R. Hemodynamic effects of physical training in essential hypertension. Acta Cardiol 32:121–133, 1977.

22. Pickering TG. Exercise and hypertension. Cardiol Clin 5(2):311–318, 1987.

23. Brorson L, Wasir H, Sannerstedt R. Haemodynamic effects of static and dynamic exercise in males with arterial hypertension of varying severity. Cardiovasc Res 12:269–275, 1978.

24. Kamid S, Wolff FW. Drug failure in reducing pressor effect of isometric handgrip stress test in hypertension. Am Heart J 86:211–215, 1973.

25. Hagberg JM. Exercise, fitness, and hypertension. In: Bouchard C, Shephard RJ, Stephens T, et al. (eds). Exercise, Fitness, and Health—A Concensus of Current Knowledge. Champaign, Ill, Human Kinetics Books, 1990.

26. Hagberg JM, Mountain SJ, Martin WH, Ehsani AA. Effects of exercise training on 60–69 year old essential hypertensives. Am J Cardiol 64:348–353, 1989.

27. Roman O, Camuzzi AL, Villalon E, Klenner C. Physical training program in arterial hypertension: A long-term prospective follow-up. Cardiology 67:230–243, 1981.

28. Sannerstedt R, Wasir H, Henning R, Werko L. Systemic hemodynamics in mild arterial hypertension before and after physical training. Clin Sci Mol Med 45:145s–149s, 1973.

29. American Heart Association. High blood pressure fact sheet. Dallas, Tex, 1988.

30. Kirkendall WM, Feinleib M, Freis ED, Mark AL. Recommendations for human blood pressure determination by sphygmomanometers (Subcommittee of the AHA Postgraduate Education Committee). American Heart Association, Dallas, Tex, 1980.

31. American College of Sports Medicine. Guidelines for Exercise Testing and Prescription. Philadelphia, Lea & Febiger, 1990.

32. Hollander W. Role of hypertension in atherosclerosis and cardiovascular disease. Am J Cardiol 38:786–798, 1976.

33. Gordon NF, Scott CB, Wilkinson WJ, et al. Exercise and mild essential hypertension—Recommendations for adults. Sports Med 10:390–404, 1990.

34. Borg GAV. Psychophysical bases of perceived exertion. Med Sci Sports Exerc 14:377–387, 1982.

35. Marble A, Krall LP, Bradley RF, et al. (eds). Joslin's Diabetes Mellitus. 12th ed. Philadelphia, Lea & Febiger, 1985.

36. Davidson MB. Diabetes Mellitus Diagnosis and Treatment. 3rd ed. New York, Churchill Livingstone, 1991.

37. Maclaren NK. Viral and immunological bases of beta cell failure in insulin-dependent diabetes. Am J Dis Child 131:1149–1154, 1977.

38. Chase HP, Jackson WE, Hoops SL, et al. Glucose control and the renal and retinal complications of insulin-dependent diabetes. JAMA 261:1155–1160, 1988.

39. Davidson MB. The case for control in diabetes mellitus (Medical Progress). West J Med 129:193–200, 1978.

40. Hanssen KF, Dahl-Jorgensen K, Lauritzen T, et al. Diabetic control and microvascular complications: The near-normoglycaemic experience. Diabetologia 29:677–684, 1986.

41. Pirart J. Diabetes mellitus and its degenerative complications: A prospective study of 4400 patients observed between 1947 and 1973. Diabetes Care 1:168–188, 1978.

42. Krall LP (ed). World Book of Diabetes in Practice. Vol. 3. New York, Elsevier Science Publishers BV, 1988.

43. Heine RJ. The insulin dilemma: Which one to use? In: Krall LP (ed). World Book of Diabetes in Practice. New York, Elsevier Science Publishers BV, 1988.

44. Kozak GP. Clinical Diabetes Mellitus. Philadelphia, WB Saunders, 1982.

45. Rybka J. Diabetes Mellitus and Exercise. ACTA Universitatis Carolinae Medica, Monograph CXVIII, 1987.

46. Vranic M, Wasserman D, Bukowiecki L. Metabolic implications of exercise and physical fitness in physiology and diabetes. In: Rifkin H, Porte D Jr (eds). Ellenberg and Rifkin's Diabetes Mellitus—Theory and Practice. 4th ed. New York, Elsevier Science, 1990.

47. Caron D, Poussier P, Marliss EB, Zinman B. The effect of postprandial exercise on meal-related glucose tolerance in insulin-dependent diabetic individuals. Diabetes Care 5:364–369, 1982.

48. Zinman B, Vranic M. Diabetes and exercise. Med Clin North Am 69:145–157, 1985.

49. Devlin JT, Hirschman M, Horton ES. Enhanced peripheral and splanchnic insulin sensitivity in NIDDM after single bout of exercise. Diabetes 36:434–439, 1987.

50. Minuk HL, Hanna AK, Marliss EB, et al. Metabolic response to moderate exercise in obese man during prolonged fasting. Am J Physiol 238:E322–E329, 1980.

51. Minuk HL, Vranic M, Marliss EB, et al. Glucoregulatory and metabolic response to exercise in obese noninsulin-dependent diabetes. Am J Physiol 240:E458–E464, 1981.

52. Bogardus C, Ravussin E, Robbins DC, et al. Effects of physical training and diet therapy on carbohydrate metabolism in patients with glucose intolerance and non-insulin-dependent diabetes mellitus. Diabetes 33:311–318, 1984.

53. Reitman JS, Vasquez B, Klimes I, Nagulesparan M. Improvement of glucose homeostasis after exercise training in non-insulin-dependent diabetes. Diabetes Care 7:434–441, 1984.

54. Ruderman NB, Ganda OP, Johnson K. The effect of physical training on glucose tolerance and plasma lipids in maturity-onset diabetes. Diabetes 28(suppl 1):89–92, 1979.

55. Saltin B, Lingärde BS, Houston M, et al. Physical training and glucose tolerance in middle-aged men with chemical diabetes. Diabetes 28:30–32, 1979.

56. Scneider SH, Amorosa LF, Khachadurian AK, Ruderman NB. Studies on the mechanism of improved glucose control during regular exercise in type 2 (non-insulin-dependent) diabetes. Diabetologia 26:355–360, 1984.

57. Trovati M, Carta Q, Cavalot F, et al. Influence of physical training on blood glucose control, glucose tolerance, insulin secretion, and insulin action in non-insulin-dependent diabetic patients. Diabetes Care 7:416–420, 1984.

58. Vranic M, Wasserman D. Exercise, fitness, and diabetes. In: Bouchard C, Shephard RJ, Stephens T, et al. (eds). Exercise, Fitness, and Health—A Consensus of Current Knowledge. Champaign, Ill, Human Kinetics Books, 1990.

59. Wallberg-Henriksson H, Gunnarsson R, Rössner S, Wahren J. Long-term physical training in female type I (insulin-dependent) diabetic patients: Absence of significant effect on glycaemic control and lipoprotein levels. Diabetologia 29:53–57, 1986.

60. Wallberg-Henriksson H, Gunnarsson R, Henriksson J, et al. Increased peripheral insulin sensitivity and muscle mitochondrial enzymes but unchanged blood glucose control in type I diabetics after physical training. Diabetes 31:1044–1050, 1982.

61. Zinman B, Zuniga-Guajardo S, Kelly D. Comparison of the acute and long-term effects of exercise on glucose control in type I diabetes. Diabetes Care 7:515–519, 1984.

62. Zinman B, Zuniga-Guajardo S, Kelly D. The effect of exercise training on glucose control in type I diabetes. Clin Invest Med 6(suppl 2):69, 1983 (abstract).

63. Kannel WB, McGee DL. Diabetes and cardiovascular disease. JAMA 241:2035–2038, 1979.

64. Leland OS. Diabetes and the heart. In: Kozak GP. Clinical Diabetes Mellitus. Philadelphia, WB Saunders, 1982.

65. Watkins PJ, Drury PL, Taylor KW. Diabetes and Its Management. 4th ed. Oxford, Blackwell Scientific Publications, 1990.

66. Kannel WB. Lipids, diabetes and coronary artery disease: Insights from the Framingham study. Am Heart J 110:1100–1107, 1985.

67. Harrower ADB, Clarke BF. Experience of coronary care in diabetes. Br Med J 1:126–128, 1976.

68. Smith JW, Marcus FE, Serokman R. Prognosis of patients with diabetes mellitus after acute myocardial infarction. Am J Cardiol 54:718–721, 1984.

69. Lichstein E, Kuhn LA, Goldberg E, et al. Diabetic treatment and primary ventricular fibrillation in acute myocardial infarction. Am J Cardiol 38:100–102, 1976.

70. Jarrett RJ (ed). Diabetes and Heart Disease. New York, Elsevier Science Publishers BV, 1984.

71. Nesto RW. Diabetes and heart disease. In: Krall LP (ed). World Book of Diabetes in Practice. New York, Elsevier Science Publishers BV, 1988, pp 256–259.

72. Baum GL, Wolinsky E (eds). Textbook of Pulmonary Diseases. Boston: Little, Brown, 1989.

73. Fujita Y, Kawaji K, Knamori A, et al. Relationship between age-adjusted heart rate and anaerobic threshold in estimating exercise intensity in diabetics. Diabetes Res Clin Pract 8:69–74, 1990.

74. Foster C, Jacobson MM, Pollock ML. Exercise for the diabetic patient. In: Pollock ML, Schmidt DH (eds). Heart Disease and Rehabilitation. 2nd ed. New York, John Wiley & Sons, 1986.

75. Leon AS. Patients with diabetes mellitus. In: Franklin BA, et al. (eds). Exercise in Modern Medicine. Baltimore, Williams & Wilkins, 1989.

76. Clements RS Jr, Bell DSH. Diabetic neuropathy—Peripheral and autonomic syndromes. Postgrad Med 71:50–67, 1982.

77. Ewing DJ. Cardiac autonomic neuropathy. In: Jarrett RL (ed). Diabetes and Heart Disease. New York, Elsevier Science Publishers BV, 1984.

78. Sweny P, Farrington K, Moorhead JF. The Kidney and Its Disorders. Oxford, Blackwell Scientific Publications, 1989.

79. O'Rourke RA, Brenner BM, Stein JH (eds). The Heart and Renal Disease. New York, Churchill Livingstone, 1984.

80. Jahn HA, Schohn DC, Schmitt RL. The heart in renal disease. In: Cheng TO (ed). The International Textbook of Cardiology. New York, Pergamon Press, 1986, pp 988–1009.

81. Gutman RA, Stead WW, Robinson RR. Physical activity and employment status of patients on maintenance dialysis. N Engl J Med 304:309–313, 1981.

82. Goldberg AP, Geltman EM, Gavin JR III, et al. Exercise training reduces coronary risk and effectively rehabilitates hemodialysis patients. Nephron 42:311–316, 1986.

83. Harter HR, Goldberg AP. Endurance exercise training—An effective therapeutic modality for hemodialysis patients. Med Clin North Am 69:159–175, 1985

84. Painter PL, Nelson-Worel JN, Hill MM, et al. Effects of exercise training during hemodialysis. Nephron 43:87–92, 1986.

85. Shalom R, Blumenthal JA, Williams RS, et al. Feasibility and benefits of exercise training in patients on maintenance dialysis. Kidney Int 25:958–963, 1984.

86. Zabetakis PM, Gleim GW, Pasternack FL, et al. Long-duration submaximal exercise conditioning in hemodialysis patients. Clin Nephrol 18:17–22, 1982.

87. Hanson P, Ward A, Painter P. Exercise training for special patient populations. J Cardiopulmonary Rehabil 6:104–112, 1986.

88. Kettner A, Goldberg A, Hagberg J, et al. Cardiovascular and metabolic responses to submaximal exercise in hemodialysis patients. Kidney Int 26:66–71, 1984

89. Goldberg AP, Geltman EM, Hagberg JM, et al. Therapeutic benefits of exercise training for hemodialysis patients. Kidney Int Suppl 16:303–309, 1983.

90. Ross DL, Grabeau GM, Smith S, et al. Efficacy of exercise for end-stage renal disease patients immediately following high-efficiency hemodialysis: A pilot study. Am J Nephrol 9:376–383, 1989.

91. Burke E, Germaine MJ, Hartzog R, et al. Physiological responses to submaximal exercise in chronic renal failure, on and off hemodialysis. Med Sci Sports Exerc 15:157, 1983 (abstract).

92. Painter P, Messer D, Hanson P, et al. Exercise capacity in hemodialysis, CAPD, and renal transplant patients. Nephron 42:47–51, 1986.

93. Painter P, Zimmerman SW. Exercise in end-stage renal disease. Am J Kidney Dis 7:386–394, 1986.

94. Miller TD, Squires RW, Gau TG, et al. Graded exercise testing and training after renal transplantation: A preliminary study. Mayo Clin Proc 62:773–777, 1987.

95. Scott JP, Hay IFC, Higenbottam TW, et al. Hypertensive exercise responses in ciclosporin-treated normotensive renal transplant recipients. Nephron 56:143–147, 1990.

96. Kallero KS. Mortality and morbidity in patients with intermittent claudication as defined by venous occlusion plethysmography. A ten-year follow-up study. J Chronic Dis 34:455–462, 1981.

97. Eldridge JE, Hossack KF. Patterns of oxygen consumption during exercise testing in peripheral vascular disease. Cardiology 74:236–240, 1987.

98. Hansen JE, Sue DY, Oren A, Wasserman K. Relation of oxygen uptake to work rate in normal men and men with circulatory disorders. Am J Cardiol 59:669–674, 1987.

99. Hiatt WR, Nawaz D, Regensteiner JG, Hossack KF. The evaluation of exercise performance in patients with peripheral vascular disease. J Cardiopulmonary Rehabil 12:525–532, 1988.

100. Boyd CE, Bird PJ, Teates CD, et al. Pain free physical training in intermittent claudication. J Sports Med 24:112–122, 1984.

101. Creasy TS, McMillan PJ, Fletcher EWL, et al. Is percutaneous transluminal angioplasty better than exercise for claudication?—Preliminary results from a prospective randomised trial. Eur J Vasc Surg 4:135–140, 1990.

102. Dahllöff AG, Holm J, Schersten T. Exercise training of patients with intermittent claudication. Scand J Rehabil Med Suppl 9:20–26, 1983.

103. Hiatt WR, Regensteinier JG, Hargarten ME, et al. Benefit of exercise conditioning for patients with peripheral arterial disease. Circulation 81:602–609, 1990.

104. Jonason T, Ringqvist I, Öman-Rydberg A. Home-training of patients with intermittent claudication. Scand J Rehabil Med 13:137–141, 1981.

105. Larsen OA, Lassen NA. Effect of daily muscular exercise in patients with intermittent claudication. Lancet 2:1093–1095, 1966.

106. Mannarino E, Pasqualini L, Menna M, et al. Effects of physical training on peripheral vascular disease: A controlled study. Angiology 40:5–10, 1989.

107. Ruell PA, Imperial ES, Bonar FJ, et al. Intermittent claudication—The effect of physical training on walking tolerance and venous lactate concentration. Eur J Appl Physiol 52:420–425, 1984.

108. Ersnt E, Matrai I. Intermittent claudication, exercise and blood rheology. Circulation 76:1110–1114, 1987.

109. Schteingart DE. Obesity. In: Kelley WN (ed-in-chief).

110. Pi-Sunyer FX. Obesity. In: Wyngaarden JB, Smith LH (eds). Cecil Textbook of Medicine. 18th ed. Philadelphia, WB Saunders, 1988, pp 1219–1228.

111. Vobecky JS, Vobecky J, Shapcott D, Demers P-P. Nutrient intake patterns and nutritional status with regard to relative weight in early infancy. Am J Clin Nutr 38:730–738, 1983.

112. Rolland-Cachera M-F, Deheeger M, Pequignot F, et al. Adiposity and food intake in young children: The environmental challenge to individual susceptibility. Br Med J 296:1037–1038, 1988.

113. Hampton MC, Huenemann RL, Shapiro LR, Mitchell BW. Caloric and nutrient intakes of teen-agers. J Am Diet Assoc 50:385–396, 1967.

114. Braitman LE, Aldin EV, Stanton JL. Obesity and caloric intake: The National Health and Nutrition Examination Survey of 1971–1975 (HANES I). J Chronic Dis 38:727–732, 1985.

115. Lincoln JE. Caloric intake, obesity, and physical activity. Am J Clin Nutr 25:390–394, 1972.

116. Maxfield E, Konish F. Patterns of food intake and physical activity in obesity. J Am Diet Assoc 49:406–408, 1966.

117. Miller WC, Lindeman AK, Wallace J, Niederpruem ST. Diet composition, energy intake, and exercise in relation to body fatness in men and women. Am J Clin Nutr 52:426–430, 1990.

118. Oscai LB, Brown MM, Miller WC. Effect of dietary fat on food intake, growth, and body composition in rats. Growth 48:415–424, 1984.

119. Oscai LB, Miller WC, Arnall DA. Effect of dietary sugar and of dietary fat on food intake and body fat composition in rats. Growth 51:64–73, 1987.

120. Fordyce-Baum MK, Langer LM, Mantero-Atienza E, et al. Use of an expanded-whole-wheat product in the reduction of body weight and serum lipids in obese females. Am J Clin Nutr 50:30–36, 1989.

121. Miller WC. Diet composition, energy intake, and nutritional status in relation to obesity in men and women. Med Sci Sports Exerc 23:280–284, 1991.

122. Rossner S, Zweigbergk DV, Ohlin A, Ryttig K. Weight reduction with dietary fibre supplements—Results of two double-blinded randomized studies Acta Med Scand 222:83–88, 1987.

123. Bjorntorp P, Yang M. Refeeding after fasting in the rat: Effect on body composition and food efficiency. Am J Clin Nutr 36:444–449, 1982.

124. Blackburn GL, Wilson GT, Kanders BS, et al. Weight cycling: The experience of human dieters. Am J Clin Nutr 49:1105–1109, 1989.

125. National Institutes of Health Concensus Development Panel on the Health Implications of Obesity. Health implications of obesity. Ann Intern Med 103:147–151, 1985.

126. Keys A. Overweight, obesity, coronary heart disease and mortality. Nutr Rev 38:297–307, 1980.

127. Sorlie P, Gordon T, Kannel WB. Body build and mortality: The Framingham study. JAMA 243:1818–1831, 1980.

128. Alexander JK. The cardiomyopathy of obesity. Prog Cardiovasc Dis 27:325–334, 1985.

129. Alexander JK. Obesity and cardiac performance. Am J Cardiol 14:860–865, 1964.

Textbook of Internal Medicine. Philadelphia, JB Lippincott, 1989.

130. Alexander JK. Obesity and the circulation. Mod Concepts Cardiovasc Dis 32:799–803, 1963.
131. Franklin B, Buskirk E, Hodgson J, et al. Effects of physical conditioning on cardiorespiratory function, body composition and serum lipids in relatively normal-weight and obese middle-aged women. Int J Obes 3:97–109, 1979.
132. Gwinup G. Effect of exercise alone on the weight of obese women. Arch Intern Med 135:676–680, 1975.
133. Kukkonen K, Rauramaa R, Siitonen O, Hänninen O. Physical training of obese middle-aged persons. Ann Clin Res 14(suppl 34):80–85, 1982.
134. Weltman A, Matter S, Stamford BA. Caloric restriction and/or mild exercise: Effects on serum lipids and body composition. Am J Clin Nutr 33:1002–1009, 1980.
135. Warwick PM, Garrow JS. The effect of addition of exercise to a regimen of dietary restriction on weight loss, nitrogen balance, resting metabolic rate and spontaneous physical activity in three obese women in a metabolic ward. Int J Obes 5:25–32, 1981.
136. Hill JO, Sparling PB, Shields TW, Heller PA. Effects of exercise and food restriction on body composition and metabolic rate in obese women. Am J Clin Nutr 46:622–630, 1987.
137. Oscai LB, Holloszky JO. Effects of weight changes produced by exercise, food restriction, or overeating on body composition. J Clin Invest 48:2124–2128, 1969.
138. Pavlou KN, Steffee WP, Lerman RH, Burrows BA. Effects of dieting and exercise on lean body mass, oxygen uptake, and strength. Med Sci Sports Exerc 17:466–471, 1985.
139. Hammer RL, Barrier CA, Roundy ES, et al. Calorie-restricted low-fat diet and exercise in obese women. Am J Clin Nutr 49:77–85, 1989.
140. Van Dale D, Saris WHM, Schoffelen PFM, Hoor FT. Does exercise give an additional effect in weight reduction regimens? Int J Obes 11:367–375, 1987.
141. Pavlou KN, Krey S, Steffee WP. Exercise as an adjunct to weight loss and maintenance in moderately obese subjects. Am J Clin Nutr 49:1115–1123, 1989.
142. Bray GA. Exercise and obesity. In: Bouchard C, Shephard RJ, Stephens T, et al. (eds). Exercise, Fitness, and Health—A Concensus of Current Knowledge. Champaign, Ill, Human Kinetics Books, 1990, pp 497–510.
143. Leon AS, Conrad J, Hunninghake DB, Serfass R. Effects of a vigorous walking program on body composition, and carbohydrate and lipid metabolism of obese young men. Am J Clin Nutr 33:1776–1787, 1979.
144. Chang RW. Cardiac manifestations of SLE. Clin Rheum Dis 8:197–206, 1982.
145. Hoffman BI. Cardiac manifestations. In: Katz WA (ed). Diagnosis and Management of Rheumatic Diseases. 2nd ed. Philadelphia, JB Lippincott, 1988, pp 198–203.
146. Doherty NE, Siegel RJ. Cardiovascular manifestations of systemic lupus erythematosis. Am Heart J 110: 1257–1265, 1985.
147. Cheng TO (ed). The International Textbook of Cardiology. New York, Pergamon Press, 1986.
148. Hurst JW, Schlant RC (eds). The Heart, Arteries and Veins. 7th ed. New York, McGraw-Hill Information Services, 1990.
149. Scoggin CH. Pulmonary manifestations. In: Katz WA (ed). Diagnosis and Management of Rheumatic Diseases. 2nd ed. Philadelphia, JB Lippincott, 1988, pp 204–210.
150. Segal AM, Calabrese LH, Ahmed M, et al. The pulmonary manifestations of systemic lupus erythematosus. Semin Arthritis Rheum 14:202–224, 1985.
151. Dickey BF, Myers AR. Pulmonary manifestations of collagen-vascular diseases. In: Fishman AP (ed). Pulmonary Diseases and Disorders. New York, McGraw-Hill, 1988, pp 645–666.
152. Gray IR. Cardiovascular manifestations of collagen vascular disease. In: Julian DG (ed). Diseases of the Heart. Toronto, Baillière Tindall, 1989, pp 1397–1403.
153. Wolff SM. Polyarteritis nodosa group. In Wyngaarden JB, Smith LH (eds). Cecil Textbook of Medicine. 18th ed. Philadelphia, WB Saunders, 1988, pp 2028–2030.
154. Katz WA (ed). Diagnosis and Management of Rheumatic Diseases. 2nd ed. Philadelphia, JB Lippincott, 1988.
155. Fishman AP (ed). Pulmonary Diseases and Disorders. New York, McGraw-Hill, 1988.
156. Goldman AP, Kotler MN. Heart disease in scleroderma. Am Heart J 110:1043–1046, 1985.
157. LeRoy EC. Scleroderma (systemic sclerosis). In: Kelly WN, Harris ED Jr, Ruddy S, Sledge CB (eds): Textbook of Rheumatology. 2nd ed. Philadelphia, WB Saunders, 1985, pp 1183–1205.
158. Celli BR, Rassulo J, Corral R. Ventilatory muscle dysfunction in patients with bilateral idiopathic diaphragmatic paralysis: Reversal by intermittent external negative pressure ventilation. Am Rev Respir Dis 136:567–585, 1986.
159. Prakash UBS. Neurological diseases. In: Baum GL, Wolinsky E (eds). Textbook of Pulmonary Diseases. Boston, Little, Brown, 1989, pp 1409–1435.
160. Chimowitz MI, Mancini GBJ. Asymptomatic coronary artery disease in patients with stroke—Prevalence prognosis, diagnosis, and treatment. Curr Concepts of Cerebrovasc Dis Stroke (American Heart Assoc.) 26:23–27, 1991.
161. Hertser NR, Young JR, Beven EG, et al. Coronary angiography in 506 patients with extracranial cerebrovascular disease. Arch Intern Med 145:849–852, 1985.
162. Bradley WG, Daroff RB, Fenichel GM, Marsden CD (eds). Neurology in Clinical Practice. Boston, Butterworth-Heinemann, 1991.
163. Massery M. Respiratory rehabilitation secondary to neurological deficits: Understanding the deficits. In: Frownfelter DL. Chest Physical Therapy and Pulmonary Rehabilitation, An Interdisciplinary Approach. 2nd ed. Chicago, Year Book Medical Publishers, 1987, pp 499–528.
164. Nev HC, Connolly JJ, Schwertley FW, et al. Obstructive, respiratory dysfunction in parkinsonian patients. Am Rev Respir Dis 95:33–47, 1967.
165. Mehta AD, Wright WB, Kirby B. Ventilatory function in Parkinson's disease. Br Med J 1:1456–1457, 1978.
166. Bateman DN, Cooper RG, Gibson GJ, et al. Levodopa dosage and ventilatory function in pulmonary disease. Br Med J 283:190–191, 1980.
167. Nakano KK, Bass H, Tyler H, Carmel RJ. Amyotrophic lateral sclerosis: A study of pulmonary function. Dis Nerv System 37:32–35, 1976.
168. Gracey DR, McMichan JC, Divertie MB, Howard FM Jr. Respiratory failure in Guillain-Barré syndrome: A 6-year experience. Mayo Clin Proc 57:742–746, 1982.
169. Gibson TC. The heart in myasthenia gravis. Am Heart J 90:389–396, 1975.

170. Perloff JK. Cardiac involvement in heredofamilial neuromyopathic diseases. Cardiovasc Clin 4:333–344, 1972.
171. Perloff JK, DeLeon AC, O'Doherty D. The cardiomyopathy of progressive muscular dystrophy. Circulation 33:625–648, 1966.
172. Schaumburg HH. Diseases of the peripheral nervous system. In: Wyngaarden JB, Smith LH (eds). Cecil Textbook of Medicine. 18th ed. Philadelphia, WB Saunders, 1988, pp 2258–2268.
173. Moorman JR, Coleman RE, Packer DL, et al. Cardiac involvement in myotonic muscular dystrophy. Medicine 64:371–387, 1985.
174. Perloff JK, Stevenson WG, Roberts NK, et al. Cardiac involvement in myotonic muscular dystrophy (Steinert's disease): A prospective study of 25 patients. Am J Cardiol 54:1074–1081, 1984.
175. Harding AE, Hewer RL. The heart disease of Friedreich's ataxia: A clinical and electrocardiographic study of 115 patients, with an analysis of serial electrocardiographic changes in 30 cases. Q J Med 208:489–502, 1983.
176. Pentland B, Fox KAA. The heart in Friedreich's ataxia. J Neurol Neurosurg Psychiatry 46:1138–1142, 1983.
177. Stover DE. Pulmonary toxicity. In: DeVita VT, Hellman S, Rosenberg SA (eds). Cancer—Principles and Practice of Oncology. 3rd ed. Philadelphia, JB Lippincott, 1989, pp 2162–2169.
178. Torti FM, Lum BL. Cardiac toxicity. In: DeVita VT, Hellman S, Rosenberg SA (eds). Cancer—Principles and Practice of Oncology. 3rd ed. Philadelphia, JB Lippincott, 1989, pp 2153–2162.
179. Watchie J, Coleman CN, Raffin TA, et al. Minimal long-term cardiopulmonary dysfunction following treatment for Hodgkin's disease. Int J Radiat Oncol Biol Phys 13:517–524, 1987.
180. Carmel RJ, Kaplan HS. Mantle irradiation in Hodgkin's disease—An analysis of technique, tumor irradiation and complications. Cancer 37:2813–2825, 1976.
181. Myers CE, Kinsella TJ. Cardiac and pulmonary toxicity. In: DeVita VT, Hellman S, Rosenberg SA (eds). Cancer—Principles and Practice of Oncology. 2nd ed. Philadelphia, JB Lippincott, 1985, pp 2022–2032.
182. Praga C, Beretta G, Vigo PL, et al. Adriamycin cardiotoxicity: A survey of 1273 patients. Cancer Treat Rep 63:827–834, 1979.
183. Pratt CB, Ransom JL, Evans WE. Age-related Adriamycin cardiotoxicity in children. Cancer Treat Rep 62:1381–1384, 1978.
184. Haupt HM, Hutchins GM, Moore GW. Ara-C lung: Noncardiogenic pulmonary edema complicating cytosine arabinoside therapy of leukemia. Am J Med 70:256–261, 1981.
185. Braunwald E (ed). Heart Disease—A Textbook of Cardiovascular Medicine. 3rd ed. Philadelphia, WB Saunders, 1988.
186. Hellenbrand W, Brown J, Covitz W, et al. Cardiovascular performance in sickle cell disease. Circulation 68(suppl 3):163, 1983.
187. Kupari M, Volin L, Soukas A, et al. Cardiac involvement in bone marrow transplantation: Electrocardiographic changes, arrhythmias, heart failure and autopsy findings. Bone Marrow Transplant 5:91–98, 1990.
188. Bearman SI, Petersen FB, Schor RA, et al. Radionuclide ejection fractions in the evaluation of patients being considered for bone marrow transplantation: Risk for cardiac toxicity. Bone Marrow Transplant 5:173–177, 1990.
189. Steinherz LJ, Steinherz PG, Tan CTC, et al. Cardiac toxicity 4 to 20 years after completing anthracycline therapy. JAMA 266:1672–1677, 1991.
190. Stover DE, White DA, Romano PA, et al. Spectrum of pulmonary diseases associated with the acquired immune deficiency syndrome. Am J Med 78:429–437, 1985.
191. Silver MA, Macher AM, Reichert CM, et al. Cardiac involvement by Kaposi's sarcoma in acquired immune deficiency syndrome (AIDS). Am J Cardiol 53:983–985, 1984.
192. Gallantino ML. Cardiopulmonary complications in AIDS patients. In: Payton O (ed). Manual of Physical Therapy. New York, Churchill Livingstone, 1989, pp 685–695.
193. Matthews EC Jr, Gardin JM, Henry WL, et al. Echocardiographic abnormalities in chronic alcoholics with and without overt congestive heart failure. Am J Cardiol 47:570–578, 1981.
194. Schwartz D, Thompson M. Do anorectics get well? Current research and future needs. Am J Psychiatry 138:319–323, 1981.
195. Moodie DS. Anorexia and the heart. Postgrad Med 82:46–61, 1987.
196. Casper RC. The pathophysiology of anorexia nervosa and bulimia nervosa. Ann Rev Nutr 6:299–316, 1986.
197. Schocken DD, Holloway JD, Powers PS. Weight loss and the heart—Effects of anorexia nervosa and starvation. Arch Intern Med 149:877–881, 1989.

Suggested General Readings

Bouchard C, Shephard RJ, Stephens T, et al. (eds). Exercise, Fitness, and Health—A Concensus of Current Knowledge. Champaign, Ill, Human Kinetics Books, 1990.
Julian DG, Camm AJ, Fox KM, et al. (eds). Diseases of the Heart. Toronto, Baillière Tindall, 1989.
Kelley WN (ed-in-chief). Textbook of Internal Medicine. Philadelphia: JB Lippincott, 1989.
Wasserman K. Cardiopulmonary limitations in exercise. In: Cheng TO (ed). The International Textbook of Cardiology. New York, Pergamon Press, 1986, pp 1088–1097.
Wilson JD, Braunwald E, Isselbacher KJ, et al. (eds). Harrison's Principles of Internal Medicine. 12th ed. New York, McGraw-Hill, 1991.
Wyngaarden JB, Smith LH (eds). Cecil Textbook of Medicine. 18th ed. Philadelphia, WB Saunders, 1988.

SECTION 3

DIAGNOSTIC TESTS AND PROCEDURES, SURGICAL INTERVENTIONS, MONITORING AND SUPPORT EQUIPMENT

8 CARDIAC TESTS AND PROCEDURES

INTRODUCTION

Objective information on the patient's cardiovascular system is derived from data obtained from laboratory studies and from diagnostic tests and procedures. Physical therapists must be able to identify and interpret the results of medical tests and procedures to enable them to assess the status of their patients' cardiovascular systems. This chapter provides the basis for an understanding of the importance and impact of medical tests that may be ordered to facilitate the achievement of a correct diagnosis, aid in the prevention of complications, develop information to determine a prognosis, identify subclinical disease states, and assist in the monitoring of the progress of treatments.

The tests and procedures that are discussed in this chapter include specific laboratory studies (e.g., for cardiac enzymes, cholesterol and triglycerides, and complete blood count), **echocardiography, Holter monitoring,** exercise testing, **coronary angiography** and **ventriculography, ergonovine stimulation, positron-emission tomography (PET),** and **multigated acquisition or angiogram (MUGA) imaging.** Electrocardiography is a separate diagnostic evaluation that is covered in Chapter 9.

327

CLINICAL LABORATORY STUDIES

Laboratory studies provide important information regarding the clinical status of the patient. The laboratory tests that are specific to the patient with cardiac dysfunction measure the serum enzymes, blood lipids (triglycerides and cholesterol), complete blood count, **coagulation** profile (prothrombin time), electrolyte levels, **blood urea nitrogen (BUN)** and **creatinine** levels, and serum glucose levels.

Serum Enzymes

Evaluation of specific serum enzyme levels contributes to a definitive diagnosis of myocardial necrosis and in some cases to an assessment of the degree of myocardial damage or the effectiveness of **reperfusion**. When damage has occurred to the myocardial tissue, cellular integrity is lost and intracellular cardiac enzymes are released into the circulation. These enzymes are released at a variable rate and are cleared by the kidney and other organs. Their presence can be measured by serum blood tests. However, owing to their variable release and clearing rate, their absence does not rule out the possibility of myocardial injury.

The enzymes that are diagnostic of cardiac injury include

- **creatine phosphokinase (CPK)**
- **lactic dehydrogenase (LDH)**
- **aspartate aminotransferase (AST)** (formerly called SGOT)

More specifically, **isoenzymes,** which are different chemical forms of the same enzyme, have been found to be most conclusive of specific muscle cell necrosis. Creatine phosphokinase has three isoenzymes (MB, MM, BB), of which the CPK-MB fraction is most conclusive for myocardial injury (MM is most conclusive for skeletal muscle damage and BB for brain injury). CPK-MB is considered abnormal if its serum level is greater than 3% (Table 8–1).[1] Serial CPK-MB levels have been correlated with infarct size and prognosis. However, CPK-MB may also be ele-

TABLE 8–1. Cardiac Enzymes			
	Normal Serum Level Values (IU)*	Onset of Rise (hr)	Time of Peak Rise (hr)	Return to Normal (days)
---	---	---	---	---
CPK	55–71†	3–4	33	3
LDH	127‡	12–24	72	5–14
SGOT	24	12	24	4

*1 IU is the amount of enzyme that will catalyze the formation of 1 μmol of substrate per minute under the conditions of the test.
†CPK MB, 0%–3%
‡LDH-1, 14%–26%
(Reprinted from Smith AM, Theirer JA, Huang SH. Serum enzymes in myocardial infarction. Am J Nurs 73[2]:277, 1973. Used with permission. All rights reserved. Copyright 1973 The American Journal of Nursing Company.)

vated after cardiac surgery and cardiopulmonary resuscitation (especially if the person was **defibrillated**) and has been found to be abnormally elevated in patients undergoing **thrombolysis** with **streptokinase** (see Chapter 12) or **tissue plasminogen activator.**[2]

Lactic dehydrogenase has five isoenzymes, of which LDH-1 is most conclusive for myocardial injury. Normally LDH-2 exceeds LDH-1 activity. Myocardial infarction results in LDH-1 activity exceeding LDH-2.[1] More specifically, a ratio of LDH-1 to LDH-2 that is greater than 1.0 is strongly suggestive of myocardial infarction. The other LDH isoenzymes are increased with heart failure, renal failure, and the like.

Enzyme and isoenzyme levels increase within the first 36 hours after myocardial injury, reaching their individual peaks at different rates (see Table 8–1).[3] Investigation indicates that marked elevation in CPK enzyme levels occurs whenever thrombolytic medications (e.g., streptokinase and tPa) are used to lyse clots. Clinically, an early or a secondary peak in CPK levels followed by a more rapid decline in the CPK-MB levels is strongly suggestive of reperfusion after thrombolytic therapy.[4]

Blood Lipids

Elevation in blood lipid levels (**hyperlipidemia**) is considered a major risk factor contributing to coronary artery disease.[5] The concentrations of serum cholesterol and triglycerides are the blood lipids of concern. The American Heart Association defines elevated blood cholesterol levels as being higher than 200 milligrams per 100 milliliters; however, the more stringent recommendations suggested by Castelli define 180 milligrams per 100 milliliters as the upper end of normal.[6] Elevated cholesterol levels are associated with ingestion of excess amounts of saturated fat and cholesterol as well as with hereditary influences. Elevated triglyceride levels are defined as being higher than 150 milligrams per 100 milliliters. Elevated triglyceride levels are associated with increased carbohydrate ingestion and often preclude diabetes mellitus. Often, measurements of cholesterol and triglyceride levels that are taken at the time of acute injury are inaccurate. Such measurements are most accurate when obtained before a myocardial injury or a few weeks after an injury.

Clinical laboratory reports are improved by giving a breakdown of the component parts of the total cholesterol. Current information now lists the **high-density lipoprotein (HDL)** and **low-density lipoprotein (LDL)** levels as well as the ratio of total cholesterol to HDL. Research has shown that the absolute values of total cholesterol or HDL cholesterol are of less importance than the ratio of total cholesterol to HDL cholesterol in establishing an individual's relative risk for developing coronary artery disease (Table 8–2). An increased ratio of total cholesterol to HDL cholesterol identifies a person at an increased risk for development of coronary artery disease.[7] High levels of LDL (higher than 130 mg/100 ml) also increase a person's relative risk of developing coronary artery disease.

Complete Blood Count

The physical therapist should evaluate the complete blood count for three components: hemoglobin and hematocrit values and white blood cell count. Hemoglobin plays a major role in the transport of oxygen throughout the body, and the hematocrit (the amount of the blood that is cells) is a significant indicator of the viscosity of the blood. Hemoglobin values are reported as a

TABLE 8–2. Total Cholesterol to High-Density Lipoprotein (HDL) Cholesterol Values

Total Cholesterol/HDL	Risk of Heart Disease
Men	
3.43	½ Average
4.97	Average
9.55	2× Average
23.39	3× Average
Women	
3.27	½ Average
4.44	Average
7.05	2× Average
11.04	3× Average

(Reproduced with permission from Gordon T, Castelli WP, Hjortland MC, et al. Diabetes, blood lipids, and the role of obesity in coronary heart disease risk for women. Ann Intern Med 87:393, 1977.)

concentration in the blood (in grams per 100 milliliters of blood). The normal range of hemoglobin for females is 12 to 16 grams per 100 milliliters, and for males it is 14 to 18 grams per 100 milliliters.[1] Low levels of hemoglobin cause the myocardium to work harder to transport adequate oxygen to the tissues (even when the body is at rest) by increasing the cardiac output. The lower limit value for hematocrit is 37 grams per 100 milliliters for females and 42 grams per 100 milliliters for males.[1] Elevated hematocrit levels suggest that the flow of blood to the tissues may be impeded because of an increase in the viscosity of the blood. Elevated levels of white blood cells indicate that the body is responding to infection.

Coagulation Profiles

Coagulation profiles have become an important component of the patient's record because of the use of thrombolytic agents to dissolve clots in the early stages of infarction. **Prothrombin time** and **partial thromboplastin time** measure the coagulation of the blood. Streptokinase or tissue plasminogen activator infusion is a means of dissolving clots that may block a coronary artery and induce a myocardial infarction.

These thrombolytic agents are most commonly administered intravenously but can also be injected directly into the coronary arteries. After the initial infusion of thrombolytics is begun, an intravenous infusion of heparin is started. As a result, prothrombin time and partial thromboplastin time must be monitored closely to determine the therapeutic ranges of anticoagulation.[1]

Electrolytes

All electrolyte levels should be observed when evaluating the laboratory results because disturbances in the electrolytes may affect the patient's performance. Sodium (Na^+), potassium (K^+), and carbon dioxide (CO_2) are the most important electrolytes to monitor. Hydration state, medications, and disease can affect these values. Patients receiving diuretics (e.g., for hypertension, heart failure) should have their sodium and potassium levels monitored carefully, because some diuretics act on the kidney at sites in the renal tubules and collecting ducts where these electrolytes are allowed to diffuse out to or are absorbed back from the blood stream. Dangerously low levels of potassium (<3.5 mEq/L) can cause serious, life-threatening arrhythmias. Dangerously high levels of potassium (>5.0 mEq/L) can affect the contractility of the myocardium. Low levels of carbon dioxide can cause an **alkalotic** state, muscle weakness, and dizziness.[1]

Blood Urea Nitrogen and Creatinine

The BUN and creatinine values can be found on the same laboratory form as that reporting the electrolytes and cholesterol. The normal range for the BUN is 8 to 23 milligrams per deciliter; an elevated BUN can be an indication of heart failure or renal failure. The BUN value is unsuitable as a single measure of renal function, and therefore the creatinine value should also be noted. Normal serum creatinine levels are lower than 1.5 milligrams per deciliter. The BUN to creatinine ratio is often used to differentiate renal failure, with a ratio of more than 15 considered to be abnormal.

Serum Glucose

Lastly, serum glucose is measured when a typical laboratory sample of blood is collected. The normal value for serum glucose is 120 milligrams per 100 milliliters of blood. If this level is elevated, it indicates a surplus of glucose in the blood. An elevated serum glucose value is suggestive of a **prediabetic** state and warrants further testing for diabetes, such as the administration of a **glucose tolerance test.**

ECHOCARDIOGRAPHY

Echocardiography is a noninvasive procedure that uses pulses of reflected ultrasound to evaluate the functioning heart. A transducer that houses a special crystal emits high-frequency sound waves and receives their echoes when placed on the chest of the patient. The returning echoes, reflected from a variety of intracardiac surfaces, are displayed on the ultrasonographic equipment.

Echocardiography has an advantage over other cardiac diagnostic tests because the technique is completely noninvasive. The transducer is placed in the third to fifth intercostal space near the left sternal border. The transducer is then tilted at various angles so that the sound waves can scan the segments of the heart (Fig. 8–1).

Important information can be obtained from the echocardiogram, including the size of the ventricular cavity, the thickness and integrity of the interatrial and interventricular septums, the functioning of the valves, and the motions of individual segments of the ventricular wall. Assessment of the performance of the heart muscle itself, especially the regional functioning of the left ventricle, is a valuable application of echocardiography as is an evaluation of a variety of signs and symptoms. Echocardiography can quantify volumes of the left ventricle, estimate an ejection fraction, and analyze motion of the

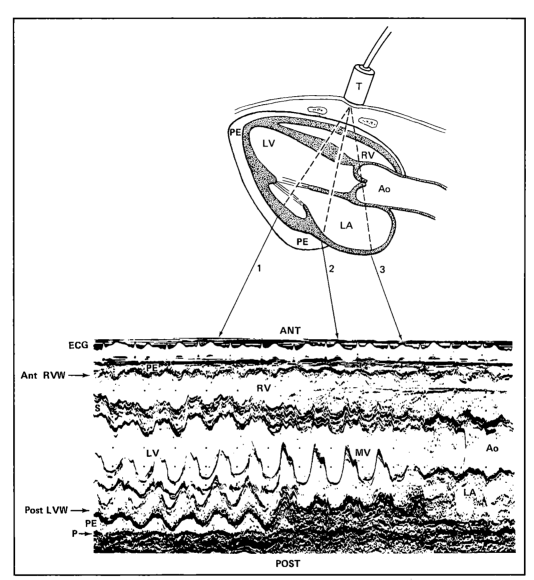

Figure 8-1.

Echocardiography is a noninvasive diagnostic tool in which the transducer is placed directly over the heart. The scan through the heart is depicted in *A*. The echocardiographic movement patterns that arise from the corresponding anatomic structures are illustrated in *B*. LV, left ventricle; PE, pericardial effusion; T, transducer; RV, right ventricle; Ao, aorta, LA, left atrium; ANT, anterior; ECG, electrocardiogram; Ant RVW, anterior right ventricular wall; MV, mitral valve; Post LVW, posterior left ventricular wall; POST, posterior; P, pericardium. (Adapted from Sokolow M, McIlroy M, Cheitlin M, et al. Clinical Cardiology. 5th ed. East Norwalk, Conn, Appleton & Lange, 1990, p 96.)

valves and the heart muscle. Specific problems that can be evaluated with the echocardiogram include

- **pericardial effusion**
- **cardiac tamponade**
- **idiopathic congestive cardiomyopathy**
- hypertrophic cardiomyopathy
- mitral valve regurgitation
- mitral valve prolapse
- aortic regurgitation
- aortic stenosis
- vegetation on the valves
- intracardiac masses
- ischemic heart muscle
- left ventricular aneurysm
- ventricular thrombi
- proximal coronary disease
- congenital heart disease

Problems exist with the image quality of standard echocardiograms owing to such confounding factors as pulmonary disease, obesity, and chest deformities. A new technique called **transesophageal echocardiography** has solved these problems and allows an improved view of the heart and mediastinum to be examined. Transesophageal echocardiography allows for improved visualization of cardiac structures and function and is valuable in the intraoperative and perioperative monitoring of left ventricular performance as well as the evaluation of surgical results.[8-11]

Two-dimensional echocardiographic studies during exercise, immediately after exercise, or both is a current noninvasive method to evaluate ischemia-induced wall motion abnormalities. In addition to treadmill or bicycle exercise, atrial pacing or the use of pharmacologic agents provides an "artificial exercise" situation from which two-dimensional echocardiographic studies can identify the presence and location of ischemia-induced abnormalities in the ventricular wall.[12]

HOLTER MONITORING

Holter monitoring consists of continuous 24-hour electrocardiographic monitoring of a patient's heart rhythm, which is essential to the diagnosis and management of episodes of cardiac arrhythmias and corresponding symptoms. Holter monitoring tracings must be reliable to capture, recognize, and reproduce any abnormality in heart rhythm, particularly those that threaten life or cardiac hemodynamics.

Indications for use of the Holter monitor include identifying symptoms possibly caused by arrhythmias (e.g., dizziness, **syncope,** shortness of breath at rest as well as with activity), describing the arrhythmias noted with activity (frequency and severity), and evaluating antiarrhythmia therapy and pacemaker functioning. A

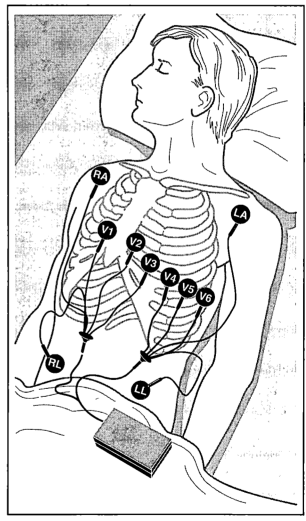

Figure 8-2.

Holter monitoring is transcutaneous, with multiple leads to record heart rhythm for 24 hours.

common practice is to perform Holter monitoring routinely before discharging any patient who has had a myocardial infarction, because arrhythmias are commonly associated with coronary disease, ischemia, and injury.

The patient's heart rhythm is monitored by means of a transcutaneous tape recorder applied to the patient's chest wall via multiple leads and electrodes (Fig. 8–2). The patient wears the Holter monitor for 24 hours while performing normal activities (except bathing). All of the patient's activities as well as any symptoms that may be felt during the 24 hours are documented by the patient. Once the recorder is removed from the patient, the tape is processed by reproducing the recording on computer or paper for visual inspection. The physician then interprets the results and plans the treatment accordingly. Repeat Holter monitoring may be necessary once treatment has been initiated to evaluate the effectiveness of the treatment.

It is the responsibility of the physical therapist working with a patient who is wearing or has worn a Holter monitor to obtain the interpretation of the results of the Holter monitor to determine if modifications are needed in the patient's activities. For example, patients with life-threatening arrhythmias recorded by the Holter monitor should not begin physical therapy activity until treatment for the arrhythmia is initiated or modified. Increasing frequency of arrhythmias or more serious (life-threatening) arrhythmias developing with activity also require further evaluation by the physician.[13]

EXERCISE TESTING

Exercise testing is a noninvasive method of measuring cardiovascular and pulmonary responses to increased activity. Originally exercise testing was used to measure functional capacity or to evaluate abnormalities of coronary circulation. Currently exercise testing is used for a variety of patient management problems, including

- evaluation of chest pain suggestive of coronary disease
- evaluation of **atypical chest pain**

- determination of prognosis and severity of coronary artery disease
- evaluation of the effects of medical or surgical therapy or intervention
- evaluation of arrhythmias
- evaluation of hypertension with activity
- assessment of **functional capacity**
- screening to provide an exercise prescription
- providing motivation for a lifestyle change to reduce the risk of developing coronary artery disease

Exercise testing involves systematically and progressively increasing the oxygen demand and evaluating the responses to the increased demand. The technique varies with different modes of exercise chosen and different protocols used by the examiner. Formal exercise testing involves the following modes of exercise:

- walking up and down steps
- exercising on a stationary bicycle
- using arm or wheelchair ergometry
- walking or jogging on a treadmill at variable speeds and inclines

Informal testing is performed to screen for exercise programs, sometimes on a group basis, and includes such tests as the 12-minute walk, Cooper's 12-minute run, the pulse recovery test, or the 1.5-mile run (Fig. 8–3).[14–16]

Safety is a key consideration in exercise testing, and among the most important determinants of safety are the knowledge and experience of the examiner conducting the test. The American College of Sports Medicine has published guidelines that document the knowledge and skills required for exercise testing, including a description of situations in which the involvement or presence of a physician during testing may be necessary.[17] Ellestad and Stuart published a survey of more than 500,000 exercise tests, which suggested an overall mortality rate of 0.5 per 10,000 tests and a morbidity rate of 9 per 10,000.[18]

Exercise testing by nonphysician health care professionals has been performed for more than 30 years, although the American Heart Association Committee on Stress Testing did not endorse the idea of "experienced paramedical personnel" as able to perform the tests until 1979.[19] In 1987 Cahalin published a report on the safety of test-

12-Minute Walking/Running Test
(distance (miles) covered in 12 minutes)

Fitness Category		Age (years)					
		13–19	20–29	30–39	40–49	50–59	60+
I. Very poor	(men)	<1.30*	<1.22	<1.18	<1.14	<1.03	<.87
	(women)	<1.0	<0.96	<0.94	<0.88	<0.84	<.78
II. Poor	(men)	1.30–1.37	1.22–1.31	1.18–1.30	1.14–1.24	1.03–1.16	0.87–1.02
	(women)	1.00–1.18	0.96–1.11	0.95–1.05	0.88–0.98	0.84–0.93	0.78–0.86
III. Fair	(men)	1.38–1.56	1.32–1.49	1.31–1.45	1.25–1.39	1.17–1.30	1.03–1.20
	(women)	1.19–1.29	1.12–1.22	1.06–1.18	.99–1.11	0.94–1.05	0.87–0.98
IV. Good	(men)	1.57–1.72	1.50–1.64	1.46–1.56	1.40–1.53	1.31–1.44	1.21–1.32
	(women)	1.30–1.43	1.23–1.34	1.19–1.29	1.12–1.24	1.06–1.18	0.99–1.09
V. Excellent	(men)	1.73–1.86	1.65–1.76	1.57–1.69	1.54–1.65	1.45–1.58	1.33–1.55
	(women)	1.44–1.51	1.35–1.45	1.30–1.39	1.25–1.34	1.19–1.30	1.10–1.18
VI. Superior	(men)	>1.87	>1.77	>1.70	>1.66	>1.59	>1.56
	(women)	>1.52	>1.46	>1.40	>1.35	>1.31	>1.19

Figure 8–3.

The 12-minute walk/run test, which identifies fitness category for the distance covered in 12 minutes. (From Cooper K. The Aerobic Ways. New York, Bantam Books, 1981.)

ing as performed by physical therapists with advanced clinical competence (see Performance Evaluation for Independent Exercise Testing).[20] In 10,577 tests performed, the mortality rate was 0.9 per 10,000 and the morbidity rate was 3.8 per 10,000.

Factors that enhance the safety of exercise testing include the use of an informed consent to be signed by the patient (Fig. 8–4), the knowledge of when to exclude a patient from proceeding with an exercise test, the knowledge of when to terminate an exercise test, the knowledge and skills to react to an abnormal response or situation, and the availability of appropriate equipment and supplies to manage an emergency (e.g., **defibrillator,** emergency medications, **intubation,** suctioning equipment).

Physical therapists wishing to conduct exercise tests on individuals older than 40 years or on persons who are at moderate to high risk of developing coronary artery disease should expect to obtain the required knowledge and skills in advanced training or in clinically supervised post-professional education. However, all physical therapists should understand the procedures involved in exercise testing and interpretation of the test results because one of the major purposes of these tests is the development of exercise prescriptions. Exercise prescriptions are

based on the results of the exercise test and other pertinent information (see Performance Evaluation for Independent Exercise Testing).

Exercise Testing Equipment

Clinical monitoring tools used during exercise testing traditionally include continuous electrocardiographic monitoring, periodic blood pressure and heart rate (this can be extracted from the electrocardiogram [ECG] recording; see Chapter 9), patient reported or demonstrated symptoms, and heart and lung sounds. In some testing laboratories expired gas analysis permits the assessment of oxygen uptake during the test (Fig. 8–5). Multiple-lead ECG monitoring is used to depict the electrical activity of the heart. Detection of both arrhythmias and ischemia can be made from the ECG. A detailed discussion of the interpretation of ECG data and a description of arrhythmias are presented in Chapter 9.

Protocols for Exercise Testing

Most institutions adopt a standard protocol to facilitate comparisons of the test subject's re-

Performance Evaluation for Independent Exercise Testing

	Points	Score		Points	Score
I. Pretest Preparation and Assessment of Patient			E. Makes correct decision regarding need for post-test follow-up of patient	10	—
A. Adequate preparation in terms of having necessary materials and information (knowledge of testing protocols/guidelines)	5	—	F. Adequate supervision and instruction of electrocardiograph technician during the test	5	—
B. Consistently obtains *all* necessary information from patient's medical record	5	—	**III. Test Interpretation**		
C. Seeks additional information directly from referring physician when necessary	5	—	A. Demonstrates consistent accuracy in interpretation, assessment of physical work capacity/functional aerobic impairment, and summary remarks/recommendations	55	—
D. Consistently completes a thorough patient interview and physical examination	5	—			
E. Accurately assesses the medical data base and results from the patient interview and physical examination	21	—	B. Completes test interpretation within allotted time and adequately supervises electrocardiograph technicians to ensure compliance with testing schedule	5	—
F. Checks for proper calibration of testing instrumentation and correct functioning of emergency equipment	5	—			
			TOTAL 176		
II. Test Performance			**IV. Ability to Respond to Life-threatening Situations**		
A. Consistently makes correct judgments regarding the conducting of the test	10	—	To test independently, the therapist must have:		—
B. Consistently obtains accurate data before, during, and after the test	30	—	A. Clearance from the medical director of the exercise testing laboratory to take definitive action in event of an emergency		
C. Accurately uses above information to determine test end points	10	—	B. Current American Heart Association certification in Advanced Cardiac Life Support		—
D. Accurately uses above information to determine point at which postexercise monitoring can be discontinued	5	—			

(From Irwin SI, Techlin JS. Cardiopulmonary Physical Therapy. 2nd ed. St. Louis, CV Mosby, 1990, p 141.)

sponses from test to test session as well as for comparisons among other subjects. Standard testing procedures require a 12-lead ECG to be obtained before any test to rule out any acute ischemia or injury before testing. The patient's ECG is continuously monitored during the test. Standard procedure is to monitor a minimum of three leads during the test. Other pretest proce-

dures include assessment of the patient's risk factor history (see Chapter 3); assessment of the patient's symptom history; and assessment of the patient's resting blood pressure, heart rate, and heart and lung auscultation.

When exercise is initiated, the workload is increased in accordance with a specific protocol. The patient's heart rate and blood pressure (and

Informed Consent for an Exercise Test (Sample)

1. *Explanation of the Exercise Test*
   You will perform an exercise test on a cycle ergometer or a motor-driven treadmill. The exercise intensity will begin at a level you can easily accomplish and will be advanced in stages, depending on your fitness level. We may stop the test at any time because of signs of fatigue or you may stop when you wish because of personal feelings of fatigue or discomfort.

2. *Risks and Discomforts*
   There exists the possibility of certain changes occurring during the test. They include abnormal blood pressure, fainting, disorder of heart beat, and in rare instances, heart attack or death. Every effort will be made to minimize these through the preliminary examination and by observations during testing. Emergency equipment and trained personnel are available to deal with unusual situations which may arise.

3. *Benefits to be Expected*
   The results obtained from the exercise test may assist in the diagnosis of your illness or in evaluating what type of physical activities you might engage with no or low hazards.

4. *Inquiries*
   Any questions about the procedures used in the exercise test or in the estimation of functional capacity are encouraged. If you have any doubts or questions, please ask us for further explanations.

5. *Freedom of Consent*
   Your permission to perform this exercise test is voluntary. You are free to deny consent if you so desire.

   I have read this form and I understand the test procedures that I will perform. I consent to participate in this test.

   _____
   Signature of Patient

   _____   _____
   Date   Witness   .

   Questions: _____

   _____

   Response: _____

   _____

   Physician signature: optional.

Figure 8–4.
Signing an informed consent form is one of the safety precautions taken with exercise testing. (From American College of Sports Medicine. Guidelines for Exercise Testing and Prescription. 3rd ed. Philadelphia, Lea & Febiger, 1988. Used with permission.)

in some tests, the expired gases) are periodically monitored throughout the test and during the recovery period. Most tests are symptom limited and, as such, are terminated at the request of the patient or on the identification of an abnormality in one or more of the parameters being measured. The patient is monitored continuously during the recovery period until the pretest values are achieved. A written report documenting and interpreting the results is prepared following the test.

Maximal and Submaximal Stress Testing

The protocols that are used are described as either maximal or submaximal; the distinction between them being the termination point of the test. **Submaximal** tests are terminated on achievement of a predetermined end point (unless symptoms otherwise limit completion of the test). The predetermined end point may be either the achievement of a certain percentage of the patient's predicted maximal heart rate (PMHR) (e.g., 75% of PMHR) or the attainment of a certain workload (e.g., 2.5 mph, 12% grade). A special subset of submaximal testing is *low-level testing*, performed on patients during the recuperative phase after myocardial injury or coronary bypass surgery.

Maximal stress tests usually use the end point of the predicted maximal heart rate or terminate when a patient is limited by symptoms. Maximal stress testing is employed to measure functional capacity as well as to diagnose coronary artery disease. The protocol for testing involves performing a progressive workload until the patient perceives an inability to continue because of some limiting symptom such as shortness of breath, leg fatigue, or chest discomfort.

Exercise tests also may be described as intermittent or continuous. *Intermittent* testing intersperses progressive workloads with short rest periods to give the subject time to recover and decrease the effect of peripheral fatigue. *Continuous* tests utilize incrementally progressive workloads until the test is terminated because of patient symptoms or a defined end point.

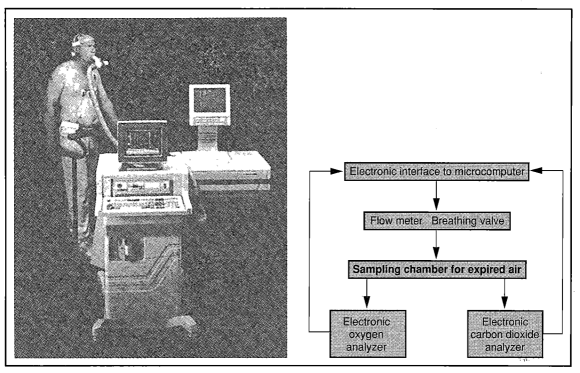

Figure 8-5.
Oxygen uptake during the exercise test can be measured directly from oxygen analyzers. (Adapted from McArdle WD, Katch FI, Katch VL. Exercise Physiology. 3rd ed. Philadelphia, Lea & Febiger, 1991. Photograph used by permission of Sensormedics, Yorba Linda, Calif.)

Contraindications to Testing

Essential to safe testing is knowing who should *not* be tested. Thoroughly evaluating the patient before testing reveals any **contraindications** to testing. Absolute contraindications to maximal stress testing include the following:

- Recent myocardial infarction (less than 4-6 weeks after the myocardial infarction for a maximal, symptom-limited test) in most clinical settings
- Acute **pericarditis** or **myocarditis**
- Resting or **unstable angina**
- Serious ventricular or rapid atrial arrhythmias (e.g., ventricular tachycardia, couplets, atrial fibrillation, or atrial flutter)
- Untreated second- or third-degree heart block
- Overt congestive heart failure (pulmonary rales, third heart sound, or both)
- Any acute illness

In addition to absolute contraindications, the general clinical status of the patient must be considered before determining whether the stress test is contraindicated. The following relative contraindications should be considered on an individual basis:

- **Aortic stenosis**
- Known left main coronary artery disease (or its equivalent)
- Severe hypertension (defined as systolic blood pressure higher than 165 mm Hg at rest, diastolic blood pressure higher than 110 mm Hg at rest, or both)
- **Idiopathic hypertrophic subaortic stenosis**
- Severe depression of the ST segment on the resting ECG
- Compensated heart failure

Testing Protocols

The most commonly used protocols in testing involve the use of either the stationary bicycle or the treadmill. Blood pressure is easier to auscultate on the stationary bicycle than on the treadmill. The bicycle also takes up less room, requires less coordination to operate, and is less expensive than the treadmill. The greatest disadvantage of the stationary bicycle, however, is that bicycling is not a daily functional activity for most persons. Therefore, patients develop muscular fatigue faster because they are using muscle groups that are not as "trained" as the muscles used for walking. Such patients do not achieve their best results, because the maximal heart rate may be well below what is considered diagnostic (85% of predicted maximal heart rate).[21] A widely used bicycle testing protocol is displayed in Figure 8–6.[22] This protocol may be employed intermittently (meaning that rests are incorporated between each work stage) rather than continuously because of the peripheral fatigue that de-

velops. Also, the workloads may be reduced by half for females or severely deconditioned individuals.

The treadmill is relatively large, requires a patient to have balance and coordination, and is extremely noisy, making the auscultation of blood pressure very difficult. However, because walking is a functional activity, the muscles do not fatigue as rapidly as they do with cycling, and therefore the treadmill is considered to have greater diagnostic benefits. The two most common treadmill protocols are the **Bruce exercise test protocol** and the **Balke exercise protocol**. The Bruce protocol (Table 8–3) is probably most widely used in the clinical setting of hospitals because it provides normative data in the form of a nomogram to calculate functional aerobic impairment (Fig. 8–7). Previous studies have reported limitations in the ability of the functional

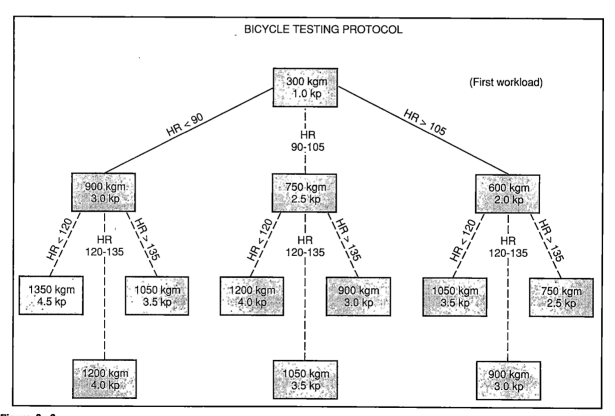

Figure 8–6.

A branching bicycle testing protocol. HR, heart rate. (Adapted from Golding LA, Myers CR, Slinning WE [eds]. The Y's Way to Physical Fitness. Rev. ed. Chicago, The YMCA of the USA, 1982, p 535, with permission of the YMCA of the USA, 101 N. Wacker Dr., Chicago IL 60606.)

TABLE 8–3. Bruce Treadmill Protocol

Stage	Time (min)	Speed (mph)	Grade	MET*
I	3	1.7	10%	4–5
II	3	2.5	12%	6–7
III	3	3.4	14%	8–10
IV	3	4.2	16%	11–13
V	3	5.0	18%	14–16
VI	3	6.0	20%	17–19

*1 MET, resting metabolic rate = 3.5 ml of oxygen per kilogram of body weight per minute.

(From Ellestad MH, Myrvin H. Stress Testing Principles and Practice. Philadelphia, FA Davis, 1986.)

The starting speed of the Bruce protocol is 1.7 miles per hour, which is a fairly comfortable speed for all. However, because of the rapid increases in speed and the fact the subject starts on a 10% grade, the average time a nontrained subject actually exercises during the test is between 6 and 12 minutes. In comparison, the Balke protocol (Fig. 8–8) starts at a speed of 3.3 miles per hour, which is often too fast for a deconditioned patient or an older individual, but the subject starts on a level surface and only gradually is an incline added during the protocol. The gradual workload increments allow closer attainment of a steady state at each stage and facilitate the measurement of true maximal oxygen consumption. However, the Balke protocol requires a longer time to perform owing to the gradual addition of the incline. The Balke protocol is used more widely with athletes, especially with runners, because runners typically do not train on steep inclines and because this protocol allows the athlete to attain a steady state in a shorter period of time.

aerobic impairment nomogram to predict functional capacity. The preferred method of predicting functional capacity is via the maximal workload performed on the treadmill test. According to Froelicher, a true test of aerobic capacity is best limited to a total exercise time of 10 minutes because of the endurance factor, which becomes significant after 10 minutes of exercise.[23]

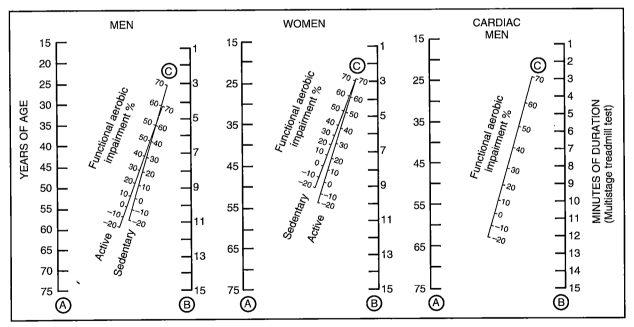

Figure 8–7.

Nomograms for evaluating functional aerobic impairment (FAI) of men, women, and cardiac men according to age and by duration of exercise on the Bruce protocol for sedentary and active groups. To find the FAI, identify age (in years) in the left column and identify duration of time on the Bruce treadmill protocol in the right column. With a straight edge, line up the two points and read where the straight edge intercepts the FAI nomogram for either active or sedentary. (Reproduced with permission from Bruce RL, Kusumi F, Hosmer D. Maximal oxygen intake and nomographic assessment of functional aerobic impairment in cardiovascular disease. Am Heart J 85:545–562, 1973.)

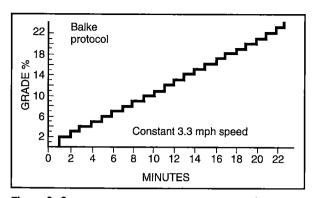

Figure 8–8.

The Balke treadmill protocol.

Special Protocols

Thallium Stress Testing

The use of a radioactive nuclear marker for detection of myocardial perfusion defects has provided clinicians with an even greater body of information than that obtained from the standard exercise test. Current practice involves injecting radioactive thallium during peak performance on an exercise test. Following the injection of the nuclear marker, a minute of exercise is required to circulate the marker. After the marker has circulated, the patient is returned to a supine position and passed under a nuclear scanner for the purpose of evaluating perfusion of the heart immediately after exercise. The subject then returns 3 to 4 hours after the exercise test to again lie under a nuclear scanner to evaluate perfusion of the heart during the delayed postexercise period of time (Fig. 8–9).

Indications for uses of thallium injection with stress testing include detection of myocardial infarction and transient myocardial ischemia. Myocardial areas supplied by narrowed coronary arteries may demonstrate normal thallium uptake at rest but when injected with thallium during exercise may show decreased concentration compared with that of normally perfused areas. This finding indicates perfusion defects that may not have been demonstrated on the ECG during the exercise test. If a region has no thallium at rest and does not change after injection during exercise, myocardial infarction, scarring, or both is

assumed to have occurred in that particular region. The **thallium exercise stress test** appears to be more sensitive than exercise electrocardiography in identifying patients with coronary disease. It is for this reason that thallium exercise tests are prescribed frequently for patients who have undergone percutaneous transluminal coronary angioplasty.

Low-level Exercise Testing

Low-level exercise testing is usually performed when patients have experienced a myocardial infarction recently or have undergone coronary artery bypass graft surgery. Such tests have been performed as early as 5 days after myocardial infarction or surgery[24] but are more likely to be performed just before or immediately after discharge from the hospital following an acute event. Some physicians prefer to wait up to 2 weeks after the cardiac event before administering the low-level exercise test.

Low-level exercise testing may be useful in predicting the subsequent course of a myocardial infarction or bypass surgery as well as for identifying the **high-risk patient.** High-risk patients exhibit an increased risk of morbidity or mortality as a result of myocardial ischemia or poor ventricular function. The high-risk patient needs more immediate intervention and should not be treated as a typical patient in a cardiac rehabilitation program. After the high-risk patient is identified, the decision on optimal medical management or surgical intervention is more easily made.

Many factors have been studied from the results of the low-level exercise test to determine the most outstanding variable for identifying high-risk patients. Exercise-induced ST-segment depression of 2.0 millimeters or greater on low-level exercise tests has been identified as the single most valuable indicator of prognosis after myocardial infarction according to the regression analysis by Davidson and DeBusk.[25] In addition, early onset of ST-segment depression is related to increased incidence of coronary events. Starling and co-workers[26] demonstrated a significantly increased risk of death after myocardial infarction when both ST-segment depression and

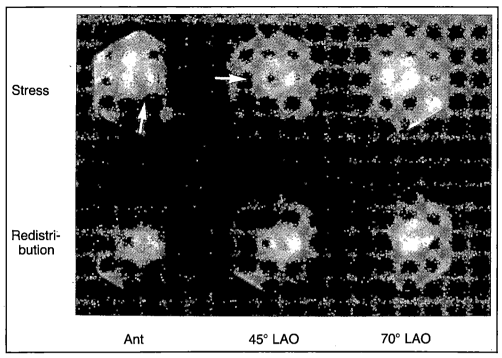

Figure 8-9.

Stress-redistribution thallium scintigram of a patient with reversible apical and distal inferior perfusion defect on the anterior view and a partially reversible septal defect on the 45-degree left anterior oblique (LAO) view. There is a decreased right ventricular thallium uptake on the 45-degree LAO view and increased pulmonary thallium uptake on the anterior view. (From Lyons, K. Cardiovascular Nuclear Medicine. East Norwalk, Conn, Appleton & Lange, 1988, p 121. Photograph by Steven A. Reisman, M.D.)

angina were produced during low-level exercise testing in the early period after a myocardial infarction. Exercise-induced angina alone was associated with subsequent coronary artery bypass surgery.[27,28] Other variables of minor prognostic significance after myocardial infarction include inappropriate blood pressure response, maximum heart rate achieved, and maximum systolic blood pressure achieved.[29,30]

Low-level exercise testing can also provide information useful for optimal medical management after myocardial injury or surgery, including treatment for angina, arrhythmias, or hypertension. Exercise-induced arrhythmias on a low-level exercise test may be an indication for therapeutic management before hospital discharge. The incidence of sudden death has been reported to be 2.5 times higher in patients manifesting ventricular arrhythmias during low-level exercise testing.[31] Poor performance, such as lim-ited exercise duration, has been highly correlated with increased incidence of heart failure and is associated with increased mortality.[32]

Because of its great prognostic and therapeutic value, low-level testing is often used for screening patients who wish to participate in cardiac rehabilitation programs.[33] Activity levels for patients during rehabilitation in the home or hospital setting can be prescribed on the basis of the results of the low-level exercise test.

However, not all patients are appropriate candidates for low-level exercise testing. Safety of exercise testing early after myocardial infarction has been a topic of debate because of the traditional medical belief that a recently damaged myocardium is prone to further injury, including rupture, **aneurysm,** extension of infarction, or susceptibility to serious arrhythmias.[34] However, the safety of properly conducted exercise testing was documented as early as 1973.[35] Knowledge

TABLE 8–4. Contraindications to Low-level Testing

Unstable angina or angina pectoris at rest
Severe heart failure (overt left ventricular failure on exam
   with pulmonary rales and S3 heart sound)
Serious arrhythmias at rest
Second- or third-degree heart block
Disabling musculoskeletal abnormalities
Valvular heart disease
Blood pressure >180/105
Patient refuses to sign consent form

(From Starling MR, Crawford MH, et al. Predictive value of early postmyocardial infarction modified treadmill exercise testing in multivessel coronary artery disease detection. Am Heart J 102[2]:169, 1981.)

of and adherence to contraindications for testing optimize the safety of exercise testing (Table 8–4).[21]

Institutions vary in the choice of an exercise testing protocol for low-level testing. However, a progressively increasing workload from 2 METs (Metabolic Equivalent Tables, a multiple of the resting metabolic rate) to approximately 6 METs is often used. Among the protocols for low-level exercise testing, the modified Naughton and modified Sheffield-Bruce protocols appear to be the ones most widely chosen (Tables 8–5, 8–6).

Low-level exercise testing soon after myocardial infarction is a safe, noninvasive method for evaluating the functional capacity for physical activity; for detecting arrhythmias, angina, and hypertensive responses with exercise; for determining optimal medical management; and for predicting the risk of subsequent cardiac events.

TABLE 8–5. Modified Naughton Treadmill Protocol

	Time (min)							
	0	3	6	9	12	15	18	21
Speed (mph)	2	2	2	2	2	3	3	3
Percent grade	3.5	7	10.5	14	17.5	12.5	15	17.5
MET	3	4	5	6	7	8	9	10

MET, resting metabolic rate.

TABLE 8–6. Modified Sheffield-Bruce Submaximal Protocol

Stage	Speed (mph)	Grade (%)	Time (min)
1	1.7	0	3
2	1.7	5	3
3	1.7	10	3
4	2.5	12	3

Safety in Exercise Testing

The physical therapist must have a clear understanding of the rationale for terminating a low-level exercise test. The specific criteria for termination vary from one institution to another, but the general criteria include

- an oxygen consumption level of 17.5 milliliters of oxygen per kilogram (6 METs)
- 70% to 75% of age-predicted maximal heart rate achieved
- fatigue or dyspnea
- maximal heart rate of 120 to 130 beats per minute
- frequent (nine or more per minute) unifocal or **multifocal** premature ventricular contractions, paired premature ventricular contractions, or ventricular tachycardia
- ST-segment depression of 1.0 to 2.0 mm
- claudication pain
- dizziness
- decrease in systolic blood pressure of 10 to 15 mm Hg below peak value
- hypertensive blood pressure (systolic > 200, diastolic > 110)
- level 1 (out of 4) angina

Both the patient and the discharging physician benefit when a predischarge exercise test is conducted.[33] The test can facilitate the distinction between chest wall and angina pain. In addition, improvement in exercise performance following a myocardial infarction has been related to improvement in the patient's self-confidence following a successful, uneventful predischarge exercise test.

Maximal exercise testing and testing of high-risk patients or postmyocardial injury patients should be done in a setting in which emergencies can be managed expertly and efficiently. Appropriate equipment, which includes emergency medications and intravenous, intubation, and suctioning materials, should be present and updated when necessary. A direct current defibrillator should be available and functioning properly. Persons performing the testing should be certified in **Advanced Cardiac Life Support,** taught by the American Heart Association, and well trained in emergency cardiac response techniques such as **defibrillation.** Written protocols describing emergency procedures to be followed should be available to all testing personnel. These can be adopted from the American Heart Association's guidelines for advanced cardiac life support.[36]

Terminating the Testing Session

The person administering the exercise test must observe the patient and the ECG monitor during the test continuously to decide when the test should be terminated. Guidelines for termination of the test are similar for all tests and include the following:

- Increasing frequency or pairing of premature ventricular complexes
- Development of ventricular tachycardia
- Rapid atrial arrhythmias, including atrial fibrillation or atrial flutter, with uncontrolled ventricular response rates
- Development of second- or third-degree heart block
- Increased angina pain (level 2 on a scale of 1 to 4)
- Hypotensive blood pressure response (20 mm Hg or greater decrease)
- Extreme shortness of breath
- Dizziness, mental confusion, or lack of coordination
- Severe ST-segment depression. The American College of Sports Medicine recommends termination when the ST segment is depressed 2.0 millimeters or more, although some testing personnel may proceed when changes of greater magnitude are demonstrated as long as there is no evidence of other abnormal responses.[17]

- Observation of the patient reveals pale and clammy skin (**pallor** and **diaphoresis**)
- Extremely elevated systolic or diastolic blood pressure, or both, which may or may not be associated with symptoms
- On achievement of predicted maximal heart rate; it is usually safe to proceed with the test beyond the predicted maximal heart rate if the patient is able and willing to continue and if other indications to terminate the test are absent.[21]
- Presence of leg fatigue or leg cramps or claudication pain
- Patient request for termination of test

Differences in criteria for termination of a low-level exercise test are listed earlier and specify different maximal heart rates, ST-segment depression, level of angina, and amount of blood pressure change allowed.

Interpretation of Results

Once the test is concluded, the results are written on a worksheet to provide data for the interpretation (Fig. 8–10). The following parameters are necessary for a thorough interpretation:

- Exercise time completed (and protocol used)
- Limiting factors (reason for termination)
- Presence or absence of chest pain at peak exercise: usually defined as positive, negative, or atypical for angina or extreme shortness of breath
- Maximal heart rate achieved
- Blood pressure response
- Arrhythmias: description of which type developed and when they occurred
- ST-segment changes: usually described as positive, negative, equivocal, or indeterminate for ischemia
  - positive: 1.0 millimeter or greater horizontal or downsloping ST-segment depression (Fig. 8–11)
  - equivocal: more than 0.5 but less than 1.0 millimeter horizontal or downsloping ST-segment depression or more than 1.5 millimeter upsloping depression
  - negative: less than 0.5 millimeter horizontal or downsloping ST-segment depression[21]

Name ___John Doe_____ Date _____

Age __45__   Sex __M__   Height __5'10"__   Weight __190 lb.__

Diagnosis _____   Reason for test __chest pains__

Protocol __Bruce__

Time of test __8 AM__   Time last cigarette _____   Time last meal __12__

Medications __None__   Time last dose _____

Physician _____

RESULTS

12-Lead ECG interpretation __Normal__

Minutes completed __7.05__   Limiting factor(s) __Leg fatigue__

Rest HR __84__   Rest BP __140/96__   Heart sounds __Normal__

Maximum HR __170__   Maximum BP __190/102__

BP Response __Diastolic hypertension throughout__

Chest pain __None__

Summary of ST segment changes __Negative for ischemia__

Summary of arrhythmias __Rare PAC throughout__

Physical work capacity __Poor, 30% below predicted functional aerobic impairment__

Remarks/recommendations __Patient needs an exercise program to decrease blood pressure and improve functional aerobic impairment.__

Interpreted by _____ Date _____

Figure 8-10.

Worksheet for interpretation of exercise test results. (From Scully R, Barnes ML. Physical Therapy. Philadelphia, JB Lippincott, 1989, p 537.)

- indeterminate: unable to measure the ST segment accurately because of the presence of any of the following: bundle branch block, medication (if patient is taking digoxin [Lanoxin]), resting ST changes on the ECG, or cardiac hypertrophy
- Heart sounds: notation of pretest and post-test sounds and description of any change
- Functional aerobic impairment: can be determined from a nomogram if the Bruce treadmill protocol is used. This value is compared with normal values to determine impairment in functional capacity (physical work capacity).
- R wave changes: amplitude changes are considered to give additional diagnostic information in interpreting exercise test results. The normal response to exercise is a decrease in R wave amplitude. If no change or an increase in R wave amplitude occurs with exercise, the

patient with coronary artery disease is considered to be at an increased risk for developing a cardiac problem in the future (Fig. 8-12).[37]
- Maximal oxygen consumption (Vo_{2max}) can be calculated using formulas if not directly measured during the test (Fig. 8-13); however, this method is not very accurate.

The final summary of the exercise test should define whether the outcome of the test is normal or abnormal; if the outcome is abnormal, the summary should provide reasons why. Although the physical therapist may not actually perform the stress test, obtaining the interpretation of the results provides valuable data for developing an exercise prescription. The interpretation also provides valuable information regarding safety during exercise for the patient.

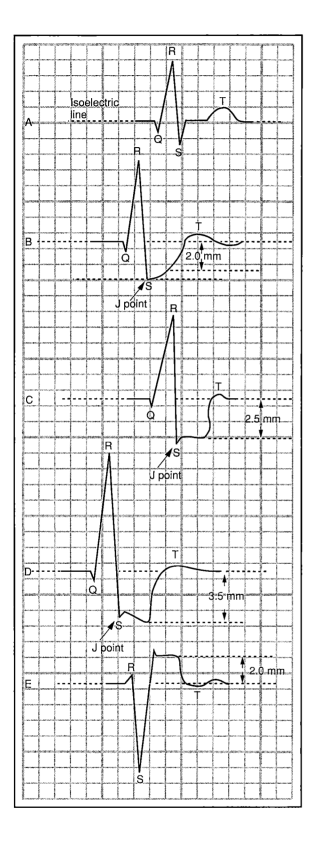

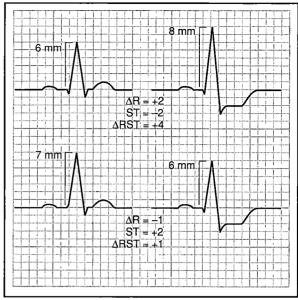

Figure 8–12.

Calculation of index (RST) in two patients with ST-segment depression and R wave increased and decreased. (From Bonoris PE, et al. Evaluation of R wave amplitude changes versus ST-segment depression in stress testing. Circulation 57[5]:904–910, 1973. Reproduced by permission of the American Heart Association.)

Prognostic Value of Maximal Exercise Testing

Maximal exercise testing is used as a noninvasive screening method for the detection of coronary disease. Its diagnostic accuracy in determining coronary disease is limited by the fact that it is a noninvasive test and therefore only reflects gross metabolic and electrical changes in the heart. Nonetheless, studies evaluating the specificity and sensitivity of stress testing have suggested that in appropriately chosen populations, it can be very helpful in identifying coronary disease and defining its severity.[21] **Sensitivity** is the measure of the reliability of stress testing in

Figure 8–11.

ST-segment changes. *A*, normal segment; *B*, slowly upsloping ST-segment depression; *C*, horizontal ST-segment depression; *D*, downsloping ST-segment depression; *E*, horizontal ST-segment elevation.

Treadmill:

$$\dot{V}o_2 \ (ml/kg^{-min}) = \text{Velocity (m/min)}$$
$$\times 1.78 \ (ml \ O_2/kg/m) \times (\% \ \text{grade} + .073)$$

(mph converts to m/min by

$$\frac{1609/m/min}{60 \ min/m} = 26.8m \ min/mph)$$

Figure 8–13.

Calculation of maximal oxygen consumption (max Vo₂) indirectly via formula.
+

identifying the presence of disease. **Specificity** is the measure of the reliability of stress testing in identifying the population without disease. In general, testing demonstrates greater sensitivity and specificity in males over the age of 40 than in females. Females generally demonstrate a greater percentage of **false-negative** results, but it is beyond the scope of this chapter to describe the predictive values for every potential population. However, to aid clinical judgment in predicting the risk of developing coronary artery disease, one can use Bayes' theorem to assist in predicting sensitivity and specificity of testing.[38]

The value of diagnostic stress testing is tempered by the amount of variability among examiners conducting the test. Problems with testing include amount of encouragement given to the patient, a lack of strict adherence to protocols, use of handrail support, and interpretation of ST-segment deviation and symptoms.[23]

Despite its acknowledged potential limitations, several studies have attempted to identify specific single parameters or combinations of variables that might identify a group of patients with more severe disease.[21] Ischemia, reflected by ST-segment depression, that occurs during the early stages of an exercise test has been correlated with more severe disease than ischemia that occurs at peak exercise. Goldschlager and co-workers reported an increased incidence of subsequent myocardial infarction in a group of patients who exhibited ST-segment depression at light workloads.[39] The severity of coronary disease has also been correlated with the length of

recovery time (postexercise rest) for ST segment to return to normal.

Other subsets of patients have been identified who demonstrate certain signs and symptoms that suggest a greater risk for the subsequent development of a cardiac event. The signs and symptoms that have increased prognostic value include ST-segment depression, bradycardic heart rate responses, presence of angina, and maximal systolic blood pressure attained. Ellestad identified a population with more serious prognosis of disease when the magnitude of ST-segment depression was considered.[21] In addition, a subset of persons at high risk for progression of angina, myocardial infarction, or death was identified by Ellestad. Persons with normal ST segments at peak effort who achieved maximal heart rates considerably below their predicted pulses (bradycardic heart rate response or **chronotropic** incompetence) demonstrated high risk of progression of angina, myocardial infarction, or death. The tendency was to describe the test results as normal because the patients in Ellestad's study did not demonstrate ischemic ST-segment changes.

The presence of angina pain gives added significance when the patient demonstrates ST-segment depression during exercise. Ellestad described a subset of patients at double the risk of a subsequent coronary event when angina and ST-segment depression occurred together, as compared with patients without angina but with ST-segment depression (silent ischemia).[21]

The incidence of sudden death is increased in the following subset of patients:

● Those unable to exceed a maximal systolic blood pressure of 130 mm Hg
● Those with increased frequency and severity of arrhythmias during testing[40]

Calculating a probability score from the combination and weighing of clinical variables from the exercise test identifies the subsets of individuals at greater risk for coronary events. Many institutions are in the process of developing multiple variable analyses to increase the predictive value of exercise testing.[41] However, the use of thallium injection at peak performance also increases the information gained from the test, as well as increasing the sensitivity of the test.

CARDIAC CATHETERIZATION: CORONARY ANGIOGRAPHY AND VENTRICULOGRAPHY

Cardiac catheterization is an invasive procedure that provides extremely valuable information for the diagnosis and management of patients with cardiac disease. The general goal of cardiac catheterization is to obtain objective information that can

- establish or confirm a diagnosis of cardiac dysfunction or heart disease
- demonstrate the severity of coronary artery disease or valvular dysfunction
- determine guidelines for optimal management of the patient, including medical and surgical management as well as a program of exercise

The data obtained from the cardiac catheterization are as follows:

- Cardiac output
- Shunt detection
- Angiography: coronary and ventriculography
- Left and right heart pressures (hemodynamics)
  - right atrial (normal = 0 to 4 mm Hg)
  - right ventricle (normal = 30/2)
  - pulmonary artery (normal = 30/10)
  - pulmonary artery wedge (normal = 8 to 12 mm Hg)
  - left ventricular end-diastolic (normal = 8 to 12 mm Hg)
- Ventricular ejection fraction (estimated)

Specific determinations that can be made as a result of cardiac catheterization include

- the presence of severity of coronary artery disease (degree of stenosis)
- the presence of left ventricular dysfunction or aneurysm or both
- the presence of valvular heart disease and the severity of the dysfunction, including aortic valve stenosis or regurgitation, mitral valve stenosis or regurgitation or prolapse, tricuspid valve dysfunction, or pulmonic valve dysfunction
- the presence of pericardial disease

- the presence of myocardial disease, including cardiomyopathy
- the presence of congenital heart disease

Procedure for Cardiac Catheterization

Cardiac catheterization involves the insertion of a catheter into the cardiovascular system to measure pressures or perform angiography (anatomic evaluation). The specific procedure includes catheterizing the right or left sides of the heart, contrast angiography, and sometimes revascularization with drugs or pacing. The procedure is invasive and is performed in a special room in the radiology department or in a special laboratory. The patient undergoing the procedure is awake but under sedation. A catheter is inserted into either the brachial artery or the femoral artery, depending on the cardiologist's expertise with an individual technique. The catheter is then passed into the great vessels and then into the great chambers under fluoroscopic control. Pressures are measured in the chambers across the valves, and cardiac output is measured to assess the competency of the valves and the function of the cardiac muscle. Finally, radiopaque contrast medium is injected into the chambers and then into the orifices of the coronary arteries (and in some cases into the aorta itself). The passage of the contrast medium is followed and filmed for closer evaluation of the integrity of the arteries and the myocardium when the procedure is completed (Fig. 8–14).

Interpreting the Test Results

On completion of the cardiac catheterization, the cardiologist reviews the films to assess the ventricular function and the severity of coronary artery stenosis. The degree of stenosis in each arterial segment is graded during the review of the film, with total occlusion graded as 100% (Fig. 8–15). One of the problems with interpreting the cardiac catheterization film is the fact that angiography is only two dimensional. Another problem concerns reliability: the film inter-

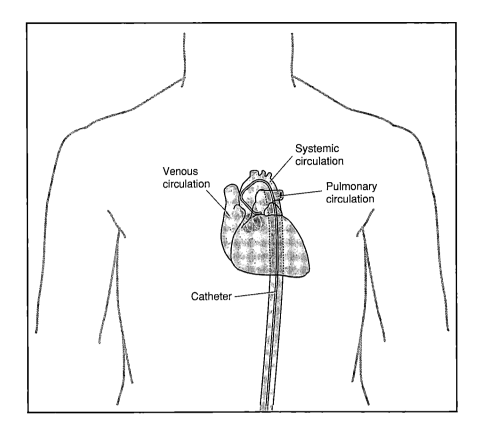

Figure 8–14.

The cardiac catheterization procedure involves the passage of a catheter through the great vessels so that radiopaque contrast medium can be injected into the orifices of the coronary arteries.

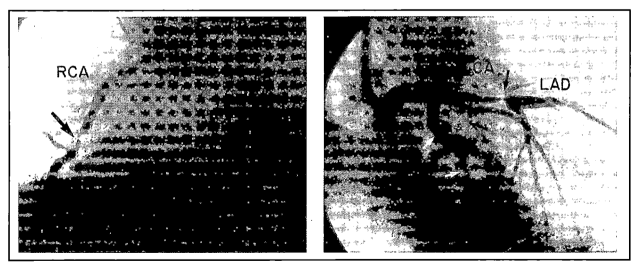

Figure 8–15.

The degree of stenosis in each arterial segment is graded during review of the film, with total occlusion graded as 100%. The arrows point to areas of occlusion. LAD, left anterior descending artery; LCA, left coronary artery; CX, circumflex artery. (Reproduced with permission from Braunwald E [ed]. Harrison's Principles of Internal Medicine. 12th ed. New York, McGraw-Hill, 1991, p 883.)

pretation relies either on a person's subjective judgment or on a computer to measure the degree of stenosis. However, cardiac catheterization has greater sensitivity in detecting disease than other noninvasive procedures previously presented.

Controversy exists over the indication for performing cardiac catheterization. Some critics in the medical field believe that the catheterization technique is overused and that less invasive procedures should be used before catheterization.[42,43] However, others note that coronary angiography is the only test that provides information about the actual site, extent, and severity of obstruction in coronary artery disease. Cardiac catheterization has greater predictive accuracy in assessment of coronary artery disease than exercise testing. It also may be used to confirm diagnoses from other noninvasive tests. Cardiac catheterization must be performed before any surgical intervention. Common practice demonstrates that coronary angiography and ventriculography are being performed on the majority of patients following acute myocardial infarction to assess severity of disease and amount of ventricular dysfunction resulting from the infarction. Cardiac catheterization results are very important in determining the entire clinical picture of the patient.

ERGONOVINE STIMULATION

Coronary artery spasm has been demonstrated to play a role in the manifestation of ischemic heart disease. To document coronary artery spasm, one must demonstrate significant or total narrowing of a segment in an artery that may or may not have partial arteriosclerotic narrowing. If increased narrowing of the artery occurs and the narrowing is relieved with the administration of a vasodilator, then coronary artery spasm has been documented. Spasm is rarely documented with coronary angiography (3%).[44] Therefore, because angiography does not frequently induce the spasm, ergonovine stimulation has become an important diagnostic test for coronary spasm.

Procedure for Ergonovine Stimulation

Ergonovine stimulation is used when coronary spasm is suspected, particularly in a patient with documented electrocardiographic changes during symptoms or with documented ischemic episodes and a normal coronary angiographic study. The test has a high degree of sensitivity and specificity for coronary vasospasm.[45,46]

Ergonovine stimulation is performed in the cardiac catheterization laboratory or in the coronary care unit (if previous angiography studies have demonstrated normal coronary arteries). Either incremental doses of ergonovine are given by intravenous injections or a single bolus of ergometrine is given while a patient is monitored continuously for electrocardiographic or hemodynamic changes (particularly ST-segment elevation or major heart rate and blood pressure changes) (Fig. 8–16). The patient is monitored throughout the injections until a maximal dosage is given or until the patient experiences symptoms.

When ergonovine stimulation is performed in the cardiac catheterization laboratory, repeat angiography is performed when symptoms or changes on the ECG develop; treatment with vasodilators is initiated after spasm is documented. In the coronary care unit, the patient is treated with vasodilators when the ECG changes or when the patient complains of symptoms. When a positive response occurs to ergonovine stimulation, the patient is managed with medications that reduce or prevent the occurrence of spasm (see discussion of calcium channel blockers in Chapter 12).

POSITRON EMISSION TOMOGRAPHY

Positron emission tomography is a nuclear technique that provides visualization and direct measurement of metabolic functioning, including glucose metabolism, fatty acid metabolism, and blood flow of the heart. As the technique requires specialized technologic equipment and

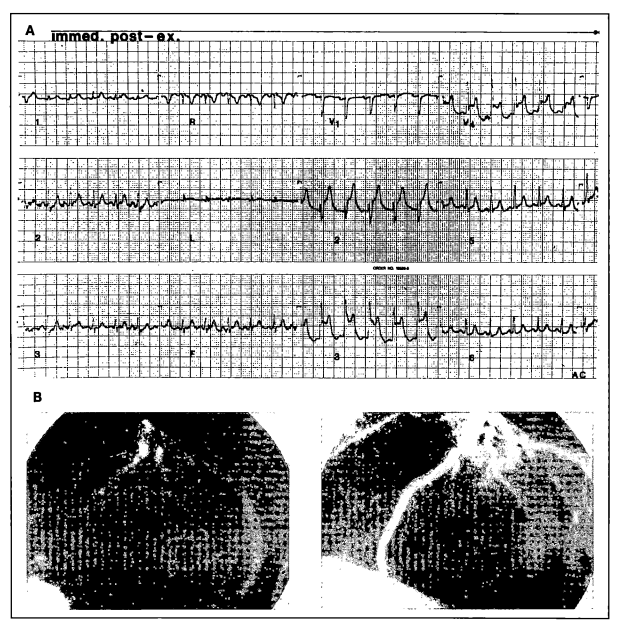

Figure 8-16.

Exercise-induced ST-segment elevation in variant angina. *A*, Exercise electrocardiogram (ECG) of a 45-year-old man with exertional, rest, and nocturnal angina. The rest ECG is normal. During exercise, ST-segment elevation is present in the anterior leads, suggesting anterior wall ischemia and left anterior descending (LAD) artery obstruction. *B*, Coronary arteriogram of the same patient. The left coronary artery *(left panel)* is normal except for a 40% obstruction in the proximal LAD *(arrow)*. A septal perforator is seen running behind the LAD. The patient developed spontaneous chest pain with anterior ST-segment elevation, similar to that present during exercise. Repeat angiography *(right panel)* shows the LAD totally obstructed *(arrow)* at the previous site of the minimal lesion and distal to the origin of the septal perforator, which is now seen clearly. The coronary artery spasm was relieved by sublingual nitroglycerin, and further arteriography showed that the 40% obstruction in the LAD remained unchanged. ST-segment elevation during exercise in this patient was probably caused by exercise-induced coronary artery spasm similar to that seen during spontaneous chest pain and not by a severe fixed coronary lesion. (From Dunn RF, Kelly TD. Exercise-induced ST-segment elevation. Primary Cardiology Supplement to Hospital Physician 1:A-79-A-90, 1982. Reprinted with permission from Turner White Communications, Inc.)

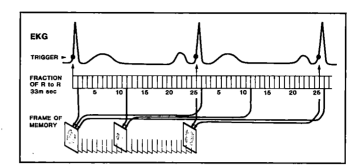

Figure 8-17.

The R-R interval is partitioned into multiple frames. An average R-R interval is calculated by the system and that time length is divided into equal intervals. (From Lyons K. Cardiovascular Nuclear Medicine. East Norwalk, Conn, Appleton & Lange, 1988, p 18.)

highly trained personnel to perform, it is not available at many hospitals, and the procedure is extremely expensive. However, it is a method of evaluating the myocardium dynamically but without having the patient exercise on a treadmill or bicycle.

Procedure for Positron Emission Tomography

Positron emission tomography testing requires administration of **dipyridamole** to cause vasodilation of the coronary arteries while the patient is at rest but the heart rate is accelerated via medication. The myocardium can then be evaluated in three dimensions to identify impairment in coronary blood flow.

This technique has advantages over thallium stress testing because it can detect jeopardized but viable myocardium.[43,47] During thallium testing, the patient is required to exercise to obtain this information. Patients can safely undergo positron emission tomography from 2 to 10 days after infarction or when any question of impedance of flow is involved. With the invention of thrombolytic medications to decrease infarct size, this technique has great advantages in evaluating the effectiveness of the thrombolysis technique because positron emission tomography testing can be performed so early after infarction.[48]

Stress testing performed with other pharmacologic intervention has been introduced recently, including the use of adenosine, dipyridamole, and dobutamine. The technique is the same in that the patient is not required to exercise to

increase the work on the heart, yet the myocardial blood flow can be effectively evaluated.

MULTIGATED ACQUISITION IMAGING

Multigated acquisition imaging or gated pool imaging is a noninvasive technique to calculate left ventricular ejection fraction. The information gathered in this study is obtained from the electrical activity of the heart using an electrocardiograph. Multigated acquisition imaging obtains multiple individual ejection fractions knowing the heart rate and R-R intervals on the electrocardiogram and then measures the emptying curves of the heart via computer (Fig. 8-17). This technique has advantages over others in that it is noninvasive and can therefore be used on critically ill cardiac patients (e.g., those with heart failure) when other more invasive tests such as catheterization would be dangerous.[49-52]

SUMMARY

- The laboratory tests that are specific to the patient with cardiac dysfunction measure the serum enzymes, blood lipids (triglycerides and cholesterol), complete blood count, coagulation profile (prothrombin time), electrolyte levels, BUN and creatinine levels, and serum glucose levels.
- The enzymes that are diagnostic of cardiac injury include: creatine phosphokinase, lactic dehydrogenase, and aspartate aminotransferase.
- Clinically, an early or a secondary peak in

CPK levels followed by a more rapid decline in the CPK-MB levels is strongly suggestive of reperfusion following thrombolytic therapy.

- Sodium, potassium, and carbon dioxide are the most important electrolytes to monitor. Hydration state, medications, and disease can affect the electrolyte levels.
- Important information can be obtained from the echocardiogram, including the size of the ventricular cavity, the thickness and integrity of the interatrial and interventricular septa, the functioning of the valves, and the motions of individual segments of the ventricular wall.
- Indications for use of the Holter monitor include identifying symptoms possibly caused by arrhythmias (e.g., dizziness, syncope, shortness of breath at rest as well as with activity), describing the arrhythmias noted with activity (frequency and severity), and evaluating antiarrhythmia therapy and pacemaker functioning.
- Most tests are symptom limited and, as such, are terminated at the request of the patient or when an abnormality is identified in one or more parameters being measured.
- Indications for uses of thallium injection with stress testing include detection of myocardial infarction and transient myocardial ischemia.
- Low-level exercise testing may be useful for predicting the subsequent course of a myocardial infarction or bypass surgery as well as for identifying the high-risk patient.
- Exercise-induced ST-segment depression of 2.0 millimeters or greater on low-level exercise tests has been identified as the single most valuable indicator of prognosis after myocardial infarction.
- Low-level exercise testing can also provide information useful for optimal medical management after myocardial injury or surgery, including treatment for angina, arrhythmias, or hypertension.
- Although the physical therapist may not actually perform the stress test, obtaining the interpretation of the results provides valuable data for developing an exercise prescription.
- Sensitivity is the measure of the reliability of stress testing to identify the presence of disease. Specificity is the measure of the reliability of stress testing to identify the population without disease.
- Specific determinations that can be made as a result of cardiac catheterization include (1) severity of coronary artery disease (degree of stenosis); (2) left ventricular dysfunction or aneurysm or both; (3) valvular heart disease and the severity of the dysfunction, including aortic valve stenosis or regurgitation, mitral valve stenosis or regurgitation or prolapse, tricuspid valve dysfunction, or pulmonic valve dysfunction; (4) pericardial disease; (5) myocardial disease including cardiomyopathy; and (6) congenital heart disease.
- Ergonovine stimulation is used when coronary spasm is suspected, particularly in a patient with ECG-documented changes during symptoms or with documented ischemic episodes and a normal coronary angiographic study.
- Positron emission tomography is a nuclear technique that provides visualization and direct measurement of metabolic functioning including glucose metabolism, fatty acid metabolism, and blood flow of the heart without the patient performing exercise.
- Multigated acquisition imaging or gated pool imaging is a noninvasive technique to calculate left ventricular ejection fraction.

References

1. Jacobs DS, Kasten BL, DeMott WR, Worlfson WL. Lab Test Handbook. Cleveland, Lexicomp/Mosby, 1988.
2. Karmazyn M. Reduction of enzyme release from reperfused ischemic hearts by steroidal and nonsteroidal prostaglandin synthesis inhibitors. Prostaglandins Leukot Med 11(3):299–315, 1983.
3. Smith AM, Theirer JA, Huang SH. Serum enzymes in myocardial infarction. Am J Nurs 73(2):277, 1973.
4. White HD, Cross DB, Williams BF, Norris RM. Safety and efficacy of repeat thrombolytic treatment after acute MI. Br Heart J 64(3):177–181, 1990.
5. Pollock ML, Schmidt DH. Epidemiologic Insights into Atherosclerotic Cardiovascular Disease from the Framingham Study in Heart Disease and Rehabilitation. 2nd ed. New York, John Wiley and Sons, 1986.
6. Castelli WP. Cholesterol and lipids in the risk of coronary artery disease—the Framingham Heart Study. Can J Cardiol 4(suppl A):5A–10A, 1988.
7. Gordon T, Castelli WP, Hjortlan MC, et al: Diabetes, blood lipids, and the role of obesity in coronary heart disease for women. Ann Intern Med 87:393, 1977.
8. Gentile R. Clinical usefulness of a new echocardiographic window: The transesophageal approach. Medicina (Firenze) 10(4):411–415, 1990.
9. Pedersen WR, Walker M, Olson JD, et al. Value of transesophageal echocardiography as an adjunct to transthoracic echocardiography in evaluation of native and prosthetic valve endocarditis. Chest 100(2):351–356, 1991.
10. Orihashi K, Hong YW, Chung G, et al. New applications of two dimensional transesophageal echocardiography in cardiac surgery. J Cardiothorac Vasc Anesth 5(1):33–39, 1991.

11. Font VE, Obarski TP, Klein AL, et al. Transesophageal echocardiography in the critical care unit. Cleve Clin J Med 58(4):3315–3322, 1991.
12. Kelly WN. Textbook of Internal Medicine. Vol. 1. Philadelphia, JB Lippincott, 1989.
13. Bigger JT, Weld F, Rolnitzky L. Prevalence, characteristics and significance of ventricular tachycardia detected with ambulatory electrocardiographic recording of late hospital phase of acute myocardial infarction. Am J Cardiol 48(5):815, 1981.
14. Cooper KH. The Aerobics Way. New York, Bantam Books, 1981.
15. McGavin CR, Gupta SP, McHardy GJR. Twelve minute walking tests for assessing disability in chronic bronchitis. Br Med J 1:822–823, 1976.
16. Jones NL, Cambell EJ. Clinical Exercise Testing. 2nd ed. Philadelphia, WB Saunders, 1982.
17. American College of Sports Medicine. Guidelines for Exercise Testing and Prescription. 4th ed. Philadelphia, Lea & Febiger, 1990.
18. Ellestad MH, Stuart RJ. National survey of exercise stress testing facilities. Chest 77:94, 1980.
19. Ellestad MH, Wan MKC. Standards for adult exercise testing laboratories. The Exercise Standards Book. Dallas, American Heart Association, 1979.
20. Cahalin LP, Blessey R, Cummer D, Simard M. The safety of exercise testing performed independently by physical therapists. J Cardiopulm Rehab 7(6):269, 1987.
21. Ellestad MH. Stress Testing Principles and Practice. Philadelphia, FA Davis, 1986.
22. Golding LA, Myers CR, Sinning WE. Y's Way to Physical Fitness. 3rd ed. Champaign, Ill, Human Kinetics, 1989.
23. Froelicher VF. Exercise and the Heart. Clinical Concepts. 2nd ed. Chicago, Year Book Medical Publishers, 1987.
24. Blessey RL. Aerobic capacity and cardiac catheterization results in 13 patients with exercise bradycardia. Med Sci Sports Exerc 8:50, 1976 (abstract).
25. Davidson DM, DeBusk RJ. Prognostic value of a single exercise test 3 weeks after uncomplicated myocardial infarction. Circulation 61:236–242, 1980.
26. Starling MR, Crawford MH, Kennedy GT, et al. Predictive value of early post-myocardial infarction modified exercise testing in multivessel coronary artery disease detection. Am Heart J 102(2):169, 1981.
27. Schwartz K, Turner J, Sheffield L, et al. Limited exercise testing soon after MI (correlation with early coronary and left ventricular angiography). Ann Intern Med 94(6):727, 1981.
28. Fuller C, Razner A, Verani M, et al. Early post myocardial infarction treadmill stress testing. Ann Intern Med 94:734, 1981.
29. Savnamki KI, Anderson D. Early exercise test in the assessment of long term prognosis after acute MI. Acta Med Scand 209:185, 1981.
30. Weld F, Chu K, Bigger J, Rolnitzky L. Risk stratification with low level exercise testing two weeks after acute MI. Circulation 64(2):306–314, 1981.
31. Theroux P, Waters D, Halphen C, et al. Prognostic value of exercise testing soon after myocardial infarction. N Engl J Med 301(7):341, 1979.
32. Firth BG, Lange RA. Pathophysiology and management of primary pump failure. In: Gersh BJ, Rahimtoola SH (eds). Acute Myocardial Infarction. New York, Elsevier, 1991.
33. Ibsen H, Kjoller E, Styperck J, et al. Routine exercise ECG three weeks after acute myocardial infarction. Acta Med Scand 198:463, 1975.
34. Ross J. Hemodynamic changes in acute MI. In: The Myocardium Failure and Infarction. New York, HP Publishing, 1974, p 261.
35. Ericsson M, Granath A, Ohlsen P, et al: Arrhythmias and symptoms during treadmill testing three weeks after myocardial infarction in 100 patients. Br Heart J 35:787, 1973.
36. McIntyre KM, Lewis AJ. Textbook of Advanced Cardiac Life Support. Dallas, American Heart Association, 1983.
37. Poyatos ME, Lerman J, Estrada A, et al. Predictive value of changes in R-wave amplitude after exercise in coronary heart disease. Am J Cardiol 54(10):1212, 1984.
38. Diamond GA, Forrester JS. Analysis of probability as an aid in the clinical diagnosis of coronary artery disease. N Engl J Med 300:1350, 1979.
39. Goldschlager H, Selzer Z, Cohn K. Treadmill stress tests as indicators of presence and severity of coronary artery disease. Ann Intern Med 85:277, 1976.
40. Bruce RA, DeRouen T, Peterson DR, et al. Noninvasive predictors of sudden death in men with coronary heart disease. Am J Cardiol 39:833, 1977.
41. Weiner DA, Ryan TJ, McCabe GH, et al. Prognostic importance of a clinical profile and exercise test in medically treated patients with coronary artery disease. J Am Coll Cardiol 3(3):772, 1984.
42. Ross J Jr, Fisch C. Guidelines for coronary angiography. J Am Coll Cardiol 10:935, 1987.
43. Beller GA, Gibson RS: Sensitivity, specificity and prognostic significance of noninvasive testing for occult or known coronary disease. Prog Cardiovasc Dis 29:241, 1987.
44. Maseri A. Role of coronary artery spasm in symptomatic and silent myocardial ischemia. J Am Coll Cardiol 9:249, 1987.
45. Igarashi Y, Yamazoe M, Shibata A. Effect of direct intracoronary administration of methylergonovine in patients with and without variant angina. Am Heart J 121(4[pt. 1]):1094–1100, 1991.
46. Khoshio A, Miyakoda H, Fukuiki M. Significance of coronary artery tone assessed by coronary responses to ergonovine and nitrate. Jpn Circ J 55(1):33–40, 1991.
47. Chan SY, Brunken RC, Buxton DB. Cardiac positron emission tomography: The foundations and clinical applications. J Thorac Imaging 5(3):9–19, 1990.
48. Berman DS, Kiat H, Van Train KF, et al. Comparison of SPECT using technetium-99m agents and thallium-201 and PET for the assessment of myocardial perfusion and viability. Am J Cardiol 66(13):72E–79E, 1990.
49. Ben-David Y, Shefer A, Weiss AT, et al. Early postoperative assessment of coronary artery bypass surgery using nuclear left ventriculography and atrial pacing. Thorac Cardiovasc Surg 31(6):377–381, 1983.
50. Gunnar WP, Martin M, Smith RF, et al. The utility of cardiac evaluation in the hemodynamically stable patient with suspected myocardial contusion. Am Surg 57(6):373, 1991.
51. Yang DC, Jain CU, Patel D, et al. Use of i.v. radionuclide total body arteriography to evaluate arterial bypass shunts—a new method—a review of several cases. Angiology 41(9[pt.1]):745–752, 1990.
52. Gottlieb SO, Gottlieb SH, Achuff SC, et al. Silent ischemia on Holter monitoring predicts mortality in high risk post infarction patients. JAMA 259:1030, 1988.

9 ELECTROCARDIOGRAPHY

INTRODUCTION

Understanding the electrocardiogram (ECG) requires a basic understanding of the electrophysiology and anatomy of the heart and conduction system (see Chapters 1 and 2), an appreciation of the ECG wave forms (both their normal and abnormal presentations in different leads), and a certain amount of practice in the systematic review of 12-lead and single-lead ECG rhythm strips. After reading this chapter the therapist should be able to determine whether an ECG tracing represents a benign or a life-threatening situation and be able to begin to make appropriate clinical decisions based on this determination. Further information regarding the ECG and more advanced arrhythmia detection should be researched in texts devoted entirely to electrocardiography.

One comment should be made about nomenclature before beginning the discussion of electrocardiography. *Dysrhythmia* is the most accurate term to describe a heart rhythm that is abnormal, because the prefix *dys* means "bad" or "difficult." However, researchers do not use this term widely but rather favor the term *arrhythmia*,

355

which means "without rhythm" or "no rhythm." In keeping with current usage, this chapter and text use arrhythmia throughout to refer to abnormal rhythm.

BASIC ELECTROPHYSIOLOGIC PRINCIPLES

The ECG is inscribed on specially ruled paper. It represents the electrical impulses of the heart and provides valuable information regarding the heart's function. The cardiac muscle provides the ECG with information as a result of differentiation of cell types found in the myocardium. The four types of monocytes that comprise the muscle include the typical working myocytes, which respond to the electrical stimulus to contract and pump the blood; nodal myocytes, which have the highest rate of rhythmicity but slow impulse-conduction rates; transitional myocytes, which conduct impulses twice as fast as nodal cells; and Purkinje's cells, which have a low rate of rhythmicity yet a high rate of conductivity.

Electrical stimulation makes the cell membrane more permeable to the flow of ions. As there is a predominance of potassium (K^+) on the inside of the cell and sodium (Na^+) on the outside, the electrical stimulation makes the membrane more permeable to the sodium ions so that they flow inward, creating a change in the resting state of the cells of the cardiac muscle from a negative to a positive charge on the interior. This sodium flow is referred to as the *fast channel*. The potassium ions then start to flow outward. The potassium flow is referred to as the *slow channel*. The electrical stimulation of the specialized cells that cause contraction is called **depolarization** (Fig. 9–1). As the cell becomes positive on the interior, the myocardial cells are stimulated to contract. When the potassium ion flow outward exceeds the sodium flow inward, repolarization begins. During **repolarization,** the myocardial cells return to a negative interior and a positive exterior, and muscle relaxation occurs.[1] When the wave of depolarization is moving toward a positive electrode located on the skin, the ECG records a simultaneous upward deflection (Fig. 9–2).

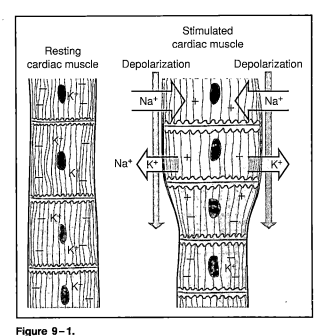

Figure 9–1.

Electrical stimulation to the cardiac muscle cell membrane causes depolarization. With depolarization the membrane is more permeable to sodium ions, allowing them to flow inward and creating a positive charge on the inside.

Cardiac muscle has three unique properties: **automaticity, rhythmicity,** and **conductivity.** Cardiac muscle cells are able to discharge an electrical stimulus without stimulation from a nerve, as is typical in all other muscle cells, demonstrating the property of automaticity. Rhythmicity is the regularity with which such pacemaking activity occurs. Cardiac muscle cells can therefore "automatically" discharge an electrical stimulus. This is particularly noticeable in the **sinoatrial (SA) node,** which is the primary pacemaker and has the most amount of automaticity of the cardiac cells.

However, other cardiac cells may discharge at any time owing to this property of automaticity, creating abnormal rates or rhythms (as in premature beats). The SA node has a normal innate automatic firing rate between 60 and 100 beats per minute. The **atrioventricular (AV) node** has an inherent firing rate of 40 to 60 beats per minute and begins to act as the pacemaker if the SA node is not functioning properly. The His-

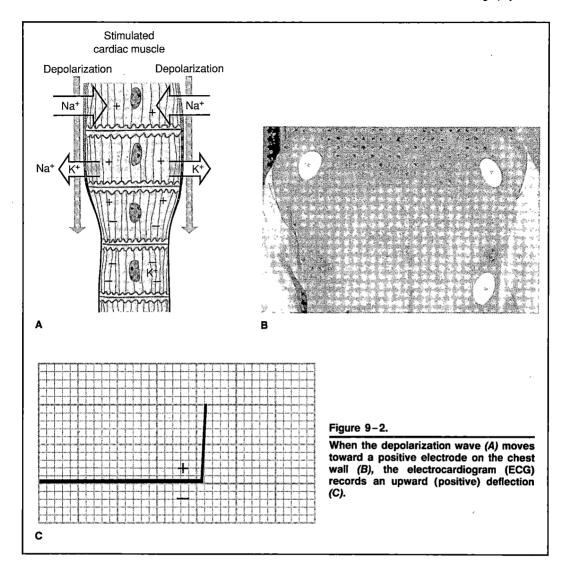

A

B

C

Figure 9-2.

When the depolarization wave (A) moves toward a positive electrode on the chest wall (B), the electrocardiogram (ECG) records an upward (positive) deflection (C).

Purkinje portions of the specialized conduction system have an inherent firing rate of 30 to 40 beats per minute.

Cardiac muscle cells also have the ability to spread impulses to adjoining cells very quickly (the property of conductivity). The rapid spread can be visualized when one considers how fast the cells must depolarize and repolarize at a heart rate of 200 beats per minute. Rapid arrhythmias such as supraventricular tachycardia and slow rates due to AV blocks are examples of problems with conductivity. See Chapter 2 for further discussion of the myocytes.

THE AUTONOMIC NERVOUS SYSTEM

The autonomic nervous system has a major influence on reflex cardiac activity as a result of two counterbalancing forces: the sympathetic and the parasympathetic divisions. The effects of the two divisions determine the delicate balance between excitation and depression of cardiac activity, which can be altered in favor of one or the other by numerous physiologic and pathologic factors and in a variety of situations. The sympathetic division is equated with acceleration, and the parasympathetic division is equated with deceleration or braking.

Sympathetic Division

The sympathetic division discharges norepinephrine (noradrenalin) from its terminal nerve branches in the atria and ventricle, resulting in an excitation of the rate of impulse formation and the velocity of impulse propagation and an increase in the force of contractile fibers. The sympathetic division acts on both the SA node and the AV node as well as on the ventricle. In addition, the sympathetic division can stimulate the adrenal gland to secrete norepinephrine and epinephrine into the bloodstream. The direct action on the heart of these hormones is equal to the direct stimulation of the terminal nerve branches in the heart. Increased sympathetic activity increases the heart rate, the conduction velocity throughout the AV node, the contractility of the heart muscle, and the irritability of the heart. In addition, automaticity may increase, which can alter the normal sinus rhythm.

Parasympathetic Division

The parasympathetic division discharges acetylcholine from the terminal nerve branches. The vagus nerve is the main component of the parasympathetic division in control of the heart, and it acts primarily on the SA node as a general inhibitor on the rate of impulse formation and conduction velocity. Increased parasympathetic activity slows the heart rate and acts to slow the conduction through the AV node. Decreased parasympathetic activity increases the heart rate, the conduction through the AV node, and the irritability of the heart. Therefore, the effect of acetylcholine and the effects of vagal stimulation

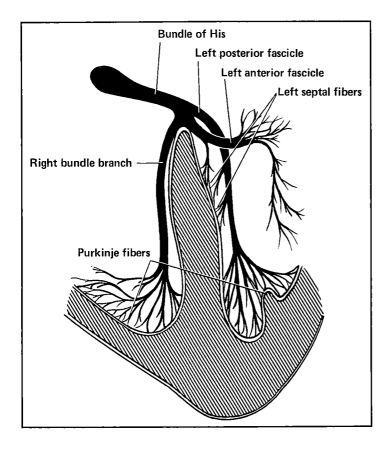

Figure 9–3.

The conduction system. The pathway of electrical activity begins at the sinoatrial node and spreads to Purkinje's fibers. (Reproduced with permission from Goldman MJ. Principles of Clinical Electrocardiography. 10th ed. Los Altos, Calif, Lange Medical Books, 1979.)

depress the automaticity and conductivity of the heart. See Chapter 2 for further discussion.

THE CONDUCTION SYSTEM

The conduction system is composed of myocytes arranged in a pathway that spreads the electrical activity throughout the four chambers (2 atria, 2 ventricles) (Fig. 9–3). The primary pacemaker that initiates the electrical impulse for the cardiac muscle is the SA node, located in the right atrium near the posterior surface and adjacent to the entry of the superior vena cava. The impulse then spreads throughout the right atrium via intra-atrial pathways and to the left atrium via **Bachmann's bundle.** The wave of atrial depolarization is represented on the ECG as the P

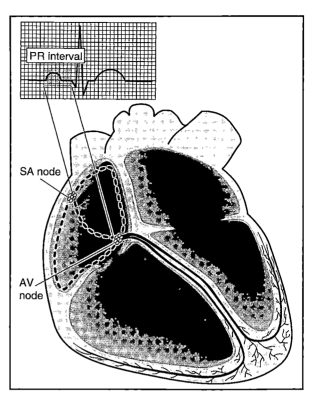

Figure 9–5.

When the spread of depolarization reaches the atrioventricular node, a slight delay occurs. The electrocardiogram records this as the P–R interval.

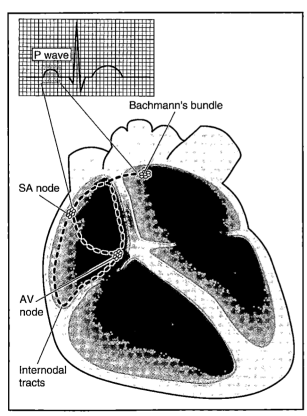

Figure 9–4.

Atrial depolarization is depicted on the electrocardiographic tracing as the P wave. The impulse is spread to the left atrium via the Bachmann's bundle.

wave. Therefore, the P wave represents atrial depolarization electrically and is normally associated with atrial contraction mechanically (Fig. 9–4). Following the spread of depolarization through the atria, the impulse then reaches the AV node, also called the junctional node, which is located near the intraventricular septum in the inferior aspect of the right atrium just superior to the tricuspid valve. The AV node delays the conduction of the electrical impulse from the atria for one tenth of a second (seen on the ECG as the isoelectric line after the P wave and before the QRS complex), allowing for the mechanical contraction of the atria to eject blood into the ventricles. This is known as the **atrial kick.** The ECG depicts this delay as the P–R segment (Fig. 9–5). The P–R segment is also considered to be the isoelectric line. The impulse then passes from the AV node into the His's bundle and then to the bundle branches. The bundle branches consist of a left and right division and are located in the interventricular septum (Fig. 9-6).

The right bundle branch is responsible for depolarization of the right ventricle, and the left bundle branch, which has an anterior fascicle and a posterior fascicle, is responsible for the depolarization of the left ventricle. The electrical impulses spread down the bundle branches and terminate in Purkinje's fibers, which are very small fibers and are numerous. These fibers penetrate the myocardium and stimulate muscle contraction from the apex upward toward the base of the heart in a "wringing" action. The ECG records the electrical stimulus of ventricular depolarization as the QRS complex (Fig. 9-7). The QRS complex represents ventricular depolarization and is normally followed closely by ventricular contraction. The ECG tracing may demonstrate a variety of QRS waveforms, depending on the pathologic condition or the location of the

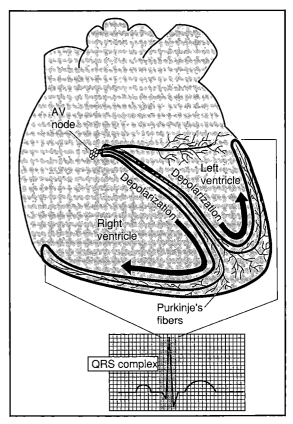

Figure 9-7.

Ventricular depolarization occurs when the electric impulse reaches Purkinje's fibers. The electrocardiogram depicts ventricular depolarization in the QRS complex.

electrode, but they are generally referred to as the QRS complex regardless of the configuration. Figure 9-8 shows the various forms of QRS complexes that may be seen on an ECG. Repolarization begins when ventricular contraction ends.

Following the QRS complex, a slight pause is noted. This pause is called the ST segment and is defined as the flat piece of isoelectric line that starts at the end of the QRS complex and ends at the beginning of the T wave (Fig. 9-9). The ventricle is initiating repolarization during the ST-segment phase of the ECG. This segment has very important predictive value and is discussed later.

Repolarization is completed with the ending of the T wave. The T wave represents the ventricu-

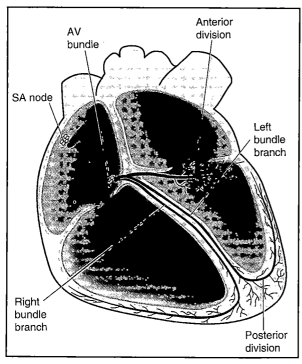

Figure 9-6.

The bundle branches, consisting of a left and right division, are located within the interventricular septum. The left bundle branch has both an anterior and a posterior division.

Figure 9-8.

Possible QRS complexes. Each individual's electrocardiographic tracing is different.

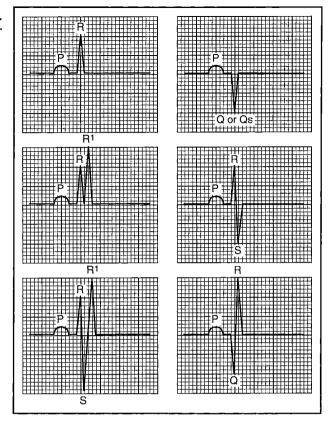

lar repolarization. Because no mechanical contraction is occurring, the T wave is strictly an electrical phenomenon that records the return of potassium inward and that of sodium outward and the change in the polarization of the cell.

THE ELECTROCARDIOGRAM RECORDING

The electrocardiogram is recorded on ruled graph paper, with the smallest divisions (or squares) being 1 millimeter long and 1 millimeter high. The height (positive deflection) or depth (negative deflection) measures the voltage as 0.1 millivolt per millimeter (Fig. 9-10). Time is represented on the graph paper by 0.04 second between each small square and 0.2 second between the large squares (Fig. 9-11) when the paper speed is set at 25 mm per second. Exact time is important to note on the ECG to determine the

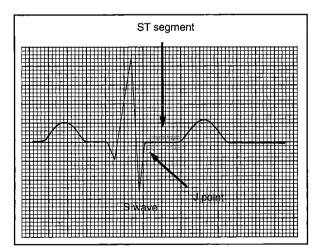

Figure 9-9.

The ST segment on the electrocardiogram tracing begins at the end of the S wave and ends at the beginning of the T wave. Notice the J point, which classically is defined as the point at which the thin line of the QRS tracing turns into a thick line. The J point is also the beginning of the ST segment and is often used when the ST segment is aberrant.

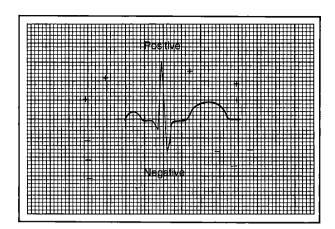

Figure 9-10.

The positive or negative deflections on the electrocardiogram tracing represent voltage. Each small square is 1 mm in height.

duration of the complexes (e.g., QRS duration) and the intervals (e.g., P-R interval) as well as to identify the heart rates and arrhythmias.

The standard 12-lead ECG consists of tracings from six limb leads and six chest leads. The six limb leads are I, II, III, aVR, aVL, and aVF. Each limb lead records from a different angle, provid-

ing a different view of the same cardiac activity. Therefore, the tracings from the various leads look different because the electrical activity is monitored from different positions. The six chest leads of the ECG are V_1, V_2, V_3, V_4, V_5, and V_6 and are monitored from six electrodes placed on the chest wall. The ECG tracing from the chest

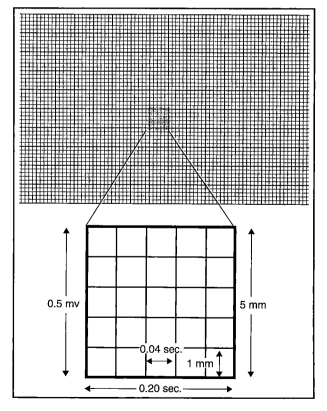

Figure 9-11.

Electrocardiogram paper displays time on the horizontal axis. Each small box represents 0.04 second, and each large box represents 0.20 second. The vertical axis changes are measured in millimeters. Each small box represents 1 mm, each large box represents 5 mm.

leads (V_1 to V_6) shows gradual changes in all the waves, as seen in Figure 9–12. Leads V_1 and V_2 are placed over the right side of the heart, and V_5 and V_6 are placed over the left side of the heart. Leads V_3 and V_4 are placed over the ventricular septum (Fig. 9–13). Figure 9–14 shows a picture of a standard 12-lead ECG with normal tracings in each of the leads, and the location of the leads on the tracing.

Four elements are specifically assessed on a 12-lead ECG tracing:

- Heart rate
- Heart rhythm
- **Hypertrophy**
- **Infarction**

A single-lead tracing, often called a *rhythm strip*, is assessed for heart rate, rhythm, and presence of arrhythmias. If hypertrophy, ischemia, or infarction is suspected, a 12-lead ECG should be obtained.

HEART RATE

The heart rate can be determined from the ECG recording by a variety of methods, includ-

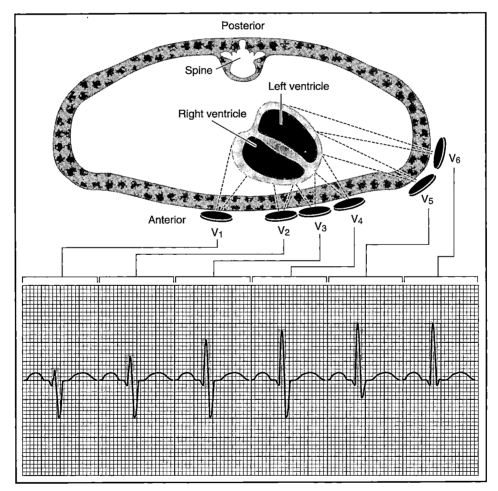

Figure 9–12.

The electrocardiographic tracing from the chest leads (V_1–V_6), showing the gradual changes that occur with the R and S waves.

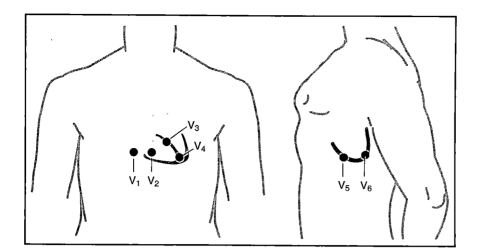

Figure 9–13.

Leads V_1 and V_2 are placed over the right side of the heart. Leads V_3 and V_4 are located over the interventricular septum. Leads V_5 and V_6 demonstrate changes on the left side of the heart.

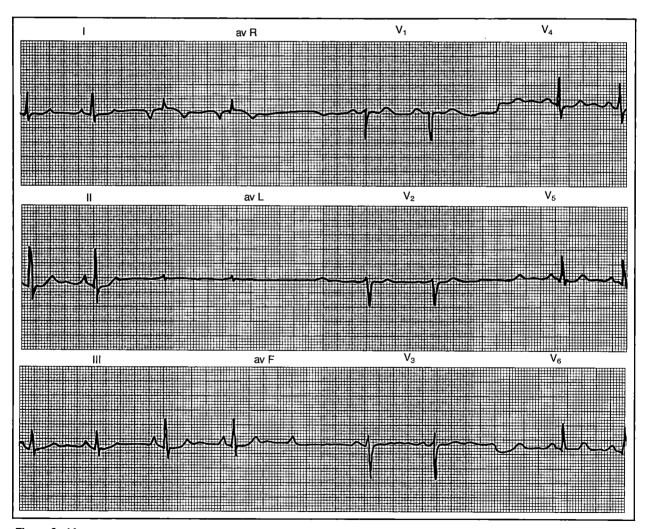

Figure 9–14.

A normal 12-lead electrocardiogram tracing. Notice that avR is the only lead in which the P wave, QRS complex, and T wave are all negative.

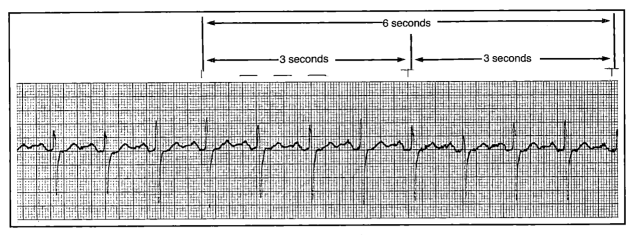

Figure 9-15.
The heart rate can be determined by identifying 6 seconds on the electrocardiogram paper and counting the number of QRS complexes in the 6-second strip. The number of QRS complexes in 6 seconds multiplied by 10 gives the heart rate for 1 minute. The heart rate in the illustrated tracing is 84.

ing obtaining a 6-second tracing, measuring specific R waves, and counting the number of large boxes (5 mm or 0.2 sec in length).

Six-Second Tracing. The investigator obtains an ECG recording that is 6 seconds in length (Fig. 9-15). The number of QRS comlexes found in the 6-second recording is then multiplied by 10 to determine the heart rate per minute.

Number of QRS complexes in a 6-second recording × 10 = heart rate per minute

R Wave Measurement. An alternative method of measuring heart rate is by identifying a specific R wave that falls on a heavy black line (large box line; Fig. 9-16). For each heavy black

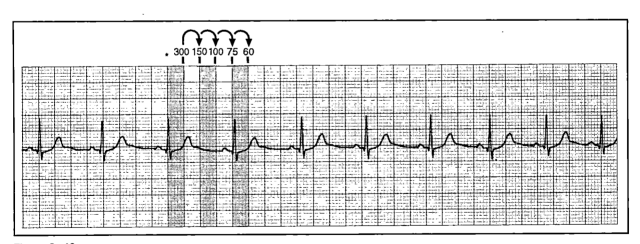

Figure 9-16.
Another method of determining heart rate is to first find a specific R wave that falls on a heavy black line (see *). Then, count off "300, 150, 100, 75, 60, 50" for each heavy black line that follows until the next R wave falls. To find the specific rate, determine the difference in rate between the dark lines that encircle the R wave (for example 300 − 150 = 150), and divide this number by 5 (the number of small boxes between the dark lines). Between 150 and 300 the distance between each small box is worth 30 beats. Between 100 and 150 the distance between each small box is worth 10 beats. This method assists in identifying a more accurate heart rate.

line that follows this R wave until the next R wave occurs the therapist counts 300, 150, 100, 75, 60, 50. Where the next R wave falls in this counting method gives the actual heart rate. To utilize this method, one must be able to memorize the specific numbers for the successive dark black lines to determine rapid heart rates from the graph paper. The one problem with R wave measurement for determining heart rate is that it cannot be used with irregular heart rhythms. For a more accurate estimate, the number of QRS complexes in a 30-second strip must be counted and then multiplied by 2.

$$\text{Number of QRS complexes in a 30-second strip} \times 2 = \text{heart rate per minute}$$

Counting Boxes. The third method of obtaining the heart rate from the graph paper is to count the number of large boxes (5 mm or 0.2 sec in length) between the first QRS complex and the next QRS complex. The number of large boxes is then divided into 300 to obtain an estimate of the heart rate.

$$300 \div \text{Number of large boxes between the first QRS complex and the next QRS complex} = \text{heart rate per minute}$$

A more accurate measurement of the heart rate can be made by counting the number of small boxes (1 mm or 0.04 sec in length) between the QRS complexes and then dividing this number into 1500. This method requires much greater time to perform heart rate interpretation (Fig. 9–17).

$$\text{Number of small boxes between QRS complexes} \div 1500 = \text{heart rate per minute}$$

HEART RHYTHM

The 12-lead ECG is used primarily for determining ischemia or infarction as well as for comparing previous ECG recordings for an individual. However, for simple detection of rate or rhythm disturbances, single-lead monitoring is the appropriate choice. Single-lead monitoring

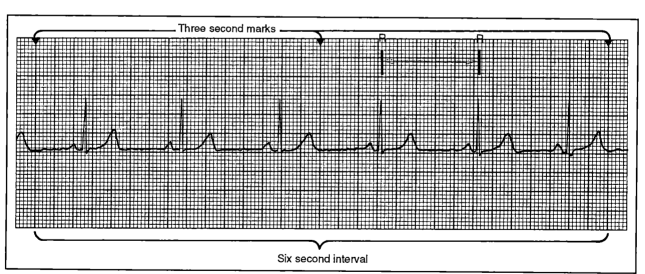

Figure 9–17.

Another method of determining heart rate is to count the number of large boxes between two R waves and divide this number into 300. Or, for greater accuracy, count the number of large boxes between the R waves, multiply this number by 5 (the number of small boxes per large box), and divide this number into 1500. (From Wiederhold R. Electrocardiography: The Monitoring Lead. Philadelphia, WB Saunders, 1989, p 47.)

via telemetry is the most common practice in stepdown intensive care units and cardiopulmonary rehabilitation programs. Single-lead monitoring is limited to detection of rate and rhythm disturbances; it *cannot* detect ischemia owing to the inability to calibrate radiotelemetry. Hardwire systems are frequently used in the intensive care unit or cardiac care unit and should be calibrated appropriately. These systems can record **ischemia.** Twelve-lead ECG monitoring is used when ischemia is suspected or when a change in condition is noted.

To determine heart rate and rhythm from single-lead monitoring, the normal waveforms and intervals must be understood (Fig. 9–18). The waveforms that represent depolarization of the myocardium have been labeled P, QRS, T, and U. A systematic approach to waveforms and interval measurement should be undertaken when reviewing cardiac rhythm. A systematic approach to the assessment of the cardiac cycle for rhythm and rate disturbances involves the following:

1. Evaluate the P wave. (Is it normal and upright, and is there a P wave before every QRS? Do all the Ps look alike?)

2. Evaluate the P–R interval. (Normal duration is 0.12–0.20 sec.)

3. Evaluate the QRS complex. (Do all QRS complexes look alike?)

4. Evaluate the QRS interval. (Normal duration is 0.06–0.10 sec.)

5. Evaluate the T wave. (Is it upright and normal in appearance?)

6. Evaluate the R to R wave interval. (Is it regular?)

7. Evaluate the heart rate (6-second strip if regular rhythm; normal rate is 60–100 beats per minute.)

8. Observe the patient, and evaluate any symptoms. (Does the observation, symptoms, or both correlate with the arrhythmia?)

Normal Wave Forms

The P wave is normally rounded, symmetric, and upright, representing atrial depolarization. A P wave should occur before every QRS complex.

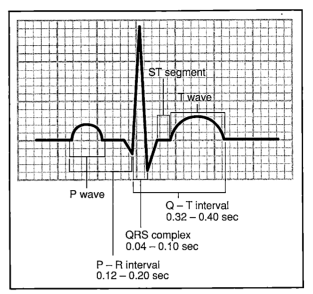

Figure 9–18.

The normal electrocardiogram tracing. The P–R interval measures between 0.12 and 0.20 second. The normal duration of the QRS complex is 0.04 to 0.10 second. The normal duration of the Q–T interval is 0.32 to 0.40 second.

The P–R interval is the interval that starts at the beginning of the P wave and ends at the beginning of the QRS complex; the portion following the P wave is also defined as the isoelectric line. The P–R interval is normally 0.12 to 0.20 second (or up to five small squares on the ECG paper). This period of time represents the atrial depolarization and the slowing of electrical conduction through the AV node.

The QRS complex follows the P–R interval and has multiple deflections and may have numerous variations, depending on the lead that is being monitored (see Fig. 9–8 for variations in the QRS complexes). The QRS complex begins at the end of the P–R interval and appears as a thin line recording from the ECG stylus, ending normally with a return to the baseline. The QRS duration reflects the time it takes for conduction to proceed to the Purkinje fibers and for the ventricles to depolarize. The normal duration is 0.04 to 0.10 second.

The ST segment follows the QRS complex, beginning where the ECG tracing transforms from a thin line to a thicker line and terminating at the beginning of the T wave. The ST segment

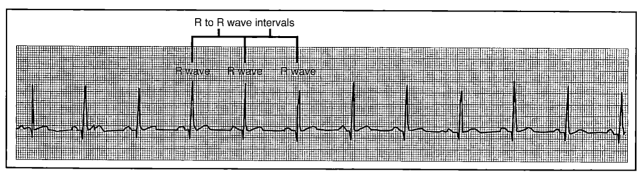

Figure 9–19.

Electrocardiogram tracing demonstrating R to R intervals. R to R intervals are evaluated for regularity of rhythm.

should be represented as an isoelectric line along the same line (if measured with a ruler) as the P–R interval or the baseline. The T wave follows the ST segment and should be rounded, symmetric, and upright. The T wave represents ventricular repolarization.

The Q–T interval (from the beginning of the QRS complex until the end of the T wave) normally measures between 0.32 to 0.40 second if a normal sinus rhythm is present. The Q–T interval usually is not measured unless drug toxicity is suspected. Occasionally a U wave may follow the T wave, but its cause and clinical value are essentially unknown.

Finally, the R to R interval is reviewed throughout the rhythm strip to assess regularity of rhythm (Fig. 9–19). Normal rhythm requires a regular R to R interval throughout; however, a discrepancy of up to 0.12 second between the shortest and the longest R to R interval is acceptable for normal respiratory variation. Occasionally single-lead monitoring may be affected by artifact, which could include

- muscle tremors or movement (including anything from sneezing and coughing to actual physical movement)
- loose electrodes
- 60-cycle electrical interference

In most cases of artifact interference, the R to R interval is regular throughout, and the interference is seen between the R waves (Fig. 9–20).

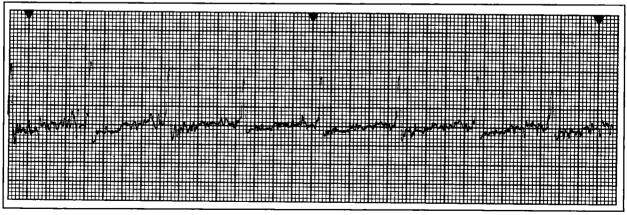

Figure 9–20.

Electrocardiogram tracing of normal sinus rhythm with artifact in between the R waves. (From Wiederhold R. Electrocardiography: The Monitoring Lead. Philadelphia, WB Saunders, 1989, p 50.)

If the R to R intervals are all regular, a 6-second strip or the counting down from 300 method can be employed to determine heart rate. Normal heart rate is between 60 and 100 beats per minute. If the R to R intervals are irregular (and greater than the acceptable range of 0.12 second for respiratory variation), a 30- to 60-second strip may be needed to determine the heart rate and the frequency or seriousness of the arrhythmia, or both.

BASIC INTERPRETATION OF HEART RHYTHM

The key to the basic interpretation of heart rhythm in the clinical setting involves using the systematic approach as presented earlier, correlating the interpretation with the history and the signs and symptoms of the patient and then deciding if the rhythm is benign or life threatening. If the decision is that the rhythm is truly benign, then the patient does not require ECG monitoring. If the rhythm is relatively benign, then occasional ECG monitoring may be necessary, or at least physiologic monitoring of the heart rate and blood pressure should be employed. If the arrhythmia is determined to be life threatening, ECG monitoring as well as physiologic monitoring should be carried out. In some cases the patient may not be a candidate for any activity or procedure until the arrhythmia is controlled.

For each of the following cardiac rhythms an ECG recording is provided along with a description of the features of each rhythm. In addition, possible etiologic factors as well as signs and symptoms that may be associated with the rhythm are explained. Treatment is discussed only so that the reader may develop an increased understanding of the whole picture of arrhythmias and their control. It should *not* be inferred that the physical therapist is responsible for the treatment of arrhythmias.

Normal Sinus Rhythm

The normal cardiac rhythm is termed *normal sinus rhythm* and begins with an impulse originating in the SA node with conduction through the normal pathways for depolarization. Parasympathetic stimulation generally slows the rate, and sympathetic stimulation increases the rate. Figure 9–21 illustrates normal sinus rhythm. The characteristics of NSR include the following:

- All P waves are upright, normal in appearance, and identical in configuration; a P wave exists before every QRS complex.
- The P–R interval is between 0.12 and 0.20 second.
- The QRS complexes are identical.
- The QRS duration is between 0.04 and 0.10 second.
- The R to R interval is regular (or if irregular, the difference between shortest and longest intervals is less than 0.12 second).
- The heart rate is between 60 and 100 beats per minute.

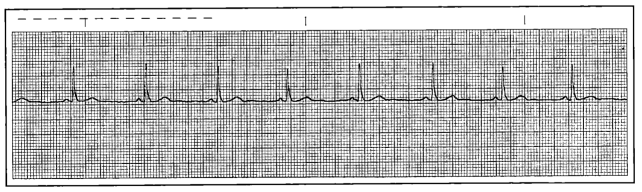

Figure 9–21.

Electrocardiogram tracing of normal sinus rhythm with a rate of approximately 62 beats per minute.

Sinus Bradycardia

Sinus bradycardia differs from normal sinus rhythm only in the rate, which is less than 60 beats per minute (Fig. 9-22). The characteristics of sinus bradycardia include the following:

- All P waves are upright, normal in appearance, and identical in configuration; a P wave exists before every QRS complex.
- The P-R interval is between 0.12 and 0.20 second.
- The QRS complexes are identical.
- The QRS duration is between 0.04 and 0.10 second.
- The R to R interval is regular throughout.
- The heart rate is less than 60 beats per minute.

Signs, Symptoms, and Causes

Sinus bradycardia is normal in well-trained athletes because of their enhanced stroke volume. It is also common in individuals taking beta-blocking medications. Sinus bradycardia may occur because of a decrease in the automaticity of the SA node or in a condition of increased vagal stimulation, such as suctioning or vomiting. Sinus bradycardia has been seen in patients who have traumatic brain injuries with increased intracranial pressures and in patients with brain tumors. Sinus bradycardia may also be present in the presence of second- or third-degree heart block; therefore, close evaluation of the P-R interval and the P to QRS ratio is necessary to rule out heart block.

Usually individuals with sinus bradycardia are asymptomatic unless a pathologic condition exists, at which time the individual may complain of **syncope,** dizziness, angina, or diaphoresis. Other arrhythmias may also develop.

Treatment

No treatment is necessary unless the patient is symptomatic. If the patient has symptoms, atropine may be used, and in some cases a temporary pacemaker may be implanted.

Sinus Tachycardia

Sinus tachycardia differs from normal sinus rhythm in rate only, which is greater than 100 beats per minute (Fig. 9-23). The characteristics of sinus tachycardia include:

- All P waves are upright, normal in appearance, and identical in configuration; a P wave exists before every QRS complex.
- The P-R interval is between 0.12 and 0.20 second.
- The QRS complexes are identical.

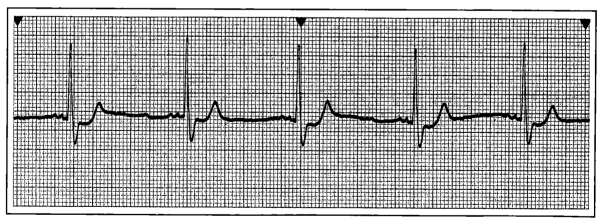

Figure 9-22.

Electrocardiogram tracing illustrating sinus bradycardia with a rate of approximately 50 beats per minute. (From Wiederhold R. Electrocardiography: The Monitoring Lead. Philadelphia, WB Saunders, 1989, p 189.)

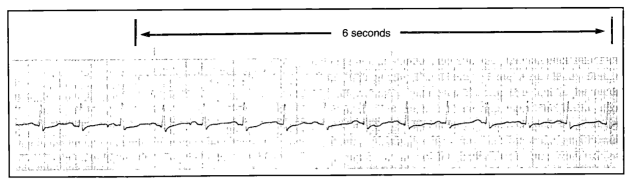

Figure 9-23.

Electrocardiogram tracing illustrating sinus tachycardia (heart rate approximately 105 beats per minute).

- The QRS duration is between 0.04 and 0.10 second.
- The R to R interval is regular.
- The heart rate is greater than 100 beats per minute.

Signs, Symptoms, and Causes

Sinus tachycardia is typically benign and is present usually in conditions in which the SA node automaticity is increased (increased sympathetic stimulation). Examples of conditions that induce sinus tachycardia include pain; fear; emotion; exertion (exercise); or any artificial stimulants such as caffeine, nicotine, amphetamines, and atropine. Sinus tachycardia is also found in situations in which the demands for oxygen are increased, including fever, congestive heart failure, infection, anemia, hemorrhage, myocardial injury, and **hyperthyroidism.** Usually individuals with sinus tachycardia are asymptomatic.

Treatment

Treatment for sinus tachycardia involves elimination (or treatment) of the underlying cause or, in some cases, the initiation of beta-blocker medication therapy.

Sinus Arrhythmia

Sinus arrhythmia is classified as an irregularity in rhythm in which the impulse is initiated by the SA node but with a phasic quickening and slowing of the impulse formation. The irregularity is usually caused by an alternation in vagal stimulation (Fig. 9-24). The characteristics of

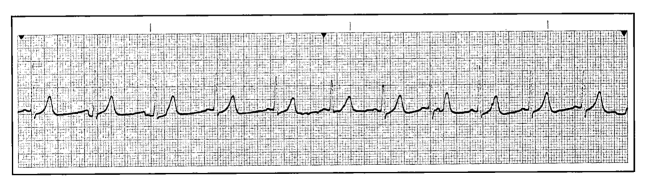

Figure 9-24.

Electrocardiogram tracing showing sinus arrhythmia. Notice the varying R to R interval. In the first 3 seconds, the R to R intervals appear long, and in the second 3 seconds the intervals appear shorter.

sinus arrhythmia include the following:

- All P waves are upright, normal in appearance, and identical in configuration; a P wave exists before every QRS complex.
- The P–R interval is between 0.12 and 0.20 second.
- The QRS complexes are identical.
- The QRS duration is between 0.04 and 0.10 second.
- The R to R interval varies throughout.
- The heart rate is between 40 to 100 beats per minute.

Signs, Symptoms, and Causes

The most common type of sinus arrhythmia is related to the respiratory cycle, with the rate increasing with inspiration and decreasing with expiration. This type of arrhythmia is usually found in the young or elderly at rest, and it disappears with activity. The other type of sinus arrhythmia is nonrespiratory and therefore is not affected by the breathing cycle. Nonrespiratory sinus arrhythmia may occur in conditions of infection, medication administration (particularly toxicity associated with digoxin or morphine), and fever.[2]

Treatment

The respiratory type of sinus arrhythmia is benign and does not require any treatment. The nonrespiratory type should be evaluated for the underlying cause, and then this cause should be treated.

Sinus Pause or Block

Sinus pause or **sinus block** occurs when the SA node fails to initiate an impulse, usually for only one cycle (Fig. 9–25). The characteristics of sinus pause and block include the following:

- All P waves are upright, normal in appearance, and identical in configuration; a P wave exists before every QRS complex.
- The P–R interval of the underlying rhythm is 0.12 to 0.20 second.
- The QRS complexes are identical.
- The QRS duration is between 0.04 and 0.10 second.
- The R to R interval is regular for the underlying rhythm, but occasional pauses are noted.
- The heart rate is usually 60 to 100 beats per minute.

Signs, Symptoms, and Causes

Sinus pause or block can occur for a number of reasons, including a sudden increase of parasympathetic activity, an organic disease of the SA node (sometimes referred to as sick sinus syndrome), an infection, a rheumatic disease, severe ischemia or infarction to the SA node, or a

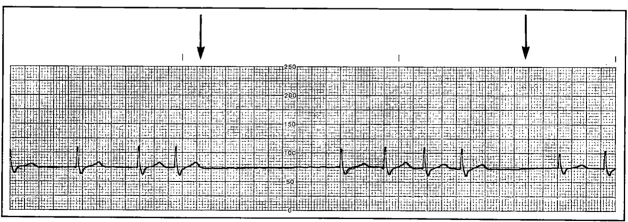

Figure 9–25.

Electrocardiogram tracing of sinus pause or block (arrows).

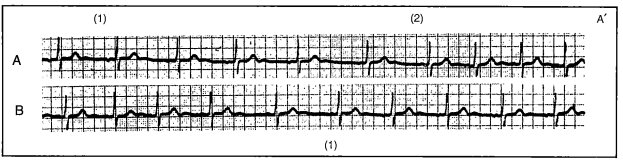

Figure 9-26.

Electrocardiogram tracing illustrating a wandering atrial pacemaker. This is a continuous recording in which B follows directly after A'. Notice that as the heart rate increases, the P waves become upright (2) and then gradually become inverted as the heart rate slows (1). (From Andreoli KG, Fowkes VH, Zipes DP, Wallace AC. Comprehensive Cardiac Care. 4th ed. St. Louis, CV Mosby, 1979.)

case of digoxin toxicity.[1] If the pause or block is prolonged or occurs frequently, the cardiac output is compromised, and the individual may complain of dizziness or syncope episodes.

Treatment

Treatment should be initiated when the patient is symptomatic. It involves treatment of the underlying cause, which may include reduction of digoxin, removal of vagal stimulation, and possibly treatment with atropine or implantation of a permanent pacemaker.

Wandering Atrial Pacemaker

The pacemaking activity in **wandering pacemaker** shifts from focus to focus, resulting in a rhythm that is very irregular and without a consistent pattern. Some of the impulses may arise from the AV node (Fig. 9-26). The characteristics of wandering pacemaker include the following:

- P waves are present but vary in configuration; each P wave may look different.
- A P wave exists before every QRS complex.
- The P-R intervals may vary but are usually within the normal width.
- The QRS complexes are identical in configuration.
- The QRS duration is between 0.04 and 0.10 second.

- The R to R intervals vary.
- The heart rate is usually less than 100 beats per minute.

Signs and Symptoms

The cause is usually an irritable focus; however, the discharge of the impulse and the speed of discharge vary within the normal range. This type of arrhythmia is seen in the young and in the elderly and may be caused by ischemia or injury to the SA node, congestive heart failure, or an increase in vagal firing.[3] Usually this arrhythmia does not cause symptoms.

Treatment

This arrhythmia may lead to **atrial fibrillation,** which may require treatment; otherwise no treatment is necessary.

Atrial Arrhythmias

Premature Atrial Complexes

A premature atrial complex is defined as an ectopic focus in either atria that initiates an impulse before the next impulse is initiated by the SA node (Fig. 9-27). The characteristics of premature atrial complexes include the following:

- The underlying rhythm is sinus rhythm.

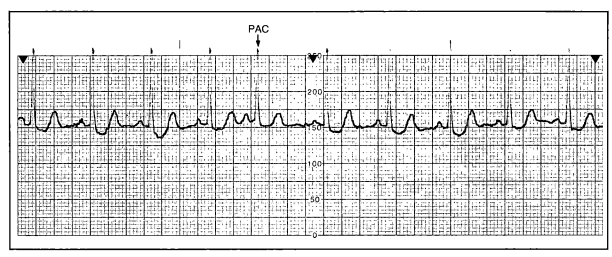

Figure 9-27.

Electrocardiogram tracing showing premature atrial complex (PAC) *(arrow)*.

- Normal complexes have one P wave and one QRS wave configuration.
- The P wave of the early beat is noticeably different from the normal Ps.
- Depending on the heart rate, the P wave of the early beat may be buried in the previous T wave.
- The QRS complex involved in the early beat should look similar to the other QRS complexes.
- All PR intervals are 0.12 to 0.20 second.
- All QRS durations are between 0.04 and 0.10 second.
- Often a pause follows the premature atrial complex, but it may not be compensatory.

Signs, Symptoms, and Causes

Causes of premature atrial complexes include emotional stress, nicotine, caffeine, alcohol, hypoxemia, infection, myocardial ischemia, rheumatic disease, and atrial damage. There may be no signs or symptoms associated with premature atrial complexes unless the pulse is palpated and the irregularity noticed.

Treatment

If the frequency of the premature atrial complexes is low, no treatment is required unless there are hemodynamic consequences. When the frequency is increased, supraventricular tachycardia or atrial fibrillation may develop.[4]

Atrial Tachycardia

The definition of **atrial tachycardia** is three or more premature atrial complexes in a row. Usually the heart rate is greater than 100 and may be as fast as 200 beats per minute (Fig. 9-28). The characteristics of atrial tachycardia include the following:

- P waves may be the same or may look different.
- P waves may not be present before every QRS complex.
- The P-R intervals vary but should be no greater than 0.20 second.
- The QRS complexes should be the same as the others that originate from the SA node.
- The QRS duration is generally between 0.04 and 0.10 second.
- The R to R intervals vary.
- The heart rate is rapid, being greater than 100 and possibly up to 200 beats per minute.

Signs, Symptoms, and Causes

The causes of atrial tachycardia include the causes of premature atrial complexes as well as

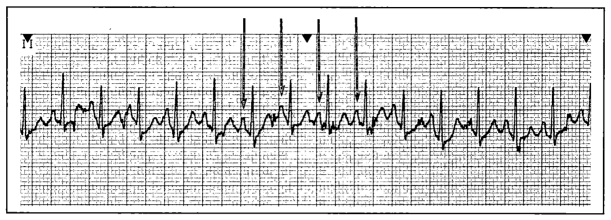

Figure 9-28.

Electrocardiogram tracing showing atrial tachycardia. Note the presence of P waves *(arrows)* despite the fast rate (approximately 145 beats per minute).

those of severe pulmonary disease with hypoxemia, pulmonary hypertension, and altered pH. Atrial tachycardia is often found in patients with chronic obstructive pulmonary disease. Symptoms may develop owing to a compromised cardiac output if prolonged, thereby causing dizziness, fatigue, and shortness of breath.[1]

Treatment

Treatment for atrial tachycardia involves treatment of the underlying cause (if the patient is hypoxemic or if pH is altered); performance of autonomic maneuvers such as Valsalva's, breath holding, and coughing; and prescription of medications such as beta blockers, verapamil, and digoxin.

Paroxysmal Atrial Tachycardia

Paroxysmal atrial tachycardia is the sudden onset of atrial tachycardia or repetitive firing from an atrial focus. The underlying rhythm is usually normal sinus rhythm, followed by an episodic burst of atrial tachycardia that eventually returns to sinus rhythm. The episode may be extremely brief but can last for hours. The rhythm starts and stops abruptly (Fig. 9-29). The characteristics of paroxysmal atrial tachycardia include the following:

● P waves may be present but may be merged with the previous T wave.
● The P-R intervals may be difficult to determine but are less than 0.20 second.

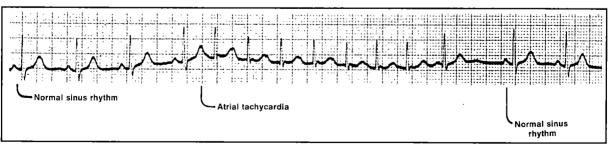

Normal sinus rhythm

Atrial tachycardia

Normal sinus rhythm

Figure 9-29.

Electrocardiogram tracing illustrating paroxysmal atrial tachycardia. (From Phillips RE, Feeney MK. The Cardiac Rhythms. 3rd ed. Philadelphia, WB Saunders, 1990, p 154.)

- The QRS complexes are identical unless there is aberration.
- The QRS duration is between 0.04 and 0.10 second.
- The R to R intervals are usually regular and may show starting and stopping of the paroxysmal atrial tachycardia.
- The ST segment may be elevated or depressed, yet the magnitude of change is not diagnostically reliable.
- The heart rate is very rapid, often greater than 160 beats per minute.

Signs, Symptoms, and Causes

The causes of paroxysmal atrial tachycardia can include emotional factors; overexertion; hyperventilation; potassium depletion; caffeine, nicotine, and aspirin sensitivity; rheumatic heart disease; mitral valve dysfunction, particularly **mitral valve prolapse;** digitalis toxicity; and pulmonary embolus.[1] The clinical description of paroxysmal atrial tachycardia is a sudden racing or fluttering of the heart beat. If paroxysmal atrial tachycardia continues beyond 24 hours, it is considered to be sustained atrial tachycardia. If the rapid rate continues for a period of time, other symptoms may include dizziness, weakness, and shortness of breath (possibly even due to hyperventilation).

Treatment

Treatment includes determining the underlying cause (often in young females this would require evaluation for mitral valve prolapse); discontinuation of medications; performance of autonomic stimulation including Valsalva's maneuver, breath holding, and coughing or gagging; and, if prolonged, treatment with medications such as verapamil or beta blockers. **Carotid massage** is often performed but only in the presence of ECG monitoring.

Atrial Flutter

Atrial flutter is defined as a rapid succession of atrial depolarization caused by an ectopic focus in the atria that depolarizes at a rate of 250 to 350 times per minute. As only one ectopic focus is firing repetitively, the P waves are called flutter waves and look identical to one another, having a characteristic "sawtooth" pattern (Fig. 9–30). The characteristics of atrial flutter include the following:

- P waves are present as flutter waves having a characteristic "sawtooth" pattern.
- There is more than one P wave before every QRS complex.

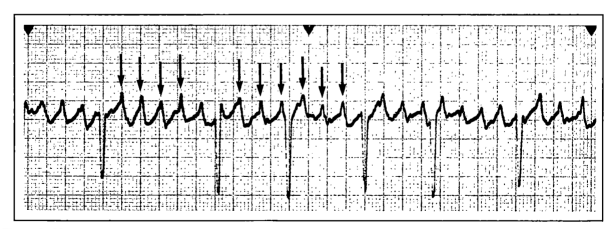

Figure 9–30.

Electrocardiogram tracing of atrial flutter waves (arrows), with a variable block. (From Wiederhold R. Electrocardiography: The Monitoring Lead. Philadelphia, WB Saunders, 1988, p 218.)

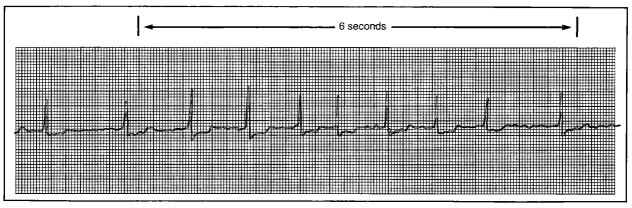

Figure 9-31.

Electrocardiogram tracing of atrial fibrillation, with a ventricular response of 80 beats per minute. Notice the lack of P waves and the irregularly irregular rhythm.

- The atrial depolarization rate is 250 to 350 times per minute.
- The QRS configuration is usually normal and identical in configuration, but usually there is more than one P wave for every QRS complex.
- The QRS duration is 0.04 to 0.11 second.
- The R to R intervals may vary depending on the atrial firing and number of P waves before each QRS complex. The conduction ratios may vary from 2 to 1 up to 8 to 1.
- The heart rate varies.

Signs, Symptoms, and Causes

Atrial flutter can be caused by numerous pathologic conditions, including rheumatic heart disease, mitral valve disease, coronary artery disease or infarction, stress, drugs, renal failure, hypoxemia, and pericarditis to name the most common causes.[5] As the rate of discharge from the **ectopic** focus is rapid, the critical role is played by the AV node, which blocks all the impulses from being conducted. Therefore, there may be an irregular rhythm associated with atrial flutter. This rhythm is usually not considered to be life threatening and may even lead to atrial fibrillation. Usually no symptoms are present, and the cardiac output is not compromised unless the ventricular rate is too fast or too slow.

Treatment

Treatment for atrial flutter includes medications (digoxin, verapamil, or beta blockers are the more common drugs of choice) or **cardioversion** with the defibrillator paddles at 10 to 50 watts.

Atrial Fibrillation

Atrial fibrillation is defined as an erratic quivering or twitching of the atrial muscle caused by multiple ectopic foci in the atria that emit electrical impulses constantly. None of the ectopic foci actually depolarizes the atria, so no true P waves are found in atrial fibrillation. The AV node acts to control the impulses that initiate a QRS complex; therefore, a totally irregular rhythm exists. Thus, the AV node determines the ventricular response by blocking impulses or allowing them to progress forward. This ventricular response may be normal, slow, or too rapid (Fig. 9-31). The characteristics of atrial fibrillation include the following:

- P waves are absent, thus leaving a flat or wavy baseline.
- The QRS duration is between 0.04 and 0.10 second.
- The R to R interval is characteristically defined as irregularly irregular.
- The rate varies but is called "ventricular response."

Signs, Symptoms, and Causes

Numerous factors may play a part in causing atrial fibrillation, including advanced age, congestive heart failure, ischemia or infarction, cardiomyopathy, digoxin toxicity, drug use, stress or pain, rheumatic heart disease, and renal failure. Atrial fibrillation presents problems for two reasons. Without atrial depolarization the atria do not contract. The contraction of the atria is also referred to as the atrial "kick." This atrial kick forces the last amount of volume to flow into the ventricles during diastole. The amount of volume that is forced into the ventricles because of atrial contraction provides up to 30% of the cardiac output. Therefore, without atrial contraction, the cardiac output is decreased up to 30%.[6]

In individuals with atrial fibrillation with heart rates (or ventricular response rates) lower than 100, the decrease in cardiac output is usually not a problem. However, as the individual exercises or if the ventricular response is greater than 100 at rest, the cardiac output may be diminished and signs of decompensation may occur. Atrial fibrillation is therefore considered relatively benign if the ventricular response is less than 100 at rest, but physiologic monitoring should be performed with exercise to assess cardiac output compensation. However, individuals who have atrial fibrillation with a ventricular response greater than 100 at rest should have physiologic monitoring during all activities, and any activity should be engaged in cautiously.

The other problem with atrial fibrillation is the potential for developing mural thrombi because of the coagulation of blood with fibrillating atria. Mural thrombi may lead to **emboli** (30% of all patients with atrial fibrillation develop emboli), so **anticoagulant** therapy is usually initiated.

The classic sign of atrial fibrillation is a very irregularly irregular pulse. Symptoms occur only if the ventricular response is too rapid, which causes cardiac output decompensation.

Treatment

The treatment for atrial fibrillation usually involves pharmacologic control (e.g., digoxin, verapamil, antiarrhythmic therapy) or cardioversion.

If a specific cause is identified, then treatment for that cause should be initiated.

Nodal or Junctional Arrhythmias

Premature Junctional or Nodal Complexes

Premature junctional complexes are premature impulses that arise from the AV node or junctional tissue. For reasons that are not understood, the AV node becomes irritated and initiates an impulse that causes an early beat. Premature junctional complexes are very similar to premature atrial complexes except for the fact that an inverted, an absent, or a retrograde (wave that follows the QRS) P wave is present (Fig. 9–32). The characteristics of premature junctional complexes include the following:

● Inverted, absent, or retrograde P waves are present.
● The QRS configurations are usually identical.
● The QRS duration is between 0.04 and 0.10 second.
● The R to R interval is regular throughout except when the premature beats arise.
● The heart rate is usually normal (between 60 and 100 beats per minute).

Signs, Symptoms, and Causes

Some of the causes of premature junctional complexes include decreased automaticity and conductivity of the SA node or some irritability of the junctional tissue. Pathologic conditions include cardiac disease and mitral valve disease.[2] Usually no symptoms or signs are present.

Treatment

Usually no treatment is required because there are no symptoms of clinical significance.

Junctional (or Nodal) Rhythm

Junctional rhythm occurs when the AV junction takes over as the pacemaker of the heart.

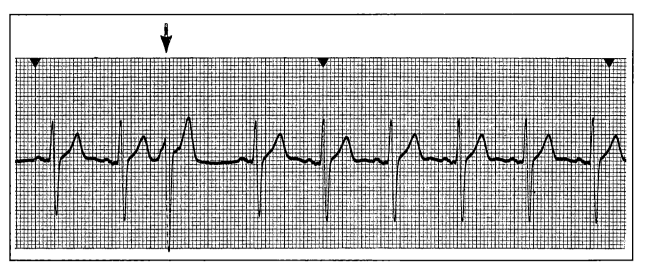

Figure 9-32.

Electrocardiogram tracing of premature junctional (or nodal) complex. The arrow points to the isolated premature beat, which has a QRS complex of normal width. The beat comes early, however, and the P wave is absent. (From Wiederhold R. Electrocardiography: The Monitoring Lead. Philadelphia, WB Saunders, 1989, p 61.)

Junctional rhythm may be considered an escape rhythm (Fig. 9-33). The characteristics of junctional rhythm include the following:

- Absence of P waves before the QRS complex, but a retrograde P wave may be identified.
- The QRS complex has a normal configuration.
- The QRS duration is between 0.04 and 0.10 second.

- The R to R intervals are regular.
- The ventricular rate is between 40 and 60 beats per minute.

Signs, Symptoms, and Causes

Causes of junctional rhythm include a failure of the SA node to act as the pacemaker in conditions such as sinus node disease or increase in

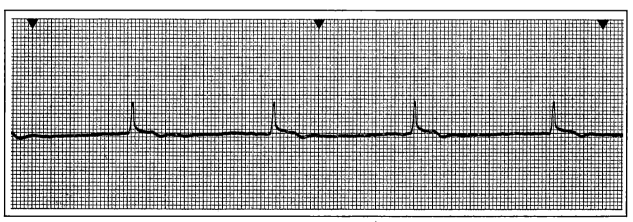

Figure 9-33.

Electrocardiogram tracing showing junction rhythm with a rate of 38 beats per minute. (From Wiederhold R. Electrocardiography: The Monitoring Lead. Philadelphia, WB Saunders, 1989, p 80.)

vagal tone, digoxin toxicity, and infarction or severe ischemia to the conduction system (typically right coronary artery disease). Symptoms are present only if the heart rate is too slow, which causes a compromise in the cardiac output.

Treatment

Treatment consists of identifying the cause and treating it if possible. If the rate becomes too slow (50 beats per minute or less) then the patient may develop symptoms of cardiac output decompensation, dizziness, and fatigue. In the case of symptoms and slower heart rates, the treatment involves medication to increase the rate (usually atropine or isoproterenol) or pacemaker insertion.

Nodal (Junctional) Tachycardia

Junctional tachycardia develops because the AV junctional tissue is acting as the pacemaker (as in junctional rhythm), but the rate of discharge is accelerated. The onset of increase in rate of discharge may be sudden, or it may be of long standing (Fig. 9–34). The characteristics of junctional tachycardia include the following:

- P waves are absent, but retrograde P wave may be present.
- The QRS configurations are identical.
- The QRS duration is between 0.04 and 0.10 second.
- The R to R interval is regular.
- The rate is usually greater than 100 beats per minute.

Signs, Symptoms, and Causes

Causes of junctional tachycardia include **hyperventilation,** coronary artery disease or infarction, postcardiac surgery, digoxin toxicity, myocarditis, caffeine or nicotine sensitivity, overexertion, and emotional factors. When the rate is extremely rapid, the individual may experience symptoms of cardiac output decompensation.[1] Symptoms include dizziness, shortness of breath, and fatigue.

Treatment

Treatment involves identifying the cause and treating it. Digoxin is given if the underlying cause is not digoxin toxicity. Vagal stimulation may be employed or pharmacologic therapy initiated (verapamil or beta blockers).

HEART BLOCKS

First-Degree Atrioventricular Heart Block

First-degree AV block occurs when the impulse is initiated in the SA node but is delayed on the way to the AV node; or it may be initiated in the AV node itself, and the AV conduction time is prolonged. This results in a lengthening of the P–R interval only (Fig. 9–35).

The characteristics associated with first-degree AV block include the following:

- A P wave is present and with normal configuration before every QRS complex.
- The P–R interval is prolonged (greater than 0.20 second).
- The QRS has a normal configuration.
- The QRS duration is between 0.04 and 0.10 second.
- The R to R intervals are regular.
- The heart rate is usually within normal limits (60 to 100 beats per minute) but may be lower than 60 beats per minute.

Signs, Symptoms, and Causes

Causes of first-degree AV block include coronary artery disease, rheumatic heart disease, infarction, and reactions to medication (digoxin or beta blockers). First-degree AV block is a relatively benign arrhythmia as it exists without symptoms (unless severe bradycardia exists in conjunction with first-degree AV block); however, it should be monitored over time because it may progress to higher forms of AV block.

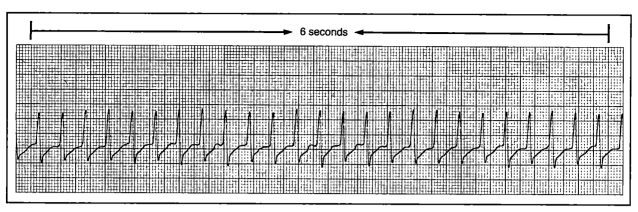

Figure 9-34.

Electrocardiogram tracing of junctional tachycardia. Note the absence of P waves, which would make this an illustration of atrial tachycardia.

Treatment

Usually treatment is not warranted unless the AV block is due to reactions to medication, in which case the medication is withheld.

Second-Degree Atrioventricular Block, Type I

Second-degree AV block, type I (Wenckebach's or Mobitz I heart block), is a relatively benign, transient disturbance that occurs high in the AV junction and prevents conduction of some of the impulses through the AV node. The typical appearance of **type I (Wenckebach's) second-degree block** is a progressive prolongation of the P-R interval until finally one impulse is not conducted through to the ventricles (no QRS complex following a P wave). The cycle then repeats itself (Fig. 9-36).

The characteristics of second-degree type I include the following:

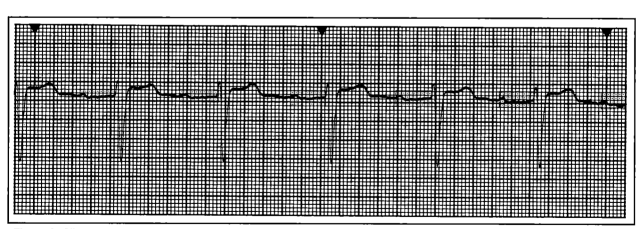

Figure 9-35.

Electrocardiogram tracing of first-degree atrioventricular block (P-R interval measures to approximately 0.32 second) with sinus bradycardia. (From Wiederhold R. Electrocardiography: The Monitoring Lead. Philadelphia, WB Saunders, 1989, p 87.)

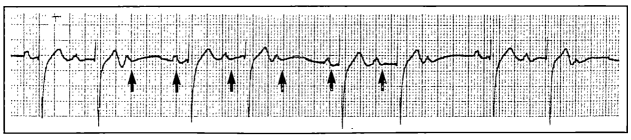

Figure 9-36.

Electrocardiogram tracing showing type I second-degree heart block (Wenckebach's). The arrows identify the P waves. Notice the progressive lengthening of the P-R interval until finally a P wave exists without a QRS complex. (From Phillips RE, Feeney MK. The Cardiac Rhythms. 3rd ed. Philadelphia, WB Saunders, 1990, p 255.)

- Initially a P wave precedes each QRS complex, but eventually a P wave may stand alone (conduction is blocked).
- Progressive lengthening of the P-R interval occurs in progressive order.
- As the P-R interval increases, a QRS complex will be dropped.
- This progressive lengthening of the P-R interval followed by a dropped QRS complex occurs in a repetitive cycle.
- The QRS configuration is normal, and the duration is between 0.04 and 0.10 second.
- Because of the dropping of the QRS complex, the R to R interval is irregular (regularly irregular).
- The heart rate varies.

Signs, Symptoms, and Causes

Causes of Wenckebach's heart block include right coronary artery disease or infarction, digoxin toxicity, and beta blocker medication. Usually the individual with type I second-degree AV block is asymptomatic.

Treatment

Treatment is usually unnecessary because most often the individual is without symptoms and without cardiac output compromise. In rare cases, either atropine or isoproterenol have been given, or a temporary pacemaker is inserted.[7] This type of AV block rarely progresses to higher forms of AV block.

Second-Degree Atrioventricular Block, Type II

Second-degree AV block, **type II (Mobitz II)**, is defined as nonconduction of an impulse to the ventricles without a change in the P-R interval. The site of the block is usually below His's bundle and may be a bilateral bundle branch block (Fig. 9-37).

The characteristics of second-degree AV block type II include the following:

- A ratio of P waves to QRS complexes that is greater than 1 to 1 and may vary from 2 to 4 P waves for every QRS complex.
- The QRS duration is between 0.04 and 0.10 second.
- The QRS configuration is normal.
- The R to R intervals may vary depending on the amount of blocking that is occurring.
- The heart rate is usually below 100 and may be below 60 beats per minute.

Signs, Symptoms, and Causes

Second-degree AV block type II occurs with myocardial infarction (especially when the left anterior descending coronary artery is involved), with ischemia or infarction of the AV node, or with digoxin toxicity. Patients may be symptomatic when the heart rate is low and when cardiac output compromise is present.[3]

Treatment

Treatment usually involves pacemaker insertion, but for immediate relief of symptoms atro-

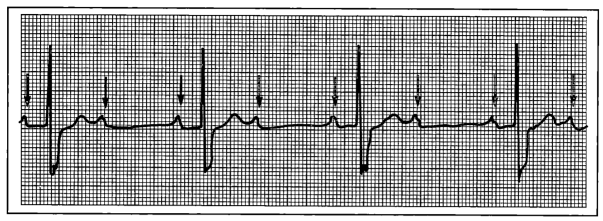

Figure 9-37.

Electrocardiogram tracing of type II second-degree heart block (Mobitz II) with a heart rate of 37 beats per minute. Note the two P waves for every QRS complex.

pine or isoproterenol may be used. The danger with type II second-degree AV block is the possibility of progression to complete heart block (third-degree AV block), which is a life-threatening condition.

Third-Degree Atrioventricular Block

In **third-degree (complete) AV block** all impulses that are initiated above the ventricle are *not* conducted to the ventricle. In complete heart block the atria fire at their own inherent rate (SA node firing or ectopic foci in the atria), and a separate pacemaker in the ventricles initiates all impulses. However, there is no communication between the atria and the ventricles and thus no coordination between the firing of the atria and the firing of the ventricles, creating complete independence of the two systems (Fig. 9-38).

The characteristics of complete heart block include the following:

● P waves are present, regular, and of identical configuration.

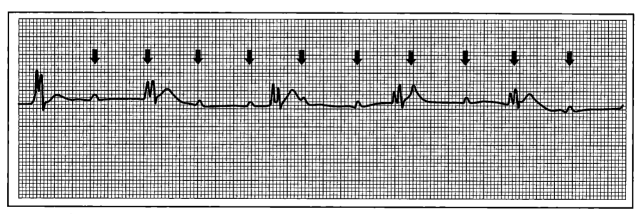

Figure 9-38.

Electrocardiogram tracing showing third-degree heart block, also known as complete heart block. Notice how the P waves have their own regular rhythm (see *arrows*) without interrupting the rhythm of the QRS complex. There is no communication between atrial firing and ventricular firing.

- The P waves have no relationship to the QRS complex because the atria are firing at their own inherent rate.
- The QRS complexes are regular in that the R to R intervals are regular.
- The QRS duration may be wider than 0.10 second if the latent pacemaker is in the ventricles.
- The heart rate depends on the latent ventricular pacemaker and may range from 30 to 50 beats per minute.

Signs, Symptoms, and Causes

The causes of complete heart block usually involve acute myocardial infarction, digoxin toxicity, or degeneration of the conduction system. If a slow ventricular rate is present, then the cardiac output often is diminished, and the patient may complain of dizziness, shortness of breath, and possibly chest pain.

Treatment

Treatment for complete heart block involves permanent pacemaker insertion, with atropine and isoproterenol injection or infusion used in the acute situation. Complete heart block is a medical emergency.

Ventricular Arrhythmias

Premature Ventricular Complexes

Premature ventricular complexes (PVCs) occur when an ectopic focus originates an impulse from somewhere in one of the ventricles. The ventricular ectopic depolarization occurs early in the cycle before the SA node actually fires. A PVC is easily recognized on the ECG because the impulse originates in the muscle of the heart, and these myocardial cells conduct impulses very slowly compared with specialized conductive tissue. Therefore, the QRS complex is classically described as a wide and bizarre looking QRS without a P wave and followed by a complete compensatory pause (see Fig. 9–38). Premature ventricular complexes may come in patterns (e.g., every third or fourth beat, paired together) or may be isolated. Premature ventricular beats may be identical, or they may look different. All these factors affect the seriousness of the PVCs and also affect the clinical decision-making process and treatment. See illustrations of PVCs: Unifocal (Fig. 9–39), multifocal (Fig. 9–40), frequent (bigeminy) (Fig. 9–41), R on T (Fig. 9–42), paired (Fig. 9–43), and triplet (Fig. 9–44).

The characteristics of PVCs include the following:

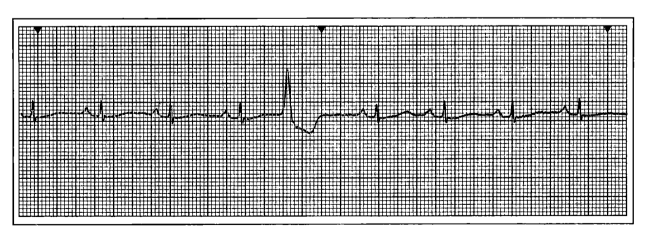

Figure 9–39.

Electrocardiogram tracing of an isolated premature ventricular complex. (From Wiederhold R. Electrocardiography: The Monitoring Lead. Philadelphia, WB Saunders, 1989, p 62.)

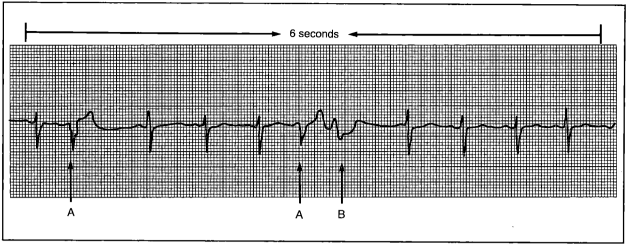

Figure 9-40.

Electrocardiogram tracing of multifocal premature ventricular complexes. Note the QRS complex of A and the difference in configuration of the QRS complex of B.

- An absence of P waves in the premature beat, with all other beats usually of sinus rhythm.
- The QRS complex of the premature beat is wide and bizarre and occurs earlier than the normal sinus beat would have occurred.
- The QRS duration of the early beat is greater than 0.10 second.
- The ST segment and the T wave often slope in the opposite direction from the normal complexes.

- The PVC is generally followed by a **compensatory pause.**
- The PVC is called bigeminy when every other beat is a PVC, trigeminy when every third beat is a PVC, and so on.
- The PVC is called unifocal if all PVCs appear identical in configuration.
- The PVCs are called **multifocal** if more than one PVC is present and the two do not appear similar in configuration.

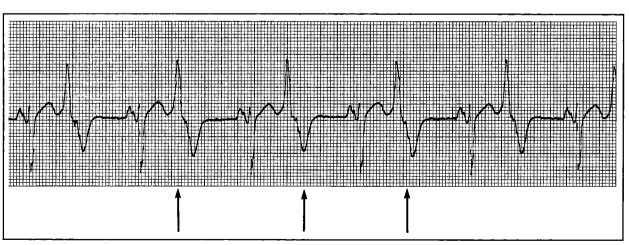

Figure 9-41.

Electrocardiogram tracing showing bigeminy (premature ventricular complexes every other beat). Arrows depict premature complexes.

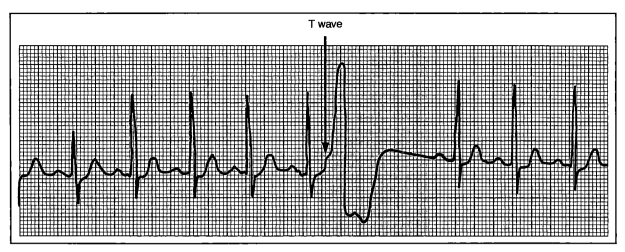

Figure 9-42.

Electrocardiogram tracing of R on T premature ventricular complex (PVC). Notice the arrow depicts a PVC that *begins* from the top of the T wave of the preceding beat. This can be extremely dangerous, because the premature beat is firing during the refractory period and could lead to ventricular tachycardia or fibrillation.

- The PVC is paired or a couplet if two PVCs are together, a triplet or VTACH if three are together in a row.
- The PVC is **interpolated** if it falls between two normal sinus beats that are separated by a normal R to R interval.

Signs, Symptoms, and Causes

The causes of PVCs are numerous. Isolated PVCs may be present owing to caffeine or nicotine sensitivity, stress, overexertion, or electrolyte imbalance (particularly **hypokalemia** or **hyperkalemia**). Premature ventricular complexes are also common in the presence of ischemia; cardiac disease; overdistention of the ventricle, as in congestive heart failure or **cardiomyopathy;** acute infarction; irritation of the myocardium or its vessels, as in cardiac catheterization; chronic lung disease and hypoxemia; and as a result of pharmacologic therapy (procan, quinidine, or digoxin toxicity).

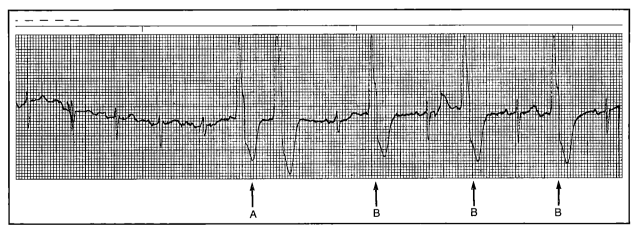

Figure 9-43.

Electrocardiogram tracing of paired premature ventricular complexes (PVCs) (*A*). In addition, unifocal PVCs are present after paired PVCs (*B*).

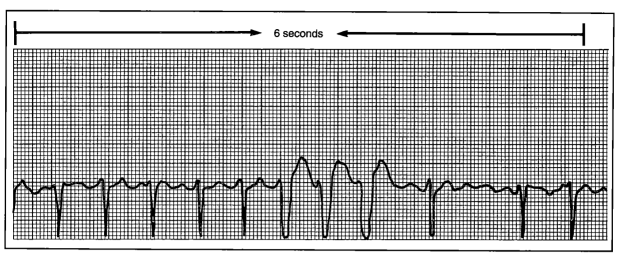

Figure 9–44.

Electrocardiogram tracing of a triplet, otherwise known as a three-beat ventricular tachycardia.

Individuals may experience symptoms with PVCs if they are frequent or more serious in nature because they may affect the cardiac output. A skipped beat can be palpated when checking a pulse. (A PVC feels like a pause or skip in the regular rhythm that usually is followed by a stronger beat.) The PVC may also be felt because of the decreased preload with the PVC beat, which is followed by a long compensatory pause that allows increased filling time of the ventricle and therefore an increased preload for the beat following the premature beat and subsequently an increased stroke volume. This increased stroke volume is usually what is felt in the previously asymptomatic individual and is often a concern. With increased frequency of PVCs, the filling time of the ventricles decreases, which leads to a decreased preload and subsequently a decreased stroke volume. Symptoms associated with PVCs include anxiety (particularly with a new onset of arrhythmias); however, if the arrhythmias are more frequent, cardiac output may decrease, and therefore shortness of breath and dizziness may occur.

Treatment

The treatment for PVCs depends on the underlying cause, the frequency and severity of the PVCs, and the symptoms associated with them. The frequency and the type of evidence for them

indicate the seriousness of the patient's condition and help to determine the clinical decision. Premature ventricular complexes are considered to be serious, or possibly life threatening, when they

● are paired together (see Fig. 9–43)
● are multifocal in origin (see Fig. 9–40)
● are more frequent than 6 per minute
● land directly on the T wave (see Fig. 9–42)
● are present in triplets or more (see Fig. 9–44)

Premature ventricular complexes are considered to be serious or life threatening because they may indicate increased irritability of the ventricular muscle and may progress to **ventricular tachycardia** or **ventricular fibrillation**—two medical emergencies.

Although PVCs may be benign, a full cardiac evaluation should be performed to rule out underlying disease in the individual who demonstrates a sudden onset of them.[6] If the individual has a history of arrhythmias, if these arrhythmias are asymptomatic, and if their frequency or seriousness does not change, then treatment is unwarranted. If the arrhythmias produce symptoms or appear to be more frequent either throughout the day or with increased activity, then further evaluation and possibly treatment is warranted. If an individual with chronic lung disease has a new onset of PVCs it may indicate hypoxemia, and supplemental oxygen may be necessary. Otherwise, after all the underlying causes are evaluated, antiarrhythmic medications may be warranted. Antiarrhythmic medication therapy is not always effective and can even produce arrhythmias. See Chapter 12 for more information on the pharmacologic management of PVCs.

Ventricular Tachycardia

Ventricular tachycardia is defined as a series of three or more PVCs in a row. Ventricular tachycardia occurs because of a rapid firing by a single ventricular focus with increased automaticity (Fig. 9–45). The characteristics of ventricular tachycardia include the following:

- P waves are absent.
- Three or more PVCs occur in a row.
- The QRS complexes of the ventricular tachycardia are wide and bizarre.
- The ventricular rate of ventricular tachycardia is between 100 and 250 beats per minute.

Signs, Symptoms, and Causes

Causes of ventricular tachycardia include ischemia or acute infarction, coronary artery disease, hypertensive heart disease, and reaction to medications (digoxin or quinidine toxicity). Occasionally it occurs in athletes during exercise (possibly due to electrolyte imbalance). Ventricular tachycardia indicates increased irritability as well as an emergency situation because cardiac output

is greatly diminished, as is the blood pressure. Symptoms usually involve lightheadedness and sometimes syncope. A weak, thready pulse may be present. The individual may become disoriented if ventricular tachycardia is sustained. Ventricular tachycardia can progress to ventricular fibrillation and death.

Treatment

Treatment usually is an immediate pharmacologic injection (lidocaine, bretylium tosylate [bretylol], or procainamide [pronestyl]) or cardioversion or **defibrillation.** Ventricular tachycardia is often considered a medical emergency.

Ventricular Tachycardia: Torsades de Pointes

Torsades de pointes is a unique configuration of ventricular tachycardia called the "twisting of the points" (Fig. 9–46). Torsades de pointes is often associated with a prolonged QT interval (greater than 0.5 second). The name relates to its presentation by twisting around the isoelectric line. This arrhythmia characteristically occurs at a rapid rate and terminates spontaneously.

Signs, Symptoms, and Causes

This type of ventricular tachycardia has been identified only in individuals receiving antiar-

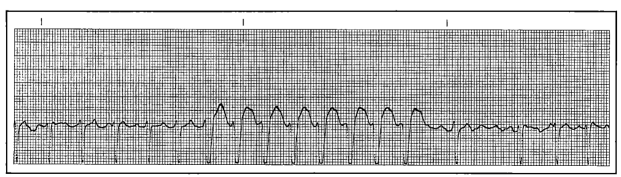

Figure 9–45.

Electrocardiogram tracing showing ventricular tachycardia.

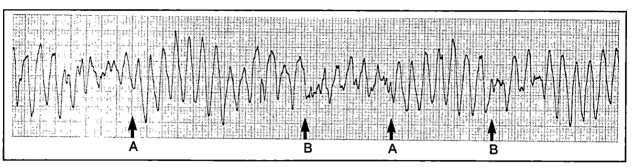

Figure 9-46.

Electrocardiogram tracing showing torsades de pointes. The arrows depict the beginning and ending of the "twisting of points." *A* depicts the beginning, and *B* depicts the end before the turning. (From Phillips RE, Feeney MK. The Cardiac Rhythms. 3rd ed. Philadelphia, WB Saunders, 1990, p 393.)

rhythmic therapy and for whom the medication is toxic. As cardiac output is severely diminished and as this arrhythmia often converts to ventricular fibrillation this condition is considered a medical emergency.[1] The individual who remains conscious with this arrhythmia may be extremely lightheaded or near syncope.

Treatment

Treatment is usually cardioversion.

Ventricular Fibrillation

Ventricular fibrillation is defined as an erratic quivering of the ventricular muscle resulting in no cardiac output. As in atrial fibrillation, multiple ectopic foci fire, creating asynchrony. The ECG results in a picture of grossly irregular up and down fluctuations of the baseline in an irregular zigzag pattern (Fig. 9-47).

Signs, Symptoms, and Causes

The causes of ventricular fibrillation are the same as those of ventricular tachycardia because ventricular fibrillation is usually the sequel to ventricular tachycardia.

Treatment

Treatment is defibrillation as quickly as possible followed by cardiopulmonary resuscitation,

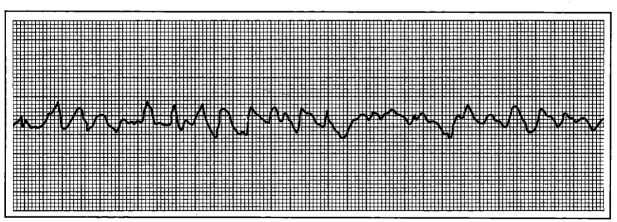

Figure 9-47.

Electrocardiogram tracing showing ventricular fibrillation (coarse).

supplemental oxygen, and injection of medications. However, if the tracing appears to be ventricular fibrillation and the patient does not have a long-term history of recurrent ventricular tachycardia or ventricular fibrillation, and the patient is able to carry on a conversation, the therapist should assume this is probably only lead displacement creating artifact.

OTHER FINDINGS ON A 12-LEAD ELECTROCARDIOGRAM

Hypertrophy

Hypertrophy refers to an increase in thickness of cardiac muscle or chamber size. Signs of atrial hypertrophy can be noted by examining the P waves of the ECG for a diphasic P wave in the chest lead V_1, or a voltage in excess of 3 millivolts. Signs of right ventricular hypertrophy are noted by changes found in lead V_1 that include a large R wave and an S wave smaller than the R wave. The R wave becomes progressively smaller in the successive chest leads (V_2, V_3, V_4, V_5). Hypertrophy of the left ventricle creates enlarged QRS complexes in the chest leads in both height of the QRS (R wave) and depth of the QRS (S wave). In left ventricular hypertrophy a deep S wave occurs in V_1 and a large R wave in V_5. If when the depth of the S wave in V_1 (in mm) is added to the height of the R wave in V_5 (in mm) the resulting number is greater than 35, then left ventricular hypertrophy is present (Fig. 9–48).

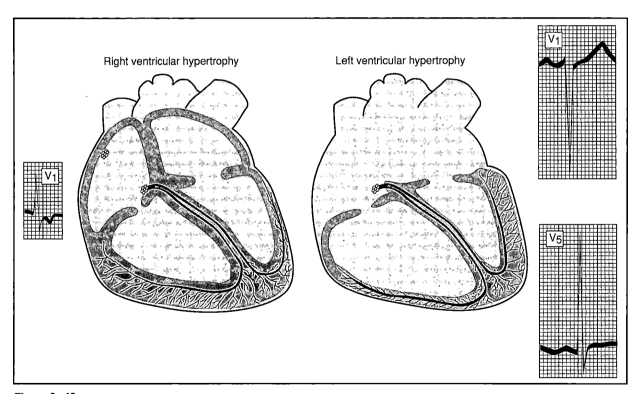

Figure 9–48.

Hypertrophy is determined by looking at voltage in V_1 and V_5. *Right* ventricular hypertrophy is defined as a large R wave in V_1, which gets progressively smaller in V_2, V_3, and V_4; normally there is a very small R wave and a large S wave in V_1. *Left* ventricular hypertrophy is defined as a large S wave in V_1 and a large R wave in V_5 that have a combined voltage of greater than 35 mm.

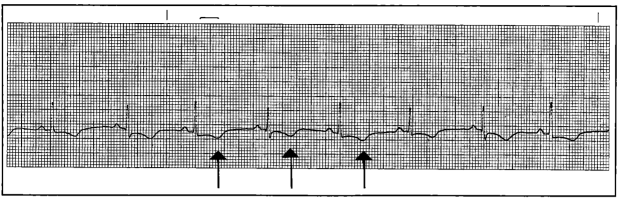

Figure 9-49.

Electrocardiogram tracing showing an inverted T wave, often indicating ischemia *(arrows)*.

Ischemia, Infarction, or Injury

A review of an ECG to detect ischemia, infarction, or injury is performed in a variety of situations, including following any episode of chest pain that brings a patient to the physician's office or to the hospital, during hospitalization, during a follow-up examination after a cardiac event, or before conducting an exercise test. The difference between ischemia and infarction is covered in great detail in Chapter 3. In simplistic terms, ischemia literally means reduced blood and refers to a diminished blood supply to the myocardium. This can occur because of occlusion of the coronary arteries from vasospasm, atherosclerotic occlusion, thrombus, or a combination of the three. Infarction means cell death and results from a complete occlusion of a coronary artery. Injury indicates the acuteness of the infarction. As a result of ischemia, injury, or infarction, conduction of electrical impulses is altered, and therefore depolarization of the muscle changes. As the ECG records the depolarization of the cardiac muscle, changes occur on the ECG in the presence of ischemia, infarction, or injury. The location of the ischemia, infarction, or injury is determined according to the specific leads of the ECG that demonstrate an alteration in depolarization.

Ischemia is classically demonstrated on the 12-lead ECG with T wave inversion or ST-segment depression. The T wave may vary from a flat configuration to a depressed inverted wave (Fig. 9-49). The T wave is an extremely sensitive indication of changes in repolarization activity within the ventricles.[8] Transient fluctuations in the T wave can be observed in numerous situations and must be associated with the activity and symptoms to determine if the abnormality is ischemic. For an individual who comes to a physician's office because of an episode of chest pain, T wave inversion may be the only noticeable abnormality. If the individual took nitroglycerin while at the office and the pain disappeared before the ECG was administered, abnormalities may be absent owing to the resolution of the ischemic event.

The location of the ST segment (that portion of the ECG tracing beginning with the end of the S wave and ending with the beginning of the T wave) is another indication of ischemia or injury. Elevation of the ST segment above the baseline when following part of an R wave indicates acute injury (Fig. 9-50). In the presence of acute infarction, the ST segment elevates and then later returns to the level of the baseline (within 24-48 hours).[8] ST-segment elevation may also occur in the presence of a ventricular aneurysm (a ballooning out of the ventricular wall, usually following a large amount of damage to the ventricular wall). The ST elevation with ventricular aneurysm never returns to the isoelectric line,

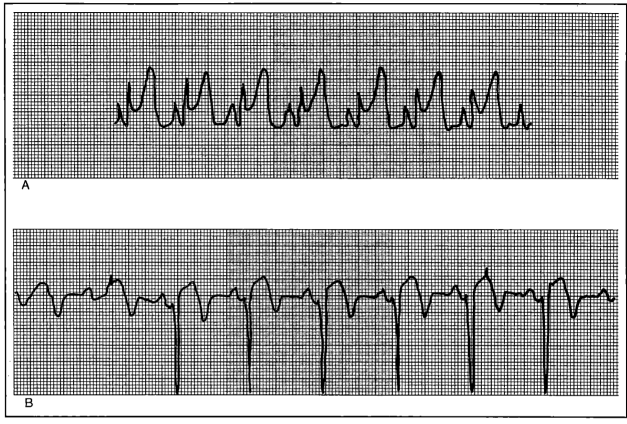

Figure 9-50.

An ST-segment elevation following part of the R wave indicates acute injury (*A*). An ST-segment elevation following a large Q wave does not always indicate injury but often the presence of a ventricular aneurysm (*B*).

and the configuration differs somewhat. The ST-segment elevation in ventricular aneurysm usually follows a large Q wave and not an R wave of the QRS complex (see Fig. 9-50). If the ECG records the presence of ST-segment elevation in the presence of acute onset of chest pain (within hours), a cardiac emergency exists and immediate treatment is indicated.

The ECG may demonstrate ST-segment depression while the patient is at rest in the presence of chest pain or of suspected coronary ischemia. The ST-segment depression in this situation represents **subendocardial infarction** and also requires immediate treatment. A subendocardial infarct is an acute injury to the myocardial wall, but it does not extend through the full thickness of the ventricular wall. Instead, the injury is only to the subendocardium (Fig. 9-51).

This ECG sign is extremely significant, because it indicates that a transmural infarction could be pending. Research has shown that an individual diagnosed with a subendocardial infarction is at extremely high risk for another infarction (this time **transmural**) within 6 weeks.[9]

Other situations may precipitate ST-segment depression. ST-segment depression in the absence of suspected ischemia or angina may be caused by digitalis toxicity (see Chapter 12 for discussion of digitalis toxicity).

ST-segment depression that develops during exercise, as seen during exercise testing, is defined as an ischemic response to exercise, and following rest it should return to the isoelectric line. This is an abnormal response to exercise that indicates an impaired coronary arterial supply during the exercise. This type of ischemic response should be further evaluated to determine the extent of the coronary artery involvement (see Chapter 8).

During myocardial injury, the affected area of muscle loses its ability to generate electrical impulses, and therefore alterations in the initial portion of the QRS complex occur. The cells are dead and cannot depolarize normally, which results in an inability to conduct impulses. Therefore, as ST-segment elevation or depression is diagnostic for acute infarction, the presence of a significant Q wave is also diagnostic for infarction, but the date of the infarction is not able to be determined simply by studying the ECG. The date of the infarction is determined by the patient's report of symptoms. The Q wave is the first downward part of the QRS complex (not preceded by anything else), and small Q waves may be present normally in some leads. When the Q wave is 0.04 second in duration wide (one small square on the ECG tracing) or is one third the size (height and depth included) of the QRS

complex, the Q wave is considered to be *significant* and indicative of a pathologic condition (it persists as a permanent electrocardiographic "scar" from infarction [Fig. 9–52]). Therefore, any scan of the ECG should include a check for the presence of significant Q waves to identify previous infarction.

The leads that demonstrate the presence of T wave inversion, ST-segment changes, or Q waves identify the location of the ischemia, injury, or infarction. The presence of significant Q waves in the chest leads, particularly in V_1, V_2, V_3, and V_4, indicates an infarction in the anterior portion of the left ventricle. When only V_1 and V_2 are involved, these infarctions are often called "septal" infarctions because they primarily affect the interventricular septum. Anterior infarctions are easy to recognize if one remembers that the chest leads are placed on the anterior aspect of the left ventricle (Fig. 9–53). Referring back to Chapter 1, remember that because the left anterior descending artery primarily supplies the anterior

Figure 9–51.

An ST segment on a resting 12-lead electrocardiogram (ECG) often is indicative of subendocardial injury. *A*, Normal tracing and normal ventricular wall. *B*, Subendocardial ischemia with an ECG tracing of T wave inversion. *C*, Subendocardial injury with ST-segment depression on the ECG.

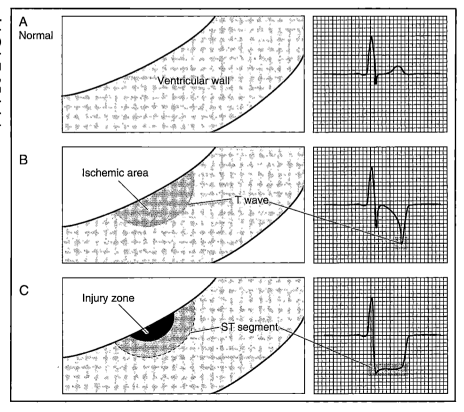

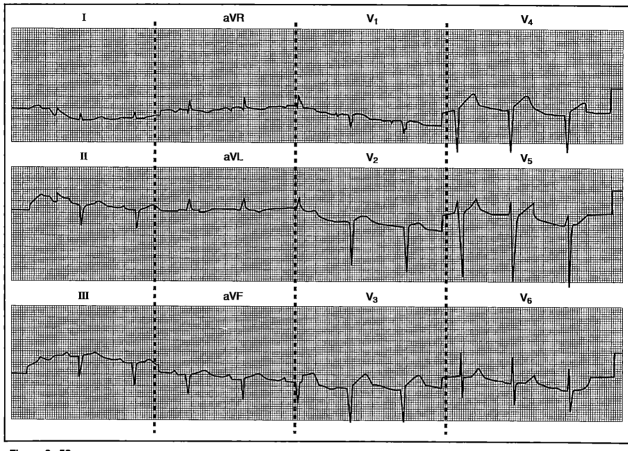

Figure 9-52.

A significant Q wave is defined as a minimum of one small square wide and one third the size of the QRS. In this electrocardiogram tracing, notice the Q waves in leads II, III, and aVF and in V_2, V_3, and V_4.

aspect of the heart, an anterior infarction infers an occlusion somewhere in the left anterior descending artery.

An inferior infarction is identified by significant Q waves in leads II, III, and aVF (Fig. 9-54). Inferior infarctions are also referred to as *diaphragmatic infarctions* because the inferior wall of the heart rests on the diaphragm. Given that the right coronary artery primarily supplies the inferior aspect of the myocardium, an inferior infarction infers an occlusion somewhere in the right coronary artery. A lateral infarction demonstrates Q waves in leads I and aVL (Fig. 9-55). Because the circumflex artery supplies primarily the lateral and posterior aspects of the myocar-

dium, an occlusion of the circumflex artery is suspected in a lateral infarction.

Probably the most difficult infarction to detect is the posterior infarction because none of the 12 leads is directly measuring the posterior aspect of the heart. Only two leads detect posterior infarcts — V_1 and V_2 — as they measure the direct opposite wall (anterior). Therefore, the direct opposite ECG tracing of an anterior infarction in V_1 and V_2 should be the ECG tracing of the posterior infarction. An anterior infarction demonstrates a significant Q wave in V_1 and V_2 with ST-segment elevation. The mirror image of this is seen in Figure 9-56, which demonstrates a large R wave in V_1 or V_2 and ST-segment depression.

Given that the posterior aspect of the myocardium may be supplied by either the right coronary artery or the circumflex artery, a posterior infarction may indicate a problem in either one of these arteries. If changes in the lateral leads (e.g., I, aVL) also exist, then the circumflex artery is probably involved. However, if changes in the inferior leads exist (e.g., II, III, aVR) as well as posterior changes, then the right coronary artery is probably involved.[8]

Caution should be taken when evaluation of an ECG for an infarction is performed in the presence of left bundle branch block.[8] Identification of significant Q waves can be difficult if the conduction is delayed throughout the myocardium on the left side. Conduction may be de-

layed through the myocardium owing to dysfunctions in the conduction system that are secondary to genetic defect, injury, or infarction. An example of conduction delay with bundle branch block occurs when a block of the impulse occurs in the right or left bundle branch. A bundle branch block creates a delay of the electrical impulse to the side that is blocked, creating a delay in the depolarization of the myocardium that would have received the blocked impulse. When the left and right sides do not depolarize simultaneously, a widened QRS appearance is seen on the ECG tracing and sometimes two R waves. In the case of left bundle branch block, the left side of the myocardium demonstrates delayed depolarization, thereby allowing the

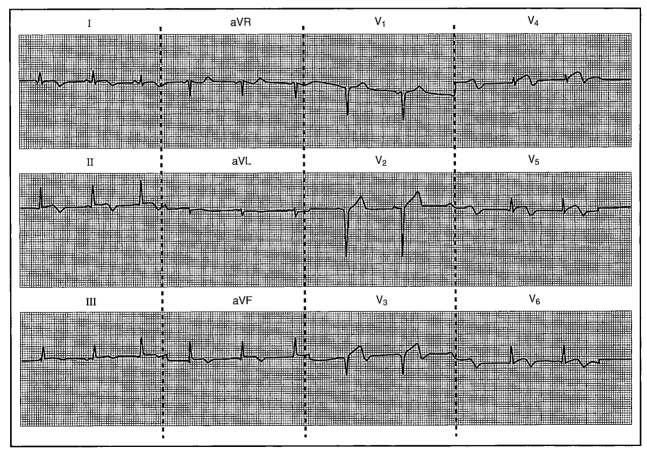

Figure 9–53.

A 12-lead electrocardiogram tracing demonstrating an anterior infarction. Note the significant Q waves in V_1, V_2, and V_3 and the inverted T waves throughout many other leads.

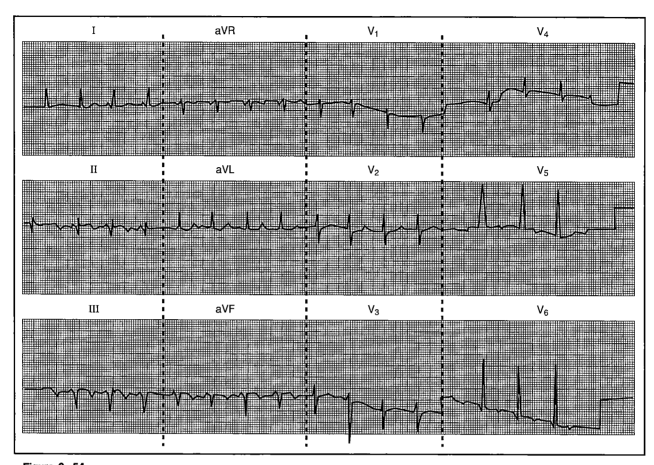

Figure 9-54.

A 12-lead electrocardiogram tracing demonstrating an inferior infarction. Notice the significant Q waves in leads II, III, and aVF.

right side of the myocardium to depolarize first and hiding any possible significant Q waves coming from the left ventricle (Fig. 9-57).

Acute **pericarditis** is a condition that causes ECG changes that differ from those caused by ischemia and infarction. These ECG changes are important to mention because they assist in the diagnosis of the condition. Acute pericarditis, defined as an inflammation of the pericardial sac, is often a complication following myocardial infarction and open heart surgery. Pericardial pain is usually intense but can closely mimic angina in location. The pain is usually aggravated or re-lieved by respiration and change of position. The ECG findings include ST-segment elevation, P-R interval depression, late T wave inversion, and atrial arrhythmias (often supraventricular tachy-cardia) (Fig. 9-58). The symptoms as well as the ECG changes are often all that is needed for diagnosis. In addition, a **pericardial rub** may be present during auscultation of the heart sounds.

Other abnormalities may exist on the ECG, including pacemaker functioning (Fig. 9-59), which is discussed in Chapter 11, and axis deviation. These abnormalities are beyond the scope of this chapter.

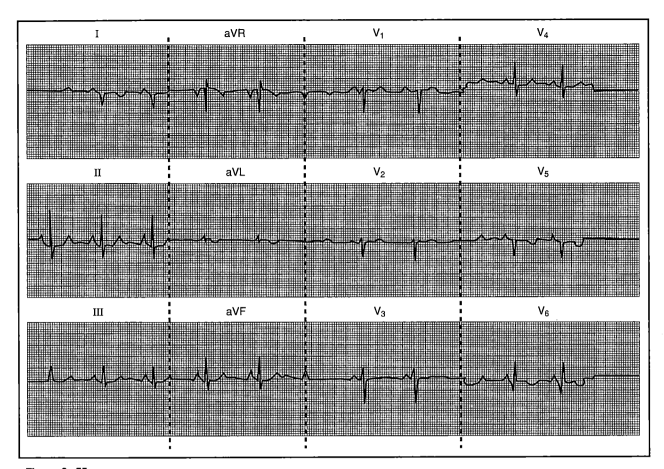

Figure 9-55.

A 12-lead electrocardiogram tracing demonstrating a lateral infarction. Notice the significant Q waves in I, V_5, and V_6, with inverted T waves in aVL as well.

CASE STUDIES

CASE 1

A 68-year-old man has a history of an acute myocardial infarction 7 months previous. He subsequently underwent coronary artery bypass graft surgery exactly 1 month after the myocardial infarction. It is now 6 months since his surgery, and he is symptom free. His goal is to return to his previously active lifestyle, so he was referred for an evaluation and exercise program.

On evaluation, his heart rate is 70, blood pressure is 124/84, and ECG is normal sinus rhythm. During the exercise treadmill test, he exercised at 2.5 miles per hour with 12% grade but complained of dizziness at 4.5 minutes of the exercise test. His heart rate was 110 and blood pressure was 130/78. The ECG rhythm showed a sudden onset of PVCs and a run of ventricular tachycardia. After the exercise was terminated, his rhythm slowed down to frequent PVCs and then normal sinus rhythm.

CASE 2

A 75-year-old woman suffered a hip fracture and underwent a surgical procedure with hip pin-

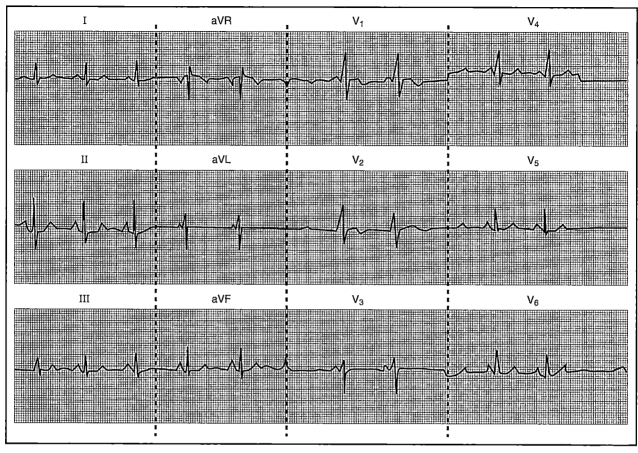

Figure 9-56.

A 12-lead electrocardiogram tracing demonstrating a posterior infarction. Notice the large R waves in V_1 and V_2 and the inverted T waves in the same leads.

ning. Two days after the patient's operation the physical therapy order was for progressive ambulation with walk using toe-touch gait. The patient had not been out of bed since before the fall. On evaluation, an irregular irregular heart beat was palpated. The ventricular response was approximately 100. Resting blood pressure was 110/70. On sitting, her blood pressure fell to 100/60 and heart rate (still irregular irregular) increased to 120. On standing, the patient complained of dizziness, and her blood pressure dropped to 90/60; her heart rate increased (still irregular irregular) to 140. The patient was returned to bed, and the physician notified. The physician left orders for the patient to spend more time sitting in a chair, so on the next visit

the physical therapist brought a telemetry monitor and attached electrodes to see the patient's rhythm. The monitor indicated that the patient had atrial fibrillation, with a ventricular response of 100 while lying supine. On sitting, heart rate again increased and blood pressure fell; the rhythm demonstrated atrial fibrillation, with a ventricular response of 120.

CASE 3

A 21-year-old female physical therapy student was sitting in class listening to a lecture and reported that her heart was racing away and that

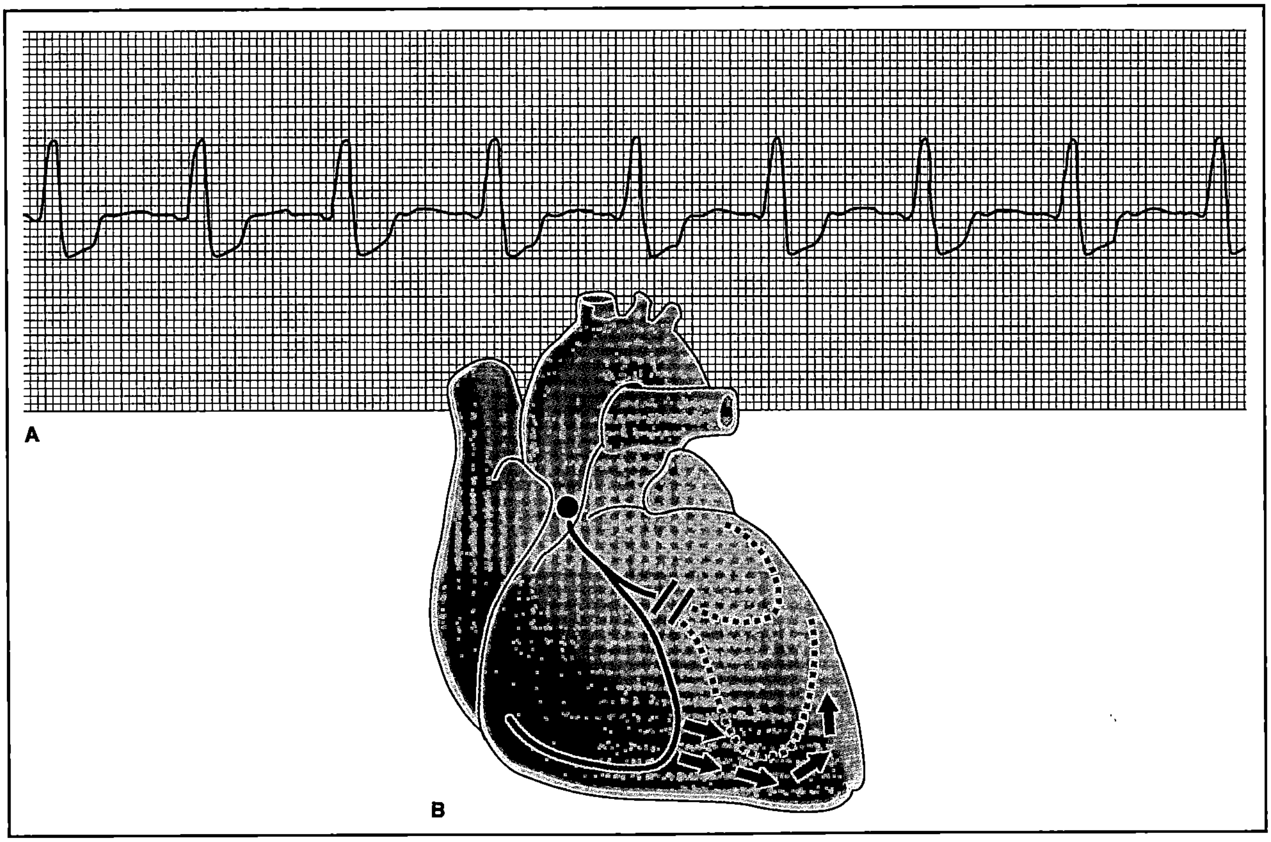

A

B

Figure 9-57.

A, A rhythm strip demonstrating a bundle branch block. Note the widened QRS interval. *B*, A left bundle branch block.

Figure 9-58.

The 12-lead electrocardiogram illustrates acute pericarditis. Note the upward concavity of the ST segment *(1)* and the notching at the junction of the QRS and ST segments *(2)*. (From Abedin Z, Conner R. 12 Lead ECG Interpretation: The Self-Assessment Approach. Philadelphia, WB Saunders, 1989, p 206.)

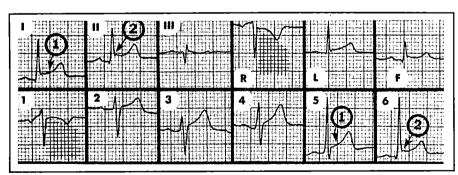

she felt slightly lightheaded. The student had never had any real illnesses or any history of cardiac problems. When the same symptoms occurred a second time she informed one of the faculty, who happened to have an ECG monitor in her office. The student was told to wear the ECG monitor to her next class. Fortunately, the student had the same recurring symptoms, and the monitor recorded a run of paroxysmal atrial tachycardia. On auscultation of heart sounds, the student was found to have a midsystolic click. The student was referred for a full cardiac evalua-

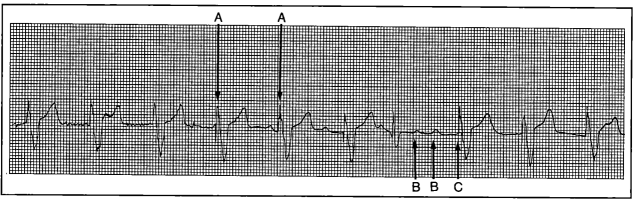

Figure 9-59.

Electrocardiogram tracing showing a demand-type pacemaker set at 72 beats per minute. The pacemaker is firing where the arrows are pointing to straight vertical lines (*A*). The arrows pointing from below show the atria firing twice but without ventricular response (*B*). Therefore, the pacemaker initiated a beat at (*C*).

tion following the documented episode. The student was found to have benign mitral valve prolapse and was told to monitor episodes for frequency of occurrence and symptoms.

SUMMARY

- Four cell types exist in the myocardium: working or mechanical cells, nodal cells, transitional cells, and Purkinje's cells.
- Depolarization of the cell membrane allows the influx of sodium ions into the cell and the efflux of potassium ions.
- As the cell becomes positive on the interior, the myocardial cells are stimulated to contract (called excitation coupling).
- On the ECG, the wave of depolarization is recorded as an upward deflection when moving toward a positive electrode (located on the skin).
- The cardiac muscle has three properties: automaticity, rhythmicity, and conductivity.
- The autonomic nervous system has a major influence on the cardiac system. Stimulation of the sympathetic division increases the heart rate, conduction velocity, and contractile force, and stimulation of the parasympathetic division (acting primarily via the vagal nerve) slows the heart rate and the conduction through the AV node.
- The conduction system involves the spread of

a stimulus via the SA node (primary pacemaker), internodal pathways, AV node, His's bundle, bundle branches, and Purkinje's fibers.

- The ECG records the electrical activity of the heart on ruled graph paper. Time is represented on the horizontal axis, and each small square is 0.04 second. Voltage is recorded on the vertical axis, and each small square is 1 mm.
- A standard 12-lead ECG consists of six limb leads and six chest leads, each recording the electrical activity from a different angle and providing a different view of the same activity in the heart.
- The ECG is reviewed to identify four areas that require interpretation: heart rate, heart rhythm, hypertrophy, and infarction.
- Numerous methods can be employed to measure heart rate from the ECG tracing, but often the 6-second strip method is the easiest if the rhythm is regular.
- Hypertrophy is detected on a 12-lead ECG by looking at the waveforms, particularly at the P wave and QRS complex for the voltage (greater than 3 mV) or configuration.
- Left ventricular hypertrophy is present if the depth of the S wave in V_1 plus the height of the R wave in V_5 is greater than 35 mm.
- In the presence of acute injury, the ST segment is elevated above the isoelectric line and gradually returns to the level of the isoelectric line over a period of 24 to 48 hours.

- In ventricular aneurysm, the ST segment remains elevated and does not return to the isoelectric line over time.
- ST-segment depression at rest associated with chest pain may indicate acute injury to the subendocardial wall.
- ST-segment depression that develops during exercise is an ischemic response to activity and following rest should return to the baseline.
- The presence of a significant Q wave is diagnostic for an infarction, but the date of the infarction cannot be determined from the ECG.
- A significant Q wave is 1 mm wide or one third the size of the QRS complex.
- A 12-lead ECG is used primarily for determining ischemia or infarction. Single-lead monitoring is employed for evaluating heart rate or rhythm.
- The location of the infarction is determined by the leads on the 12-lead ECG that demonstrate changes.
- The presence of significant Q waves in V_1 through V_4 indicates an anterior infarction and probable involvement of the left anterior descending coronary artery.
- The presence of significant Q waves in II, III, and aVF indicates an inferior infarction and probable involvement of the right coronary artery.
- A systematic approach should be taken when evaluating the rhythm strip. All the waveform configurations should be evaluated, as well as the P–R intervals, the QRS intervals, the R to R intervals, and the rate to assess the rhythm disturbance.
- Following identification of the rhythm disturbance, an assessment of signs and symptoms should be undertaken, after which a clinical decision can be made regarding the amount of monitoring the individual will need with activity as well as the safety of activity.

References

1. Cohen M, Fuster V. Insights into the pathogenetic mechanisms of unstable angina. Haemostasis 20(suppl 1):102–112, 1990.
2. Schaper J, Schaper W. Time course of myocardial necrosis. Cardiovasc Drugs Ther 2(1):17–25, 1988.
3. Bekn Haim SA, Becker B, Edoute Y, et al. Beat to beat electrocardiographic morphology variation in healed myocardial infarction. Am J Cardiol 68(8):725–728, 1991.
4. Phillips RE, Feeney MK. The Cardiac Rhythms: A Systematic Approach to Interpretation. 3rd ed. Philadelphia, WB Saunders, 1990.
5. Scheidt S. Basic Electrocardiography: Leads, Axes, Arrhythmias. New Jersey, CIBA Clinical Symposia, 1983.
6. Berne RM, Levy MN. Cardiovascular Physiology. 6th ed. St. Louis, Mosby–Year Book, 1992.
7. Grauer K, Curry RW. Clinical Electrocardiography: A Primary Care Approach. 2nd ed. Boston, Blackwell Scientific Publishers, 1992.
8. Abedin Z, Conner RP. 12 Lead ECG Interpretation: The Self-Assessment Approach. Philadelphia, WB Saunders, 1989.
9. Valle BK, Lemberg L. Non-Q wave versus nontransmural infarction. Heart Lung 19(2):208–211, 1990.

Suggested Readings

Dubin D. Rapid ECG Interpretation. 3rd ed. Tampa, Fla, Cover Publishing, 1974.

McIntyre K, Lewis J (eds). Textbook of Advanced Cardiac Life Support. Dallas, American Heart Association, 1983.

Grauer K, Curry RW. Clinical Electrocardiography: A Primary Care Approach. 2nd ed. Boston, Blackwell Scientific Publications, 1992.

Abedin Z, Conner RP. 12 Lead ECG Interpretation: The Self-Assessment Approach. Philadelphia, WB Saunders, 1989.

Andreoli KG, Fowkes VH, Zipes DP, Wallace AC. Comprehensive Cardiac Care. 7th ed. St. Louis, CV Mosby, 1987.

Marriott HJL. Practical Electrocardiography. 8th ed. Baltimore, Williams & Wilkins, 1988.

Bean DY. Introduction to ECG Interpretation. Rockville, Md, Aspen Publishers, 1987.

Fenstermacher K. Dysrhythmia Recognition and Management. Philadelphia, WB Saunders, 1989.

Fisch C. Electrocardiography of Arrhythmias. Philadelphia, Lea & Febiger, 1990.

Wiederhold R. Electrocardiography: The Monitoring Lead. Philadelphia, WB Saunders, 1988.

10 PULMONARY DIAGNOSTIC TESTS AND PROCEDURES

INTRODUCTION

This chapter introduces several of the diagnostic tests and procedures commonly utilized in the assessment of patients with pulmonary disease. Although the tests and procedures described in this chapter are not necessarily performed by physical therapists, they nonetheless provide them with invaluable information. To apply this information to the planning, implementation, and monitoring of patient treatments, physical therapists must have a fundamental understanding of chest imaging, pulmonary function testing, bronchoscopy, arterial blood gas analysis, oximetry, and bacteriologic and cytologic tests. The

incorporation of this information in the evaluative process is discussed in Chapter 14.

CHEST IMAGING

Over the past decade there has been an explosion of progress in the area of chest imaging. Largely as a result of new technologies but also because of refinements in older techniques, several imaging options are now available in addition to the standard "plain film" radiograph. It is certainly beyond the scope of this text to present all the abnormal chest findings that are identifiable by these imaging techniques. Rather, the

403

information in this chapter is intended to assist in the development of a framework on which to build an understanding of these imaging techniques. A basic knowledge of how the images are produced and of what they display can facilitate physician-therapist dialogue and enhance physical therapy treatment planning.

Roentgen Rays

Roentgen rays are produced whenever high-speed electrons undergo sudden deceleration. Electrons flowing through a wire in a vacuum-sealed cathode tube are focused to strike a small area on a positively charged anodal plate, resulting in the emission of roentgen rays. Traveling at the same speed as light, roentgen rays have a very high frequency and a relatively short wavelength. These rays are not reflected back like light rays; instead they penetrate matter and are invisible. Certain phosphors become fluorescent when excited by roentgen rays, and these may be placed on fluorescent screens that are superimposed over photographic film to make a roentgen ray cassette. Typically, a patient is placed between a roentgen ray source and a cassette (Fig. 10–1). When the rays penetrate the tissues of the patient, they stimulate the fluorescent screen to emit light, which exposes the film. Because scattered radiation reduces subject contrast, several different scatter reduction techniques (e.g., grids, air-gap, moving slits) are used to decrease the incidence of scattered roentgen rays striking the film cassette.[1-4] The radiograph thus produced is also referred to as a **roentgenogram** after Wilhelm Konrad Roentgen, who received the first Nobel Prize for Physics in 1901 for his work in defining the major properties of roentgen rays and the conditions necessary for their production. It was Roentgen who coined the term *x ray.*

Radiographs

Despite the newer technologies, in most clinical settings the standard radiograph remains the predominant medium by which anatomic ab-

normalities resulting from pathologic processes within the chest are assessed. Consequently, a significant portion of this chapter is devoted to the chest radiograph. The newer technologies often contribute valuable confirmatory or differential diagnostic information to that already obtained from a chest radiograph and are discussed in lesser detail later in this chapter.

Chest radiographs provide a static view of the anatomy of the chest, and as such, they may be used to screen for abnormalities, to provide a baseline from which subsequent assessments can be made, or to monitor the progress of a disease process or treatment intervention. The principal objects shown on a chest radiograph are air, fat, water, tissue, and bone. Air in the lungs produces a low tissue density and allows greater roentgen ray penetration, resulting in a dark image on a radiograph—**radiolucency.** At the opposite extreme is bone, which, because it is denser, allows fewer roentgen rays to penetrate and results in a white image on a radiograph—**radiopacity.** Depending on the densities and thicknesses of the numerous structures in the chest, the roentgen rays penetrating a patient are variably absorbed and create "shadows" on the film. Several other factors also affect the image depicted on a radiograph but are beyond the scope of this chapter. Therefore, the reader is referred to standard radiology texts for more detailed information.

The standard chest radiograph, as typically obtained in a radiology department, is routinely taken in two views: **a posteroanterior (PA) view,** with the patient in the standing position with the front of the chest facing the film cassette (Fig. 10–2); and a **left lateral view** (Fig. 10–3), unless the pathologic process is known to be present on the right side of the chest (in which case a right lateral view would be obtained). The lateral view is extremely helpful in localizing the position of an abnormality, because in the PA view the upper and middle lobes of the lung override portions of the lower lobes. Other views that may be obtained include

- the **decubitus views,** which are taken to confirm the presence of an air-fluid level in the lungs or a small pleural effusion. Depending

Figure 10-1.

Relationship of the patient to the film cassette and roentgen ray source for a standard posteroanterior radiograph.

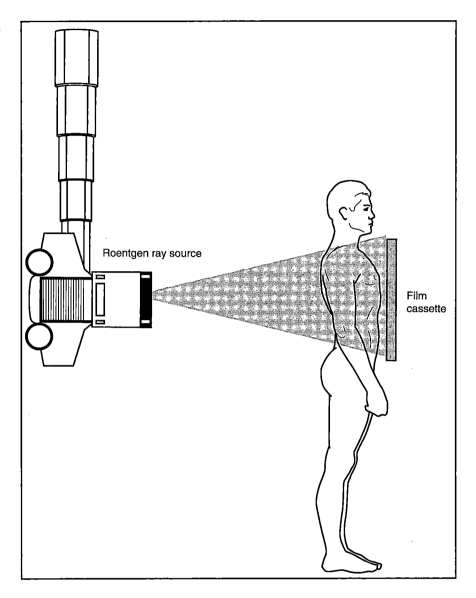

Roentgen ray source

Film cassette

on the location of the suspected pathologic condition, the patient is placed in the supine, prone, or right or left side-lying position.

- the **lordotic view,** used to visualize the apical or mid (right middle lobe or left lingular segments) regions of the lungs or specifically to screen for pulmonary tuberculosis, which typically manifests itself in the apical regions. The roentgen ray source is lowered and angled upward, and the patient may or may not be tipped slightly backward.

- the **oblique views,** taken to detect pleural thickening, to evaluate the carina, or to visualize the heart and great vessels. The patient stands at an angle of 45 to 60 degrees to the film with either the left or right anterior, or the left or right posterior, chest against the film cassette (anterior or posterior oblique views, respectively).

- the **anteroposterior (AP) view,** taken at the patient's bedside when the patient is too ill to travel to the radiology department. AP radio-

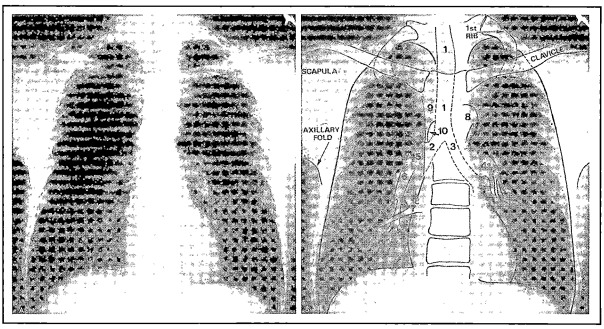

Figure 10-2.

A, Normal chest radiograph—posteroanterior view. *B*, Same radiograph as in *A*, with the normal anatomic structures labeled or numbered: 1, trachea; 2, right mainstem bronchus; 3, left mainstem bronchus; 4, left pulmonary artery; 5, pulmonary vein to the right upper lobe; 6, right interlobular artery; 7, vein to right middle and lower lobes; 8, aortic knob; 9, superior vena cava; 10, ascending aorta. (From Fraser RG, Paré JAP, Paré PD, et al. Diagnosis of Diseases of the Chest. Vol 1. 3rd ed. Philadelphia, WB Saunders, 1988, pp 287, 288.)

graphs are obtained with the patient supine, semirecumbent, or sitting upright against the film cassette and facing the machine. When the film is taken in the supine position, the abdominal contents tend to elevate the hemidiaphragms; the pulmonary blood flow is redistributed; and the mediastinal structures appear larger (Fig. 10-4).

The potential interpreter of radiographs is presented with several challenges, among these being the two-dimensional representation of three-dimensional objects and the limited greyscale "shadow" depiction of the various organs, tissues, and pathologic processes. Although it may be more likely that the clinician will have access to a radiologist's report rather than to the actual radiograph, many clinical settings offer the therapist direct access to the patient's chest radiographs. Consequently, therapists should be familiar with the manner in which chest radiographs are assessed.

Examining Chest Radiographs

There is no single "best" method for examining chest radiographs; nevertheless, a systematic approach should be utilized. Rau and Pierce[5] and Cookson and Finlay[6] recommend starting at the center of the film and working outward toward the soft tissues. Kersten[7] and Freundlich and Bragg[8] suggest a body system approach to examining chest films (the method described in what follows), starting with an examination of the bones and soft tissues, including the abdomen; the mediastinum from the larynx to the abdomen; the cardiovascular system; the hila; and finally the lung fields themselves. Independent of the method of examination, the mediastinum and hila are typically assessed for abnormal vasculature or mass lesions, the heart for changes in shape or position, and the lungs for abnormal increased density or lucency. By convention, frontal chest radiographs should be viewed as if the patient's right side were on the therapist's left side—as if two people were "shaking hands." The left lateral chest radiograph should be viewed as if the patient's left side were facing the therapist; the reverse is true for the right lateral view.

In the body systems approach to examining chest radiographs, the overall adequacy of the image should be addressed first. The optimal radiograph should be taken with the patient holding a deep inspiration. Furthermore, the entire chest should be visible on the radiograph (see Fig. 10–2). Then the following should be considered in turn:

1. **Bones and soft tissues:** The size, shape, and symmetry of the bony thorax should be considered; the vertebral bodies should be faintly visible through the mediastinal shadow, and all of the other bones of the thorax should be included on the radiograph. To determine whether the patient is rotated to either side, the medial ends of each clavicle should be checked to see that they are equally distant from the spinous processes of the vertebral bodies (if the patient is rotated, the distances between the medial ends of the clavicles and the spinous processes are unequal). In a PA film the clavicles often appear to be lower than in an AP film. Because of the position of the shoulders, the medial aspect of the scapulae are typically lateral to and outside the lung fields in a PA film, whereas in an AP film, the medial borders may appear as vertical or oblique lines within the lung fields.

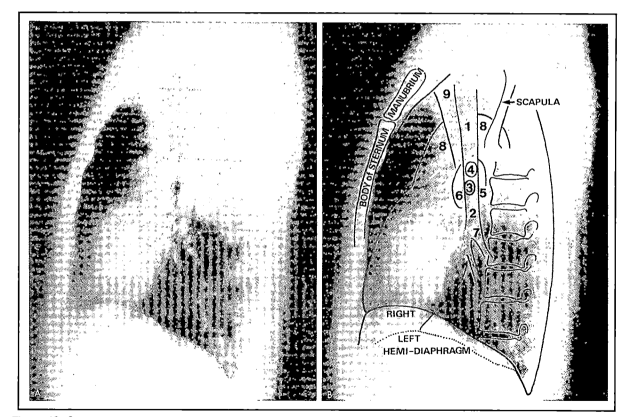

Figure 10–3.

A, Normal chest radiograph—lateral view. *B*, Same radiograph as in *A*, with the normal anatomic structures labeled or numbered: 1, trachea; 2, right intermediate bronchus; 3, left upper lobe bronchus; 4, right upper lobe bronchus; 5, left interlobar artery; 6, right interlobar artery; 7, junction of the pulmonary veins; 8, aortic arch; 9, brachiocephalic vessels. (From Fraser RG, Paré JAP, Paré PD, et al. Diagnosis of Diseases of the Chest. Vol. 1. 3rd ed. Philadelphia, WB Saunders, 1988, pp 289, 290.)

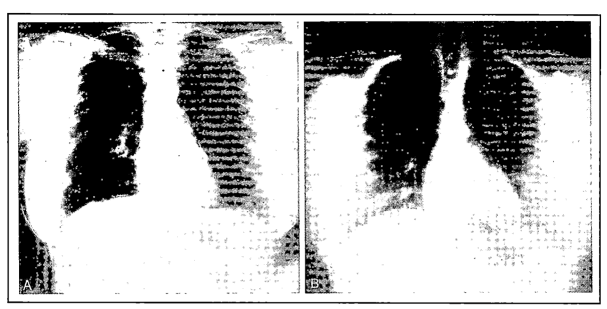

Figure 10-4.

Comparison of posteroanterior (*A*) and anteroposterior (*B*) radiographic views of the same 30-year-old woman. (From Kersten LD. Comprehensive Respiratory Nursing: A Decision Making Approach. Philadelphia, WB Saunders, 1989, pp 408, 409.)

The various densities of the soft tissues (e.g., skin, subcutaneous fat, and muscle) normally blend together—the **summation effect.** The width of the intercostal spaces should be considered because widened intercostal spaces may be indicative of increased thoracic volume (the best way to gain an appreciation of the normal intercostal space width is to review normal chest radiographs).

The two hemidiaphragms should appear as rounded, smooth, sharply defined shadows; the dome of the right hemidiaphragm is normally 1 to 2 centimeters higher than the left. The diaphragm is said to be *elevated* if during a deep inhalation fewer than nine ribs are visible above the level of the domes; it is *depressed* if more than ten ribs are visible. Where the hemidiaphragms meet the chest wall at their lateral aspects, the **costophrenic angles** are formed. The costophrenic angles are moderately deep, and they are approximately equal in size on the two sides. Opacification of the costophrenic angle is indicative of either pleural thickening (if the change has occurred over many months or years) or pleural effusion (if the change has occurred

recently). Medially, the hemidiaphragms normally form a cardiophrenic angle where they meet the borders of the heart.

2. **Mediastinum, trachea, and cardiovascular system:** The size of the mediastinum varies with body size, being long and narrow in tall, thin persons and short and wide in short, stocky persons. Regardless of size, the borders of the mediastinum are generally as outlined in Figure 1-23. The trachea normally appears as a vertical translucent shadow superimposed on the mediastinal shadow in the midline, overlying the cervical vertebrae. In most cases, tracheal deviation from the midline position suggests that the patient is rotated. However, pathologic conditions can also result in tracheal deviation. For example, a large pneumothorax can push the trachea toward the contralateral side of the chest, or a massive atelectasis can pull the trachea toward the ipsilateral side of the chest. Visualization of the tracheal shadow is particularly important if the patient is intubated (has an endotracheal tube in place), because proper positioning of the endotracheal tube is determined by the proximity of its distal end to the tracheal bifurcation. The tip

of a properly placed endotracheal tube should be about 2 inches above the carina when the patient's head is in the neutral position.

The heart and great vessels occupy the lower two thirds of the mediastinum, giving the mediastinum a characteristic profile. Two distinct curves should be noted on the right side of the cardiovascular shadow. The first, formed entirely by the right atrium, begins at the right cardiophrenic angle and proceeds superiorly. The inferior vena cava can often be seen entering the right atrium, inferiorly. The second curve is formed by the ascending aorta and the superior vena cava. On the left side, there are typically four curves of importance. The first curve is formed by the transverse arch and descending aorta before it passes behind the main pulmonary artery, which makes the next curve. The third curve may not be visible and denotes the site of the left atrial appendage. The border of the left ventricle extends downward to the diaphragm, forming the fourth curve.

3. **The hila:** The hila are formed by the root of the lungs (comprising the pulmonary blood vessels, the bronchi, and a group of lymph nodes) at approximately the T4 to T5 level. The hila appear as poorly defined areas of variable density in the medial part of the central portion of the lung fields. The left hilum is partially obscured by the overlying shadow of the heart and great vessels, and it lies at a slightly higher level than the right hilum.

4. The **lung fields:** Although the lobes of the lung normally cannot be distinguished, knowledge of lobar and segmental anatomy is crucial to an assessment of the lung fields. The left and right upper lobes and the right middle lobe lie superiorly and anteriorly within the thoracic cavity, and the lower lobes occupy the posteroinferior aspects. Although the medial segment of the right middle lobe is in contact with the right border of the heart and the lingular segments of the left upper lobe are in contact with the left border of the heart, the lobes overlap each other considerably so that a clear localization of each lobe is not possible in the PA or the AP view alone. A lateral view is essential to delineate accurately the lobes of the lungs and their various bronchopulmonary segments.

The **silhouette sign** (present when the normal line of demarcation between two structures is partially or completely obliterated) may be used to localize lesions within the lung fields.[9] In the critical care setting, life-support and monitoring equipment can complicate the interpretation of a chest radiograph, as demonstrated in Figure 10–5.

The airways outside the mediastinum are not usually visible on a chest radiograph because of their thin walls and air-filled lumina. However, the pulmonary arteries and veins can frequently be seen as they branch and taper outward toward the periphery until they disappear in the outer third of the lung fields. By observing serial films, these **vascular markings** can be described as unchanged, increased, or decreased. Increased vascular markings are indicative of venous dilation, whereas decreased vascular markings may indicate hyperinflation of the lungs.

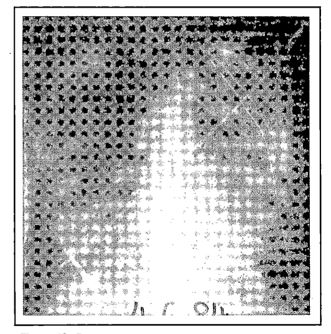

Figure 10–5.

Anteroposterior radiographic view of a patient with adult respiratory distress syndrome, illustrating the complications introduced by the additional shadows of life-support and monitoring equipment. (From Dantzker DR. Cardiopulmonary Critical Care. 2nd ed. Philadelphia, WB Saunders, 1991, p 370.)

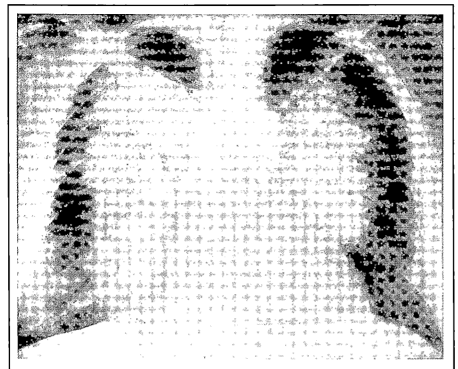

Figure 10–6.

An example of the alveolar pattern of pulmonary edema in a 59-year-old man, 48 hours after a massive myocardial infarction. (From Fraser RG, Paré JAP, Paré PD, et al. Diagnosis of Diseases of the Chest. Vol. 3. 3rd ed. Philadelphia, WB Saunders, 1990, p 1917.)

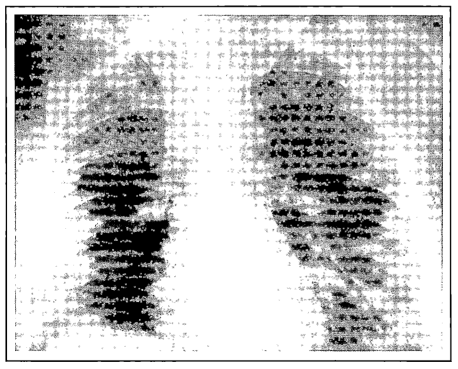

Figure 10–7.

An example of the interstitial pattern that signifies interstitial thickening secondary to an inflammatory process. (From Fraser RG, Paré JAP, Paré PD, et al. Diagnosis of Diseases of the Chest. Vol. 3. 3rd ed. Philadelphia, WB Saunders, 1990, p 1941.)

Specific lung lesions are assessed by observing the lung fields for any abnormal density that obliterates the vascular markings or that alters the distribution of the densities within the lung fields. Lastly, the lung fields should be assessed for any abnormal patterns of radiopacity. If present, these abnormal patterns are typically described as either **alveolar patterns** or **interstitial patterns,** and they may be localized independently or diffuse or coexistent. Alveolar patterns are sometimes described as "fluffy infil-

trates"; they represent a pathologic process within the distal airways, for example, pulmonary edema or alveolar pneumonia (Fig. 10–6). In contrast, interstitial patterns represent interstitial thickening, for example, inflammation (Fig. 10–7). Interstitial disease may also assume the appearance of fine diffuse nodules throughout the lungs. If they are of uniform size, they are called miliary nodules. The pattern of increased pulmonary vascularity often strongly resembles the interstitial pattern.

Some neonatal pulmonary diseases have unique radiographic appearances. Nevertheless the same general principles of radiologic assessment that are used in the assessment of older children and adults apply. To this end, the assessment must determine whether the problem is in the lungs, the heart, the mediastinum (distinct from the heart), or the thoracic wall. The level of the right hemidiaphragm defines normal lung volume in the neonate, and it should be at about the level of the eighth or ninth thoracic vertebra.[5]

Regardless of the source of the information that details the results of a radiographic chest examination, the data provided can be invaluable to the physical therapist in facilitating the choice and planning of treatment interventions and in the subsequent evaluation of treatment efficacy. Several additional chest imaging techniques can provide the clinician with information on which decisions regarding treatment planning or efficacy may be made. Several of these are described briefly.

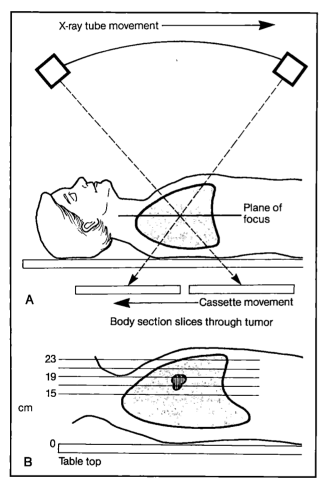

Figure 10–8.

Obtaining a tomographic image of the chest: *A,* One of many focal planes that comprise a tomographic image of the chest, obtained as the radiographic source and the film cassette are moved. *B,* An example of several focal planes that isolate an area of disease. (From Kersten LD. Comprehensive Respiratory Nursing: A Decision Making Approach. Philadelphia, WB Saunders, 1989, p 413.)

Tomography

Standard tomography, or sectional radiography, involves the curvilinear movement of the roentgen ray source and the film or screen system in opposite directions about the patient (Fig. 10–8). The shadow of the selected plane remains stationary on the moving film while the shadows of all other planes are obliterated by their relative displacement. Linear tomography is generally used to enhance the evaluation of pathologic processes in the lung parenchyma, hila, and mediastinum.[4] Standard tomography has been obviated somewhat by newer imaging techniques such as computed tomography and ultrasound. However, standard tomography remains particularly useful for detecting calcifications or cavities suspected in the shadows of conventional radiographs.[6]

Computed Tomography

The introduction of the **computed tomography (CT)** scanner in 1972 has been touted as the single greatest advance in radiography since the discovery of roentgen rays. Computed tomography, or digital chest radiography, involves a narrow beam of roentgen rays moved across the field of examination in such a way as to define successive adjacent columns of tissue—a process called **translation.** Another pass is then made at a different angle, the new angle being referred to as a **rotation.** The process is repeated many times, with subsequent digitization of each analog image into a numeric form by means of computer-based processing. Each digital image is an array (matrix) of numbers, each number representing a single element of the picture (pixel) and the value of the number defining the degree of brightness or darkness of that particular point in the image. Several digital images are then manipulated mathematically to produce a summated image for diagnostic interpretation.

Magnetic Resonance Imaging

Magnetic resonance imaging (MRI) involves the interaction of stimulated hydrogen nuclei and a strong magnetic field. An MRI scanner produces a gradient magnetic field in the region of the body to be imaged. The hydrogen nuclei tend to align themselves with the magnetic field and resonate at a frequency that is proportional to the strength of the magnetic field. There is a gradient of nuclear resonance proportional to the gradient of the magnetic field—magnetic resonance. The patient is then exposed to a radio signal that stimulates those nuclei whose magnetic resonance is the same as the frequency of the radio signal. These stimulated nuclei reemit the radio signal, which is "picked up" by an antenna in the MRI scanner and digitally recorded by a computer—isolating a "slice of tissue" in much the same manner as that for a CT image. As soon as the reemitted signal is recorded, a new gradient is produced in a perpendicular plane to the original slice and this new slice is stimulated and recorded. The original gradient is then restored. This excitation and retrieval process is repeated many times with the transverse gradient being applied at a slightly different angle each time.[10] The data thus obtained may be manipulated mathematically to produce a final enhanced image for interpretation, an example of which is shown in Figure 10–9. Unfortunately, MRI is currently of limited utility in the evaluation of pathologic processes in the parenchyma because the expanded lungs have an insufficient density of protons (hydrogen nuclei) for the generation of a magnetic resonance signal.[11] However, MRI is indicated for the evaluation of chest wall processes that may involve bone, muscle, fat, or pleura.

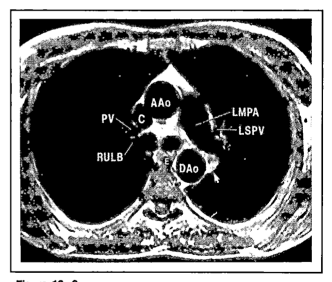

Figure 10–9.

An example of a magnetic resonance image of the chest showing normal anatomy at the level of the carina. RULB, right upper lobe bronchus; PV, right superior pulmonary vein; C, superior vena cava; AAo, ascending aorta; DAo, descending aorta; E, esophagus; LMPA, left main pulmonary artery; LSPV, left superior pulmonary vein. (From Naidich DP, Zerhouni EA, Siegelman SS. Computed Tomography and Magnetic Resonance of the Thorax. 2nd ed. New York, Raven Press, 1991, p 239.)

Bronchography

Contrast bronchography involves the opacification of the bronchial tree by the installation of contrast medium so that the radiographic shadows of the airways may be studied.[4,12] **Bronchograms** permit the study of normal and variant anatomy and of gross pathologic changes in the bronchial wall and lumen. A bronchogram demonstrating bronchiectasis of the left lower lobe bronchi is shown in Figure 10-10.

Ventilation and Perfusion Scans

Several different tests can be used to measure the gas distribution in the lungs. To measure the regional distribution of ventilation in the lungs the patient breathes xenon gas (^{133}Xe). The test is usually performed with the patient in a sitting or supine position. The patient is asked to inhale a normal tidal volume from a closed system containing a specific volume or concentration of xenon, and then to refrain from exhaling for several seconds while photoscintigrams — ventilation scans — are made over the lung field. To determine the rate of equilibrium of the gas in the lungs, serial photoscintigrams are made over a 10- to 15-minute period with the use of a rebreathing technique. Finally, to determine the washout rate of the xenon gas, the patient is returned to atmospheric breathing while serial photoscintigrams are made.

To measure the regional distribution of pulmonary blood flow in the lungs, the patient is injected intravenously with radioactive iodine (^{131}I) and serial photoscintigrams — perfusion scans — are made over the lung fields as the blood perfuses the lungs.

Although they may be performed as separate tests, ventilation and perfusion scans ($\dot{V}/\dot{Q}$ scans) provide the maximum amount of information when used together. Such information describes how the alveolar ventilation and pulmonary perfusion are matched in the patient. In the normal person, the $\dot{V}/\dot{Q}$ scans show greater ventilation and perfusion in the bases of the lung and less ventilation and perfusion in the apices. Ventilation and perfusion scans that illustrate normal and abnormal findings are shown in Figure 10-11.

BRONCHOSCOPY

The advent of the fiberoptic bronchoscope has decreased the necessity and usefulness of contrast bronchography markedly by permitting the

Figure 10-10.

Bronchogram in posteroanterior (A) and lateral (B) projections of the left lower lobe bronchi demonstrating the typical dilatations of bronchiectasis. (From Paré JAP, Fraser RG. Synopsis of Diseases of the Chest. Philadelphia, WB Saunders, 1983, p 560.)

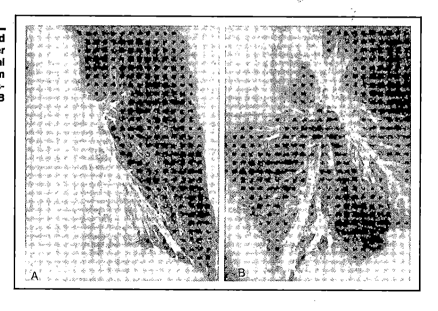

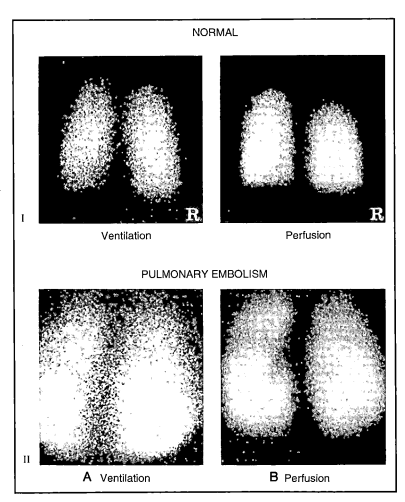

NORMAL

Ventilation   Perfusion

PULMONARY EMBOLISM

A Ventilation   B Perfusion

Figure 10–11.

Examples of ventilation-perfusion scans. *I*, normal ventilation-perfusion scan; *II*, ventilation-perfusion scan of a patient with a pulmonary embolism showing a normal ventilation scan (*A*) and an abnormal perfusion scan (*B*). (From Fraser RG, Paré JAP. Diagnosis of Diseases of the Chest. Vol. 1. 2nd ed. Philadelphia, WB Saunders, 1977, pp 234, 235.)

direct visualization of previously inaccessible areas of the bronchial tree. The typical appearance of the segmental origins within each lobe is depicted in Figure 10–12.

PULMONARY FUNCTION TESTING

Pulmonary function tests provide the clinician with information about the integrity of the airways, the function of the respiratory musculature, and the condition of the lung tissues themselves. A thorough evaluation of pulmonary function involves several tests that measure lung volumes and capacities, gas flow rates, gas diffusion, and distribution. Based on the results of pulmonary function tests, pulmonary diseases may be classified into three basic categories: obstructive, restrictive, or combined. A working knowledge of the principal tests and an ability to interpret their findings is an essential prerequisite to the planning and implementation of effective interventions.

Tests of Lung Volume and Capacity

The basic lung volumes and capacities are defined in Chapter 2. With the notable exception of the residual volume (RV) and therefore the functional residual capacity (FRC) and total lung capacity (TLC), lung volumes are measured by

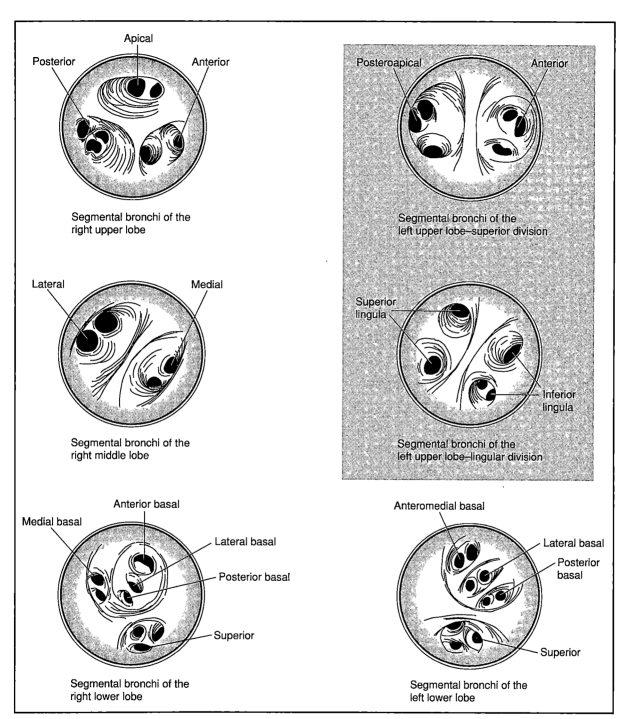

Figure 10–12.

Typical bronchoscopic views of the segmental bronchi of each lung.

means of simple spirometry. Spirometers may be of the traditional manual waterseal type, or they may be electronic computerized devices (e.g., pneumotachometers). In either case, a graphic tracing—called a *spirogram*—of the lung volumes is typically produced to facilitate interpretation of the measurements (Fig. 10–13).

Many spirometric measurements can be accurately taken at the bedside using relatively uncomplicated equipment (Fig. 10–14), whereas others must be made using the equipment found in a pulmonary function laboratory (Fig. 10–15). In either setting, the patient should be positioned in an upright sitting posture, and a nose clip should be used. The patient should breathe normally into the spirometer (or other appropriate instrument) through a tight-fitting mouthpiece until a normal rhythm is established. The following is a brief description of the manner in which the spirometrically determined volumes and capacities are measured.

- **Tidal volume (VT):** The total volume of air (V) moved during either inhalation or exhalation over a specific period of time (usually 1 min) is measured and then divided by the ventilatory rate (f): $V_T = V/f$. The average healthy adult's V_T is around 500 milliliters (± 100 ml), but because there is a great deal of variability within the normal population, measurements outside the normal range (400–600 ml) do not necessarily indicate the presence of a disease process.
- **Inspiratory reserve volume (IRV):** This is a component of the inspiratory capacity. It is not usually measured during spirometry because it is not a significant clinical measurement of lung mechanics.[13]
- **Expiratory reserve volume (ERV):** The patient is asked to exhale maximally after a few normal breaths. The normal ERV is approximately 1000 milliliters, but restrictive disease processes (refer to Chapter 5) typically result in a reduced ERV.
- **Vital capacity (VC):** The patient first inhales

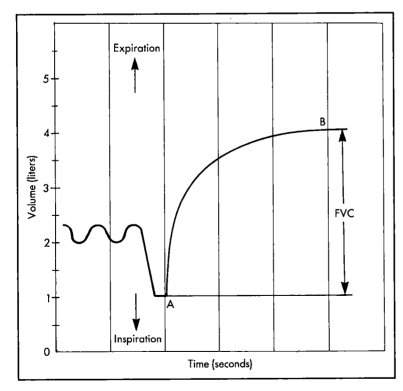

Figure 10–13.

Typical spirogram obtained as a patient exhales forcefully. (From Ruppel G. Manual of Pulmonary Function Testing. St. Louis, CV Mosby, 1986, p 28. Courtesy of Warren E. Collins, Inc., Braintree, Mass.)

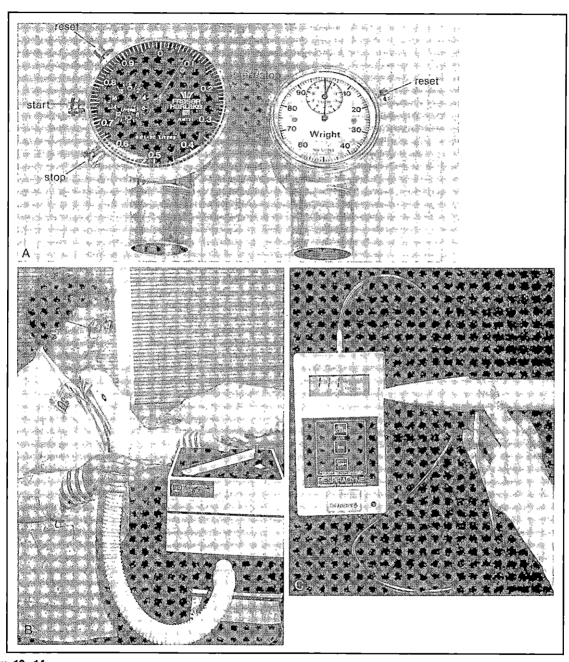

Figure 10-14.

Examples of several different spirometers that can be used to conduct simple spirometric measurements at a patient's bedside. *A*, The Fraser-Harlake *(left)* and the Wright *(right)* respirometers; *B*, SMI I spirometer; *C*, Respiradyne spirometer. (From Kersten LD. Comprehensive Respiratory Nursing: A Decision Making Approach. Philadelphia, WB Saunders, 1989, pp 386, 387.)

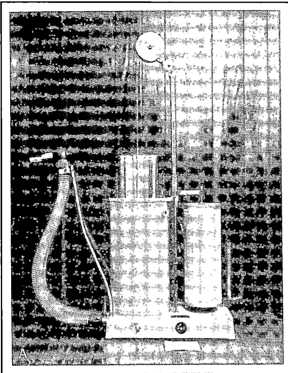

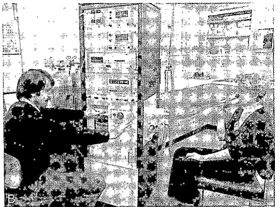

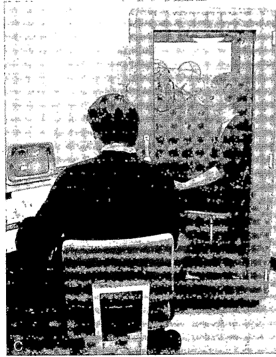

Figure 10–15.

Typical pulmonary function testing equipment found in a pulmonary function laboratory. *A*, A water-seal spirometer with counterweight pulley; *B*, computerized pulmonary function system; *C*, whole body plethysmograph. (*A* from Ruppel G. Manual of Pulmonary Function Testing. St. Louis, CV Mosby, 1986, p 124. Courtesy of Warren E. Collins, Inc., Braintree, Mass. *B* and *C* from Kersten LD. Comprehensive Respiratory Nursing: A Decision Making Approach. Philadelphia, WB Saunders, 1989, pp 372, 373.)

as deeply as possible and then exhales fully, taking as much time as is necessary to exhale completely. The normal VC ranges between 4000 to 5000 milliliters, representing approximately 80% of the TLC, but normal values can vary significantly, depending on age, gender, and test position. Although the VC may be normal in the early to moderate stages of obstructive lung disease, it is generally reduced in severe obstructive lung diseases. Restrictive diseases, too, may cause the VC to be decreased.

● **Inspiratory capacity (IC):** The patient is asked to inhale maximally following a normal exhalation. The IC normally varies between 3000 and 4000 milliliters, but it varies widely in the normal population. The IC should represent about 75% to 80% of the VC and around 55% to 60% of the TLC. Although normal values can be registered by patients who have obstructive or restrictive lung diseases, the IC is generally reduced in both disease states. Increases in the IC usually indicate poor initial patient participation.

As mentioned earlier, the RV cannot be measured directly with simple spirometry, and, in fact, most pulmonary function tests actually measure the FRC (by using the formula RV = FRC − ERV, the RV is then calculated).[7,13,14] The three most commonly used methods for determining the FRC and RV are

● the **helium dilution method (closed-circuit method):** Following a normal exhalation, the patient is connected to a closed spirometer system and breathes a known volume and concentration of helium (He) until an equilibrium is reached (carbon dioxide is eliminated through a carbon dioxide absorbent, and oxygen is added at a rate equal to the oxygen consumption). Once equilibrium is reached, the FRC is calculated from the change in helium concentration in the spirometer (e.g., the larger the patient's lung volume, the less the helium concentration in the spirometer). It normally takes less than 5 minutes for equilibrium of the helium between the patient and the spirometer to occur; however, in patients with severe obstructive disease it can take up to 30 minutes.

● the **nitrogen washout method (open-circuit method):** As in the helium dilution test, the patient is connected to the system at the end of an exhalation. The nitrogen (N_2) concentration in the lungs is in equilibrium with the atmosphere—approximately 79%—so that as the patient inhales pure oxygen from the spirometer, the nitrogen is "washed out" of the lungs. Because the volume of nitrogen washed out of the lungs by breathing pure oxygen is proportional to the person's end-expiratory lung volume, by measuring the volume and the nitrogen percentages of the exhaled gas, the FRC is determined. The nitrogen washout method typically takes about 7 minutes to complete.

● **body plethysmography:** The plethysmograph is an airtight chamber in which the patient sits; pressure transducers measure pressure both at the airway (mouthpiece) and in the chamber. The patient is placed in a plethysmograph, connected to the mouthpiece, and asked to breathe normally. At end-inspiration and end-expiration no airflow occurs, and the alveolar pressure is equal to the airway pressure at that time. At a specific time (end-expiration, for example) the shutter is occluded, and the various volume and pressure values are measured. Because the body plethysmography method of FRC determination actually measures the total amount of gas in the thorax, the values obtained may be larger than those from either the helium dilution or the nitrogen washout techniques (any difference between the measurements is an estimate of the volume of poorly ventilated regions of the lungs).

The TLC is the sum of the VC and the RV and is the only individually diagnostic parameter in spirometry. It is always elevated in obstructive lung diseases and reduced in chronic restrictive lung diseases. Certain acute disorders, such as pulmonary edema, atelectasis, and consolidation, will also cause a reduction in TLC.

Tests of Gas Flow Rates

Tests that measure airflow rates during forced breathing maneuvers provide important information relating to the actual function of the lungs, the degree of impairment, and often the general location (e.g., large airways, small airways) of the problem. The basic measures of airflow rates include the following:

- **Forced vital capacity (FVC):** This is the maximum volume of gas the patient can exhale as forcefully and as quickly as possible. It is measured by having the patient exhale as forcefully and as quickly as possible into a spirometer or pneumotachometer. The patient should breathe in maximally and exhale as quickly as possible. The FVC is highly dependent on the amount of force used by the patient in early expiration at volumes near TLC. Therefore, it may be necessary to coach the patient to achieve a maximum expiratory effort. A normal spirographic tracing of an FVC is shown in Figure 10–12. As seen in Figure 10–16, the FVC is generally reduced in both obstructive and restrictive diseases; the primary difference between the curve in the patient with restrictive disease as compared with that of the patient with obstructive disease is the slope of the curve. The FVC is less than the normal slow VC when airway collapse and air trapping are present. Furthermore, by analyzing the FVC with respect to the volume of air exhaled per unit of time and the relationship of expiratory flow to lung volume, inferences may be made about the localization of any problem.

- **Forced expiratory volume in 1 second (FEV$_1$):** The FEV$_1$ is the volume of air that is exhaled during the first second of the FVC, reflecting the airflow in the large airways. Although other timed forced expiratory volumes (e.g., FEV$_{0.5}$, FEV$_2$, or FEV$_3$) may be used to evaluate the mechanics of breathing, the FEV$_1$ has been called the most useful parameter for the assessment of respiratory impairment or disease progression in obstructive disease.[7] The utility of the FEV$_1$ measurement is exemplified by the simple relationship between it and the associated degree of obstruction:

> Little or no obstruction: FEV$_1$ > 2.0 L to normal
> Mild to moderate obstruction: FEV$_1$ between 1.0 and 2.0 L
> Severe obstruction: FEV$_1$ < 1.0 L

This volume may also be expressed as a percentage of the FVC exhaled in 1 second (FEV$_{1\%}$). Normally, 75% of the FVC should be

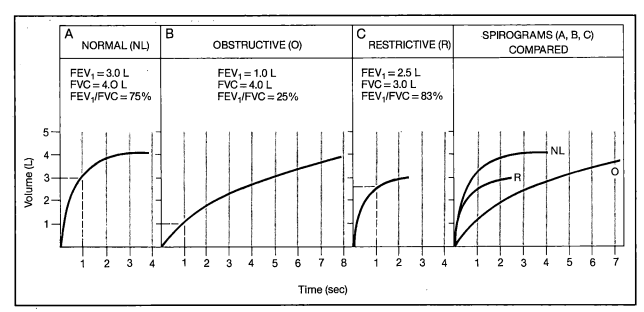

Figure 10–16.

Examples of spirograms comparing the results of forced expiratory breathing maneuvers in normal lungs (NL), lungs with obstructive pulmonary disease (O), and lungs with restrictive pulmonary disease (R). (From Kersten LD. Comprehensive Respiratory Nursing: A Decision Making Approach. Philadelphia, WB Saunders, 1989, p 376.)

exhaled within 1 second. An $FEV_{1\%}$ of more than 80% or 90% indicates restrictive disease, whereas a reduced $FEV_{1\%}$ indicates airway obstruction. Petty[15] suggests that patients with an $FEV_{1\%}$ of less than 60% have increased morbidity and mortality when compared with patients whose values are more than 75%.

Of course, age exerts an influence on both the FVC and the FEV_1. After the late twenties to mid thirties, a progressive decline in the FEV_1 of from 20 to 50 milliliters per year can be expected in normal persons; adults with chronic obstructive lung disease can expect a decline of as much as 50 to 80 milliliters per year.[16,17]

● **Forced midexpiratory flow (FEF_{25-75}):** This measurement used to be called the maximal midexpiratory flow rate. It is the volume of air exhaled over the middle half of the FVC divided by the time required to exhale it. The normal FEF_{25-75} is approximately 4 liters per second (240 L per min). The FEF_{25-75} reflects airflow in the small peripheral airways and may therefore be more sensitive than the FEV_1 in detecting differences between smokers and nonsmokers.[18] However, although the FEF_{25-75} has proved to be effective in detecting the presence of changes in lung function, it has not proved to be a particularly satisfactory parameter for use in quantifying the changes because it depends on the FVC.

Numerous additional indices of lung mechanics are frequently presented on pulmonary function test reports. Among them are

● **forced expiratory flow, 200–1200 ($FEF_{200-1200}$):** The $FEF_{200-1200}$ is the average expiratory flow during the early phase of exhalation. Specifically, it is a measurement of the flow for 1 liter of expired gas immediately following the first 200 milliliters of expired gas. The normal $FEF_{200-1200}$ is usually greater than 5 liters per second (300 L/min).
● **maximum voluntary ventilation (MVV):** The MVV is the maximum volume of a gas a person can move during 1 minute (previously called the maximum breathing capacity). The patient is asked to breathe as deeply and as rapidly as possible for 10, 12, or 15 seconds; the volume expired is extrapolated to yield the flow rate in liters per minute. The normal value for adult males is about 160 to 180 liters

per minute; it is slightly lower in adult females. In restrictive lung disease the MVV value may be normal or only slightly reduced. Normal values vary by as much as 25% to 30%; therefore, only major reductions in the values are clinically significant. However, the American College of Chest Physicians suggests that if the MVV does not equal the FEV_1 multiplied by 35, the test results are invalid owing to poor patient effort.[19]

● **peak expiratory flow (PEF):** The PEF is the maximum flow that occurs at any point in time during the FVC. Normal peak flows average 9 to 10 liters per second. The reliability of PEF as a clinical tool for evaluation of lung mechanics is limited because of the initial high flows that can occur even in obstructive disorders. Decreased peak flows reflect nonspecific mechanical problems of the lung, patient cooperation, and effort.
● **airway resistance (Raw):** The Raw is the driving pressure necessary to move a volume of gas in a specific period of time. Mathematically, it is the ratio of the driving pressure to the flow. The most common method of measuring the airway resistance is body plethysmography. Typically, the patient is instructed to pant at V_T between 100 to 200 milliliters at a frequency usually greater than 100 breaths per minute. While the patient is breathing, an electronic shutter momentarily closes, creating a no-flow situation, and the alveolar pressure is determined. Normal airway resistance is between 0.5 and 2.5 cm $H_2O \cdot L^{-1} \cdot s^{-1}$, measured at a standardized flow of 0.5 $L \cdot s^{-1}$. The Raw decreases with increasing lung volumes, primarily because of the increasing airway caliber. Any factor (e.g., edema, bronchial secretions, bronchoconstriction, or vascular congestion due to inflammation) that reduces the caliber of the airway causes an increase in airway resistance. A loss of lung elastance (increased compliance) also causes an increase in airway resistance because of the loss of radial support in the region of the small airways. Therefore, disorders such as asthma, emphysema, and bronchitis cause increases in airway resistance.
● **compliance (C):** Compliance refers to the volume change in the lung per unit of pressure change; it is a measure of the distensibility of the chest, the lungs, or both. To measure the compliance of the lungs (C_L), the patient is

asked to swallow a balloon catheter. The catheter is positioned in the lower third of the esophagus and is connected to a manometer for measurement of pressure. Pressure changes are then plotted against various lung volumes. Normal C_L is approximately 0.2 L $\cdot$ cm^{-1} H$_2$O. The lung-thorax compliance (C_{LT}) is measured with body plethysmography. By serial reduction of pressures within the chambers and measurement of the resulting changes in volume, a pressure-volume curve can be plotted. Normal C_{LT} is approximately 0.1 L $\cdot$ cm^{-1} H$_2$O. From these two values, thoracic compliance (C_T) can be calculated.

The various tests of breathing mechanics are measured again 5 to 20 minutes (the time depends on the specific drug and its dosage) after the administration of a bronchodilator (e.g., isoproterenol or isoetharine). In normal persons, or in persons with pure restrictive processes, the before and after bronchodilator measurements should not differ. In persons with obstructive disease, bronchodilators are used primarily to measure the reversibility of the obstruction. Airway obstruction is said to be reversible when there is a 15% or greater increase in the post-bronchodilator values for at least two of the following three parameters: FVC, FEV$_1$, and FEF$_{25-75}$.[20] However, because no data were presented to substantiate this recommendation, the criteria for determining a significant response may vary widely among physicians.

Tests of Diffusion

The diffusing capacity of the lung (D_L or $D_{L_{CO}}$) is the amount of gas entering the pulmonary blood flow per unit of time relative to the difference between the partial pressures of the gas in the alveoli and in the pulmonary blood. The D_L is not so much a measure of pulmonary mechanics as it is a measure of the integrity of the functional lung unit. The D_L is expressed in millimeters per minute per millimeter of mercury (ml/min/mm Hg). Carbon monoxide is normally employed to measure D_L because it has an affinity for hemoglobin nearly 210 times greater than that of oxygen. As long as the patient's hemo-

globin is normal, all the alveolar carbon monoxide should bind to hemoglobin and the partial pressure of carbon monoxide in the plasma should be zero. Several tests can be used to measure D_L, but the single-breath technique is most commonly used.[7,21] In this test the patient is asked to exhale as much as possible, then to inhale a deep breath of a 0.3% carbon monoxide and 10% helium gas mixture, hold this breath for 10 seconds, and then exhale. The amount of carbon monoxide that diffuses into the patient's lungs is the difference between the concentration of carbon monoxide in the alveolar gas at the end of the 10-second interval and the beginning concentration. Normal diffusing capacity of carbon monoxide is approximately 25 to 30 ml/min/mm Hg.

There may be many causes for an abnormal D_L, but a reduced D_L is the result of three key factors:

● Decreased quantity of hemoglobin per unit volume of blood
● Increased "thickness" of the alveolar-capillary membrane
● Decreased functional surface area available for diffusion

Loss of surface area has been identified as the primary factor.

Additional Tests of Gas Exchange

In addition to the specific tests of lung volume and capacity, gas flow rates, or diffusion, measurements or calculations of other gas exchange variables (Table 10–1) are helpful in diagnosing the many causes of exertional dyspnea, evaluating the extent of functional impairment, or evaluating the effect of medical, surgical, or rehabilitative therapy.

The reader is warned, however, that without an appreciation of the conditions under which a specific gas volume may have been determined, significant errors may be made when interpreting the significance of the volume. For example, tradition dictates that lung volumes are reported at body temperature saturated with water vapor at

TABLE 10–1. Typical Gas Exchange Variables		
Variable	**Symbol**	**Definition**
Respiratory frequency	f	Number of complete breaths per unit of time
Tidal volume	V_T	Volume of air moved during either inhalation or exhalation over a specific period of time (usually 1 min)
Minute ventilation	$\dot{V}_E$	Volume of air exhaled per unit of time
Carbon dioxide output	$\dot{V}_{CO_2}$	Volume of carbon dioxide exhaled per unit of time
Oxygen uptake	$\dot{V}_{O_2}$	Volume of oxygen consumed per unit of time
Gas exchange ratio	R	Ratio of $\dot{V}_{CO_2}$ to $\dot{V}_{O_2}$
Ventilatory equivalent for carbon dioxide or oxygen	$\dot{V}_E/\dot{V}_{CO_2}$ or $\dot{V}_E/\dot{V}_{O_2}$	Ventilatory requirement for a given metabolic rate
Oxygen pulse	$\dot{V}_{O_2}/HR$	Amount of oxygen consumed per heart beat

ambient pressure (BTPS). Most commonly, though, lung volumes are measured with the gas fully saturated with water vapor at ambient temperature and pressure (ATPS). It becomes necessary, therefore, to convert from one condition to the other. The following formula is used to convert volume from ATPS to BTPS:

$$\dot{V}_E\langle L/min, BTPS\rangle = \dot{V}_E\langle L/min, ATPS\rangle$$
$$\times \frac{\langle 273 + 37\rangle}{273 + T} \times \frac{P_B - P_{H_2O} \langle at\ T\rangle}{P_B - 47}$$

where T is ambient temperature, body temperature is 37°C, P_{H_2O} at 37° is 47 mm Hg, and P_B is barometric pressure.[22] Additionally, some gas exchange variables (e.g., oxygen uptake) necessitate conversion from BTPS to standard temperature and pressure, dry (STPD); that is, 273°K, barometric pressure = 760 mm Hg, and no water vapor present. The following formula can be used to convert BTPS values to STPD:

$$\dot{V}_E\langle L/min, STPD\rangle = \dot{V}_E\langle L/min, BTPS\rangle$$
$$\times \frac{273}{273 + 37} \times \frac{P_B - 47}{760}$$

Flow-Volume Loop

The flow-volume loop or curve is not so much a pulmonary function test as a way of graphically representing the events that occur during forced inspiration and expiration. The flow-volume procedure simply records flow against volume on an X–Y recorder. Following a period of normal, quiet breathing, the patient is instructed to perform a maximal inspiratory maneuver, to hold this breath for 1 to 2 seconds, to do an FVC maneuver, and then to do another maximal inspiratory maneuver. A normal flow-volume loop is shown in Figure 10–17.

The initial portion of the expiratory loop is effort dependent; however, after the first third of the expiratory curve, the curve is effort independent and reproducible. The highest point on the expiratory curve denotes the **peak expiratory flow rate (PEFR)**. The line that connects the PEFR and the end of expiration at the RV is normally straight. However, this effort-independent portion is altered by both restrictive and obstructive processes. Values for the FVC, FEV_1, peak flow, and so on should be the same as those obtained by conventional spirometric methods.

The flow-volume loop of patients with minimal to mild small airway obstructive lung disease looks essentially normal except for a slight "scooped out" appearance at the end of expiration. As the disease progresses, the PEFR becomes noticeably reduced and the scooping becomes more pronounced (see Fig. 10–17). The inspiratory portion of the curve is more sensitive to central airway obstruction, whereas the expiratory portion of the curve is more sensitive to peripheral airway obstruction. The restrictive lung disease processes show near-normal peak expiratory flow volume (FEV_t) when compared with the percentage of FVC (%FEV_t/FVC).

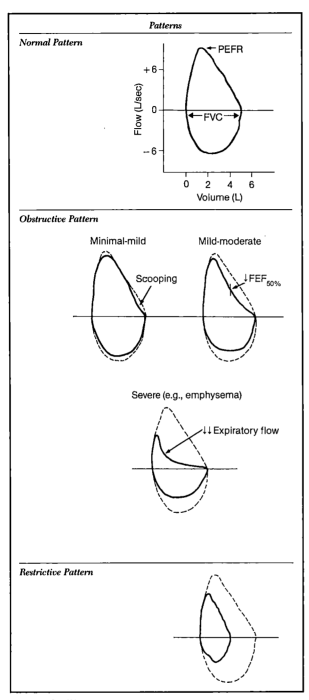

Figure 10–17.

Examples of flow-volume loop patterns for normal lungs, lungs with obstructive pulmonary disease, and lungs with restrictive pulmonary disease. The dashed lines represent the boundaries of the normal flow-volume loop. (Adapted from Kersten LD. Comprehensive Respiratory Nursing: A Decision Making Approach. Philadelphia, WB Saunders, 1989, p 382.)

INTERPRETATION OF BASIC PULMONARY FUNCTION TEST RESULTS

Pulmonary function test results are almost universally presented in columns of predicted, observed, and percent predicted values. The predicted values (derived from a variety of nomograms) are those that would normally be anticipated on the basis of the patient's age (volumes decrease with age), gender (males have larger volumes than females), height (tall individuals have larger volumes than short individuals), weight, and race (native American Indians, blacks, and orientals have as much as 12% to 14% lower volumes than whites).[14,19,23] Children pose a unique challenge to prediction because their development is phasic; thus specific nomograms are used for the pediatric population.[24] The observed values are those actually attained by the patient. The percent predicted values are derived by dividing the observed values by the predicted values. Generally, there should be more than 20% difference between observed and predicted values before they are considered abnormal. The generalized effects of obstructive or restrictive diseases are shown in Table 10–2.

The following points should be kept in mind when interpreting the results of pulmonary function tests:

- Determine whether the results are normal.
- Determine whether the results are indicative of obstructive or restrictive disease.
- If the problem is obstructive in nature, determine its reversibility.
- Consider the history and physical examination along with serial pulmonary function tests (if available) to determine disease progression.
- Be suspicious of test results if there are signs of poor patient effort.

BLOOD GAS ANALYSIS

Blood gas analysis is crucial to the assessment of problems related to acid-base balance, ventilation, and oxygenation. Samples for blood gas analysis may be obtained from any number of sites representing different regions of the vascular bed:

TABLE 10-2. Typical Effect of Obstructive or Restrictive Disease on Spirometric and Airflow Volume Measurements

Measurement	Obstructive	Restrictive
Tidal volume (VT)	N or ⇑	N or ⇓
Inspiratory capacity (IC)	N or ⇓	N or ⇓
Expiratory reserve volume (ERV)	N or ⇓	N or ⇓
Vital capacity (VC)	N or ⇓	⇓
Forced vital capacity (FVC)	N or ⇓	⇓
Residual volume (RV)	N or ⇑	N or ⇓
Functional residual capacity (FRC)	N or ⇑	N or ⇓
Total lung capacity (TLC)	N or ⇑	⇓
Forced expiratory volume in 0.5 sec (FEV$_{0.5}$)	⇓	N
Forced expiratory volume in 1 sec (FEV$_1$)	⇓	N
Forced expiratory volume in 2 sec (FEV$_2$)	⇓	N
Forced expiratory volume in 3 sec (FEV$_3$)	⇓	N
Forced expiratory flow rate between 200 ml and 1200 ml (FEF$_{200-1200}$)	⇓	N or ⇓
Forced expiratory flow rate between 25% and 75% FVC (FEF$_{25-75}$)	⇓	N or ⇓
Maximal voluntary ventilation (MVV)	⇓	N or ⇓
Peak expiratory flow (PEF)	N or ⇓	N or ⇓

● *Arterial*—either from a needle puncture or an indwelling cannula in a peripheral artery
● *Venous*—from a peripheral venous puncture or catheter
● *Mixed venous*—from a pulmonary artery catheter

Unless otherwise specified, a blood gas sample is presumed to be arterial in origin. Arterial blood gases are frequently used to monitor the condition of patients in the critical care setting and to help modify respiratory interventions. A typical report of an arterial blood gas analysis contains the following measurements: arterial pH, partial pressures of carbon dioxide (Pa$_{CO_2}$) and oxygen (Pa$_{O_2}$), oxygen saturation (Sa$_{O_2}$), bicarbonate concentration (HCO$_3^-$), and **base excess (BE)**. Although the immediate utility of arterial blood gases for the physical therapist may have been supplanted by the pulse oximeter, a systematic approach to a more detailed and complete interpretation of acid-base, ventilatory, or oxygenation status should not be overlooked, particularly with respect to ventilator-dependent patients.

Normal Values

The laboratory normal values for pH and Pa$_{CO_2}$ (7.40 and 40 mm Hg, respectively) represent the statistically determined mean values from a large representative sample population. The laboratory normal range may vary from institution to institution based on the particular laboratory's established normal range—on whether 1 or 2 standard deviations (SD) define the range. The narrower pH range of 7.38 to 7.42 and Pa$_{CO_2}$ range of 38 to 42 mm Hg represents 1 SD from the normal values. The wider pH range of 7.35 to 7.45 and Pa$_{CO_2}$ range of 35 to 45 mm Hg represents 2 SD from the normal values. For the purposes of this chapter, the normal range for pH is 7.35 to 7.45 and for Pa$_{CO_2}$ is 35 to 45 mm Hg, depending on posture, age, obesity, and the like.[14,25] An even broader "clinically acceptable range" has been promoted by some clinicians.[25] Table 10-3 presents the normal values and normal ranges for arterial blood gas parameters.

TABLE 10−3. The Generally Accepted Normal Ranges (±2 SD) for Arterial Blood Gas Values

	pH	P_{CO_2}	P_{O_2}	HCO_3^-	BE	%Sat
Normal value	7.40	40	97	24	0	—
Normal range	7.35−7.45	35−45	>80	22−28	±2	>95%

Adequacy of Alveolar Ventilation

The adequacy of alveolar ventilation is directly reflected by the Pa_{CO_2}. Given a normal Pa_{CO_2} value of 40 mm Hg, **alveolar hyperventilation** is indicated by a Pa_{CO_2} that is less than normal, and alveolar hypoventilation is indicated by a Pa_{CO_2} that is greater than normal. When a patient's Pa_{CO_2} is greater than 50 mm Hg, the condition is called **ventilatory failure.** Ventilatory failure can be diagnosed only on the basis of the Pa_{CO_2} level, but its severity is determined from the extent of the accompanying acidemia and the rapidity of the change in pH. Sudden pH changes hinder cellular function to a greater degree than do gradual changes. Kersten[7] suggests that when acuity or chronicity are masked by the presence of mixed disorders, the patient's level of alertness should be used as an indicator. Sudden (acute) changes in pH are more often associated with a loss of alertness and coma than are gradual (chronic) pH changes.

The events leading to ventilatory failure can occur relatively rapidly in patients who are acutely ill, or over a period of days or weeks in patients with chronic lung disease, as they decompensate, that is, become unable to meet the demands for the increased minute ventilation needed to maintain adequate gas exchange. Because no reliable means exist to predict a patient's ability to avert decompensation with any certainty, monitoring of their ventilatory status is mandatory. Such monitoring consists of ongoing assessment of pH, Pa_{CO_2}, and the signs and symptoms that suggest an increased work of breathing. Cardiopulmonary monitoring equipment is discussed in Chapter 11, and specific physiologic monitoring techniques are discussed in Chapter 14. To determine the nature and se-verity of illness with accuracy, an assessment of the relationship between arterial pH and arterial carbon dioxide tension is necessary.

Acid-Base Balance

The assessment of blood pH provides insight to the nature and magnitude of respiratory and metabolic disorders. In general terms, the pH describes the balance between blood acids and blood bases. Specifically, it indicates the concentration of hydrogen ions (H^+) in the blood. To review, acids give up hydrogen ions in a solution; bases accept hydrogen ions from a solution.

The two types of acids found in the body— volatile and nonvolatile—are regulated by the lungs and the kidneys. Volatile acids alternate readily from liquid to gaseous states. The lungs regulate volatile acids, primarily represented by carbonic acid in the blood, via the excretion of carbon dioxide. Nonvolatile acids (e.g., lactic acid or keto acid) cannot change to gases and must, therefore, be excreted by the kidneys. The principal source of nonvolatile acids is from dietary intake (organic and inorganic acids), and although the liver is where most of these nonvolatile acids are metabolized, the kidneys regulate their excretion from the body.[26] The kidneys are also primarily responsible for regulation of the major blood base—bicarbonate (HCO_3^-). Bicarbonate is responsible for 60% to 90% of the extracellular buffering of nonvolatile acids (buffers act to prevent extreme fluctuations in hydrogen ion concentration so that cellular metabolism is not hampered). Hemoglobin accounts for approximately 85% of nonbicarbonate buffering action (phosphate and serum proteins are the other nonbicarbonate buffers).

Henderson-Hasselbalch Equation

By looking at one specific component—the carbonic acid to bicarbonate ion relationship—a complete analysis of acid-base balance is possible, because the amount of hydrogen ion activity resulting from the dissociation of carbonic acid is controlled by the interrelationship of all the blood acids, bases, and buffers.[25] The Henderson-Hasselbalch equation defines pH in terms of this relationship:

$$pH = pK + \log \frac{[HCO_3\text{-}]}{[H_2CO_3]}$$

where pH is the negative log of hydrogen ion concentration ($-\log[H^+]$) and pK equals 6.1 (pK is a constant representing the pH at which a solute is 50% dissolved; its mathematical derivation, and that of pH, exceed the scope of this chapter). In terms of clinically derived variables, the Henderson-Hasselbalch equation can be expressed as follows:

$$pH = pK + \log \frac{[HCO_3\text{-}]}{s \times Pa_{CO_2}}$$

where $s = 0.03$ and is the solubility coefficient for carbon dioxide. In plasma, the concentration of dissolved carbon dioxide (dCO_2) is about 1000 times greater than the concentration of carbonic acid because the catalyzing enzyme **carbonic anhydrase** does not exist in the plasma. Because it is extremely difficult to distinguish between dCO_2 and H_2CO_3, for convenience, their respective concentrations are added together and the sum is referred to as the *total* dissolved carbon dioxide in the blood. Thus, substitution of $s \times Pa_{CO_2}$ for carbonic acid is permitted because the partial pressure of carbon dioxide (Pco_2) times its solubility coefficient yields the total carbon dioxide dissolved. Essentially then, the Pco_2 can be considered to be equivalent to the plasma H_2CO_3 plus the dCO_2. Although this total dissolved carbon dioxide in the plasma is a very small portion of the total carbon dioxide content of the blood, it is extremely important because it exerts the pressure that determines the pressure gradient controlling the movement of carbon dioxide into or out of the blood.[7,25,26]

Acid-Base Terminology

Since the normal human blood pH is 7.4, a pH of less than 7.4 is defined as **acidemia**. The process causing the acidemia (whatever it may be) is called **acidosis**. From the Henderson-Hasselbalch equation, there are only two ways in which acidemia can occur:

● There can be a low HCO_3^-—called **metabolic acidosis**
● There can be a high Pa_{CO_2}—called **respiratory acidosis** (synonymous terms are alveolar hypoventilation and hypercapnea)

Similarly, a pH greater than 7.4 is defined as **alkalemia,** and the process causing it is called **alkalosis**. There are also only two ways in which alkalemia can occur:

● There can be a high HCO_3^-—called **metabolic alkalosis**
● There can be a low Pa_{CO_2}—called **respiratory alkalosis** (alternatively called alveolar hyperventilation or hypocapnea)

These four acid-base states constitute the **primary acid-base disorders,** and each elicits a *compensatory* response. For example, if some disease were to cause a decreased HCO_3^- (a primary metabolic acidosis), the body's response would be an attempt to decrease the Pa_{CO_2} (a compensatory respiratory alkalosis) to return the pH toward its normal value.

In this manner, respiratory compensation for primary metabolic disorders begins in a matter of seconds by means of alveolar hyperventilation or hypoventilation. The kidneys compensate for primary respiratory disorders by retaining or excreting bicarbonate and hydrogen ions. However, unlike the rapidity with which respiratory compensatory activity exhibits its effect, the renal compensatory process requires 12 to 24 hours to effect significant pH change.

The relationships described in the Henderson-Hasselbalch equation permit us to identify "quickly" any of the four primary disorders based on pH and carbon dioxide changes. If the normal inverse relationship between pH and Pa_{CO_2} is maintained, the primary problem is most likely to be respiratory in nature; if the relationship is not maintained, the primary problem is most likely to be metabolic. This generalization holds true in most situations, even when combined respiratory and metabolic changes occur at the same time. However, in the face of combined disorders with large Pa_{CO_2} changes, one must keep in mind that the Pa_{CO_2} may preferentially reflect the respiratory component instead of equally reflecting combined respiratory and metabolic bicarbonate changes. Because this makes separating metabolic and respiratory components more difficult, an additional parameter that reflects the metabolic component must be considered. The BE is such a parameter. The BE is a measure of the deviation of the concentration of nonvolatile acids from normal (defined as a pH of 7.40 and a Pa_{CO_2} of 40). As such, the BE is a true nonrespiratory measurement that reflects the concentration of bicarbonate in the body. The normal range of the BE is ± 2 mEq $\cdot$ L^{-1}.

When breathing room air, the normal Pa_{O_2} is 80 to 100 mm Hg (see Chapter 2).[7,25] The normal newborn infant (range of 40–70 mm Hg) and persons older than 60 years of age are exceptions to this rule of thumb (in general, for every year over 60 years of age subtract 1 mm Hg from the normal minimally acceptable Pa_{O_2} of 80 mm Hg; this guideline does not apply to persons older than 90 years of age). When the arterial oxygen tension is less than normal, a condition called **hypoxemia** is said to exist.

Interpreting Arterial Blood Gas Data

The reader cannot expect to interpret very unusual arterial blood gas data without a great deal of practice and clinical experience. Nonetheless, an orderly approach to the assessment of arterial blood gases permits the majority of blood reports to be analyzed. Interpretation of arterial blood gas data involves a few basic processes:

- Assessment of ventilatory status
- Assessment of oxygenation and hypoxemic status

Assessment of the Ventilatory Status

The first step in the assessment of a patient's ventilatory status is to determine whether the pH value reflects acidemia or alkalemia. The second step is to classify the pathophysiologic state of the ventilatory system on the basis of the relationship between the pH and the Pa_{CO_2} values. This step determines whether the blood gas values represent a primary respiratory or a primary metabolic disorder. If the normal inverse relationship between pH and Pa_{CO_2} is preserved, the primary disorder is likely to be respiratory in nature; if it is not, the primary disorder is probably metabolic. The third step is to determine the adequacy of alveolar ventilation on the basis of the Pa_{CO_2} value:

- Less than 30 mm Hg = alveolar hyperventilation
- Between 30 and 50 mm Hg = adequate alveolar ventilation
- Greater than 50 mm Hg = ventilatory failure

The following sample pH and Pa_{CO_2} values are offered to illustrate the steps just described (the reader should not attempt to correlate these values with any clinical situation).

1. **pH 7.26**
   Pa_{CO_2} (mm Hg) 56
   From step 1, we see that the pH value represents acidemia. From step 2, we see that the normal inverse relationship between pH and Pa_{CO_2} is maintained; thus, the values probably represent a primary respiratory acid-base disorder—respiratory acidosis. From step 3, we see that the Pa_{CO_2} represents ventilatory failure.

2. **pH 7.56**
   Pa_{CO_2} (mm Hg) 44
   From step 1, we see that the pH value represents an alkalemia. From step

2, we see that the normal inverse relationship between pH and Pa_{CO_2} is not maintained; thus, the values probably represent a primary metabolic acid-base disorder—metabolic alkalosis. From step 3, we see that the Pa_{CO_2} indicates adequate alveolar ventilation.

The final step in the assessment of ventilatory status is the determination of the extent of the respiratory and metabolic components of the disorder. The action taken depends on whether the primary problem is respiratory or metabolic. If the primary problem is respiratory, we calculate an "expected" pH and classify the problem on the basis of acuity. To do this, take the following steps:

1. Determine the absolute value of the difference between the reported Pa_{CO_2} and 40.
2. Divide this number by 100.
3. Subtract half of this value from 7.40 if the reported Pa_{CO_2} is more than 40; add the entire value to 7.40 if the reported Pa_{CO_2} is less than 40.
4. Classify the problem as "acute" if the reported pH is the same as or farther from normal than the expected pH; classify the problem as "chronic" if the reported pH is closer to normal than the expected pH.

For example, in our assessment of the first set of pH and Pa_{CO_2} values, we concluded that they represented a respiratory acidosis. Next, we classify the acuity of the problem in accordance with the previously listed steps:

1. $56 - 40 = 16$
2. $16 \div 100 = 0.16$
3. $7.40 - 0.08 = 7.32$ (because the reported Pa_{CO_2} is more than 40)

Because the reported pH is farther from normal than the expected pH, we classify the problem as acute. Thus, from our assessment of the arterial pH and the P_{CO_2} values, we conclude that they

represent an **acute respiratory acidosis.** In fact, because the Pa_{CO_2} is greater than 50 mm Hg, we call this problem **acute ventilatory failure.**

If the primary problem is metabolic, we classify the problem on the basis of the relationship between the pH and the Pa_{CO_2}. The problem is classified as "uncompensated" if the reported pH is outside the normal range and the reported Pa_{CO_2} is within the normal range; it is classified as "partially compensated" if both the reported pH and the Pa_{CO_2} are outside the normal range; or it is classified as "compensated" if the reported pH is within the normal range and the reported Pa_{CO_2} is outside the normal range. For example, in our assessment of the second set of pH and Pa_{CO_2} values, we concluded that they represented a metabolic alkalosis. Our next step is to classify the problem on the basis of the relationship between the pH and the Pa_{CO_2} values. Because the pH is outside the normal range and the Pa_{CO_2} is within the normal range, we conclude that the problem is an **uncompensated metabolic alkalosis.** The extent of the metabolic problem is inferred from the base excess or deficit. To calculate the base excess or deficit, take the following steps:

1. Calculate the expected pH.
2. Subtract the expected pH from the reported pH (if the value is positive, it is called *base excess*; if the value is negative, it is called *base deficit*).
3. Multiply this number by 100.
4. Calculate the base excess or deficit by taking two thirds of this number.

For example, from the second set of pH and Pa_{CO_2} values, we calculate the BE to be:

1. $44 - 40 = 4$
   $4 \div 100 = 0.04$
   $7.40 - 0.02 = 7.38$ (because the reported Pa_{CO_2} is more than 40)
2. $7.56 - 7.38 = 0.18$ (since the number is positive, it represents a BE)
3. $0.18 \times 100 = 18$
4. $18 \times \frac{2}{3} = 12$

Thus, the BE = 12 mEq/L, suggesting a fairly significant metabolic alkalosis because the normal BE is ± 2 mEq/L. Table 10–4 summarizes the classification nomenclature typically used to describe acid-base disorders.

Assessment of the Oxygenation and Hypoxemic Status

The oxygenation status of a patient is assessed by determining the extent to which the observed Pa_{O_2} is above or below the normal range. Generally, as long as a patient's Pa_{O_2} is within the normal range, arterial oxygenation is considered to be acceptable. If a patient's Pa_{O_2} is between 60 to 80 mm Hg, the patient is said to be mildly hypoxemic; if it is between 40 to 60 mm Hg, moderately hypoxemic; and if it is less than 40 mm Hg, severely hypoxemic. Hypoxemia is not an absolute indicator of cellular **hypoxia** — a condition of inadequate cellular oxygenation — because other factors, such as hemoglobin level and capillary circulation, must also be considered. However, hypoxemia strongly suggests tissue hypoxia and necessitates further evaluation.

Quite frequently, patients require supplemental oxygen in the course of their medical treatment. When a patient is receiving supplemental oxygen, the adequacy of arterial oxygenation is assessed on the basis of the fraction of inspired oxygen. As a general rule, the fraction of inspired oxygen (FI_{O_2}) multiplied by 500 approximates the arterial oxygen tension expected. If that tension is not present, one may assume that the patient is hypoxemic. For example, consider two patients, each with a Pa_{O_2} of 95 mm Hg. Patient 1 is breathing room air, so we conclude that the Pa_{O_2} represents adequate oxygenation and no hypoxemia. Patient 2, on the other hand, is receiving supplemental oxygen and has an FI_{O_2} of 0.30 (30% oxygen). If this patient's arterial blood were being oxygenated normally, we would anticipate a Pa_{O_2} in the neighborhood of 150 mm Hg. Thus, we can reasonably conclude that this patient is hypoxemic.

OXIMETRY

Oximetry is a descriptive term for the various technologies available for measuring oxyhemoglobin saturation. The modern pulse oximeter involves a light-emitting diode (LED), a photodiode signal detector, and a microprocessor. The LED alternately emits red and infrared light hundreds of times per second; the microprocessor compares the signals received by the signal detector and calculates the degree of oxyhemoglobin saturation based on the intensity of transmitted light at the detector. Most units display a digital oxyhemoglobin saturation ($O_2Hb\%$) that is brought up to date every few seconds.

CYTOLOGIC AND HEMATOLOGIC TESTS

As part of the diagnostic process, many cytologic and hematologic tests are often performed on patients with pulmonary disease. These tests are helpful in the identification of disease-

TABLE 10–4. Nomenclature for Evaluating and Classifying Acid-Base Disorders		
pH	Pa_{CO_2}	Status
>7.50	<30 mm Hg	Acute alveolar hyperventilation
7.40–7.50	<30 mm Hg	Chronic alveolar hyperventilation
7.30–7.40	<30 mm Hg	Compensated metabolic acidosis
<7.30	<30 mm Hg	Partially compensated metabolic acidosis
>7.50	35–45 mm Hg	Metabolic alkalosis
7.35–7.45	35–45 mm Hg	Normal
<7.30	35–45 mm Hg	Metabolic acidosis
>7.50	>50 mm Hg	Partially compensated metabolic alkalosis
7.30–7.50	>50 mm Hg	Chronic ventilatory failure
<7.30	>50 mm Hg	Acute ventilatory failure

TABLE 10-5. Examples of Some Microbial Classification Systems

Taxonomy	Structure	Habitat	Morphology
Viruses	Capsid	Obligate intracellular	Isometric, helical
Bacteria		Extracellular or facultative intracellular	
Chlamydiae*	Prokaryote	Obligate intracellular	Spherical (cocci), rod-shaped (bacilli), spiral (spirochete)
Mycoplasmas*		Extracellular†	
Rickettsiae*		Obligate intracellular	
Fungi	Eukaryote	Extracellular or facultative intracellular	
Protozoa		Extracellular, facultative, or obligate intracellular	

* Sometimes classified as bacteria.
† Other habitats possible.

causing organisms and in monitoring the body's responses to them.

Cytologic tests are used to identify specific microorganisms that may cause disease. Several classification schemes, often used simultaneously, describe the various microorganisms identified by cytologic testing. Microorganisms are frequently described

- taxonomically
- according to their structure (e.g., viruses have a simple central core of DNA or RNA encapsulated by a protein coat; prokaryotes have discrete cell walls, but lack nuclear membranes; eukaryotes have distinct cellular and nuclear membranes)
- with respect to their habitat (e.g., **obligate intracellular parasites** require specific cell types or cellular organelles for reproduction; **facultative parasites** can replicate either outside or inside cells; and **extracellular parasites** only reproduce outside the cell)
- morphologically (e.g., spherical, rod-shaped, spiral) (Table 10-5 gives some examples)
- on the basis of their staining characteristics (e.g., gram-negative, gram-positive, acid-fast)

Numerous microorganisms can normally be found on the skin or mucous membranes of the nasopharynx, oropharynx, and upper airway. Indigenous microbes are often referred to as **normal flora** (Table 10-6). The host organism is said to be **colonized** if the parasitic microbes cause no injury to the host's cells and infected if the microbes are present below the host cells' external integument. Some parasites share a **symbiotic** relationship with the host (e.g., vitamin B_{12} is produced by bacteria in the ileum); some are **pathogenic,** interfering with the host's integrity and function; and some are **commensal,** having no deleterious effects on a "healthy" host but becoming opportunistically pathogenic in a compromised host. The extent to which a patho-

TABLE 10-6. Common Upper Respiratory Tract Commensal Bacteria, Fungi, Protozoa, and Viruses

Gram-Positive Cocci	Gram-Positive Rods	Gram-Negative Cocci	Gram-Negative Rods	Fungi	Protozoa	Viruses
Streptococci	*Actinomyces*	*Veillonella*	*Pseudomonas*	*Candida*	*Trichomonas*	With the exception of herpes simplex, viruses are typically pathogenic
Staphylococci	*Corynebacterium*	*Neisseria*	*Haemophilus*	*Aspergillus*	*Selenomonas*	
	Lactobacilli		*Fusobacterium*			
			Bacteroides			

gen interferes with a host's function depends on the virulence and number of the offending microbes: some organisms are invariably pathogenic, their identification always signifying disease, whereas others are facultative, capable of colonization or infection, depending on the state of the host's natural chemical and physical barriers.[27,28] Respiratory infections are typically divided into two groups: upper respiratory tract infection or lower respiratory tract infection. Rhinoviruses account for the majority of upper respiratory infections, although any of the commensal organisms may become pathogenic.

The tracheobronchial tree below the level of the true vocal cords is normally sterile or only minimally colonized. Lower respiratory tract infections are commonly caused by viruses, bacteria, protozoa, and fungi (Table 10–7 lists common pathogens of the lower respiratory tract). Microorganisms typically reach the lungs by inhalation, but occasionally they are transported via the blood from another infected site. Unfor-

tunately, many medical treatments and procedures (e.g., immunosuppressive or cytotoxic therapy, intubation, catheterization, or surgical intervention) provide an opportunity for the entry of infectious agents.

Definitive diagnosis of respiratory infections depends on the isolation of specific pathogens from pulmonary secretions or the detection of pathogen-specific antibodies. Microscopic examination and culturing can proceed once appropriate specimens have been collected. Specimens are most often obtained by expectoration, but invasive techniques for specimen collection range from nasotracheal suctioning to open-lung biopsy. Expectorated sputum is the most frequently collected specimen for the diagnosis of pneumonia.[29] However, the utility of such specimens is controversial because the lower respiratory tract secretions are frequently contaminated by upper respiratory tract flora, making interpretation difficult. For this reason, before obtaining an expectorated specimen for culture, it is a good idea to instruct the patient to remove any dentures and to rinse the mouth with water.

Microscopic examination with various stains broadly indicates what sort of organisms are present in the specimen, but culturing is the definitive step. Culturing entails placing the specimen in a variety of cultural media in the presence and absence of oxygen and carbon dioxide and at different temperatures for varied lengths of time. Antimicrobial therapy is not automatically initiated at the presence of a pathogen — colonization must be distinguished from infection. However, antimicrobial therapy is often initiated when the signs and symptoms of infection are recognized, even before a specific pathogen has been identified. Once a pathogen is identified, its sensitivity to various antimicrobial agents is assessed so that the antimicrobial therapy can be appropriately directed. Refer to Chapter 13 for information regarding pulmonary pharmacologic agents.

Hematologic tests also aid greatly in the assessment of cardiopulmonary disease. Typical tests include arterial blood gases (described previously), electrolyte analysis, complete blood counts, and coagulation studies. The complete blood count imparts information about the num-

TABLE 10–7. Common Pathogens of the Lower Respiratory Tract

	Pathogens
Viruses	Influenza A
	Influenza B
	Adenoviruses
	Respiratory syncytial virus
	Parainfluenza viruses
Bacteria	*Streptococcus pneumoniae*
	Staphylococcus aureus
	Haemophilus influenzae
	Enterobacteriaceae
	Klebsiella pneumoniae
	Pseudomonas aeruginosa
	Legionella (all species)
	Mycoplasma pneumoniae
	Chlamydia (all species)
Fungi	*Coccidioides immitis*
	Histoplasma capsulatum
	Blastomyces dermatitidis
	Aspergillus (all species)
	Cryptococcus neoformans
	Candida (all species)
Protozoa	*Pneumocystis carinii* (uncertain taxonomy)

(From Washington JA. Infectious disease aspects of respiratory therapy. In: Burton GG, Hodgkin JE, Ward JJ [eds]. Respiratory Care: A Guide to Clinical Practice. 3rd ed. Philadelphia, JB Lippincott, 1991, p 400.)

TABLE 10−8. Normal Values for a Complete Blood Cell Count

Test	Males	Females
Red blood cell	4.8 to 6.0 × 10⁶/cubic mm	4.1 to 5.1 × 10⁶/cubic mm
Hemoglobin	13 to 16 g/dL or g%	12 to 14 g/dL or g%
Hematocrit	40%−54%	37%−47%
White blood cell	5000−10,000/cubic mm	
Platelets	200,000−350,000/cubic mm	

ber of red blood cells, the hemoglobin level, the proportion of the blood that is cells (hematocrit), the number and composition of white blood cells, and the platelet count. Coagulation studies evaluate the tendency of the blood to clot.

Tables 10–8 and 10–9 present normal values for the various components of a complete blood count. A less than normal quantity of hemoglobin, a low red blood cell count, or a low hematocrit value is indicative of anemia and suggests that the oxygen-carrying capacity will be decreased. Conversely, an increase in the quantity of hemoglobin, red blood cell count, or hematocrit value is indicative of polycythemia. An increased white blood cell count (leukocytosis) is frequently associated with a bacterial infection, whereas, a decreased white blood cell count (leukopenia) may indicate leukemia, but radiation or chemotherapy can also yield this result. An increased neutrophil count is sometimes a first indication of the body's response to inflammation or bacterial infection. An increase in the level of immature neutrophils (bands)—called a leftward shift of neutrophils—is an indication of the body's stress response (the greater the shift, the greater the stress). Eosinophilia (an increased number of eosinophils) is usually an indication

of an allergic response. Viral infections often result in an increase in the number of lymphocytes. An increased number of monocytes is typical of a chronic infection. An increased number of basophils is frequently associated with some myeloproliferative disorder. Platelets are integral to a normal coagulation process; too few platelets can result in small skin hemorrhages, but too many can increase the likelihood of thrombosis.

In general, four tests are used in an evaluation of the blood's tendency to clot:

● Bleeding time
● Platelet count
● Partial thromboplastin time
● Prothrombin time

The bleeding time measures the rate of formation of a platelet thrombus; a normal bleeding time is up to 6 minutes. The partial thromboplastin time measures the overall rate of both the intrinsic and common pathways (normal partial thromboplastin time is 32 to 70 sec), and the prothrombin time measures the rate of the extrinsic and common pathways (normal PT is 12 to 15 sec). Together, the prothrombin time and the partial thromboplastin time detect more than 95% of coagulation abnormalities.

TABLE 10−9. Differential of White Blood Cell Count

Neutrophils	50%−75%
	Segments: 90%−100% of total neutrophils
	Bands: 0%−10% of total neutrophils
Eosinophils	2%−4%
Basophils	<0.5%
Lymphocytes	20%−40%
Monocytes	3%−8%

SUMMARY

In this chapter, various chest imaging techniques have been considered and a method for examining chest radiographs has been discussed. Likewise, several tests of pulmonary function and their interpretation were considered. Lastly, cytologic and hematologic tests were briefly discussed. It is hoped that this information, together with that in Chapter 14, will facilitate the interpretation of evaluative findings.

- The standard radiograph is the predominant medium by which anatomic abnormalities arising from pathologic processes within the chest are assessed.
- The standard chest radiograph is typically taken in two views: posteroanterior and left lateral.
- Dark areas on a chest radiograph are termed *radiolucent;* light areas are called *radiopaque.*
- In a "body systems" approach to the analysis of a chest radiograph, the examiner should examine (1) the bones and soft tissues; (2) the mediastinum, trachea, and cardiovascular system; (3) the hila; and (4) the lung fields.
- A tomogram (sectional radiograph) differs from a standard radiograph because tomography involves the curvilinear movement of the roentgen-ray source and the imaging medium in opposite directions about the patient.
- A magnetic resonance image is produced in much the same manner as a CT image, except that a gradient magnetic field is used to align the protons of the target tissue, and then radio signals are used to stimulate them to create an image.
- Magnetic resonance imaging is currently limited to evaluation of chest wall (bone, muscle, fat, or pleura) processes because the expanded lungs have an insufficient density of protons for the generation of an adequate image from which to evaluate pathologic processes of the parenchyma.
- To obtain a bronchogram, the bronchial tree is opacified by the instillation of a contrast (radiopaque) medium as a radiographic or tomographic image is produced.
- Bronchograms permit the study of gross pathologic changes in the walls and lumina of the bronchial tree.
- Ventilation/perfusion scintillography $(\dot{V}/\dot{Q}$ scan) is used to evaluate the regional distribution of gas and blood flow in the lungs.
- The fiberoptic bronchoscope makes the direct visualization of the bronchial tree clinically possible.
- Pulmonary function tests provide information about the integrity of the airways, the function of the respiratory musculature, and the condition of the lung tissues themselves. Generally, these tests involve the assessment of lung volumes and capacities, gas flow rates, diffusion, and gas exchange.
- Pulmonary diseases are classified into three basic categories on the basis of pulmonary function testing: obstructive, restrictive, or combined.
- The three most commonly used methods for the determination of FRC and RV are the helium dilution (closed-circuit) method, the nitrogen washout (open-circuit) method, and body plethysmography.
- When expressed as a percentage of the FVC, the volume of air exhaled in the first second of the maneuver (FEV_1) is one of the most useful parameters in the assessment of respiratory impairment.
- An FEV_1 of more than 80% or 90% indicates the presence of restrictive disease, whereas an FEV_1 of 60% or less suggests the existence of obstructive disease with an increased morbidity and mortality.
- Blood gas analysis (arterial, venous, or mixed venous) allows the assessment of problems related to acid-base balance, ventilation, and oxygenation. By convention, unless otherwise specified, a blood gas sample is presumed to be arterial in origin.
- The normal pH of the blood is 7.40; a pH of less than 7.40 is defined as *acidemia;* and a pH of more than 7.40 is defined as *alkalemia.* Any process that causes acidemia is called an *acidosis,* and any process that causes alkalemia is called an *alkalosis.*
- The adequacy of alveolar ventilation is directly reflected by the Pa_{CO_2}. *Alveolar hyperventilation* is indicated by a Pa_{CO_2} that is less than normal, and *alveolar hypoventilation* is indicated by a Pa_{CO_2} that is greater than normal. When a patient's Pa_{CO_2} is greater than 50 mm Hg, the condition is called *ventilatory failure.*
- A patient's oxygenation status is assessed by determining the extent to which the observed Pa_{O_2} is above or below the normal range (generally accepted as being between 80 to 100 mm Hg, when breathing room air).
- Numerous cytologic tests are used to identify specific microorganisms that may cause disease. A cytologic sample is said to be *infected* if the parasitic microbes are present below the host cells' integument; it is *colonized* if the parasitic microbes present cause no injury to the host's cells.
- The complete blood count imparts information

about the number of red blood cells, the hemoglobin level, the hematocrit, the number and composition of white blood cells, and the platelet count.

References

1. Sheldon RL, Dunbar RD. Systematic analysis of the chest radiograph. In: Scanlan CL, Spearman CB, Sheldon RL (eds). Egan's Fundamentals of Respiratory Care. 5th ed. St. Louis, CV Mosby, 1990.
2. Michaelson F, Koons HV, Weckstein ML, Victor LD. Fundamentals. In: Victor LD (ed). An Atlas of Critical Care Chest Roentgenography. Rockville, Md, Aspen Systems, 1985, pp 7–11.
3. Cameron JR, Alter AJ, Wochos JF. Optimization of Chest Radiography. Proceedings of a Symposium. Rockville, Md, US Department of Health and Human Services, 1980.
4. Mintzer RA. Chest Imaging: An Integrated Approach. Baltimore, Williams & Wilkins, 1981.
5. Rau J, Pierce D. Understanding Chest Radiographs. Denver, Multimedia Publishing, 1984.
6. Cookson, JB, Finlay DBL. Essential Chest Radiography. Oxford, Heinemann Medical Books, 1988, pp 1–14.
7. Kersten LD. Comprehensive Respiratory Nursing: A Decision Making Approach. Philadelphia, WB Saunders, 1989.
8. Freundlich IM, Bragg DG. A Radiologic Approach to Diseases of the Chest. Baltimore, Williams & Wilkins, 1992.
9. Felson B, Weinstein A, Spitz H. Principles of Chest Roentgenology—A Programmed Text. Philadelphia, WB Saunders, 1965.
10. Olendorf W, Olendorf W. MRI Primer. New York, Raven Press, 1991, pp 9–39.
11. Naidich DP, Zerhouni EA, Siegelman SS. Computed Tomography and Magnetic Resonance of the Thorax. 2nd ed. New York, Raven Press, 1991.
12. Simon G. Principles of Chest X-ray Diagnosis. 3rd ed. London, Butterworth & Company, 1971.
13. Youtsey JW. Basic pulmonary function measurement. In: Scanlan CL, Spearman CB, Sheldon RL (eds). Egan's Fundamentals of Respiratory Care. 5th ed. St Louis, CV Mosby, 1990, pp 374–395.
14. Clausen JL. Pulmonary Function Testing Guidelines and Controversies. London, Grune & Stratton, 1984.
15. Petty TL. Office Spirometry for the Assessment of Pulmonary Disease. New York, Breon Laboratories, 1980.
16. Fletcher CM, Peto R. The natural history of chronic airflow obstruction. Br Med J 1:1645–1648, 1976.
17. Burrows B, Cline MG, Knudson RJ, et al. A descriptive analysis of the growth and decline of the FVC and FEV$_1$. Chest 83:717–724, 1983.
18. Allen GW, Sabin S. Comparison of direct and indirect measurement of airway resistance. Am Rev Respir Dis 104:61–71, 1971.
19. American College of Chest Physicians. Statement on spirometry—a report of the section on respiratory pathophysiology. Chest 83:547–550, 1983.
20. Report of the Committee on Emphysema. American College of Chest Physicians. Criteria for the assessment of reversibility in airways obstruction. Chest 65:552–553, 1974.
21. Bates DV. Respiratory Function in Disease. 3rd ed. Philadelphia, WB Saunders, 1989.
22. Wasserman K, Hansen JE, Sue DY, Whipp BJ. Principles of Exercise Testing and Interpretation. Philadelphia, Lea & Febiger, 1987.
23. Schoenberg JB, Beck GJ, Bouhuys A. Growth and decay of pulmonary function in healthy blacks and whites. Respir Physiol 33:367–393, 1978.
24. Polgar G, Promadhat V. Pulmonary Function in Children: Techniques and Standards. Philadelphia, WB Saunders, 1971.
25. Shapiro BA, Harrison RA, Cane RD, Templin R. Clinical Application of Blood Gases. 4th ed. Chicago, Year Book Medical Publishers, 1989.
26. Chenevey B. Overview of fluids and electrolytes. Nurs Clin North Am 22:749–759, 1987.
27. Robbins SL, Cotran RS, Vinay K. Pathologic Basis of Disease. 4th ed. Philadelphia, WB Saunders, 1989.
28. Purtilo DT. A Survey of Human Diseases. Menlo Park, Calif, Addison-Wesley, 1978.
29. Washington JA. Infectious disease aspects of respiratory therapy. In: Burton GG, Hodgkin JE, Ward JJ (eds). Respiratory Care: A Guide to Clinical Practice. 3rd ed. Philadelphia, JB Lippincott, 1991.

11 THORACIC SURGICAL PROCEDURES, MONITORING, AND SUPPORT EQUIPMENT

INTRODUCTION

In addition to the pathologic conditions that have already been discussed in Chapters 3 through 7, an almost unlimited number of surgical procedures can have a significant impact on the functioning of and interaction between the cardiovascular and pulmonary systems. Therefore, because an appreciation for the extent and involvement of surgical incisions is beneficial when planning and implementing therapeutic interventions for postoperative patients, the first part of this chapter introduces the reader to the most commonly used thoracic incisions. The second part of the chapter introduces the equipment commonly used for the monitoring and life support of patients who have cardiovascular or pulmonary disease. Although it is true that some of

the monitoring and life-support equipment is often restricted to the confines of the critical care unit, it should be understood that much of it is also used extensively with patients in long-term rehabilitation, outpatient, and home-care settings.

CARDIOVASCULAR AND THORACIC SURGICAL PROCEDURES

Surgical Approaches

Individual surgeons develop preferences for particular surgical approaches based on their particular experiences and training. Thus, posterolateral and lateral thoracotomy incisions are

437

most commonly used for lung resection procedures, although a median sternotomy may be employed occasionally (e.g., when lung resection is combined with a cardiac procedure).[1] Cardiac procedures are performed almost exclusively through a median sternotomy, although the great vessels sometimes are approached via a thoracotomy incision. Procedures that involve the pericardium or epicardium (e.g., pericardial biopsy, epicardial pacemaker insertion) are typically accomplished through a subxiphoid incision. Diaphragmatic procedures are commonly performed through either a lateral thoracotomy or a thoracoabdominal incision.

Posterolateral Thoracotomy

In preparation for a **posterolateral thoracotomy**, patients are generally positioned one-quarter turn from prone (operative side elevated) with the uppermost arm elevated forward, flexed at the elbow, and placed beside the head. The typical posterolateral thoracotomy incision extends downward from a point midway between the spine of the fourth thorcic vertebra and the scapula in a gently curving arch around the tip of the scapula to the fifth or sixth intercostal space at the anterior axillary line (Fig. 11–1). The serratus anterior is divided close to its muscular attachment in an effort to preserve its function and to avoid the long thoracic nerve. The pleural space is most often entered via an incision through the intercostal muscles at the fifth intercostal space, although a specific pathologic condition may dictate entry via another intercostal space.

Anterolateral Thoracotomy

Patients are positioned one-quarter turn from supine (operative side elevated) with the uppermost arm flexed at the elbow and placed beneath the back (retracting the latissimus dorsi muscle) in preparation for an **anterolateral thoracotomy.** The submammary incision curves from the fourth or fifth intercostal space at the midaxillary line to the midclavicular or parasternal region (Fig. 11–2). The pectoralis major is incised, and fibers of the serratus anterior are separated (with female patients, it is sometimes necessary for the surgeon to reflect the breast superiorly).

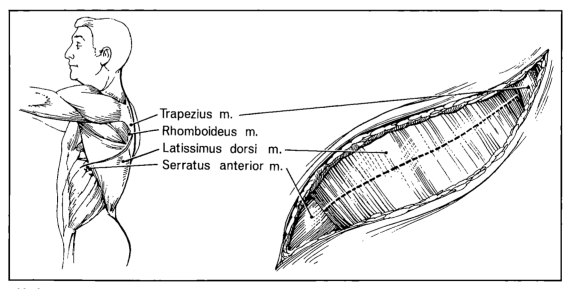

Trapezius m.
Rhomboideus m.
Latissimus dorsi m.
Serratus anterior m.

Figure 11–1

The posterolateral thoracotomy incision. This incision is often used for lung resection procedures or for procedures involving the descending thoracic aorta. (From Cooley DA. Techniques in Cardiac Surgery. 2nd ed. Philadelphia, WB Saunders, 1984, p 16.)

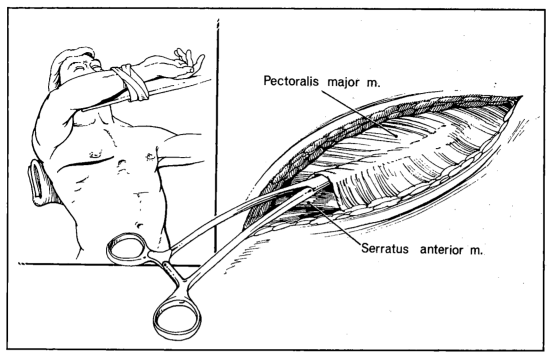

Pectoralis major m.

Serratus anterior m.

Figure 11–2

The anterolateral thoracotomy incision. This incision is not used as often as the posterolateral approach, but it is used for some cardiac procedures, pulmonary resections, and esophageal procedures. (From Cooley DA. Techniques in Cardiac Surgery. 2nd ed. Philadelphia, WB Saunders, 1984, p 14.)

Lateral Thoracotomy

Patients are placed in sidelying position, operative side up, with the arm abducted, flexed at the elbow, and rotated in preparation for a **lateral thoracotomy** (excessive abduction or rotation, which might cause stretching of the brachial plexus, is avoided). There are several variations of the lateral thoracotomy incision, although it generally begins near the nipple line and extends toward the scapula (Fig. 11–3). The latissimus dorsi muscle is not incised; instead, it is retracted either anteriorly or posteriorly, and the fibers of either the serratus anterior or the intercostal muscles between the serratus interdigitations are incised to gain access to the appropriate intercostal space (most often the fourth, fifth, or sixth). Postoperative scapular winging is avoided by careful preservation of the long thoracic nerve.

Axillary Thoracotomy

An **axillary thoracotomy** is sometimes used for apical **bleb** resection or dorsal sympathectomy. Patients are placed in a sidelying position with the arm flexed at the elbow, abducted 90 degrees at the shoulder, and rotated as for a lateral thoracotomy. From the edge of the pectoralis major, anteriorly, the incision extends posteriorly within the second intercostal space to the edge of the latissimus dorsi.

Median Sternotomy

A **median sternotomy** is probably the most frequently used incision for cardiothoracic operations.[1,2] In preparation for a median sternotomy, the patient is placed in the supine position. The initial skin incision usually begins in the midline

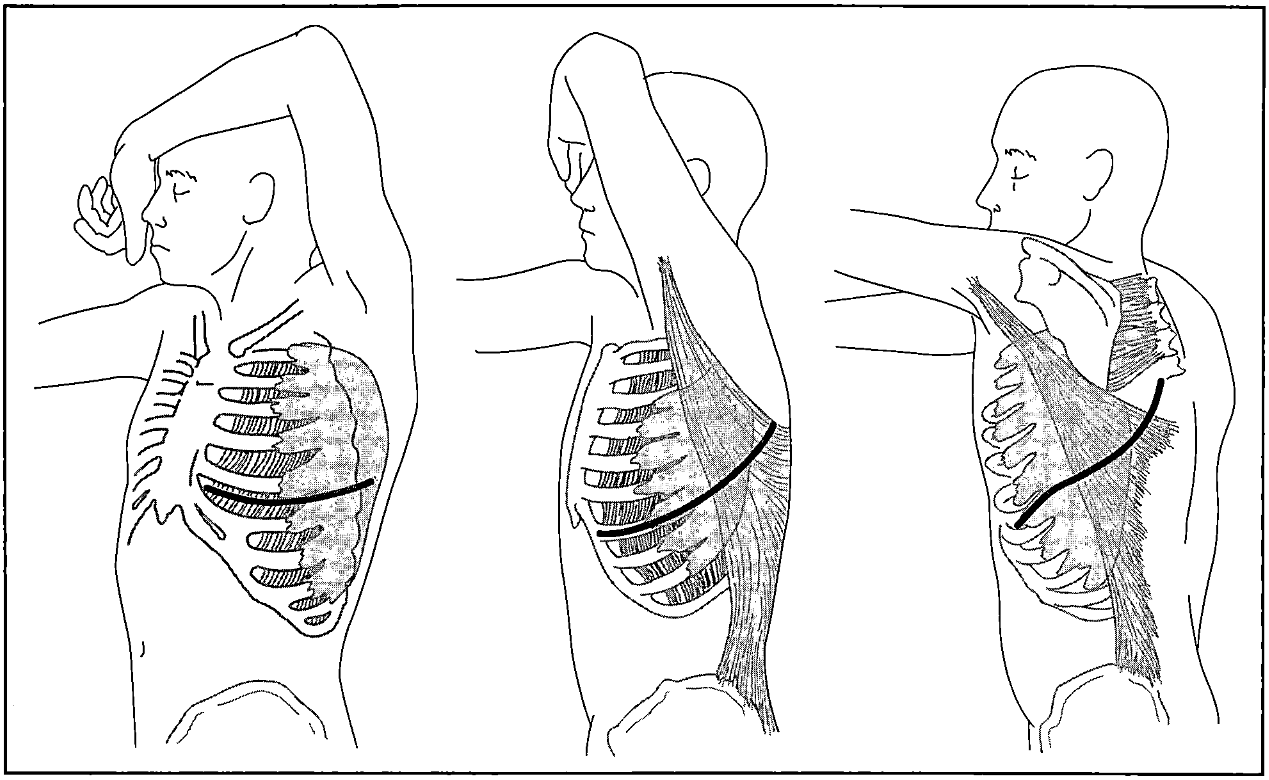

Figure 11–3

The lateral thoracotomy incision. This incision is often used because it spares the latissimus dorsi (the muscle does not have to be divided) while providing access for pneumonectomy, lobectomy, or wedge resection procedures. (Redrawn with permission from Alley RD. In: Cooper F [ed]. The Craft of Surgery. Vol. 1. Boston, Little, Brown & Co, 1964, p 197.)

inferior to the suprasternal notch and extends below the xiphoid (Fig. 11–4A). The sternum is divided along its midline in a series of steps, and a sternal retractor is used to hold the incision open (Fig. 11–4B). At the end of the surgical procedure, the sternum is generally closed with stainless steel sutures either through or around the sternum, and the wound is closed in layers (Fig. 11–4C).

Thoracoabdominal Incisions

A **thoracoabdominal incision** permits procedures on the diaphragm, esophagus, biliary tract, right lobe of the liver, spleen, adrenal gland, and kidney, as well as placement of portacaval shunts. In preparation, patients are positioned supine with the operative side rotated upward 30

to 45 degrees, the buttocks and back elevated, and the arm on the operative side extended anteriorly as in a posterolateral thoracotomy. The incision usually extends from the eighth or ninth intercostal space at the posterior axillary line to the midline of the abdomen, transecting the latissimus dorsi, serratus anterior, external oblique, and rectus abdominis muscles (Fig. 11–5).

Specific Surgical Procedures

A description of all of the possible cardiovascular or thoracic surgical procedures is well beyond the scope of this chapter. However, because cardiovascular and thoracic surgical procedures are so prevalent, a few procedures deserve attention.

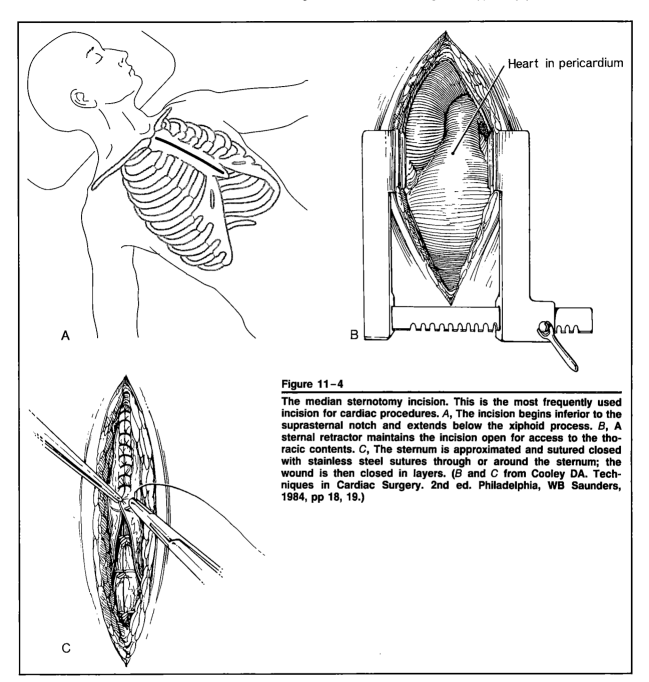

Heart in pericardium

Figure 11-4

The median sternotomy incision. This is the most frequently used incision for cardiac procedures. *A,* The incision begins inferior to the suprasternal notch and extends below the xiphoid process. *B,* A sternal retractor maintains the incision open for access to the thoracic contents. *C,* The sternum is approximated and sutured closed with stainless steel sutures through or around the sternum; the wound is then closed in layers. (*B* and *C* from Cooley DA. Techniques in Cardiac Surgery. 2nd ed. Philadelphia, WB Saunders, 1984, pp 18, 19.)

Percutaneous Revascularization Procedures

As discussed in Chapter 3, coronary arterial atherosclerotic disease can produce occlusive plaques that, in turn, compromise coronary arte- rial blood flow to such an extent that coronary arterial revascularization procedures become nec- essary to preserve myocardial integrity. Three procedures are discussed: angioplasty, arthrec- tomy, and stenting. Common to each of these procedures is the introduction (under fluoro-

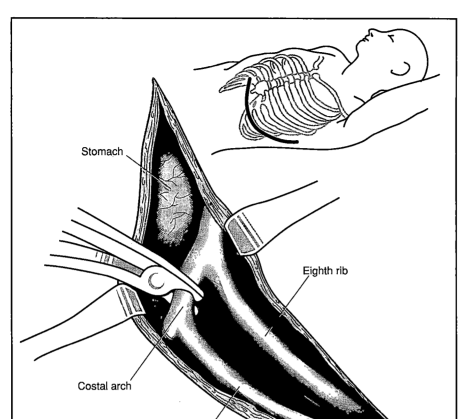

Figure 11–5

The thoracoabdominal incision. This incision is used for procedures involving the diaphragm, the upper abdomen, or the retroperitoneal space. (Redrawn from Waldhausen JA, Pierce WS. Johnson's Surgery of the Chest. 5th ed. Chicago, Year Book Medical Publishers, 1985, p 59.)

Stomach

Eighth rib

Costal arch

Ninth rib

scopic guidance) of a balloon-equipped catheter, via a peripheral arterial access site (e.g., femoral artery), into the coronary arterial tree to the site of the stenotic lesion. The procedure is successful if the lumen remains patent when the catheter is withdrawn and there is no ensuing angiospasm. The return of blood flow to the distribution of the previously occluded artery is immediately checked by means of an angiogram (see Chapter 9). None of the procedures is completely risk free; the arterial wall can be perforated when the lesion is penetrated, or it can rupture when the balloon is inflated.[3–6] Therefore, it is not uncommon to have a cardiac surgical suite held in reserve for the emergency remediation of any complications. Generally, however, no significant postoperative movement restrictions are associated with the procedure—patients can be ambulatory within a matter of hours following the procedure. Patients are rarely hospitalized for more than 2 to 3 days, if that long. In fact, many patients are tested, on an outpatient basis, to determine the extent of the resolution of preprocedure electrocardiographic ischemic changes and referred for outpatient cardiac rehabilitation within that time frame.

A **percutaneous transluminal coronary angioplasty (PTCA)** may be performed when a stenotic lesion is not too large, that is, when it does not completely occlude the lumen of the coronary artery. The atherosclerotic lesion is penetrated, and the balloon at the distal aspect of the catheter is inflated—compressing the central portion of the lesion outward against the wall of the artery (Fig. 11–6A). This process may be repeated with successively larger catheters to increase the lumen size as much as possible. A **directional coronary arthrectomy (DCA)** may be performed instead of, or in conjunction with, a percutaneous transluminal coronary angioplasty.[7] This procedure involves the introduction of an arthrectomy catheter through the stenotic lesion of a coronary artery. The cutter housing at

the distal end of the catheter has a longitudinal opening on one side and an inflatable balloon on the other. The opening is positioned so that it faces the atheroma, and the balloon is inflated so that the housing is fixed against the arterial wall, displacing the atheroma into the housing opening. The cutter is then activated and advanced, pushing an excised specimen into the distal part of the housing (Fig. 11–6B). Technologic ad-

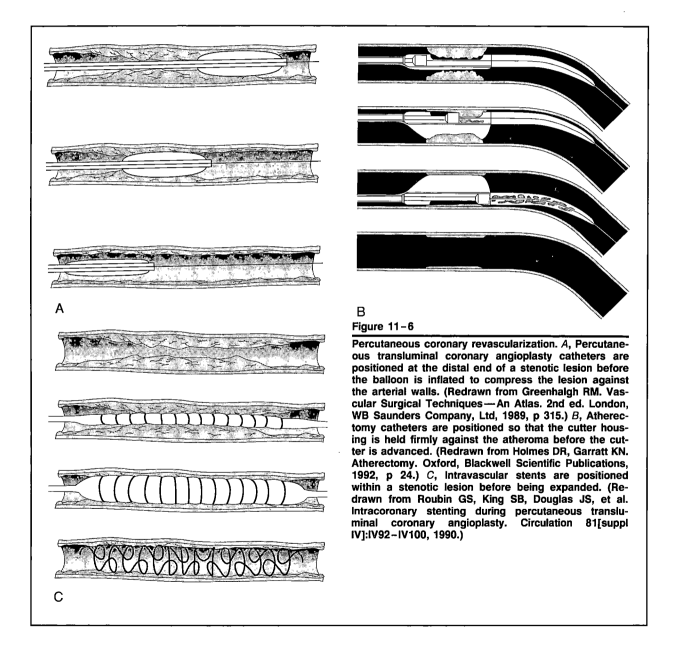

Figure 11–6

Percutaneous coronary revascularization. *A*, Percutaneous transluminal coronary angioplasty catheters are positioned at the distal end of a stenotic lesion before the balloon is inflated to compress the lesion against the arterial walls. (Redrawn from Greenhalgh RM. Vascular Surgical Techniques—An Atlas. 2nd ed. London, WB Saunders Company, Ltd, 1989, p 315.) *B*, Atherectomy catheters are positioned so that the cutter housing is held firmly against the atheroma before the cutter is advanced. (Redrawn from Holmes DR, Garratt KN. Atherectomy. Oxford, Blackwell Scientific Publications, 1992, p 24.) *C*, Intravascular stents are positioned within a stenotic lesion before being expanded. (Redrawn from Roubin GS, King SB, Douglas JS, et al. Intracoronary stenting during percutaneous transluminal coronary angioplasty. Circulation 81[suppl IV]:IV92–IV100, 1990.)

vances have reached the point that atherectomies may now be performed using laser-tipped catheters also. The placement of **endoluminal stents** is another means of coronary revascularization that is gaining clinical acceptance.[8] Stents are tiny springlike devices introduced into a stenotic lesion in an effort to increase the intravascular luminal diameter (Fig. 11–6C).

Coronary Artery Bypass Graft

When a coronary arterial atherosclerotic lesion progresses to such an extent that the artery becomes completely occluded, or when the lesion is not amenable to percutaneous transluminal coronary angioplasty or directional coronary arthrectomy, a **coronary artery bypass graft** (CABG) may have to be performed to revascularize the myocardium. Vascular grafts are often procured from either or both of the saphenous veins (Fig. 11–7), but the left internal mammary artery can also be diverted for use in a coronary revascularization procedure. Following a median sternotomy, the site or sites of coronary arterial blockage are located and isolated. When a saphenous venous graft is used, it is cut to the appropriate length and desired shape before being anastomosed above and below the occlusion (Fig. 11–8). If the internal mammary artery is used in the revascularization procedure, it is anastomosed below the level of the occlusive lesion (Fig. 11–9). Once grafting is completed, the tissue layers are approximated and the wound is closed.

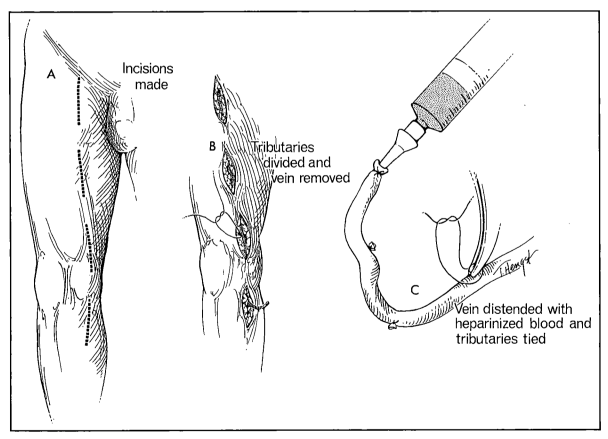

Figure 11–7

Procurement of saphenous vein grafts for use in coronary artery bypass surgery. (From Cooley DA. Techniques in Cardiac Surgery. 2nd ed. Philadelphia, WB Saunders, 1984, p 225.)

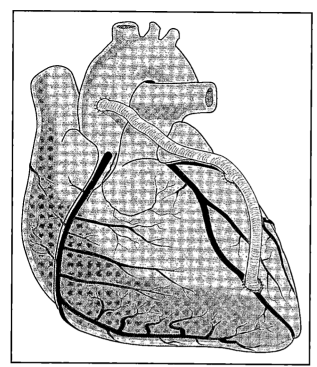

Figure 11–8

Saphenous vein grafts are anastomosed above and below the level of the occlusive lesion after they are cut to the appropriate length and desired shape.

Pacemaker Implantation

A cardiac pacemaker is an electronic pulse generator used to create an artificial action potential for the purpose of controlling some types of cardiac arrhythmias. Pacemakers may be used as a temporary measure to control transient arrhythmias during myocardial infarction or following cardiac surgery when vagal tone (parasympathetic stimulation) is often increased. Chronic arrhythmias (e.g., second- or third-degree heart blocks or recurrent tachyarrhythmias) may require the surgical implantation of a permanent pacemaker. The American College of Cardiology has published guidelines that discuss specific electrocardiographic indications for pacemaker implantation.[9] However, the criteria actually applied often vary from institution to institution.[10] Nevertheless, the general indications involve sinoatrial nodal disorders (e.g., bradyarrhythmias), atrioventricular nodal disorders (e.g.,

complete heart block, Mobitz type II arrhythmia), or tachyarrhythmias (e.g., supraventricular tachycardia, frequent ventricular ectopy) that result in hemodynamic embarrassment (signs and symptoms such as lightheadedness, fainting, blurred vision, slurred speech, confusion, or weakness) due to inadequate cardiac output. (See Chapter 9 for more information about cardiac arrhythmias and their appearance on electrocardiogram [ECG].)

Cardiac pacemakers are able to initiate myocardial depolarization by creating an electrical voltage difference between two electrodes, thus initiating an artificial depolarization spike. Figure

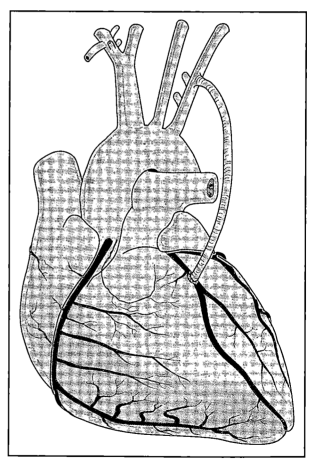

Figure 11–9

Internal mammary arterial grafts are anastomosed below the level of the occlusive lesion. (Redrawn from Waldhausen JA, Pierce WS. Johnson's Surgery of the Chest. 5th ed. Chicago, Year Book Medical Publishers, 1985, p 480.)

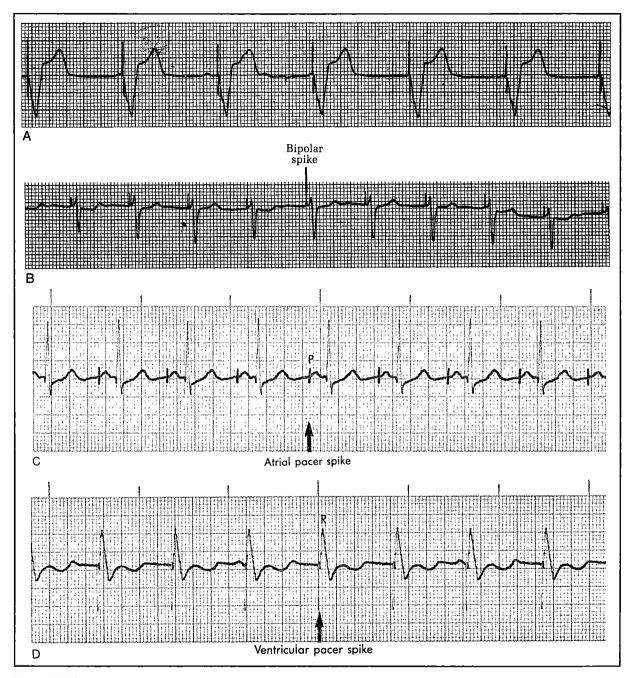

Figure 11-10

Appearance of pacemaker rhythms on electrocardiogram. *A*, Typical unipolar pacemaker spikes precede each ventricular complex. *B*, Bipolar pacemaker spikes are small (or invisible). (*A* and *B* from Conover MB. Understanding Electrocardiography. 5th ed. St. Louis, CV Mosby, p 389.) *C*, Atrial pacemaker rhythm. *D*, Ventricular pacemaker rhythm. *E*, Sequential (atrial and ventricular) pacemaker rhythm. (*C*, *D*, and *E* from Atwood S, Stanton C, Storey J. Introduction to Basic Cardiac Dysrhythmias. St. Louis, CV Mosby, 1990, pp 115, 116, 117.)

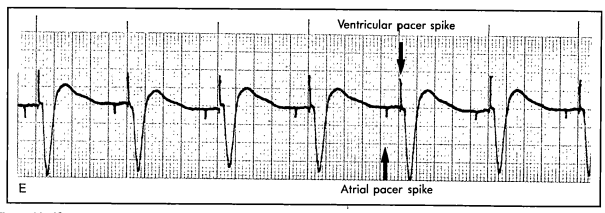

Ventricular pacer spike

Atrial pacer spike

E

Figure 11-10

Continued

11-10 shows typical ECG tracings of atrially and ventricularly paced rhythms. Cardiac pacemakers employ electrical conduction configurations that are classified as being either unipolar or bipolar (Fig. 11-11). **Unipolar pacing systems** use one electrode that is in direct contact with the cardiac tissue; the second, or anodal, electrode is usually the metal housing of the pacemaker, which is located at some point distant to the myocardium. **Bipolar pacing systems** use two electrodes that are in close proximity to each other where they make contact with the myocardium.

Rechargeable power sources for cardiac pacemakers are no longer employed, and it is highly unlikely that a pacemaker operating from a mercury-zinc power source is in operation today.

Figure 11-11

Pacemaker electrode configurations. *A*, Unipolar electrode. *B*, Bipolar electrode.

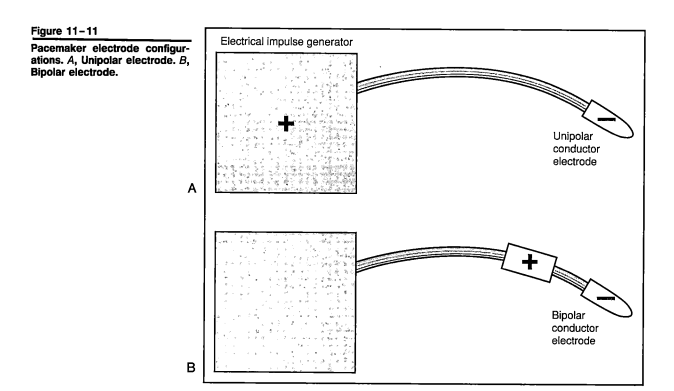

Electrical impulse generator

Unipolar conductor electrode

A

Bipolar conductor electrode

B

The vast majority of pacemakers in current clinical use operate from lithium-chemistry power sources, although "nuclear" (radioactive plutonium) pacemakers have been available for more than 15 years. On an actuarial basis, the 50% survival point (the battery half-life) of modern lithium–chemistry-powered pacemakers is greater than 6 years. According to Bilitch and co-workers in 1987,[11] 88% of nuclear-powered pacemakers were operational after 12 years of use.

Regardless of the electrode configuration, cardiac pacing leads are of two primary types:

● **Endocardial leads** are placed inside the right atrium, the right ventricle, or both via a transvenous route.
● **Epicardial leads** are attached directly to the surface of the right atrium or the right or left ventricle.

No matter which type of electrode is used, the pacing lead is constructed of multiple strands of conductive material so that, unlike monofilament conductors, it can withstand repeated flexure without breaking. The importance of this aspect of pacing lead construction is made abundantly clear when one considers that if a patient's heart is paced at a constant rate of 68 beats per minute, the lead flexes 35,765,280 times per year.

Endocardial lead placement can be made by means of *transvenous* (technically *pervenous* because the leads go through the vessel, not across it) insertion via the subclavian, internal jugular, or cephalic venous routes. However, the preferred route of insertion for permanent endocardial leads is via the left cephalic vein, with the impulse generator being placed in an infraclavicular pocket (Fig. 11–12).[12] The tips of these transvenous electrodes are placed in direct contact with the interior surface of either the right atrium or right ventricle, or both.

Epicardial implantation is usually accomplished during a cardiac surgical procedure. Sometimes conductive suture electrodes are sewn into the exterior myocardial wall for temporary pacing; however, in most cases electrodes are screwed, hooked, or sewn onto the myocardial surface for permanent pacing. For temporary external pacing, conductive lead wires frequently exit the

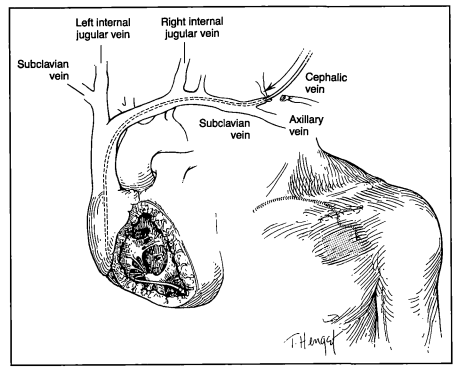

Left internal jugular vein
Right internal jugular vein
Subclavian vein
Cephalic vein
Subclavian vein
Axillary vein

Figure 11–12

An endocardial electrode may be inserted transvenously (left cephalic vein depicted here) into the right atrium or ventricle and connected to a permanent pacemaker that is placed in an infraclavicular pocket. (Adapted from Cooley DA. Techniques in Cardiac Surgery. 2nd ed. Philadelphia, WB Saunders, 1984, p 79.)

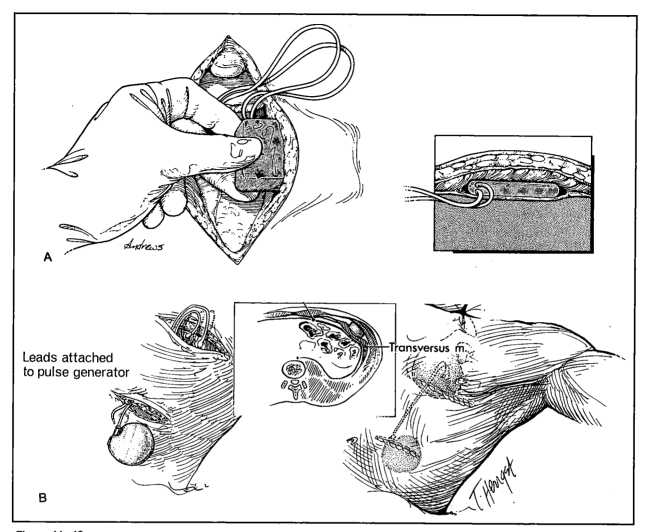

Figure 11-13

Alternative locations for pacemakers. *A*, A subxiphoid pocket. *B*, A transthoracic pocket. (From Cooley DA. Techniques in Cardiac Surgery. 2nd ed. Philadelphia, WB Saunders, 1984, pp 76, 78.)

chest from small subxiphoid incisions. For permanent pacing, the impulse generator may be placed in a subxiphoid rectus sheath pocket (Fig. 11-13*A*). If for some reason (e.g., abdominal infection, primary thoracic entry via median sternotomy) the subxiphoid approach cannot be or is not used, a transthoracic approach may be employed (Fig. 11-13*B*).

The field of cardiac pacing has expanded explosively, creating the need for a uniform means of communicating information regarding the characteristics of a particular device. The capabil-

ities of current pacing devices—which include telemetry; programmability; and antibradyarrhythmia, antitachyarrhythmia, and adaptive-rate pacing—far surpass those of devices from just a few years ago. In response to the need for a simple conversational code to describe such pacing devices, the North American Society of Pacing and Electrophysiology (NASPE) and the British Pacing and Electrophysiology Group (BPEG) collaborated to devise a generic pacemaker code, the *NBG Code*.[13] The five-position NBG Code has gained widespread clinical acceptance and is

TABLE 11–1. The NBG Pacemaker Code

Pacing Location	Sensing Location	Response to Pacing	Programmability/Modulation	Antitachyarrhythmia Function
O = None No antibradyarrhythmia stimulation	N = None No bradyarrhythmia detecting capability	O = None No response	O = None No programmability; no rate modulation	O = None No antitachyarrhythmia capability
A = Atrium	A = Atrium Detects spontaneous atrial depolarizations	I = Inhibited Inhibits a pending stimulus when a spontaneous depolarization is detected	S = Simple programmable Capable of either or both rate and output adjustment	P = Pacing Low-energy stimulus used to interrupt tachyarrhythmia
V = Ventricle	V = Ventricle Detects spontaneous ventricular depolarizations	T = Triggered Detection produces an immediate stimulus in the same chamber	M = Multiprogrammable Can be programmed more extensively	S = Shock High-energy stimulus used to interrupt tachyarrhythmia (e.g., cardioversion or defibrillation)
D = Dual Atrium and ventricle can be stimulated to control bradyarrhythmia	D = Dual Detects spontaneous depolarizations independently in the atrium and the ventricle	D = Dual Can simultaneously inhibit and trigger a stimulus	C = Communicating Can be extensively programmed and has some "telemetry" capability	D = Dual Has both low- and high-energy capability
S = A or V Manufacturer's designation to indicate that either chamber is acceptable for pacing by a single chamber pacemaker	S = A or V Manufacturer's designation to indicate that a single-chamber pacemaker may be used in either chamber		R = Rate modulation Can automatically control rate by measuring one or more other physiologic variables	

(From Bernstein AD, Camm AJ, Fletcher RD, et al. The NASPE/BPEG generic pacemaker code for antibradyarrhythmia and adaptive-rate pacing and antitachyarrhythmia devices. PACE 10:795, 1987.)

summarized in Table 11–1. The first position of the code provides a classification of the possible stimulation sites for antibradyarrhythmia pacing. The second position classifies the pacemaker's ability to "sense" either atrial or ventricular spontaneous depolarizations, or both. The third position indicates what the pacemaker does if it detects a spontaneous depolarization. The fourth position indicates the programmability or rate modulation capabilities of the pacemaker. The fifth position, if used, indicates the pacemaker's ability to prevent tachyarrhythmia. In many instances, however, only the first three positions of the NBG Code are used in clinical conversation. For example, a pacemaker that can stimulate both the atrium and the ventricle, can sense spontaneous depolarizations independently in the atrium and the ventricle, can inhibit a pending stimulus in the chamber in which a spontaneous depolarization was sensed, and at the same time can trigger a ventricular stimulation (after an appropriate interval) in response to sensing a spontaneous atrial depolarization is called a DDD pacemaker. Likewise, a pacemaker that stimulates only the ventricle, can sense spontaneous depolarizations only in the ventricle, and can inhibit a pending stimulus when a spontaneous depolarization is sensed is called a VVI pacemaker. Clearly, the NBG Code facilitates the exchange of a great deal of information in a very concise format. With a basic understanding of the NBG Code, the physical therapist treating a patient with a pacemaker can anticipate the patient's cardiac response capabilities for myriad situations.

Drainage Tube Placement

Following a thoracic surgical procedure, tubes are typically placed through the chest wall to drain the affected body cavity. Although any tube penetrating the chest wall could be termed a *chest tube*, this term is generally reserved for the description of **intrapleural drainage tubes** —tubes that drain the intrapleural space—or **mediastinal drainage tubes**—tubes that drain the mediastinum. Most chest tubes are multifenestrated, and all are made of an inert material. Like endotracheal tubes, chest tubes have radio-

paque markers to facilitate their localization on chest radiographs. Chest tubes and drainage collection systems permit the amount of drainage and intrathoracic blood loss to be monitored, and they provide a means by which the presence of any air leaks can be verified (Fig. 11–14).

Whenever a thoracotomy or median sternotomy is performed, the pleural cavity, mediastinum, or both is generally drained by the placement of one or more chest tubes connected to underwater seal or suction. These chest tubes drain pleural or mediastinal fluids and air with expansion of the lung. Intrapleural tubes are inserted into the second or third intercostal space (ICS) at the midclavicular line to drain air. To drain fluids, they are usually inserted at the fourth or fifth intercostal space at the anterior axillary line (sometimes as low as the eighth or ninth intercostal space at the midaxillary line). The tube's tip is advanced several inches into the pleural space; the distal end of the drainage tube may or may not be attached to a sealed drainage collection system, which may or may not be attached to suction. Posteriorly placed intrapleural tubes are not often used because they are easily kinked; they are also very uncomfortable for the patient. Mediastinal chest tubes are commonly inserted via subxiphoid incisions that are distinct from the sternotomy incision. Chest tubes normally pass obliquely through the chest wall rather than directly through at a right angle (see Fig. 11–14A). The clinician is cautioned against tipping the collection system so as not to compromise the water seal. Because disconnection of intrapleural tubes can result in collapse of the lung, all chest tubes should be treated as if they were intrapleural drainage tubes so that proper precautions are never neglected. Nonetheless, the presence of chest drainage tubes should not preclude the patient's participation in physical therapy activities.

Much like intrapleural tubes, intra-abdominal drainage tubes are used to eliminate air or fluid from the abdominal cavity. Intra-abdominal tubes may simply drain into a collection bag by gravity or be connected to a vacuum device (e.g., Jackson-Pratt drainage tubes). Bladder drainage tubes are also common in the critical care setting. They are usually attached to "urinary catheter

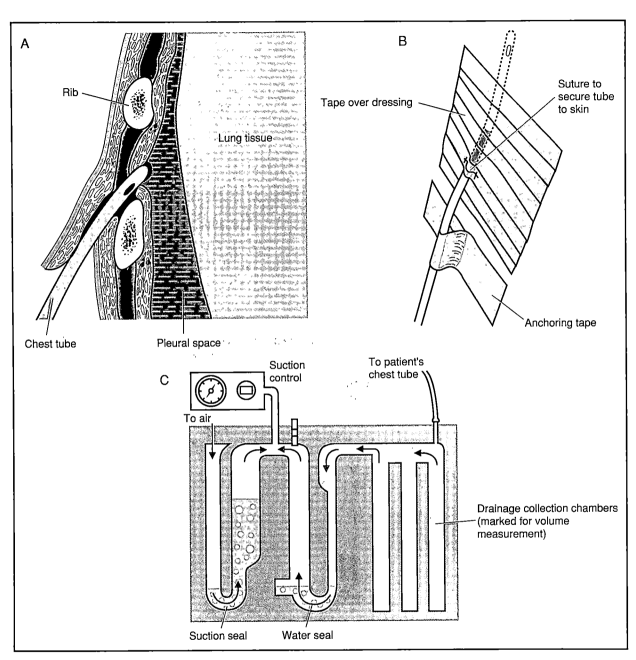

Figure 11-14

Chest drainage tubes may be placed to eliminate fluids, air, or both from the pleural or mediastinal spaces. *A*, A pleural tube being inserted into the pleural space. *B*, Once positioned, the drainage tube is sutured to the skin and covered with an occlusive dressing. *C*, Chest drainage tubes are typically connected to a collection device that may or may not be attached to suction. (*C* redrawn from Kersten LD. Comprehensive Respiratory Nursing. Philadelphia, WB Saunders, 1989, p 776.)

bags," which are also frequently used with general acute care patients as well.

Tracheostomy

In the medical and surgical management of various pathologic conditions, it sometimes becomes necessary to perform a **tracheostomy**. There are several reasons for choosing a tracheostomy (e.g., prolonged mechanical ventilation, airway protection or maintenance), and these generally dictate whether the procedure will be temporary or permanent. A few surgeons prefer to perform a *cricothyroidotomy* instead of a tracheostomy. In either case, the surgery is generally a planned procedure with the patient intubated from above.

In preparation for a tracheostomy, the patient is placed in the supine position, and the neck is slightly hyperextended. The initial incision is made in the region of the third tracheal ring, and, whether by a transverse[14] or vertical incision,[15] the thyroid isthmus is divided and the trachea is exposed. The third (and if necessary the second and fourth also) tracheal ring is divided, and a tracheostomy tube is inserted (Fig. 11–15).

Figure 11–15

A tracheostomy is performed on an intubated patient. *A*, The initial incision is made over the third tracheal cartilage; the muscles are separated; and the thyroid isthmus is divided. *B*, The third, and if necessary the second and fourth, tracheal cartilage is incised and divided. *C*, The tracheostomy tube is inserted. (Redrawn from Grillo HC. Tracheostomy and its complications. In: Sabiston DC. Davis-Christopher Textbook of Surgery. 12th ed. Philadelphia, WB Saunders, 1981, p 2060.)

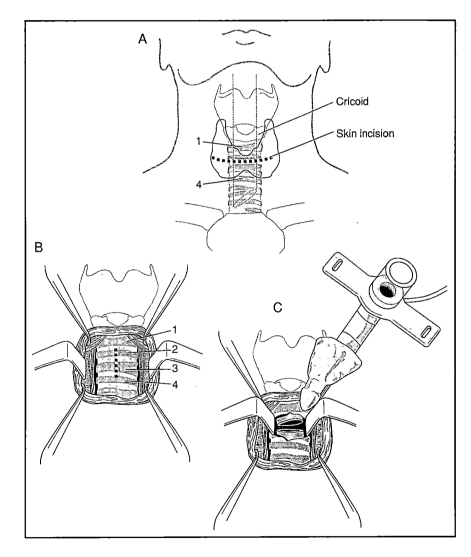

MONITORING AND LIFE-SUPPORT EQUIPMENT

Pressure-recording, volume-collecting, electrical, or flow-sensing instruments are frequently used to measure those physiologic variables that may indicate a patient's level of homeostasis. Much of the equipment is electronic and consists of some or all of the following basic components:

- A device to detect the physiologic event
- An amplifier to increase the magnitude of the signal from the sensor
- A recorder or meter to display the resultant signal

Many variables must be considered in the process of clinical physiologic monitoring, but in regard to subsequent life-support interventions the principal areas of concern include hemodynamic, electrocardiographic, and ventilatory components.

Hemodynamic Monitoring and Life Support

Hemodynamic monitoring generally involves observing or calculating, and then assessing, some specific cardiovascular pressures. In addition to the stethoscope and sphygmomanometer, a pressure transducer, pressure transmission tubing, and a pressure monitor-recorder are frequently used, especially in the intensive care unit. A typical transducer, shown in Figure 11–16, is basically a strain gauge consisting of sensor wires attached to the undersurface of a diaphragm. The diaphragm is covered with a dome that connects the transducer via pressure transmission tubing to a cannulated vessel. The dome, the tubing, and the catheter are filled with a heparinized saline solution that produces a continuous fluid column. The dome contains a thin, separating membrane that acts as an interruption between the fluid column and the diaphragm. Deformation of the diaphragm in response to vascular pressure changes causes a relative stretch or compression of the sensor wires, thus impeding or enhancing electrical flow, respectively. When calibrated in relation to the stan-dard anatomic reference level at which the catheter tip is assumed to rest (the phlebostatic point—usually at the level of the right atrium when the patient is in the supine position), this fluid-filled monitoring system should be accurate to within 1 mm Hg.[16]

The presence of the various catheters and tubes associated with hemodynamic monitoring should not be considered a contraindication to physical therapy intervention because the assessment of hemodynamic and pulmonary function at the patient's bedside has become standard in the care of the critically ill. Therefore, knowledge of normal hemodynamic values, and the implications of deviations from normal, is essential to the implementation of physical therapy treatment plans. Normal values for the cardiovascular hemodynamic parameters commonly monitored are listed in Table 11–2.

Arterial Pressures

Arterial blood pressure is the result of the rate of flow of blood (cardiac output) through and against the resistance of the circulatory system (systemic vascular resistance). In the acutely ill patient with cardiopulmonary disease, a low stroke volume and excessive peripheral vasoconstriction may make **Korotkoff's sounds** (the sounds heard over an artery when blood pressure is determined by the auscultatory method) impossible to hear. Therefore, rather than applying a blood pressure cuff, an intra-arterial pressure monitoring device is used to provide continuous measurement of systolic, diastolic, and mean pressures (see Fig. 11–16). Additionally, the indwelling arterial catheter provides a convenient route of access for arterial blood sampling to assess ventilatory efficacy.

The systolic blood pressure (the maximum systolic left ventricular pressure) reflects the compliance of the large arteries and the total peripheral resistance. In the normal adult, systolic pressure is usually about 120 mm Hg, ranging from 90 to 140 mm Hg, although it normally increases with age. Regardless of age, systolic blood pressure should be expected to increase with exertion in a fairly linear fashion. In fact, increases of 7 to 8

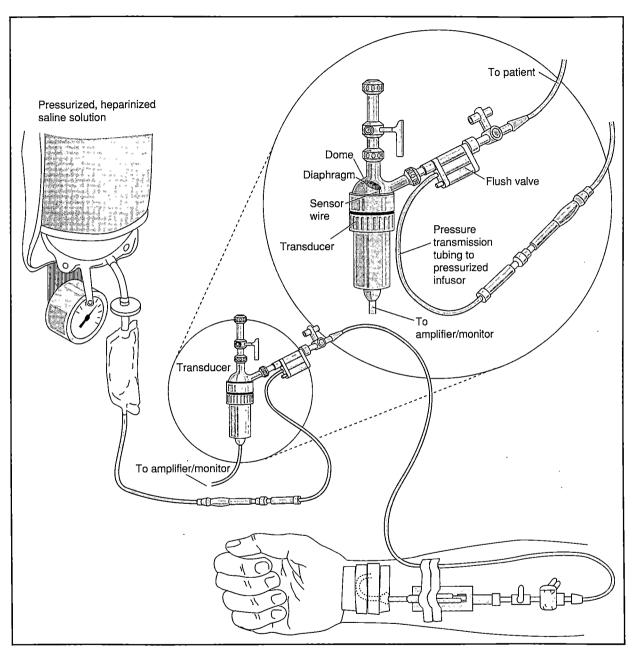

Figure 11-16

Indwelling arterial catheter, connecting tubing, and pressure transducer. (Redrawn from Darovic GO. Hemodynamic Monitoring: Invasive and Noninvasive Clinical Application. Philadelphia, WB Saunders, 1987, pp 113, 86.)

TABLE 11–2. Common Hemodynamic Parameters

Parameter	Common Acronym	Normal Values
Arterial blood pressures	BP	
Systolic	SBP	90–140 mm Hg
Diastolic	DBP	60–80 mm Hg
Right atrial pressure	RAP	0–8 mm Hg (mean)
Right ventricular pressures		
Systolic	RVs	15–30 mm Hg *or*
End-diastolic	RVEDP	0–8 mm Hg
Pulmonary artery pressures	PAP	
Systolic	PAs	15–30 mm Hg
Diastolic	PAd	5–15 mm Hg
Pulmonary artery wedge pressure	PWP, PCWP	4–15 mm Hg (mean)
Left atrial pressure	LAP	4–12 mm Hg (mean)
Left ventricular pressures		
Systolic	LVs	100–140 mm Hg
End-diastolic	LVEDP	4–12 mm Hg
Calculated Values		
Mean arterial pressure $\dfrac{SBP + (2 \cdot DBP)}{3}$	MAP or $\overline{BP}$	70–110 mm Hg
Mean PAP $\dfrac{PAs + (2 \cdot PAd)}{3}$	$\overline{PAP}$	8–20 mm Hg
Systemic vascular resistance $\dfrac{MAP - RAP}{\dot{Q}} \cdot 80$	SVR	800–1200 dynes $\cdot$ sec^{-1} $\cdot$ cm^{-1}
Pulmonary vascular resistance $\dfrac{\overline{PAP} - PWP}{\dot{Q}} \cdot 80$	PVR	<100 dynes $\cdot$ sec^{-1} $\cdot$ cm^{-1} *or* ⅙ SVR

mm Hg per metabolic equivalent (commonly abbreviated MET) increase in work rate intensity are not uncommon.[17] Nevertheless, it is generally considered unsafe if the systolic blood pressure exceeds 225 to 230 mm Hg. If the systolic blood pressure falls or fails to increase as workload increases, it may be assumed that the functional reserve capacity of the heart has been exceeded. If these situations develop, activity should be curtailed or terminated.[16–18]

The diastolic blood pressure is the lowest point of declining pressure resulting from the runoff of blood from the proximal aorta to the peripheral vessels, and it reflects the velocity of the runoff and the elasticity of the arterial system. Because the duration of the diastolic period of the cardiac cycle is directly related to the heart rate, the longer the period of diastole, the more the diastolic pressure falls. The diastolic blood pres-

sure normally ranges from 60 to 80 mm Hg, though it increases somewhat with the aging process. It does not change much during repetitive, rhythmic-type activities involving the lower extremities, such as bicycling, walking, or running. However, during upper extremity exercise or isometric exercise involving any muscle group, the diastolic blood pressure normally increases. Activity should be curtailed or halted if the diastolic blood pressure exceeds 130 mm Hg.[16–18]

The **mean arterial pressure (MAP)** is the average pressure tending to push blood through the circulatory system, and it reflects the tissue perfusion pressure. The MAP is closer to the diastolic than the systolic pressure because the duration of diastole is greater than that of systole. The MAP, therefore, is not a true arithmetic mean of systolic and diastolic pressures. The normal MAP varies between 70 and 110 mm Hg;

it is useful clinically because it yields one number that relates to cardiac output and systemic vascular resistance. A MAP of less than 60 mm Hg indicates an inadequate tissue perfusion pressure. A normal arterial pressure tracing is depicted in Figure 11–17; the dicrotic notch signifies the closure of the pulmonic valves, heralding the onset of the diastolic phase.

Right Atrial Pressure

In the 1950s, the right atrial pressure (central venous pressure) was estimated by measuring the vertical distance from the sternal angle to the level of the pulsating blood in one of the neck veins. In the 1960s, central venous catheters were developed, which allowed central venous pressures to be measured directly from the proximal superior vena cava by a water manometer. The term *right atrial pressure* (RAP) more correctly describes the anatomic and physiologic origins of what traditionally has been referred to as the central venous pressure. The advent of modern electronics has permitted the continuous monitoring of RAP to assess cardiac function and intravascular fluid status. Additionally, the catheter may be used as a route for medication or fluid administration, blood sampling, and emergency placement of a temporary pacemaker.

Although it was originally believed that central venous pressure was a reliable reflection of both right and left ventricular filling pressures, it is now recognized that generally these two pressures are poorly correlated as a result of the indirect temporal relationship of left ventricular dysfunction and RAP. Normally, the mean RAP is less than 5 mm Hg, though it ranges from zero to 8 mm Hg.[16,19,20] Elevated RAP may result from fluid overload, right ventricular failure, tricuspid valve insufficiency, or chronic left ventricular failure. Low RAP may be indicative of hypovolemia and dehydration. Subclavian and jugular insertion sites are most common for this catheter and should not be an impediment to physical activity.

Pulmonary Artery Pressures

Although the introduction of RAP monitoring in the early 1960s was a breakthrough in direct bedside monitoring of cardiac function, flow and pressure abnormalities distal to the RAP catheter render meaningful evaluation of left ventricular filling pressures impossible. Thus, the development of the flow-directed, balloon-tipped pulmonary artery catheter in the 1970s permitted bedside assessment of left ventricular function. The modern pulmonary artery catheter permits the direct measurement of right atrial and pul-

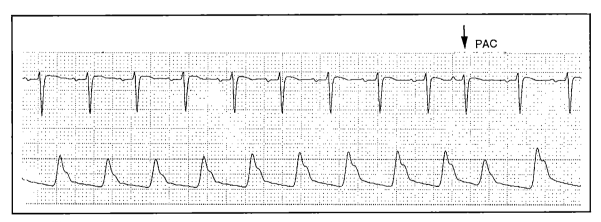

Figure 11–17

Electrocardiogram and arterial pressure tracings. Note the effect of a premature atrial complex on the pressure tracing (sinus tachycardia at rate between 110 and 120).

monary arterial pressures; the determination of mixed venous oxygen saturation, cardiac output, or both; the calculation of systemic and pulmonary vascular resistance (PVR); and the pacing of the atrium, ventricles, or both. The pulmonary artery catheter is typically introduced via a central venous access point (e.g., internal jugular or subclavian veins) and passes from the vena cava into the right atrium, through the right atrioventricular (tricuspid) valve into the right ventricle, through the pulmonic valve, and into the pulmonary artery (Fig. 11–18).

Because the left ventricular end-diastolic pressure (LVEDP) reflects the compliance of the left ventricle, it is the primary indicator of left ventricular performance. The LVEDP is difficult (even risky) to measure and is not monitored clinically; direct measurement of LVEDP is performed in the angiography laboratory as part of the coronary catheterization procedure. Fortuitously, though, the pressures in the left ventricle and in the left atrium are equal at the end of diastole because the mitral valve is still open (in the absence of a pathologic condition in the mitral valve). Moreover, because there are no valves in the pulmonary venous system, the pressures in the pulmonary veins, the pulmonary capillaries, and the pulmonary artery are also equal at the end of diastole. Thus, the pulmonary artery end-diastolic (PAd) pressure is equal to the LVEDP (normally less than 12 mm Hg) in the absence of a pathologic condition. However, if the pulmonary vascular resistance is elevated (as with pulmonary embolism, hypoxia, chronic lung disease, or other dead space–producing pathologic conditions), the pulmonary artery pressure reflects the high pulmonary vascular resistance instead of the LVEDP. In such situations, the pulmonary capillary wedge pressure (normally less than 12 mm Hg) is monitored intermittently. Note that during this monitoring, the balloon is inflated, thus "wedging" the catheter into a branch of the pulmonary artery. For this reason, it is important to keep in mind that patients should not be engaged in treatment if the catheter is in the wedge position, because the possibility of rupturing the pulmonary artery is very real.

When treating patients who are being monitored using pulmonary arterial lines, recognition of the normality of the potential waveforms is the key to deciding whether it is advisable to perform physical therapy. A RAP waveform should be recognizable when RAPs are being monitored; likewise, it should be possible to recognize a pulmonary arterial waveform when pulmonary artery pressures are being monitored. Normal wave configurations for right atrial, right ventricular, pulmonary artery, and pulmonary artery wedge pressures are shown in Figure 11–19. Generally, it is *not* normal to see a right ventricular or a wedge waveform when the catheter is properly positioned. If the clinician thinks that the catheter may be positioned improperly, physical therapy should be withheld until the correct catheter position is confirmed.

Cardiac Output

The amount of blood ejected with each contraction of the heart is called the *stroke volume* (SV). The amount of blood pumped by the heart per unit of time is termed the *cardiac output* ($\dot{Q}$), and unless an intracardiac shunt is present, the output of both the right and left ventricles is essentially the same. The normal resting $\dot{Q}$ is 4 to 8 liters per minute (L/min), and the normal SV ranges from 60 to 130 ml.[16,18] Cardiac output normally increases as activity increases. However, pathologic conditions can greatly affect $\dot{Q}$ and can impinge on an individual's homeostatic tolerance.

The $\dot{Q}$ is generally determined clinically by the **thermodilution method**. A cold bolus of saline is injected into the right atrium via the proximal lumen of a flow-directed, thermal-sensitive catheter; the resultant temperature change is sensed by a thermistor near the tip of the catheter located in the pulmonary artery. A temperature-time curve is constructed, and the $\dot{Q}$ is calculated.[21] The mean SV is calculated by dividing the cardiac output by the ventricular rate over a specific period of time. Conditions such as an arterial-venous fistula, anoxia, and Paget's disease may ultimately decrease the peripheral vas-

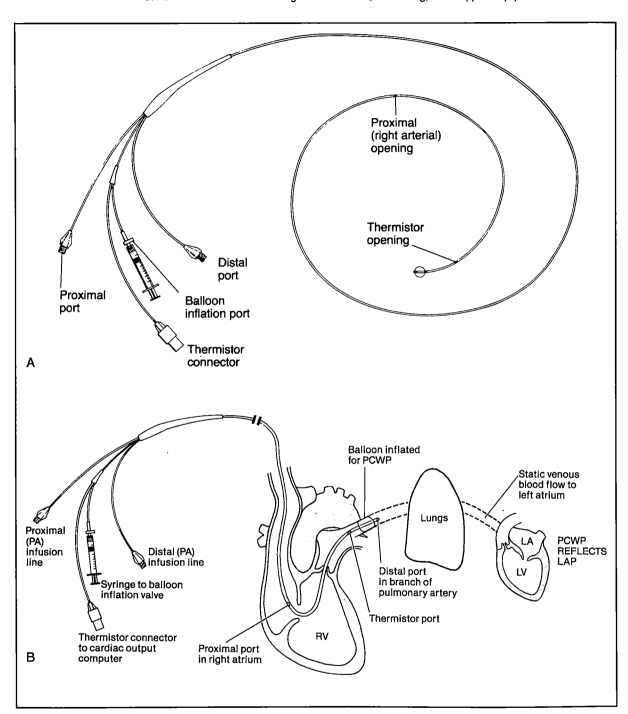

Figure 11–18

Pulmonary arterial catheter. *A,* Typical multilumen pulmonary artery catheter. (From Darovic GO. Hemodynamic Monitoring: Invasive and Noninvasive Clinical Application. Philadelphia, WB Saunders, 1987, p 140.) *B,* The pulmonary artery catheter passes through the right atrium and ventricle to rest in the pulmonary artery. (From Kersten LD. Comprehensive Respiratory Nursing. Philadelphia, WB Saunders, 1989, p 758.)

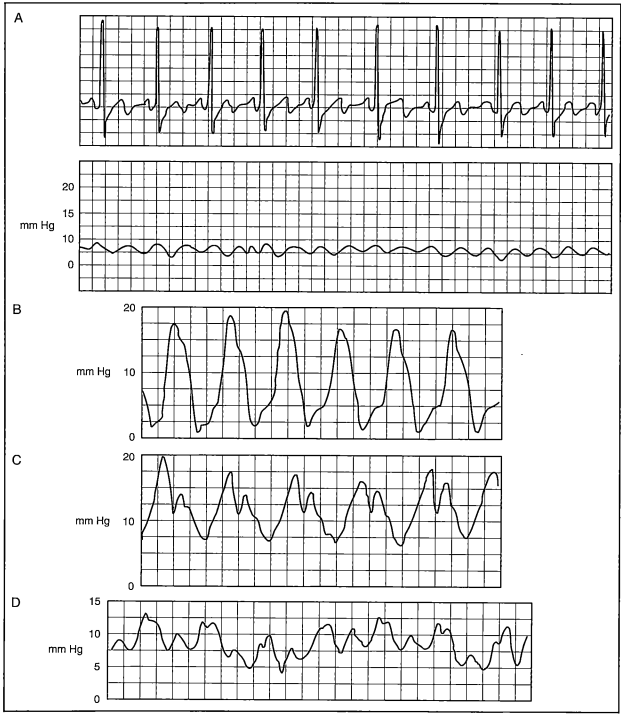

Figure 11-19

Normal right heart pressure tracings. *A,* Electrocardiogram and concurrent right atrial pressure tracings. *B,* Right ventricular pressure waveform, normally observed only when the catheter is initially inserted. *C,* Pulmonary arterial pressure waveform. *D,* Capillary wedge pressure waveform.

cular resistance and increase cardiac output by increasing venous return to the heart. Conversely, conditions that result in decreased blood volume reduce the venous return to the heart, decreasing $\dot{Q}$.

Unfortunately, simple $\dot{Q}$ measurements do not take into account an individual's specific needs with respect to actual body size. For this reason, the **cardiac index**—the cardiac output per square meter of body surface area—is often reported. The normal cardiac index for adults is approximately 3.0 L/min/m². A cardiac index of less than 2.2 L/min/m² is considered diagnostic of **cardiogenic shock**.[18] Cardiogenic shock is a condition in which the blood supply to the body tissues is insufficient because of inadequate $\dot{Q}$.

Mixed Venous Oxygen Saturation

The supply of oxygen to the tissues depends on $\dot{Q}$, hemoglobin level, and arterial oxygen saturation. Dissolved oxygen diffuses out of the capillaries and into the cells because of the pressure gradient that exists between them.[22] The partial pressure of oxygen in the blood (Po_2) is normally 100 mm Hg at the arteriolar end of the capillary bed and about 5 mm Hg at the cell, so oxygen diffuses into the cells according the gradient. By the time the blood reaches the venous end of the capillary bed, the PvO_2 (partial pressure of oxygen, venous) is about 40 mm Hg. Because the oxygen bound to the hemoglobin in the blood replenishes the dissolved oxygen that diffused out to the cells, the low PvO_2 causes oxygen to dissociate from hemoglobin, as described by the oxyhemoglobin dissociation curve. Venous blood, therefore, is about 75% saturated with oxygen.[23]

The amount of oxygen returning to the heart is called the *venous oxygen reserve*. When tissue demands for oxygen increase—as with exercise or increased metabolic rate resulting from a fever —the normal physiologic response is to increase oxygen supply and preserve the venous oxygen reserve. The oxygen supply is normally increased through an increase in $\dot{Q}$ and expiratory minute ventilation ($\dot{V}E$). Some patients (those with hypoxemia, anemia, heart failure, or heart failure

and pulmonary edema) cannot increase their oxygen supply in response to demand. When supply fails to meet demand, the venous oxygen reserve is affected because the tissues extract what they need as long as there is oxygen bound to the hemoglobin to replenish the dissolved oxygen taken by the cells. If the cellular demand for oxygen cannot be met, anaerobic metabolism ensues and lactic acidosis may result.

Mixed venous blood represents the average of venous blood from all parts of the body. Venous blood is considered to be mixed when it has reached the pulmonary artery. The oxygen saturation of mixed venous blood is normally 60% to 80%. Because changes in oxygen saturation are prompted by changes in the Po_2, and because venous saturation (SvO_2) is decreased only when oxygen supply fails to meet demand, it is clear that SvO_2 might be a sensitive indicator of oxygen supply-demand status. The pulmonary artery catheter permits monitoring of $S\overline{v}O_2$, thus allowing for evaluation of the tissue's need for oxygen and the adequacy with which that need is being met. The designation for a pulmonary artery blood sample is customarily denoted by "$\overline{v}$," which signifies a mixed venous sample in contrast to a sample from some peripheral venous site (e.g., $S\overline{v}O_2$ vs. SvO_2).

The presence of hemodynamic monitoring lines should alert the clinician to be aware of the signs of intolerance of treatment that are commensurate with the level of acuity that necessitated the placement of the monitoring line or lines. For example, a patient who needs a pulmonary arterial line is generally less hemodynamically stable than a patient who does not.

The clinical skills of observation and assessment should dictate clinical action. Attention should be paid to the trends demonstrated by hemodynamic variables, rather than to the value of any single parameter. Paying attention only to the values displayed on a bedside monitor and comparing them with normative standards without regard for the entire picture increases the likelihood of taking inappropriate action. For example, if a patient's pulmonary artery systolic pressure (as displayed on a bedside monitor) were 22 mm Hg in the supine position with activity, a clinician might decide that more aggressive bed mobility activities were warranted. Accordingly, the clinician might proceed to sit the patient at the edge of the bed to concentrate on breathing control and balance. If the hypothetic patient's right atrium were then 18 inches above the transducer because, as is customary, the transducer level was not readjusted, the pulmonary artery systolic pressure displayed on the bedside monitor would be 36 mm Hg higher than the actual value. This is because, for every inch that the phlebostatic point is located above or below the level of the transducer, an error of approximately 2 mm Hg is introduced in the pressure displayed on a bedside monitor (either falsely high or low, respectively). Thus, if the clinician failed to take into account the effect of the change in the patient's position with respect to the transducer, and if the displayed pulmonary artery systolic pressure were 55 mm Hg, the clinician could misinterpret the reading as being suggestive of a significantly hypertensive response. The clinician might conclude that the patient was not tolerating the position change and prematurely return the patient to the supine position. This error could be compounded if the clinician then informed the physician that the patient could not tolerate the upright sitting position because of the development of a pulmonary artery systolic pressure of 55 mm Hg (instead of the actual acceptable value of 19 mm

Hg). Because an error of as little as 6 mm Hg could result in significant errors in the medical therapeutic response, the clinician in such a situation should (1) move the transducer to the new level of the phlebostatic point or (2) note that value displayed with the phlebostatic point in the new position and make judgments in accordance with the new number (assuming there are no other indications of the patient's intolerance) to minimize the chances of misinterpretation.

Intra-aortic Balloon Counterpulsation

Sometimes, as the result of either pathologic insult or surgical intervention, patients become so hemodynamically unstable that **intra-aortic balloon counterpulsation** is used to augment the diastolic blood pressure and to increase coronary blood flow. The balloon is usually inserted into one of the femoral arteries and advanced until the balloon tip is just below the level of the left subclavian artery orifice (Fig. 11–20; intra-aortic balloon counterpulsation is also discussed in Chapter 4). When activated, the balloon is deflated during left ventricular systole — lowering left ventricular systolic pressure — and inflated during diastole — increasing diastolic pressure and coronary blood flow. The timing for balloon

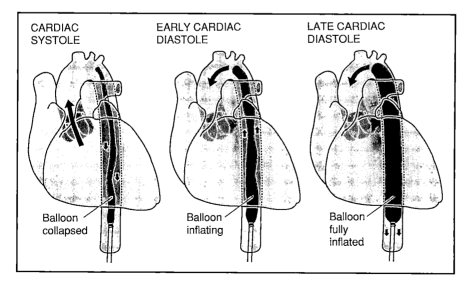

CARDIAC SYSTOLE

Balloon collapsed

EARLY CARDIAC DIASTOLE

Balloon inflating

LATE CARDIAC DIASTOLE

Balloon fully inflated

Figure 11–20

The intra-aortic balloon counterpulsation device is positioned in the descending aorta just below the orifice of the left subclavian artery. (Redrawn from Waldhausen JA, Pierce WS. Johnson's Surgery of the Chest. 5th ed. Chicago, Year Book Medical Publishers, 1985, p 273.)

TABLE 11–3. Pulmonary Function Parameters Readily Obtainable at the Bedside		
Parameter	**Common Acronym**	**Definition**
Respiratory frequency	f	Number of breaths per minute
Tidal volume	V_T	Volume of air inhaled or exhaled with each normal resting breath
Minute ventilation	$\dot{V}_E$	Volume of air exhaled per minute
Vital capacity	VC Nonforced or timed	Volume of air that can be expelled from the lungs following full inspiration
Forced vital capacity	FVC	Volume of air that can be quickly and forcibly expelled from the lungs following full inspiration
Forced expiratory volume per unit time	FEV_t	Volume of air that can forcibly be exhaled per unit of time (e.g., FEV_1 = volume in 1 second)
Peak expiratory flow	PEF	Highest flow rate attained in a forced expiratory maneuver
Maximal/inspiratory force or negative inspiratory force	MIF or NIF	Greatest negative pressure achieved during an inspiratory effort

inflation is based on either the R wave of the ECG or the patient's arterial pressure pulse. As long as hip flexion for the involved limb is kept below 70 degrees, the patient can usually participate in bed mobility and range of motion activities.

Electrocardiographic Monitoring

The ECG is a graphic representation of the electrical activity of the heart. An electrocardiographic tracing demonstrates depolarization and repolarization of the atria and ventricles, although atrial repolarization is masked by ventricular depolarization. The position of the positive (recording) electrode in relation to the spread of the electrical impulse is referred to as the *lead*. By convention, there are 12 electrocardiographic leads: 3 standard limb leads, 3 augmented limb leads, and 6 precordial leads.

In the critical care unit, patients are routinely monitored using one of several possible leads for heart rate and rhythm. A standard 12-lead ECG is requested for definitive analysis if irregularities are newly noted. Basic electrocardiographic interpretation is discussed in Chapter 9. The reader is referred to additional sources for more in-depth discussion of the technical aspects of ECG interpretation (e.g., Conover,[24] Dubin,[25] Brown and Jacobson[26]).

Ventilatory Monitoring and Life Support

Bedside Pulmonary Function Measurement

Respiratory physical therapy interventions are designed to promote bronchial hygiene, improve breathing efficiency, or promote physical reconditioning. To this end, the therapists involved may need to perform bedside pulmonary function testing or monitoring to ascertain treatment efficacy. Table 11–3 lists some of the parameters that may be measured at the bedside using relatively small and portable volume-collecting or flow-sensing devices. Additional tests may be performed at the bedside, but they require more sophisticated equipment. Nomograms specifically developed for the patient population being tested should be consulted before drawing conclusions regarding the results of pulmonary function tests.[27,28] However, it is generally accepted that pulmonary function results should be within 80% and 120% of predicted values. Particularly when considering weaning a patient from mechanical ventilation, bedside spirometry or pulmonary function testing is indispensable. Several parameters, reflecting oxygenation status, ventilatory mechanics, respiratory muscle strength, and ventilatory demand, may predict weaning success.[29–32]

Oxygenation may be inferred from several clinically obtainable measurements. An acceptable SaO_2 (arterial oxygen saturation) and PaO_2 (partial pressure of oxygen, arterial) with an FiO_2 less than or equal to 0.5 is often cited as a criterion guideline preparatory to weaning attempts, as long as the PaO_2 to FiO_2 ratio is greater than 200 mm Hg.[30] The literature on oxygenation criteria for weaning generally predates the widespread use of **positive end-expiratory pressure (PEEP)** in the treatment of adult respiratory distress syndrome, but a PEEP of less than or equal to 7.5 cm H_2O is desirable before the initiation of weaning.

Ventilatory mechanics are probably best inferred in most cases by the inspiratory capacity (IC). A tidal volume (VT) of at least 5 milliliters per kilogram and a static system compliance greater than 30 ml/cm H_2O may be predictive of weaning success.[29,30] Likewise, a vital capacity (VC) of at least 15 milliliters per kilogram or a negative (maximal) inspiratory force (NIF or MIF) of more than 20 cm H_2O, or both, has been suggested as a suitable predictor.

The patient's ability to meet ventilatory demand may be inferred from VE, dead space to tidal volume ratio (VD to VT), and CO_2 production (VCO$_2$). A VE of less than 10 liters per minute, for a $PaCO_2$ of 40 mm Hg, is one parameter that is highly predictive of successful weaning.[32]

Monitoring the forces generated by the respiratory muscles is important because these muscles are the only skeletal muscles on which life is directly dependent. For the respiratory muscles, which work primarily in terms of elastic and resistive loads, force-length and force-velocity relationships are inferred from measurements of pressure (force developed, divided by surface area over which it acts), changes in volume (inferring changes in length), and flow-rate of volume change (inferring velocity). Thus, respiratory muscle strength may be inferred from the MIF, IC or VC, peak flow rate, or forced expiratory volume in 1 second (FEV$_1$).

Airway Adjuncts

An **oral pharyngeal airway** (Fig. 11–21A) is a semirigid tube of plastic or rubber shaped to fit the natural curve of the soft palate and tongue. It is used to hold the tongue away from the back of the throat and maintain airway patency. The oral airway may also be used as a bite block. The **nasal pharyngeal airway** (Fig. 11–21B) is a soft latex or rubber tube inserted through one of the nares. It follows the wall of the nasopharynx and oropharynx to the base of the tongue. The nasal airway is generally better tolerated because it is less likely to stimulate a gag in the semiconscious or alert patient. However, the clinician is cautioned that when nasal airways are left in place for prolonged periods of time, interference with normal sinus drainage may occur. Nonetheless, when properly utilized, both the oral and the nasal airways may reduce mucosal trauma by providing a pathway for suctioning of the hypopharynx.

An endotracheal tube (Fig. 11–21C), an artificial airway inserted into the trachea, is made of silicone rubber or polyvinyl chloride and is generally disposable. An **oral endotracheal tube** is inserted via the mouth, and a **nasal endotracheal tube** is inserted via the nose; the specific rationale for using each type of tube may vary regionally. Regardless of the route, endotracheal intubation is usually undertaken as a last resort when other means of airway management have or are likely to fail. There are four primary reasons for employing endotracheal intubation:

- Upper airway obstruction
- Inability to protect the lower airway from aspiration
- Inability to clear secretions from the lower airways
- Need for positive pressure mechanical ventilatory assistance

The addition of a radiopaque line extending the length of the tube or a marker at the distal end of the tube facilitates location of the endotracheal tube by radiograph. Endotracheal tubes are beveled at their distal ends, and they are usually labeled near their proximal ends with the manufacturer's name, tube type, and internal diameter (ID) in millimeters.

Unfortunately, there is no clear standard for reporting tube sizes. Instead of ID size, French size and Jackson size may be reported (for an

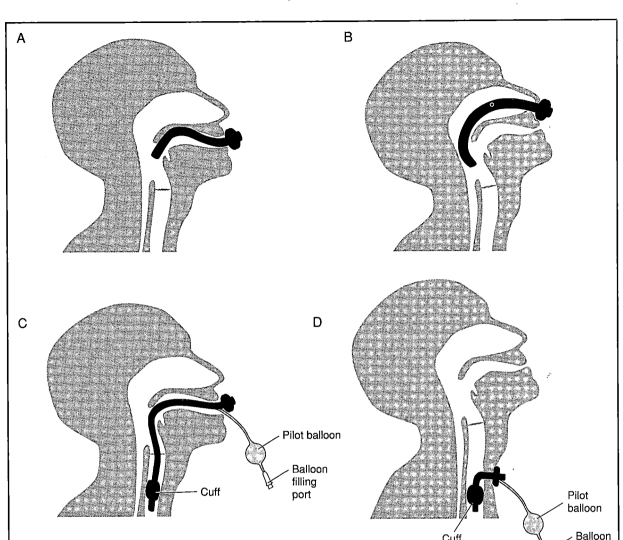

Figure 11-21

Airway adjuncts. A, Oral pharyngeal tube. B, Nasal pharyngeal tube. C, Oral endotracheal tube. D, Tracheostomy tube. (Redrawn from Kersten LD. Comprehensive Respiratory Nursing. Philadelphia, WB Saunders, 1989, p 630.)

approximate conversion of ID size to French size, multiply the ID size by 4).[20] The reader is referred to Caldwell and Sullivan's discussion for more information.[33]

Adult endotracheal tubes normally have low-pressure, large-volume inflatable cuffs at their distal ends. Inflating the cuff stabilizes the endotracheal tube and seals the airway so that only air can move through the tube. A pilot balloon, attached to the tube that inflates the cuff, provides an indication of whether the cuff is inflated. Neonatal and pediatric endotracheal tubes generally do not have cuffs. A standard 15-millimeter adapter or universal adapter is attached at the proximal end of the endotracheal tube to facilitate connection to mechanical ventilators, manual resuscitation bags, or other respiratory maintenance devices.

A **tracheostomy tube** (Fig. 11–21D) is an artificial airway inserted into the trachea via a tracheostomy below the level of the vocal cords. A tracheostomy may be performed for several reasons, but it is not normally an emergency procedure. In the critical care setting, tracheostomy usually follows prolonged endotracheal intubation to minimize tracheal or vocal cord injury. The tracheostomy tube is short (2 to 6 inches long) but otherwise similar to an endotracheal tube except that it is not beveled at its distal end. An external flange near the proximal end of the tube is usually labeled with the manufacturer's name and internal or external diameter in millimeters. The flange stabilizes the tube in the trachea and acts as a base from which the tube may be secured to the patient's neck. Some tracheostomy tubes have a removable inner cannula to facilitate cleaning of the tube. Because several types of special-use tracheostomy tubes are manufactured, the clinician should be aware of the type of tube being used with the patient so that any special precautions can be noted. For example, the fenestrated tube has a hole cut into the superior aspect of the outer cannula, which permits utilization of the upper airway with the tube in place if the inner cannula is removed.

Although most tracheostomy tubes are cuffed, in many situations the cuff is deflated. For example, when assessing the patient's ability to protect the lower airway during swallowing, the cuff may be deflated. If the cuff is ever found deflated, the clinician is advised to inquire first whether the cuff should be inflated or deflated before taking any action. The cuff should *not* be inflated or deflated capriciously; dire consequences for the patient may result. Specialized texts or clinical experts can provide further details regarding inflation and deflation of tracheostomy cuffs.

The use of a **tracheostomy button** (Fig. 11–22) may be an intermediate step between mechanical ventilation and spontaneous breathing in the process of weaning a patient from mechanical ventilatory support. It permits utilization of the upper airway for spontaneous ventilation while providing a means of maintaining the tracheostomy stoma as a direct access route to the lower airway until the patient no longer re-

quires assistance to clear bronchial secretions or breathe.

Mechanical Ventilation

The two primary reasons that mechanical ventilation might be instituted for a patient are ventilatory failure and hypoxemia. Positive-pressure ventilation is used in the critical care setting. The positive pressure from the ventilator provides the force that delivers gas into the patient's lungs by increasing intrathoracic pressure to expand the chest wall. The termination of gas flow allows the chest wall to recoil to the resting position and thus to exhale the gas. Mechanical ventilators are generally classified according their cycling mechanism, that is, the method used to stop the inspiratory phase and initiate the expiratory phase. Basically, there are three types of mechanical ventilators:

- Pressure cycled (e.g., Bird series,* Bennett series†)
- Volume cycled (e.g., Bear series,‡ Bennett MA series,† Monaghan 225,§ Ohio CCV-2‖)
- Time cycled (e.g., Engstrom,¶ Emerson series,** Siemens Servo series,†† Bourns BP200,‡ Bird Babybird*)

More sophisticated ventilators that employ computer and microprocessor technology (e.g., Bear 5,‡ Bennett 7200,† Hamilton‡‡), which do not lend themselves to simple classification, are gaining favor clinically.

---

* Bird Products Corporation, 3101 E. Alejo Rd., Palm Springs CA 92262.
† Puritan Bennett Corporation, 12655 Beatrice Street, Los Angeles CA 90066.
‡ Bourns-Bear Medical Systems, Inc., 2085 Rustin Ave., Riverside CA 92507.
§ Monaghan Medical Corporation, Franklyn Bldg., Rte 9 North, P.O. Box 978, Plattsburgh NY 12901.
‖ Ohmeda, 303 Ohmeda Drive, P.O. Box 7550, Madison WI 53707.
¶ Engstrom, 600 Knight's Bridge Parkway, Lincolnshire IL 60069.
** J. H. Emerson Co., 22 Cottage Park Ave., Cambridge MA 02140.
†† Siemens-Elma Ventilator Systems, 2360 N. Palmer Drive, Schaumburg IL 60195.
‡‡ Hamilton Medical Inc., P.O. Box 30008, Reno NV 89520.

Figure 11-22

Tracheostomy button. (Adapted from Kersten LD. Comprehensive Respiratory Nursing. Philadelphia, WB Saunders, 1989, p 660.)

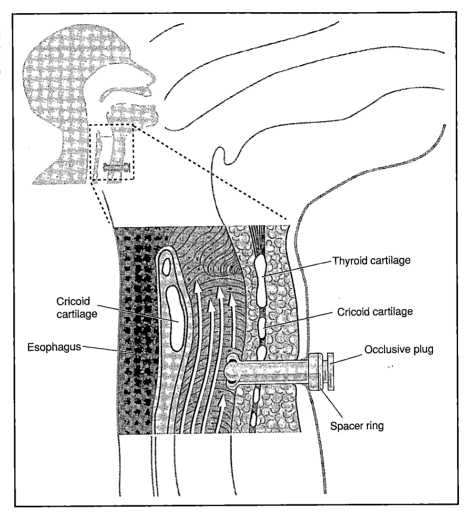

Thyroid cartilage

Cricoid cartilage

Cricoid cartilage

Esophagus

Occlusive plug

Spacer ring

Knowledge of the basic ventilator setup and settings prepares the clinician to monitor the patient more appropriately. The tubing and equipment connecting the patient to the ventilator is called the **circuit**. The circuit generally consists of tubing and valves that attach to a mask or a mouthpiece or directly to an endotracheal or a tracheostomy tube. In some institutions, an additional port in the terminal end of the circuit permits suctioning while maintaining the integrity of the circuit, which obviates the need to disconnect the endotracheal tube from the circuit. During the performance of various bronchial hygiene procedures, or simply to facilitate positioning for patient comfort, the circuit may need to be dis-

connected from the patient. Disconnection may mean simply removing a mask or mouthpiece, as would be done with the termination of an intermittent positive-pressure breathing (IPPB) treatment, or it may involve disengaging the circuit from an endotracheal or a tracheostomy tube in conjunction with hyperoxygenation. This latter effort necessitates stabilizing the endotracheal or tracheostomy tube while the circuit is removed, taking care to ensure that the patient is not inadvertently extubated (endotracheal or tracheostomy tube removed), and then ventilating the patient manually with a self-inflating resuscitation bag (a procedure that is discussed later).

By convention, there are several methods of

providing mechanical ventilation to the patient. Controlled ventilation is the provision of positive-pressure breaths at a set rate without regard for patient participation. Assist or assist-control ventilation is the provision of positive-pressure breaths at a set rate, unless the patient triggers the machine by creating a negative inspiratory force less than the preset threshold pressure of the machine. In this case, the machine delivers a positive-pressure breath at the rate established by the patient's efforts. **Intermittent mandatory ventilation (IMV)** or **synchronized intermittent mandatory ventilation (SIMV)** is the provision of a preset number of ventilator breaths in conjunction with a source of gas from which the patient may spontaneously breathe. In the IMV mode, the mandatory breath is delivered at a preset rate regardless of the phase of the patient's spontaneous efforts. In the SIMV mode, the mandatory breath is initiated by the patient's spontaneous inspiratory effort. **Pressure support ventilation (PSV)** is the augmentation of the inspiratory phase of a patient's spontaneous ventilatory efforts with a preset amount of positive pressure. Figure 11–23 shows the pressure curves generated by various ventilatory modes and some of the airway maneuvers.

Mechanical ventilation is frequently associated with a veritable alphabet soup of acronyms and terms that are used to describe various airway

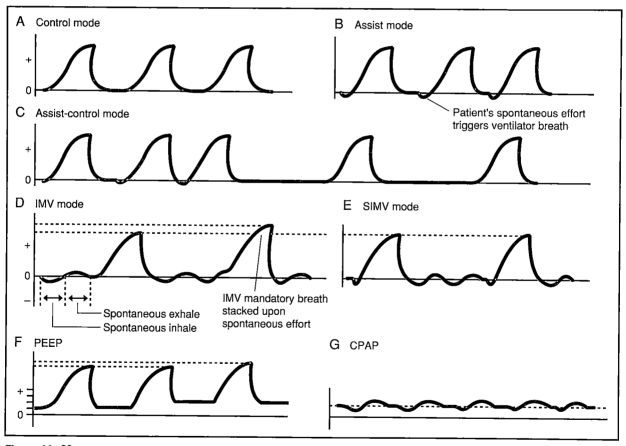

Figure 11–23

Pressure waves produced by several different modes of mechanical ventilation. *A*, Control mode. *B*, Assist mode. *C*, Assist-control mode. *D*, Intermittent mandatory ventilation (IMV) mode. *E*, Synchronized intermittent mandatory ventilation (SIMV) mode. *F*, Positive end-expiratory pressure (PEEP). *G*, Continuous positive airway pressure (CPAP) (see text for details). (Adapted from Kersten LD. Comprehensive Respiratory Nursing. Philadelphia, WB Saunders, 1989, p 712.)

maneuvers that augment or modify a patient's ventilatory status. These include the following:

- **Inspiratory hold**—a maneuver in which either the preset pressure or predetermined volume is reached and held for some period of time before exhalation is initiated
- **Positive end-expiratory pressure**—a thresholdlike resistance applied after exhalation that permits the circuit pressure to drop to a set level above atmospheric pressure
- **Expiratory retard**—an orificial resistance applied to exhalation whereby the circuit pressure is permitted to drop slowly to atmospheric as the expiratory gas flow ceases
- **Continuous positive airway pressure (CPAP)**—the application of an elevated baseline pressure (greater than atmospheric) from which a patient spontaneously breathes

Supplemental Oxygen-Delivery Devices

Physical therapists working with patients in the intensive care unit often come into contact with at least two types of oxygen systems. In the intensive care unit, patients' mechanical ventilators or other supplemental oxygen devices are connected to the hospital's bulk oxygen system outlets at the bedside. However, for transport or ambulation, portable oxygen tanks or cylinders are needed. This section considers the portable systems, such as cylinders or liquid oxygen canisters, that permit oxygen to accompany a patient away from the bedside.

Compressed oxygen that is stored in tanks or cylinders is a common method of supplying oxygen for portable or out-of-hospital needs. By convention, these cylinders are green and are labeled "Oxygen." When full, an oxygen cylinder exerts about 2200 pounds per square inch (psi) of pressure. A pressure regulator reduces the high pressures from the gas in the cylinder to a lower working pressure, usually 50 psi, before the gas enters the flowmeter. The flowmeter measures and controls the flow of oxygen to the patient. Although cylinders vary in size, the most common are an E cylinder (in the hospital or outpatient setting) and an H cylinder (in the home-care setting). When full, E cylinders con-

tain approximately 620 liters of oxygen and H cylinders about 6900 liters. Depending on the liter flow needed for the specific delivery device, the clinician can calculate the amount of time left at the given flow rate by using the following formula:

$$\frac{\text{psi} \times k}{\text{flow rate}} = \text{minutes}$$

where psi = pounds per square inch (read from the regulator dial), and k = cylinder constant (3.14 for an H tank; 0.28 for an E cylinder).

Portable liquid oxygen systems are in common use outside the hospital setting because of their relatively greater capacity and lighter weight. Under very high pressure, oxygen liquefies. As a liquid, oxygen occupies 1/860 the volume of gas at standard atmospheric pressure. A typical liquid oxygen system provides oxygen for approximately 8 hours at a flow rate of 2 liters per minute and weighs less than 10 pounds; an E cylinder lasts about 5 hours at a similar flow rate and weighs about 17 pounds.[17]

The gases used for therapeutic purposes are stored with all water vapor removed, that is, 100% dry. Depending on the gas flow rate, the frequency or duration of use, and the patient's state of hydration, the lack of humidity could irritate the mucosa of the pulmonary passageways. At low flow rates (less than 4 L · min^{-1}), humidification of the gases may not be necessary. At flow rates of less than 10 L · min^{-1}, simple humidifiers (Fig. 11–24) may be used to add sufficient humidity to make the gas comfortable. When the upper airway is bypassed—for example, when the patient has a tracheostomy tube in place or is intubated—the gas must be heated to increase its capacity to carry water vapor. Heated humidifiers are often used when flow rates exceed 10 L · min^{-1} or when the upper airway is bypassed. Aerosolized water is another means by which medical gases may be humidified. Aerosols are produced by nebulizers (Fig. 11–25), of which there are many types.[34]

Oxygen administration devices include nasal cannulas, masks, tents, hoods, and incubators. The **nasal cannula** is used with low oxygen flow rates between 1 and 6 L · min^{-1} (see Fig. 11–

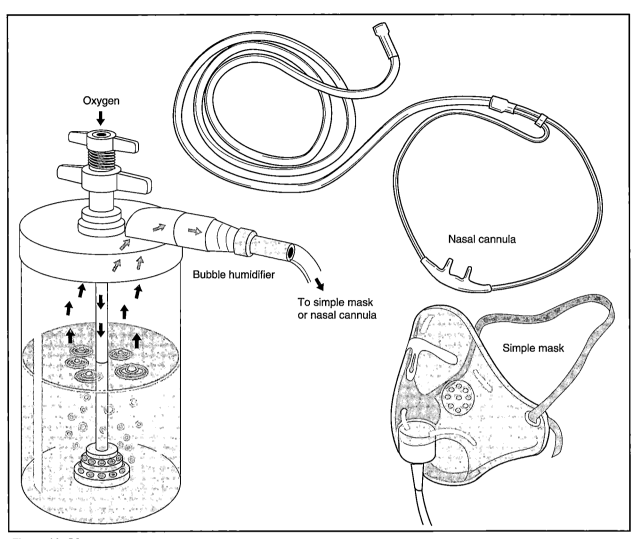

Figure 11-24

Low-flow supplemental oxygen delivery devices and flow-by humidifier. (Redrawn from Kersten LD. Comprehensive Respiratory Nursing. Philadelphia, WB Saunders, 1989, pp 608, 609.)

24). Whether a humidifier is used in conjunction with a nasal cannula may depend on individual physician preference. However, at flow rates exceeding $3 \; L \cdot min^{-1}$ the nasal mucosa may become dried and irritated with sustained use of nonhumidified gas. An accurate fraction of inspired oxygen (FI_{O_2}) cannot be delivered with a nasal cannula because respiratory rate, V_T, and anatomic V_D are so variable among patients. As Table 11-4 shows, it is assumed that the approximate FI_{O_2} is increased by 4% with each 1 liter per minute increase in oxygen flow rate.

The delivery of an accurate and consistent FI_{O_2} requires that the flow of gas be sufficient to exceed the patient's peak inspiratory flow demand, which generally requires higher flow rates than can be tolerably achieved by nasal cannula. Therefore, masks are used. Several different types of masks are used for administering medical gases.

Simple Mask. The **simple mask** (see Fig. 11-24) is designed to provide a flow of gas into a face piece that fits over the patient's nose and mouth. Some simple masks also include a diluter to add room air and thus increase the total gas flow as the oxygen flows into the mask. The oxygen percentage that can be delivered with a simple mask ranges from 35% to 55%, at flow rates of 5 to 10 L · min⁻¹ (for adults). As is true with nasal cannulas, whether a humidifier is used in conjunction with a simple mask may depend on individual physician preference. However, at oxygen concentrations exceeding 30%, the nasal and oral mucosa may become dried and irritated with sustained use of nonhumidified gas.

Aerosol Mask. The **aerosol mask** (see Fig. 11–25) was originally designed for the administration of aerosolized medications. However, these masks are used widely for the administration of controlled percentages of oxygen at flow rates slightly greater than those for simple masks (10 to 12 liters per minute), to exceed the patient's inspiratory demand. Typically, aerosol

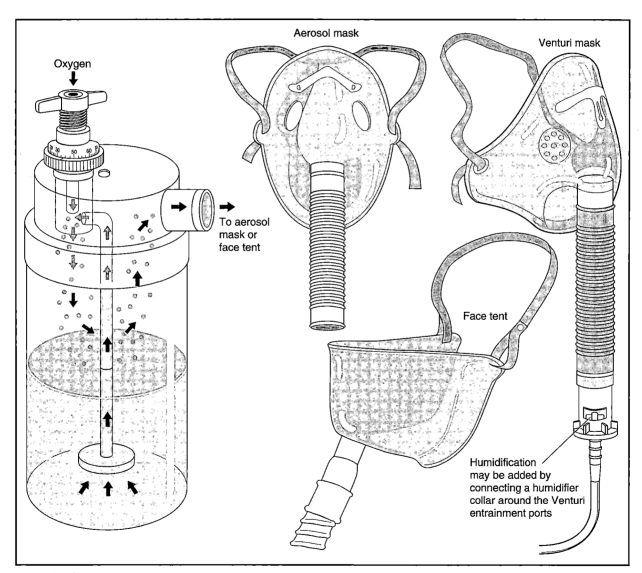

Figure 11–25

High-flow supplemental oxygen delivery devices and aerosol nebulizer. (Redrawn from Kersten LD. Comprehensive Respiratory Nursing. Philadelphia, WB Saunders, 1989, pp 581, 585.)

TABLE 11-4. Approximate FIO_2 Achieved with Different Oxygen Delivery Devices

Device	Oxygen Flow Rate	FIO_2
Nasal cannula (estimated FIO_2, assuming normal $\dot{V}E$)		
	1 L/min	0.24
	2 L/min	0.28
	3 L/min	0.32
	4 L/min	0.36
	5 L/min	0.40
	6 L/min	0.44
Simple mask		
	5-6 L/min	0.35
	6-7 L/min	0.45
	7-10 L/min	0.55
Aerosol mask		
	10-12 L/min	0.35-1.0
		(depends on setting)
Venturi mask (O_2 flow rates are minimums to be used with specific-sized orifice for desired FIO_2)		
	4 L/min	0.24*
	4 L/min	0.28*
	6 L/min	0.31
	8 L/min	0.35*
	8 L/min	0.40*
	10 L/min	0.50

* FIO_2 depends on the size of the orifice or the entrainment ports; these vary among manufacturers.

masks are employed in conjunction with a nebulizer to humidify the gas. The FIO_2 is regulated between 35% and 100% by means of an adjustable air entrainment port on the nebulizer. Increasing the FIO_2 setting closes the entrainment port and decreases the dilution of the oxygen.

Venturi Mask. The **Venturi mask** (see Fig. 11-25) generally provides a greater flow of gas to a patient by entraining room air through a side port. The FIO_2 is selected by changing either the size of the orifice through which oxygen is delivered or the size of the entrainment ports and adjusting the oxygen flow rate. Venturi masks operate by application of Bernouilli's principle: oxygen enters the larger flexible tubing via a narrowed orifice, creating a relative negative pressure within the tubing, which pulls room air through the entrainment ports. These masks may or may not be humidified. Table 11-4 details the oxygen flow rates and the FIO_2 delivered by Venturi masks (different manufacturers' devices may provide different FIO_2s).

Oxygen Tent, Oxygen Hood, and Incubator. In the pediatric setting, oxygen tents, hoods, or incubators are frequently used. In an **oxygen tent**, the FIO_2 attained depends on the incoming gas flow, the canopy volume, and the degree to which the tent is sealed. Tents generally envelop the patient's upper torso or entire body. Continuous oxygen monitoring is necessary because patient care requires entering the tent. This, therefore, alters the FIO_2. Ice reservoirs are often incorporated for temperature control. An **oxygen hood**, a small plastic enclosure placed over the patient's head, permits nursing care or other treatment without hindering oxygen therapy. An **incubator** may be used for similar reasons as an oxygen tent, but it generally provides for warming instead of cooling of the environment.

Other Mechanical Devices

Additional equipment that does not readily fall in the previously discussed categories includes incentive spirometers and resistive breathing devices, mechanical percussors, manual resuscitators, and negative-pressure ventilators. Although they might be more correctly termed adjuncts to treatment, these devices are frequently employed by physical therapists in the treatment of patients with respiratory dysfunction.

Incentive Spirometry and Inspiratory Resistance Devices

Approximately six to nine times an hour, the normal adult takes a deep inhalation, or sigh, that approaches the total lung capacity. In a pattern of shallow breathing, without periodic deep breaths, yawns, or sighs, a gradual alveolar collapse develops that, if not corrected or reversed, can lead to gross **atelectasis**. Trauma, disease, and surgical procedures all contribute to such abnormal patterns of breathing. Additionally, an inadequate IC inhibits the patient's cough strength. For example, a patient may alter the respiratory patterns, avoiding prolonged inspiratory efforts, coughing, or both as a result of incisional pain or muscle weakness. Therefore, breathing exercises that incorporate sustained maximal inspiratory efforts with coughing assistance techniques may be indicated.

The **incentive spirometer** is designed to provide patients with immediate visual feedback regarding achievement of preset goals while they perform sustained maximal inspiratory maneuvers. This visual input, it is hoped, encourages patients to continue to use the unit and to work toward increasing their maximal inspiratory effort. Two types of incentive spirometers are commonly used in the clinic: flow and volume spirometers (Fig. 11–26).[34]

Figure 11–26

Flow- and volume-incentive spirometers. (Redrawn by permission of Sherwood Medical, St. Louis, Mo.)

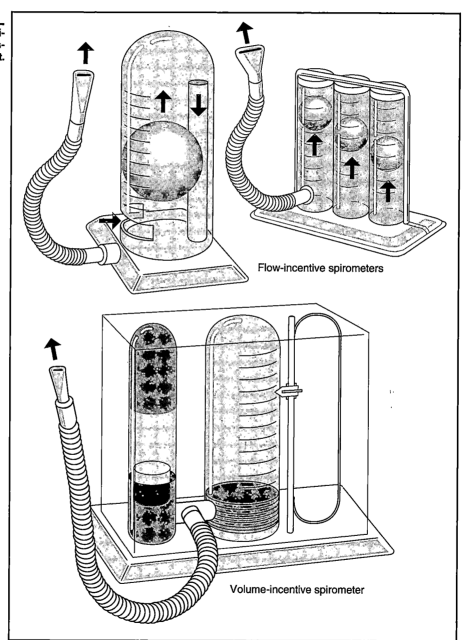

Flow-incentive spirometers

Volume-incentive spirometer

Flow incentive spirometers are flow dependent. Generally, they consist of one or more chambers containing a table tennis–like ball. Inhalation elevates the ball, or balls, and keeps it floating as long as the flow of air is of sufficient magnitude. Unfortunately, a very brisk flow rate pulls the ball to the top of the chamber with a relatively low-volume breath. Alternately, a breath with an especially slow flow rate may achieve total lung capacity without moving the ball.

Volume incentive spirometers permit the selection of preset volumes that indicate directly whether the actual volume is achieved. The commonly used volume spirometers have a bellows or piston that registers the volume achieved. The clinician adjusts an indicator to the desired inspiratory goal.

Although the patient is encouraged to use either incentive spirometer independently, neither device should be placed at the patient's bedside without first providing the patient with proper instruction for its use. Several brands of incentive spirometers are commercially available.

Physical therapists are unique in their ability to assess and intervene in the rehabilitation of unused muscles. Although it is easy to see the atrophy of arm or leg muscles following the removal of a plaster cast and to appreciate that the prolonged disuse of these muscles may predispose them to weakness and rapid fatigue, too often this same association is not made with reference to the respiratory muscles following prolonged mechanical ventilatory support. A fundamental principle of exercise training is to work a muscle to the point of fatigue and then allow it to rest.

In a study on respiratory muscle strengthening and endurance training in which patients with chronic obstructive pulmonary disease (COPD) utilized 3- to 5-second maximal inspiratory efforts in conjunction with expiratory maneuvers at 20% increments over their VC ranges for strength training, and ventilation to exhaustion three to five times daily for endurance training, Leith and Bradley[35] showed that strength trainers increased maximal inspiratory pressures by 55% and that endurance trainers increased their ability to sustain hyperpnea from 81% to 96% of their pretraining maximal voluntary ventilation (largest volume that can be breathed per minute with voluntary effort—MVV) while increasing their maximal voluntary ventilation by 14%. In another investigation, Gross and colleagues[36] reported that an 8-week regimen of 30 minutes of daily inspiratory resistance training by quadriplegic patients resulted in a 21.5% increase in mean maximal inspiratory force. Thus, resistive inspiratory training may be a beneficial treatment tool (see Chapter 16 for more details).

Mechanical Percussors

Percussion and vibration, as employed in the performance of a bronchial hygiene regimen, constitute a significant portion of the treatment time. Judiciously applied, these methods have been shown to augment the mobilization and elimination of excessive secretions. Yet, as many therapists can attest, these techniques can be difficult to learn and quite fatiguing if not performed properly. Electrically or pneumatically powered mechanical percussors are commercially available to ameliorate these difficulties. However, the efficacy of these mechanical adjuncts are as highly dependent on their proper use as are the manual techniques. Although it may be true that these devices conserve the therapist's energy, they eliminate an often overlooked and underrated nonverbal communication system between therapist and patient—touch.

Manual Resuscitators

Sometimes the therapist must disconnect the patient from the mechanical ventilator for a prolonged period of time (e.g., transfer or ambulation training, endotracheal suctioning). In such instances, the patient will require ventilatory assistance from a manual resuscitator. Several manufacturers produce manual resuscitators, and the valve systems of each are unique. Some occasions call for the use of portable, battery-powered mechanical ventilators. Clinicians should become thoroughly familiar with the equipment needed by their patients.

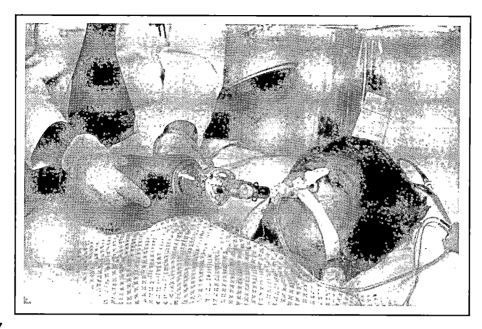

Figure 11–27

Self-inflating manual resuscitation bag being used to manually ventilate an intubated patient. (From Kersten LD. Comprehensive Respiratory Nursing. Philadelphia, WB Saunders, 1989, p 630.)

Manual resuscitation bags (Fig. 11–27) are self-inflating; when compressed, they deliver a volume of gas to the patient by means of one-way valves. When the bag is compressed, gas enters the valve and pushes the diaphragms against the exhalation ports. The flow of gas then opens the inhalation valve, permitting gas to flow to the patient. When flow from the bag ceases and exhalation begins, exhaled gas from the patient pushes the inhalation valve closed and opens the diaphragms, allowing gas to flow out the exhalation ports. The bag intake port may be fitted with an oxygen reservoir system to deliver oxygen-enriched breaths. Manual resuscitation bags may be used to stimulate or mimic a cough, to augment V_T and supplement oxygen for intubated and nonintubated patients, or to do both.

Negative-Pressure Ventilators

Finally, mention should be made of a negative-pressure ventilator—the **cuirass**. Basically, the cuirass is a rigid shell that encloses the pa-

tient's anterior thorax so that subatmospheric pressure can be exerted within the shell. A vacuum cleaner–like pump generates the negative pressure. The shells are usually made individually for each patient, although prefabricated shells are available. The cuirass is probably not used more widely because

- it tends to be noisy
- provision of patient care may be hampered
- regulation of inspiratory to expiratory ratios is difficult

These units are useful, however, for providing augmentation to patients with weakened respiratory musculature who are able to breathe spontaneously. Additionally, ventilatory mechanics are more normal than they are with positive-pressure machines, and many patients do not require a tracheostomy. Patients who require intermittent or periodic ventilatory assistance (e.g., patients suffering from Guillain-Barré syndrome, amyotrophic lateral sclerosis) may benefit from such ventilators.

SUMMARY

- The numerous surgical procedures that may be performed on the cardiovascular or pulmonary systems are generally made via any of three approaches (or modifications thereof): thoracotomy incisions are most commonly used for lung resection procedures; most cardiac procedures are performed through a median sternotomy; procedures involving the diaphragm, pericardium, or epicardium are commonly performed through a thoracoabdominal incision.

- Cardiac revascularization procedures are among the most common of cardiothoracic surgical procedures. They may be performed percutaneously (e.g., angioplasty, atherectomy, stenting) or transthoracically (e.g., bypass grafting). Either approach is associated with its own postprocedure movement precautions.

- If, as the result of disease or trauma, the heart is unable to generate an adequate cardiac output, cardiovascular life support equipment is frequently employed to stimulate or augment cardiac function. Pacemaker devices generate an artificial electrical stimulus to supplant or replace the heart's native rhythm of depolarization. Intra-aortic balloon counterpulsation may be used to augment coronary arterial blood flow and diastolic blood pressure.

- Chest drainage tubes (e.g., intrapleural or mediastinal) are usually employed following cardiothoracic surgical procedures or chest trauma, or when metabolic disorders so disrupt vascular permeability and osmotic pressures that fluid collects within the thoracic cavity. Their presence should not preclude the patient's participation in physical therapy activities.

- Airway adjuncts (e.g., oral or nasal pharyngeal airways, nasal or oral endotracheal tubes, tracheostomy tubes) are used to (1) facilitate the removal of excess secretions from the pharynx, trachea, or large proximal airways; (2) prevent the aspiration of oral or gastric contents into the lungs; and (3) provide access for the administration of mechanical ventilatory support and supplemental oxygen.

- Bedside hemodynamic monitoring entails the observation and periodic recording of various vascular pressures (e.g., peripheral arterial, right atrial, pulmonary arterial) and volumes (e.g., cardiac output). Changes in the various parameters can provide insights regarding the patient's cardiovascular responses to physical therapy intervention.

- Bedside pulmonary function monitoring (e.g., simple spirometry, arterial blood gas analysis) provides information that is helpful in the assessment of the patient's ventilatory mechanics, respiratory muscle strength, ventilatory demand, and oxygenation status. Several of these parameters may be helpful in predicting the success of weaning from mechanical ventilatory support.

References

1. Kittle CF. Thoracic incisions. In: Baue AE (ed). Glenn's Thoracic and Cardiovascular Surgery. 5th ed. East Norwalk, Conn, Appleton & Lange, 1991.
2. Julian OC, Lopez-Belio M, Dye WS, et al. The median sternal incision in intrathoracic surgery with extracorporeal circulation: A general evaluation of its use in heart surgery. Surgery 42:753–761, 1957.
3. Dick RJ, Popma JJ, Muller DW, et al. In-hospital costs associated with new percutaneous coronary devices. Am J Cardiol 68:879–885, 1991.
4. Warner M, Chami Y, Johnson D, Cowley MJ. Directional coronary atherectomy for failed angioplasty due to occlusive coronary dissection. Catheterization and Cardiovascular Diagnosis 24:28–31, 1991.
5. Rowe MH, Hinohara T, White NW, et al. Comparison of dissection rates and angiographic results following directional atheyerectomy and coronary angioplasty. Am J Cardiol 66:49–53, 1990.
6. Mansour M, Carrozza JP, Kuntz RE, et al. Frequency and outcome of chest pain after two new coronary interventions (atherectomy and stenting). Am J Cardiol 69:1379–1382, 1992.
7. Hinohara T, Selmon MR, Robertson GC, et al. Directional atherectomy. New approaches for treatment of obstructive coronary and peripheral vascular disease. Circulation 81(suppl 3):IV79–IV91, 1990.
8. Kuntz RE, Safian RD, Levine MJ, et al. Novel approach to the analysis of restenosis after the use of three new coronary devices. J Am Coll Cardiol 19:1493–1499, 1992.
9. Frye RL, Collins JJ, DiSanctis RW, et al. Guidelines for permanent cardiac pacemaker implantation. J Am Coll Cardiol 4:434–442, 1984.
10. Bernstein AD. Classification of cardiac pacemakers. In: El-Sherif N, Samet P. Cardiac Pacing and Electrophysiology. 3rd ed. Philadelphia, WB Saunders, 1991, pp 494–503.
11. Bilitch M, Hauser RG, Goldman BS, et al. Performance of implantable cardiac rhythm management devices. PACE 10:389–398, 1987.
12. Reul GJ. Implantation of permanent cardiac pacemaker. In: Cooley DA. Techniques in Cardiac Surgery. 2nd ed. Philadelphia, WB Saunders, 1984, pp 75–81.

13. The NASPE/BPEG generic pacemaker code for anti-bradyarrhythmia and adaptive-rate pacing and antitachy-arrhythmia devices. PACE 10:794–799, 1987.
14. Sabiston DC, Spencer FC. Gibbon's Surgery of the Chest. 4th ed. Philadelphia, WB Saunders, 1983.
15. Astrachan DI, Sasaki CT. Tracheotomy. In: Baue AE (ed). Glenn's Thoracic and Cardiovascular Surgery. 5th ed. East Norwalk, Conn, Appleton & Lange, 1991, pp 603–614.
16. Darovic GO. Hemodynamic Monitoring. Philadelphia, WB Saunders, 1987, pp 83–212.
17. Blair SN, Painter P, Pate RR, et al. (eds). Resource Manual for Guidelines for Exercise Testing and Prescription. Philadelphia, Lea & Febiger, 1988, pp 126–129, 212–214.
18. Dalie EK, Schroeder JS. Techniques in Bedside Monitoring. 4th ed. St Louis, CV Mosby, 1989, pp 88–217.
19. Cohen M, Michel TH. Cardiopulmonary Symptoms in Physical Therapy Practice. New York, Churchill Livingstone, 1988, pp 27, 85.
20. Kersten LD. Comprehensive Respiratory Nursing. Philadelphia, WB Saunders, 1989, p 756.
21. Forrester JS. Thermodilution cardiac output determination with a single flow-directed catheter. Am Heart J 83:306–311, 1972.
22. Guyton AC. Textbook of Medical Physiology. 8th ed. Philadelphia, WB Saunders, 1991, pp 118–147, 422–443.
23. White KM. Completing the hemodynamic picture: SvO_2. Heart Lung 14:272–280, 1985.
24. Conover MB. Understanding Electrocardiography. 5th ed. St. Louis, CV Mosby, 1988, pp 75–301.
25. Dubin D. Rapid Interpretation of EKG's. 4th ed. Tampa, Fla, Cover Publishing, 1989, pp 48–157.
26. Brown KR, Jacobson S. Mastering Dysrhythmias: A Problem-Solving Guide. Philadelphia, FA Davis, 1988, pp 3–36.
27. American College of Chest Physicians. Statement on spirometry—A report of the section on respiratory pathophysiology. Chest 83:547–550, 1983.
28. Zapletal A, Samánek M, Paul T. Lung Function in Children and Adolescents—Methods, Reference Values. Basel, Switzerland, S Karger AG, 1987, pp 114–218.
29. Pierson DJ. Weaning from mechanical ventilation in acute respiratory failure: Concepts, indications, and techniques. Respiratory Care 28:646–660, 1983.
30. Jung RC. Weaning criteria for patients on mechanical respiratory assistance. West J Med 131:49, 1979.
31. Hodgkin JE, Gray LS, Burton GG. Techniques of ventilator weaning. In: Burton GG, Hodgkin JE (eds). Respiratory Care. 2nd ed. Philadelphia, JB Lippincott, 1984, pp 648–655.
32. Sahn SA, Lakshminarayan S. Bedside criteria for discontinuation of mechanical ventilation. Chest 63:1002–1005, 1973.
33. Caldwell S, Sullivan K. Artificial Airways. In: Burton G, Hodgkin J (eds). Respiratory Care—A Guide to Clinical Practice. Philadelphia, JB Lippincott, 1984.
34. McPherson SP. Respiratory Therapy Equipment. 3rd ed. St Louis, CV Mosby, 1985, pp 269–583.
35. Leith DE, Bradley M. Ventilatory muscle strength and endurance training. J Appl Physiol 41:508–516, 1976.
36. Gross D, Riley E, Grassino A, et al. Influence of resistive training on respiratory muscle strength and endurance in quadriplegia. Am Rev Respir Dis 117(suppl):343, 1978 (abstract).

SECTION
PHARMACOLOGY 4

12 CARDIAC MEDICATIONS

INTRODUCTION

"Pharmacology can be broadly defined as the science dealing with interactions between living systems and molecules, especially chemicals introduced from outside the system. . . . A drug . . . [is] . . . any small molecule that, when introduced into the body, alters the body's

481

function by interactions at the molecular level."[1] By strict definition, therefore, a drug may both cause disease (e.g., environmental chemicals and hazardous wastes) as well as treat and prevent disease (e.g., medical pharmacology). More specific to this discussion is the role of drugs within a medical setting to prevent, treat, and identify cardiovascular disease.

Although medications have significantly broadened the management of cardiovascular dysfunction, "a drug cannot impart a new function to a cell . . . it modulates ongoing function."[2] The impact of pharmacologic management for the patient with a cardiovascular disorder cannot be underestimated. The responsibility of the physical therapist in treating any individual is to understand the effects and potential side effects of the individual's drug regimen as well as the drugs' influence on the outcome of the physical therapy intervention. This chapter presents the pharmacologic clinical management of the most common cardiovascular dysfunctions.

To appreciate the impact and complexity of drug management, a few supportive concepts should be introduced. Drugs may be prescribed by their generic or trade name. Generic prescriptions incorporate the name of the chemical substance or substances that make up the drug; the trade name (brand name) is the name that the individual drug company assigns to its own product. In this chapter, the generic name appears first, the trade name or names follow in parentheses, for example, **verapamil** (Calan, Isoptin).

The goal of drug therapy is to prescribe the appropriate medication for the individual's needs with the expectation that the medication is delivered to the site of action in adequate strength (therapeutic level) to elicit the appropriate clinical response. The foundation of this goal rests on two broad concepts, **pharmacokinetics** and **pharmacodynamics.**[3] Pharmacokinetics addresses how the drug is absorbed, how much of the drug is available to be delivered to the target site or sites **(bioavailability),** how the drug is distributed, and how the drug is metabolized and excreted. Pharmacodynamics deals with the mechanism of the drug action and the relationship between the drug concentration and the clinical effect[4] (Fig. 12–1).

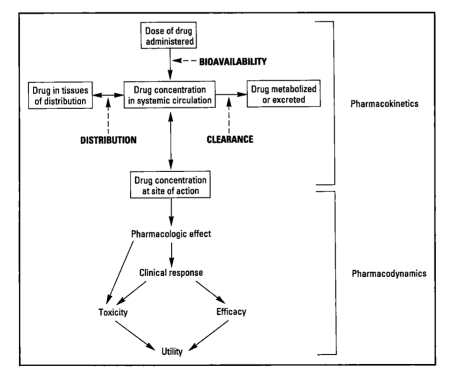

Figure 12–1.

Schematic representation of the pharmacokinetic and pharmacodynamic processes. (From Katzung BG [ed]. Basic and Clinical Pharmacology. 5th ed. East Norwalk, Conn, Appleton & Lange, 1992, p 29.)

PHARMACOKINETICS

Drugs may be administered to the body through different access routes; the two most common are by mouth or by injection. By mouth (oral or p.o.) is also known as **enteral,** indicating that the drug enters the gastrointestinal system before it enters the circulation. Injection is one form of **parenteral** administration, a nongastrointestinal (i.e., nonenteral) route. Parenteral routes bypass the absorption within the gastrointestinal system. See Table 12–1 for examples of drug routes.

Bioavailability

The route of administration affects the bioavailability of the drug and the length of time it takes the drug to work. Drugs taken by mouth are absorbed from the stomach and intestine and then pass through the liver (portal circulation) before reaching the systemic circulation. The active drug may be partially inactivated if it is metabolized in the liver or gastrointestinal system. This partial inactivation as a result of metabolic processes is known as the **first pass effect.** The greater the first pass effect, the less bioavailability of the drug. The liver is the principal organ of drug metabolism and therefore the principal organ for first pass effect.

Parenteral routes by definition bypass the gastrointestinal system, and although there may be some first pass effect through the lungs, the bioavailability is greater and the onset of action is faster than with enteral medications. Because of their fast onset of action, parenteral medications, particularly those using the intravenous and **sublingual** routes, are a key component in the management of hemodynamic stability in emergency and critical care settings. Drugs administered through sublingual routes enter the circulation through the systemic veins that drain the highly vascular oral mucosa and do not pass through the gastrointestinal system or portal circulation. **Nitroglycerin** is perhaps the most widely used sublingual medication. **Lidocaine** (Xylocaine) and **morphine** are two critical care drugs that are given intravenously because of their extensive first pass effects.

TABLE 12–1. Common Routes of Drug Administration

Route	Comments
Parenteral	No gastrointestinal absorption
	Fast acting
Injection	Valuable in emergencies
	May cause pain and tissue damage at injection site
intravenous (IV)	May deliver a high concentration of drug quickly
subcutaneous (SubQ)	Self-administered
intramuscular (IM)	
intrathecal (spinal)	
intraperitoneal	
Buccal (sublingual)	
Inhalational	Quick delivery of drug to bronchi and alveoli for local effect
	Gaseous anesthetic
	Useful with drugs that vaporize quickly
Enteral	Absorbed through the gastrointestinal system
By mouth (p.o.)	Convenient
tablets or capsules	Most common
enteric coated	Effective absorption
sustained release	Usually most economical
chewable	
Liquid	Effective with children
oral solutions	
elixir	
Rectal	May have local or systemic effects
	Effective when gastrointestinal upset precludes use of oral
Transdermal	Slowly absorbed, prolongs blood levels

(Adapted from Gilman AG, Goodman LS, Rall TW, Murad F [eds]. Goodman and Gilman's The Pharmacologic Basis of Therapeutics. 7th ed. New York, Macmillan, 1985, pp 3–10; and Katzung BG [ed]. Basic and Clinical Pharmacology. 4th ed. East Norwalk, Conn, Appleton & Lange, 1989.)

Distribution

After the drug is absorbed into the bloodstream, the next phase of pharmacokinetics occurs: the distribution of the drug throughout the body by means of the circulatory system. Drug distribution may be general or restricted, depending on the ability of the drug to pass through particular cell membranes and on the permeability of the capillaries for the particular drug. Differential distribution may occur as a result of one of the following: drug binding to proteins (especially plasma protein), difficulty of drugs crossing the blood-brain barrier of the central nervous system, or storage of drugs within body tissues (particularly adipose and muscle tissues). Drugs bind to proteins both in the tissues and in the plasma; the most common plasma proteins are **albumin** and **alpha₁-acid-glycoprotein.** As a result of the protein-drug binding, the drug is unavailable to bind with its receptor sites and therefore is unable to exert its pharmacologic effect. Although protein-drug binding is a reversible and dynamic process, it may temporarily limit drug distribution.

Clearance

"Clearance of a drug is the rate of elimination by all routes relative to the concentration of drug in any biologic fluid."[3] Routes of elimination are through the renal, biliary, and pulmonary systems and through fecal matter. The kidneys serve as the most important route for overall drug elimination, whereas the lungs are the major organs for the excretion of gaseous substances. A dysfunction within any of these systems or an inadequate circulatory system to distribute the unbound drug interferes with the clearance of the drug from the body. Drug toxicity may occur if clearance is impeded (e.g., by kidney dysfunction) because the drug level increases. Insufficient drug levels may result if the drug is cleared too rapidly, as it is with diarrhea or vomiting.

Half-life

The time it takes for the plasma concentration of the drug to be reduced by 50% is known as the **half-life.** Half-life serves as a rough indicator of the length of time the effects of the medication will last. The longer the half-life, the longer the effect of the drug.

The frequency of the administration of medication is influenced by half-life; some medications must be taken four times a day (qid) to be most effective; others may be taken only once (qd), twice (bid), or three times a day (tid). Pa-

tients should not try to manipulate the timing of their medications once a routine has been established. Medications need to be taken at regular intervals; a delay in taking the medication, for example, waiting until after a physical therapy appointment, only delays the onset and effectiveness of the medication. In some instances, once a medication schedule has been interrupted, such as a delay in taking pain medications, the usual dosage may be insufficient for patient comfort, and a larger dosage may be necessary. An example of different half-lives can be seen with two commonly used cardiac medications, **digoxin** (Lanoxin) and **propranolol** (Inderal). The half-life of digoxin is 36 hours; that of propranolol is only 3 to 6 hours.

Dosage

In deciding the appropriate dosage of a drug, four variables must be considered:

- The amount of drug to be administered at one time
- The route of administration
- The interval between doses
- The period of time over which drug administration is to be continued[3]

Drugs may be administered by two common methods: continuous input or intermittent doses. Sustained release by mouth and infusions by intravenous or subcutaneous routes are examples of continuous input. The continuous insulin pump is an example of a subcutaneous continuous infusion; intravenous nitroglycerin given temporarily during the acute stages of myocardial ischemia is an example of an intravenous continuous infusion. Medications given at certain time intervals throughout the day by any route are examples of intermittent doses.

PHARMACODYNAMICS

Pharmacodynamics helps us to understand the critical role of drug receptors. Drugs do not have isolated effects on isolated tissues. Drug receptors are located throughout the body; therefore, the drug affects all of the receptors specific to the drug's structure. Pharmacokinetics is affected by many factors, not the least of which is individual metabolism. Any disease or dysfunction of the gastrointestinal system, liver, and kidneys can influence the bioavailability and clearance of the drug. Nutritional habits, use of antacids and laxatives, as well as the natural process of aging itself may also alter an individual's response to a particular drug regimen by affecting both the bioavailability of the drug through altered metabolism and the drug clearance through the gastrointestinal and renal systems.

Drug receptors are cellular macromolecules that are generally, but not exclusively, cellular proteins. The best identified protein receptors are regulatory proteins that mediate the actions of neurotransmitters, hormones, and autacoids—a local hormone-like substance that includes histamines, polypeptides (e.g., angiotensin, bradykinin), and prostaglandins. Besides regulatory proteins, other common drug receptors are enzymes, transport proteins, and structural proteins. The drug and its receptor form a complementary relationship, likened to a lock and key. Receptors may have biochemical functions common to many cells, and, as a result, no drug produces a single effect or affects only a specific tissue. Drugs therefore have primary effects, secondary effects, and side effects. In choosing the appropriate drug, an individual's tolerance to the drug is determined not only by the primary effect, but, just as importantly, by the impact of the secondary and side effects. An example of such a drug-receptor relationship that has generalized systemic effects is that of digitalis and the sodium-potassium pump. Because of digitalis's widespread effects on many types of tissue, varied side effects and a low threshold for toxicity can exist for this powerful drug.

Drugs are selective regarding the type of receptor to which they are attracted but cannot be absolutely specific to a single effect or to a type of tissue. Selectivity means that when a certain concentration of the drug exists, the drug is preferentially attracted to one group or a subgroup of receptors. An example of selectivity can be seen within a very common group of cardiac drugs, the beta blockers. The receptors for the beta blockers (the subgroups beta$_1$ and beta$_2$) are found within the autonomic nervous system. The drug **atenolol** (Tenormin) is a selective beta blocker, affecting only the beta$_1$ receptors; propranolol (Inderal) is a nonselective beta blocker, affecting both beta$_1$ and beta$_2$ receptors.

Agonists and Antagonists

Drugs can be broadly classified as agonists or antagonists. An **agonist** is a drug that initiates a sequence of physiologic and biochemical changes within the cell. An **antagonist** acts as an inhibitor of agonistic activity by inactivating the receptor. A drug may be a complete or partial agonist or antagonist. Many cardiac drugs serve their function by acting as antagonists (e.g., beta-adrenergic antagonists [beta blockers] and calcium channel antagonists [calcium channel blockers]).

Receptors

Although drug receptors are found in many cells of the body, the most common sites for cardiac drug-receptor interactions are the autonomic nervous system (Table 12–2), the kidneys, and the vascular smooth muscle. Other sites such as the central nervous system for the management of hypertension and the blood cells for their role in clotting and lysis are also critically important for achieving cardiovascular stability.

Autonomic Nervous System

Understanding the autonomic nervous system requires a thorough review of its anatomy; please refer to Chapter 1 for more complete detail. The autonomic nervous system contains two divisions; the sympathetic and the parasympathetic nervous systems. One of the distinctions between the two is their postganglionic neurotransmitter substance: acetylcholine in the parasympathetic system and norepinephrine in the sympathetic system. As a result of their neurotransmitters, the receptors of the parasympathetic nervous system are known as **cholinergic,** and the receptors of

TABLE 12–2. Autonomic Receptor Types

Name	Typical Locations
Cholinoceptors Muscarinic[1] M_1	Central nervous system neurons, sympathetic postganglionic neurons, some presynaptic sites
Muscarinic[1] M_2	Myocardium, smooth muscle, some presynaptic sites
Nicotinic	Autonomic ganglia, skeletal muscle neuromuscular end-plate, spinal cord
Adrenoceptors Alpha$_1$	Postsynaptic effector cells, especially smooth muscle
Alpha$_2$	Presynaptic adrenergic nerve terminals, platelets, lipocytes, smooth muscle
Beta$_1$	Postsynaptic effector cells, especially heart; lipocytes, brain, presynaptic noradrenergic nerve terminals
Beta$_2$	Postsynaptic effector cells, especially smooth muscle
Dopamine	Brain and postsynaptic effectors, especially vascular smooth muscle of the splanchnic and renal vascular beds. Presynaptic receptors on nerve terminals, especially in the heart, vessels, and gastrointestinal system

[1]Assignment of muscarinic receptor subtypes is still tentative (Eglen, 1986). (From Katzung BG [ed]. Basic and Clinical Pharmacology. 5th ed. East Norwalk, Conn, Appleton & Lange, 1992, p 75.)

the sympathetic are known as **adrenergic**. The two subdivisions of the adrenergic receptors are the alpha and beta adrenoceptors. Both alpha and beta receptors are responsive to the **catecholamines**: norepinephrine, released at the local level from the sympathetic postganglionic fibers, and epinephrine, released from the adrenal medulla into the circulatory system. The sensitivity of each receptor to catecholamines differs, as does the location and action of each receptor. When alpha receptors in the vascular smooth muscle are stimulated, contraction occurs; when beta receptors are stimulated in the vascular smooth muscle, relaxation occurs. Both alpha and beta receptors are divided further into alpha$_1$ and alpha$_2$ and beta$_1$ and beta$_2$ (Table 12–3). Use of beta-adrenergic antagonists (beta blockers) has formed a cornerstone in the management of coronary artery disease over the past 30 years. Drug research is in progress regarding the new and expanding role for alpha receptors, both alone or in combination with beta receptors.

Sympathomimetics are a group of drugs whose activity mimics the activity of the endogenous chemicals of the sympathetic nervous system (particularly the catecholamines epinephrine, norepinephrine, and dopamine). Sympathomimetics are also known as adrenergic agonists. **Sympatholytic** drugs block the action of the sympathetic nervous system and are also known as adrenergic antagonists.

Cholinergic receptors are either **muscarinic** or **nicotinic**. The site of action for muscarinic receptors is on autonomic effector cells; within the heart the receptors are in the atria and sinoatrial and atrioventricular nodes. The site of action for nicotinic receptors is the end plates of skeletal muscle and autonomic ganglion cells. Cholinergic receptors have minimal direct clinical influence on the cardiovascular system from a pharmacologic point of view. Compared with the expansive impact of the adrenergic receptors, the pharmacologic impact of cholinergic receptors is significantly less.

TABLE 12–3. Distribution of Adrenoceptor Subtypes

Type	Tissue	Actions
Alpha$_1$	Most vascular smooth muscle (innervated)	Contraction
	Pupillary dilator muscle	Contraction (dilates pupil)
	Pilomotor smooth muscle	Erects hair
	Rat liver	Glycogenolysis
	Heart	Increase force of contraction
Alpha$_2$	Postsynaptic central nervous system adrenoceptors	Probably multiple
	Platelets	Aggregation
	Adrenergic and cholinergic nerve terminals	Inhibition of transmitter release
	Some vascular smooth muscle (noninnervated)	Contraction
	Fat cells	Inhibition of lipolysis
Beta$_1$	Heart	Increase force and rate of contraction
	Fat cells	Activate lipolysis
Beta$_2$	Respiratory, uterine, and vascular smooth muscle	Promote smooth muscle relaxation
	Skeletal muscle	Promote potassium uptake
	Human liver	Activate glycogenolysis

(From Katzung BG [ed]. Basic and Clinical Pharmacology. 4th ed. East Norwalk, Conn, Appleton & Lange, 1989, p 98.)

TABLE 12–4. Effects of Direct-Acting Cholinoceptor Stimulants

Organ	Response
Eye	
Sphincter muscle of iris	Contraction (miosis)
Ciliary muscle	Contraction for near vision
Heart	
Sinoatrial node	Decrease in rate (negative chronotropy)
Atria	Decrease in contractile strength (negative inotropy)
	Decrease in refractory period
Atrioventricular node	Decrease in conduction velocity (negative dromotropy)
	Increase in refractory period
Ventricles	Small decrease in contractile strength
Blood vessels	Dilation (via EDRF)
Arteries	Constriction (high dose direct effect)
Veins	Dilation (via EDRF)
	Constriction (high dose direct effect)
Lung	
Bronchial muscle	Contraction (bronchoconstriction)
Bronchial glands	Stimulation
Gastrointestinal tract	
Motility	Increase
Sphincters	Relaxation
Secretion	Stimulation
Urinary bladder	
Detrusor	Contraction
Trigone and sphincter	Relaxation
Glands	
Sweat, salivary, lacrimal, nasopharyngeal	Secretion

EDRF = endothelium releasing factor.
(From Katzung BG [ed]. Basic and Clinical Pharmacology. 5th ed. East Norwalk, Conn, Appleton & Lange, 1992, p 86.)

Stimulation by cholinergic activating drugs (e.g., acetylcholine) through the muscarinic receptors results in decreased contractility and heart rate and a reduction in peripheral vascular resistance. Stimulation by cholinergic blocking drugs (e.g., atropine) through the muscarinic receptors results in increased heart rate. Nicotinic receptor stimulation of the autonomic ganglia has sympathetic-like effects on the cardiovascular system and may result in tachycardia and hypertension. Blocking of the nicotinic receptors' influence on the cardiovascular system decreases arteriolar and venomotor tone, thereby decreasing both blood pressure and venous return. Cholinergic drugs that simulate parasympathetic activity are known as **parasympathomimetic** or cholinergic agonists; conversely, drugs that block cholinergic activity are known as **parasympatholytic** or cholinergic antagonists (Table 12–4).

Kidney

Drug receptor sites within the kidneys are found within the proximal tubule, collecting tubule and ducts, and Henle's loop. Refer to the section on antihypertension drugs and to Figure 12–7 for the site of action and the effect of specific drugs.

Vascular Smooth Muscle

Receptors within vascular muscle appear to be the site of action for nitrates and calcium channel blockers.

PHARMACOLOGIC MANAGEMENT

Management of cardiac dysfunction often involves the prescription of a multifaceted drug regimen that must be dynamic in its ability to respond to an individual's needs. Long-term use of certain drugs may cause a desensitization of the receptor to that drug such that the dosage may need to be altered, the drug replaced, or an additional drug prescribed to supplement the initial drug. The cost of drugs often influences which drug (generic or trade) or class of drugs is prescribed when a choice is available. Patient compliance is also influenced by drug cost; some patients choose to decrease the frequency of their medications "to save money" or avoid taking the drug at all. Patients are often unaware of the consequences of self-regulation of medications; many cardiac drugs cannot be stopped abruptly without significant deleterious effects. Previously tolerated drugs may become a problem following the flu, gastrointestinal upset, or change in metabolism.

The awareness of all health care professionals that a drug cannot work unless it is taken as prescribed should sensitize prescribers of drugs to the issues that contribute to noncompliance: cost of drug, difficulty in following a complicated drug regimen, poorly tolerated side effects, and undesirable interactions with other prescribed medications are just a few examples. Often a drug that is poorly tolerated may be exchanged for a similar drug that produces the same clinical effect but with less troublesome side effects to the patient.

ANTI-ISCHEMIC DRUGS

Dramatic changes have taken place during the latter part of the twentieth century in the pharmacologic management of ischemic heart disease. With the introduction of beta blockers, calcium channel blockers, thrombolytic agents, and the critical care regimen of **vasopressors** and positive **inotropes,** hemodynamic stability has been established in many individuals who formerly might have led the lifestyle of the "cardiac cripple" at best or faced death at worst. Coronary artery disease still exists, however, holding the unfortunate distinction of being the number one cause of death in the United States. Present drug therapy is limited to dealing with the sequelae of this ravaging disease and not its prevention. Perhaps with aggressive lifestyle changes and frugal management of blood lipid levels, the twenty-first century will render a discussion such as this obsolete.

Physiology

The heart is an oxygen-dependent organ whose energy needs are met by aerobic metabolism. Oxygen is delivered to the myocardium and conducting tissues via the coronary arteries. Adequate myocardial oxygen supply is dependent on many factors, most particularly the coronary blood flow, the oxygen-carrying capacity of blood, and the anatomy of coronary arteries (especially the lumen diameter). When myocardial oxygen demand (MVo_2) increases, such as with exercise, myocardial oxygen supply is increased by an increase in coronary blood flow.

Myocardial oxygen demand is affected by afterload, systolic wall tension, wall thickness, contractile state, preload, heart rate, and left ventricular volume and diameter. Although many factors influence myocardial oxygen demand, MVo_2 may be clinically assessed as the product of heart rate and systolic blood pressure. This clinical method for MVo_2 assessment is called the double product or **rate-pressure product.**

Pathophysiology

Unlike striated muscle, the myocardium can function without adequate oxygen for only a relatively short period of time. The myocardium receives its oxygen through coronary blood flow. When coronary blood flow is inadequate to meet the myocardial oxygen demands, the tissue becomes **ischemic.** Demand is increased under conditions that increase heart rate, blood pressure, or both: exercise; increased systemic vascular resistance; high output states such as pregnancy, fever, and increased thyroid function; anemia; emotional stress; and anxiety are but a few examples.

The supply of oxygenated blood to the myocardium can be decreased when arterial oxygen content is decreased **(hypoxemia)** or lumen size is reduced. The most common cause of decreased supply is coronary artery disease. The atherosclerotic plaque associated with coronary artery disease reduces lumen size and therefore blood flow. Lumen diameter may also be decreased as a result of smooth muscle spasm within the walls of the coronary artery; spasm may occur in the presence or absence of coronary artery disease.

In an acute myocardial infarction, a thrombus may form at the site of the atherosclerotic lesion and further occlude the lumen. Three steps are necessary for thrombus formation[5]:

- A conducive surface (such as damaged intravascular endothelium) on which the thrombus can form
- A sequence of platelet-mediated events: platelet adhesion, followed by platelet aggregation, followed by release of agents further stimulating platelet aggregation and vasoconstriction

● Activation of the clotting mechanism and the formation of fibrin

A clot is made up of insoluble fibrin filaments that join together to form a durable mesh. Fibrin comes from the protein fibrinogen that is produced in the liver and present in the plasma. Fibrinogen is a stable structure and only converts to fibrin under the influence of **thrombin.**

Thrombin comes from **prothrombin,** a normal protein constituent of plasma. The formation of thrombin from prothrombin requires a highly complex, integrated network. Adequate calcium, phospholipids, and at least seven plasma proteins (factor XI, factor XII, factor IX, factor VIII, factor X, factor V, factor XIII) are necessary for thrombin formation. Also required is the interaction of **thromboplastin,** released by the injured tissue, with factor X[6] (Fig. 12–2A). The role of platelets and the clotting factors necessary for the formation of thrombin are referred to as intrinsic clotting factors; the role of tissue thromboplastin is referred to as an extrinsic clotting factor.

Under normal conditions, the process of lysing a blood clot takes place over many days. The plasma enzyme plasmin actively digests the fibrin, fibrinogen, and prothrombin.[6] Plasmin, however, must first be activated by its precursor, plasminogen (Fig. 12–2B).

Pharmacologic Intervention

Pharmacologic management of myocardial ischemia involves the reestablishment of a balance between myocardial oxygen supply and myocardial oxygen demand. Drugs that either decrease heart rate or systemic blood pressure decrease myocardial oxygen demand. Drugs that increase arterial lumen size by decreasing either coronary arterial spasm or thrombus increase myocardial oxygen supply. At present, no drug exists that directly decreases a fixed atherosclerotic lesion. Reduction of risk factors for coronary artery disease and directed lipid management with or without the use of drugs have been postulated to result in a regression of coronary plaque.

Decreasing Myocardial Oxygen Demand

Current practice includes the use of beta blockers, calcium channel blockers, and nitrates to decrease MVo_2 by decreasing peripheral vascular resistance, decreasing venous return (preload), decreasing heart rate, or a combination of the three.

Beta Blockers (Table 12–5). Beta-adrenergic antagonists compete with the catecholamines epinephrine and norepinephrine for beta receptor binding sites, thereby preventing the catecholamines from binding. Beta-antagonist activity may be complete (without catecholamine stimulation) or partial (some catecholamine stimulation). Of the two beta subtypes, $beta_1$ receptors are found primarily in the myocardium and have an equal affinity for epinephrine and norepinephrine; $beta_2$ receptors are also found in the myocardium (especially the atria), but comparatively more are within the peripheral circulation and bronchi, and they have a higher affinity for epinephrine. Inhibition of catecholamine stimulation by beta blockers affects the cardiovascular system by decreasing heart rate, decreasing contractility, decreasing cardiac output, and decreasing blood pressure.

Drugs that block both $beta_1$ and $beta_2$ receptors are referred to as nonselective; drugs that block $beta_1$ receptors are referred to as cardioselective or $beta_1$ selective. Patients with disease

TABLE 12–5. Beta-Adrenergic Antagonists: Beta Blockers

Category	Generic (Trade)
Nonselective	Propranolol (Inderal)
	Timolol (Blocadren)
	Nadolol (Corgard)
	Pindolol (Visken)
	Labetalol (Normodyne)
Beta₁ selective	Metropolol (Lopressor)
	Atenolol (Tenormin)
	Acebutolol (Sectral)
	Esmolol (Brevibloc)
	Alprenolol
Beta₂ selective	Butoxamine
Alpha and beta antagonists	Labetalol (Normodyne, Trandate)

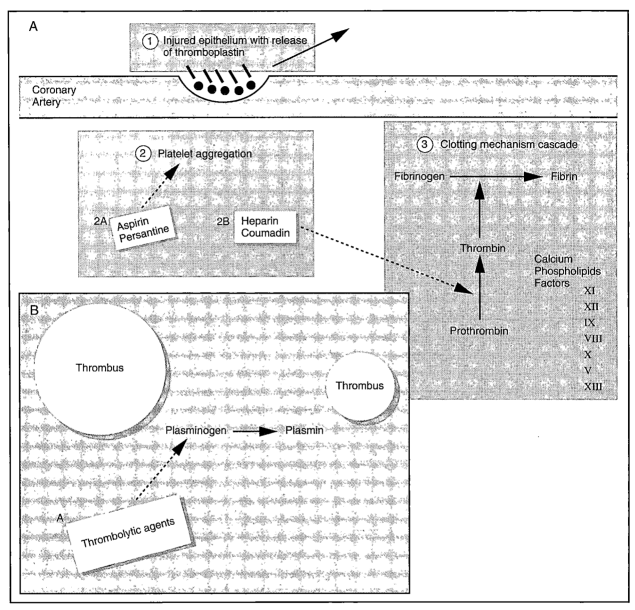

Figure 12-2.

A, Clot formation. The three steps for clot formation within the coronary artery: (1) injured epithelium with release of tissue thromboplastin, (2) platelet aggregation, and (3) clotting mechanism. Site of action of drugs: (A) aspirin and persantine—antiplatelet agents; (B) heparin and coumadin—anticoagulants. *B*, Clot lysis. Site of action of drugs: (A) thrombolytic agents.

processes involving the peripheral circulation and bronchi (the sites of beta$_2$ receptors) pose a challenging problem in drug management when they require beta blockers. Beta$_1$-selective drugs rather than a nonselective beta blocker are usually pre-scribed to avoid the vasoconstriction effects of beta$_2$ antagonists. Because no currently available beta$_1$-selective antagonist is able to avoid completely interactions with beta$_2$ receptors, there are some beta$_2$ effects[7]; therefore, patients with chronic obstructive pulmonary disease or peripheral vascular disease may have their noncardiac symptoms worsened by the use of beta blockers. Caution must be exercised in the prescription of beta blockers as with all drugs. At present, the class of $beta_2$-selective antagonists is limited to the drug butoxamine, which has little cardiovascular effect except to inhibit an increase in both heart rate and smooth muscle relaxation.

In a relatively newer class of drugs, beta blockers may combine with alpha-adrenergic blockers. This combination results in a decrease in systemic vascular resistance without a compensatory increase in heart rate. The alpha blocking component causes vasodilation and thus results in decreased systemic vascular resistance. The beta-blocking component suppresses the compensatory rise in heart rate that would be expected with alpha blockade alone and therefore also limits the increase in MV_{O_2}. This class of drugs, of which **labetalol** (Normodyne, Trandate) is an example, is used primarily for hypertension control.

Side Effects of Beta Blockers. The potential side effects associated with the use of beta blockers are varied. "Three major mechanisms . . . (of side effects) . . . are through (1) central nervous penetration (dreams), (2) smooth muscle spasm (bronchospasm and cold extremities), and (3) exaggeration of the cardiac therapeutic actions (bradycardia, heart block, excess negative inotropic effect with heart failure)."[8] $Beta_1$-selective drugs such as atenolol (Tenormin) should have fewer peripheral side effects of bronchospasm, cold extremities, worsening claudication, and sexual dysfunction than nonselective drugs like propranolol (Inderal). Beta blockers also may cause fatigue, insomnia, masking of symptoms of hypoglycemia in diabetic patients, impaired glucose tolerance, **hypertriglyceridemia,** and decreased high-density lipoprotein (HDL) cholesterol. **Pindolol** (Visken) and **acebutolol** (Sectral), however, do not appear to decrease HDL cholesterol.

Clinical Considerations. The popularity of beta blockers as part of an anti-ischemic regimen cannot be disputed. Beta blockers, however, have also been used in the treatment of the following conditions: cardiac arrhythmias; glaucoma; hy-

perthyroidism; mitral valve prolapse; and various neurologic disorders, such as migraine headaches, alcohol withdrawal, and anxiety. Awareness of the potential side effects of beta blockade for these patient populations is certainly clinically relevant. As with patients with peripheral vascular disease and chronic obstructive pulmonary disease, the use of $beta_1$-selective drugs may also be preferred for patients with diabetes. $Beta_2$ receptors of the liver activate glycogenolysis; use of a $beta_1$-selective drug minimizes the suppression of this critical function. Poor tolerance of one beta blocker does not mean that all beta blockers will be poorly tolerated; experimentation and trial and error are credible clinical tools in assessing the compatibility of the drug with the patient.

Because beta blockers are negative inotropes, patients with decreased contractility (particularly if the ejection fraction is below 35%) are generally not appropriate candidates for this drug. If a patient on a beta blocker begins to complain of dyspnea, ankle or extremity edema, orthopnea, or other signs of heart failure, the appropriate physical therapy intervention is to avoid treatment until the primary physician has been notified. Once the patient has stabilized and is medically cleared to continue with physical therapy, treatment should begin slowly and patient tolerance should be assessed on an ongoing basis.

Beta blockers decrease both resting and exercise heart rates. Before prescribing aerobic exercise for a patient on beta blockers, it is necessary to know the results of the patient's performance on an exercise tolerance test given with the same drug and dosage that the patient is presently taking. There does not appear to be a reliable relationship between heart rate and drug dosages among individual drugs. A patient who was changed from propranolol (Inderal) to metropolol (Lopressor) has a different exercise heart rate response on each drug and may therefore need a new exercise prescription, a new exercise tolerance test, or both.

A potentially interesting relationship may exist between weight control and beta blockers. Fat cells have $beta_1$ receptors, which, when stimulated, activate **lipolysis.** With beta blockade, lipolysis is inhibited. Clinical observation has been that patients on beta blockers have a difficult time achieving weight loss. Whether this is owing to decreased metabolism, fatigue, lipocyte inhibition, or some other factor or combination of factors remains to be seen.

Calcium Channel Blockers. Calcium channel blockers do not fit exclusively into either category of decreasing myocardial oxygen demand or increasing myocardial oxygen supply; they influence both. For the structure of this chapter only, calcium channel blockers are discussed under the section regarding increasing myocardial oxygen supply; its effects on myocardial oxygen demand as well as supply are discussed at that time.

Nitrates. First synthesized in 1846, nitroglycerin and its analogues are perhaps one of the oldest anti-ischemic medications. This group of drugs is unusually selective, that is, the effect of nitrates is almost exclusively on smooth muscle cells, in particular on vascular smooth muscle. Nitroglycerin acts in at least three ways:

- as a venodilator, decreasing venous return (preload)
- as an arteriodilator, thus decreasing afterload
- as a relaxant for coronary artery smooth muscle, thus possibly increasing coronary blood supply

The possibility that nitrates may also redistribute blood flow to ischemic subendocardial tissue has been postulated.[9] The major contribution to anti-ischemia from nitroglycerin, however, comes from its decrease of myocardial demand, specifically in its ability to decrease venous return and left ventricular filling pressures. Besides their use for anti-ischemia, nitrates may also be prescribed for the management of congestive heart failure by decreasing preload and for the control of diastolic hypertension.

Many different preparations of nitrates are available. Routes of administration and duration of action vary widely among the preparations, from the immediate- and short-acting sublingual nitroglycerin to the slow release, longer-acting transdermal patch (Table 12–6).

Clinical Considerations. Perhaps the side effect of nitrate therapy most troublesome to patients is headache, particularly with the short-acting sublingual tablet and in the "adjustment" stage when a long-acting transdermal patch is started. Other potential side effects resulting from the vasodilator action are

- hypotension
- reflex tachycardia
- flushing of the skin
- nausea and vomiting

Because hypotension may accompany the use of nitrates, it may be recommended that patients who are taking sublingual nitroglycerin for the first time sit down. If a patient in the physical therapy clinic takes a sublingual nitroglycerin tablet either before or as a result of a physical therapy intervention, it is important to reevaluate both the intervention and the patient (e.g., heart rate, blood pressure) before making a decision to continue. Use of prophylactic sublingual nitroglycerin is sometimes recommended before exercise, but this decision must be by physician order and cannot be decided solely by the physical therapist and patient. Patients should also be told to store nitroglycerin in a dark glass jar and to keep it tightly closed; once the jar is opened the tablets lose their potency. Unused sublingual nitroglycerin should be discarded within 3 months of opening unless suggested otherwise by the manufacturer. Active sublingual nitroglycerin gives a burning sensation when placed under the tongue. If the nitroglycerin does not "burn," the effect of the drug may be substantially reduced. Nitroglycerin is also available in the form of a lingual spray, which has a longer shelf life than the sublingual preparations.

Long-acting nitrates may cause a nitrate tolerance to develop, such that the drug receptors become desensitized. Use of interval dosage, with nitrate-free times, may prolong receptor site sensitivity. Patients must be informed that they are not to alter their prescribed drug schedule without consulting their health care provider. Nitrates must be given along their prescribed route; for example, taking sublingual nitroglycerin orally markedly decreases its effectiveness.

Increasing Myocardial Oxygen Supply

Pharmocologic interventions to increase myocardial oxygen supply in coronary artery disease

TABLE 12–6. Nitrate Preparations

Generic	Category (Trade or Common Name)	Comments: Duration
Amyl nitrate inhalation	(Aspirol, Vaporole)	10 sec–10 min
Nitroglycerin (glyceryl trinitrate)	(Nitro-Bid, Nitrostat, others)	
sublingual		1½ min–1 hr peak: 2 min
spray		Effects apparent in 5 min: duration unknown
percutaneous ointment		3–4 hr
oral; sustained release		8–12 hr
intravenous		During infusion and 30 min after infusion
transdermal patch	(Nitrodur)	Initial reports up to 24 hr (not confirmed)
	(Transderm-Nitro)	As above
	(Nitrodisc)	As above
Isosorbide dinitrate	(Isordil, Sorbitrate)	
sublingual		5–60 min
oral		15 min–4 hr
chewable		2 min–2½ hr
oral, sustained release		reported 2–6 hr free from angina
Pentaerythritol tetranitrate		
sublingual	(Peritrate)	10–30 min
oral	(Pentrinitrol)	30 min–12 hr
oral	(Pentafin)	4–5 hr
sustained release	(Vasitol)	30 min–12 hr
Erythrityl tetranitrate		
oral	(Tetranitrol)	30 min–4 hr
oral	(Erythrol tetranitrate)	30 min– 2–4 hr
sublingual	(Cardilate)	5 min– 2–4 hr

(Adapted from Opie LH [ed]. Drugs for the Heart. 2nd expanded ed. Philadelphia, WB Saunders, 1987, pp 22–23; and Hahn AB, Barkin RL, Oestrrich, SJK, Pharmacology in Nursing. 15th ed. St. Louis, CV Mosby, 1982, p 595.)

are limited. Although calcium channel blockers and nitrates may have secondary effects of coronary vasodilation and calcium channel blockers can decrease coronary artery spasm, no direct way exists to increase coronary blood flow in the presence of ischemic heart disease. Over the past decade, the management of an acute myocardial infarction has broadened to include the use of thrombolytic agents.

Thrombolytic Agents. The purpose of these drugs is to acutely destroy (lyse) or decrease the blood clot (thrombus) formation that occurs within the coronary artery at the time of the myocardial infarction. In doing so, some coronary blood flow within the affected area is maintained, and reduction in infarction size may be possible. Use of thrombolytic therapy is reserved for a selected group of patients. Although protocols may vary among institutions, general guidelines are that thrombolytic agents should be given within 3 to 4 hours from the onset of myocardial ischemia and with evidence of ST

elevation on the electrocardiogram (ECG).[10] For certain patients, thrombolytic treatment may be effective up to 6 hours after the onset of ischemic symptoms if there is persistent ST elevation with symptoms yet no evidence of extensive Q wave development on the ECG.[10] The patient should have no history of bleeding abnormalities, cerebral vascular events, or uncontrolled hypertension. Even under ideal conditions, only 75% of patients are successfully *reperfused* with thrombolytic therapy and of those that are reperfused, 10% to 20% experience early reocclusion.[10] Thrombolytic agents facilitate the conversion of plasminogen to plasmin, and therefore clot lysis can occur quickly rather than over a period of days.

Streptokinase (Kabikinase, Streptase), **urokinase** (Abbokinase), and **alteplase recombinant tPA** (Activase, t-PA) are examples of thrombolytic agents presently used in the United States. Other drugs undergoing study are **anisoylated plasminogen streptokinase activator complex**

(APSAC, Eminase), and single-chain urokinase plasminogen activator (SCU-PA, prourokinase). Streptokinase liberates plasmin from plasminogen. It is not fibrin specific and therefore produces systemic lysis. In contrast, t-PA is fibrin specific, thereby causing less systemic effects than streptokinase. Clinically, however, no significant difference in the risk of serious bleeding complications has been identified among the thrombolytic agents.[11]

Clinical Considerations. Care must be taken with thrombolytic agents to avoid situations of potential tissue trauma such as venipunctures, manual shaving, resistive exercises, or soft tissue injury because the patient's blood clotting ability is markedly altered during this period. Cardiac rehabilitation physical therapy, including progressive ambulation, may proceed within established acceptable guidelines.

Although thrombolytic agents may limit the amount of myocardial tissue damage, the use of these agents is not without risk. Thrombolytic agents are not absolutely tissue specific; therefore, systemic bleeding may occur as well as lysis of the coronary thrombus. Potential undesirable side effects include

- cerebral vascular accidents
- genitourinary bleeding
- gastrointestinal bleeding

Ventricular arrhythmias are common within the acute time frame following thrombolysis and are believed to be in response to tissue reperfusion and do not therefore require prolonged antiarrhythmic management.

Antiplatelet Agents. Antiplatelet agents are given prophylactically to prevent thrombus formation by decreasing the platelets' ability to adhere and aggregate at the site of the injury. Commonly used agents for this purpose are **salicylic acid** (aspirin, ASA) and **dipyridamole** (Persantine).

Anticoagulants. **Anticoagulants** are used prophylactically to prevent blood clot formation. These agents inhibit the formation of thrombin and therefore negate the influence of thrombin on fibrinogen. Anticoagulants may also be used when a thrombus is already formed to prevent emboli. Commonly used agents are **heparin**

(Liquaemin Sodium) and **warfarin** (Coumadin). Table 12–7 summarizes common drugs and their sites of action.

Calcium Channel Blockers. There are two sources of calcium:

- intracellular calcium, stored within the sarcoplasmic reticulum
- extracellular calcium, stored within the plasma

Different tissue types have an affinity for the different sources of calcium. Smooth muscle in both the coronary arteries and peripheral vascular system and in the sinoatrial and atrioventricular nodes is more dependent on extracellular calcium; striated muscle, myocardium, and coronary veins have a primary affinity for intracellular calcium.

Calcium plays a key role in muscular contraction. The process of muscular contraction requires the availability of actin, myosin, troponin, tropomyosin and calcium. In order for actin and myosin to form cross bridges, calcium must bind with **troponin**. Troponin, when not bound to calcium, inhibits coupling of actin and myosin. In the absence of calcium, troponin is free to inhibit the actin-myosin interaction, thereby inhibiting contraction. Calcium channel blockers block the entrance of calcium into the cell from the extracellular stores. Calcium channel blockers therefore prevent smooth muscle contractions within the coronary artery (i.e., coronary spasm).

Calcium channel blockers were initially used as part of an anti-ischemic regimen because of their ability to decrease vasospasm in the coro-

TABLE 12–7. Common Drugs and Site of Action

Anticoagulants
 Heparin sodium (Heparin): decreases thrombin activity, thereby preventing formation of stable clot (A 2d)
 Warfarin sodium (Coumadin): decreases prothrombin activity (A 2d)

Antiplatelets: decrease platelet aggregation (A 1b)
 Acetylsalicylic acid (aspirin)
 Dipyridamole (Persantine)

Thrombolytic Agents: facilitate the conversion of plasminogen to plasmin
 Streptokinase (Streptase)
 Urokinase (Abbokinase)
 Alteplase recombinant tPa (Activase)

nary arteries. In addition to that primary role, specific calcium channel blockers are now also used for

● arrhythmia control, particularly supraventricular tachycardia
● blood pressure control
● reducing the incidence of reinfarction in patients with non–Q wave infarcts
● treatment of postinfarction angina (Table 12–8).

(See the following sections on drug management of hypertension and arrhythmia for further discussion.)

"Calcium channel antagonists have made a substantial contribution to the patients with ischemic heart disease. For patients with postinfarction ischemic syndromes, the addition of a calcium channel antagonist to the medical regimen can often provide salutary effects."[11] Myocardial ischemia causes an influx of calcium ions into the cell. This increase in intracellular calcium elevates the cellular metabolic rate, which, in turn, elevates myocardial oxygen demand. Ischemia increases the energy demand on tissue that already has compromised perfusion. When calcium channel blockers are used for postinfarction ischemia, potential infarction size may be decreased.

Clinical Considerations. Although calcium channel blockers are relatively safe drugs with few serious side effects, these medications may have negative inotropic properties at high doses; therefore, clinical observation for heart failure is warranted. **Orthostatic hypotension** often occurs in the initiation and regulation of dosages of **nifedipine** (Procardia), so the clinician should be sensitized to watching for orthostatic signs and symptoms when initiating an increase in activity orders or when assisting the patient out of bed for the first time.

HEART FAILURE

"In the United States, an estimated 400,000 individuals develop heart failure annually: it is thus the most common inpatient diagnosis of patients older than 65 years. . . . The most common causes of congestive heart failure in the United States are as follows: (1) coronary artery disease with destruction of contractile muscle tissue, (2) systemic hypertension, (3) chronic alcoholism, (4) diabetes mellitus, (5) idiopathic dilated cardiomyopathy, (6) valvular heart disease."[12]

Heart failure may be chronic, low level, and easily managed by oral medications over a period of years. Heart failure may also be acute and life threatening, requiring the use of parenteral medications to maintain an adequate cardiac output. The medical management of heart failure includes preload reduction with diuretics, venodilators, or angiotensin converting enzyme (ACE) inhibitors; increased inotropy with cardiac glycosides, sympathomimetics, or bipyridines; and afterload reduction with arteriodilators, calcium channel blockers, or ACE inhibitors.

Physiology

For a more complete review of cardiovascular physiology, please refer to Chapter 2. The following serves only as a brief review of key concepts influential in the drug management of heart failure.

The heart is a pump, the function of which is to provide oxygenated blood to all parts of the body. The amount of blood that the heart is able

TABLE 12–8. Calcium Channel Blockers

Generic (Trade)	Common Usage*	Comments/ Side Effects
Nifedipine (Procardia, Adalat)	Blood pressure control	—
Verapamil (Isoptin, Calan)	Supraventricular arrhythmias	Flushing
Diltiazem (Cardizem)	Ischemic heart disease	Peripheral edema Constipation‡
Nicardipine (Cardene)	Blood pressure control	Orthostatic hypotension† Headache
Isradipine (DynaCirc)	Similar to nifedipine but may have less reflex tachycardia	Dizziness Tachycardia

*Prevention of coronary spasm is common to all.
†Especially nifedipine.
‡Especially verapamil and diltiazem.

to pump per minute is called the cardiac output. Cardiac output is directly affected by stroke volume (the amount the ventricle pumps out with each heart beat) and the heart rate (the number of heart beats per minute). The factors that influence stroke volume are preload, afterload, and contractility. Preload—the filling pressure of the left ventricle (left ventricular end diastolic pressure)—is influenced by venous return and the distensibility of the left ventricle. Afterload—the resistance against which the left ventricle contracts—is influenced by arterial pressure and resistance across the aortic valve. Contractility (inotropy)—the ability of the myocardial muscle to contract—is dependent on adequate amounts of calcium, sodium, and potassium to facilitate cellular depolarization and actin-myosin interaction. Drugs that increase myocardial contractility are known as positive inotropes and drugs that decrease contractility as negative inotropes.

Pathophysiology

Heart failure occurs when the heart is unable (i.e., fails) to provide sufficient cardiac output to serve the needs of the body. Heart failure occurs, therefore, because of an inadequate heart rate, stroke volume, or both or, more specifically, because of failure of their components: rhythm, preload, afterload, or contractility. A few clinical examples of situations that may induce heart failure are

- arrhythmias
- increased preload associated with fluid overload
- increased afterload as seen with hypertension
- significant loss of contractile tissue such as with a myocardial infarction
- significant decrease in contractility as a result of ischemia

There are many degrees of heart failure, from mild (compensated), in which the symptoms of decreased cardiac output are apparent only with moderate activity, to severe (uncompensated), in which the heart fails to provide adequate cardiac output even at rest. Heart failure may progress from mild to severe and therefore requires dynamic, ongoing reevaluation and aggressive pharmacologic intervention as determined by the degree of hemodynamic compromise. Heart failure, however, may also remain mild over a period of years, hemodynamically well controlled with medications and without further progression.

Pharmacologic Intervention

Drug management of heart failure attempts to address the underlying cause of the failure and to maintain an adequate cardiac output. Initial treatment of mild heart failure involves regulating fluids, decreasing preload, and improving contractility through oral medications. As the hemodynamic compromise progresses and the clinical picture worsens, medical management broadens to include afterload reduction, parenteral medications, oxygen, and sedation (to decrease anxiety and metabolic energy) (see Table 12–15). The five categories of drugs commonly used for the management of heart failure are

- diuretics
- positive inotropes
- vasodilators
- ACE inhibitors
- morphine (Table 12–9)

Diuretics

As a first-line drug for the management of heart failure, diuretics decrease circulating blood volume, thereby decreasing preload. Diuretics encourage **diuresis** and influence water and electrolyte balance by inhibiting sodium and water reabsorption. The influence on diuresis is dependent on the site of action of the drug within the kidneys. The strongest diuretics are those that act at Henle's loop; the milder diuretics are those that act on the proximal tubules and the collecting tubules and ducts. The most common diuretic for symptomatic heart failure is the loop diuretic **furosemide** (Lasix), which, besides sodium inhibition, also inhibits the movement of potassium and chloride across the plasma membrane of the ascending Henle's loop.

TABLE 12–9. Pharmacologic Management of Heart Failure

Category	Generic (Trade)	Side Effects/Comments
	Diuretics	
Thiazide Thiazide-like Loop Potassium sparing Osmotic Combination	See Table 12–12	
	Positive Inotropes	
Cardiac glycosides Digitalis	Digitoxin (Crystodigin) Digoxin (Lanoxin) Deslanoside (Cedilanid-DIV)	Toxicity common
Sympathomimetics Beta$_1$	Dobutamine (Dobutrex) Prenalterol (investigational)	Arrhythmias
Nonselective beta	Epinephrine (Adrenalin Chloride) Isoproterenol (Isuprel)	Tachycardia
Dopaminergic	Dopamine (Intropin, Dopastat)	Myocardial ischemia similar to beta
Mixed alpha and beta	Norepinephrine (Levophed)	May cause dangerous decrease in peripheral blood flow
Bipyridines	Amrinone (Inocor; parenteral)	Nausea and vomiting Thrombocytopenia Ventricular ectopy Liver abnormalities
	Vasodilators	
Venodilators Nitrates Arteriolar	See Table 12–6 Hydralazine (Apresoline) Minoxidil (Loniten)	Hydralazine:tachycardia Palpitations, orthostatic hypotension, rebound hypotension Fluid retention Both hydralazine and minoxidil should be used with a beta blocker and diuretic. Minoxidil is useful when renal failure accompanies heart failure.
	Nifedipine (Procardia) Diazoxide (Hyperstat IV)	See Table 12–8
Combined arteriolar and venodilator	Sodium nitroprusside (Nipride)	Rapid onset of action, delivery via infusion pump May result in excess hypotension, metabolic acidosis, and arrhythmias
	Angiotensin-Converting	
Enzyme Inhibitor	Captopril (Capoten) Enalapril (Vasotec) Lisinopril (Prinivil, Zestril)	Hypotension Renal failure Neutropenia Skin rashes Taste disturbances
	Analgesic	
	Morphine sulfate (Morphine, MS Contin)	Used in acute pulmonary edema

Diuretics that produce only mild diuresis are not adequate for moderate to severe heart failure. The subsequent section on antihypertension drugs provides an expanded list of diuretics and their sites of action (see Fig. 12–8; Table 12–12).

Positive Inotropes

Three categories of drugs increase contractility: cardiac glycosides, sympathomimetics, and bipyridines.

Cardiac Glycosides. One of the oldest classes of cardiac medications, cardiac glycosides is represented by the drug **digitalis.** Digitalis is available in several different preparations, the most common of which are **digitoxin** (Crystodigin) and digoxin (Lanoxin, Lanoxicaps). Digoxin appears to be the more commonly used of the two preparations, perhaps owing to its comparatively shorter half-life and therefore decreased risk of toxicity. Digitalis increases contractility by inhibiting the sodium-potassium-ATPase enzyme, which normally provides the energy for the sodium-potassium pump (NA$^+$-K$^+$ pump). The Na$^+$-K$^+$ pump expels Na$^+$, accumulated during depolarization, from the cell and brings in K$^+$ during repolarization. By binding to the enzyme, digitalis inhibits the active transport of sodium and potassium, thereby increasing intracellular sodium. An increase in intracellular sodium results in an ionic exchange of intracellular sodium for extracellular calcium (Ca^{++}). The resultant increase in intracellular calcium stimulates large quantities of calcium to be released from the sarcoplasmic reticulum and to be available for excitation-contraction. Myocardial contractility is therefore increased as a result of increased calcium. Patients in chronic heart failure who experience limited hemodynamic compromise are commonly managed with digitalis.

Diuretics and digitalis are frequently prescribed together as successful agents for the management of chronic heart failure. In the setting of heart failure, particularly with ventricular dilation, myocardial contraction is often inefficient and results in an increase in myocardial oxygen demand. Diuretics reduce preload with resultant improvement in the ventricular length-tension relationship. This improved mechanical advantage allows more actin and myosin to interact, and contractility becomes more energy efficient. Myocardial oxygen demand is reduced, and heart failure improves.

Besides its positive inotropic effects, digitalis also has both negative **chronotropic** (decreased heart rate) and negative **dromotropic** (conduction delay) action; the dromotropic effect being primarily on the atrioventricular conduction system. The bradycardic and delayed atrioventricular node conduction effect of digitalis is especially useful in the treatment of atrial fibrillation (see the subsequent section on antiarrhythmic drugs).

Digitalis toxicity may occur for a variety of reasons. The more common causes are

- the interaction of digitalis with other drugs
- decreased renal function
- altered gastrointestinal absorption

Examples of drugs known to interact in this manner with digitalis are **quinidine** (various preparations and trade names, Duraquin, Cardioquin), **amiodarone** (Cordarone), verapamil (Calan, Isoptin), potassium-sparing diuretics, and antibiotics. Antacids, a high-fiber diet, and chemotherapeutic agents may decrease the bioavailability of digitalis. The typical patient with digitalis toxicity is usually elderly, in **atrial fibrillation,** with underlying heart disease of many years, abnormal renal function, and concomitant pulmonary disease.

Signs and symptoms of digitalis toxicity include

- gastrointestinal problems—anorexia, nausea, vomiting, diarrhea
- neurologic problems—malaise, fatigue, vertigo, colored vision (especially green or yellow halos around lights), insomnia, depression, facial pain
- cardiologic problems—palpitations, arrhythmias, syncope
- hematologic problems—high digoxin levels especially with low potassium and altered blood urea nitrogen (BUN) and creatinine.

Sympathomimetics. Drugs that bind to the adrenoceptors and partially or completely mimic the actions of epinephrine or norepinephrine are known as sympathomimetics. The use of sympathomimetics, given parenterally in the treatment of heart failure to optimize cardiac output, is reserved for hemodynamically compromised patients within a critical care setting (see Tables 12–9, 12–12, and 12–16).

Stimulation of beta$_1$ adrenoceptors of the myocardium results in an increased calcium influx into myocardial cells with resultant electrical and mechanical influences: increased sinus node firing, enhanced atrioventricular conduction, and increased myocardial contractility. Stimulation of beta$_2$ adrenoceptors causes dilation of smooth muscles of the bronchi and blood vessels, with myocardial effects similar to those of beta$_1$. Pharmacologic stimulation of beta$_1$ and beta$_2$ agonist receptors in a failing heart therefore increases contractility, and beta$_2$ stimulation decreases afterload by its peripheral arterial vasodilatory effect. Use of these drugs is limited to acute interventions in a critical care setting because prolonged use of beta stimulators may lead to receptor desensitization and decreased inotropy. Unwanted ventricular arrhythmias may develop in response to the increased myocardial oxygen cost from pharmacologically induced improved contractility. Increased myocardial oxygen cost may further aggravate ischemia.

Examples of beta agonist adrenoceptors are the following: selective beta$_1$: **dobutamine** (Dobutrex), **norepinephrine (Levophed),** prenalterol; nonselective beta$_1$ and beta$_2$: epinephrine (Adrenalin Chloride), **isoproterenol** (Isuprel). Relatively selective beta$_2$ agonists are used primarily in the management of respiratory dysfunctions.

Another category of sympathomimetic agonists is **dopamine** (Intropin). Dopamine stimulates beta$_1$ myocardial receptors, D-1 (dopamine) vascular receptors, and alpha vascular receptors. Dopamine is used when heart failure is accompanied by systemic hypotension because it acts as both a positive inotrope (via beta$_1$ receptors) and a vasopressor (via alpha receptors). The combined beta and alpha effect increases cardiac output through increased contractility and increases blood pressure through peripheral vascular vasoconstriction as well as increased cardiac output. At low doses, dopamine (via its D-1 receptors) causes selective vasodilation and therefore increased blood flow to the renal, cerebral, coronary, and mesenteric arterial beds.

Dopamine (Intropin) and dobutamine (Dobutrex) are often used together in the management of heart failure with accompanying hypotension. Although both are potent beta-adrenergic agonists, dobutamine has no alpha-adrenergic stimulation and therefore cannot increase blood pressure through vasoconstriction, whereas dopamine is able to do so. Moderate doses of both drugs, when given together, have been demonstrated to maintain arterial blood pressure, decrease pulmonary artery wedge pressure, and increase contractility.

Bipyridines. As a group, bipyridines act as positive inotropes and vasodilators. They are often recommended for the treatment of heart failure that has failed to respond to other drug management. The inotropic effect of these drugs differs from that of the previous two drugs in that bipyridines increase myocardial contractility without altering the Na^+-K^+ pumping mechanism (as does digoxin) or stimulating the adrenoceptors (as does dopamine). Bipyridines increase intracellular calcium influx by inhibition of the **cyclic nucleotide phosphodiesterase.** Amrinone (Inocor) is presently the only U.S. Food and Drug Administration–accepted drug within this class. Amrinone is relatively specific for myocardial and vascular smooth muscle because its vasodilatory effects are balanced between preload and afterload. Overall effects of amrinone are an increase in cardiac output, reduction in preload, and decrease in afterload. In preload reduction, as measured by decreased pulmonary artery wedge pressure, amrinone is more effective than dopamine (Intropin) or dobutamine (Dobutrex); as a positive inotrope and vasodilator, it is intermediate between nitroprusside (Nipride) and dobutamine. Milrinone, an investigational bipyridine, has been shown in one long-term study to increase morbidity and mortality of patients with severe heart failure; mortality was reported to have increased by 30%.[13] At this time, this drug has not been accepted by the Food and Drug Administration.

Vasodilators

Both arterial and venous vasodilators are used in the management of heart failure as afterload and preload reducers, respectively. Arterial vaso-dilators are useful only when arterial hypoten-sion is not present. Arterial vasodilators decrease afterload, which decreases left ventricular myo-cardial oxygen demand. Reduction in preload may also decrease myocardial oxygen demand by decreasing ventricular volume, thus improving the length-tension relationship of the myocardial fibers. The improvement allows for a greater actin-myosin interaction and more effective con-tractility. Myocardial oxygen demand may be re-duced as the efficiency of the contraction im-proves. Ischemia may be decreased as myocardial oxygen demand is decreased.

Drugs that exhibit vasodilator properties are the following:

- smooth muscle relaxants such as nitroglycerin, nitroprusside (Nipride), and **hydralazine** (Apresoline)
- calcium channel blockers
- morphine
- ACE inhibitors
- alpha-adrenergic antagonists (see Tables 12–9 and 12–12)

Alpha antagonists are primarily used for the management of hypertension rather than heart failure. Reflex tachycardia and a compensatory increase in blood volume with long-term use have been identified as potential detrimental side effects of alpha antagonists. **Prazosin** (Minipress) and **terazosin** (Hytrin) are examples of alpha$_1$ antagonists (see Table 12–12).

Venodilators. Nitrates reduce the preload via venodilation. Nitrates are available in many forms, including topical, sublingual, and oral. Please refer to the previous section on anti-ischemic drugs and Table 12–6 for further dis-cussion.

Arteriodilators. Hydralazine (Apresoline) and **minoxidil** (Loniten) decrease afterload by de-creasing arterial resistance. Potential side effects are many with hydralazine when it is used alone; therefore, prudent clinical practice recom-mends combination therapy with a diuretic and a beta blocker. Please refer to the section on anti-hypertension drugs and Table 12–12 for further discussion.

Combined Arteriolar and Venous. Nitroprus-side (Nipride) affects both arterial resistance and venous capacitance. When it is given parenter-ally, it has a rapid onset of action and is effective in the treatment of severe heart failure with or without **cardiogenic shock.**

Calcium Channel Blockers

Calcium channel blockers work by relaxing the smooth muscle within the arterial walls, which results in a decreased afterload. Nifedipine is the most potent peripheral vasodilator of the calcium channel blockers. Please refer to the sections on anti-ischemic and antiarrhythmic drugs and to Table 12–8 for further discussion.

Angiotensin-Converting Enzyme Inhibitors

When cardiac output is decreased, such as with symptomatic heart failure, perfusion of the renal artery is also decreased. Decreased renal perfusion stimulates the release of **renin** from the afferent arteriole of the glomerulus. Renin, along with a renin substrate, forms **angiotensin I,** which converts into **angiotensin II** (see Fig. 12–9). "This reaction is catalyzed by angiotensin converting enzyme (ACE), which is located in many organs, including the lung, the luminal membrane of vascular epithelial cells, and the **juxtaglomerular** apparatus itself."[14] Angiotensin II has two key effects: an increase in systemic vascular resistance owing to its potency as a va-soconstrictor and an increase in extracellular vol-ume owing to renal sodium and water reten-tion.[14] When the reaction of angiotensin I to angiotensin II is inhibited, the effects of angio-tensin II are significantly limited.

Angiotensin-converting enzyme inhibitors are used in the management of heart failure to de-crease the excess intravascular volume that occurs as a result of sodium and water retention. A decrease in volume decreases preload. A de-crease in preload in a failing heart decreases myocardial oxygen demand and may improve contractility (refer to sections on diuretics and antihypertensive drugs). Commonly used ACE inhibitors for heart failure are

- **captopril** (Capoten)
- **enalapril** (Vasotec)
- **lisinopril** (Zestril) (see Tables 12–9 and 12–12)

Morphine

The use of morphine in the treatment of severe heart failure has proved invaluable for both its analgesic and its hemodynamic effects. Morphine decreases preload via marked venodilation and exhibits mild arterial vasodilation. The anxiety and effort of dyspnea associated with severe heart failure appear to improve with the administration of morphine.

Clinical Considerations

The importance of recognizing the side effects of all drugs has previously been stated and yet bears repetition. In the case of digoxin (Lanoxin), for example, the side effects may be perceived initially by the patient as "just not feeling well"; the correlation of those feelings to the specific drug may go unnoticed. Many patients seen by physical therapists for noncardiac reasons are taking digoxin. Any new patient complaint should be evaluated in light of its relationship to digoxin and reported to the physician. If patients are on digoxin because of atrial fibrillation, the physical therapist must recognize that they will have an irregular pulse. In addition, an atrial fibrillation with a ventricular response at rest greater than 110 beats per minute warrants evaluation before continuing with an exercise program. Resting pulses should be taken for a full minute when atrial fibrillation or any other rhythm disturbance is present owing to the irregularity of the rhythm.

Signs and Symptoms

For the therapist who is seeing a patient on an outpatient basis, the signs and symptoms of going into heart failure may be subtle over a period of days; therefore, the therapist should be alerted to any dyspnea, ankle swelling, or both or the presence of an S3 heart sound as possible signs of heart failure. If new bilateral ankle edema is present, the patient should not be exercised until a physician is contacted and the situation clarified or remedied. In the case of severe heart failure warranting parenterally delivered vasopressors and positive inotropes to maintain an appropriate cardiac output at rest, progressive exercise is not suggested until the patient is hemodynamically stable. Maintaining good alveolar expansion, joint protection and energy conservation techniques (e.g., arms supported on pillows for activities of daily living to decrease upper extremity energy requirements), and low-level activity are possible treatment interventions when warranted. As stroke volume decreases, heart rate compensatorily rises to prevent cardiac output from falling further. Therefore, when the patient has tachycardia at rest it is inappropriate to begin an exercise program without clear direction and mutual understanding of the treatment goals from all members of the health care team.

Patients on diuretics may also become dehydrated because of excess diuresis. Their complaints may be of lightheadedness, weakness, fatigue, or an irregular pulse. Symptoms may be more pronounced when standing as compared with sitting or lying down. Clinical signs may be resting tachycardia and postural hypotension. Patients should not participate in an exercise regimen until the situation has been stabilized and the patient has appropriately rehydrated (and replaced electrolytes if needed) under a physician's guidance.

ANTIARRHYTHMIC AGENTS

Disturbances in cardiac rhythm are known as arrhythmias. They are the result of irregularities in heart pacemaker or conduction tissue function. Arrhythmias present a broad spectrum of clinical consequences: they may be benign and remain undetected throughout life or prove fatal upon initial presentation (e.g., sudden death). Arrhythmias are recognized clinically as irregularities in the rhythm of the heartbeat on palpation, auscultation, or ECG tracing. They are labeled according to the anatomic origin of the abnormal beat (e.g., atrial, nodal, or ventricular), their frequency (e.g., tachycardia or bradycardia), and their relationship to the previous beat (e.g., premature or late).

Electrolyte imbalances, drug toxicity, excessive nicotine or caffeine ingestion, emotional stress, **hyperthyroidism,** or **mitral valve prolapse** syndrome can all produce arrhythmias. On correction of these conditions, persistent cardiac rhythm disturbances that are hemodynamically significant require drug therapy. The focus of antiarrhythmic therapy, therefore, is to maintain adequate cardiac output in the presence of pacemaker or conduction tissue pathology.

Physical therapists must be alert to the etiology and presence of arrhythmias, their hemodynamic consequences, and the efficacy of the antiarrhythmic agent prescribed. Drugs suppress arrhythmias (abnormal impulse formation or conduction) by altering cell membrane permeability to specific ions, for example, sodium and calcium. Although exercise may be responsible for production of arrhythmias, electrolyte imbalances and toxic level of antiarrhythmic drugs are other nondisease states that may be arrhythmogenic.

Physiology

To understand how antiarrhythmic agents suppress rhythm disturbances, it is necessary to review the unique characteristics of normal myocardial pacemaker and conduction system functioning. See Chapter 9 for an in-depth discussion of cardiac arrhythmias. Inherent myocardial properties of automaticity, excitability, and conduction depend on the resting polarity of pacemaker (nodal) and myocardial conduction tissue (Purkinje's fibers). Refer to Chapter 2 for further information. This specialized conduction system is able to initiate, respond to, and conduct a stimulus as long as an adequate transmembrane potential exists. Resting cell polarity depends on two factors:

● The membrane permeability to sodium, calcium, potassium, and chloride ions

● The duration between action potentials (diastole)

The cardiac action potential is thought to result from an orderly and sequential change in membrane permeability to various ions. The characteristic time course has been described by phases and separated into "fast" and "slow" responses (Fig. 12–3). Whereas membrane permeability to sodium alone is felt to be responsible for the rapid upstroke of phase 0 depolarization found in normal atrial and ventricular contractile cell action potential, membrane permeability to both calcium and sodium are responsible for the slow phase 0 depolarization of sinus and atrioventricular nodal cell action potential. Repolarization via the "fast" channels can be described by three phases:

● Phase 1 is the early rapid phase and depends on membrane permeability to chloride.
● Phase 2 is the plateau phase affected by calcium and potassium movement across the membrane.
● Phase 3 is the final rapid phase of repolarization, primarily influenced by membrane permeability to potassium.

These three phases of repolarization cannot be distinguished clearly in cells with slower action potentials (see Fig. 12–3B). Phase 4 is the period of diastole and is constant in many atrial and ventricular contractile cells that rest indefinitely until stimulated. However, sinus node, atrioventricular node, and Purkinje's fibers have a unique ability to spontaneously depolarize and self-excite by achieving a threshold at which more rapid depolarization occurs.

Both myocardial contractile and conduction tissue are refractory to restimulation when the cell membrane is still depolarized. When the membrane is partially repolarized (phase 3), excitation becomes possible but not usual, and the cell is in a "relative" refractory state (see Fig. 12–3).

Pathophysiology

The action potential and the diastolic interval between action potentials are affected by changes in the

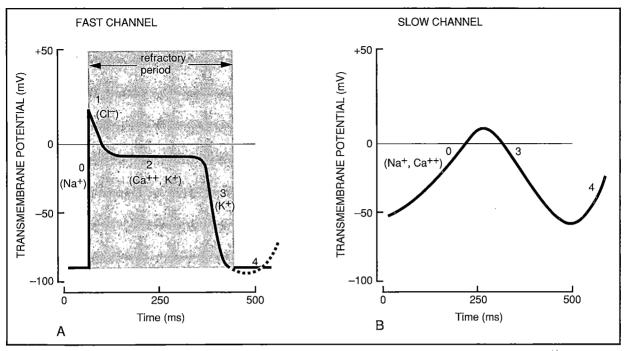

Figure 12-3.

Schematic representation of phases of action potential (AP) in fast and slow depolarization. The primary ion movement responsible for AP is noted at each phase. *A,* Fast response AP (black) begins with a relatively greater negativity and has a rapid rate of depolarization and a plateaued repolarization. This AP is found in ordinary atrial, ventricular, and Purkinje's fibers. Purkinje's fibers demonstrate a fast depolarization phase (0) but also have similar phase 4 diastole characteristics of self-excitation as in the slow channel (red dotted line). *B,* Slow response AP (red) begins with a less negative voltage and has a slower depolarization phase (0). Repolarization lasts longer and exhibits a slow, spontaneous depolarization during phase 4 diastole. This AP is found in sinoatrial and atrioventricular nodal cells.

• maximum diastolic potential
• slope of phase 4 depolarization
• threshold potential required to depolarize the cell[15]

Figure 12-4*A, B,* and *C* demonstrate slowing of the heart rate by changes in any of these three action potential parameters. Numerous cardiac conditions, including cell hypoxia, ischemia, scarred tissue, and medications can alter these parameters and can cause some cardiac cells that normally have fast action potentials to become faster or much slower, and slow action potentials to respond faster or slower than normal. When any of these alterations in the action potential occur, slow, fast, or escape rhythms may become manifest. For example, if sinoatrial node cells have an excess of potassium **(hyperkalemia),** the resting polarity is greater than normal (more

negativity). Consequently, more sodium has to enter the cell to fully depolarize the membrane, and more sodium has to leave the cell to complete repolarization. This excess of sodium and potassium creates a longer interval before the occurrence of another action potential, as illustrated in Figure 12-4*A.* Each heart beat reflects the mechanical event triggered by the electrical conduction of an action potential. Hence, a longer period between action potentials is seen clinically as a slower heart rate. Additionally, if the interval is long enough, pacemaker cells in the atrioventricular node may depolarize spontaneously, producing an "escape" action potential or a premature nodal heart beat. Similarly, if normal cell membrane integrity is disturbed and sodium permeability increases, cells may depolarize and repolarize more rapidly, causing an increase in heart rate.

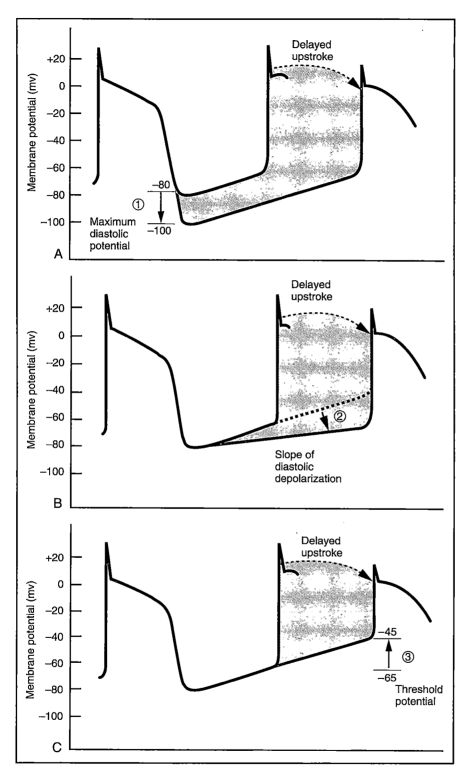

Figure 12-4.
Determinants of action potential rate and diastolic interval, as seen in Purkinje's fibers. The rate can be slowed (and the interval lengthened; shaded area) by three diastolic mechanisms. *A*, More negative maximum diastolic potential. *B*, Reduction of the slope of diastolic depolarization. *C*, More positive threshold potential. (Adapted from Katzung BG [ed]. Basic and Clinical Pharmacology. 5th ed. East Norwalk, Conn, Appleton & Lange, 1992, p 169.)

In addition to the changes in the action potential, variability in the duration of the refractory period of the action potential can cause arrhythmias. In certain conditions, diseased myocardial cells repolarize and conduct slower than neighboring healthy myocardial cells, enabling "reentry" to occur. Reentry, a common cause of rhythm disturbances, occurs when one impulse reenters and excites areas of the heart that have already been stimulated by the original impulse (Fig. 12–5). For reentry to occur, there must be

- some obstacle blocking normal impulse conduction
- another "avenue" for the impulse to be conducted through the tissue (unidirectional block)
- sufficient time for the impulse to travel via this alternative "avenue" (that is, long enough so that after the impulse passes through this tissue, the surrounding tissue will have repolarized and will be able to "accept" the impulse)

When these three conditions exist, the single or repetitive conduction of a "secondary" pacemaker occurs and is manifested clinically as a premature beat or a series of premature beats. Disease conditions such as myocardial ischemia with resultant hypoxia can cause partial depolarization and "unidirectional" block, providing the setting for reentrant rhythms. The slower repolarization rate of such disease tissue slows the reentrant impulse so that healthy surrounding tissue is no longer refractory and can respond to stimulation by this "secondary" pacemaker, subsequently making the healthy tissue refractory to the primary pacemaker.

Reentry is probably responsible for many cardiac arrhythmias, including atrial and ventricular flutter and fibrillation, supraventricular tachycardia involving accessory pathway or nodal reentry, and many ventricular tachycardias.[16] New technology enables precise identification of the origin and physiology of the reentrant rhythm. With this knowledge, physicians can plan treatment with more accuracy, including pharmacologic alteration of the action potential.

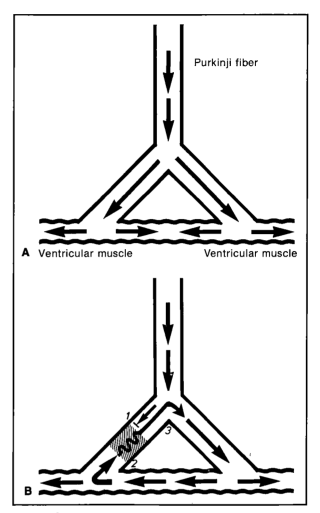

Figure 12–5.

Conduction pathway. *A*, Normal conduction pathway of a depolarization wave through a Purkinje fiber to ventricular muscle. The depolarization wave arrives simultaneously at all portions of ventricular muscle and then extinguishes. *B*, Reentry circuit model with unidirectional block. The depolarization wave is blocked at the ischemic zone (1); however, it is able to depolarize the ventricular muscle from the opposite direction (2). By the time the impulse passes through this ischemic area, the healthy muscle is repolarized and responds to this impulse (3) before the next impulse can be generated from the SA node. Drugs can abolish the arrhythmia by improving forward conduction at 1 or by preventing conduction at 2. (Modified from Tyndall A. A nursing perspective of the invasive approach to treatment of ventricular arrhythmias. Heart Lung 12:6, 1983; reproduced from Cohen M, Michel T. Cardiopulmonary Symptoms in Physical Therapy Practice. New York, Churchill Livingstone, 1988, p 161.)

Pharmacologic Intervention

Suppression of arrhythmias by pharmacologic intervention can be complex. Although antiarrhythmic agents can reverse lethal rhythms, it is unclear that these drugs promote longevity. They can depress cardiac inotropy and may even produce arrhythmias owing to their effect on the action potential (arrhythmogenic). Antiarrhythmic agents act to inhibit abnormal impulse formation or conduction by altering cell membrane permeability to specific ions. The exact interaction of antiarrhythmics with various ionic channels is not well understood. As discussed in Chapter 2, current theory proposes the existence of activation and inactivation "gates," which control the flow of sodium, calcium, potassium, and chloride ions depending on stimulation. Classification of antiarrhythmic drugs according to their effects on the action potential of myocardial and pacemaker cell gates is found in Table 12–10. Significant overlapping of drug properties exists across all categories. For purposes of clarity, those classes acting primarily on the ionic channels to stabilize the membrane (classes 1 and 4), are discussed first. Beta blockers, which also appear in this classification, are discussed next (class 2), and lastly, class 3 drugs, which have properties of the previous classes, are presented. Additionally, two classes of antiarrhythmics, beta blockers and calcium channel blockers, are not only effective in the treatment of arrhythmias, but also are used as anti-ischemic and antihypertensive agents (as is discussed elsewhere in this chapter).

Membrane Stabilizers

Class 1 Drugs. Class 1 drugs primarily affect the fast sodium channel and act like local anesthetics. Subclasses A, B, and C all significantly block the sodium channel of depolarized cells, but vary in the degree of sodium channel block in normal cells. Similarly, class 1 drugs prolong the refractory period of depolarized cells but vary in their effect on normal cells. Prolongation of the refractory period of diseased tissue inhibits reentry by creating bidirectional block in these cells (see Fig. 12–5). Lidocaine (Xylocaine), a class 1B agent, facilitates propagation of the original (sinoatrial) stimulus by shortening the **refractory period** of normal cell action potentials while slowing or completely blocking the potential reentrant stimulus in diseased tissue. Lidocaine is a very effective drug for ventricular arrhythmia management in the early hours of an acute myocardial infarction when ischemic cells are in varied states of polarization. In this clinical setting, combinations of abnormal conduction and abnormal impulse formation are often responsible for many postinfarction arrhythmias.

In general, class 1 drugs are very effective in the treatment of ventricular tachycardia (VT). They may be useful in the treatment of supraventricular tachycardia (SVT), with class 1A being the most effective. The ECG of a patient on a class 1 antiarrhythmic drug may exhibit a prolongation of the QRS duration, with a normal or prolonged P–R interval.

Class 2 Drugs. Class 2 antiarrhythmic agents —beta blockers—do not directly affect the cell membrane. They indirectly alter the action potential by blocking sympathetic excitation of the heart to control cardiac rhythm disturbances. They are especially indicated for the treatment of supraventricular and ventricular arrhythmias that occur in the postmyocardial infarction period and arrhythmias that occur during exercise. Beta blockers are prescribed cautiously owing to their negative inotropic activity. Patients taking beta blockers may have a prolongation of the P–R interval on their ECG tracing.

Class 3 Drugs. The class 3 drugs act primarily to prolong the refractory period of cardiac tissue, thereby slowing repolarization and making it more difficult for myocardial cells to respond to stimulation. They may be effective in both SVT and VT. Amiodarone (Cordarone), one of the two drugs currently in this class, has properties of class 1A, 2, 3, and 4 agents. Its use is limited owing to its potent adverse side effects, because it is deposited in every organ of the body.

Class 4 Drugs. Class 4 drugs primarily block the slow calcium channel. Like class 1 drugs, they prolong the refractory period and decrease pacemaker activity of depolarized cells. The ECG of a patient on calcium channel blockers may show a prolonged P–R interval and no effect on

TABLE 12–10. Classification of Antiarrhythmic Drugs

Category	Physiologic Effect*	Drug generic (trade)	Comments
	Class 1		
Membrane depressants (sodium channel blockers)	Depolarized cells: ↑ Na⁺ channel block ↑ Refractory period ↓ Pacemaker activity		
1A	Normal cell: ↑ Na⁺ channel block ↑ Refractory period	Quinidine (Biquin, Kinidin, Durules) Disopyramide (Norpace, Rythmodan) Procainamide (Pronestyl) Imipramine (investigational)	Gastrointestinal side effects Urinary retention effect Lupus erythematosus Used as an antidepressant
1B	Normal cell: No effect	Lidocaine (Xylocaine) Mexiletine (Mexitil) Phenytoin (Dilantin) Tocainide (Tonocard) Moricizine (Ethmozine)†	Signs of central nervous system abnormality may indicate toxicity
1C	Normal cell: ↑↑ Na⁺ channel block ∅, ↑ Refractory period	Encainide (Enkaid) Flecainide (Tambocor) Propafenone (Rythmol)	Defibrillation problems, arrhythmogenic during exercise
	Class 2		
Beta adrenoceptor blockers	Depolarized cell: ∅ Effect on Na⁺ channel ↑ Refractory period Normal cell: Variable effect	See beta blocker Table 12–5	Sotolol (investigational); also has Class 3 properties
	Class 3		
Refractory period alterations	↑↑↑ Refractory period ↓ Pacemaker activity Sympatholytic	Amiodarone (Cordarone) Bretylium tosylate (Bretylol)	Has properties of Classes 1A, 2, and 4 May transiently increase pacemaker activity
	Class 4		
Calcium channel blockers	All cells: ↑↑↑ Ca⁺⁺ channel blockade Depolarized cells: ↑ Na⁺ channel block ↑ Refractory period ↓ Pacemaker activity Sympatholytic	See calcium channel blocker Table 12–8	Verapamil (Isoptin, Calan), is most effective in this group for treatment of supraventricular tachycardia

*General effect on action potential; individual agents may differ slightly.
†Controversial classification; acts like 1C as well.

the QRS complex. Verapamil (Isoptin, Calan), demonstrates the most antiarrhythmic properties in this class and is significantly more effective in the treatment of SVT than of VT.

Digitalis

Digitalis, not found in the above classification, is a cardiac glycoside and may also be used in arrhythmia management. In the normal heart, it directly depresses vagal tone (parasympathetic nervous system), whereas in the failing heart, it depresses adrenergic action (sympathetic nervous system); both actions result in slowing the heart and depressing conduction through the atrioventricular node. Hence, digitalis can be used to prevent conduction of atrial arrhythmias into the ventricles. Digitalis administration, however, can predispose an individual to arrhythmias, owing to its action on the electrophysiologic properties of the heart. Commonly used in the treatment of congestive heart failure, digitalis "poisons" (inhibits) the sodium-potassium pump (review previous section in this chapter). This causes excessive calcium to accumulate in the cell, along with intracellular sodium. Although this increased calcium enhances myocardial cell contraction, thereby ameliorating heart failure, the increased sodium causes a decrease in intracellular potassium. As intracellular potassium falls, maximal diastolic membrane potential decreases (less negativity), and the slope of phase 4 depolarization increases (see Fig. 12–4). The resultant increase in automaticity and ectopic activity can increase the likelihood of arrhythmias. Hence, whether prescribed for heart failure or management of rapid atrial heart rates, serum digitalis concentration and electrolyte levels should be monitored carefully.

Clinical Considerations

Pharmacologic management of arrhythmias is most successful when approached in a systematic fashion. First, adequate documentation of the arrhythmia is made by clinical evaluation, electrocardiogram, or electrophysiologic study. Assessment of hemodynamic compromise, consequences, and symptom prevalence in an emergency or long-term care setting are considered. Second, once a drug is chosen, its efficacy is evaluated by clinical and electrocardiographic observation with possible electrophysiologic study. Third, the adequacy of the dosage is measured by determination of drug concentration in the blood. Intolerance to antiarrhythmic agents and drug toxicity are common problems. Current prescription of antiarrhythmics is empirical, and several agents may need to be tried before one is found that is both effective and well tolerated by the patient. Rapid advances in electrophysiologic study and testing have helped verify the effectiveness of certain agents. Additionally, as this technology progresses, new combinations of drugs are developed (several are currently undergoing investigation) (see Table 12–10).

TABLE 12–11. Associations of Arrhythmias with Exercise
Normal cardiovascular system
Coronary artery disease
Mitral valve prolapse
Left ventricular trabeculations
Digitalis
Hypokalemia
Cardiomyopathy
Left ventricle outflow obstruction
Aortic stenosis
Hypertrophic cardiomyopathy
Long–QT interval syndromes
Idiopathic
Quinidine induced
Phenothiazine induced
Proarrhythmias due to antiarrhythmic drugs (Flecainide)
Pulmonary disease

(From Froelicher V, Marcondes G. Manual of Exercise Testing. St. Louis, CV Mosby, 1989, p 303.)

Health professionals responsible for monitoring the exercise response of patients on antiarrhythmic agents should understand the basis of arrhythmia production and suppression. Exercise is commonly the culprit in the production of arrhythmias (Table 12–11). However, abnormal electrolyte levels or toxic levels of a drug may be responsible for cardiac rhythm disturbances. A medication prescribed to inhibit arrhythmias can in fact become arrhythmogenic if safe serum levels are exceeded.

ANTIHYPERTENSIVE THERAPY

Although surveys vary, an estimated 10% to 15% of North Americans have arterial hypertension (defined elsewhere in text).[17,18] Of those who obtain medical treatment, most are prescribed diet or exercise or drug therapy, or a combination of these. The goal of hypertensive therapy is to prevent the negative effects of chronic blood pressure elevation. Sustained hypertension results in increased morbidity and mortality associated with renal failure, coronary disease, and stroke. Owing to the absence of symptoms from high blood pressure and the numerous side effects of available drug agents, noncompliance with therapy is common. Further risk of noncompliance is created by the frequent use of multiple drugs to control blood pressure.

Physiology

A number of physiologic factors combine to create normotension in the cardiovascular system. At any one moment, several mechanisms interact to maintain adequate pressure in the circulation to allow vital systems to function. Carotid baroreceptors and kidney sensors detect changes in blood pressure and trigger appropriate alterations in cardiac output and peripheral vascular resistance to maintain normotension. These alterations are regulated at three anatomic sites: the arterioles, the postcapillary venules, and the heart. A fourth site, the kidneys, acts to control blood pressure by regulating intravascular volume (cardiac preload). The sympathetic nervous system and **humoral** mechanisms, that is, renin-angiotensin-aldosterone system, continuously control the interaction of simultaneous changes at each site, influencing compensatory mechanisms between anatomic sites (Fig. 12–6).

Pathophysiology

In the majority of individuals with hypertension, the threshold of stimulation of both the **baroreceptors** and the renal blood volume-pressure control systems is "set" too high.[17,18] This causes a delay in the initiation of central and peripheral changes involved in the maintenance of normotension. Once baroreceptors are stimulated, the sympathetic nervous system and the kidneys usually respond normally. However, just as in normotensive individuals, if one anatomic site is "blocked" for some reason (e.g., pathology, drug), other sites compensate to maintain a blood pressure level that no longer stimulates the baroreceptors. When this baseline blood pressure level is pathologically elevated, another of the remaining three anatomic sites of blood pressure regulation warrants blocking. Hence several pharmacologic agents are used to "limit" multiple normal physiologic blood pressure control mechanisms. The use of several

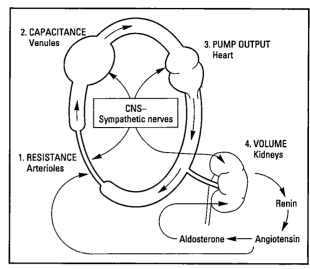

Figure 12–6.

Anatomic sites of blood pressure control. (From Katzung BG [ed]. Basic and Clinical Pharmacology. 5th ed. East Norwalk, Conn, Appleton & Lange, 1992, p 140.)

agents also allows lower dosages of each agent and hence fewer side effects from each drug.

Pharmacologic Intervention

Antihypertensive drugs can be classified by their principal site of action:

● Diuretics, which act on kidneys to reduce volume
● Those that act to limit sympathetic nervous system activity
● Vasodilators (arterial and venous)
● Those that act on the renin-angiotensin-aldosterone system at the kidney

At present, no drug has been found effective and safe in directly altering baroreceptor activity.

Diuretics

Alterations in intravascular blood volume have a significant effect on blood pressure. Diuretics, the most commonly prescribed antihypertensive agents, act to reduce circulating volume and thereby lower blood pressure. Acting at various sites along the renal tubule or Henle's loop, diuretics alter the reabsorption of sodium, consequently affecting the retention of water (Fig. 12–7). Furosemide (Lasix), a **"loop" diuretic,** acts on the medullary ascending limb of Henle's loop and has the greatest diuresing effect. Carbonic anhydrase inhibitors, acting on the proximal tubules, and potassium-sparing diuretics, acting on the collecting tubules and ducts, are the most mild diuretics. The **sulfonamide diuretics** (thiazides and thiazide-like drugs) have moderate diuretic effects. These act on the cortical ascending limb of Henle's loop and the distal tubule. Thiazides are a frequently prescribed diuretic; however, they have been associated with hyperlipidemia when administered in high doses.

Clinical Considerations. The physician may choose to prescribe diuretic therapy from a long list of agents (Table 12–12). The choice of diuretic depends on the severity of the hypertension and the drug's side effects. The potency of the drug is dependent on its site of action in the **nephron** (see Fig. 12–7). Combinations of diuretics can be prescribed to treat hypertension. Caution should be used when patients taking diuretics are encouraged to participate in aerobic exercise. Volume reduction and electrolyte disturbances can predispose the exercising individual to hypotension or arrhythmias, respectively. Hypokalemia can be a serious consequence of diuretic therapy when potent agents are prescribed. Usually potassium supplementation is prescribed to prevent a potentially unstable electrolyte environment. Hyperkalemia may occur with potassium-sparing diuretics.

Drugs Acting on the Sympathetic Nervous System

Blood pressure is influenced by sympathetic nervous system regulation of cardiac output and peripheral vascular resistance. Pharmacologic agents can be used to alter sympathetic nervous

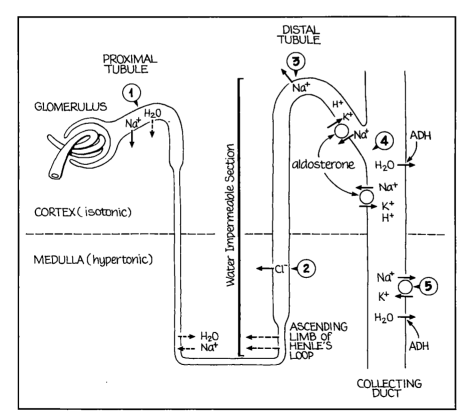

Figure 12–7.

Sites of action of diuretic agents in the nephron: (1) carbonic anhydrase inhibitors; osmotic diuretics; (2) "loop" diuretics; (3) sulfonamide diuretics; (4) aldosterone antagonists; (5) potassium-sparing diuretics. (From Marquez-Julio A, Whiteside C. Diuretics. In: Kalant H, Roschlau W, Sellers M [eds]. Principles of Medical Pharmacology. 4th ed. New York, Oxford University Press, 1985.)

TABLE 12–12. Antihypertensive Agents

Category	Generic (trade) Name	Comments
	Diuretics	
High ceiling (loop)	Bumetanide (Bumex, Burinex) Ethacrynic acid (Edecrin) Furosemide (Lasix, Furomide, Dryptal) Frusemide (Frusetic, Frusid) Piretanide (Arlix)	Mild to severe hypokalemia may occur with diuretics, necessatating K⁺ supplementation.
Sulfonamide (thiazide and thiazide-like)	Hydrochlorothiazide* (HydroDIURIL, Esidrix, Oretic, Direma) Chlorothiazide (Diuril, Saluric) Quinethazone (Hydromox, Aquamox) Bendroflumethiazide (Naturetin) Methylclothiazide (Duretic, Enduron, Aquatensen) Polythiazide (Renese) Trichlormethiazide (Naqua, Metahydrin) Metolazone (Zaroxylin, Mykrox, Diulo) Indapamide (Lozol, Natrilix) Chlorthalidone* (Hygroton) Bendrofluazide (Aprinox, Centyl, others) Benzthiazide (Aquatag, Exna, Hydrex) Cyclothiazide (Anhydron [discontinued]) Hydroflumethiazide (Diurcardin, Hydrenox, Saluron) Cyclopenthiazide (Navidrex)	Hyperkalemia may occur with K⁺-sparing agents.
Carbonic anhydrase inhibitors	Acetazolamide (Diamox)	
Potassium-sparing	Spironolactone (Aldactone, Alatone) Triamterene (Dyrenium, Dytac) Amiloride (Midamor) Potassium canrenoate (Spiroctan-M)	
Osmotic	Mannitol (Osmitrol)	

Combination diuretics	Hydrochlorothiazide and:
	Triamterene (Dyazide, Maxzide)
	Spironolactone (Aldactazide)
	Amiloride hydrochloride (Moduretic, Moduret)
	Frusemide and:
	    Amiloride (Frumil)
	    Triamterene (Frusene)	

	Sympathetic Nervous System Inhibition	
Central nervous system acting	Clonidine (Catapres) Methyldopa (Aldomet)	May have side effects of sedation, mental depression, and sleep disturbances.
Ganglion blocking	Trimethaphan (Arfonad) Mecamylamine (Inversine) Reserpine (Serpasil)	
Postganglion blocking	Guanethidine (Ismelin Sulfate) Guanadrel (Hylorel)	May cause hypotension that is increased with exercise and upright posture.
Alpha₁-adrenergic blocking	Prazosin (Minipress) Phenoxybenzamine (Dibenzyline) Terazosin (Hytrin) Trimazosin (Cardovar) Phentolamine† (Regitine)	Prazosin is both a venous and an arterial dilator.
Beta-adrenergic blocking	See beta blockers, Table 12–5	

Table continued on following page

TABLE 12–12. Antihypertensive Agents *Continued*

Category	Generic (trade) Name	Comments
	Vasodilators	
Venodilators	Nitrates (see Table 12–6)	Hydralazine and Minoxidil are used for outpatient, long term, therapy, while nitroprusside and diazoxide are parenteral agents, used in emergent conditions; Ca^{++} channel blockers are used in both acute and chronic conditions.
Arteriolar dilators	Hydralazine (Apresoline) Minoxidil (Loniten) Diazoxide (Hyperstat IV) Calcium channel blockers (see Table 12–8)	
Combination arteriolar and venodilator	See alpha$_1$-adrenergic blockers, above Nitroprusside (Nipride)	Nitroprusside is preferred over IV alpha$_1$-adrenergic blockers.
	Angiotensin-Converting Enzyme Inhibitor	
	Captopril (Capoten) Enalapril (Vasotec) Lisinopril (Zestril, Prinivil)	Severe hypotension in some patients who are hypovolemic due to diuretics, salt restriction, or gastrointestinal fluid loss.

*Diuretic agents most commonly used and least expensive.
†Blocks alpha$_2$ receptors also; given by intravenous infusion, it has a rapid action, lasts only minutes, and is expensive.

system activity to control blood pressure in the following ways (see Table 12–12):

- Centrally acting compounds reduce neural transmission from vasopressor centers in the brainstem, inhibiting vasoconstriction.
- Ganglionic blockers limit vasoconstriction that is normally mediated by norepinephrine released at autonomic ganglia. However, parasympathetic nervous system inhibition occurs with these drugs also.
- Postganglionic blockers inhibit norepinephrine release from postganglionic adrenergic neurons in the heart and vessels, thereby reducing cardiac output and limiting vasoconstriction.
- Blocking alpha adrenoceptors in arterioles and venules prevents vasoconstriction normally induced by norepinephrine; hence, peripheral vascular resistance is reduced.
- Blocking beta adrenoceptors in heart and juxtaglomerular cells responsible for the release of renin limits cardiac output and vasoconstriction, respectively.

Clinical Considerations. A typical second drug group used to control hypertension when a mild diuretic alone is ineffective is the beta-adrenergic blocking agents (see Table 12–5). If these drugs cannot be prescribed because of their negative inotropy or chronotropy, vasomotor center-acting agents typically can be used. Potential side ef-

fects and frequency of drug administration are also considered in making decisions about the appropriate sympathetic nervous system inhibition therapy for hypertension.

Vasodilators

This group of antihypertensive drugs acts directly on vascular smooth muscle cells to reduce peripheral vascular resistance (arterial dilation) or venous return to the heart (venous dilation). Systolic hypertension can be treated effectively with arterial dilators. Hydralazine (Apresoline), minoxidil (Loniten), and diazoxide (Hyperstat IV) are examples of arterial dilators. Calcium channel blockers reduce blood pressure by preventing actin and myosin coupling, thereby promoting vascular smooth muscle dilation as well (discussed earlier in this chapter). Venodilators are especially effective in the treatment of diastolic hypertension because they reduce cardiac preload and end-diastolic pressure (see Table 12–12). Sodium nitroprusside (Nipride) is both a venous and arterial dilator.

Vasodilators can be administered orally or intravenously for rapid treatment of hypertension. However, compensatory mechanisms elicit increased sympathetic nervous system activity, including tachycardia, reflex vasoconstriction, and elevated plasma renin. For these reasons, vasodilators are usually used in combination with beta blocking or other sympathetic nervous system–inhibiting drugs to limit hypertension. In addition, simultaneous diuretic therapy can limit fluid retention caused by the compensatory increase in aldosterone associated with the use of vasodilators.

Angiotensin-Converting Enzyme Inhibitors

The renal cortex is stimulated to produce renin when it detects a drop in renal artery pressure or stimulation by the sympathetic nervous system or a reduction in sodium. Renin reacts to form angiotensin I, and in the presence of a converting enzyme, angiotensin I forms angiotensin II (Fig. 12–8). This latter substance is a potent vasoconstrictor that promotes sodium retention and causes aldosterone production, all factors that result in blood pressure elevation. Captopril (Capoten), enalapril (Vasotec), and lisinopril (Zestril) act as ACE inhibitors to prevent the formation of angiotensin II. Hence ACE inhibitors lower blood pressure primarily by lowering peripheral vascular resistance. Unlike vasodilators, ACE inhibitors do not result in reflex sympathetic nervous system activity. Studies provide strong evidence of the efficacy of ACE inhibitors in blood pressure management in patients with depressed ejection fraction, further accounting for their escalating utilization.[11]

PHARMACOLOGIC MANAGEMENT OF LIPID DISORDERS

In 1985 a turning point occurred in the awareness and management of lipid disorders in the United States. In that year the National Institutes of Health Consensus Conference concluded what many practioners had believed for years: elevated blood cholesterol levels, especially low-density lipoprotein (LDL), were associated with premature coronary heart disease, and, most important for clinical practice, lowering the LDL levels decreased the risk of developing coronary

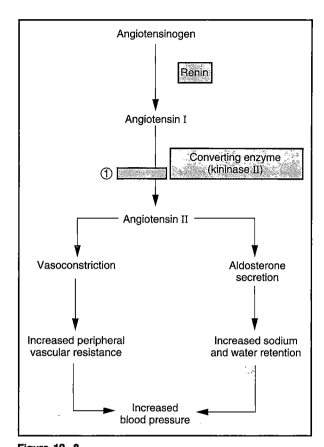

Figure 12–8.

Site of action of captopril (Capoten) blockade at 1. (Adapted from Katzung BG [ed]. Basic and Clinical Pharmacology. 5th ed. East Norwalk, Conn, Appleton & Lange, 1992.)

heart disease. The panel recommended guidelines for treatment, including dietary and pharmacologic interventions as well as screening programs to identify persons at risk. Since that time people have become familiar with the terms *good cholesterol, bad cholesterol,* and *saturated fat,* not only from the medical establishment but also from the media, food corporations, and fast-food restaurants. Thus, early detection of lipid abnormalities has improved because of advances within the medical community and as a result of consumer education.

Cholesterol is a naturally occurring fatlike substance that is found within various tissues of the body: cell membranes, hormones, and plasma. Approximately 93% of all cholesterol is found in cell membranes, and the other 7% circulates within the blood plasma. A relatively small amount of the circulating cholesterol is used by the adrenals and gonads for hormone synthesis, and another small proportion is used by peripheral cells in building and maintaining membranous structures. Cholesterol is transported in the blood within a lipdid molecule, which in turn is carried by *lipoproteins*. Therefore, because cholesterol is attached to the lipoproteins within the blood, assessment of cholesterol abnormalities involves lipoprotein assessment.

Three specific lipoproteins carry blood cholesterol:

- Low-density lipoproteins
- High-density lipoproteins
- Very low density lipoproteins (VLDL)

Triglycerides, a glycerol molecule with three fatty acid chains, contains only about one fifth cholesterol; the cholesterol of triglycerides is carried on the VLDL lipoprotein. Current research indicates that increased LDL and decreased HDL cholesterol are associated with the development of atherosclerosis and coronary artery disease.

Hypercholesterolemia is defined as elevated plasma cholesterol concentration greater than 240 milligrams per deciliter with normal triglycerides; HDL deficiency is identified as an HDL cholesterol level less than 35 milligrams per deciliter with normal VLDL and LDL. Five types of lipid abnormalities exist currently and are described in Table 12–13.

Drug therapy is recommended after at least a 6-month trial of diet in all patients with LDL cholesterol levels higher than 190 milligrams per deciliter, with the goal of reducing LDL cholesterol levels to less than 160 milligrams per deciliter. Drug therapy is also recommended after dietary therapy in patients with LDL cholesterol levels higher than 160 milligrams per deciliter if coronary heart disease or two or more risk factors for coronary heart disease are present, with the goal of reducing the LDL cholesterol level to less than 130 milligrams per deciliter. Medications used for lipid reduction include anion exchange resins, niacin, fibric acid derivatives, HMG CoA reductase inhibitors, fish oils, and probucol.[19] The goal of lipid management is to decrease lipid levels by a combination of diet, exercise, and medications as needed to attain acceptable levels. See Table 12–14 for drug management.

TABLE 12–13. Lipid Abnormalities

Type I:	Normal total cholesterol
	Increased triglycerides
	? Low HDL
Type II:	
IIa:	Increased total cholesterol
	Increased LDL
	Normal triglycerides
IIb:	Increased LDL
	Increased VLDL
	Increased total cholesterol
	Increased triglycerides
Type III:	Increased LDL
	Increased total cholesterol
	Increased triglycerides
Type IV:	Increased triglycerides
	Increased VLDL
	Normal cholesterol
Type V:	Increased triglycerides
	Increased cholesterol
	Increased VLDL

HDL, high-density lipoprotein; LDL, low-density lipoprotein; VLDL, very low density lipoprotein.

Side Effects

The adverse effects of lipid-lowering drugs include

- gastrointestinal distress (e.g., constipation, diarrhea, nausea)
- liver function abnormalities
- skin rashes (especially with niacin)
- increased bleeding time (fish oils)

TABLE 12–14. Classifications of Lipid-Lowering Drugs

Anion Exchange Resins

Cholystyramine (Questran)
Colestipol (Colestid)

Primary Effect:

Decreases LDL
  (a) binds intestinal bile, causing fecal excretion of bile acids
  (b) increases LDL receptor activity

TABLE 12–14. Classifications of Lipid-Lowering Drugs *Continued*

Useful in Treating:

Type IIa, Type IIb

Fibric Acid Derivatives
Clofibrate (Atromid-S)
Gemfibrozil (Lopid)
Fenofibrate (not available in U.S.)

Primary Effect:

Decreases triglycerides
(a) reduces ability of free fatty acids to form triglycerides
(b) increases intravascular breakdown of VLDL

Secondary Effect:

(a) increases activity of lipoprotein lipase

Useful in Treating:

Type IIa, Type IIb; Type III; Type IV; Type V

HMG - CoA Reductase Inhibitor
Lovastatin (Mevacor)
Pravastatin

Primary Effect:

Decreases LDL
(a) increases LDL receptor activity
(b) inhibits cholesterol synthesis

Secondary Effect:

Increases HDL

Useful in Treating:

Type IIa, Type IIb; Type III

Nicotinic Acid

Niacin

Primary Effect:

Decreases LDL, decreases triglycerides
(a) reduces hepatic synthesis of VLDL
(b) decreases plasma levels of free fatty acids

Secondary Effect:

Increases HDL

Useful in Treating:

Type IIa, Type IIb; Type III; Type IV; Type V

Probucol (Lorelco)

Primary Effect:

Decreases LDL
(a) combines with LDL and enhances LDL catabolism

Deleterious Effect:

Decreases HDL

Fish Oils

Omega-3 fatty acid (many over-the-counter varieties, e.g., SuperEPA)

Primary Effect:

Decreases triglycerides

LDL, low-density lipoprotein; VLDL, very low density lipoprotein; HDL, high-density lipoprotein.
(From Rakel R. Conn's Current Therapy 1993. Philadelphia, WB Saunders, 1993, p 548.)

Lovastatin may contribute to headaches, sleep disturbances, decreased sleep duration, fatigue, and muscle cramping. **Pravastatin,** another HMG-CoA reductase inhibitor, does not cross the blood-brain barrier as does lovastatin and therefore may have less effect on the central nervous system.

Clinical Considerations

Because of the potential for worsening glucose levels, niacin and fish oils are not recommended for the diabetic patient. Liver enzyme levels should be checked within the first 6 weeks and again at 3- and 6-month intervals as needed for patients on lovastatin, niacin, and gemfibrozil. General fatigue, achiness, and abdominal discomfort may accompany elevated lipid levels. Patients who exercise and take lovastatin often complain of muscle achiness and should be evaluated for possible drug-induced side effects and exercise intolerance.

CARDIAC DRUGS USED IN CRITICAL CARE

Many pathologic conditions warrant observation and management in the critical care setting. The hemodynamic instability caused by an underlying pathologic condition often requires quick responsiveness by the medical staff. Administration of appropriate pharmacologic agents and close monitoring of their effects can significantly alter the outcome of therapy. Numerous cardiovascular conditions may be responsible for systemic compromise. Common etiologies include

● acute myocardial ischemia or infarct
● congestive heart failure and pulmonary edema
● cardiac structural abnormalities
● cardiac conduction system disease

Clinical presentations of these cardiac dysfunctions may include

● hypoxia
● pain
● alterations in blood pressure (e.g., hypertension or hypotension)

- alterations in heart rate
- heart rhythm abnormalities

Whenever possible, drug therapy is directed at removal of the underlying pathologic condition, for example, thrombolysis (discussed elsewhere in this chapter). In addition to providing the patient with oxygen to help reverse hypoxia, pharmacologic therapy may focus on the manipulation of the autonomic nervous system to alter hemodynamics favorably. Drug agonists and antagonists of the parasympathetic and sympathetic nervous systems are used to induce changes in vasomotor tone, cardiac inotropy, and chronotropy. Cardiac output may be further improved by the administration of antihypertensive agents (those acting independent of the autonomic nervous system) and antiarrhythmic drugs. Elimination of pain, induction of sedation, and prevention of the complications of bedrest may also be addressed with drug therapy in the critical care setting.

Pharmacologic management of the patient in the cardiac critical care setting is often guided by invasive measurement as well as by symptoms. For example, to prescribe a vasodilator, the physician must closely monitor left ventricular filling pressures (preload) and cardiac output. Patients with dyspnea and high-filling pressures might benefit from venodilators to reduce preload, whereas patients with fatigue and low cardiac output might benefit from arteriodilators to improve forward output.[20] Table 12–15 categorizes hemodynamic indices found in acute myocardial infarction and suggests guidelines for use of pharmacologic agents in this setting.

Oxygen

Although oxygen is not frequently thought of as a drug, it should be thought of as a drug, and it warrants a brief discussion in the context of pharmacologic considerations in cardiac critical care. Tissue hypoxia caused by disturbances in cardiac output can rarely be improved by the administration of oxygen. However, oxygen therapy is usually beneficial when concomitant hypoxemia exists.[21] Pulmonary edema, often a finding with congestive heart failure, can hinder oxygen diffusion in the lung, thereby decreasing arterial oxygen content. The administration of oxygen may help limit the severity of hypoxemia and consequent tissue hypoxia. In addition, when hemoglobin concentration is reduced, as in anemia or in conditions that cause hemoglobin to **desaturate,** the administration of oxygen is considered beneficial. Oxygen delivery systems are discussed in Chapter 10.

Agents That Affect the Autonomic Nervous System

The autonomic nervous system exerts significant control over cardiovascular function. A

TABLE 12–15. Suggested Therapeutic Interventions in Relation to Hemodynamic Indices Found in Acute Myocardial Infarction

Hemodynamic Category	Cardiac Output	Left Ventricular Filling Pressure	Suggested Therapy
Normal	Normal	Normal	Observation
Hypovolemia	Decreased	Decreased or Normal	Volume replacement
Pulmonary congestion	Normal	Raised	Diuretics
Left ventricular failure			
Moderate	Decreased	Raised	Afterload reducing agents, with or without diuretics
Severe (cardiogenic shock)	Markedly decreased	Raised	Circulatory assist (counterpulsation) Afterload reducing agents Use of inotropic agents if other measures do not increase cardiac output*

*E.g., dopamine (Intropin, Dopastat), dobutamine (Dobutrex).
(Adapted from Sokolow M, McIlroy M, Cheitlin M. Clinical Cardiology. 5th ed. East Norwalk, Conn, Appleton & Lange, 1990.)

complex system of feedback loops coordinates reflex responses of the sympathetic and the parasympathetic nervous systems. Transmission of impulses from the autonomic portion of the central nervous system to the effector organ to be stimulated occurs via neurotransmitter substances. As discussed in the introduction, most preganglionic fibers, and all parasympathetic nervous system postganglionic fibers release *acetylcholine.* Most sympathetic nervous system postganglionic fibers release norepinephrine (noradrenaline). These substances, or catecholamines, can be partially or completely mimicked by pharmacologic agents (e.g., sympathomimetics, parasympathomimetics, or sympathetic or parasympathetic nervous system agonists). Similarly,

receptors in the effector organ can be partially or completely blocked by pharmacologic agents (e.g., adrenoceptor or cholinoceptor blocking agents or sympathetic or parasympathetic nervous system antagonists).

When negative alterations in mean arterial blood pressure are sensed, **adrenoceptors** and **cholinoceptors** are stimulated. Appropriate modification of peripheral vascular resistance and cardiac output are orchestrated (Fig. 12–9). In a critically ill cardiac patient, pharmacologic agents can act on the autonomic nervous system receptors to help bring about a hemodynamic stability and an effective cardiac output. By fine manipulation of the degree of vasodilation, vasoconstriction, or cardiac inotropy, an adequate mean arte-

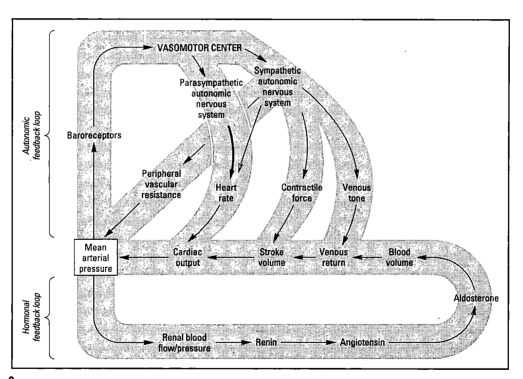

Figure 12–9.

Autonomic and hormonal control of cardiovascular function. Note that at least two feedback loops are present, the autonomic nervous system loop and the hormonal loop. In addition, each major loop has several components. Thus, the sympathetic nervous system directly influences four major variables; peripheral vascular resistance, heart rate, force, and venous tone. The parasympathetic directly influences heart rate. Angiotensin II directly increases peripheral vascular resistance (not shown), and the sympathetic nervous system directly increases renin secretion (not shown). Because these control mechanisms are designed to maintain normal blood pressure, the net feedback effect of each loop is negative in that it tends to compensate for the change in arterial blood pressure that evoked the response. Thus, decreased blood pressure due to blood loss would be compensated for by increased sympathetic outflow and renin release. Conversely, elevated pressure due to the administration of a vasoconstrictor drug would cause reduced sympathetic outflow and renin release, and increased parasympathetic (vagal) outflow. (From Katzung BG [ed]. Basic and Clinical Pharmacology. 5th ed. East Norwalk, Conn, Appleton & Lange, 1992, p 76.)

rial blood pressure can be established with drug therapy. Table 12–16 lists drugs that act as agonists or antagonists to the sympathetic and parasympathetic nervous systems to control blood pressure. Because of the reflex nature of the feedback "loop" of the autonomic nervous system, the effects of these agents are monitored closely. Although some drugs are receptor selective, some act on multiple receptor sites. Often drugs are used in combinations in an attempt to reduce or augment certain hemodynamic responses, which further emphasizes the importance of medical observation. Epinephrine (Adrenalin Chloride), for example, is both an alpha-adrenergic agonist and a beta-adrenergic agonist; clinically, however, it usually acts only as a beta agonist.

Antihypertensive Agents

In addition to manipulating the autonomic nervous system with drugs to manage arterial blood pressure in critical care, physicians can also prescribe other antihypertensive agents. Sodium nitroprusside (Nipride), a potent peripheral vasodilator, and intravenous nitroglycerin are frequently used. The intravenous nitroglycerin produces a slightly greater reduction in preload and a slightly lesser reduction in afterload as compared with those of sodium nitroprusside.[22] Although both agents are effective in reducing blood pressure, the intravenous nitroglycerin is the emergency drug of choice in the treatment of congestive heart failure associated with ischemic heart disease. Sodium nitroprusside is the paren-

TABLE 12–16. Drugs Affecting the Autonomic Nervous System: Agents Commonly Used in Critical Care

Autonomic Nervous System Receptor	Action	Agonist generic (trade)	Antagonist generic (trade)
		Adrenoceptor	
Alpha$_1$	Contraction of vascular smooth muscle	Phenylephrine (Neo-Synephrine) Methoxamine (Vasoxyl)	See antihypertensives, Table 12–12 (alpha$_1$ blockers)
Alpha$_2$	Contraction of vascular smooth muscle Platelet aggregation	Clonidine (Catapres) Alpha-methyl-norepinephrine	Tolazoline (Priscoline) Yohimbine (Yohimex)
Combined alpha$_1$ and alpha$_2$		Epinephrine* (Adrenalin Chloride) Norepinephrine† (Levophed)	Phentolamine (Rogitine)
Beta$_1$	Increase force and rate of cardiac contraction	Norepinephrine† (Levophed) Dobutamine (Dobutrex) Prenalterol (investigational)	See beta blockers, Table 12–5
Beta$_2$	Relaxation of vascular, respiratory smooth muscle	Albuterol (Proventil, Ventolin) Terbutaline (Brethine) Metaproterenol (Alupent, Metaprel)	See beta blockers, Table 12–5
Combined beta$_1$ and beta$_2$		Isoproterenol‡ (Isuprel) Epinephrine* (Adrenalin Chloride)	See beta blockers, Table 12–5
Dopaminic	Vasodilation	Dopamine (Intropin)	
		Cholinoceptor	
Muscarinic	Decreases rate and force of atrial contraction	Acetylcholine (Miochol)	Atropine (Isopto Atropine)
	Decreases peripheral vascular resistance	Edrophonium§ (Tensilon)	

*Epinephrine is also called adrenalin; it acts primarily as a beta agonist.
†Norepinephrine is also called noradrenalin or levarterenol.
‡Isoproterenol is also called isoprenaline.
§This is not a direct-acting agonist; rather it acts indirectly by inhibiting acetylcholinesterase, thereby increasing acetylcholine.

teral treatment of choice for hypertension emergencies.

As discussed earlier in this chapter, diuretics act to reduce central venous pressures by decreasing venous return. Furosemide (Lasix) is a potent, rapidly acting diuretic, often administered parenterally in the emergency treatment of pulmonary congestion in the presence of left ventricular dysfunction.

Antiarrhythmic Agents

Life-threatening arrhythmias are commonly treated in cardiac critical care units. In addition to electrical cardioversion of unstable rhythms, pharmacologic intervention is the mainstay of medical treatment. Lidocaine (Xylocaine) is the drug of choice for the suppression of ventricular ectopy in critically ill patients. It is used both **prophylactically** for patients with acute myocardial ischemia · and therapeutically for patients suffering ventricular tachycardia or fibrillation. In emergencies, it is delivered as a bolus injection that is followed by subsequent continuous intravenous infusion.

When lidocaine (Xylocaine) cannot control ventricular arrhythmias, **procainamide** (Pronestyl) can be useful. **Bretylium tosylate** (Bretylol), a class 3 antiarrhythmic, has been used in the treatment of ventricular fibrillation when lidocaine, procainamide, and electrical defibrillation fail. Verapamil (Isoptin, Calan), a calcium channel blocker (class 4 antiarrhythmic), is the drug of choice for the management of supraventricular tachycardia not requiring **cardioversion.**

Finally, digitalis may be used to control the ventricular response rate to atrial flutter or fibrillation. Unfortunately, it may cause significant toxicity and adverse drug interactions in critically ill patients. Although digitalis may successfully convert **paroxysmal supraventricular tachycardia** to normal sinus rhythm, it may alternatively convert atrial flutter to atrial fibrillation. Digitalis's effects on contractility are less potent than those of sympathomimetic parenteral inotropes, such as dobutamine (Dobutrex) or norepinephrine (Levophed), and therefore typically are not used for this purpose in critical care.

Other Pharmacologic Agents Used in Critical Care

Other pharmacologic agents frequently used in critical care include anticoagulants, such as heparin (Liquaemin Sodium), sedatives to reduce agitation and anxiety, and analgesics. Morphine sulfate, included in this last group, is the drug of choice for management of myocardial ischemic pain. However, it is also very useful in the treatment of acute cardiogenic pulmonary edema. It is a potent vasodilator and acts to increase venous capacitance as well as to relieve pulmonary congestion.

As patients become hemodynamically stable, the prescription of many of the potent drugs described in this section is discontinued and replaced by oral medications. Readers interested in additional information regarding drugs used in critical care are encouraged to refer to the *Textbook of Advanced Cardiac Life Support* published by the American Heart Association.

CARDIAC PHARMACOLOGY IN THE GERIATRIC POPULATION

All drugs, not just those prescribed for cardiac problems, may have altered pharmacokinetics and pharmacodynamics in the elderly. Normal aging involves changes in body composition and function (Table 12–17). Specifically, decreases in renal function and altered blood flow (as in coronary artery disease and congestive heart failure) are responsible for adverse or suboptimal reactions to cardiac drugs. The elderly also exhibit increased sensitivity to the toxic effects of cardiac drugs such as antiarrhythmics, digitalis, or beta blockers. Other disease states such as liver or nutritional deficiencies, which often accompany aging, can alter the effectiveness of cardiac drug therapy. In addition, numerous socioeconomic and practical considerations can affect the degree of compliance by the elderly with these drug regimens.

TABLE 12–17. Average Changes in Body Composition and Function with Age	
	Change from Age 20 to Age 80 (%)
Body fat/total body weight	+35
Plasma volume	−8
Plasma albumin	−10
Plasma globulin	−10
Total body water	−17
Extracellular fluid (from age 20 to age 65)	−40
Conduction velocity	−20
Cardiac index	−40
Glomerular filtration rate	−50
Vital capacity	−60
Cardiac output	−30–40
Splanchnic and renal blood flow	−40

(From Kalant H, Roschlau W, Sellers M. Principles of Medical Pharmacology. 4th ed. New York, Oxford University Press, 1985, p 68.)

Alteration in Pharmacokinetics

Elderly patients may have difficulty with absorption, distribution, or metabolism of cardiac drugs. Effective drug elimination is dependent on adequate renal function. The typical age-related decline in kidney competency significantly increases the likelihood of drug accumulation and subsequent toxicity. This problem of drug accumulation is especially relevant with regard to the older patient's cardiac conduction system. The elderly are more susceptible to arrhythmias. Positive inotropes, such as digitalis, and antihypertensive agents, such as diuretics, can be particularly dangerous. These drugs alter electrolytes involved in conduction tissue depolarization. Inadequate drug elimination and consequent accumulation can cause cardiac irritability and a higher incidence of arrhythmias.

Therapeutic Indications

Cardiovascular drugs are used for treatment of the same conditions in the elderly as in other age groups. However, the significance of lowering cholesterol in an older population is still unclear. At this time, it appears prudent to reduce lipid levels in both primary and secondary prevention of coronary artery disease, and anticholesterolemic agents may be prescribed.

Socioeconomic Issues

As with most drugs, the effectiveness of cardiovascular agents depends on numerous practical concerns. Elderly patients often demonstrate difficulty with full compliance with drug prescriptions. In addition to financial concerns, they may have several physicians prescribing drugs and no one monitoring the effects of drug combinations. Patients may get confused and forget a dose. When elderly patients feel good, they may choose to discontinue taking the drug, or the side effects themselves may discourage patients from taking the drug. Although these issues may occur in younger age groups, the elderly are especially susceptible to these problems. Dementia or physical inability may also hamper adequate utilization of cardiovascular drugs. Seemingly simple items such as reading drug labels, removing bottle caps, or distinguishing pill color can present major obstacles to visually impaired or physically disabled elderly patients. Drug holders with the day of the week written on each compartment may improve compliance with medications.

Safe and effective use of cardiovascular agents in the geriatric population can be enhanced by knowledgeable health care providers and educated patients and family members. Drug regimens should be simplified whenever possible, with small initial doses and progressive titration until a therapeutic response is reached. Additionally, when working with the older patient, the medical team should remain alert to adverse drug reactions and interactions, taking care to avoid provoking a drug reaction that would be worse than the disease itself.

CARDIAC PHARMACOLOGY IN THE NEONATE AND PEDIATRIC POPULATIONS

Although many pharmacologic agents used to treat adult cardiac conditions are also used to treat **neonate** and pediatric patients, the younger population's response may demonstrate significant clinical differences. The immature organism can demonstrate unpredictable responses because of the unique pharmacokinetic and pharmacodynamic reactions found during each stage of development. Additionally, most cardiac drug activity has been studied in adults, and the paucity of controlled research on the immature patient causes further concern regarding optimal drug therapy in this population.

Alteration in Pharmacokinetics

Adequate plasma concentrations of a drug can be influenced by proper administration and absorption of the agent. Newborns absorb drugs more slowly than children, whereas children may have difficulty swallowing medicines. Drugs delivered intravenously bypass the absorption process; however, choosing the intravenous route increases the risks of fluid overload. The relative intolerance of infants to the volumes of fluid needed to carry a drug warrants slower rates of infusion and at times negligible concentrations if the drug is eliminated at the same rate.

As the infant develops, changes in body composition and plasma protein binding capacity affect the distribution of a drug. Total body water decreases as adipose tissue increases and fluid shifts between body compartments. Drugs are less avidly bound to plasma proteins in neonates and infants than in children and adults. Development of the liver and kidneys affects metabolism and elimination of a drug, with both organs showing decreased function at birth. However, infants and young children may metabolize drugs faster than adults.

Alteration in Pharmacodynamics

The ability of the infant or child to respond to adequate concentrations of a cardiac drug is influenced by structural concerns that are unique to the developing organism.[23,24] Although not well studied in humans, fetal and newborn puppies and lambs exhibit (1) stiffer, less compliant ventricles; (2) smaller myocardial cells (adjusted for weight and size); and (3) a higher proportion of noncontractile to contractile tissue (e.g., mitochondria to **myofilaments**) as compared with the adult. Sympathetic nervous system innervation of the heart and periphery are decreased at birth and continue to develop during the first few months of life. Infants and young children have a higher baseline heart rate; this, in combination with a lower stroke volume, which has a limited ability to increase, means that the ways to improve cardiac output with drugs may be impaired.

Therapeutic Indications

Cardiac conditions in pediatric populations that warrant pharmacologic intervention usually include heart failure, blood pressure abnormalities, and arrhythmias. Digoxin (Lanoxin), a commonly used inotrope, is better tolerated in infants and young children than in adults, and usually achieves a satisfactory response at lower doses (normalized for weight and size). Other inotropes frequently used include isoproterenol (Isuprel), dopamine (Intropin, Dopastat), and dobutamine (Dobutrex). Because the immature heart is limited in its ability to increase stroke volume, inotropic agents may be less effective in it than in an adult heart. Therefore, increases in cardiac output may depend on drug-induced increases in heart rate.

Vasodilators such as sodium nitroprusside (Nipride) and nitroglycerin (Nitro-Bid, Nitrostat, and others) are often used in treating patients with severe congestive cardiomyopathy and postcardiac surgery patients. They are used with special caution in newborns owing to the immature peripheral vascular resistance mechanisms of the sympathetic nervous system and the consequent enhanced risks of hypotension.

Drug therapy for pediatric patients parallels therapy for adults. The same agents are used for the same physiologic abnormalities. The immature heart, lungs, and systemic vascular structures require individualized therapeutic regimens. Understanding the progressive nature of the organism's development and the exact stage of maturity greatly influences the clinical efficacy of cardiac pharmacotherapy for this population.

TABLE 12–18. Oral Hypoglycemic Agents Used in Diabetic Management

Generic Name	Brand Name
First generation	
Tolbutamide	Orinase
Chlorpropamide	Diabinese
Tolazamide	Tolinase
Acetohexamide	Dymelor
Second generation	
Glyburide	Micronase, Diabeta
Glipizide	Glucotrol

(From Rakel R [ed]. Conn's Current Therapy 1990. Philadelphia, WB Saunders, 1990, p 499.)

PHARMACOLOGIC MANAGEMENT OF DIABETES

Pharmacologic management for the diabetic patient includes the use of either oral hypoglycemic agents or insulin (Tables 12–18 and 12–19). Patients with impaired insulin production, insulin resistance, or both are placed on oral agents; patients with chronic insulin deficiency or absence of endogenous insulin production from the beta cells of the pancreas are managed with insulin.

Clinical Considerations

One of the important components of a safe exercise program is avoidance of exercise-induced hypoglycemia. Signs and symptoms of hypoglycemia include

- weakness
- **diaphoresis**
- mental confusion
- muscle rigidity

For patients with coronary artery disease, angina or an anginal equivalent may occur. In insulin-dependent diabetics, hypoglycemia may occur during or immediately following the exercise session or hours after the session has ended as the muscles are replenishing their energy stores. Knowledge of the type of insulin that a person is taking and avoidance of exercise during its peak effect is crucial to avoid augmentation of exercise-induced hypoglycemia (see Table 12–19). During the beginning days of an exercise program, insulin-dependent patients should monitor their blood glucose both before and after exercise to understand their individualized response to exercise. Patients should make certain that their blood sugar is appropriate before starting exercise and may need to take a supplemental snack within the 60 to 90 minutes before beginning (Table 12–20). Patients should be encouraged to carry a readily available carbohydrate source, for example, hard candy or jelly beans, and to meet with a nutritionist for specific diet instruction. It is prudent for any physical therapy department that treats insulin-dependent patients to have easy access to juice and sugar.

TABLE 12–19. Types of Insulin

Insulin	Modifier	Onset* (hr)	Peak* (hr)	Duration* (hr)
Short acting				
Regular	None	0.5–1.0	2–5	5–8
Semilente	Zinc	1.0–1.5	3–8	8–16
Intermediate acting				
NPH	Protamine	1–1.5	6–14	18–28
Lente	Zinc	1–2.5	6–14	18–28
Long acting				
PZI	Protamine, zinc	4–8	None	24–36
Ultralente	Zinc	4–8	None	24–36

*Considerable interindividual variation for these times.
NPH, neutral protamine Hagedorn; PZI, protamine zinc insulin.
(From Rakel R [ed]. Conn's Current Therapy 1990. Philadelphia, WB Saunders, 1990, p 500.)

TABLE 12–20. General Guidelines for Making Food Adjustments for Exercise

Type of Exercise and Examples	If Blood Glucose Is:	Increase Food Intake By:	Suggestions of Food to Use
Exercise of short duration and of low to moderate intensity (walking a half mile or leisurely bicycling for less than 30 minutes)	Less than 100 mg/dL	10 to 15 g of carbohydrate per hour	1 fruit or 1 starch/bread exchange
	100 mg/dL or above	Not necessary to increase food	
Exercise of moderate intensity (1 hour of tennis, swimming, jogging, leisurely bicycling, golfing, etc.)	Less than 100 mg/dL	25 to 50 g of carbohydrate before exercise, then 10 to 15 g per hour of exercise	1/2 meat sandwich with a milk or fruit exchange
	100 to 180 mg/dL	10 to 15 g of carbohydrate	1 fruit or 1 starch/bread exchange
	180 to 300 mg/dL	Not necessary to increase food	
	300 mg/dL or above	Don't begin exercise until blood glucose is under better control	
Strenuous activity or exercise (about 1 to 2 hours of football, hockey, racquetball, or basketball games; strenuous bicycling or swimming; shoveling heavy snow)	Less than 100 mg/dL	50 g of carbohydrate, monitor blood glucose carefully	1 meat sandwich (2 slices of bread) with a milk and fruit exchange
	100 to 180 mg/dL	25 to 50 g of carbohydrate, depending on intensity and duration	1/2 meat sandwich with a milk or fruit exchange
	180 to 300 mg/dL	10 to 15 g of carbohydrate	1 fruit or 1 starch/bread exchange
	300 mg/dL or above	Don't begin exercise until blood glucose is under better control	

(Reprinted, with permission, from Franz MJ, Norstrom RD, Norstrom J. Diabetes Actively Staying Healthy [DASH]: Your Game Plan for Diabetes and Exercise, Minneapolis, International Diabetes Center, 1990; Wayzata, Minn, DCI Publishing, pp 112–113.)

Patients whose blood sugar level is greater than 250 milligrams per deciliter should not exercise because blood sugar will not decrease but may in fact worsen. Blood sugar levels of greater than 250 milligrams per deciliter are often accompanied by the presence of **ketones** in the urine. When this occurs, exercise is absolutely contraindicated until improved glycemic control has been established.

Patients should be reminded not to inject insulin into muscle but into subcutaneous tissue. Exercise of a limb that has received an insulin injection should be avoided for at least 60 to 90 minutes or until the peak effect of the insulin has been reached. Exercising the limb sooner than that may cause the insulin effect to peak prematurely because the increased blood flow associated with exercise facilitates the entry of insulin into the blood. As with all patients, adequate fluid intake is important before, during, and after exercise beyond 30 minutes in duration.

Awareness that blisters from ill-fitting footwear may lead to prolonged healing and may develop complications is sufficient reason to instruct patients to choose footwear wisely. Within the physical therapy department, avoiding situations that may bruise the patient is very important for all patients but particularly for diabetic patients. Patients with diabetic **retinopathy** should avoid any head-down position or situation that would cause a blood pressure reading of greater than 180 mm Hg systolic. **Peripheral neuropathy** may make walking on uneven surfaces unsafe for the patient, and routine activities of daily living may be cumbersome and difficult.

Hypoglycemia may also occur in the non-insulin-dependent diabetic patient, although this is not seen as frequently as it is in insulin-dependent patients.

PHARMACOLOGY AND HEART TRANSPLANTATION

Survival after **orthotopic heart transplantation** has improved dramatically since the first procedure was performed in 1967. Advances in drug specificity have played a major role in the current 1-year survival rate, which exceeds 80%.[25] Rejection and infection have been the primary precursors of early mortality in this population. A combination of improved techniques used to monitor and detect early rejection and newer **immunosuppressive** pharmacologic agents may account for this reduction in morbidity and mortality. Clinical and laboratory research continues in an attempt to identify agents that act on specific components of the **immune system** while leaving other systems unaffected. Thus far, no one drug satisfies this goal. Medical centers vary considerably in their pharmacologic protocols for the heart transplant population.

Immune Mechanism

The immune system is a complex network of humoral and cellular functions that protect human beings from foreign substances **(antigens).** This system is stimulated when a heart is implanted in a patient with end-stage heart disease, because the recipient's immune system recognizes the donor heart as foreign.

Lymphocytes, mononuclear cells that circulate in the blood and lymph, interact with foreign substances to protect the body from invasion. Two types of lymphocytes, T cells and B cells, mediate cellular and serologic immunity, respectively. Current immunosuppressive therapy limits organ rejection by interfering with lymphocyte development, activation, and proliferation.

Pharmacologic Intervention

Corticosteroids

Corticosteroids were the first group of drugs to be recognized as having lympholytic properties.

Prednisone is the most commonly used immunosuppressor in this drug class. It is **cytotoxic** to certain subsets of T cells and further suppresses **antibody, prostaglandin,** and **leukotriene** synthesis, all important components of the immune system. Because precursor lymphoid (stem) cells are sensitive to prednisone, the primary response of lymphocyte formation may also be diminished. Unfortunately, long-term use of **steroids** has been implicated in morbidity, including **osteoporosis** and poor healing. The development of additional immunosuppressive agents (as discussed later) has enabled heart transplant recipients to be maintained on lower doses of steroids, thereby reducing the incidence of their negative side effects.

Cyclosporine

Before **cyclosporine** (Sandimmune) began to be used for immunosuppression of patients undergoing heart transplantation, 1-year survival rates were at best 65%.[25] Cyclosporine use, either alone or in combination with prednisone, has resulted in a lower incidence of rejection and infection in this population.[26] This agent appears to act at an early stage in stem cell differentiation to block T cell activation. It does not appear to affect already converted lymphoblasts. The lymphocytes it does affect recover their normal function after the drug is eliminated from the system.

Although cyclosporine appears to be impressive as a highly selective agent that is effective against a subpopulation of lymphocytes, it has a considerable number of side effects. Besides promoting **lymphoma,** cyclosporine causes **nephrotoxicity** and consequent hypertension. Elevated blood pressure due to cyclosporine is usually well controlled by one or two agents, such as ACE inhibitors and beta blockers.[25]

Azathioprine

Azathioprine (Imuran) interferes with the wave of lymphocyte proliferation that occurs after the antigen stimulates the immune system. It is especially effective against T cells but can also block serologic immune responses. Toxicity to azathioprine results in bone marrow depression and hepatic dysfunction. Gastrointestinal disorders may occur at higher doses.

Antilymphocyte Antibodies

Several medical centers regularly use **antilymphocytic globulin, antithymocytic globulin,** or both for immunosuppression. Injection of animal (e.g., horse, rabbit) with human lymphocytes provokes the animal's immune mechanism to form antibodies to human lymphocytes. The animal's antilymphocytic globulin can then be injected into the transplant recipient, which ultimately causes cytotoxic destruction of the recipient's lymphocytes. Using these agents does increase the risk of cancer, however, because of the suppression of the normal defense system against carcinogens. Another antibody, OKT3, (a monoclonal antibody), has been found effective in blocking both cytotoxic activity of human T cells and the generation of other T cell function.

CASE STUDIES

CASE 1 – Anti-ischemia and Lipid Management, Part A

Mr. H is a 52-year-old business executive who underwent a routine physical examination for business insurance reasons. At the time of the physical, he stated that he was feeling fine. On further questioning, he acknowledged that his weekly tennis game was getting a bit slow; in fact he needed to switch from playing singles to playing doubles because he found himself becoming more easily winded. Mr. H attributed this to being out of shape, having slowly gained 20 pounds over the last 5 years and having been unable to give up his one pack per day cigarette habit. Blood pressure on the day of the physical was 148/100; the patient stated that he was a little nervous. Random, nonfasting cholesterol total was 270; patient was instructed to have a fasting lipid profile within the week. It was rec-

ommended that Mr. H have a baseline exercise tolerance test (ETT), to which he agreed.

Mr. H underwent a treadmill ETT using the Bruce protocol; total duration 5 minutes 30 seconds, at which time the test was stopped because Mr. H complained of difficulty breathing and chest heaviness. Vital signs at maximum work capacity were a heart rate of 170, blood pressure of 180/100. The ECG was interpreted as positive for ST depression at a heart rate of 160 and a blood pressure of 170/100. Mr. H was told that his ETT was positive for ischemia and that the medical recommendation at the time was to begin aggressive lifestyle and health habit alterations, including beginning a moderate exercise routine, quitting smoking, and getting nutritional counseling. Patient also began taking atenolol and was instructed in the use of sublingual nitroglycerin (NTG).

Mr. H was next seen 2 years later when he came to the emergency department with a chief complaint of chest heaviness unrelieved by nitroglycerin. Patient had been doing yard work when the discomfort first appeared about 2 hours earlier. Mr. H took NTG at the time of the discomfort, but he noted it didn't burn. (The bottle had been opened originally 2 years ago.) In the emergency department, Mr. H's ECG was significant for marked ST elevation in the inferior leads. Medical evaluation determined that Mr. H would be an appropriate candidate for thrombolytic therapy, and he was begun on the hospital's streptokinase protocol and, as soon as he was pain free, was admitted to the coronary care unit.

In the coronary care unit, the patient continued to follow the streptokinase protocol, including the use of continuous infusion heparin. Patient ruled in for a small inferior myocardial infarction; ejection fraction by cardiac ultrasound was 45%. Mr. H was begun on cardiac rehabilitation by physical therapy on hospital day 2. Patient did well with activity progression and appeared to understand and agree with discharge instructions. Mr. H was discharged on atenolol and diltiazem and was given a new prescription for NTG. Predischarge ETT was negative for ischemia at a heart rate of 110 beats per minute; Mr. H was given a follow-up appointment for maximal ETT in 6 weeks.

CASE 1, Part B

Mr. H called his physician to state that he was having recurrent chest discomfort 4 weeks after the inferior myocardial infarction was treated with streptokinase. Chest discomfort usually occurred while Mr. H was taking his 20-minute walk, but during the previous evening the discomfort came while he was eating. All symptoms were relieved with NTG. Physician ordered an ETT (modified Bruce protocol) for that day. Test was stopped at 2½ minutes when the ECG showed significant ST depression in leads II, III, and aVF at a heart rate of 80 beats per minute. Patient felt his usual chest discomfort, which was relieved with NTG. Mr. H was sent for an emergency cardiac catherization, which was significant for an 80% occlusion in the right coronary artery (RCA) and 30% to 50% lesions in the circumflex. Patient underwent percutaneous transluminal coronary angioplasty of the RCA. Discharge medications included persantine, diltiazem, and atenolol. Predischarge blood work indicated that Mr. H's lipid profile was as follows: total cholesterol 265, LDL 190, HDL 20, and triglycerides 275. Type IIb hyperlipoproteinemia was diagnosed, and Mr. H was begun on mevacor. Mr. H admitted that he had not followed through with the recommendations for either smoking cessation or nutritional counseling in the past but was determined to do so this time.

Mr. H was seen for regularly scheduled physician visits throughout the following year. He was compliant with diet, exercise, and smoking cessation and had lost 30 pounds. Resting heart rate was 54 beats per minute, blood pressure was 90/60. Physician decreased both the atenolol and diltiazem by half. A repeat lipid profile was scheduled for 3 months, and the patient was told to come off the mevacor.

Three months later, a fasting lipid profile showed the following: total cholesterol 160, HDL 45, LDL 90, triglycerides 125. Mr. H had lost another 10 pounds and was exercising for 50 minutes, four times a week within his training heart rate range; he stated that he never felt better in his life. Mr. H underwent a modified Bruce ETT; his duration was 14 minutes 20 seconds, and his maximum vital signs were heart rate 145 beats per minute and blood pressure 170/70. Test was negative for ischemia at that level.

CASE 2 – Antiarrhythmic

Mr. J is a 52-year-old businessman who was admitted to the coronary care unit after complaining of 2 hours of substernal chest pain, nausea, and diaphoresis. His ECG was consistent with an inferior wall myocardial infarction. Thirty minutes after his arrival in the coronary care unit he developed frequent unifocal premature ventricular contractions, bigeminy, couplets, and several short runs (5 beats) of ventricular tachycardia. A bolus of lidocaine (Xylocaine) was administered, and an intravenous drip was started. Forty-eight hours after admission, the lidocaine was discontinued. No further ventricular ectopy was noticed, and long-term antiarrhythmic therapy was not necessary.

CASE 3 – Antiarrhythmic

Mr. P is a 68-year-old retired dentist who began to notice occasional "flutters" in his chest accompanied by slight dizziness. He had suffered an anterolateral wall myocardial infarction 8 years earlier and had been taking isordil, atenolol, and diltiazem. He checked his pulse when he had these episodes, and it felt "as if his heart stopped beating after every second beat." He called his physician, who ordered a 24-hour Holter monitor. A review of the Holter showed multifocal premature ventricular contractions in bigeminy and trigeminy; rare couplets were also recorded. He was given a prescription for quinidine. Two days after starting this medication, Mr. P noticed gastrointestinal symptoms of diarrhea and slight nausea. He was switched to procainamide and experienced no further distress. Ten months after the initiation of this drug, he noticed a return of his "flutter" symptoms and lightheadedness. The Holter monitor now showed frequent couplets and nonsustained ventricular tachycardia. Also, he began complaining of arthralgias and stopped his regular exercise program. Procainamide was discontinued, and he was admitted to the hospital. He underwent exercise thallium testing to rule out the possibility of ischemia-induced ectopy. The test was negative for ischemia; however dyskinesis of the anterior and anteroapical walls was noted, which was consistent with aneurysm. During subsequent electrophysiologic testing, ventricular tachycardia was provoked and required defibrillation to regain normal sinus rhythm. He was begun on mexiletine and was retested when serum levels were therapeutic. Ventricular tachycardia was no longer inducible, and Mr. P was discharged on mexilitine and told to resume his normal activities and participate in a monitored cardiac rehabilitation program.

CASE 4 – Critical Care

Mrs. S is a 72-year-old woman who arrived in the emergency department with mild symptoms of fatigue, shortness of breath, and recent (1-day) history of diaphoresis and nausea. An anterior wall myocardial infarction (MI) was diagnosed, but Mrs. S denies ever experiencing chest pain.

Her past medical history includes two silent MIs, insulin-dependent diabetes mellitus for 22 years, obesity, cigarette abuse, sedentary lifestyle, arthritis, and cataracts (right worse than left). Mrs. S is a widow and lives in a second-floor apartment. Her son lives on the first floor, and he is trying to convince his mother to move downstairs.

On day three after admission, Mrs. S developed severe respiratory distress and was transferred to the critical care unit for management of pulmonary edema and congestive heart failure. Her inderal was discontinued, and she was started on oxygen, intravenous morphine, and furosemide (Lasix). Her cardiac output dropped, consistent with cardiogenic shock. Invasive monitoring allowed hemodynamic observation as intravenous dobutamine and nitroglycerin were added to her pharmacologic regimen. Potassium was given orally. Her symptoms resolved; however, it

took 5 days to wean her from intravenous support and on to oral medications. She left the critical care unit on oxygen, Isordil, digitalis, Lasix, and an ACE inhibitor. After 6 days of symptom-free, graded ambulation, Mrs. S was transferred to a rehabilitation facility for further endurance training. A cardiac catheterization was postponed until she gained strength or became symptomatic.

SUMMARY

● Abnormal cardiac impulse formation or conduction can be treated by altering cell membrane permeability to specific ions (e.g., sodium, calcium).
● Although exercise may be responsible for production of arrhythmias, an electrolyte imbalance or toxic levels of antiarrhythmic drugs may also be responsible.
● Drugs used to treat hypertension act by altering kidney, autonomic nervous system, and peripheral vessel activity to reduce circulating volume, promote vasodilation, and inhibit vasoconstriction and cardiac inotropy.
● Diuretics can predispose the exercising individual to hypotension or arrhythmias owing to volume reduction or electrolyte disturbances, respectively.
● Cardiac drugs used in critical care settings typically act by altering the sympathetic and parasympathetic nervous systems and are used cautiously with hemodynamic monitoring.
● Although patients of all ages can be treated with most cardiac drugs, an awareness of the unique alterations in pharmacokinetics in the very young or the elderly patient is essential.
● Drugs have primary effects, secondary effects, and side effects.
● Selectivity means that when a certain concentration of the drug exists, the drug is preferentially attracted to one group or subgroup of receptors.
● An agonist (drug) is one that facilitates activity within a cell; an antagonist (drug) inhibits agonist activity.
● Triple therapy for coronary artery disease involves the use of beta blockers, calcium channel blockers, and nitrates.
● Beta blockers are not used when the ejection fraction is less than 35%.

- Pharmacologic management of heart failure includes the use of diuretics, positive inotropes, venodilators, arteriodilators, calcium channel blockers, ACE inhibitors, and, in severe failure, morphine.
- Digoxin toxicity is relatively common and may include nausea, arrhythmias, and light sensitivity.
- Drug management for hyperlipoproteinemia is influenced by the type of lipid dysfunction present.
- Rebound hypoglycemia may occur hours after exercise-induced hypoglycemia.

References

1. Katzung BG. Introduction. In: Katzung BG (ed). Basic and Clinical Pharmacology. 4th ed. East Norwalk, Conn, Appleton & Lange, 1989.
2. Ross EM, Gilman AG. Pharmacodynamics: Mechanisms of drug action and the relationship between drug concentration and effect. In: Gilman AG, Goodman LS, Rall TW, Murad F (eds). Goodman and Gilman's The Pharmacologic Basis of Therapeutics. 7th ed. New York, Macmillan, 1985, p 35.
3. Benet LZ. Pharmacokinetics: Absorption, distribution and elimination. In: Katzung BG (ed). Basic and Clinical Pharmacology. 4th ed. East Norwalk, Conn, Appleton & Lange, 1989, p 29.
4. Blaschke TF, Nies AS, Mamelok RD. Principles of therapeutics. In: Gilman AG, Goodman LS, Rall TW, Murad F (eds). Goodman and Gilman's The Pharmacologic Basis of Therapeutics. 7th ed. New York, Macmillan, 1985, pp 50–53.
5. Opie LH, Gersh BJ. Antithrombotic agents: Platelet inhibitors, anticoagulants, and fibrinolytics. In: Opie LH (ed). Drugs for the Heart. 2nd ed. Philadelphia, WB Saunders, 1987, p 163.
6. Conley CL. Hemostasis. In: Mountcastle VB. Medical Physiology. 13th ed. St. Louis, CV Mosby, 1974, p 1040.
7. Hoffman BB. Adrenoceptor-blocking drugs. In: Katzung BG (ed). Basic and Clinical Pharmocology. 4th ed. East Norwalk, Conn, Appleton & Lange, 1989, p 112.
8. Opie LH, Sonnenblick EH, et al. Beta-blocking agents. In: Opie LH (ed). Drugs for the Heart. 2nd ed. Philadelphia, WB Saunders, 1987, p 9.
9. Needleman P, Corr PB, Johnson EM. Drugs used for the treatment of angina: Organic nitrates, calcium channel blockers, and beta-adrenergic antagonists. In: Gilman AG, Goodman LS, Rall TW, Murad F (eds). Goodman and Gilman's The Pharmacologic Basis of Therapeutics. 7th ed. New York, Macmillan, 1985, pp 808–810.
10. Dec GW, O'Gara PT, Curfman GD. Acute myocardial infarction. In: Rakel R (ed). Conn's Current Therapy 1990. Philadelphia, WB Saunders, 1990, p 266.
11. O'Gara PT, Dec WG, Curfman GD. Acute myocardial infarction. In: Rakel R (ed). Conn's Current Therapy 1991. Philadelphia, WB Saunders, 1991.
12. Francis GS. Congestive heart failure. In: Rakel R (ed). Conn's Current Therapy 1990. Philadelphia, WB Saunders, 1990, p 242.
13. Packer M, Carver JR, Rodeheffer RJ. Effect of oral milrinone on mortality in severe chronic heart failure. N Engl J Med 325:1468–1475, 1991.
14. Rose BD. Pathogenesis of essential hypertension. In: Rose BD. Pathophysiology of Renal Disease. 2nd ed. New York, McGraw-Hill, 1987, pp 475–476.
15. Hondeghen L, Mason J. Agents used in cardiac arrhythmias. In: Katzung BG (ed). Basic and Clinical Pharmacology. 4th ed. Appleton & Lange, East Norwalk, Conn, Appleton & Lange, 1989.
16. Katzung B, Scheinman M. Drugs used in cardiac arrhythmias. In: Katzung BG (ed). Clinical Pharmacology. East Norwalk, Conn, Appleton & Lange, 1988–1989.
17. Zsoter T. Pharmacotherapy of hypertension. In: Kalant H, Roschlau W, Sellers E. Principles of Medical Pharmacology. 4th ed. New York, Oxford University Press, 1985.
18. Benowitz M, Bourne H. Anti-hypertensive agents. In: Katzung BG (ed). Basic and Clinical Pharmacology. 4th ed. East Norwalk, Conn, Appleton & Lange, 1989.
19. Schaeffer EJ. Hyperlipoproteinemia. In: Rakel R (ed). Conn's Current Therapy 1990. Philadelphia, WB Saunders, 1990.
20. Katzung B, Parmley W. Cardiac glycosides and other drugs used in congestive heart failure. In: Katzung BG (ed). Basic and Clinical Pharmacology. 4th ed. East Norwalk, Conn, Appleton & Lange, 1989.
21. Albert J, Rippe J. Manual of Cardiovascular Diagnosis and Therapy. 3rd ed. Boston, Little, Brown, 1988.
22. Textbook of Advanced Cardiac Life Support. Dallas, American Heart Association, 1987.
23. Notterman D. Pediatric pharmacology. In: Chernow B (ed). Essentials of Critical Care Pharmacology. 2nd ed. Baltimore, Williams & Wilkins, 1989.
24. MacLeod S, Radde I. Textbook of Pediatric Clinical Pharmacology. Littleton, Mass, PSG Publishing Company, 1985.
25. Copeland J. Teaching conference in clinical cardiology. University of Miami, School of Medicine, February 19–22, 1991.
26. Salmon S. Immunopharmacology. In: Katzung BG (ed). Basic and Clinical Pharmacology. 4th ed. East Norwalk, Conn, Appleton & Lange, 1989.

Suggested Readings

Andries E, Stroobandt R (ed). International Congress Series 724, Amsterdam Proceedings of the Workshop on Cardiac Arrhythmias (Mallorca, October 18–19, 1985), Excerpta Medica, 1986.

Chernow B (ed). Essentials of Critical Care Pharmacology. 2nd ed. Baltimore, Williams & Wilkins, 1989.

Chung E. Manual of Cardiac Arrhythmias. Stoneham, Mass, Butterworth-Heinemann, 1986.

Conn PM, Gebhardt GF. Essentials of Pharmacology. Philadelphia, FA Davis, 1989.

Dunagan MR. Manual of Medical Therapeutics. 26th ed. Boston, Little, Brown, 1989.

Gilman AG, Goodman LS, Rall TW, Murad F (eds). Goodman and Gilman's The Pharmacological Basis of Therapeutics. 7th ed. New York, Macmillan, 1985.

Hahn AB, Barkin RL, Oestreich SJ. Pharmacology in Nursing. 15th ed. St. Louis, CV Mosby, 1982.

Harvey AM, Johns RJ, McKusick VA, et al. Principles and Practice of Medicine. 22nd ed. East Norwalk, Conn, Appleton & Lange, 1988.

Kalant H, Roschlau W, Sellers E. Principles of Medical Pharmacology. 4th ed. New York, Oxford University Press, 1985.

Katzung BG (ed). Basic and Clinical Pharmacology. 4th ed. East Norwalk, Conn, Appleton & Lange, 1989.

Learning to Live Well with Diabetes. Minneapolis, DCI Publishing, 1987.

MacLeod S, Radde I. Textbook of Pediatric Clinical Pharmacology. Littleton, Mass, PSG Publishing Company, 1985.

Mountcastle VB. Medical Physiology. 13th ed. St. Louis, CV Mosby, 1974.

Opie LH. Drugs for the Heart. 2nd ed. Philadelphia, WB Saunders, 1987.

Rakel R (ed). Conn's Current Therapy 1991. Philadelphia, WB Saunders, 1991.

Simonson W. Medications and the Elderly. Rockville, Md, Aspen Systems Corporation, 1984.

Sokolow M, McIlroy M, Cheitlin M. Clinical Cardiology. 5th ed. East Norwalk, Conn, Appleton & Lange, 1990.

West JB. Physiological Basis of Medical Practice. 11th ed. Baltimore, Williams & Wilkins, 1985.

LAWRENCE P. CAHALIN
H. STEVEN SADOWSKY

13 PULMONARY MEDICATIONS

INTRODUCTION

This chapter discusses medications that are commonly used in the treatment of pulmonary disorders. The information regarding pharmacokinetics and pharmacodynamics presented in the preceding chapter is equally applicable to pulmonary pharmacology. Several groups of pulmonary medications are used in the treatment of pulmonary diseases: bronchodilators, anti-inflammatory agents, decongestants, antihistamines, antitussives, mucokinetics, respiratory stimulants and depressants, paralyzing and antimicrobial agents. Regardless of the group within which a particular medication may be classified, the rationale for its prescription centers on four basic goals:

- Promotion of bronchodilation or relief of bronchoconstriction or both
- Facilitation of the removal of secretions from the lungs
- Improvement of alveolar ventilation, oxygenation, or both
- Optimization of the breathing pattern

The relative importance of each of these goals depends on the specific disease process and the respiratory problem or problems that result from it.

BRONCHODILATOR THERAPY

Bronchodilators are the most often used drugs in the treatment of pulmonary disease.[1] Therefore, they are considered before the other drug groups. However, a brief discussion of the mechanisms of **bronchoconstriction,** or airway narrowing, facilitates an understanding of the actions of bronchodilator drugs.

The bronchial smooth muscle fibers that cover the airways of the lungs involuntarily constrict in response to various types of irritation. The resultant bronchospasm plays a major role in the pathophysiology of most obstructive pulmonary diseases. Bronchoconstriction can be attributed to any or all of three primary pathologic factors: abnormal bronchomotor tone (bronchospasm), inflammation, and mechanical obstruction.[2] With the elimination of overt mechanical obstruction, the control of bronchomotor tone and inflammation becomes the significant component of airway management in the treatment of patients with pulmonary disease. Only after constricted airways are dilated can mucociliary transport, re-

531

moval of secretions, and subsequent alveolar ventilation and oxygenation take place.

Mechanisms of Bronchoconstriction

Normal bronchomotor tone is the result of a balance between adrenergic and cholinergic influences (Fig. 13-1).[3] When this balance is disrupted (e.g., by disease or allergy), bronchoconstriction results. The characteristic findings in acute bronchoconstriction are bronchospasm, production of mucus, vascular engorgement, and submucosal inflammatory edema. The mechanisms of bronchoconstriction are exquisitely demonstrated when asthma is chosen as a model (see Chapter 6 for more information about asthma). In asthma, and possibly in other pulmonary disorders, an imbalance in autonomic nervous system activity causes a predominant parasympathetic influence, increasing bronchomotor tone and resulting in narrowing of bronchial and bronchiolar passages.[4]

Other receptors in the connective tissue of the airways (e.g., mast cells) and the blood are also stimulated to release mediator substances (Fig. 13-2). This response is called **inflammation,**

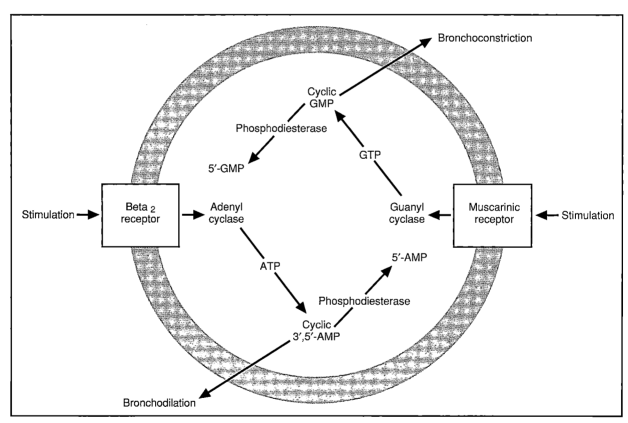

Figure 13-1.

Normal bronchomotor tone is the result of a balance between adrenergic and cholinergic influences mediated through the intracellular nucleotides cyclic adenosine 3',5'-monophosphate (cyclic AMP) and cyclic guanosine monophosphate (cyclic GMP). Adrenergic stimulation of the appropriate receptor catalyzes (via adenyl cyclase) the conversion of adenosine triphosphate (ATP) to cyclic AMP, eliciting relaxation of the affected bronchial smooth muscle. Cyclic AMP is metabolized by phosphodiesterase. Cholinergic stimulation of the appropriate receptor catalyzes (via guanyl cyclase) the conversion of guanosine triphosphate (GTP) to cyclic GMP, eliciting contraction of the affected bronchial smooth muscle. Cyclic GMP is metabolized by phosphodiesterase.

Figure 13-2.

Typical sequence of events that comprise the inflammatory, allergic reaction associated with asthma.

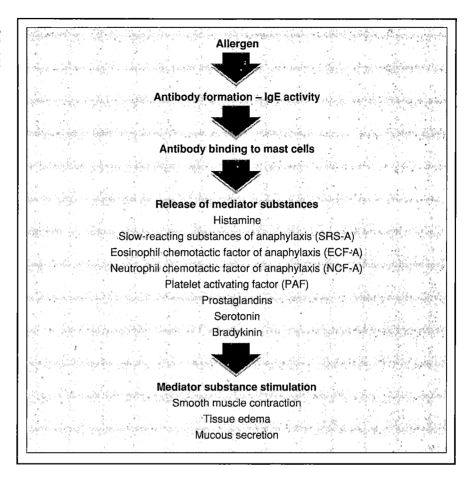

Allergen

Antibody formation – IgE activity

Antibody binding to mast cells

Release of mediator substances
Histamine
Slow-reacting substances of anaphylaxis (SRS-A)
Eosinophil chemotactic factor of anaphylaxis (ECF-A)
Neutrophil chemotactic factor of anaphylaxis (NCF-A)
Platelet activating factor (PAF)
Prostaglandins
Serotonin
Bradykinin

Mediator substance stimulation
Smooth muscle contraction
Tissue edema
Mucous secretion

and it plays a significant role in the production of bronchoconstriction in the vast majority of respiratory disorders.[1,2,4] The mediator substances originate from the plasma or adjacent cells or from the damaged tissue and are associated with at least eight major events:

● Changes in vascular flow and caliber
● Changes in vascular permeability
● Leukocytic (e.g., neutrophils, monocytes, eosinophils, lymphocytes, and basophils) exudation
● Clustering of leukocytes along the capillary endothelial cells at the site of injury—*margination*
● Adherence of the leukocytes to the endothelial surface at the site of injury—*sticking*
● Leukocytic insinuation between endothelial cells—*emigration*
● Unidirectional migration of polymorphonu-

clear leukocytes from the bloodstream to the site of injury in response to released attractants—*chemotaxis*
● *Phagocytosis*[2,4,5]

Although macrophages, leukocytes, and neutrophils assist in the elimination of an invading agent by means of phagocytosis, it is the action of the lymphocytes that is probably most significant. In fact, lymphocytes have been identified as the "cornerstones of the immune process."[2,4]

Invading organisms (e.g., bacteria) or other irritants (e.g., allergens) are referred to as **antigens**. Antigens stimulate the different types of lymphocytes stored in the lymph nodes to produce two mediator substances: antibodies or sensitized lymphocytes (Fig. 13-3). **Antibodies** are produced by an interaction between antigens and B lymphocytes; they are also referred to as **im-**

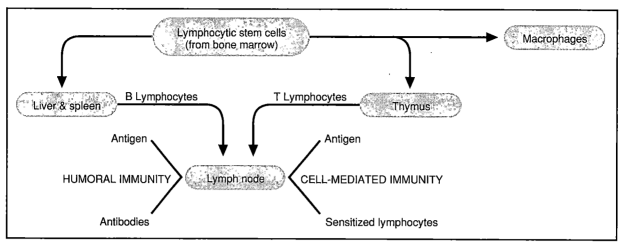

Figure 13-3.

Acquired immunity. The formation of antibodies (immunoglobulins) results from the interaction of antigens with B lympho-cytes and initiates the humoral immune response. The formation of lymphokines results from the interaction of antigens with T lymphocytes and initiates the cell-mediated immune response.

munoglobulins, because many reside in the gamma globulin fraction of the blood.[4] Antibodies are generally grouped into five major classes: IgA, IgE, IgG, IgM, and IgD; the first four of these have been identified in respiratory secretions.[1,2,4] Lymphokines (sensitized lymphocytes) are produced through an interaction of antigens with T lymphocytes and are responsible for a variety of actions including the activation of macrophages (by the production and release of *macrophage-activating factor*), the inhibition of leukocyte migration (by the production and release of *leukocyte inhibitory factor*), and the destruction of susceptible target cells *(lymphotoxic effect)*.[2,4]

The humoral response is the result of antigen-antibody interaction, which causes the release of chemical mediators from mast cells and leukocytes—a type I hypersensitivity reaction (Table 13-1). This immediate reaction is apparently related to IgE antibody activity and occurs within 10 to 20 minutes. The cell-mediated response takes approximately 48 hours to develop and is most likely due to antigen-lymphokine interaction, which causes attracted macrophages to release specific enzymes that produce inflammation—a type IV sensitivity reaction.[2,4] These differences are important because

the methods of treatment may differ depending on the type of interaction. Antigen-antibody interactions are treated with agents that act rapidly, such as glucocorticoids, whereas antigen-lymphokine interactions can be treated with agents that act less rapidly and that may have side effects that are less profound.

Principles of Bronchodilator Therapy

The primary goal of bronchodilator therapy is to manipulate the autonomic nervous system via two opposing nucleotides: cyclic adenosine monophosphate (cAMP) and cyclic guanosine monophosphate (cGMP) (Fig. 13-4).[1,2,4,6] Cyclic adenosine monophosphate facilitates smooth muscle relaxation and inhibits mast cell degranulation to cause bronchodilation. Cyclic guanosine monophosphate facilitates smooth muscle contraction and may enhance mast cell release of histamine and other mediators to cause bronchoconstriction. In the lungs, the effects of cAMP or cGMP can be attributed to

- cholinergic stimulation (muscarinic receptors, predominantly), which increases cGMP and enhances bronchoconstriction

TABLE 13–1. Hypersensitivity Reactions in the Lung

Type	Name	Antibodies Involved	Main Mechanism	Reaction Time	Example of Disease
I	Immediate hypersensitivity reaction	IgE IgE in some individuals	Antigen-antibody reaction causes release of chemical mediators from mast cells and basophils	10 to 20 min lasting 1 to 2 hr	Anaphylactic reaction, asthma, hay fever
II	Cytotoxic reaction	IgG IgM	Antibody (primarily IgG) reacts directly with a cell surface antigen to produce cellular damage (autoimmune response)	Variable	Autoimmune diseases, e.g., Goodpasture's syndrome
III	Immune complex–mediated reaction	IgG IgM	Lysosomal enzyme release or production of toxic metabolites by polymorphonuclear lymphocytes causes bronchial wall inflammation. Mast cells release mediator substances	Usually 4 to 8 hr, lasting 24 to 96 hr	Asthma (delayed onset), hypersensitivity pneumonitis, systemic lupus erythematosus
IV	Cell-mediated delayed reaction	No antibody identified; involves sensitized T lymphocytes (type of white blood cell)	Antigen binds with T cells and results in liberation of lymphokines (mediators). Attracted macrophages release hydrolytic enzymes and cause inflammation.	48 hr	Granulomatous diseases, such as tuberculosis; lymphokines may induce inflammatory reaction in any chest disease with a hypersensitivity reaction.

(From Kersten LD. Comprehensive Respiratory Nursing: A Decision Making Approach. Philadelphia, WB Saunders, 1989, p 103.)

● adrenergic stimulation: beta$_2$ receptor stimulation, which produces an increase in cAMP and bronchodilation; alpha$_1$ receptor stimulation, which produces a decrease in cAMP and enhances vasoconstriction or bronchoconstriction)[7,8]

However, as previously mentioned, in asthma and possibly in other pulmonary disorders, sympathetic activity appears to be less because of a predominant parasympathetic influence. The three main effects of enhanced parasympathetic influence are heart rate slowing, bronchial constriction, and increased exocrine gland secretion.[1,2,4] Clearly, these effects may be deleterious to a patient with pulmonary disease. Consequently, autonomic-active agents are often used in the pharmacologic treatment of patients with pulmonary disease. Beta-adrenergic agonists, some prostaglandins, methylxanthines, and glucocorticoids may be given to increase cAMP and to promote bronchodilation. Alpha-adrenergic antagonists, glucocorticoids, cholinergic antagonists, and cromolyn sodium may be given to inhibit cGMP or to enhance cAMP. The common autonomic-active bronchodilating agents, methylxanthines, cromolyn sodium, and glucocorticoids are listed in Table 13–2 and discussed in the following section.

Drugs That Promote Bronchodilation

Drugs that stimulate the adrenergic receptors are frequently referred to as **sympathomimetics** (adrenergic), and those that inhibit adrenergic receptors are referred to as **sympatholytics** (antiadrenergic). Similarly, drugs that stimulate the cholinergic receptors are referred to as **parasympathomimetics** (cholinergic), and those that inhibit cholinergic receptors are called **parasympatholytics** (anticholinergic). The actions and adverse effects of the principal bronchodilators are here reviewed, specifically the autonomic-active agents (adrenergic sympathomimetics and parasympatholytics), methylxanthines, corticosteroids, and cromolyn sodium.

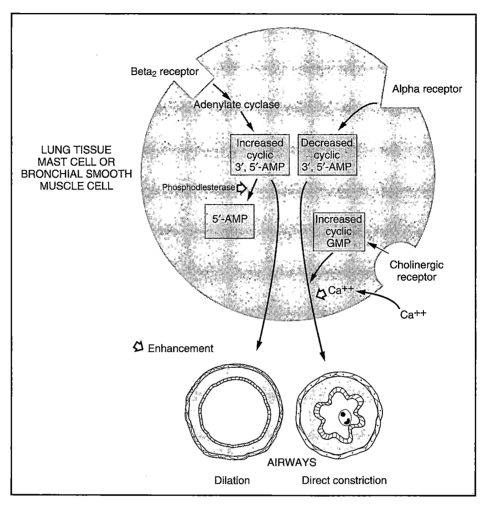

Figure 13-4.

A, Factors influencing adrenergic and cholinergic mediation of bronchomotor tone. **B,** Pharmacologic control of broncho-motor tone and the allergen-induced release of chemical mediators. Stimulation of beta$_2$ receptors by sympathomimetic agents (e.g., isoproterenol) facilitates dilation. Glucocorticoids, methylxanthines (e.g., theophylline), and some prostaglandins enhance the bronchodilator effect of beta$_2$ adrenergic stimulation. However, glucocorticoids and alpha sympatholytic

Sympathomimetics

Sympathomimetic drugs may be selective or nonselective in their activity. Selective medications react with specific receptors, whereas nonselective medications react with several receptors. The response to these drugs depends on the relative intensity of the receptor reaction, the route of administration, and the dosage of the particular drug. Recall that

● alpha receptors are distributed within the peripheral and bronchial smooth muscle, the

myocardium, and the mucosal blood vessels, but they are most abundant in the peripheral smooth muscle.
● beta$_1$ receptors are more abundant in cardiac tissue, although they are also present in mucosal blood vessels.
● beta$_2$ receptors predominate in the bronchial smooth muscle, though they are also found in peripheral smooth muscle and skeletal muscle.

Epinephrine (Adrenalin Chloride) and *ephedrine* typify general, nonselective sympathomimetics. Epinephrine has a short duration of action, dem-

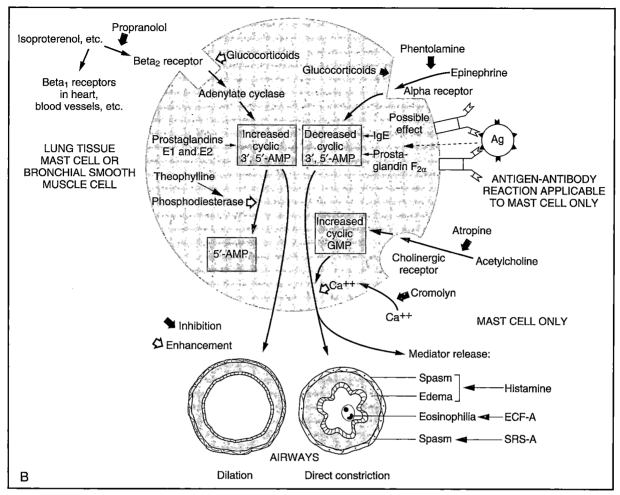

Figure 13-4. *Continued*

drugs (e.g., phentolamine) inhibit the alpha-adrenergic contribution to bronchoconstriction. Similarly, parasympatholytics (e.g., atropine) inhibit cholinergic bronchoconstrictive influences. Cromolyn retards the release of mediators by inhibiting calcium ion movement into unstable mast cells, thereby preventing bronchoconstriction. (Adapted from Townley RG. Pharmacologic blocks to mediator release: Clinical application. Adv Asthma Allergy 2:7, 1975.)

onstrating moderate alpha-receptor activity, strong beta$_1$-receptor activity, and moderate beta$_2$-receptor activity. Ephedrine has a long duration of action, exhibiting mild alpha-receptor activity and moderate beta$_1$- and beta$_2$-receptor activity. Thus, in the treatment of bronchoconstriction, peripheral vascular constriction and cardiac stimulation may result from the alpha and beta$_1$ effects. Other adverse reactions include agitation, sweating, headache, and nausea.

Clearly, then, drugs that have no alpha-receptor activity and more specific beta$_2$-receptor

activity are desirable for bronchodilator therapy. *Isoproterenol*, a drug with questionable, weak alpha-receptor activity and strong beta$_1$- and beta$_2$-receptor activity, is the most commonly prescribed nonspecific beta sympathomimetic. Selective beta$_2$ stimulation is preferable, because beta$_2$-specific agents affect the lungs without affecting the heart. Beta$_2$-specific agents produce bronchiolar dilatation via relaxation of bronchial smooth muscle as well as dilating effects of increased cAMP levels. *Isoetharine, terbutaline* (which have weak beta$_1$-receptor activity and

TABLE 13–2. Primary Bronchodilator Agents

Drug Group	Action	Effect	Side Effects
Beta sympathomimetics	Increase cAMP, decrease intracellular calcium concentrations, thus relaxing smooth muscle	Bronchodilation	Tremor, palpitations and tachycardia, headache, nervousness, dizziness, nausea, hypertension
Methylxanthines	Increase cAMP, block the decrease of cAMP	Bronchodilation	Agitation, tachycardia, headache, palpitations, dizziness, hypotension, chest pain, nausea, possibly diuresis
Alpha sympatholytics	Block the decrease of cAMP	Bronchodilation	Agitation, tachycardia, headache, palpitations, dizziness, hypotension, chest pain, nausea, possibly diuresis
Parasympatholytics	Block parasympathetic stimulation, which prevents an increase in cGMP, allowing cAMP to increase; block the activity of the enzyme phosphodiesterase, which prevents the degradation of cAMP	Prevent bronchoconstriction	Central nervous system stimulation with low doses but depression with high doses; delirium, hallucinations, decreased gastrointestinal activity
Glucocorticoids	Decrease inflammatory response	Bronchodilation	Cushingoid appearance; obesity; growth suppression; hyperglycemia and diabetes, mood changes, irritability, or depression; thinning of skin; muscle wasting; osteoporosis; hypertension; immunosuppression
Cromolyn sodium	Prevents influx of calcium ions, thus blocking mast cell release of mediators responsible for bronchoconstriction	Bronchodilation	Throat irritation, hoarseness, dry mouth, cough, chest tightness, bronchospasm

cAMP, cyclic adenosine monophosphate; cGMP, cyclic guanosine monophosphate.

moderate beta$_2$-receptor activity), *albuterol*, and *bitolterol* (which each have weak beta$_1$-receptor activity and strong beta$_2$-receptor activity) are the most commonly prescribed beta$_2$-specific sympathomimetics.[8,9] The adverse effects of the beta$_2$ sympathomimetics are similar to those of the nonspecific beta sympathomimetics and include tremor, palpitations, tachycardia, headache, nervousness, dizziness, nausea, and hypertension.[4,9,10] The nonspecific beta sympathomimetic drugs also elicit inotropic (enhanced myocardial contractility) and chronotropic (enhanced heart rate) effects. The major sympathomimetic drugs are listed in Table 13–3.

Sympatholytics

Because the effects of alpha stimulation include vasoconstriction and bronchoconstriction, the pharmacologic reduction of alpha stimulation via **alpha sympatholytics** is certainly warranted for patients with pulmonary disease. Alpha sym-

patholytic action inhibits the decrease of cAMP associated with the antigen-antibody reaction, allowing bronchodilation to occur. The agent most commonly used for this purpose is *phentolamine*, which, although exhibiting some of the same adverse effects as those seen with beta sympathomimetics, generally elicits a less adverse reaction because direct stimulation of the sympathetic nervous system does not occur.[11] The most common side effects associated with the administration of alpha sympatholytics are nausea and dizziness.

Parasympatholytics

The lungs receive a rich supply of parasympathetic innervation via the vagus nerve.[12] The role of the parasympatholytics is similar to that of alpha sympatholytics in that it is the "lytic" action (inhibitory effect) that produces the desired effect of bronchodilation.[4] Blocking parasympathetic stimulation prevents an increase in cGMP

TABLE 13–3. Major Sympathomimetic Drugs

Drug	Route of Administration	Time to Onset of Action	Duration of Action	Clinical Uses
Epinephrine	Subcutaneous	≈5 min	1–2 hr	Acute bronchospasm; also topical vasoconstrictor, vasopressor, intracardiac stimulant; increase blood sugar
	Nebulized (Vaponefrin)	1–5 min	1–3 hr	
	Inhaler (Medihaler-Epi)	1–5 min	1–3 hr	
Ephedrine	Oral	≈1 hr	≈4 hr	Frequently combined with other bronchodilator agents; often used as a decongestant
Isoproterenol	Nebulized (Isuprel) Inhaler (Isuprel Mistometer, Medihaler-Iso)	2–5 min	≈2 hr	Acute bronchospasm; also cardiac stimulant, pressor agent
	Intravenous (Isuprel)	Immediate	As long as infusion continues	
Isoetharine	Nebulized (Bronkosol) Inhaler (Bronkometer)	≈5 min	2–3 hr	Acute bronchospasm
Terbutaline	Subcutaneous (Brethine, Bricanyl IV)	5–15 min	2–4 hr	Acute bronchospasm
	Nebulizer	5–30 min	4–6 hr	
	Inhaler (Brethaire)	5–30 min	4–6 hr	
Albuterol (salbutamol)	Inhaler (Proventil, Ventolin)	Within 15 min	4–6 hr	Acute bronchospasm
Bitolterol	Inhaler (Tornalate)	Within 15 min	5–8 hr	Acute bronchospasm

and, therefore, produces a relative increase in the amount of cAMP and promotes the relaxation of bronchial smooth muscle.[13–15] Historically, the agent most commonly used for this purpose was the muscarinic antagonist *atropine.* However, because atropine is readily absorbed into the systemic circulation, it is frequently associated with adverse reactions, including

- stimulation of the central nervous system with low doses or depression with high doses
- delirium
- hallucinations
- decreased gastrointestinal activity

The newer drug *ipratropium (Atrovent)* is poorly absorbed into the systemic circulation and, therefore, is associated with fewer side effects.[16]

Methylxanthines

The intracellular level of cAMP can be enhanced if the process of its degradation by the enzyme phosphodiesterase can be inhibited. By blocking the inactivation of cAMP, bronchodila-

tion is facilitated. The group of drugs that most significantly inhibits the action of phosphodiesterase is the **methylxanthines.** Furthermore, evidence indicates that methylxanthines may also enhance diaphragmatic contractility.[17,18] The most commonly used methylxanthine is *theophylline (Theo-Dur)*, which is associated with a variety of side effects, including

- agitation
- tachycardia
- headache
- palpitations
- dizziness
- hypotension
- chest pain
- nausea
- possible diuresis

Cromolyn Sodium (Disodium Cromoglycate)

Research in England in the 1960s on an extract of a Mediterranean plant resulted in the discovery of *cromolyn sodium*, which is known by the brand names *Intal* and *Aarane.* Cromolyn is used prophylactically in cases of chronic asthma because it prevents the immediate hypersensitivity reaction (also known as type I reaction). Recall from earlier discussions that immediate hypersensitivity reactions are controlled by mast cells via the release of specific mediators (e.g., histamine, lymphokines, bradykinin, among many others) that produce bronchoconstriction and various other signs and symptoms, for example, mucous secretion, mucosal swelling, and dyspnea. Cromolyn sodium does not prevent the activation of mast cells and the subsequent release of specific mediators that results from the coupling of IgE with an allergen.[4] However, the late-phase reaction in an acute asthma episode (which can cause severe airway obstruction 4 to 6 hours after initial bronchoconstriction) can be prevented by the administration of cromolyn sodium.[19] Specifically, cromolyn prevents the influx of calcium ions into the mast cells, blocking the degranulation process of these cells, and thereby inhibiting the further release of mediators that cause bronchoconstriction. Thus, although cromolyn has no effect on the mediators released from the antigen-antibody reaction of an acute asthma attack, it prevents later bronchoconstriction prophylactically by impairing the release of mediators.[19] It seems that cromolyn is quite benign; its most common side effects include

- dry mouth and throat
- airway irritation
- possible bronchospasm

Glucocorticoids

The adrenal cortex synthesizes cholesterol and secretes two major corticosteroids: the mineralocorticoids and the glucocorticoids. Although there is some controversy as to the exact mechanism, glucocorticoids are postulated to suppress the process of IgE-mediated bronchoconstriction and to block or inhibit a variety of mediator substances.[1,2,4,20] Even though glucocorticoids are not classified as primary bronchodilators, they are known to have the following general effects[20,6]:

- Inhibition of the migration of leukocytes and mast cells

- Reduction of stickiness and margination of polymorphonuclear leukocytes
- Potentiation of catecholamine activity
- Reduction of tissue stores of histamine and other mediators
- Suppression of kinin activity, resulting in constriction of the microvasculature
- Stabilization of mast cell membranes
- Improvement of cardiac contractility (inotropy)
- Reduction of phosphodiesterase activity

It is because of their profound anti-inflammatory actions that glucocorticoids are considered the drugs of first choice during an acute attack of asthma.

The most commonly used glucocorticoids in the treatment of bronchoconstriction are summarized in Table 13–4.[1,2,4] The route of administration of corticosteroids is important because the incidence of side effects can be affected tremendously by the route: the more localized the area of administration, the less likely the chance of systemic reaction. During episodes of severe bronchoconstriction, glucocorticoids are usually administered intravenously *(methylprednisolone)*. However, for prolonged use, an oral *(prednisone)* or inhalational route *(dexamethasone sodium phosphate, beclomethasone dipropionate, triamcinolone acetonide, flunisolide)* is used, although the inhalational route is preferred because it is associated with fewer side effects.[21]

Most of the adverse effects of glucocorticoid therapy are dosage dependent and take a few days or weeks to manifest themselves. However, some side effects are unavoidable; reactions span the spectrum from merely unpleasant to danger-

TABLE 13–4. Common Glucocorticoids

Drug	Brand Name	Route of Administration
Prednisone	Many	Intravenous, oral
Hydrocortisone	Solu-Cortef	Intravenous, oral
Methylprednisolone	Solu-Medrol	Intravenous
Dexamethasone	Decadron Phosphate Respihaler	Inhaler
Beclomethasone	Beclovent, Vanceril	Inhaler
Triamcinolone	Azmacort	Inhaler
Flunisolide	Aerobid	Inhaler

TABLE 13-5. Complications That May Be Associated with Glucocorticoid Therapy

Site	Unpleasant Effects	Dangerous Effects
Skin	Acne, hirsutism, striae, flushing, facial erythema, increased perspiration	Loss of subcutaneous tissue, poor wound healing
Vascular	Petechiae, bruising	Thromboemboli, vasculitis, periarteritis nodosa
Appearance	Fat deposition (facial mooning, buffalo hump, truncal obesity, etc.)	Stunting of growth in children
Central nervous system	Insomnia, restlessness, agitation	Altered personality, psychosis (euphoria, mania, depression, confusion), pseudotumor cerebri
Cardiovascular	Edema (due to sodium retention), nocturia	Hypertension, heart failure, arrhythmias
Metabolic	Electrolyte disturbance, calcium loss, alkalosis, negative nitrogen balance, hyperlipidemia	Diabetogenic effect, hyperosmolar nonketotic coma
Musculoskeletal	Weakness (due to myopathy, hypokalemia and wasting), osteoporosis	Vertebral and other fractures, aseptic bone necrosis of femoral and humeral heads
Endocrine	Menstrual disorders, menopausal symptoms, impotence	Hypothalamic-pituitary-adrenal axis suppression
Gastrointestinal	Nausea, vomiting, fatty liver, increased appetite, esophagitis	Increased risk of peptic ulceration (in rheumatoid arthritis), large bowel perforation, pancreatitis
Ocular	Exophthalmos, posterior subcapsular cataract, sixth-nerve palsies (diplopia)	Papilledema, increased risk of fungal and viral keratitis
Immunologic	Suppression of skin responses to antigenic tests, depression of immunologic responses	Impaired response to infections, susceptibility to dissemination of vaccinations, opportunistic infections
Fetus		Risk of teratogenicity in first trimester, possible adrenal insufficiency in newborn infant

(From Ziment I. Respiratory Pharmacology and Therapeutics. Philadelphia, WB Saunders, 1989, p 226.)

ous (Table 13-5). The primary side effects associated with steroid use include

- immunosuppression
- gastrointestinal disturbance
- emotional lability (vacillation between euphoria and depression)
- insomnia
- osteoporosis
- retardation of growth
- muscle weakness and atrophy (particularly of pelvic and shoulder girdle musculature)
- hyperglycemia
- sodium and water retention
- cushingoid effects[1,2,4,6]

ANCILLARY PULMONARY MEDICATIONS

In addition to bronchodilators, several other drug groups are frequently used in the treatment of respiratory disorders:

- Decongestants
- Antihistamines
- Antitussives
- Mucokinetics
- Respiratory stimulants and depressants
- Paralyzing and antimicrobial agents

The drug grouping may provide clues regarding the nature of the problem for which it was taken, or the problem may provide clues about the drug. For example, a patient experiencing mucosal edema may complain of feeling "stuffed up," and it may be found that that patient is taking an over-the-counter decongestant or antihistamine.

Decongestants

The common cold, allergies, and many respiratory infections have in common the symptoms of "runny nose and stuffy head." **Decongestants** are used to treat this upper airway mucosal edema and discharge. The most common decongestants are alpha-adrenergic sympathomimetics, specifically alpha$_1$ agonists.[22] These medications stimulate vasoconstriction by binding with the alpha$_1$ receptors in the blood vessels of the mucosal lining of the upper airway. The desired result is a decreased congestion in the upper airways.

Decongestants are frequently combined with other ingredients (e.g., antihistamines) as constituents of commercially available, nonprescription, over-the-counter preparations (Table 13–6). When used appropriately, these medications can be safe and effective. However, if a patient has a specific sensitivity or if the decongestant medication is improperly used, adverse effects may arise. Primary side effects include

- headache
- dizziness
- nausea
- nervousness
- hypertension
- cardiac irregularities (e.g., palpitations)

Antihistamines

Treatment of the respiratory allergic responses associated with seasonal allergies (e.g., hay fever) is one of the most common uses of **antihistamines.** Histamines play a role in the regulation of gastric secretion and the modulation of neural activity within the central nervous system by means of H$_1$ and H$_2$ receptors.[23] The H$_1$ receptors, primarily located in vascular, respiratory, and gastrointestinal smooth muscle, are specifically targeted for blockade by antihistamines (drugs that block the H$_2$ receptors are referred to as H$_2$ antagonists).[24] By blocking the H$_1$ receptors, these drugs decrease the mucosal congestion, irritation, and discharge caused by inhaled allergens. Antihistamines may also reduce the coughing and sneezing often associated with common colds.

Some of the antihistamines commonly used to treat the symptoms of hay fever and other hay fever–like allergies are listed in Table 13–7. Antihistamines are frequently combined with other ingredients, such as alpha-adrenergic sympathomimetics. The adverse effects most often attributable to antihistamines include

- sedation
- fatigue
- dizziness
- blurred vision
- loss of coordination
- gastrointestinal distress

TABLE 13–7. Common Antihistamines

Drug (Generic Name)	Drug (Brand Name)	Route of Administration
Brompheniramine	Dimetapp*	Oral
Chlorpheniramine	Chlor-Trimeton,* Sudafed,* Coricidin*	Oral
Dexbrompheniramine	Drixoral*	Oral
Dimenhydrinate	Dramamine	Oral
Diphenhydramine	Benadryl	Oral
Pheniramine	Triaminic*	Oral
Phenyltoloxamine	Sinutab*	Oral
Triprolidine	Actifed*	Oral

* Antihistamine combined with other ingredients.

Antitussives

The cough is such a common and troublesome symptom that more prescription drugs are available for the treatment of cough than for any other symptom.[25] Used to suppress the ineffective, dry, hacking cough associated with minor throat irritations and the common cold, **antitussive** agents act to correct the irritation, to block the receptors, or to increase the threshold of the cough center in the brain. They are generally indicated for short-term use only and are not indicated for coughs due to retained secretions.

TABLE 13–6. Common Decongestant Agents

Drug (Generic Name)	Drug (Brand Name)	Route of Administration
Ephedrine	Primatene tablets*	Oral
Epinephrine	Primatene Mist	Nasal spray
Oxymetazoline	Neo-Synephrine 12-Hour	Nasal spray
Phenylephrine	Neo-Synephrine	Nasal spray
Phenylpropanolamine	Triaminic,* Contac*	Oral
Pseudoephedrine	Sudafed	Oral

* Decongestant combined with other ingredients.

TABLE 13–8. Common Antitussive Agents

Drug (Generic Name)	Drug (Brand Name)	Classification
Benzonatate	Tessalon	Local anesthetic
Codeine*	Many brand names	Increases threshold in cough center
Dextromethor-phan*	Many brand names	Increases threshold in cough center
Diphenhydramine	Benadryl	Antihistamine
Hydrocodone	Triaminic Expec-torant DH	Increases threshold in cough center

* Frequently combined with other ingredients (e.g., expectorants, decongestants).

Antitussives may be classified as topical anesthetics (e.g., lidocaine), nonnarcotics (e.g., dextromethorphan, benzonatate), and narcotics (e.g., codeine, morphine); they are frequently combined with other ingredients and are offered under many brand names. The primary adverse effect of antitussive agents is sedation. However, gastrointestinal distress and dizziness may also occur. Common antitussives are listed in Table 13–8.

Mucokinetics

Drugs that promote the mobilization and removal of secretions from the respiratory tract are called **mucokinetic** agents. There are four basic types of mucokinetic agents:

● Mucolytics
● Expectorants
● Wetting agents
● Surface-active agents

Mucolytic Drugs

Mucolytic drugs disrupt the chemical bonds in mucoid and purulent secretions, decreasing the viscosity of the mucus and promoting expectoration. Administered by inhalation or direct intratracheal instillation, *acetylcysteine (Mucomyst)* is the principal mucolytic drug used today. Acetylcysteine's primary adverse effects include mucosal irritation, coughing, bronchospasm (especially in asthmatics), and nausea.

Expectorants

Expectorants increase the production of respiratory secretions, thus facilitating their ejection from the respiratory tract. Several expectorant drugs are available; among these are *guaifenesin, potassium iodide,* and *ammonium chloride.* These drugs are often combined with others and are available by many trade names. The utility of expectorant drugs is currently a topic of debate.[1] Nonetheless, in the acute care setting, expectorants may be administered as an adjunct to vigorous bronchial hygiene techniques.

Wetting Agents and Surface-Active Agents

By humidifying and lubricating secretions, **wetting agents** make expectoration easier for the patient. The diluent of choice is *half normal saline* (0.45% NaCl) delivered by either continuous aerosol or intermittent ultrasonic nebulization.[26] However, sterile water is sometimes administered via a nebulizer as an airway irritant to induce coughing and facilitate the expectoration of sputum for subsequent laboratory testing. While **surface-active agents** may stabilize aerosol droplets, and thereby enhance their efficacy as carrier vehicles for nebulized drugs, the utility of these agents is debatable.[1,6]

Respiratory Stimulants and Depressants

Any agent that increases the output of the central respiratory centers may be considered a **respiratory stimulant.** Certainly, noxious stimuli, such as pain or verbal exhortation, may result in excitation of the central nervous system and thus elicit enhanced respiratory center activity. Some drugs can also stimulate respiratory center activity—carbon dioxide, sympathomimetics, and methylxanthines—and induce an increase in ventilation. Drugs that have a specific ability to cause excitation of the central nervous system with subsequent enhanced activity of the respiratory center are called **analeptics.** Unfortunately, analeptic drugs elicit dose-dependent levels of central stimulation that can ultimately result in convulsions. Therefore, the clinical use of analeptic medications is not without controversy, but few would disagree that when respiratory failure has been aggravated by an injudicious intervention (e.g., oxygen, narcotics), respiratory stimulants serve a purpose.[27,28]

Because it stimulates respiration more than it activates the cortical or spinal neurons, *doxapram* is one of the most widely accepted analeptics.[29] Administered intravenously, it is used to prevent a rise in Pa_{CO_2} with oxygen therapy in acute ventilatory failure. It is also used in high-risk postoperative patients to prevent respiratory depression. Another drug, *medroxyprogesterone (Depo-Provera)*, is sometimes given to patients with end-stage obstructive pulmonary dysfunction to prevent nocturnal alveolar hypoventilation.[30]

Some drugs (e.g., sedatives, tranquilizers) are, to varying degrees, **respiratory depressants.** In general, patients with pulmonary disease should avoid the use of sedatives because they suppress the ventilatory drive. However, in some instances intravenous *morphine* or *diazepam (Valium)* is given to patients on mechanical ventilation if anxiety or agitation is contributing to an increased work of breathing and hindering mechanical ventilation. The tranquilizer *haloperidol (Haldol)* may be prescribed for patients who can breathe spontaneously to control agitation because it has less respiratory depressant action than other tranquilizers or sedatives.[1] Many of the drugs used in the treatment of psychiatric disorders have varying degrees of sedative effect, depressing the central nervous system and possibly leading to respiratory depression in some pa-

tients. Some antipsychotic drugs are associated with significant parasympatholytic effects, causing symptoms such as bronchoconstriction, dry mouth, blurred vision, constipation, and urinary retention.

Paralyzing Agents

Although tranquilizers can relieve muscle spasm, they do not prevent volitional muscle activity; to completely ablate muscular tone during general anesthesia, the level of anesthesia must be profound—a situation not wholly desirable. Therefore, anesthetists and anesthesiologists usually opt for lighter general anesthesia in conjunction with muscle paralyzing agents to produce the desired degree of immobilization. Paralyzing agents are also used to facilitate endotracheal intubation or to control laryngeal spasm; to treat diseases that cause neuromuscular hyperactivity (e.g., tetanus, severe intractable seizure activity); and occasionally to prevent struggling, fighting, or excessive tachypnea in patients who are being ventilated mechanically. Table 13–9 presents the neuromuscular blocking agents that are frequently used clinically.

Antimicrobial Agents

Drugs used to combat small, unicellular organisms (e.g., bacteria, viruses) that invade the body are often called **antimicrobial** agents or **antibiotics.** There are numerous pathogenic organisms (Table 13–10), so it is quite likely that

			Usual	
Drug	**Type**	**Brand Name**	**Duration of Effect**	**Adverse Reactions**
d-Tubocurarine (curare)	Nondepolarizing	Tubadil, Tubarine	Typically 45–90 min	Hyper- or hypotension, bradycardia or tachycardia
Pancuronium	Nondepolarizing	Pavulon	Up to 50 min	Mild hypertension, mild tachycardia
Succinylcholine (suxamethonium)	Depolarizing	Anectine	About 5 min	Vagal and sympathetic stimulation; associated fasciculations may cause muscle pain

TABLE 13–9. Common Paralyzing Agents

TABLE 13–10. Major Respiratory Pathogens

Organism	Associated Diseases	Comment
Gram-Positive Bacteria		
Group A *Streptococcus*	Pharyngitis, tonsillitis, sinusitis, otitis	May be present in aspiration pneumonias
Staphylococcus aureus	Sinusitis, otitis, pneumonia, lung abscess, empyema, cystic fibrosis	Many species are now penicillin-resistant
Diplococcus pneumoniae	Sinusitis, otitis, bronchitis, pneumonia, empyema	Main cause of pneumonia
Gram-Negative Bacteria		
Haemophilus influenzae	Epiglottitis, bronchitis, bronchiolitis, pneumonia, acute otitis in children	Accompanies *D. pneumoniae* in bronchitis
Pseudomonas aeruginosa	Pneumonia, lung abscess, empyema, cystic fibrosis	Common in debilitated patients
Klebsiella pneumoniae	Pneumonia, lung abscess, empyema, bronchiectasis	Uncommon cause of pneumonia at present
Escherichia coli *Proteus* species *Serratia marcescens* *Enterobacter aerogenes*	Pneumonia, lung abscess, empyema, bronchiectasis, cystic fibrosis	Opportunistic infections. Can be introduced by contaminated inhalation therapy equipment
Anaerobic Bacteria		
Bacteroides species *Streptococcus* species Others	Sinusitis, otitis, aspiration pneumonia, lung abscess, empyema	Cause foul-smelling pus; usually present in mixed infection
Mycoplasma and Viruses		
Mycoplasma pneumoniae	Pneumonia	Common in young adults and children
Adenoviruses	Common cold, pharyngitis, bronchiolitis, bronchitis, croup, pneumonia	One of commonest group of respiratory viruses
Respiratory syncytial virus	Bronchiolitis, pneumonia	Occurs in children
Influenza viruses Parainfluenza	Rhinitis, pharyngitis, laryngotracheitis, pneumonia	Cause influenza syndromes
Rhinovirus, coronavirus, etc.	Common cold	Probably major causes of colds
Mycobacteria		
Mycobacterium tuberculosis	Tuberculosis syndromes	Can cause similar diseases of lungs and other organs
Atypical mycobacteria	Tuberculosis-like syndromes	
Fungi		
Coccidioides immitis *Histoplasma capsulatum* *Blastomyces dermatitidis* *Sporotrichum schenckii* *Actinomyces israelii*	Coccidioidomycosis Histoplasmosis Blastomycosis Sporotrichosis Actinomycosis	Tend to develop in normal hosts as primary infections
Aspergillus fumigatus *Candida* species *Cryptococcus neoformans* *Nocardia* species	Aspergillosis Candidiasis (moniliasis) Cryptococcosis Nocardiosis	Tend to develop in abnormal hosts as opportunistic infections
Parasites (Protozoa)		
Pneumocystis carinii	Pneumonia	Develops in immunosuppressed hosts and in infants
Toxoplasma gondii		Seen mainly in immunologically abnormal infants

(From Ziment I. Respiratory Pharmacology and Therapeutics. Philadelphia, WB Saunders, 1989, p 341.)

many patients receiving physical therapy are taking one or more antimicrobial drugs. Unfortunately, the majority of antimicrobial agents may be as toxic to the host cells as to the infecting organisms.[6] The commonly used antimicrobial agents (Table 13–11) act by inhibiting cell wall synthesis and function (e.g., the *penicillins*, the *cephalosporins, bacitracin, vancomycin, cycloserine, polypeptides*, the antifungal *polyenes*), protein synthesis (e.g., *aminoglycosides, chloramphenicol*, the *marcolides*, the *tetracyclines*, the *lincomycins*), or nucleotide formation (e.g., *rifampin, isoniazid*). Antibacterial drugs may be classified as **bactericidal** (killing or destroying bacteria) or **bacterio-** **static** (limiting growth and proliferation of bacteria). The bactericidal or bacteriostatic characteristics of a drug may depend on the dosage of the drug, some drugs (e.g., erythromycin) being bacteriostatic at low doses and bactericidal at higher doses.

Penicillins are a mainstay in the treatment of respiratory infections. The semisynthetic pencillins have a broader spectrum of antibacterial activity than the natural penicillins.[21] The principal drawback to the use of penicillins is hypersensitivity, which manifests itself as skin rashes, hives, bronchoconstriction, or even anaphylactic reaction.

TABLE 13–11. Common Antimicrobial Agents

Group	Drug (Generic Name)	Drug (Brand Name)	Typical Use
Antibacterial drugs that inhibit cell membrane synthesis			
PENICILLINS Natural penicillins			
	Penicillin G	Bicillin, Crysticillin, Permapen, etc.	*Bacillus anthracis, Clostridium perfringens, Clostridium tetani, Corynebacterium diphtheriae*
	Penicillin V	V-Cillin, Pen•Vee K, Penapar VK, etc.	*Streptococcus pyrogenes*
Penicillinase- resistant penicillins			
	Cloxacillin	Cloxapen, Tegopen	*Staphylococcus aureus*
	Dicloxacillin	Dynapen, Pathocil	
	Methicillin	Staphcillin	
	Nafcillin	Unipen	
	Oxacillin	Bactocill, Prostaphlin	
Aminopenicillins			
	Amoxicillin	Amoxil, Polymox	
	Ampicillin	Amcill, Omnipen, Polycillin, etc.	*Escherichia coli, Proteus mirabilis, Neisseria gonorrhoeae*
	Bacampicillin	Spectrobid	
Wide-spectrum penicillins			
	Azlocillin		
	Carbenicillin	Geocillin, Geopen, Pyopen	
	Mezlocillin	Mezlin	
	Piperacillin	Pipracil	*Klebsiella pneumoniae*
	Ticarcillin	Ticar IV	
CEPHALOSPORINS First-generation			Cephalosporins generally serve as alternatives to penicillins if they prove ineffective or are poorly tolerated by the patient
	Cefadroxil	Duricef, Ultracef	
	Cefazolin	Ancef IV, Kefzol IV	
	Cephalexin	Keflex	
	Cephalothin	Keflin, Seffin	
	Cephapirin	Cefadyl	
Second-generation			
	Cefaclor	Ceclor Pulvules	
	Cefamandole	Mandol	
	Cefonicid	Monocid IV	
	Ceforanide	Precef	
	Cefotetan	Cefotan	

Cephalosporins are generally considered as alternatives to the penicillins when penicillins are not tolerated by the patient or when they are ineffective. First-generation cephalosporins are used to eradicate gram-positive cocci and some gram-negative bacteria; second-generation cephalosporins are similar in effectiveness against gram-positive cocci and are generally thought to be more effective against gram-negative bacteria; third-generation cephalosporins are effective against the greatest number of gram-negative bacteria but are of limited effectiveness against gram-positive cocci. Cephalosporins may elicit stomach cramps, diarrhea, nausea, and vomiting,

and some patients may exhibit similar hypersensitivity reactions to penicillins.

Aminoglycoside drugs have a wide spectrum of antibacterial activity; they are active against many aerobic gram-negative bacteria, against some aerobic gram-positive bacteria, and against many anaerobic bacteria. Unfortunately, this wide spectrum of activity is associated with a significant level of toxicity.[31] Nephrotoxicity and ototoxicity are the primary toxic manifestations, especially in patients who have a particular susceptibility (elderly persons, patients with liver or renal failure). The erythromycins also exhibit a broad spectrum of antibacterial activity, being ef-

TABLE 13–11. Common Antimicrobial Agents *Continued*

Group	Drug (Generic Name)	Drug (Brand Name)	Typical Use
Third-generation			
	Cefoperazone	Cefobid	
	Cefotaxime	Claforan	
	Ceftazidime	Fortaz, Tazicef	
	Cefoxitin	Mefoxin	
OTHERS			
	Bacitracin	Bacitrin ointment	
	Cycloserine	Seromycin Pulvules	
	Vancomycin	Vancocin IV, Vancoled	*Corynebacterium* species
	Antibacterial drugs that inhibit protein synthesis		
AMINOGLYCOSIDES			Often used as supplements to the penicillins
	Amikacin	Amikin	
	Gentamicin	Apogen, Garamycin	*Enterobacter aerogenes*
	Kanamycin	Kantrex, Klebcil	
	Neomycin	Neo-IM	
	Streptomycin		
	Tobramycin	Nebcin	
MACROLIDES			
	Erythromycin	ERYC, E-Mycin, etc.	
	Erythromycin estolate	Ilosone	
	Erythromycin ethylsuccinate	EES, Pediamycin	
	Erythromycin gluceptate	Ilotycin	
	Erythromycin lactobionate	Erythrocin	
	Erythromycin stearate	Erypar, Ethril	
	Triacetyloleandomycin	Tao capsules	
TETRACYCLINES			
	Tetracycline	Achromycin V, Sumycin, etc.	
	Chlortetracycline	Aureomycin	
	Doxycycline hyclate	Doxychel Hyclate, Vibramycin Hyclate, etc.	
	Oxytetracycline	Terramycin	
LINCOMYCINS			
	Lincomycin	Lincocin	
	Clindamycin	Cleocin	
OTHER			
	Chloramphenicol	Chloromycetin, etc.	

fective against many gram-positive and some gram-negative bacteria. The most common side effect of erythromycin administration is gastrointestinal distress (stomach cramps, nausea, vomiting, and diarrhea). When the tetracyclines were first introduced, they were effective against many gram-positive and gram-negative bacteria, as well as organisms such as *Chlamydia, Rickettsia*, and *Spirochaeta*. However, because tetracyclines are generally bacteriostatic, many bacterial strains have developed resistance to tetracycline and its derivatives.

There are not many effective drugs for the treatment of viral infections in humans. However, research into this area of pharmacology is in a period of ferment and discovery. Interferons represent just one of the drugs of potential pharmacologic and physiologic benefit; advancements revealed in the testing of vaccines have been encouraging. Fungal and protozoal infections have been associated historically with tropical and subtropical environments or with less developed areas of the world where sanitation and hygiene are inadequate. The incidence of these infections has become more prevalent, however, because immunoinsufficiency, acquired (AIDS) or induced (after organ transplantation), is more widespread. Therefore, the use of antifungal and antiprotozoal agents is becoming more common.

It is often very difficult to establish the causative agent in an acute pulmonary infection because transoral sputum is often contaminated, revealing mixtures of many organisms on culture. Nevertheless, the organisms *Diplococcus pneumoniae* and *Haemophilus influenzae* are generally thought to be the primary causative agents of infection of the respiratory mucosa in patients with chronic obstructive pulmonary dysfunction.[32,33] Precise diagnosis generally requires that sputum samples be obtained by transtracheal aspiration, bronchoscopy, or transpulmonary aspiration.

SUMMARY

In this chapter, we have discussed the principal groups of drugs used in the treatment of pulmonary dysfunction: bronchodilators, anti-inflammatory agents, decongestants, antitussives, mucokinetics, respiratory stimulants and depressants, paralyzing agents, and antimicrobials. Readers should refer to appropriate preceding chapters for clarification if they lack an understanding of the following:

- Normal bronchomotor tone is the result of a balance between the influences of the sympathetic and parasympathetic divisions of the autonomic nervous system.
- Bronchoconstriction is the result of abnormal bronchomotor tone (bronchospasm), inflammation, mechanical obstruction, or a combination of these.
- The primary goal of bronchodilator therapy is to manipulate the influences of the autonomic nervous system through two opposing nucleotides: cAMP and cGMP.
- Decongestants are used to treat the mucosal edema and increased mucus production that are often associated with common colds, allergies, and many respiratory infections.
- Antihistamines are often used alone or combined with other ingredients to control the production of mucus and the mucosal edema and irritation commonly associated with respiratory allergic responses.
- Antitussives are used to suppress the ineffective, dry, hacking cough associated with minor throat irritations and the common cold.
- Mucokinetics promote the mobilization and removal of secretions from the respiratory tract.
- Analeptics are used to stimulate the central nervous system and enhance respiratory center activity.
- Paralyzing agents are used to ensure the immobility of patients during surgical procedures, to facilitate endotracheal intubation, and to reduce the work of breathing in some patients who are being ventilated mechanically.
- Antimicrobial agents are used to combat microorganisms that invade the body, either by killing them or by limiting their growth and proliferation.

References

1. Kersten LD. Comprehensive Respiratory Nursing: A Decision Making Approach. Philadelphia, WB Saunders, 1989.

2. Cherniack RM, Cherniack L. Respiration in Health and Disease. 3rd ed. Philadelphia, WB Saunders, 1983.
3. Middleton E. Autonomic imbalance in asthma with special reference to beta adrenergic blockade. Adv Intern Med 18:177–197, 1972.
4. Rau JL. Respiratory Care Pharmacology. 3rd ed. Chicago: Year Book Publishers, 1989.
5. Robbins SL, Cotran RS, Kumar V. Pathologic Basis of Disease. 3rd ed. Philadelphia, WB Saunders, 1984.
6. Ziment I. Respiratory Pharmacology and Therapeutics. Philadelphia, WB Saunders, 1978.
7. Popa V. Beta-adrenergic drugs. Clin Chest Med 7:313–329, 1986.
8. Tashkin DP, Jenne JW. Alpha and beta adrenergic agents. In: Weiss EB, Segal MS, Stein M (eds). Bronchial Asthma: Mechanisms and Therapeutics. Boston: Little, Brown, 1985.
9. Patterson JW, Conolly CT, Davies DS, Dollery CT. Isoprenaline resistance and the use of pressurized aerosols in asthma. Lancet 2:426–429, 1968.
10. Orgel HA, Kemp JP, Tinkelman DG, et al. Bitolterol and albuterol metered dose aerosols: Comparison of two long-acting beta₂-adrenergic bronchodilators for treatment of asthma. J Allergy Clin Immunol 75:55–62, 1985.
11. Gross GN, Souhadra JF, Farr RS. The long-term treatment of an asthmatic patient using phentolamine. Chest 66:397–401, 1974.
12. Nadel JA, Barnes PJ. Autonomic regulation of the airways. Annu Rev Med 35:451–467, 1984.
13. Cropp GJA. The role of the parasympathetic nervous system in the maintenance of chronic airway obstruction in asthmatic children. Am Rev Respir Dis 112:599–605, 1975.
14. Orehek J, Gayrard P. Atropine effects on antigen-mediated airway constriction. Am Rev Respir Dis 116:792–793, 1977.
15. Bleecker ER. Cholinergic and neurogenic mechanisms in obstructive airways disease. Am J Med 81(suppl 5A):2–11, 1986.
16. Berry RB, Light RW. Chronic obstructive pulmonary disease. In: Rakel RE (ed). Conn's Current Therapy. Philadelphia, WB Saunders, 1988.
17. Holgate ST, Mann JS, Cushley MJ. Adenosine as a bronchoconstrictor mediator in asthma and its antago-

nism by methylxanthines. J Allergy Clin Immunol 74:302–306, 1984.
18. Isles AF, MacLeod SM, Levison H. Theophylline: New thoughts about an old drug. Chest 82(suppl):49S–54S, 1982.
19. McFadden ER Jr. Cromolyn: First-line therapy for chronic asthma? J Respir Dis 8:39–48, 1987.
20. Townley RG, Suliaman F. The mechanism of corticosteroids in treating asthma. Ann Allergy 58:1–6, 1987.
21. Ciccone CD. Pharmacology in Rehabilitation. Philadelphia, FA Davis, 1990.
22. Aviado DM. Sympathomimetic Drugs. Springfield, Ill, Charles C Thomas, 1970.
23. Douglas WW. Histamine and 5-hydroxytryptamine (serotonin) and their antagonists. In: Gilman AG, Goodman LS, Rall TW, Murad F (eds). The Pharmacological Basis of Therapeutics. 7th ed. New York, Macmillan, 1985.
24. White JP, Mills J, Eiser NM. Comparison of the effects of histamine H₁- and H₂-receptor agonists on large and small airways in normal and asthmatic subjects. Br J Dis Chest 81:155–169, 1987.
25. Burack R, Fox FJ. The New Handbook of Prescription Drugs. New York, Ballantine Books, 1975.
26. Shrake K, Oltmann T. Effective use of wetting agents, mucolytics, and bronchodilators. Respiratory Therapy 10:73–77, 1980.
27. Woolf CR. The use of "respiratory stimulant" drugs. Chest 58:49–53, 1970.
28. Bickermann HA, Chusid EL. The case against the use of respiratory stimulants. Chest 58:53–56, 1970.
29. Winnie AP. Chemical respirogenesis: A comparative study. Acta Anaesth Scand Suppl 51:1–32, 1973.
30. Skatrud JJ, Dempsey J, Iber C, Berssenbrugge A. Correction of CO₂ retention during sleep in patients with COPD. Am Rev Respir Dis 124:260–268, 1981.
31. John JF. What price success? The continuing saga of the toxic:therapeutic ratio in the use of aminoglycoside antibiotics. J Infect Dis 158:1–6, 1988.
32. Crofton J. The chemotherapy of bacterial respiratory infections. Am Rev Respir Dis 101:841–859, 1970.
33. Smith CB, Golden CA, Kanner RE, Renzetti AT. Haemophilus influenzae and Haemophilus parainfluenzae in chronic obstructive pulmonary disease. Lancet 2:1253–1255, 1976.

SECTION 5
ASSESSMENT AND TREATMENT

14 CARDIOPULMONARY ASSESSMENT

INTRODUCTION

Optimal rehabilitation depends on a thorough assessment of the entire patient to evaluate the extent of dysfunction that may affect future performance. In this chapter, the evaluative procedures used to provide information regarding specific cardiopulmonary system pathology are described. While performing the initial assessment, objective information can be obtained from a thorough review of the medical record, an interview with the patient, and an evaluation of the patient at rest (including observation and inspection, palpation, auscultation, **mediate percussion,** general muscle strength, and joint range of motion) and during activity. In addition, the physical therapist must also have a good understanding of other therapeutic regimens and concomitant problems and be able to recognize

them. On conclusion of the evaluation, the therapist should be able to interpret the evaluative findings appropriately to make a decision regarding therapeutic interventions.

MEDICAL CHART REVIEW

The purpose of the medical chart review is to extract pertinent information to develop a database on the patient. Based on the information obtained, the physical therapist performs the appropriate physical assessment and develops an optimal treatment plan. The therapist should focus the review of the medical record by identifying the following significant information:

● Diagnosis and date of event
● Symptoms on admission and since the patient's admission

553

- Other significant medical problems in the past medical history
- Current medications
- Risk factors for heart disease
- Relevant social history, including smoking, alcohol, drug use, lifestyle, support mechanisms
- Clinical laboratory data
- Radiologic studies
- Oxygen therapy and other respiratory treatment
- Surgical procedures
- Other therapeutic regimens
- Electrocardiogram and telemetry monitoring
- Pulmonary function tests
- Arterial blood gases
- Cardiac catheterization laboratory data
- Other diagnostic tests
- Vital signs
- Hospital course since admission, particularly in the patient with cardiac injury to determine whether it has been a complicated or an uncomplicated course
- Occupational history
- Home environment assessment

Diagnosis and Date of Event

The physical therapist needs to know and understand the primary diagnosis as well as any additional diagnoses made since the hospital admission or referral to determine the appropriateness of treatment and the need for monitoring of the patient's responses. Often a patient's primary diagnosis may have been the reason for admission (e.g., a fractured hip), yet a secondary diagnosis may be the reason for referral for physical therapy (e.g., pneumonia postoperatively). Any diagnosis that begins "Rule out ———" requires a thorough review of the chart to see if the diagnosis was confirmed or rejected.

The date of the event is significant, because it determines the acuteness of the situation. The date of the primary event or diagnosis is often documented in the physician's history and physical examination report; however, the date of the secondary diagnosis or subsequent events may be discovered by reviewing the physician's progress notes or orders.

Symptoms

Both cardiac and pulmonary symptoms need to be evaluated. Cardiac ischemic symptoms are those that occur anywhere above the waist; they are typically expressed on, or exacerbated by, exertion and are relieved with rest. These symptoms may be described differently by each patient. Classically, any discomfort, such as chest pain, tightness or pressure, shortness of breath, palpitations, indigestion, and burning, should be considered a cardiac symptom unless cardiac dysfunction has been ruled out. Reviewing the patient's symptoms on admission and during hospitalization provides the therapist with an awareness of those symptoms that are to be assessed as cardiac or noncardiac. During activity the therapist may be trying to reproduce those symptoms as well as observe for new ones.

Classic pulmonary symptoms are described as shortness of breath, dyspnea on exertion, audible wheezing, cough, increased work of breathing, and sputum production. The severity of the symptoms as well as the means of reproducing these symptoms are important to identify. Changes in these symptoms (e.g., worsening of symptoms versus improvement) assist the therapist in developing a plan of care that meets the patient's changing needs.

Other Medical Problems and Past Medical History

The patient's past medical history, including other medical problems, may have a bearing on the evaluation or the plan of treatment proposed by the therapist. Diagnoses other than cardiopulmonary may include orthopedic, neurologic, psychological, or **integumentary,** and these diagnoses may affect the optimal treatment plan proposed. For example, an attempt to increase the activity level of a patient with a history of rheumatoid arthritis may be limited by an orthopedic (joint) dysfunction rather than by a cardiac or pulmonary condition.

Medications

The medications the patient is currently taking are usually listed in the chart (often in the physicians' orders). In the inpatient setting, a comprehensive listing can be found on the nurses' medication cart. Knowledge of the patient's medications can provide information about the patient's present or recent past medical history and may include clues regarding treatment for hypertension, heart failure, angina, bronchospasm, infection, and the like.

Because certain medications may affect the patient's responses to exercise, the physical therapist must become familiar with the broad categories of cardiac and pulmonary medications, understand the indications for their use, and know their general side effects. For further discussion of medications and their indications and side effects see Chapters 12 and 13.

Risk Factors for Heart Disease

From the history and physical examination, one usually can determine whether the patient has any of the following major risk factors for heart disease[1]:

- Hypertension
- Smoking
- An elevated serum cholesterol or a diet high in cholesterol
- A family history of heart disease
- Stress
- A sedentary lifestyle
- Older age
- Male gender
- Obesity
- Diabetes

An awareness of the patient's risk factors enables the therapist to develop realistic goals for the patient's long-term treatment, to identify other rehabilitation team members to whom the patient should be referred, and most important, to decide on precautions to increased activity, depending on the risk for heart disease. Detailed information on the risk factors can be obtained from Chapter 3.

Relevant Social History

Self-abusive social habits, such as excessive drinking of alcohol, smoking, and use of illicit drugs, can affect the cardiopulmonary system and could affect rehabilitation. Therefore, knowledge of the patient's habits, including the length of time involved in the habit and the degree of intake, is an important component of the evaluation. Some of this information can be obtained from the history and physical, but often this information is obtained from the patient or the family.

Heavy alcohol consumption has been associated with the development of **cardiomyopathy,** and long-term cigarette smoking has been associated with the development of chronic obstructive lung disease. Drug use is one habit that may not be readily acknowledged but that may be suspected from the individual's behavior (e.g., extreme nervousness), history of sleeplessness, muscle twitching, anorexia, and nasal irritation. Currently the incidence of cocaine use in the general population is relatively high. Cocaine has serious effects on the cardiovascular system, particularly on the coronary arteries. Cocaine is known to cause severe coronary artery spasm and in some cases can precipitate acute myocardial infarction.[2-4] Cocaine use (especially crack cocaine) has been associated with an increased incidence of severe arrhythmias and in some cases sudden death.

The physician or other medical personnel treating the patient may be unaware of the patient's heavy alcohol consumption or drug addiction. Either of these conditions could prove to be an extreme problem early in the patient's hospitalization because of the symptoms and side effects of sudden withdrawal from these substances.

Clinical Laboratory Data

Laboratory data provide important objective information regarding the clinical status of the patient with cardiopulmonary dysfunction. The seriousness of the dysfunction may also be inferred from the magnitude of deviation of the values from normal. The laboratory data specific to the patient with cardiopulmonary dysfunction include the values for cardiac enzymes (creatine phosphokinase, lactate dehydrogenase, aspartate aminotransferase), blood lipids (cholesterol and triglycerides), complete blood count (specifically hemoglobin, hematocrit, white blood cell count), arterial blood gases, and culture and sensitivity, as well as the results of **coagulation** studies, electrolyte screening panels, and glucose tolerance tests. These are discussed in greater detail in Chapters 8 and 10.

Radiologic Studies

In most situations the therapist reviews the radiologic report and not the actual study films. The radiologic reports that are routinely reviewed for patients with cardiopulmonary dysfunction include chest radiographs, **computed tomography (CT)** scan, **magnetic resonance imaging (MRI)**, and **scintillography.**

The chest radiographs provide a general static assessment of pathologic conditions of the lungs and chest wall, including changes in functional lung space, pleural space, chest wall configuration, presence of fluid, heart size, and vascularization of the lungs. Information about the extent of heart failure or cardiomyopathy as well as pneumonia, restrictive lung disease, pleural effusion, and the like can be obtained from the chest radiograph.

In addition to baseline chest radiographs, patients with heart failure and acute pulmonary dysfunction can be followed with serial radiographs to monitor disease progression, effectiveness of treatment, or both. Therefore, it is important to note the date of the radiograph (particularly if the patient's status is fluctuating). Also the orientation of the chest radiograph is important to identify. The ideal chest radiograph is a posteroanterior (PA) film taken at a distance of approximately 6 feet with the patient in an upright position and performing a maximal inspiration. Portable equipment utilizing the anteroposterior (AP) orientation is used to take

chest films of patients who are too sick or unstable to be transported to the radiology department for a standard PA film. The quality of the film taken with portable equipment and using the AP orientation is generally poorer owing to the position of the patient and the patient's inability to cooperate or to perform a maximal inspiration. The therapist should keep these limitations in mind when evaluating the findings of a portable AP chest radiograph.

Oxygen Therapy and Other Respiratory Treatment

The use of supplemental oxygen should be noted along with its method of delivery (e.g., nasal cannula, face mask, **tracheostomy** collar, blow-by ventilator, or mechanical ventilator). The physical therapist must also know the amount of oxygen being delivered (e.g., 60% via mask or 2 liters via cannula). This information should be correlated with arterial blood gas analysis or hemoglobin saturation data to determine if the patient is adequately oxygenated before beginning any therapy. Depending on the arterial blood gas or saturation information, the therapist may need to use oxygen or to increase the amount of oxygen while exercising the patient (e.g., during formal exercise, activities of daily living, gait). Any patient with a resting Po_2 of less than 60 mm Hg in room air or an oxygen percentage saturation of less than 90% should be considered for supplemental oxygen. If a patient has a low Po_2 but one not below 60 mm Hg on room air or a low Po_2 on oxygen, the patient may require supplemental oxygen with exercise to prevent hypoxemia during exercise. Chapter 10 presents a method of assessing the degree of **hypoxemia** when patients are receiving supplemental oxygen.

Other respiratory treatments (e.g., aerosols, bronchodilator treatments, inspirometers) that are prescribed should be noted because these treatments can improve the patient's exercise performance if they are administered before exercise; however, they may also be extremely fatiguing to the patient and may necessitate limitations on activity immediately following treatment. The necessity for the coordination of physical therapy and respiratory treatments to optimize rehabilitation should be readily apparent. If the patient is being ventilated mechanically, the mode of ventilatory assistance, the set rate, the set volume, the peak inspiratory pressure, the fraction of inspired oxygen, the spontaneous rate, and the like should be identified. A full description of ventilators is found in Chapter 10.

Surgical Procedures

An understanding of specific surgical approaches and procedures, as well as a knowledge of the anatomy of the chest wall, is integral to the chart review process. Knowledge of the approach or procedure may be helpful in defining the physical therapy diagnosis and extent of the problem and in identifying limitations or precautions to any therapeutic procedures being planned.

It is important to understand the number of and placement of the bypass grafts as well as any complications that occurred during the procedure (e.g., whether a pacemaker was inserted) in patients who have undergone coronary artery bypass surgery. For the patient who has undergone bypass surgery with numerous vessels requiring bypass grafts or requiring left main or left main equivalent bypass, one might assume that the patient was more limited in activity before surgery. With extensive disease, patients usually have more symptoms with activity and may have had restrictions with low levels of exertion. In addition, the patient who experiences complications (such as a perioperative myocardial infarction or stroke) during or following the surgery usually has a slower recovery and may require increased activity supervision and may make slower progress.

In the patient who has undergone pulmonary surgery, the amount of lung tissue that was operated on is significant to note (e.g., **wedge resection, lobectomy,** or **pneumonectomy**), as well as the location of the incision. The greater

the amount of lung tissue that was removed, the smaller the amount of lung space is available (one would expect) to actively diffuse oxygen and carbon dioxide and therefore the greater the impairment in performance of activities.

Other Therapeutic Regimens

As a result of the patient's primary or secondary diagnoses or subsequent surgical procedures, additional therapeutic interventions could have an impact on the proposed treatment. Identification of these interventions (e.g., pacemaker implantation, intravenous or intra-arterial drug administration, **parenteral nutrition,** electrolyte replacement, or bedrest limitations) helps the physical therapist develop an appropriate treatment plan with appropriate precautions.

Electrocardiogram and Serial Monitoring

The electrocardiogram (ECG) provides valuable information regarding the state of the heart muscle and the rhythm of the heart. The ECG is used to define previous as well as current myocardial injury, hypertrophy of the heart muscle, pericardial involvement, or delays in the generation of the depolarization impulse. Serial ECG monitoring provides a historic record of the patient's cardiac injury and rhythm disturbances and allows the correlation of the history of rhythm disturbances with changes in medications or medical status. Details of the ECG and rhythm disturbances were discussed in Chapter 9.

Pulmonary Function Tests

Pulmonary function testing (PFT) is an essential component of the assessment process because abnormal PFTs indicate the effects of the pathologic condition and may provide clues regarding the patient's motivation. Measurement of PFTs is done via spirometry. Pulmonary function tests can measure static and dynamic properties of the chest and lungs as well as gas exchange. Static measurements assess the lung volumes and capacities (e.g., tidal volume, vital capacity, inspiratory reserve volume) and determine mechanical abnormalities, whereas dynamic measurements provide data on the flow rates of air moving in and out of the lungs. The dynamic properties reflect the nonelastic components of the pulmonary system and include the forced expiratory flows and volumes.

Values for PFTs are used primarily to identify a baseline of pulmonary dysfunction, as well as to follow the progression of altered respiratory mechanics in chronic lung and musculoskeletal diseases. Chapter 10 explains PFTs in greater detail.

Values for PFTs may be described as abnormal owing to the static values (volumes and capacities), the dynamic values (flow volumes and rates), or both. When patients demonstrate decreased volumes and capacities, they are exhibiting restrictive lung dysfunction. They therefore have less lung space for active diffusion of oxygen into the circulatory system and carbon dioxide out of the system. Patients with decreased dynamic values often have limitations on exercise owing to an inability to actively move large volumes of air rapidly. Treatment planning requires modifications, possibly including supplemental oxygen for patients with extremely low lung volumes or bronchodilator medication before exercise for patients with decreased flow rates or volumes.

Arterial Blood Gases

Arterial blood gases are a measurement of the acid-base and oxygenation status of patients via arterial blood sampling. Blood gas determinations can identify the effectiveness of a treatment designed to improve airway clearance and ventilation. Therefore, serial arterial blood gases are often measured to provide feedback to the medical personnel on the therapeutic regimen. Arterial blood gases are discussed in greater detail in Chapter 10.

Cardiac Catheterization Laboratory Data

Cardiac catheterization, which is an invasive diagnostic procedure, provides information about the anatomy of the coronary arteries and can provide a dynamic assessment of the cardiac muscle. In addition, information on hemodynamic measurement (e.g., estimates of ejection fraction or systolic and diastolic pressures) as well as valvular function can be obtained. Cardiac catheterizations are performed to visualize the cardiac dysfunction and to assist in the decision-making process regarding medical versus surgical management. Repeat cardiac catheterizations also provide information on the progression or, in rare cases, regression of coronary disease or valvular dysfunction.

Vital Signs

Daily recordings of vital signs are often kept in the graphics section of the chart. Vital signs such as heart rate, temperature, blood pressure, and respiration are important to review for trends as well as for the establishment of a baseline. For example, pulmonary patients with infection who are being monitored for improvement can be followed by checking temperature and in some cases respirations and heart rate. Hypertension and treatment for hypertension can be monitored daily by viewing the blood pressure recordings (keeping in mind that these have been recorded at rest and usually in the supine position).

Hospital Course

A thorough review of the medical record, including physicians' and other caregivers' notes, and the order sheets should reveal pertinent information regarding the patient's clinical course since admission. For example, patients with serious complications within the first 4 days of a myocardial infarction have a higher incidence of mortality or later serious complications. Criteria for a complicated postmyocardial infarction hospital course as defined by McNeer and co-workers include the following[5]:

- Ventricular tachycardia and fibrillation
- Atrial flutter or fibrillation
- Second- or third-degree atrioventricular block
- Persistent sinus tachycardia (>100 beats per minute)
- Persistent systolic hypotension (<90 mm Hg)
- Pulmonary edema
- Cardiogenic shock
- Persistent angina or extension of infarction

Patients who are characterized as "uncomplicated" have significantly lower morbidity and mortality rates following their initial cardiac events. A prolonged or complicated hospital course can affect an individual's activity progression owing to the effects of inactivity or bedrest.

Occupation

Identifying the type of work the patient currently performs allows for the setting of realistic goals and for developing a plan for return to work, if possible. For example, a patient who has experienced a massive complicated myocardial infarction may not be an appropriate candidate for returning to a job requiring heavy lifting and may need a referral for **vocational rehabilitation.** The earlier the referral is made, the less the chance of financial or emotional distress. In addition, if a patient requires job modifications or will be delayed in returning to work, referrals can be made to appropriate team members to assist the employer in making the changes necessary or to assist the patient with financial planning.

Home Environment and Family Situation

A supportive family is important to the success of the rehabilitation of any patient. A support system can improve a patient's ability to respond to disease, whereas a negative home environment can deter the patient's rehabilitation.[6] In addition, if the patient requires a great deal of care, the family's ability to supply this care and its financial resources should be assessed. Early assessment of the family situation and home environment as well as involvement of the family in the patient's rehabilitation provides for optimal transition to home.

INTERVIEW WITH THE PATIENT AND THE FAMILY

After a thorough chart review, the interview with the patient and the family is the next step in the physical therapist's initial evaluation. The purpose of this interview is to gather important information about the patient's present complaint, history of medical problems, report of symptoms, risk factors, perception and understanding of the problem, family situation, and goals for rehabilitation (both occupational and leisure).

Important components of the interview are the establishment of effective communication and rapport with the patient and family. Simple, open-ended questions using language easily understood by the patient and family should elicit the answers needed. For example, the therapist might ask, "What did your discomfort feel like when you were admitted to the hospital?" or "How long have you had this breathing problem?" Listening is essential for learning about the patient's problems, as well as the patient's understanding of and reaction to them. The therapist must remember that a patient with pulmonary dysfunction may have difficulty with phonation owing to shortness of breath and may have to take breaths frequently between words. Table 14–1 provides some sample descriptors and questions for assessing cardiac symptoms.

PHYSICAL EXAMINATION

The physical examination is the third step in the initial evaluation of the patient. The physical examination requires the physical therapist to use the skills of inspection, palpation, percussion, auscultation, and activity evaluation when appropriate.

TABLE 14–1. Differentiation of Nonanginal Discomforts from Angina

Stable Angina	Nonanginal Discomfort (chest wall pain)
1. Relieved by nitroglycerin (30 seconds to 1 minute)	1. Nitroglycerin generally has no effect
2. Comes on at the same heart rate and blood pressure and is relieved by rest (lasts only a few minutes)	2. Occurs any time; lasts for hours
3. Not palpable	3. Muscle soreness, joint soreness, evoked by palpation or deep breaths
4. Associated with feelings of doom, cold sweats, shortness of breath	4. Minimal additional symptoms
5. Often seen with ST-segment depression	5. No ST-segment depression

(From Irwin ST, Techlin JS. Cardiopulmonary Physical Therapy. 2nd ed. St. Louis, CV Mosby, 1990, p 124.)

Inspection

Inspection (observation) is a key component in the assessment of *any* patient, but it is extremely important in patients with cardiopulmonary dysfunction. The patient's physical appearance may change slightly as the clinical state changes. Recognition of these slight changes is essential to the day-to-day management and therapeutic treatment of patients with cardiopulmonary dysfunction. Inspection should be performed in a systematic manner, starting with the head and proceeding caudally (until the therapist has developed a degree of proficiency). In addition to the general appearance, the other specific areas that should be noted on inspection include facial expression, effort to breathe through nose or mouth, the neck, the chest in both a resting and a dynamic situation, **phonation,** cough and **sputum** production, posture and positioning, and finally the extremities.

General Appearance

The patient's level of consciousness, body type, posture and positioning, skin tone, and need for external monitoring or support equipment should be considered in an assessment of "general appearance". Obviously, a patient's level of consciousness (e.g., alert, agitated, confused, semicomatose, comatose) may have a direct impact on whether the treatment plan is understood. A comatose patient may require constant attention for positioning and prevention of pulmonary dysfunction, whereas a confused patient may not be able to follow a therapist's instructions without help. Observation of body type (e.g., obese, normal, **cachectic**) is a routine aspect of assessment that gives an indirect measure of nutrition and in some cases an indication of level of exercise tolerance. For example, a patient who is markedly obese may demonstrate a decreased exercise tolerance and an increased work of breathing owing to the restrictive effects of an excessively large abdomen pushing against the diaphragm (Fig. 14–1). By contrast, cachectic patients may also demonstrate a decreased exercise tolerance and an increased work of breathing with exercise because of weakness from muscle wasting.

Body posture and position should also be assessed to determine their impact on the pulmonary system. Kyphosis and **scoliosis** are two postures that functionally limit vital capacity and may therefore affect exercise tolerance. In addition, if a patient is assuming the **professorial position** (leaning forward on knees or on some object; Fig. 14–2) and demonstrating increased effort with breathing and increased use of accessory muscles, one might begin to assume the patient has chronic obstructive disease. Most patients with cardiopulmonary dysfunction cannot tolerate lying on a bed with the head flat and often are found lying either in the semi-Fowler's position in bed (Fig. 14–3) or sitting over the side of the bed or in a chair.

Skin tone may indicate the general level of oxygenation and perfusion of the periphery. An individual who has a general **cyanotic** look (bluish color most noticeably at lips and finger-

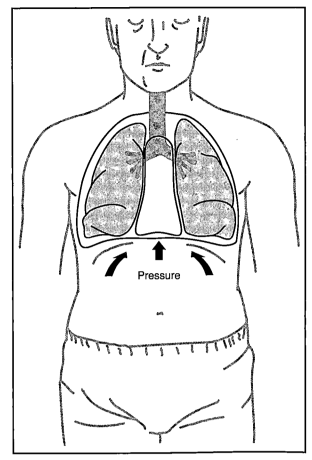

Figure 14-1.

The increased size of the abdomen in obesity (or pregnancy) restricts the full downward movement of the diaphragm during inspiration and restricts lung tissue at rest, therefore creating a restrictive effect on the lung.

nail beds) may have a low Po_2 and may be in need of supplemental oxygen.

Finally, the presence of all equipment used in managing the patient, including monitoring or support equipment, should be noted. In addition, an assessment should be made of whether the equipment is being used correctly by the patient. For example, a patient who requires supplemental oxygen may be breathing through the mouth and therefore not inhaling the oxygen appropriately and may be in a confused state, which can result in an unstable clinical situation. This patient's general appearance may be cya-

notic, when in fact the most recent blood gas values recorded on the chart with the patient on the oxygen are normal. However, if the patient forgot to put the oxygen mask on or happened to pull the mask off because of "feelings of suffocation" and became confused and agitated as well as cyanotic, the acute change the therapist may note on entering the patient's room may be reversed by simply observing that the oxygen is not being used appropriately. Quick action by the therapist may solve this unstable clinical situation. In addition, the use of a cardiac monitor, pulmonary artery catheter, or **intra-aortic balloon pump** indicates a more seriously ill patient who may have rhythm or hemodynamic disturbances (Fig. 14-4).

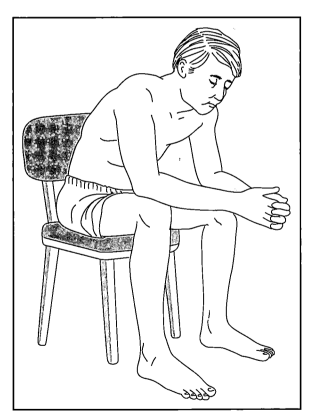

Figure 14-2.

The professorial position provides stabilization of the thorax and arms to increase the effectiveness of accessory muscles during breathing.

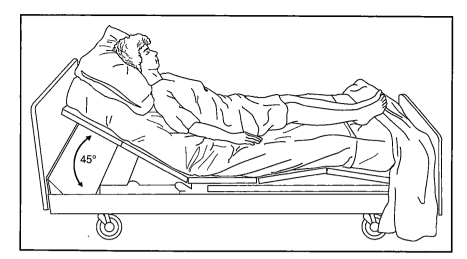

Figure 14-3.

Semi-Fowler's position. Patients with cardiopulmonary dysfunction often require the head of the bed elevated.

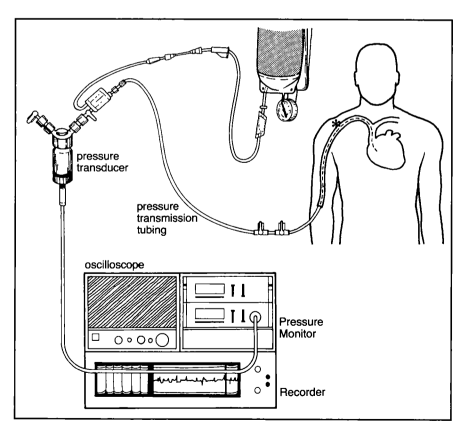

Figure 14-4.

The setup for pulmonary artery monitoring. (Redrawn from Darovic GO. Hemodynamic Monitoring. Philadelphia, WB Saunders, 1987, p 85.)

Facial Characteristics

Facial expression and effort to breathe are two characteristics that can be observed easily; both give important information for the clinical evaluation of the patient. Facial expressions of distress or fatigue may indicate a need for change in the therapeutic treatment. Facial signs of distress include nasal flaring, sweating, paleness, and focused or enlarged pupils. The effort to breathe can be evaluated not only by the facial expression of distress, but also by the degree of work put forth from the musculature of the face and neck and the movement of the lips to breathe. Pursed-lip breathing is a clinical sign of chronic obstructive lung disease, performed to alleviate the trapping of air in the lungs, and is character-

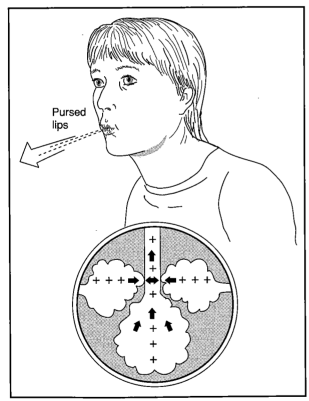

Figure 14-5.
Demonstration of pursed-lip breathing in patients with emphysema and its effects. The weakened bronchiole airways are kept open by the effects of positive pressure created by the pursed lips during expiration.

ized by the patient breathing out against lips that are mostly closed and shaped in a circular fashion (Fig. 14-5).

Evaluation of the Neck

The activity of the neck musculature during breathing and the appearance of the jugular veins should be a part of the standard patient assessment. The presence of hypertrophy or adaptive shortening of the sternocleidomastoid muscles may indicate a chronic pulmonary condition. (The sternocleidomastoid muscle is a very important accessory respiratory muscle that often hypertrophies when used excessively for breathing; Fig. 14-6). In addition, because of a chronic forward-bent posture of the head and trunk typically assumed to improve the efficiency of the breathing effort, the sternocleidomastoid muscle may adaptively shorten, and the clavicles may appear more prominent. Breathing efforts during activity may elicit more work from the neck accessory muscles to lift the chest wall up and assist in breathing during rest.

The presence of **jugular venous distension** should be assessed with the patient sitting or recumbent in bed with the head elevated at least 45 degrees. Jugular venous distention is said to be present if the veins distend above the level of the clavicles. It is an indication of increased volume in the venous system and may be an early sign of right-sided heart failure (cor pulmonale) (Fig. 14-7). In addition, the patient may have left-sided heart failure (congestive heart failure), but this distinction requires auscultation of the lungs, arterial pressure measurements, and possibly a chest radiograph.

Evaluation of the Chest: Resting and Dynamic

The resting chest is evaluated for its symmetry, configuration, rib angles, and intercostal spaces and musculature. Checking symmetry between sides and comparing anteroposterior and transverse diameters provide information regarding the chronicity of the cardiopulmonary dysfunction as well as any present pathologic condition. For example, a patient with chronic obstructive

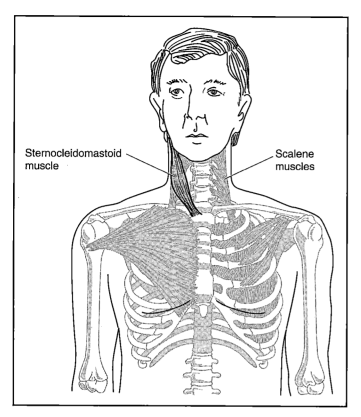

Sternocleidomastoid muscle

Scalene muscles

Figure 14-6.

The sternocleidomastoid muscles often hypertrophy in chronic obstructive pulmonary disease owing to increased work of the accessory muscles to assist with breathing.

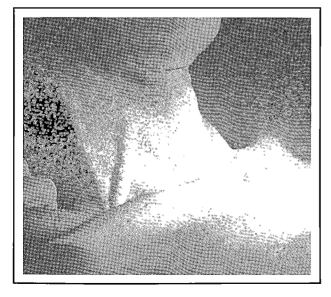

Figure 14-7.

Jugular venous distention. (From Daily EK, Schroeder JP. Techniques in Bedside Hemodynamic Monitoring. 2nd ed. St. Louis, CV Mosby, 1981.)

disease may have a hyperinflated chest, which increases the anterior to posterior diameter (more barrel-like). The normal anterior to posterior diameter is one half the size of the transverse diameter. In the chronically hyperinflated chest wall, the AP diameter may be equal to the transverse diameter (Fig. 14–8). An individual with scoliosis has asymmetry from side to side when observed from either the front or the back. Scoliosis also rotates the lungs as the scoliotic curve progresses throughout life. In addition, an individual who undergoes thoracic surgery with a lateral incision may have developed asymmetry due to pain and splinting or due to actual lung or rib loss from the surgical procedure (Fig. 14–9). Symmetry of the chest wall is also assessed dynamically with palpation of the spinous processes, ribs, and clavicles, comparing the motion from side to side and from top to bottom, anteriorly, laterally, and posteriorly.

Some congenital defects such as **pectus exca-vatum** (funnel chest) or **pectus carinatum** (pigeon chest) are important to observe, although they often have little effect on pulmonary function (Fig. 14–10). Rib angles and intercostal spaces should be observed for abnormalities that might suggest the presence of chronic disease. Normally, rib angles measure less than 90 degrees (Fig. 14–11), and they attach to the vertebrae at approximately 45-degree angles. The intercostal spaces are normally broader posteriorly than anteriorly, but chronic hyperinflation causes the rib angles to increase and the intercostal spaces to become broader anteriorly. Consequently, an increased stretch is placed on the diaphragm muscle, and it adapts by becoming flatter and thus less effective (see Fig. 14–11).

Other respiratory accessory muscles may hypertrophy as a result of chronic obstructive pulmonary disease because of the demand placed on them owing to the diminished capacity of the diaphragm muscle. The scalenes, trapezius, and

Figure 14–8.

A, A normal anteroposterior (AP) diameter. *B,* The increased AP diameter in a chronically hyperinflated chest.

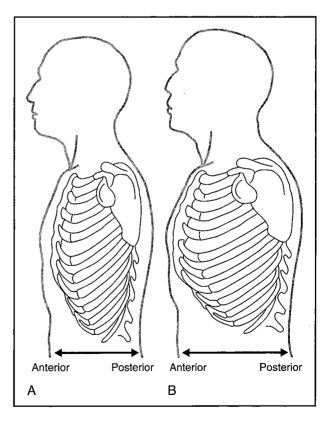

Anterior   Posterior   Anterior   Posterior

A   B

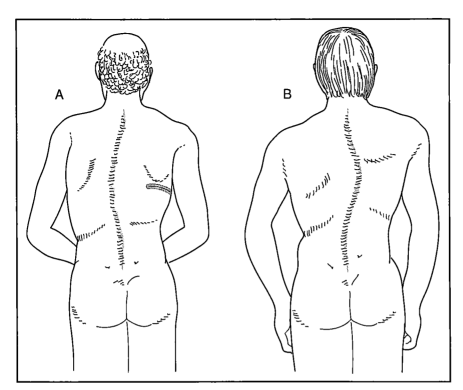

Figure 14-9.

A, Splinting postthoracic surgery (on right), demonstrating thoracic asymmetry. *B,* Thoracic asymmetry found with scoliosis.

intercostals work harder than normal when their contribution to normal resting or exercise breathing is increased. Ultimately, the muscles make adaptive changes to the increased workloads by becoming hypertrophied.

Just as the resting chest wall must be evaluated, so must the dynamic or moving chest wall. Observations of breathing patterns, rates, inspiratory to expiratory ratios, and symmetry of chest wall motion must all be made. Abnormal breathing patterns should be noted with descriptive terminology, as is presented in Table 14-2. The normal adult respiratory rate is 10 to 20 breaths per minute and can be assessed by counting the respirations for 1 full minute. Observation and palpation of the moving chest are the recommended methods, but one problem with assessing the respiratory rate is the fact that patients are often aware that respirations are being counted, and therefore they may subconsciously alter the rate.

The ratio of inspiration to expiration during the normal breathing cycle is an important consideration. The normal inspiration to expiration ratio is 1 to 2; however, in individuals with chronic obstructive pulmonary diseases, particularly with asthmatics, the ratio may be reduced to 1 to 4 owing to their inability to get rid of air in the lungs. Also, the pattern of breathing should be noted: *paradoxical breathing* occurs because of an impairment of the respiratory center's control over breathing (often found in chronic respiratory disease or neurologic insult). An example of paradoxical breathing is the individual with chronic obstructive pulmonary disease and air entrapment who must actively contract the abdominal musculature during expiration to decrease the air trapped in the lungs. The same sort of paradoxical breathing is found in an infant in respiratory distress.

Phonation, Cough, and Cough Production

Evaluation of a patient's speech also is an assessment of shortness of breath at rest. When speech is interrupted for breath, an individual is described as having dyspnea of phonation. Con-

Figure 14-10.

Congenital thoracic defects. *A,* Pectus excavatum (funnel chest), characterized by depression in the lower portion of the sternum. *B,* Pectus carinatum (pigeon chest), characterized by a displaced anterior chest and increased anteroposterior diameter.

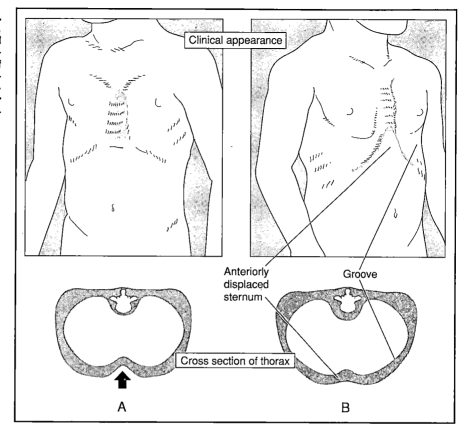

Figure 14-11.

Rib angles. *A,* Normal: measuring less than 90 degrees and attaching at the vertebrae at approximately a 45-degree angle. *B,* Abnormal: rib angles greater than 90 degrees and attaching to the vertebrae with angles greater than 45 degrees in the hyperinflated chest. Also note that the position of the diaphragm is flattened.

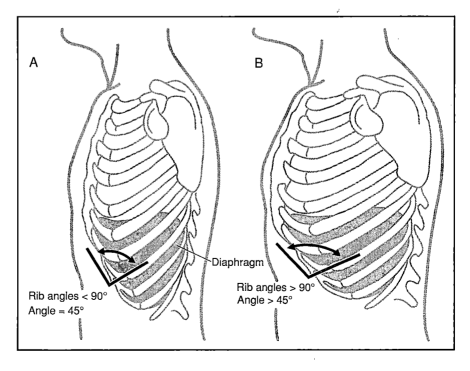

TABLE 14–2. Breathing Patterns Commonly Encountered in the Assessment of Patients with Respiratory Problems

Pattern of Breathing	Description
Apnea	Absence of ventilation
Fish-mouth	Apnea with concomitant mouth opening and closing; associated with neck extension and bradypnea
Eupnea	Normal rate, normal depth, regular rhythm
Bradypnea	Slow rate, shallow or normal depth, regular rhythm; associated with drug overdose
Tachypnea	Fast rate, shallow depth, regular rhythm; associated with restrictive lung disease
Hyperpnea	Normal rate, increased depth, regular rhythm
Cheyne-Stokes (periodic)	Increasing then decreasing depth, period of apnea interspersed; somewhat regular rhythm; associated with critically ill patients
Biot's	Slow rate, shallow depth, apneic periods, irregular rhythm; associated with central nervous system disorders like meningitis
Apneustic	Slow rate, deep inspiration followed by apnea, irregular rhythm; associated with brainstem disorders
Prolonged expiration	Fast inspiration, slow and prolonged expiration yet normal rate, depth, and regular rhythm; associated with obstructive lung disease
Orthopnea	Difficulty breathing in postures other than erect
Hyperventilation	Fast rate, increased depth, regular rhythm; results in decreased arterial carbon dioxide, tension; called "Kussmaul breathing" in metabolic acidosis; also associated with central nervous system disorders like encephalitis
Psychogenic dyspnea	Normal rate, regular intervals of sighing; associated with anxiety
Dyspnea	Rapid rate, shallow depth, regular rhythm; associated with accessory muscle activity
Doorstop	Normal rate and rhythm; characterized by abrupt cessation of inspiration when restriction is encountered; associated with pleurisy

(From Irwin ST, Techlin JS. Cardiopulmonary Physical Therapy. 2nd ed. St. Louis, CV Mosby, 1990, p 286.)

TABLE 14–3. Guidelines for Evaluating Cough

Cough Characteristics	Associated Features	Interpretation
Nonspecific	Sore throat, runny nose, runny eyes	Acute lung infection; tracheobronchitis
Productive	Preceded by an earlier, painful, nonproductive cough associated with an upper respiratory infection	Lobar pneumonia
Dry or productive	Acute bronchitis	Bronchopneumonia
Paroxysmal; mucoid or blood-stained sputum	Flulike syndrome	*Mycoplasma* or viral pneumonia
Purulent sputum	Sputum formerly mucoid	Acute exacerbation of chronic bronchitis
Productive for more than 3 months consecutively and for at least 2 years		Chronic bronchitis
Foul-smelling, copious, layered purulent sputum	Long-standing problem	Bronchiectasis
Blood-tinged sputum	Month long	Tuberculosis or fungal infection
Persistent, nonproductive		Pneumonitis, interstitial fibrosis, pulmonary infiltrates
Persistent, minimally productive	Smoking history, injected pharynx	"Smoker's cough"
Nonspecific; minimal hemoptysis	Long standing	Neoplastic disease
Nonproductive	Long standing; dyspnea	Mediastinal neoplasm
Brassy		Aortic aneurysm
Violent cough	Sudden; onset at the same time as signs of asphyxia; localized wheezing	Aspiration of foreign body
Frothy sputum	Worsens in supine position, dyspnea	Heart failure, pulmonary edema
Hemoptysis	Sudden; simultaneous dyspnea; pleural effusion	Pulmonary infarct

(Adapted by permission from Fishman AP. Pulmonary Disease and Disorders. Vol. 1. New York, McGraw-Hill, 1980.)

fusion exists in the literature as well as in the clinic, because shortness of breath and dyspnea are often used interchangeably. The definition of dyspnea is "the patient's subjective report of discomfort with breathing." Shortness of breath is thus the actual symptom observed. Therefore, the description of **dyspnea** of phonation is made by identifying how many words can be expressed before the next breath. For example, one-word dyspnea would mean that speech is interrupted for a breath between every word. Voice control can also be used to assess shortness of breath as well as strength of the musculature used in speaking and breathing, because poor voice control often indicates weak musculature in both breathing and speaking.

The strength of the patient's cough needs to be assessed, as well as the production of any secretions from the cough (if they are present). Several characteristics of the cough are essential to evaluate, including the effectiveness of the cough (strength, depth, and length of cough). For example, an individual with weak respiratory accessory muscles (e.g., one who has a high spinal cord injury) would have a very weak and therefore ineffective cough. In addition, an individual with **bronchospasm** may have a very long, drawn out **spasmodic cough** that is just as ineffective.

The secretions should be assessed and described with regard to quantity, color, smell, and consistency (Table 14–3). Normally, persons may raise 100 milliliters of mucus (clear to white) per day and not notice it.

In addition to the sputum odor, the individual's breath odor should be assessed. Foul-smelling breath may indicate an anaerobic infection of the mouth or respiratory tract, whereas an acetone breath may indicate diabetic **keto-acidosis.**

Appearance of Extremities

Observation of the fingers and toes and the calves of the legs should indicate whether long-term problems with circulation and oxygenation are present. **Digital clubbing** of the fingers and toes indicates chronic tissue hypoxia and is found in many instances of hypoxemia-

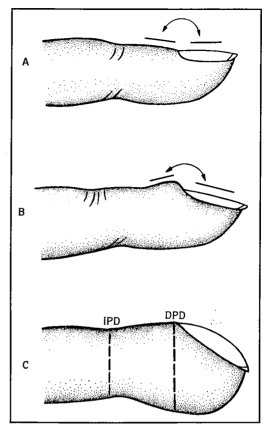

Figure 14–12.

Normal digit configuration (A) and digital clubbing (B). Note that the angle between the nail and the proximal skin exceeds 180 degrees. C, Also note that the distal phalangeal depth (DPD) is greater than the interphalangeal depth (IPD). (From Wilkins RL, Krider SJ. Clinical Assessment in Respiratory Care. St. Louis, CV Mosby, 1985.)

producing disease (Fig. 14–12). Cyanosis (blueness) of the nail beds may also indicate cardiopulmonary dysfunction, but cyanosis can be an indication of decreased circulation to these areas because of cold, vasospasm, peripheral vascular disease, or decreased cardiac output. The calves of the legs should be observed for skin color changes of blue or purple. This may be indicative of peripheral vascular insufficiency.

Auscultation of the Lungs

Auscultation is an evaluation technique used to confirm the findings of chart assessment and

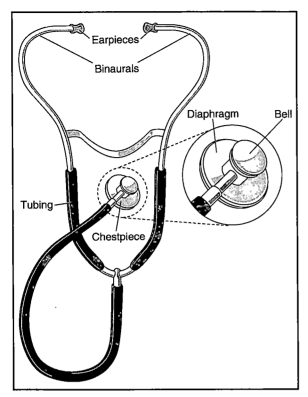

Figure 14–13.

A stethoscope, showing the diaphragm (flattened side) and the bell.

inspection as well as to rule out other cardiopulmonary dysfunction. Auscultation is also an excellent tool for reassessment of an individual's ventilation following treatment techniques to improve bronchial hygiene or regional ventilation.

Auscultation requires appropriate equipment (the stethoscope) as well as appropriate instructions to the patient and proper positioning. It is recommended that the physical therapist invest in a personal stethoscope, because stethoscopes fit different people in different ways owing to the types, sizes, and positions of the earpieces. The most appropriate choice is a stethoscope that comes with adjustable earpieces, with adequate but not excessive tubing, and with both a diaphragm (the flat side) and a bell, including a valve to turn toward either the diaphragm or the bell. Auscultation of lung sounds is performed with the diaphragm of the stethoscope preferably in a quiet environment (Fig. 14–13). Ausculta-

tion of heart sounds requires both the diaphragm and the bell and, again, a quiet environment.

For auscultation of the lung sounds, the optimal position is for the patient to be sitting to permit auscultation of the entire lung space, including both the anterior and posterior chest wall. In addition, optimal auscultation involves removal of bed clothes to expose the bare skin while the individual breathes deeply through an open mouth. Unfortunately, some of the more seriously ill patients can neither tolerate the sitting position at the time of initial visit nor perform adequate deep breaths for auscultation.

Auscultation should be performed over the entire lung space, with at least one breath auscultated in each bronchopulmonary segment. The intensity, pitch, and quality of the breath sounds should be compared between right and left and in the craniocaudal direction. Auscultation should be performed in a systematic manner, anteriorly and then posteriorly (or vice versa) (Fig. 14–14). Precautions that should be taken during auscultation are the following:

- Prevent the patient from falling if weak or if poor balance is noted.
- Prevent the patient from becoming dizzy secondary to hyperventilation by auscultating slowly between pulmonary segments.
- Maintain appropriate draping of the patient, particularly females.
- If auscultation reveals very faint or distant sounds, remind the patient to take deep breaths and to breathe in and out through the mouth so that a recheck can be done.

Lung Sound Definitions

Disagreement exists regarding the terms used to identify the auscultated lung sounds.[7] Nonetheless, lung sounds may be divided into two types: normal breath sounds and **adventitious breath sounds**. Normal breath sounds are the normal noises of breathing that can be heard with a stethoscope. They are described as vesicular and are soft, low-pitched sounds heard primarily during inspiration. During expiration low, vesicular sounds are minimal and occur only during the initial one third of exhalation. Expira-

Figure 14-14.

One method of auscultating the chest. *A,* The chest. *B,* The back. (Redrawn from Buckingham EB. A Primer of Clinical Diagnosis. 2nd ed. New York, Harper & Row, 1979.)

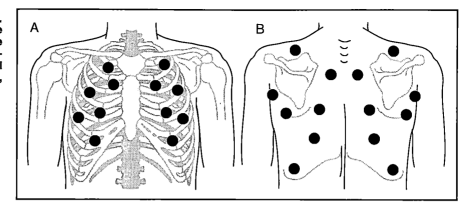

tory sounds flow directly from inspiratory sounds, without a break in the sounds.

Different breath sounds are auscultated over different portions of the tracheobronchial tree, which are also normal. **Bronchial breath sounds,** described as tubular sounds, are loud, high-pitched sounds with approximately equal inspiratory and expiratory duration. Also a pause occurs between the inspiratory and expiratory components. A third type of "normal" breath sound is heard over the junction of the mainstem bronchi with the segmental bronchi, called bronchovesicular. **Bronchovesicular breath sounds** are a softer version of bronchial sounds but differ only in that they are continuous between inspiration and expiration. Posteriorly the bronchovesicular sounds are normally heard only between the scapulae (Fig. 14-15). Table 14-4 provides a list of errors of auscultation to avoid.

These normal sounds are produced from the turbulence of airflow in the airways. The belief is that the inspiratory component of vesicular sounds is produced regionally within each lung and possibly within each lobe.[8] The expiratory component is believed to be produced in the larger airways. The fact that airflow is directed away from the chest wall during expiration might explain the fading away of the sound during expiration and the reason why only approximately the first third of expiration can be heard.

A pathologic condition in the lungs can change the transmission of the sounds. An increase in lung tissue density causes increased sound transmission. This is the reason one may hear bronchial breath sounds in areas other than the mainstem bronchi when a pathologic condition that causes **consolidation** exists. A decrease in lung tissue density, as in the emphysematous lung, would cause decreased sound transmission. Decreased sound transmission also occurs if only shallow breaths are taken or if distance of transmission between the airways and the stethoscope is increased (as in obesity, pleural effusion, or barrel chest).

TABLE 14-4. Errors of Auscultation to Avoid

Errors	Correct Technique
Listening to breath sounds through the patient's gown	Placing bell or diaphragm directly against the chest wall
Allowing tubing to rub against bed rails or patient's gown	Keeping tubing free from contact with any objects during auscultation
Attempting to auscultate in a noisy room	Turning television or radio off
Interpreting chest hair sounds as adventitious lung sounds	Wetting chest hair before auscultation if thick
Auscultating only the "convenient" areas	Asking alert patient to sit up; rolling comatose patient onto his side to auscultate posterior lobes

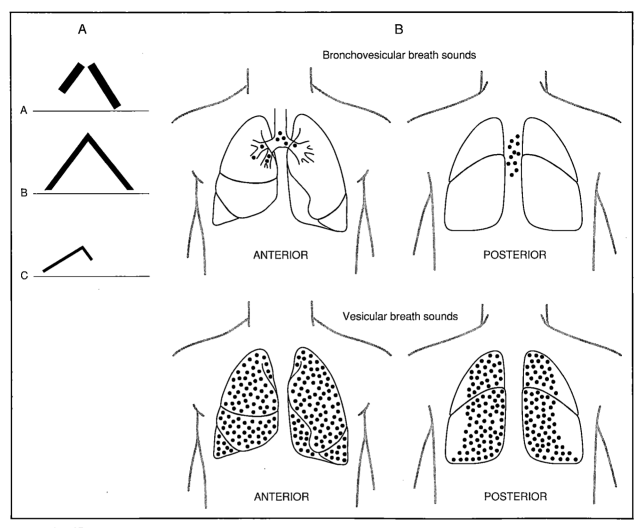

Figure 14–15.

A, Breath sound diagrams: normal tracheobronchial (A); bronchovesicular (B); vesicular (C). The upstroke represents inspiration and the downstroke expiration. The thickness of the line indicates intensity. *B*, The positions on the anterior and posterior chest walls at which normal vesicular and bronchovesicular breath sounds are identified. (Redrawn from Wilkins RL, Hodgkin JE, Lopez B. Lung Sounds: A Practical Guide. St. Louis, CV Mosby, 1988.)

When a pathologic condition of the lung is suspected because of increased or decreased transmission sounds, then further evaluative measures must be taken. **Egophony, bronchophony**, and **whispering pectoriloquy** are three techniques to further evaluate the abnormal transmission of sound. Asking a patient to say "99" or "E," or to whisper are three techniques that can be employed to assess the abnormally transmitted sounds. Egophony is demonstrated when a patient is asked to say "E" aloud, but the sound that is auscultated over the chest is "A." Bronchophony is demonstrated when a patient is asked to say "99," and the words are auscultated clearly over the entire chest. Whispering pectoriloquy is evident when a patient is asked to whisper, and the whispered words are clearly and distinctly heard through the stethescope. The relative strengths of each of the sounds auscultated when using these techniques suggest the degree of consolidation or hyperinflation of the underlying lung; stronger, louder sounds are heard in the presence of consolidative pathology, whereas weaker, softer sounds are heard in the presence of hyperinflation.

Adventitious Lung Sounds. Adventitious lung sounds are the abnormal noises heard only with a stethoscope. These can be divided into two categories: *continuous* and *discontinuous* lung sounds. The American Thoracic Society and the American College of Chest Physicians Ad Hoc Subcommittee on Pulmonary Nomenclature (ATS-ACCP) further clarified the continuous sounds as *wheezes* (previously defined as *rhonchi*) and the discontinuous adventitious lung sounds as *crackles* (previously called *rales*).[9]

Wheezes. **Wheezes** are continuous adventitious lung sounds with a constant pitch and varying duration. These sounds are most frequently heard on exhalation and are associated with airway obstruction. Some clinicians still advocate using the term **rhonchi** to describe low-pitched continuous adventitious lung sounds. The ATS-ACCP, however, recommends referring to all continuous adventitious sounds as wheezes and specifying whether they are high-pitched or low-pitched. When describing the wheeze it is extremely important to document the time of its occurrence (inspiration or expiration) because this may help to differentiate pathologic conditions.

Wheezes on expiration are most common and are often associated with airway constriction as is found in bronchospasm or when secretions are narrowing the airway. The wheeze on inspiration is not very common and indicates a more severe obstruction of the airway.[10] Wheezes may diminish or change in pitch as a result of bronchodilator treatments. The monophonic, continuous adventitious sound heard over the upper airways of a patient with upper airway obstruction (as when a peanut is lodged in a bronchus or when epiglottic interference occurs) is called **stridor** and differs from the normal wheeze in intensity and pitch.

Crackles. **Crackles** are discontinuous adventitious lung sounds that sound like brief bursts of popping bubbles. Crackles are more commonly heard during inspiration and may be associated with restrictive or obstructive respiratory disor-

ders because they can be produced via several mechanisms.[10,11,12] They may result from the sudden opening of closed airways[8-14] (Fig. 14-16) or as the result of the movement of secretions during inspiration and expiration.[15] Some clinicians still use the term **rales** for what are now called crackles.

Peripheral airways can collapse owing to atelectasis, pulmonary edema, fibrosis, or compression from pleural effusion, and often crackles auscultated with these pathologic conditions are in the latter half of inspiration. Crackles occurring in the early half of inspiration often result from the popping open of more proximal airways.[14] The closure of proximal airways may result from the weakening of bronchial and broncheolar support structures as occurs in the latter stages of chronic obstructive pathologic diseases such as bronchitis or emphysema. Crackles due to the movement of fluid or secretions within the lungs are often described as low-pitched and may be found on either inspiration or expiration or both.

Pleural Rub. Another abnormal sound that should be checked by auscultation in the lower lateral chest areas (both right and left) is a

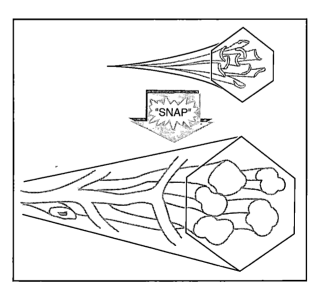

Figure 14-16.

Sudden reexpansion of collapsed peripheral airways. (Redrawn from Murphy RLH. Lung sounds. Basics of Respiratory Disease, Vol. 8, No. 4, Am Thor Soc, 1980.)

pleural (friction) rub, which may be an indication of pleural inflammation. The pleural rub sounds like two pieces of leather or sandpaper rubbing together, and it occurs with each inspiration and expiration.[10]

Evaluation of breath sounds via auscultation should be systematic, beginning with an initial description as vesicular, bronchovesicular, bronchial, diminished, or absent. With bronchial and bronchovesicular sounds, further definitive techniques such as egophony, bronchophony, and whispering pectoriloquy should be employed. If adventitious sounds are heard, they first must be defined as continuous or discontinuous. Following this distinction, descriptors such as pitch, intensity, duration, and portion of the respiratory cycle in which they occur should be used to further define the sounds. On completion of the auscultatory assessment, the therapist can interpret the sounds with regard to what they may indicate (Table 14–5).

Auscultation of the Heart

Auscultation of heart sounds requires a quiet environment and a stethoscope with a diaphragm and bell. The diaphragm is placed firmly on the skin and is used to auscultate initially the topographic areas on the chest wall, identifying high-pitched sounds. The bell accentuates lower frequency sounds, including **atrial** and **ventricular gallops,** filtering out the high-pitched sounds. Care must be taken to place the bell lightly on the skin and not to press firmly, because increased pressure causes the skin to act like a diaphragm so that low-frequency sounds cannot be heard.

Auscultation of heart sounds is a clinical skill that can be learned only by practice with auscultation on individuals with different heart sounds. The entry-level practitioner should not be expected to be competent in auscultation of *all* heart sounds. However, an entry-level practitioner should be able to perform a competent systematic auscultation of the heart and be able to note normal heart sounds and blatantly abnormal heart sounds (e.g., loud murmurs and loud atrial or ventricular gallops).

TABLE 14–5. Guidelines for the Documentation and Interpretation of Auscultated Sounds

Type of Sound	Nomenclature	Interpretation
Breath sound	Normal	Normal, air-filled lung
	Decreased	Hyperinflation in chronic obstructive pulmonary disease
		Hypoinflation in acute lung disease, e.g., atelectasis, pneumothorax, pleural effusion
	Absent	Pleural effusion Pneumothorax Severe hyperinflation Obesity
	Bronchial	Consolidation Atelectasis with adjacent patent airway
	Crackles	Secretions, if biphasic Deflation, if monophasic
	Wheezes	Diffuse airway obstruction, if polyphonic Localized stenosis, if monophonic
Voice sound	Normal	Normal, air-filled lung
	Decreased	Atelectasis Pleural effusion Pneumothorax
	Increased	Consolidation Pulmonary fibrosis
Extrapulmonary adventitious sounds	Crunch	Mediastinal emphysema
	Pleural rub	Pleural inflammation or reaction
	Pericardial rub	Pericardial inflammation

(From Irwin S, Techlin JS. Cardiopulmonary Physical Therapy. 2nd ed. St. Louis, CV Mosby, 1990, p 289.)

Auscultation of the heart requires selective listening for each component of the cardiac cycle while placing the stethoscope over the five main topographic areas for auscultation (Fig. 14–17). The five areas where sounds are best heard are

- the **aortic area:** auscultated best in the second intercostal space close to the sternum on the right of the sternum
- the **pulmonic area:** auscultated best at the second intercostal space to the left of the sternum
- the **third left intercostal space:** murmurs of both aortic and pulmonic origin are best heard here
- the **tricuspid area:** located at the lower left

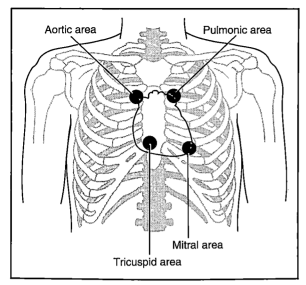

Figure 14-17.

Areas to auscultate for sounds generated from the aortic, pulmonic, tricuspid, and mitral valves. In the normal heart, the mitral area is the apical pulse point and the point of maximal impulse. (Redrawn from Leatham A. Introduction to the Examination of the Cardiovascular System. 2nd ed. Oxford, Oxford University Press, 1979, p 20. By permission of Oxford University Press.)

sternal border, approximately the fourth to fifth intercostal space
• the **mitral area (apex of heart):** located in the fifth left intercostal space, medial to the mid-clavicular line

As with breath sounds, auscultation of heart sounds should be performed in a systematic manner, such as by beginning at the aortic area and listening to both the first and second heart sounds. When listening to the sounds, the intensity and timing, as well as any splitting, extra sounds, or murmurs should be noted. The intensity varies according to the proximity to the valve and chest wall.

The first heart sound, S_1 (the *lub* of the lub-dub), is associated with the closure of the mitral and tricuspid valves and corresponds with the onset of ventricular systole. The S_1 sound is normally louder and longer and lower pitched when auscultated at the apex or even in the tricuspid region.

The second heart sound, S_2 (the *dub* of lub-

dub), is associated with the closure of the aortic and pulmonic valves and corresponds with the start of ventricular diastole. The second sound has greatest intensity when auscultated at the aortic or pulmonic regions.

Transient splitting of the first or second sound may be noted during inspiration. Splitting of the S_1 is best heard over the tricuspid region, whereas splitting of the S_2 is heard more readily over the pulmonic region. Both splitting sounds are considered to be normal and are indicative of slight timing differences between closure of the left heart valves and the right heart valves.

Abnormal Heart Sounds

Third Heart Sound. A third heart sound (S_3) occurs early in diastole while the ventricle is rapidly filling (immediately following S_2 and sounding like lub-dub-*dub*). The S_3 sound is low-pitched and must be auscultated with the bell of the stethoscope. Auscultation is often best performed with the patient laying on the left side so that the apex of the heart is closest to the chest wall. When an S_3 is heard in healthy children or young adults, it is considered to be normal and is called a *physiologic* third heart sound. When an S_3 is auscultated in an older, non-physically active person or in the presence of heart disease, it typically indicates a loss of ventricular compliance (failure), often called a ventricular gallop. In patients with suspected ventricular dysfunction, the clinician should search carefully for the presence of a ventricular gallop because it is a key diagnostic sign for congestive heart failure.

Fourth Heart Sound. The fourth heart sound (S_4) occurs late in diastole (just before S_1 and sounding like *la*-lub-dub) and is associated with atrial contraction. S_4 is also a low-pitched sound best heard with the bell of the stethoscope. S_4, otherwise known as the atrial gallop sound, is not normal and is associated with an increased resistance to ventricular filling. An S_4 is commonly heard in individuals with hypertensive cardiac disease, coronary artery disease, or pulmonary disease and is also commonly found in individuals with a history of myocardial infarction or coronary artery bypass surgery.

Murmurs

Murmurs can be very complex and difficult to understand for the entry-level practitioner. However, there are three broad classifications of murmurs that can help one understand the mechanism of the murmurs:

- Murmurs caused by high rates of flow either through normal or abnormal valves
- Murmurs caused by forward flow through a constricted or deformed valve or flow into a dilated vessel or chamber
- Murmurs caused by backward flow through a valve (regurgitation)[16]

Murmurs are classified according to their timing, quality, intensity, pitch, location, and radiation. In addition, murmurs are classified by the position of the patient in which the murmur is best heard and by the part of the respiratory cycle in which it is best heard.

Systolic and Diastolic Murmurs. Systolic murmurs are the most common and may be caused by either ejection or regurgitation. These murmurs are heard between S_1 and S_2 and are best described as a "swishing" sound associated with S_1 (instead of hearing lub-dub, one usually hears "*lush*-dub"). One of the most classic systolic murmurs is associated with aortic stenosis. The murmur heard is a high-pitched murmur, best heard at the right sternal border, second intercostal space, frequently radiating to the neck and the carotid arteries.

Other valvular dysfunction, as well as congenital defects that include atrial and ventricular defects, may produce systolic murmurs. In addition, diastolic murmurs, although uncommon, may occur. These murmurs are heard immediately following the S_2 and diminish in intensity quickly. Pathologic conditions associated with these murmurs include aortic and pulmonic regurgitation and mitral stenosis.

Another common murmur is associated with mitral valve dysfunction and is called *mitral valve prolapse*. When abnormalities exist with the chordae tendineae (as with papillary muscle rupture after a myocardial infarction or with mitral valve prolapse), clicking sounds in the middle of ventricular systole may be heard. These are referred to as *midsystolic clicks*.[17] Further discussion of murmurs is beyond the scope of this text because it is beyond the level of the entry-level practitioner.

Pericardial Friction Rub. An abnormal sound associated with each beat of the heart is known as a pericardial friction rub. It is the sign of pericardial inflammation (pericarditis). Auscultation for a pericardial friction rub is best performed with the patient in the supine position with the therapist listening over the third or fourth intercostal space along the anterior axillary line. The pericardial friction rub sounds like a "creak" with each beat and has also been described as a "leathery" sound, as if two pieces of leather were being rubbed together.[17]

Palpation

Palpation is an assessment technique employed to refine the information previously gathered from the chart review, inspection, and auscultation. The purposes of palpation are to evaluate the mediastinum (for tracheal shift), chest motion, chest wall pain, fremitus, muscle activity of the chest wall and diaphragm, and circulatory status.

The Mediastinum (Tracheal Position)

Evaluation of the mediastinum assesses tracheal shift that is due to disproportionate intrathoracic pressures or lung volumes between the two sides of the thorax. The contents of the thorax may shift toward the affected side when the lung volume or intrathoracic pressure on that side is decreased. This can happen following a lobectomy or pneumonectomy or a large degree of atelectasis. The content of the thorax may shift to the unaffected side (the contralateral side) when there is increased pressure on the same side, as happens in a pleural effusion or an untreated pneumothorax.

Palpation for such shifts is performed while the patient is sitting upright with the neck flexed slightly to allow relaxation of the sternocleidomastoid muscles, and the chin should be positioned in the midline. Palpation proceeds with the tip of the index finger being placed in the suprasternal notch, first medially to the left sternoclavicular joint, and pushed inward toward the cervical spine. Then the index finger is placed medial to the right sternoclavicular joint and pushed inward toward the cervical spine (Fig. 14–18).

When a significant shift to the unaffected side occurs, aggressive treatment is usually indicated. If the shift is due to a pneumothorax, a chest tube is usually inserted immediately. In the case of the large pleural effusion, a thoracentesis may be performed to drain the fluid or to evaluate the contents of the fluid or both. When the shift goes to the affected side in the patient after a lobectomy or pneumonectomy, the patient should be cautioned against lying on the affected side, because this would only increase the **mediastinal shift.**

Chest Motion

Palpation is performed segmentally to compare the chest wall motion over the upper, middle, and lower lobes while the patient is breathing quietly and while breathing deeply. The impor-

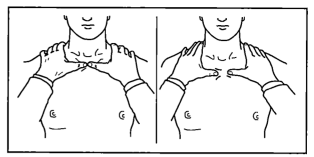

Figure 14–19.

Palpation of upper lobe motion. (Redrawn from Cherniack RM, Cherniack L. Respiration in Health and Disease. 2nd ed. Philadelphia, WB Saunders, 1972.)

tant components of the evaluation include the amount of movement of the hands, the presence or absence of symmetry of movement, and the timing of the movement (Figs. 14–19 to 14–21).

The upper chest wall expansion is evaluated by the therapist placing the palms of the hands anteriorly over the chest wall from the fourth rib upward. The fingers should be stretched upward and over the trapezius, and the thumbs should be placed together along the midline of the chest. The skin on the patient's chest may need to be mobilized to position the palms down with the thumbs touching. The patient should be asked to take a maximal inspiration, and the therapist's hands should be relaxed so that they move with the chest wall. Notation of the extent of movement and the symmetry of the move-

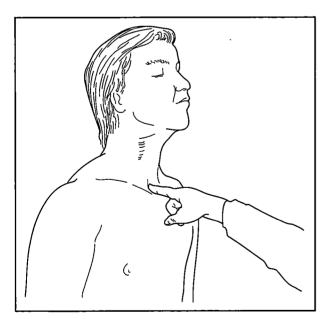

Figure 14–18.

Palpation for position of the mediastinum to evaluate for tracheal deviation.

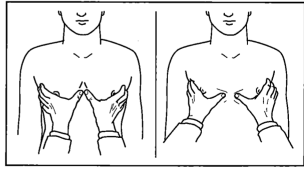

Figure 14–20.

Palpation of right middle and left lingula lobe motion. (Redrawn from Cherniack RM, Cherniack L. Respiration in Health and Disease. 2nd ed. Philadelphia, WB Saunders, 1972.)

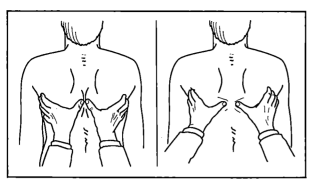

Figure 14–21.

Palpation of lower lobe motion. (Redrawn from Cherniack RM, Cherniack L. Respiration in Health and Disease. 2nd ed. Philadelphia, WB Saunders, 1972.)

ment is important (see Fig. 14–19). Chest wall motion over the right middle lobe and lingula segments of the left upper lobe is evaluated by the therapist placing the fingers laterally and over posterior axillary folds, with the palms pressed firmly on the anterior chest wall. The skin is then drawn medially until the thumbs meet at the midline. The patient should take a maximal inspiration with the therapist's hands gliding with the movement of the lobes underneath. Again, extent of movement and symmetry of movement should be documented (see Fig. 14–20).

The lower chest wall expansion is evaluated with the patient's back toward the therapist, and the therapist's fingers wrapped around the anterior axillary fold. The skin is then drawn medially until the tips of the thumbs meet at the spinal column. While a maximal inspiration is performed by the patient, the therapist should allow the hands to glide with the movement of the rib cage, and the extent of the movement as well as the symmetry should be documented (see Fig. 14–21).

Evaluation of Fremitus

Fremitus is defined as the vibration that is produced by the voice or by the presence of secretions in the airways and is transmitted to the chest wall and palpated by the hand. Palpation of fremitus is performed with the palms of the hands placed lightly on the chest wall while the patient repeats some word, such as "99," to distinguish normal vocal fremitus from the abnormal fremitus produced by secretions. Normally palpation reveals a uniform vibration throughout the entire chest wall. Increased fremitus is palpated in the presence of an increase in secretions in a particular area. Decreased fremitus indicates an increase in air in the particular area. Palpation of fremitus is especially important when auscultation has defined an area of decreased breath sounds that may be an area of consolidation resulting from secretions. When fremitus is increased, the suspicion of consolidation is supported.

Evaluation of Muscle Activity of Chest Wall and Diaphragm

Palpation is an excellent tool to evaluate the amount of accessory muscle activity used during quiet breathing. By palpating the accessory muscles, in particular the scalenes and the trapezii, an assessment of the amount of work of breathing may be made (Fig. 14–22). In addition, the extent of the diaphragmatic contribution can be assessed with the patient in the supine position (Fig. 14–23). Normal quiet breathing is mostly performed by the diaphragm, with equal and upward motion of the lower rib cage. Palpation of the anterior chest wall with the thumbs over the costal margins and thumb tips meeting at the xiphoid gives the most accurate assessment of the extent of diaphragmatic activity. With a deep inspiration the hands should travel equally apart, total circumferential diameter increasing by at least 2 to 3 inches. The extent of movement is an important part of the assessment of diaphragmatic excursion. For example, an individual with significant chronic obstructive lung disease might exhibit increased muscle activity of the respiratory accessory muscles and decreased diaphragmatic contribution to quiet breathing.

Chest Wall Pain or Discomfort

Palpation may also be performed to evaluate chest wall discomfort and should include all areas of the chest wall: anterior, posterior, and lateral regions of the thorax. Patients may often

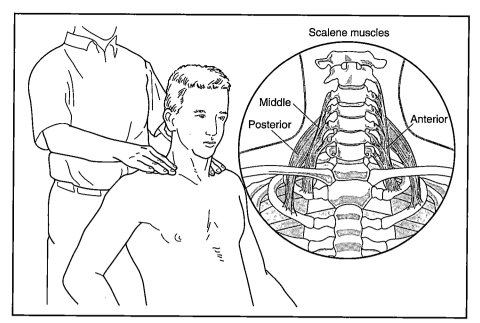

Figure 14-22.
Palpation of the activity of the scalene muscles during quiet breathing.

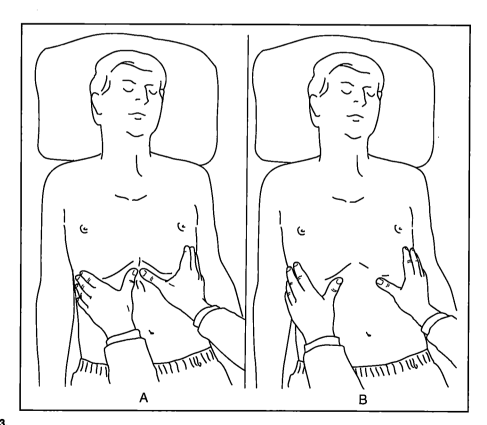

A   B

Figure 14-23.
Palpation of diaphragmatic motion. *A,* At rest. *B,* At the end of a normal inspiration. (Redrawn from Cherniack RM, Cherniack L. Respiration in Health and Disease. 2nd ed. Philadelphia, WB Saunders, 1972.)

develop musculoskeletal pain from bedrest and inactivity, which are frequently associated with diseases of the cardiopulmonary system. Musculoskeletal pain must be differentiated from anginal pain; palpation is an extremely useful tool to distinguish between the two. If chest pain is increased with deep inspiration or if it is increased or reproduced by direct point palpation, it is less likely to be of cardiac origin than of skeletal muscle origin. If a patient reports chest pain during the patient interview and can point to the exact area of pain, then palpation should be done to assess whether this pain is of musculoskeletal origin.

Evaluation of Circulation

Pulses throughout the extremities should be palpated during the initial evaluation because of the diffuse nature of atherosclerotic disease (see Chapter 3). Identification of the risk factors and symptoms of arterial disease are the two components of the history that assist in the assessment of arterial disease. Ischemic pain appears in the soft tissue served by the artery that is diseased. In addition to history taking, visual inspection for trophic changes (hair loss, muscle atrophy, dry skin, and in some cases dry gangrene or ulcers) is a valuable evaluation tool, particularly for examining individuals with moderate to severe arterial occlusion. Blood flow tests provide additional information about the degree of occlusion in the extremities. A reactive hyperemia test may be performed by sharply elevating the limbs to produce blanching. Blanching is more rapid in the partially or severely occluded extremity than in the normal extremity. In addition, palpation of pulses and skin temperature can be performed to assess perfusion of the extremities and the head and neck. Patients with diabetes or peripheral vascular disease often have diminished pulses, particularly in the hands and feet. In addition, individuals with right-sided heart failure and bilateral peripheral edema demonstrate diminished pulses in the foot and ankle. The following is a list of locations for pulse palpation:

- Brachial artery
- Radial artery
- Carotid artery
- Femoral artery
- Popliteal artery (palpated using the fingers of both hands)
- Posterior tibial artery
- Dorsalis pedis artery

The quality of the pulse should be noted, and a comparison should be made to the pulses of the opposite extremity to determine unilateral or individual differences. Pulse palpation may be difficult to quantify and does have a degree of unreliability from one clinician to the next. As a result, pulse palpation is now often supplemented by noninvasive techniques to measure blood flow such as **Doppler velocimetry.** Doppler velocimetry is particularly useful in identifying individuals with asymptomatic arterial disease or those whose pulses are severely obliterated.[18]

Mediate Percussion

Mediate percussion is the final component of the chest examination and is performed to further evaluate any abnormal findings, especially changes in lung density. In addition, percussion is also useful to evaluate the extent of diaphragmatic excursion.

Percussion is performed with the middle finger of one hand placed flat on the chest wall along the intercostal space between two ribs (usually the nondominant hand), while all other fingers are lifted off the chest wall. The other hand is positioned with the wrist in dorsiflexion, acting like a fulcrum, and the hand moving forward and back in rapid succession with the tip of the middle finger striking the nondominant middle finger on the chest wall (Fig. 14–24). Percussion usually proceeds in a cephalocaudal direction and back and forth between the left and right sides, anteriorly and posteriorly.

Three types of sounds are typically produced with percussion. A normal sound is when normal lung tissue is percussed and normal **resonance** is produced. A dull sound is produced with percussion over the liver or other dense tissue (as occurs with consolidation or tumors) and is described as a "thud." The student can

Figure 14-24.

The technique for mediate percussion.

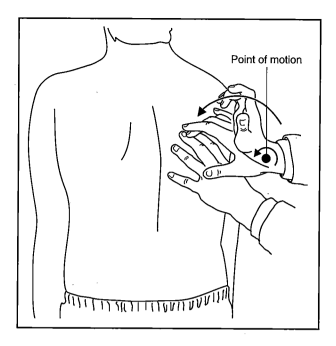

Point of motion

reproduce the dull sound by percussing on a bare thigh. A tympanic sound is loud, long, and hollow and may be heard over an empty stomach or a hyperinflated chest. Figure 14-25 shows the areas of normal, tympany, and dull sounds on a chest. Figure 14-26 demonstrates the systematic technique for evaluation of lung density.

Diaphragmatic excursion can also be assessed by percussion. The patient must be in a seated

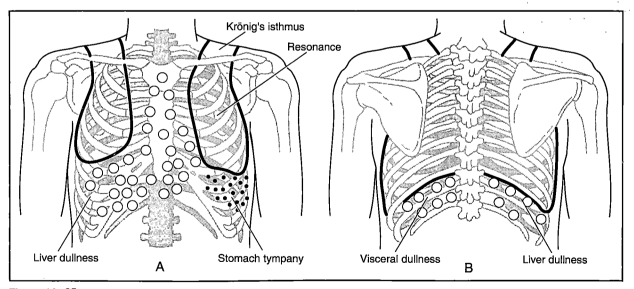

A

Krönig's isthmus

Resonance

Liver dullness   Stomach tympany

B

Visceral dullness   Liver dullness

Figure 14-25.

Normal resonance pattern of the chest. A, Anteriorly. B, Posteriorly. Also shown are areas of dullness (circles) and tympanic areas (small dots). (Redrawn from Irwin SF, Techlin JS. Cardiopulmonary Physical Therapy. 2nd ed. St. Louis, CV Mosby, 1990.)

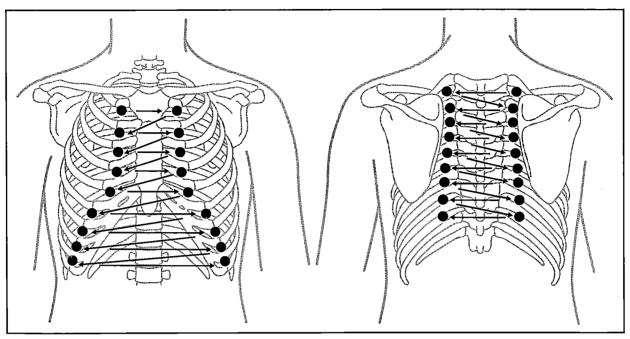

Figure 14-26.

The systematic technique for evaluation of lung density anteriorly *(A)* and posteriorly *(B)*.

position with the back exposed to evaluate diaphragmatic excursion. Percussion from the apex of the lungs to the bases of the lungs is performed while a patient is quietly breathing and a line measuring the point of demarcation between resonance to dullness is drawn on the left side and the right. After these lines are drawn, the therapist asks the patient to take a maximal inspiration and to hold this breath. At this time, the therapist continues percussion from the line downward to determine where the new point of dullness to resonance is located and draws a second line. The distance between the lines is the distance of diaphragmatic excursion. Normal excursion is 3 to 5 cm but may be extremely decreased in the patient with chronic obstructive lung disease because of hyperinflation of the chest and a flattened diaphragm (Fig. 14-27).

Activity Evaluation

Following the chest wall examination, the therapist is ready to perform an initial evaluation of the patient's responses to exercise. The activity evaluation (or self-care evaluation) is an assessment of the patient's responses to the following situations: rest (supine), sitting, standing, some type of activity of daily living (e.g., dressing lower or upper extremities, combing hair, brushing teeth), and ambulation of some distance; in some cases, **Valsalva's maneuver** is also performed (Fig. 14-28).

For patients recently recovering from a myocardial infarction, the evaluation discussed previously should be performed as soon as the patient is able to get out of bed. This often occurs as early as 1 to 2 days after an uncomplicated myocardial infarction. If the patient has not experienced a myocardial infarction but has some sort of cardiopulmonary dysfunction, this assessment is made as soon as the patient is considered stable. Patients receiving mechanical ventilatory assistance can perform these activities while still on the ventilator.

During the activity evaluation, the patient's heart rate and rhythm (via ECG telemetry if possible), blood pressure, and symptoms should be

Figure 14–27.

Evaluation of diaphragmatic excursion (normal = 3–5 cm); normal breathing (solid line), deep inspiration (broken line).

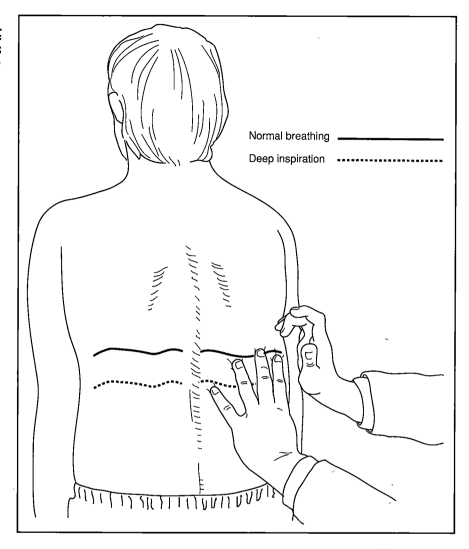

Normal breathing ——————

Deep inspiration ·····················

monitored with all activities. Heart and lung sounds should be measured before each activity and immediately following the last activity. The responses should be recorded and interpreted throughout the entire evaluation. The evaluation is terminated at anytime during the assessment that an abnormal response is identified if such response makes continuing the evaluation inappropriate or unsafe. On conclusion of the activities evaluation, an individualized program of progressive monitored ambulation is initiated if the responses were assessed as safe and appropriate. Studies have shown that the heart rate, blood pressure, and ECG responses with ambu-

lation during the activities evaluation strongly correlate with the responses that occur with the patient's daily monitored ambulation program.[19]

Heart Rate Measurement

The heart rate can be measured via palpation and is usually done via the radial pulse; it can also be measured from the ECG, either directly from a digital reading or from a recording of a 6-second ECG strip. Although an ECG recording may be more accurate, the palpation method may be more common in the clinic owing to the lack of availability of ECG equipment. Heart

SELF-CARE MONITOR

Department of Physical Therapy and Rehabilitation
Cardiac Rehabilitation Program

Patient name _____

Hospital no. _____

Risk factors   HBP _____ Family history _____ Obesity _____

             Smoking _____ Diabetes _____ Age _____

             Sedentary _____ Other _____

	HR	BP
Rest (supine)		
Sitting		
Standing		
ADL activity		
Ambulation		
Valsalva		

ECG strips

INTERPRETATION

Therapist _____ Date _____

Figure 14–28.

Self-care monitor form.

rhythm (the presence or absence of rhythm disturbances) can also be evaluated if palpated continuously for at least 1 minute but is more accurately recorded via the ECG.

The heart rate should be recorded with all activity, but the important factor is the heart rate response to activity. The normal heart rate response to any exertion is a gradual rise with an increase in work. If the individual is well trained (participates regularly in an aerobic exercise activity), the rate of heart rate rise is much more blunted (Fig. 14–29).

In addition, the heart rate achieved with activity should be compared with the predicted maximal heart rate. The predicted maximal heart rate of an individual is related to age. One method of determining the predicted maximal rate is to subtract the patient's age from 220 (220 − age). However, this method is known to underestimate the maximal heart rate in well-trained and in elderly persons. For these patients, the following two formulas are recommended: for males, $205 - \frac{1}{2}$ age; for females, $225 -$ age.[20] There-fore, if an individual were performing near maximal capacity, it is reasonable to expect heart rate to approximate predicted maximal heart rate. Normally, in the acute care setting, patients should not be working anywhere near maximal heart rate.

Abnormal heart rate responses are of three types: a very rapid rise in heart rate with increased workload, a very flat rate of rise (bradycardic response), and a decrease in palpated heart rate. Patients who demonstrate a rapid rise in heart rate generally have one of two problems: severe deconditioning or a cardiovascular condition that is limiting the stroke volume. Patients who are not taking cardiac medications and who demonstrate a very flat rate of rise in heart rate are believed to have underlying cardiovascular disease. Also, individuals who have a decrease in palpated heart rate are not actually showing a true decreased heart rate but rather a decrease in palpable heart rate. If an ECG telemetry unit were available, these individuals should be monitored, because the palpable decrease in

Figure 14–29.

Heart rate response to increased workload in a normal sedentary individual (A) versus a trained individual (B).

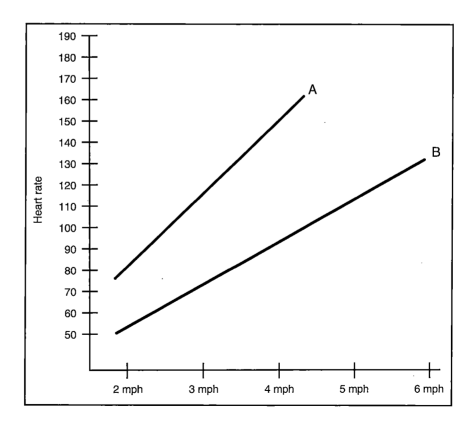

heart rate indicates an increase in arrhythmias (probably ventricular). When premature ectopic beats arise in the heart, they can often be palpated as a skip or pause in the pulse. When an increased number of pauses are palpated, it might appear to the therapist palpating the pulse that the heart rate actually decreased with exercise, when in reality the number of arrhythmias increased. If the pauses as well as the palpable beats were counted, one might not see a decrease in heart rate with exercise but rather an increase in heart rate with exercise. So, in reality, the heart rate does not decrease with exercise, but the palpated heart rate may *appear* to decrease if the number of arrhythmias increase. An increase in arrhythmias with exercise is also considered to be an abnormal response to exercise (see Heart Rhythm).

In a patient taking certain cardiac medications, specifically beta-blocking medications, a **blunted** (slower rate of rise and lower peak) **heart rate response** to exercise is anticipated and considered normal. The slower rate of rise aspect of the response is similar to that exhibited by highly trained individuals who also demonstrate a very gradual rate of rise in heart rate with increased work.

Heart Rhythm

Heart rhythm can be palpated to assess regularity during exercise, but the interpretation of any specific rhythm disturbance cannot be made without ECG monitoring. Numerous patients, with and without cardiopulmonary dysfunction, have arrhythmias, so physical therapists must be able to identify commonly observed basic and life-threatening arrhythmias as well as be able to assess the severity of these arrhythmias to make appropriate clinical decisions. Arrhythmias are discussed in Chapter 9.

Heart rhythm should remain regular with exercise; however, if an individual has arrhythmias at rest, the normal response would be a lack of change in the frequency or type of arrhythmia with an increase in activity. If a change occurs with increased activity, four factors should be considered in the clinical decision-making pro-

cess: (1) whether the arrhythmias represent a new finding, (2) whether the arrhythmias are benign or life threatening, (3) whether the patient's pharmacologic regimen may be producing the arrhythmias, and (4) the severity of the symptoms associated with the arrhythmias. Clinically, patients with occasional arrhythmias may not demonstrate serious arrhythmias with increased activity; in fact, arrhythmias may decrease or disappear with activity (as in sinus arrhythmia). In addition, arrhythmias may be well controlled by medication when the patient is at rest but not when the patient becomes active. A serious problem exists when a patient develops symptoms because of an arrhythmia or when the arrhythmia changes in character to become life threatening. Individuals who demonstrate an increasing frequency of premature ventricular ectopy with activity have been shown to have more serious coronary artery disease (two- and three-vessel disease) than individuals who do not.[21] In addition, patients who demonstrate premature ventricular ectopy at rest that disappears with activity have also been shown to have an increased incidence of coronary disease.[22]

Clinically, disturbances in heart rhythm should, at least, be monitored during an initial evaluation by means of direct palpation. When patients are known to have rhythm disturbances (either by direct palpation or history), further evaluative efforts should include ECG monitoring during activity.

Blood Pressure Measurement

Arterial blood pressure is a general indicator of the function of the heart as a pump. The arterial blood pressure is defined as the *systolic* pressure (pressure exerted against the arteries during the ejection cycle) and *diastolic* pressure (pressure exerted against the arteries during rest). Factors affecting blood pressure include cardiac output, peripheral resistance, distensibility of the arteries (vasomotor tone), volume of blood in the system, viscosity of the blood, and neural input.

Normal blood pressure in the aorta and arteries is defined as less than 140 mm Hg systolic and less than 90 mm Hg diastolic. Table 14–6

TABLE 14–6. Definition of Resting Blood Pressure

	Normal	Borderline	Hypertensive
Systolic (mm Hg)	<140	140–150	>150
Diastolic (mm Hg)	<90	90–100	>100

(American Heart Association Guidelines)

includes guidelines from the American Heart Association for normal, borderline, and hypertensive blood pressure. Blood pressure can be measured directly by means of indwelling arterial catheterization using a catheter inserted into an artery (as done in laboratory or critical care situations) or indirectly using a **sphygmomanometer**. Blood pressures are usually taken on the upper arm with the distal margin of the cuff approximately 3 centimeters above the antecubital fossa. Palpation is performed to locate the brachial artery pulse. This is the location for auscultation of the blood pressure. Following inflation of the cuff, auscultation of the first audible sound designates the systolic pressure, whereas the diastolic pressure is the value when the sounds become muffled.

The blood pressure may vary between extremities, with change of position, and with any type of activity. The changes between like extremities may reflect uneven peripheral resistance due to either differences in vasomotor tone or arterial occlusion. Changes in blood pressure with body position may reflect the influences of the vasomotor tone, the venous return, or the hydrostatic effects of gravity, or a combination of all three. Blood pressure changes associated with activity typically reflect the amount of work the heart must do to meet the metabolic demands of the activity.

Changes in blood pressure may also reflect the capability of the therapist to measure the blood pressure, because problems arise in the accurate measurement of blood pressure with activity. When a patient stops performing an activity, the direct metabolic demands decrease while the muscle activity that assists in the return of the venous blood stops. As a result, the blood pres-

sure may drop rapidly (within 15 seconds).[22] Therefore, it is essential that the physical therapist be competent in blood pressure measurement and knowledgeable regarding normal blood pressure responses to exertion in addition to being able to identify and react to abnormal responses.

Normal Responses

To understand normal responses to exercise, it is important to recognize that two key factors affect the blood pressure response: cardiac output and peripheral vascular resistance. Generally, with increased work, the cardiac output increases and the peripheral vascular resistance decreases as a result of (1) the **hypothalamic** response to increased body temperature and (2) the local effects of hydrogen ions, heat, decreased availability of oxygen, and increased carbon dioxide production on the arterioles. Thus, there is a normal increase in systolic blood pressure with increasing levels of exertion. It is important to note that adult females tend to demonstrate a slower rate of rise in the systolic pressure during exertion in contrast to adult males.

The normal diastolic response is a maximum of 10 mm Hg increase or decrease from the resting value because of the adaptive dilation of the peripheral vascular bed that occurs with exercise (Fig. 14–30). Younger persons and trained athletes may demonstrate a progressive decrease in diastolic pressure during exercise as a result of the increased peripheral vasodilation. Therefore, a fall in diastolic pressure greater than the 10 mm Hg can be considered a normal response in this population but not in older, untrained individuals.

The normal systolic and diastolic blood pressure responses to endurance activity (when an individual maintains a constant submaximal workload) are to remain constant or even to decrease slightly. This indicates that the body has achieved a steady state condition and that the central and peripheral mechanisms that adjust the blood pressure (e.g., cardiac output and peripheral vascular resistance) have accommodated to the workload.

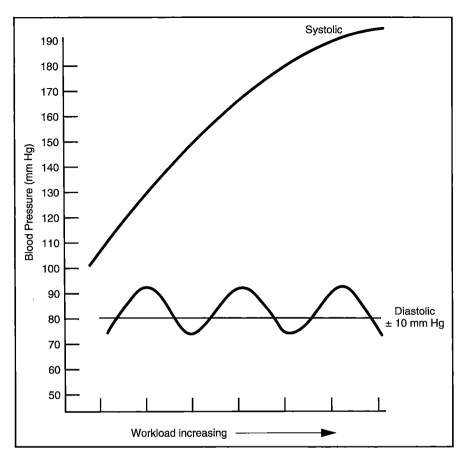

Figure 14–30.

The systolic blood pressure gradually rises with a gradual increase in workload. The diastolic blood pressure should change very little with an increase in workload (±10 mm Hg). (Redrawn from Scully R, Barnes ML. Physical Therapy. Philadelphia, JB Lippincott, 1989.)

Abnormal Responses

If one knows and understands the normal blood pressure responses to exercise, then identifying abnormal responses is simplified. Abnormalities can exist with the systolic or diastolic response or both. The abnormal responses are first defined, and then the mechanism of action and clinical implications are described.

Abnormal Systolic Responses. There are three abnormal systolic blood pressure responses to activity that are described in the literature: hypertensive, hypotensive, and blunted or flat. A hypertensive blood pressure response is one in which an individual who is normotensive at rest exhibits an abnormally high systolic blood pressure for a given level of exertion. This type of response has been associated with an increased risk for the future development of hypertension

at rest. Furthermore, this response should be distinguished from that found in an individual who is hypertensive at rest yet exhibits a normally increasing systolic blood pressure during increasing levels of exertion.[23] Although the mechanism for the hypertensive blood pressure response is not fully understood, it may be related to the following: an increased plasma concentration of **catecholamines,** an increased resistance to blood flow arising from peripheral vascular occlusive disease, or an abnormal centrally mediated resting vasomotor tone.

Exertional systolic hypotension is described as a normally rising systolic pressure at submaximal levels, followed by a sudden progressive decrease in systolic blood pressure in the face of increasing workload (Fig. 14–31); it has been highly correlated with pathologic cardiac conditions.[24] Individuals with exertional hypotension often demonstrate coronary perfusion defects on exercise thallium tests and severe coronary disease, poor ventricular function, or both as documented by coronary angiography.[24]

A blunted blood pressure response is defined as a slight increase in systolic blood pressure at low levels of exertion with a failure to rise with increasing levels of work. This definition applies only to those individuals who are not receiving pharmacologic intervention that might affect blood pressure. Failure to reach a systolic blood pressure in excess of 130 mm Hg at maximal effort in the absence of any medication that restricts the blood pressure is associated with a high risk for future sudden death.[25] However, this is equivalent to the blunted response that is seen in individuals who are receiving beta-adrenergic antagonists as part of a therapeutic pharmacologic regimen. When these medications are prescribed, the blunted blood pressure response is expected and considered normal.

A hypotensive or blunted blood pressure response indicates that either the cardiac output is failing to meet the demands of the body or that the peripheral vascular resistance is rapidly decreasing. Evidence in the literature suggests that hypotensive or blunted blood pressure responses are most often due to a failing cardiac output.[26,27] Because the cardiac output is directly dependent on stroke volume and heart rate, if the stroke volume is unable to increase appropriately for a given level of work, any increase in cardiac out-put arises solely as the result of an increase in the heart rate. In this situation, the blood pressure may rise slightly or may remain flat. Unfortunately, because of the concomitant increase in myocardial oxygen demand that accompanies an increase in heart rate, the heart is unable to maintain an increased cardiac output for any significant period of time, which results in a falling blood pressure.

When an individual is performing endurance exercise (of greater than 3–5 min in duration), a continuous rise in systolic blood pressure is considered an abnormal response. Persons who demonstrate an abnormal blood pressure response during endurance exercise typically have one of two conditions: either a high degree of ventricular wall dysfunction or a dysfunction in the ability of myocardial tissue to extract oxygen from the circulatory system.

Clinical Implications. Patients who demonstrate abnormal blood pressure responses during exercise typically suffer from coronary artery disease (e.g., have a history of angioplasty, angina, coronary bypass surgery, or myocardial infarction), moderate to severe aortic valvular stenosis, or other cardiac muscle dysfunction.[26–29]

The assessment of peak blood pressure as well as the interpretation of the blood pressure response during activity is an essential component of the initial and continuing evaluation of every patient. Although restrictions on any activity might be unnecessary, patients with abnormal

Figure 14–31.

An abnormal blood pressure response to an increase in workload. Greater than 2.5 mph workload caused the systolic blood pressure to decrease continually, demonstrating a failure of the heart muscle to meet the demands. (Redrawn from Scully R, Barnes ML. Physical Therapy. Philadelphia, JB Lippincott, 1989.)

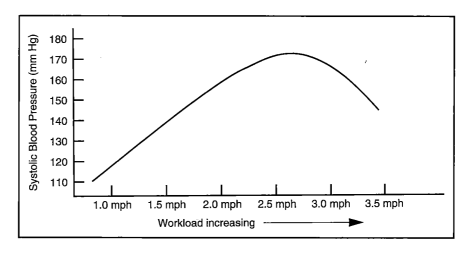

systolic blood pressure responses should be monitored closely during typical activities and especially during new exertional activities. In addition, the treatment or exercise prescription may require alterations in duration, intensity, or both. Some activities may require supervision so that the patient can perform the activity safely. Also, the patients themselves should be educated regarding their specific limitations and the signs and symptoms of overexertion when performing any activities.

Abnormal Diastolic Responses. As stated previously, a normal diastolic blood pressure response is one in which a change is no greater than 10 mm Hg; an abnormal diastolic blood pressure response would be either an increase or decrease of more than 10 mm Hg (in an untrained or older population). In addition, a sustained elevation of the diastolic blood pressure during the recovery phase of activity is considered to be abnormal.[30]

The mechanism behind the progressive rise in diastolic blood pressure is thought to be a response to the need for an increased driving pressure in the coronary arteries, which is necessary to overcome the increased resistance to flow within the coronary arteries. When blood flow through the coronary arteries is decreased below the level needed to meet the demand of the myocardium as a result of either increased vascular tone or vascular occlusion, a stimulus is created for an increased driving pressure to make the blood flow through the resistant arteries.[30] Despite a lack of research-based documentation regarding this abnormality, the physical therapist should be aware of the normal anticipated physiologic response and therefore be very sensitive to a progressive rise in diastolic pressure, interpreting this as an abnormal response. Patients who demonstrate a progressive rise in diastolic pressure usually have numerous risk factors for heart disease, are deemed high risk for or already have coronary artery disease, or have a previous history of coronary angioplasty or bypass surgery. Patients with hypertensive heart disease and compensated heart failure may also demonstrate this abnormal response.

Other Symptoms of Cardiovascular Inadequacy

The other symptoms associated with cardiovascular inadequacy are more difficult to interpret and therefore more difficult to treat. Angina, shortness of breath, and **palpitations** are the most common symptoms of patients with cardiopulmonary dysfunction. The other classic symptoms to be aware of are dizziness, **pallor,** and fatigue. The therapist, therefore, must have a thorough understanding of how to assess these symptoms.

Angina. Angina is a discomfort found anywhere above the waist but more likely in the chest, neck, or jaw and is typically described using terms such as dull ache, tightness, fullness, burning, pressure, indigestion, or neck or jaw discomfort. Classic angina is brought on by exertion or emotional upset and at times by eating; it is relieved by either rest or nitroglycerine. Angina and other chest wall or neurologic complaints are differentiated by the activity that reproduces the discomfort. Angina is reproducible only by increasing myocardial oxygen consumption (as in activity or emotion), whereas musculoskeletal pain can be reproduced by palpation or deep inspiration and expiration, and neurologic pain may follow a dermatome and exist all the time.

There are six types of "chest pain" that make the differential diagnosis of angina difficult, however. Two of these situations relate to angina and include **variant angina** (as found in the pure form called **Prinzmetal's angina**) and **preinfarction angina.**

Variant Angina. Variant angina, defined as angina produced from vasospasm of the coronary arteries in the absence of occlusive disease (i.e., the arteries are free of disease), is called Prinzmetal's angina. Individuals who experience vasospasm often develop resting chest pain, making the classic definition of angina inappropriate.[31] In the case of variant angina, an individual is more likely to have discomfort that is due to emotional upset or inspiration of cold air.

Variant angina usually responds to nitroglycerine and is typically diagnosed when nitroglycerine is found to be effective or when other long-term pharmacologic therapy is found effective. Calcium channel blockers are typically the long-term pharmacologic choice for the treatment of variant angina. These drugs retard the uptake of the calcium in the cells and therefore inhibit smooth muscle contraction of the arterial walls (see Chapters 2 and 12).

Preinfarction Angina. Preinfarction angina is defined as *unstable* angina; it occurs at rest and worsens with activity. An individual may or may not have had symptoms of classic angina before experiencing the intense and constant pain of preinfarction angina. This condition is one that requires immediate medical treatment to prevent full transmural infarction.

Although the description of angina may vary from individual to individual, the description remains constant for each individual. Therefore, once the therapist concludes that the symptoms being described constitute angina, then the patient's terms used to describe the angina should be remembered and used in all future assessments of symptoms. The other four types of chest pain in addition to angina are **pericarditis, mitral valve dysfunction, bronchospasm,** and esophageal spasm.

Pericarditis. Pericarditis is an inflammation of the pericardial sac that surrounds the heart and may actually result in a restriction of cardiac output. Patients who are suspected of having pericardial pain should be referred for immediate medical treatment and discontinued from exertional activities until the pericarditis subsides. Pericarditis produces a chest pain symptom that is constant and sharp and is described as intense and "stabbing." Pericarditis pain usually does not increase with activity but may remain constant 24 hours per day and is very intense. Associated fever and fatigue may also occur with the stabbing pain, as well as ECG changes.[32] Pericardial pain is a common symptom following coronary artery bypass surgery and occurs occasionally in the early phase following a myocardial infarction. Treatment usually includes anti-inflammatory medications.

Mitral Valve Dysfunction. Individuals with mitral valve dysfunction (mitral valve prolapse or mitral valve regurgitation) may demonstrate classic angina with exertion yet lack a suspicious risk factor profile. They tend to be younger and are free of cardiovascular occlusive disease. Auscultation of heart sounds usually reveals a systolic murmur or click. Echocardiography usually identifies mitral valve dysfunction. The classic angina pain from mitral valve dysfunction arises from the diminished blood flow resulting from the subsequent decreased cardiac output.[33]

Bronchospasm. Some patients experience exercise-induced bronchospasm, which can manifest itself as chest wall tightness or discomfort, or both, with exertion. Differentiation of exercise-induced bronchospasm from exertional angina is performed by assessing the individual's degree of difficulty in breathing. An individual experiencing exercise-induced bronchospasm usually demonstrates a greatly increased work of breathing as well as an extreme effort to take the next breath.

Esophageal Spasm. Esophageal spasm or inflammation may produce a midsternal pain that is mistaken for angina.[34] Diffuse esophageal spasm is usually idiopathic and produces a chest pain with dysphagia. Esophageal spasm is suspected when the chest discomfort develops with eating and can be diagnosed with esophageal manometry or with barium swallow. Treatment for this type of chest pain includes medication to decrease the acid reflux into the esophagus, sublingual nitroglycerin, and calcium channel blockers.[34,35]

Shortness of Breath. Shortness of breath is one of the other common symptoms found in patients with cardiopulmonary dysfunction. Shortness of breath may be due to several different physiologic mechanisms, including the equivalent of angina in individuals who cannot perceive chest pain or discomfort, as in the diabetic with peripheral neuropathy. Shortness of breath may also be due to limited cardiovascular reserve in patients with coronary disease or cardiac muscle dysfunction; pulmonary pathology with limited ventilatory reserve, diffusion, or arterial oxygen carrying capacity; and finally physiologic limitations in an individual's oxygen transport system when shortness of breath occurs during exercise. When shortness of breath does develop during the assessment, these mechanisms need to be evaluated to determine the cause of the shortness of breath and to make appropriate clinical decisions regarding progression of activity.

Palpitations. Palpitations are a common complaint of patients with cardiopulmonary dysfunction. Palpitations usually indicate arrhythmias.[36] Palpitations must be evaluated to determine the seriousness of any rhythm disturbances as well as the cause of any symptoms. Evaluation usually involves 24-hour Holter monitoring.

Dizziness. Dizziness can have several origins, including the vestibular system, vision, medications, blood pressure, and cardiac output. Dizziness is a symptom that must be evaluated with reference to the activity that produces it and then compared with the blood pressure response. If an individual becomes dizzy on standing and a blood pressure drop is noted, the condition is described as orthostatic hypotension. However, if the patient complains of dizziness with an increase in activity and a blood pressure drop is noted, this patient is defined as having exertional hypotension. Clinical decision making therefore depends on the constellation of symptoms presented by the patient and the effect the associated dizziness has on his or her activity.

Fatigue. Fatigue may also have several origins, including depression, general deconditioning, pharmacologic management and side effects, and physiologic limitation, as seen in the individual with cardiac muscle dysfunction. Therefore, fatigue should never be the only symptom the therapist uses to make a clinical decision regarding exercise prescription or progression. The cause of the fatigue may need to be investigated further if it is the only symptom limiting activity and all other responses are normal.

Monitored Activity

On completion of the full cardiopulmonary assessment, including chest examination and activity evaluation, a decision is made regarding the patient's treatment. Acute care treatment procedures are discussed in Chapter 15. However, the therapist must always remember that each treatment session becomes an assessment, particularly of responses to the treatment. Therefore, each treatment session is, in essence, a monitored activity session, requiring constant reevaluation and assessment as to the significance of the clinical findings.

CASE STUDIES

CASE 1

A 72-year-old woman who contracted polio in 1948 fell in her retirement home apartment, fracturing the proximal left femur. She was found immediately because she used her emergency call cord in her apartment.

The patient underwent open reduction internal fixation with spinal anesthesia 3 days earlier, and the physician has just ordered physical therapy for out of bed activities and ambulation with a walker.

The chart Review revealed

● a 54-year history of smoking approximately 1.5 to 2.0 packs per day
● no history of hypertension, family history of heart disease, or other major medical problems (Patient had been ambulatory with wheeled tripod walker and lives alone.)
● laboratory study results within normal limits
● chest radiograph demonstrates hyperinflated chest with few patchy areas of infiltrate in both bases

In the interview, the patient reported that she is in a lot of pain. She plans to return to extended care at the retirement home until she is able to take care of herself.

The physical exam revealed the following:

● General appearance: slight grayish color; thin, slightly underweight
● Neck: observation of hypertrophy of sternocleidomastoid muscles bilaterally; forward head, and sits in bed with the head of the bed elevated to 60 degrees
● Chest: Upward movement of chest with every breath; patient is observed to have increased

accessory muscle use, increased AP diameter, and increased respiratory rate

● Phonation, cough, and cough production: patient is observed to have moist, nonproductive, ineffective cough; phonation requires breaths between words in sentence; extremities have mild clubbing, gray-blue color with tobacco stains

● Auscultation: decreased breath sounds auscultated with coarse wheezing and wet rales on expiration in bilateral bases but slightly cleared with a cough; auscultation of the heart demonstrates loud atrial gallop with rapid heart beat

● Palpation: decreased chest wall motion palpated throughout, with palpable fremitus in bilateral bases; increased accessory muscle use including sternocleidomastoid and scalenes, with decreased diaphragmatic excursion; good pulses throughout, except bilateral dorsalis pedis

● Percussion: mild dullness to percussion noted in bases

● Activity evaluation: Patient was evaluated in supine-to-sit position only; patient could not tolerate standing owing to increased pain in left lower extremity and dizziness

● Vital signs: heart rate 100 (supine), 120 (sitting); blood pressure 110/70 (supine), 90/66 (sitting)

These findings from the cardiopulmonary assessment demonstrate an elderly female with a long-term history of smoking and signs of chronic obstructive pulmonary disease in addition to the hip fracture problem. She is at extreme risk for pneumonia. Also, the patient has a problem with orthostatic hypotension as evidenced by her vital signs. The chronic obstructive pulmonary disease and the present pulmonary condition (e.g., infiltrates in bases, retained secretions), as well as the orthostatic hypotension, will affect her activity progression.

CASE 2

The patient is a 58-year-old woman, admitted with a diagnosis of arthritis in the right knee, who underwent a total knee replacement. The patient's past medical history includes treatment for

hypertension (Tenormin, 100 mg/day), adult onset diabetes (controlled with oral insulin), and rheumatic fever as a child. Recently she has had very limited activity because of the painful right knee. The patient is markedly obese.

Since surgery the right knee has been in a continuous passive motion apparatus, but the patient has been limited to bedrest owing to numerous postoperative complications, including infections and nonhealing of the incision. The nurses are unable to get the patient out of bed owing to her weight and complaints of dizziness. The physician has ordered gait training with a walker with toe-touch weight-bearing status.

In the interview, the patient reported that she feels weak since being in bed after surgery. Her plans are to return home to her apartment. She lives alone.

The physical examination revealed the following:

● Inspection: Patient is markedly obese with good general appearance; right knee has large bandage with dark pink skin surrounding the bandage and increased edema on right

● Auscultation: reveals normal heart sounds, diminished breath sounds throughout, with crackles on inspiration throughout the bases; nonproductive dry cough

● Palpation: no abnormalities with chest motion, although diaphragmatic excursion appears limited; pulses are intact and normal throughout; patient is sensitive to touch around the right knee

● Activity evaluation: Patient requires the maximal assistance of two people (one person to move the right lower extremity) to transfer from a supine to a sitting position and the maximal assistance of two people to raise the patient to a standing position holding onto walker

● Vital signs: heart rate 66 (supine), 72 sitting, 80 standing; blood pressure 108/70 (supine), 90/66 (sitting), 80/60 (standing); patient complained of extreme dizziness with 60 seconds of standing and returned to sitting position

Patient's blood pressure response and symptoms are the major limiting factors to progression. Her weakness from bedrest and her obesity are additional factors. In addition, with the patient's history of hypertension and the current medications she is taking for hypertension, her physician should be notified before she resumes activity. Her medication may be affecting her blood pressure response to the upright position and blocking a heart rate rise.

CASE 3

The patient is a 32-year-old man who was admitted to the intensive care unit with a diagnosis of bilateral lower lobe pneumonia and was placed on a mechanical ventilator on assist-control mode. The patient had seen his physician for a chronically elevated temperature and night sweats 1 week before admission.

The chart review revealed no history of smoking. The chest radiograph demonstrated diffuse patchy infiltrates throughout the interstitium bilaterally. The physician has given orders for increased bed mobility and range of motion and out of bed activities.

The physical examination revealed the following:

- Inspection: The patient is on a volume-assist mode ventilator, alert but pale and cachectic in appearance; he appears to be in no distress at present but does initiate coughing spasmodically when his position is changed; atrophy of lower and upper extremities is apparent on observation; respiration rate is approximately 30 breaths per minute with ventilator assistance
- Auscultation: reveals crackles throughout both bases, lingula and right middle lobe; heart sounds normal but very rapid
- Palpation: has a normal chest motion and an absence of fremitus but excessive accessory muscle use; no pain elicited on palpation of the chest; circulation evaluation demonstrated normal pulses bilaterally throughout
- Activity evaluation: Patient required the assistance of one person to roll to the side and sit up in bed and move his legs over the side of the bed.
- Vital signs: heart rate 108 (supine), 130 (sit over side); blood pressure 110/70 (supine), 120/76 (sit over side); no symptoms were reported, but patient appeared to increase respiration rate with sitting and complained of fatigue after sitting for a few minutes

The patient's weakness and decreased ventilatory capacity is limiting his progress. Breathing exercises to work on increasing the depth of ventilation, strengthening, and energy conservation are recommended. Intolerance to activity is also limiting him. Progression of activity should be slow and monitored.

SUMMARY

- A thorough evaluation of the patient is essential for optimal treatment.
- Included in the cardiopulmonary assessment is a thorough chart review to identify past medical history, diagnostic studies, and current medical status.
- The physical therapist must remember that although the chart should have all of the necessary information about the patient, the optimal situation is one that allows the acquisition of pertinent information directly from the patient.
- The patient interview can shed new light on the chart information, or it can provide a completely different picture.
- Performing a physical examination of the patient provides the most accurate information regarding the patient's current cardiopulmonary status.
- The physical examination includes a thorough inspection, auscultation, palpation, percussion, and activity evaluation.
- Based on the initial assessment, a plan of treatment or exercise prescription can be developed for optimal rehabilitation.
- The assessment must be ongoing, and components of the physical examination need to be performed on a daily basis to assess the patient's status with increased activity.
- Reevaluation is just as important for the patient's progression of activity as is the initial assessment.

References

1. Kannel WB, Castelli WP, Gordon T, et al. Serum cholesterol, liproproteins, and the risk of coronary heart disease: The Framingham study. Ann Intern Med 24:1, 1971.

2. Laposata EA. Cocaine induced heart disease: Mechanisms and pathology. J Thorac Imaging 6(1):68–75, 1991.
3. Rezkalla SH, Hale S, Kloner RA. Cocaine induced heart diseases. Am Heart J 120(6):1403–1408, 1990.
4. Morris DC. Cocaine heart disease. Hosp Pract [Off] 26(9):83–92, 1991.
5. McNeer JF, Wallace AG, Wagner GS, et al. The course of acute myocardial infarction. Circulation 51:410, 1975.
6. Steinhart MJ. Depression and chronic fatigue in the patient with heart disease. Prim Care 18(2):309–325, 1991.
7. Wilkins RL, Dexter JR, Murphy RL Jr, DelBono EA. Lung sound nomenclature survey. Chest 98(4):886–889, 1990.
8. Kramin SS. Determination of the site of production of respiratory sounds by subtraction phonopneumography. Am Rev Respir Dis 122:303, 1980.
9. American College of CP & ATS Joint Committee on Pulmonary Nomenclature. Pulmonary terms and symbols. Chest 67:583, 1975.
10. Wilkins RL, Hodgkin JE, Lopez B. Lung Sounds: A Practical Guide. St. Louis, CV Mosby, 1988.
11. Piirila P, Sovijarvi AR, Kaisla T, et al. Crackles in patients with fibrosing alveolitis, bronchiectasis, COPD and heart failure. Chest 99(5):1076–1083, 1991.
12. Nath AR, Capel LH. Inspiratory crackles and the mechanical events of breathing. Thorax 29:695, 1974.
13. Forgacs P. The functional basis of pulmonary sounds. Chest 73:399, 1978.
14. Nath AR, Capel LH. Inspiratory crackles—Early and late. Thorax 29:223, 1974.
15. Murphy RLH. Discontinuous adventitious lung sounds. Semin Respir Med 6:210, 1985.
16. Ravin A. Auscultation of the Heart. Chicago, Year Book Medical Publishers, 1968.
17. Luisada AA, Portaluppi F. The Heart Sounds: New Facts and Their Clinical Applications. New York, Praeger Publishers, 1982.
18. Criqui MH, Fronek A, Klauber MR. The sensitivity, specificity and predictive value of traditional clinical evidence of peripheral arterial disease: Results from noninvasive testing in a defined population. Circulation 71(3):516–522, 1985.
19. Butler SM. Phase one cardiac rehabilitation: The role of functional evaluation in patient progression. Master's thesis. Atlanta, Emory University, 1983.
20. Cooper KH. The Aerobics Way. New York, Bantam Books, 1981.
21. Pleskot M, Pidrman V, Tilser P, et al. (Programmed ventricular stimulation in the evaluation of the clinical significance of premature ventricular contractions). Vnitr-Lek 37(6):548–556, 1991.
22. Henschel A, De La Vega F, Taylor HL. Simultaneous direct and indirect blood pressure measurements in man at rest and work. J Appl Physiol 6:506, 1954.
23. Dlin RA, Hanne N, Silverberg DS, et al. Followup of normotensive men with exaggerated blood pressure response to exercise. Am Heart J 106(2):316, 1983.
24. Hakki A, Munley BM, Hadjimiltiades J. Determinants of abnormal blood pressure response to exercise in coronary artery disease. Am J Cardiol 57:71, 1986.
25. Bruce RA, DeRouen T, Peterson DR, et al. Noninvasive predictors of sudden death in men with coronary heart disease. Am J Cardiol 39:833, 1977.
26. Frenneaux MP, Counihan PJ, Caforior AL, et al. Abnormal blood pressure response during exercise in hypertrophic cardiomyopathy. Circulation 82(6):1995–2002, 1990.
27. Pavlovic M. (Decrease in systolic blood pressure during physical exertion in stress tests). Srp-Arh-Celok-Lek 117(11–12):777–786, 1989.
28. Cavan D, O'Donnell MJ, Parkes A, et al. Abnormal blood pressure response to exercise in normoalbuminuric insulin dependent diabetic patients. J Hum Hypertens 5(1):21–26, 1991.
29. Guerrera G, Melina D, Colivicchi F, et al. Abnormal blood pressure response to exercise in borderline hypertension. A two year follow-up study. Am J Hypertens 4(3, pt 1):271–273, 1991.
30. Guyton AC, Jones CE, Coleman TG. Circulatory Physiology: Cardiac Output and Its Regulation. Philadelphia, WB Saunders, 1973.
31. Maseri A, Crea F, Kaski JC, Crake T. Mechanisms of angina pectoris in syndrome X. J Am Coll Cardiol 17:499, 1991.
32. Phillips RE, Feeney MK. The Cardiac Rhythms: A Systematic Approach to Interpretation. Philadelphia, WB Saunders, 1990.
33. Albert MA, Mukerji V, Sabeti M, et al. Mitral valve prolapse, panic disorder, and chest pain. Med Clin North Am 75(5):1119–1133, 1991.
34. Rakel RE. Conn's Current Therapy. Philadelphia, WB Saunders, 1991, pp 424–425.
35. Nevens F, Janssens J, Piessens J, et al. Prospective study on prevalence of esophageal chest pain in patients referred on an elective basis to a cardiac unit for suspected myocardial ischemia. Dig Dis Sci 36(2):229, 1991.
36. Cohen M, Michel TH. Cardiopulmonary Symptoms in Physical Therapy Practice. New York, Churchill Livingstone, 1988.

WILLIAM T. KUNTZ

15 THE ACUTE CARE SETTING

INTRODUCTION

The distinctive sound of chest percussion can be heard on the surgical floors of any hospital. To many it is the hallmark of what some clinicians call *chest physical therapy* and the sum and substance of its practice. This perception does a disservice to this very diversified and vital area of physical therapy practice. The cardiopulmo-nary physical therapist has a great deal to offer in the treatment of the acutely ill patient. A strong background in anatomy, physiology, and pathophysiology; expertise in body mechanics and positioning of patients; and skill in providing neuromuscular facilitation and other specialized manual treatment techniques make the physical therapist uniquely suited to provide treatment in this area.

597

The practice of cardiopulmonary physical therapy in the acute care hospital is both challenging and extremely rewarding. The therapist interfaces with state of the art medical technology to render treatment to acutely ill patients that has the potential to improve their cardiopulmonary status and medical condition dramatically. Mastery of the techniques practiced and application of the principles of medicine, physiology, and anatomy that are relevant in the acute care setting are simply the cornerstone of good physical therapy practice.

CLINICAL PHYSIOLOGIC MONITORING AND ITS IMPLICATIONS

There are many invasive and noninvasive methods of monitoring the physiologic and medical status of the acutely ill patient. The information provided is essential in planning, implementing, and modifying treatment rendered by the physical therapist. This section discusses the most common methods of monitoring and their implications in treatment. A table is provided delineating the normal values for the parameters measured. (See Chapter 11 for specific information on the equipment.)

Pulmonary Artery Catheter

A **pulmonary artery catheter**, also called a *Swan-Ganz catheter*, provides an immediate profile of cardiac function by measuring the pulmonary artery pressures. **Pulmonary artery pressure** and **pulmonary artery wedge pressure** are measured as well as cardiac output and **right atrial pressure** (Table 15–1 lists ranges of normal values). The pulmonary artery catheter is an invasive monitoring device, so greater care must be taken in treating a patient with a pulmonary artery catheter in place. Chest percussion should be done cautiously, and the therapist should watch for changes in the waveform or the pressures when changing the patient's position. Changes in the waveform may signal a movement of the catheter in the artery that must be corrected by repositioning the patient. The pulmonary artery wedge pressure approximates **left**

TABLE 15–1. Normal Values

Cardiac Pressures	
Pulmonary artery pressure	
Systolic	15–25 mm Hg
End diastolic	8–12 mm Hg
Mean	10–20 mm Hg
Pulmonary artery wedge pressure	4–12 mm Hg
Right atrial pressure	2–6 mm Hg
Right ventricular pressure	
Systolic	20–30 mm Hg
Diastolic	0–5 mm Hg
End diastolic	2–6 mm Hg
Left atrial pressure	5–10 mm Hg
Left ventricular pressure	
Systolic	100–120 mm Hg
End diastolic	0–12 mm Hg
Central Venous Pressure	5–12 cm H_2O
Intra-arterial Pressures	
Systolic	100–140 mm Hg
Diastolic	60–80 mm Hg
Mean	70–90 mm Hg
Cardiac Output	4–8 L/min
Arterial Blood Gases	
pH	7.35–7.45
Po_2	80–100 mm Hg
Pco_2	35–45 mm Hg
HCO_3^-	22–28 mEq/L
O_2 saturation	98%
Alveolar-Arterial Oxygen Difference ($PA_{O_2} - Pa_{O_2}$)	
Ages 21–30	5–10 mm Hg
Ages 61–75	16 mm Hg

ventricular end-diastolic pressure or left ventricular preload (the volume of blood in the ventricle before contraction). Elevation of pulmonary artery wedge pressure (and thus left ventricular end-diastolic pressure) signals an increase in preload and may be an indication of impaired left ventricular function (failure). When pulmonary artery wedge pressure rises above 12 mm Hg, the patient should not be placed in a horizontal position because venous return increases. The increased venous return increases the workload on the impaired chamber.

Arterial Line

An **arterial catheter** measures systemic blood pressure more accurately than a standard blood pressure cuff. The arterial line is commonly found in the radial artery but may also be placed in the femoral artery. The arterial line measures the arterial blood pressure. This measurement may be altered by the patient's position; for example, when the line is in the radial artery it gives an accurate reading with the wrist in an extended position. Relative or absolute flexion of the wrist produces an erroneous reading (and often triggers the alarm). Extension or hyperextension of the wrist should restore an accurate reading (Fig. 15–1). There are no contraindications for treatment of a patient with an arterial line. Blood for arterial blood gas analysis and many other laboratory tests is also drawn from this line.

Central Venous Line

The **central venous catheter** is inserted most commonly through the subclavian, internal jugular, or femoral veins. The central venous line measures right atrial pressures (it may be part of a triple lumen catheter). Rolling a patient with a central venous line to the side (particularly to a left side-lying position) may advance the line internally. The therapist should be aware that this may trigger premature ventricular complexes, in which case the patient must be rolled back to the supine position.

Electrocardiographic Telemetry

Electrocardiographic telemetry is a simple one-lead setup used to provide instantaneous information on heart rate and rhythm. The placement of the electrodes may be varied, but the configuration generally used is lead II (right arm with left leg). The patient may be attached to a bedside monitor or to a transducer or transmitter that transmits the information to a monitor in a remote location, such as the nurses' station. There are no contraindications to treating patients on telemetry; however, patients on telemetry should be observed for signs and symptoms of decompensation associated with life-threatening arrhythmias. The therapist also should consult the monitor frequently during treatment to observe changes in heart rate or rhythm that are produced by positional changes or other factors. Another consideration is that chest percussion may produce artifact on the monitor, giving false evidence of an elevated heart rate (Fig. 15–2).

Pulse Oximetry

Pulse oximetry is a noninvasive means of providing sensitive and immediate readings of heart rate and **oxygen saturation** of the blood. A sen-

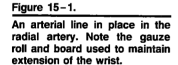

Figure 15–1.

An arterial line in place in the radial artery. Note the gauze roll and board used to maintain extension of the wrist.

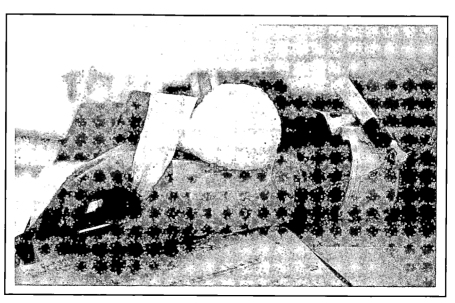

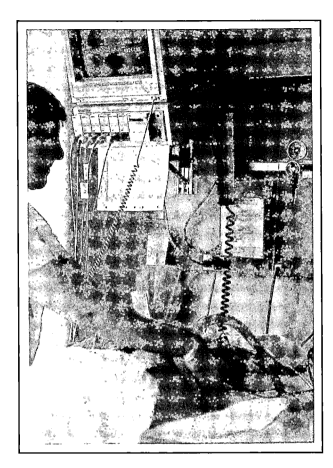

Figure 15-2.

The monitor should be observed frequently during treatment.

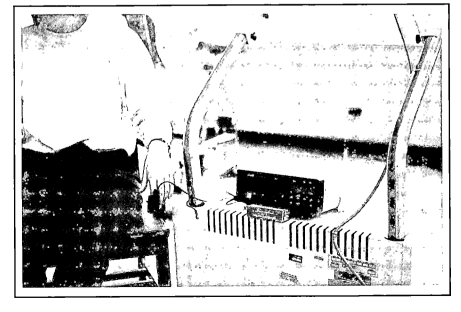

Figure 15-3.

A pulse oximeter with a finger sensor. Note display: oxygen saturation is on the left; pulse is on the right.

sor is attached to a finger or an ear lobe or over the forehead (Fig. 15-3). The information obtained is extremely useful in measuring a patient's response to exercise or positioning during treatment. A significant drop in arterial oxygen saturation may indicate that an activity is too strenuous for the patient or that cardiopulmonary function is inadequate to meet demand. The efficacy of supplemental oxygen may also be assessed as well as the efficacy of treatments such as breathing exercises and retraining.

Arterial Blood Gases

Blood drawn from an arterial line is processed and analyzed so that partial pressures of oxygen (Pa_{O_2}) and carbon dioxide (Pa_{CO_2}), concentration of bicarbonate (HCO_3^-), and oxygen saturation in the arterial blood (Sa_{O_2}) can be determined. (See Chapter 10 for more explanation.) Conditions such as **acidosis** and **alkalosis** and their causes may be easily ascertained, which may help the therapist in selecting treatment methods. For example, a patient with arterial blood gases of $Pa_{O_2} = 45$, $Pa_{CO_2} = 55$, $HCO_3^- = 24$, and $pH = 7.20$ demonstrates respiratory acidosis probably caused by hypoventilation. The therapist should emphasize postural drainage (if indicated) and breathing exercises to increase the depth of respiration. The therapist should also consider the effectiveness of the patient's supplemental oxygen system.

Chest Radiograph

A radiologist's report or an attending physician's note should be relied on for definitive interpretation of the patient's most recent chest radiograph. The information garnered in this way when combined with clinical findings helps the therapist set priorities and plan individual treatment sessions as well as indicate progress or regression and efficacy of previous treatments. For example, treatment for a patient with a recent chest radiograph showing a right lower lobe infiltrate (corroborated by clinical findings—e.g., auscultation and percussion) would be approached differently than that for a patient with a chest film finding of a cavitating lesion in the left

upper lobe. (See Chapter 10 for more detailed information on chest radiographs.)

Body Temperature

Body temperature may be indicative of the presence of a pathologic condition such as atelectasis, pneumonia, or superficial or systemic infection. Atelectasis is often accompanied by a low-grade fever (100°-101° F), whereas pneumonia or other infections may produce fevers higher than 101 degrees. The accepted values for normal temperature are 98.6 degrees F and 37.0 degrees C.

Intake and Output Measurements

A large difference in volume of fluid taken in and excreted may account for some physical findings. For example, this result may help in determining whether **rales** heard on auscultation are pulmonary in nature **(atelectatic)** or cardiogenic (congestive heart failure or fluid overload).

INTEGRATING THE INFORMATION TO FORM A CLINICAL IMPRESSION

Before seeing a patient for the first time the therapist should be familiar with the patient's medical history, both distant past and recent; the reason for hospitalization; the diagnosis and date of surgery; the type of procedure and postoperative diagnosis (if applicable); and the patient's smoking history. This information gives the clinician a general idea of what to expect and what to look for before ever seeing the patient. The information should be written down and maintained by the therapist in a format that is easily accessible during the patient's hospital stay (e.g., on a large index card).

Next, the therapist should look for recent findings such as the preoperative and most recent chest radiograph report, the body temperature, the arterial blood gas results, and the most recent physician's note. This information advises the therapist of the patient's immediate problems and helps in planning the treatment approach.

THE POSTOPERATIVE PATIENT

More than any other surgical patient, the one who has had upper abdominal or thoracic surgery is at increased risk for postoperative pulmonary complications.[1,2] These complications include atelectasis, **pulmonary edema,** lower respiratory infection (pneumonia), and ventilatory insufficiency, and they are the major causes of mortality and morbidity in this population.[3,4]

Changes in the Adult and Geriatric Lung Caused by Anesthesia and Surgery

Pulmonary gas exchange is impaired both during surgery while under general anesthesia and during the postoperative period. This impairment is the most significant effect of surgery and general anesthesia.[1] During the operation, the chest wall configuration changes as a result of muscle paralysis caused by the anesthesia. Muscle tone decreases, resulting in deformation of the chest wall. In the patient lying horizontally, these changes produce a decrease in anteroposterior diameter of the thorax and abdomen and an increase in the lateral diameter. Diaphragmatic tone is also decreased, and the resting position of this muscle shifts in a cephalad direction, which reduces the thoracic volume. These changes result in a decrease in the functional residual capacity (FRC) (generally about 20%).[3] The decreased FRC contributes to the onset of atelectasis. **Pleural pressure** exceeds atmospheric (airway) pressure in dependent lung regions. This positive pleural pressure causes collapse of small airways that are not supported by cartilage (< 1.0 mm diameter), and ventilation is thereby reduced to these regions of the lung.[2]

The effect of these changes is to increase the **intrapulmonary shunt** (perfusion of unventilated lung tissue). This leads to a greater than normal alveolar-to-arterial Po_2 difference (PA_{O_2} to Pa_{O_2}) (see Table 15–1 for normal values), causing hypoxemia. Hypoxemia is further exacerbated by a decrease in ventilation secondary to the depression of respiratory centers in the central nervous system by the general anesthesia.[1]

Inhaled anesthesia and high concentrations of oxygen temporarily alter the composition of **surfactant,** which further impairs gas exchange. These same factors also decrease tracheal mucus velocity by making the mucus more viscid.[2] The respiratory epithelium becomes dehydrated, and the function of the mucociliary escalator (that moves mucus from distal airways up to the larger airways where it can be coughed out) is impaired.[1,5]

In this postoperative period the FRC continues to decrease, and the pulmonary function of the patient takes on a restrictive pattern (see Chapter 5). Pain with resultant splinting, diaphragmatic dysfunction, and narcotics used for analgesia all reduce the patient's respiratory drive and effort. A small tidal volume, increased respiratory rate, and absence of sighing (periodic reflexive deep breaths) characterize this period.

Ciliary clearance of pulmonary secretions is impaired. The patient's immobility fosters pooling of secretions in dependent lung regions. Because of incisional discomfort, effective coughing is painful and difficult, as are position changes. This combination of factors puts the patient at great risk for lower respiratory infection. The effects of these factors peak between days 2 and 4 postoperatively.[1,3,4] Two weeks may elapse before pulmonary function returns to preoperative levels.[3]

The geriatric patient is, of course, subject to all of the aforementioned complications, in addition to the anatomic and physiologic changes in the elderly that heighten the postoperative effects and make the recovery from surgery more arduous. The elderly patient is more likely to have a long smoking history, preexisting pulmonary disease, or both. The major age-related change in the elderly lung involves a decrease in the elastic recoil brought about by a change in the proportions of elastin to collagen. Vital capacity also declines with increased age (a somewhat greater decline documented in men than in women). Ventilation distribution appears to be less uniform and efficient in the elderly. The respiratory reflexes are decreased (such as the response to **hypoxemia** whereby heart rate increases in response to decreased Pa_{O_2}). Finally, aging produces a reduction in Pa_{O_2} (on the order of 0.4 mm Hg per year).[3]

TREATMENT METHODS AND PROGRESSION

Preoperative Teaching

All patients should receive some instruction (with respect to pulmonary hygiene) before surgery. Teaching should begin with a brief discussion of the deleterious effects of anesthesia and the complications physical therapy can prevent or reverse. This should be done in general terms at a level that the patient can comprehend and in a manner that does not increase the patient's anxiety.

Some of the time spent with the patient may be taken to help resolve some of the patient's anxieties and worries by answering questions, particularly those relating to the physical therapy treatment. The therapist should allow enough time to approach the task in a relaxed, unhurried manner and should try to impart confidence to the patient.

CASE 1 – Preoperative

A referral is received for preoperative and postoperative physical therapy for Mr. Jones, a 65-year-old male, who has an admitting diagnosis of pancreatic cancer. He is scheduled for a Whipple procedure (pancreatoduodenal resection) the following day. In reviewing the chart, the therapist compiles the following information:

Past medical history:	Hypertension for 15 years controlled with patient on beta blocking medication; peptic ulcer disease
Past surgical history:	Tonsils and adenoids removed as a child
Smoking history:	Two packs per day for 30 years (60 pack years); patient stopped smoking 15 years ago
Preoperative chest radiograph:	Lungs are clear; normal chest

The impression is of an elderly male who was in relatively good health until his recent illness. A heavy but distant smoking history may predis-

pose him to postoperative complications. He will undergo an involved abdominal procedure that will leave him with a large, high abdominal incision to the right of or in the midline. The location of the surgical intervention on the pancreas and the incision predispose this patient to problems in reexpanding his right lung postoperatively. This condition may be exacerbated by a breathing pattern limited by pain, splinting, and narcotics.

Preoperative Instruction

Preoperative teaching may begin with an explanation such as this:

"Good morning, Mr. Jones. I understand that your surgery is scheduled for tomorrow." When this is confirmed, the therapist can proceed: "Dr. Thomas has asked us to work with you after the surgery, and we feel that it helps if we discuss it beforehand with you so you'll know what to expect. What we will be doing is routine at this hospital, as we work with all of Dr. Thomas's patients who have similar surgery. The general anesthesia that you'll be receiving may have some effect on your respiratory system that we will help you to prevent, as much as possible. The anesthesia is generally a depressant that slows down your need to breathe and decreases the depth of your breathing. Therefore, you won't be breathing as much or as deeply immediately after the surgery. You will find the anesthesia dehydrates you slightly, making your mucus thicker and harder to clear. The fact that you will have an incision on your abdomen will make you uncomfortable and make you have more difficulty breathing deeply or coughing to clear the mucus. We will be helping you to breathe deeper and to cough and show you ways to make the process as comfortable as possible."

Mr. Jones should then be instructed in moving from side to side in the bed and rolling to either side-lying position. Breathing exercises emphasizing rib cage expansion should be taught, incorporating diaphragmatic breathing with pursed-lip expiration. Percussion and vibration are demonstrated (so the patient is not startled postoperatively), and the patient is told the reasons these techniques are used. The patient should be taught splinted coughing to decrease the discomfort and ankle exercises to help promote circulation and prevent clotting problems postoperatively. Following these procedures, auscultation of the lungs should be performed to establish a baseline.

Postoperative Treatment

Bed Mobility

Postoperative bed mobility is performed by medical personnel until the patient is independent. The therapist is often called on to move patients in bed (especially during the immediate postoperative period). One goal of treatment is to teach patients how to move themselves comfortably or to assist them in moving themselves.

The directions that a patient most frequently has to move in bed are laterally (as a prelude to rolling), rolling to a side-lying position, moving toward the head of the bed, and eventually coming from supine to side-lying to short sitting or sitting with the legs over the side of the bed. At all times therapists should be aware of their own body mechanics, particularly when moving patients in bed. The bed should be at a comfortable working height so that the therapist can move without excessive bending which causes undue strain on the therapist's back and neck.

The bridging maneuver is taught when instructing a patient to move laterally in bed. The patient flexes the knees (when not contraindicated; see special considerations later in this chapter), raises the pelvis slightly, and, once raised, shifts the pelvis to the side opposite the side to which you wish the patient to roll. The shoulders can then be eased over. This maneuver gives the patient sufficient room to roll comfortably. Patients may need assistance with some aspects of this maneuver, such as helping to lift the pelvis or helping to shift once it is lifted. The most effective way to accomplish this is by placing yourself on the side of the bed you wish the patient to move to. When the patient begins the bridging maneuver, slip one arm underneath and around the top of the pelvis and the other slightly distal to the buttocks. The patient can be easily pulled toward you (Fig. 15–4). Direct contact with the patient's skin should be avoided. In addition, the draw sheet or incontinence pad should be kept between the therapist's hands and the patient when reaching underneath.

Rolling is best taught with the therapist on the side to which the patient is supposed to roll. Many postoperative patients cannot tolerate a supine position because it stretches out the trunk

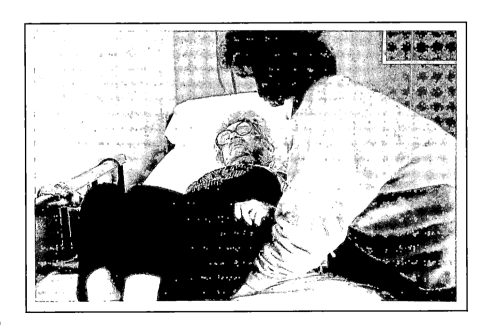

Figure 15–4.

Shifting a patient's hips to one side of the bed in preparation for rolling. Note that the therapist is suppporting her back and weight with her right knee.

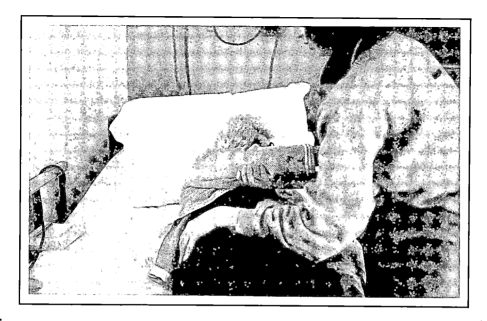

Figure 15-5.

Helping a patient roll to a side-lying position. Note that the patient is assisting in the rolling by pulling on the therapist's right arm.

and subsequently places stress on an abdominal incision. Therefore, rolling may be best performed by turning the patient while in a semi-Fowler's position (with the head of the bed elevated 20 to 30 degrees). The bed can be slowly lowered to horizontal once the patient has been rolled.

Before rolling, the patient's knees should be flexed as they were for moving laterally. The patient should be supported with the topmost arm on the therapist's arm and assisted with the other hand by gently guiding the hip (Fig. 15-5). Once rolled, the patient must be positioned completely on the side. This can be done by shifting the bottom hip posteriorly. Again, the therapist may assume a position behind the patient and, reaching underneath the pelvis, help the patient shift the hip. Once properly positioned, the patient should be able to comfortably maintain the side-lying position without holding on to the therapist or the guard rail.

Moving up in bed is best accomplished with the bed horizontal. The patient is instructed to bend the knees and exert pressure through the feet to extend the legs while the therapist assists by pulling the patient toward the head of the bed.

Coming to sit is done by rolling to a side-lying position, swinging the feet off the bed, and pushing against the bed or siderail with the topmost hand and bottom elbow.

Positioning, Pain Relief, and Relaxation

Positioning a patient for comfort can be vital in the immediate postoperative period. As previously discussed, the breathing pattern of these patients is altered by pain, anxiety, and medication. Significant changes in the rate and depth of respiration can be made simply by helping a patient become more comfortably positioned in the bed.

Generally speaking, the position of comfort for the patients at highest risk for pulmonary complications (e.g., those who have had upper abdominal or thoracic surgeries) is to have the head of the bed elevated 20 to 30 degrees and the knees and hips maintained in a slightly flexed position. With the trunk only slightly elevated

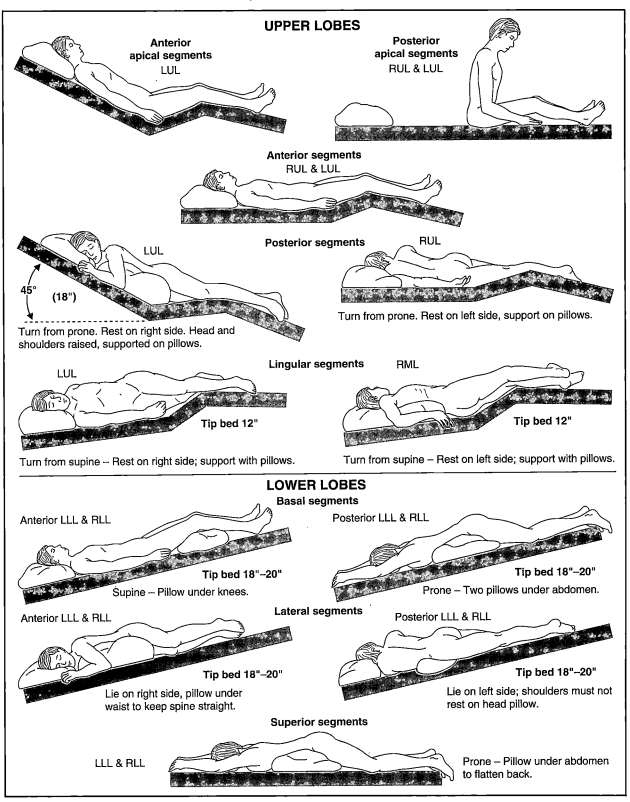

Figure 15-6.

The twelve postural drainage positions. LLL, left lower lobe; RUL, right upper lobe; LUL, left upper lobe; RLL, right lower lobe; RML, right middle lobe. (From White, GC. Basic Clinical Competencies for Respiratory Care: An Integrated Approach. Albany, NY, Delmar Publishers, 1988, Fig. 9-5. Reproduced by permission.)

the abdominal contents do not restrict diaphragmatic excursion (as would occur in a sitting position), allowing the patient deeper, more comfortable respirations. The slightly flexed position also reduces traction on an abdominal or thoracic incision. Supporting the arms or feet with soft pillows may also enhance relaxation and comfort.

Treatments should always be coordinated with the administration of pain medication. This makes the treatment more tolerable for the patient and results in increased cooperation with improved results. Generally speaking, pain medications such as morphine or meperidine (Demerol) begin to take effect within 20 minutes of administration, an ideal time frame within which to plan to administer treatment.

Relaxation is important to improve the patient's sense of well-being. Relaxation is also a key factor in changing the postoperative breathing pattern. Therefore no "right" or specific time to introduce relaxation into the treatment can be stated. Relaxation may be necessary to begin treatment by placing a patient in a comfortable position, or it may be necessary to use relaxation as a "breather" during treatment. Initially treatment may be geared strictly to comfort, relaxation, and breathing exercises (segmental expansion). This is particularly true for patients who are in the immediate postoperative phase and whose pain is not adequately relieved by analgesics. For other patients, relaxation and positioning may be more important at a later phase in their recovery as analgesics are being withdrawn.

The therapist's judgment and experience dictate when instruction in relaxation techniques may be most effective.

Postural Drainage

Postural drainage may be an essential part of postoperative care (when indicated). Placing the patient in various positions facilitates the movement of secretions with the assistance of gravity. Secretions may be moved from small to large airways and subsequently may be expelled by coughing. The anatomy and the configuration of the tracheobronchial tree are fairly consistent in every individual (see Chapter 1); therefore, specific positions are effective in draining individual lobes and segments of the lungs (Fig. 15–6). Some of these positions involve the patient being in a head-down or **Trendelenburg position**. The postoperative patient is not always stable and therefore cannot always be placed in this position. In this instance modified postural drainage is generally performed: the patient is not tipped head down, and the bed is not brought below the horizontal position. Instead, the patient remains horizontal.

Manual techniques also exist that are used by the therapist to facilitate drainage:

Percussion. The therapist's hands are held in a cupped manner (Fig. 15–7), and percussion is performed over the ribs to the patient's tolerance, generally lasting no more than 3 to 5 minutes per area of treatment. The hands may be

Figure 15–7.

Proper configuration of the hand for percussion.

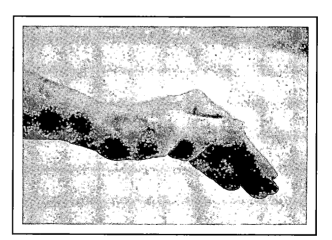

moved from posterior to anterior and inferior to superior on the chest, with percussion over the scapula or any drains and incisions avoided. Percussion is performed in a rhythmic, alternating manner, with most of the movement occurring at the wrist and not the elbow or shoulders. This position avoids fatigue of large proximal muscle groups when the technique is performed over protracted periods of time (Fig. 15–8). Percussion, when performed properly, should not leave the skin erythematous. A layer of cloth such as a gown or bedsheet may be placed to cover the skin during percussion. Percussion must be done cautiously in the presence of a pulmonary artery catheter (in some facilities it is contraindicated). Caution should also be exercised in using percussion on a patient with a history of prolonged corticosteroid treatment or one with severe osteoporosis.

The benefits of percussion must be weighed against the risks. Percussion is contraindicated in patients who have platelet counts below 20,000 (normal is > 259,000) owing to a risk of bleeding. It is also contraindicated in the presence of rib fractures (on the side with the fracture).

Vibration. Vibration is one of the most effective manual techniques to facilitate the clearance of secretions. The therapist applies gentle downward force to the thorax through the hands. Os-

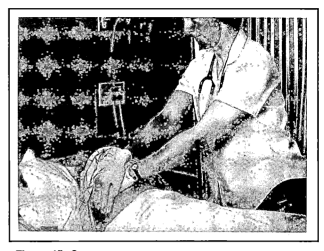

Figure 15–9.

Proper hand placement for chest vibration.

cillating movements of the hands with the downward force produce a vibration that is transmitted to the contents of the thorax. The vibration is thought to assist in moving secretions to the large airways.

In performing the technique, it is essential that the bed or treatment table be at a height at which the therapist's arms can be maintained in an extended position with the hands on the patient's thorax. Hands are placed directly on the patient's skin. The dominant hand should be on the bottom with the force applied from the shoulders down through the extended arms (Fig. 15–9). The patient is asked to take a deep inspiration, concentrating on expanding the area under the therapist's hands. The therapist applies the gentle force and oscillations as the patient exhales through pursed lips. The technique may also be used while a patient is coughing and huffing.

No contraindications exist to vibration except possibly vibrating over a rib fracture, although precautions should be taken with patients who have pulmonary artery catheters, low platelet counts, and severe osteoporosis. Vibration thus has wide and valuable use with the postoperative patient.

Shaking. The technique and theory of shaking is the same as that for vibration except that the hands are placed with the thumbs interlocking

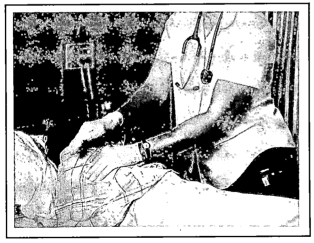

Figure 15–8.

Chest percussion. Note the correct height of the bed in relationship to the therapist's body.

and the fingers wrapped around the thorax (with the thumbs pointing toward the patient's head) (Fig. 15–10). Force is not applied uniformly throughout exhalation but is directed in gentle thrusts. The same type of precautions observed with vibration should be observed with shaking.

Suctioning. Suctioning is used to clear secretions from the nasopharynx, oropharynx, or tracheobronchial tree. As a general rule, any patient unable to clear secretions by coughing is a candidate for suctioning. Patients who are unconscious or obtunded and those with respiratory insufficiency or respiratory failure generally comprise the population of patients who are suctioned. However, owing to the trauma that may occur to the constantly suctioned tracheobronchial tree, suctioning should not be done on a routine or scheduled basis but rather only when deemed necessary. Suctioning may be more effective when it is performed following postural drainage. Specific indications include

- abnormal breath sounds (such as ronchi or wet rales) indicating the presence of secretions
- significant hypoxemia (decreased Pa_{O_2})

- respiratory distress

Great care must be taken in performing suctioning because it is an invasive procedure. Severe complications may develop, including a drop in a patient's already low Pa_{O_2} by an average of 33 mm Hg following 15 seconds of suctioning (the suction catheter evacuates not only secretions from the tracheobronchial tree but oxygen as well).[6] Preoxygenation and postoxygenation with 100% oxygen helps to minimize the effects of the reduction in Pa_{O_2} with suctioning in most patients.[6] Hypoxemia or stimulation of the vagus nerve (which innervates the trachea and carina) may cause bradycardia and premature ventricular complexes. These arrhythmias are common during suctioning of an unstable patient. Hypoxemia with resultant arrhythmias (bradycardia) and paroxysmal coughing (triggered by suctioning) may also precipitate hypotension in the patient. **Diaphoresis** and extreme changes in the patient's respiratory rate may also indicate that the hyperinflation or hyperoxygenation was ineffective. Tissue trauma caused by invagination of the airway wall into the catheter

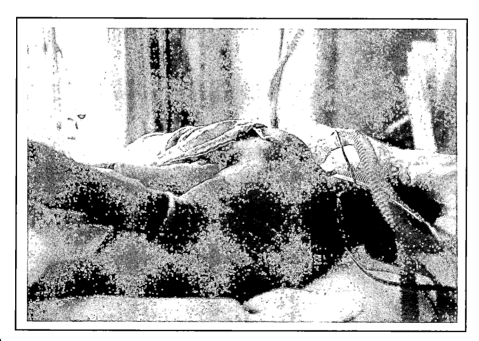

Figure 15–10.
Hand position for shaking. Note overlapped thumbs.

is a further hazard of suctioning. Tissue trauma may be minimized by using proper technique.

Equipment Required for Suctioning

- Sterile gloves
- Sterile suction catheter of appropriate size
- Continuous wall suction source with suction trap (vacuum pressure −80 to −120 mm Hg)
- Oxygen source with manual Ambu or ventilation bag
- Cardiac monitor
- Sterile basin or container
- Sterile water for cleaning catheter
- Sterile normal saline for irrigation or lavage
- Water soluble lubricant (for nasotracheal suctioning)
- Protective eyewear for person doing the suctioning

Procedure for Suctioning

1. Lay out sterile field containing gloves, catheter, and container (for sterile water).

2. Wear sterile glove on dominant hand (this hand is used to remove container and catheter, when ready, from field. Put on protective eyewear.

3. Pour sterile water into container.

4. Remove catheter and attach to suction. Hold catheter in dominant (sterile) hand; hold attachment from suction source in nonsterile hand.

5. Preoxygenate patient with 100% oxygen. An oxygen mask, nasal cannula, or ventilator may be used; however a manual Ambu or ventilation bag attached to a continuous oxygen source is best.

6. Insert catheter into airway; technique and distance of insertion vary with airway used. End point for insertion is when resistance is felt (the catheter should never be forced) or when reflexive coughing is triggered (when the catheter touches the carina). At either end point, the catheter should be withdrawn 1 centimeter before applying suction.

7. Withdraw catheter using a twirling motion between thumb and second and third fingers. At the same time, apply suction by closing the port on the proximal end of the catheter with the thumb of nonsterile hand. Do not maintain suction for more than 10 seconds.

8. Oxygenate patient with 100% oxygen.

9. Clean catheter by drawing up sterile water through it.

Helpful Hints for Suctioning. When conditions permit, suctioning is most effective when carried out by two people. One person performs the suctioning while the other performs the preoxygenation and postoxygenation. Vibration of the upper anterior thorax also makes the suctioning more effective. As the catheter is being withdrawn (while the suction is being applied), the second person vibrates over the upper airways.

In some institutions, a newer "closed-circuit" suctioning adapter for ventilator circuits is used. This eliminates the necessity for many of the sterile precautions and the additional personnel.

Incentive Spirometry

Incentive spirometry is the most widely used method for prevention and treatment of postoperative atelectasis.[7] Many different types of incentive spirometers exist, but all serve the same purpose. A consistent, maximal inspiratory effort is encouraged by the visual feedback from the instrument employed. The effectiveness of incentive spirometry is thoroughly dependent on patient effort and correct usage of the device. The patient should be instructed to exhale normally and then insert the mouthpiece and take a slow, deep inspiration. Occasionally, a nose clip may be necessary if the patient has difficulty with proper inhalation technique.

Another technique is the inhalation-hold method. The patient takes a maximal inhalation and momentarily holds the inspiration for a count of 3 to 5 seconds. This technique helps ventilate airways that are collapsed distal to an obstruction such as a mucous plug. Ventilation of obstructed airsacs is believed to occur owing to collateral ventilation through Kohn's pores (see Chapter 1). By increasing the volume in the distal airways, the cough may become more effective. An improved cough facilitates clearance of mucous plugs.

Incentive spirometry is advantageous because it is inexpensive; the equipment is disposable; and it is an easily understood method of biofeedback, making it a perfect method for independent patient use. Once the technique is mastered, the patient should continue to use it independently. The optimum usage is for six to ten deep breaths in a row per hour during waking hours.[4] For example, a patient who likes to watch television could be encouraged to use the incentive spirometer during the commercials.

Segmental Expansions

Segmental breathing exercises are also helpful to expand areas of the lungs selectively. The patient is positioned so that the area to be expanded is exposed (e.g., to expand the base of the right lung, the patient is positioned to lie on the left side) or in some cases is positioned in the postural drainage position for the particular segment in question. Expansion is facilitated with tactile and verbal cueing. For example, the therapist places a hand or hands on the patient's lower ribs (laterally or posteriorly, depending on what is indicated by auscultation) and tells the patient to "take a deep breath in through your nose. As you breathe in, raise your ribs into my hand."

Coughing

The cough is a physiologic mechanism that clears the airways of foreign material or excess secretions.

There are five processes in the cough mechanism:

- Deep inspiration
- Closure of the glottis
- Contraction of the chest wall (intercostal muscles) and abdominal muscles to increase intrathoracic and intra-abdominal pressure
- Opening of the glottis
- Forceful expulsion of air

Controlled Coughing. The postoperative patient is often reluctant or unable to cough. The process of "controlled coughing" is useful to achieve an effective cough. The patient is asked to take three deep breaths. The first two breaths are exhaled normally. With the third breath, the patient is instructed to cough firmly. The deep

breaths preceding the cough are thought to decrease atelectasis and increase the volume and thus the effectiveness of the cough.[6]

Splinted Cough. A pillow or other soft cushion held gently but firmly against the incision while coughing makes the process less painful. During the cough the patient feels the thoracic or abdominal wall pushing out, and the patient can give counterpressure with the pillow or cushion.

Huffing (Forced Expiration Technique)

Huffing is similar in concept and effect to coughing with one major difference. The mouth is kept open, keeping the glottis from closing. Air is forcefully exhaled as in coughing, but less effort from the patient is required. The technique is also taught to individuals with chronic, excessive secretions (e.g., those with bronchiectasis, bronchitis, or cystic fibrosis). It is generally felt to be less stressful to the patient and more effective in clearing the airways than constant forced coughing.[8]

Out of Bed Mobility

Early mobility is stressed as a means of preventing postoperative complications such as atelectasis and pulmonary embolism.[9] Inactivity results in shallow breathing and pooling of fluids in the extremities. Patients should be instructed in supine-to-sit transitions and bed-to-chair transfers as soon as their medical condition and pain tolerance allow. The techniques for these maneuvers are basically no different than those that are taught in the rehabilitation setting. Considerations need to be made for all lines and tubes to prevent pulling or detaching. Patient comfort should also be considered, and excessive traction on or stretching of incisions should be avoided during transitions.

Isotonic ankle exercises should be performed regularly, while patients are in bed or sitting. Ambulation (with appropriate assistive device, if necessary) should begin as soon as the physician considers the patient to be stable and ready.

SPECIFIC CONSIDERATIONS FOR SPECIFIC PROCEDURES

Cardiovascular Surgery

Certain steps in the procedure of coronary artery bypass graft surgery may result in minor complications in respiratory function. These complications are frequently observed after the operation. Topical icing used to rest the heart during surgery is associated with phrenic nerve injury. Harvesting of the internal mammary artery as a graft may have a similar effect.[4] The resulting diaphragmatic dysfunction or paralysis produces significant atelectasis or collapse of a lower lobe. The problem generally occurs with the left lung and may persist for several months. Prolonged time on the bypass pump (during surgery) may also result in diaphragmatic dysfunction.[4]

In the immediate postoperative period percussion of the upper anterior thorax should be avoided. During surgery, the sternum is bisected (a **sternotomy**) and then realigned and wired in place. While the bones are healing, a force such as percussion could cause malunion or nonunion. When absolutely necessary to facilitate clearance of secretions, vibrations should be applied bilaterally with equal force on each side of the chest. An unstable sternum may be detected by visual inspection (asymmetric movement), palpation, or the presence of sternal "click." In the presence of an unstable sternum, treatment should be discontinued until the nursing staff or the physician is notified of this situation.

Ankle exercises (ankle pumps and circles) are also important in this population to prevent venostasis, to help maintain an adequate cardiac output, and to help prevent deep vein thrombosis.

Peripheral Vascular Surgery

After arterial bypass grafts involving the extremities, certain precautions are in effect. For example, after a **femoral-popliteal (fem-pop) bypass,** the patient is not allowed to flex the hip or knee more than 90 degrees; after an **axillary-femoral bypass,** the patient is not permitted to lie on the operative side. These precautions are generally observed for about 1 month after the operation. Again, ankle isotonics are important to decrease venostasis and prevent phlebitis.

Thoracotomy

During preoperative teaching of a patient undergoing a thoracotomy, active range of motion of the shoulder on the operative side should always be measured and documented. Following the surgery, the patient has a tendency to splint on the surgical side and to keep the upper extremity relatively immobile. Elevation of the humerus puts traction on the incision and causes discomfort. If the patient does not move the shoulder through the normal range of motion, a painful frozen shoulder may ensue. Active and gentle active assistive range of motion is initiated in the immediate postoperative period with self range of motion taught to the patient. Range of motion should be returned to preoperative baseline levels on discharge from the hospital.

Patients with Chest Tubes

Movement with chest tubes in place is sometimes painful, and many patients are extremely reluctant to roll onto the side into which the chest tubes are inserted. To prevent pooling of secretions and to ensure adequate ventilation, patients should spend equal time lying on both sides. Patients with chest tubes must be rolled and positioned carefully and gently and given the information and support to help them overcome the reluctance to roll onto the chest tube. In addition, deep inspirations should be encouraged while side-lying with the chest tube elevated to facilitate full expansion and enhance chest wall mobility.

Pneumonectomy

Following resection of an entire lung (**pneumonectomy**), the patient should not be positioned with the remaining lung in the upright position for several weeks. Doing this could severely impair ventilation and cause severe tracheal shift deviation. (See Chapter 11 for more detailed information on surgical procedures.)

OXYGEN DELIVERY SYSTEMS

Because of altered postsurgical breathing patterns, many patients require supplemental oxygen to meet metabolic demands and maintain adequate arterial blood gases. Excluding mechanical ventilation, there are two basic types of oxygen delivery systems—*low-flow systems* and *high-flow systems* (see Chapter 10). Pulse oximetry is helpful in determining a need for supplemental oxygen (as are arterial blood gases) or evaluating the efficacy of a system in use. In the absence of pulse oximetry, signs and symptoms observed by the therapist aid in determining a need for oxygen. Rapid, shallow respirations, elevated heart rate at rest, and cyanosis are signs of hypoxemia. Should any of these signs develop during treatment, the treatment should be stopped, the patient returned to a position of comfort, and supplemental oxygen provided.

Oxygen masks and cannulas should be kept in place during all treatments when possible. This helps to prevent or minimize hypoxemia resulting from hypoventilation caused by positioning or splinting secondary to pain. Humidification may be added to all systems to prevent irritation of the mucosa and upper airways. Humidification also helps to thin secretions and facilitate their clearance.

UNIVERSAL PRECAUTIONS

In 1987 the Centers for Disease Control recommended that universal precautions be followed by health care practitioners to prevent transmission of the human immunodeficiency virus (HIV), hepatitis B and other blood-borne pathogens.[10] The implications of this recommendation are that all patients in a facility should be treated as potential carriers of these pathogens and that blood and body fluid precautions

TABLE 15–2. Universal Precautions

Precaution	Gown	Gloves	Mask	Glasses
Enteric	X	X		
Respiratory			X	
Strict	X	X	X	
Contact	X	X	X	
Blood and body fluid	X	X		X
Drainage/secretions	X	X		
Tuberculosis (AFB)	X		X	

AFB, Acid-fast bacilli.

should be observed in all situations in which exposure to these fluids is likely (Table 15–2).

In addition, proper and frequent hand washing (before and after each patient contact) to prevent contamination and the spread of infection remains an essential element in infection control procedures.

CASE 2–Postoperative

A Whipple procedure was performed on Mr. Jones yesterday, and the admitting diagnosis was confirmed. His epidural catheter (for pain relief) was removed this morning, and he is currently receiving morphine sulfate as needed. A postoperative chest radiograph shows significant loss of volume in the right lung. His body temperature is 100.8 degrees F at present. Arterial blood gases are not available.

Postoperative Day 1

It is 9:00 A.M., and the patient is in a postoperative or step-down unit. He is found in bed in a semi-Fowler's position, lethargic and sleepy after having received morphine sulfate for pain 20 minutes earlier.

After introducing himself to Mr. Jones, the therapist explains briefly what he is about to do. With the patient's consent, he lifts the gown just enough to uncover the incision. This is done so the location can be ascertained and any tubes or drains may be noted.

The incision is midline, and three **Jackson-Pratt drains** are in place. (These are tubes inserted into the abdomen near the surgical site. Their purpose is to drain excess fluid and thus to prevent ascites. They have an external collection chamber and may be placed on low suction.) The patient also has a Foley catheter to drain his bladder and a central venous line. The patient is receiving supplemental oxygen through a simple mist mask set at 35% oxygen. He is on electrocardiographic telemetry with a bedside monitor.

It is a good idea to begin treatment with the patient in a left side-lying position. (Many patients on postoperative day 1 are not able to tolerate a full treatment on each side. Initiating treatment in the left side-lying position facilitates reexpansion of the right lung and ensures that this would be done first.)

Treatment proceeds as follows:

1. The patient's upper lobes (anterior segments) are auscultated and found to be clear.

2. The patient is rolled to the left side-lying position, the therapist being careful not to roll onto the drains or dislodge the Foley catheter or central venous line.

3. The head of the bed is lowered to a flat position. The electrocardiographic monitor is checked continually during these movements.

4. In a left side-lying position with the bed flat, the patient's right side is auscultated. He is found to have absent breath sounds at the right base. It is also noted that the patient's respiratory rate is 22 with shallow inspirations. There is little movement of the thorax when the patient is asked to breathe deeply.

5. Segmental expansions of the right base laterally and posteriorly are performed with the therapist providing verbal and tactile cues. Hands are placed on the patient's lower rib cage: on the side for lateral costal expansion and on the back for posterior expansion. The patient is asked to breathe into the therapist's hands or to make the therapist's hands rise.

6. After three such deep breaths, three more breaths are performed with the therapist providing vibration throughout exhalation.

7. Percussion is performed for 1 minute (if indicated for secretion management) followed by three more segmental breaths with vibration.

8. The patient is taught splinted coughing, which produces a large green mucous plug.

9. The incentive spirometer is used for three deep breaths of 1000 milliliters. Auscultation reveals decreased breath sounds in the right base.

10. The patient is rolled to a right side-lying position, and the previous sequence is repeated.

11. Finally, the patient is placed in a semi-Fowler's position with the knees raised for comfort. Ankle exercises are performed in this position. The patient is instructed in independent, hourly use of the incentive spirometer.

12. If scheduling permits, this patient should be seen again in the afternoon.

For the afternoon treatment, the patient is instructed in coming to a short sitting position at the side of the bed and is assisted in transferring to a chair. Breathing exercises, splinted coughing, incentive spirometry, and ankle exercises are performed. Breathing exercises focus on segmental expansion on the right.

Postoperative Day 2

At 10:00 A.M. the patient's temperature is 101 degrees F; there is no report yet from a chest radiograph taken earlier in the day. The patient is sitting up in bed. The Foley catheter and central venous line have been removed. Electrocardiographic telemetry results show that the patient is in normal sinus rhythm with a heart rate of 98 with occasional premature ventricular contractions. Auscultation in a sitting or in a high Fowler's position reveals decreased breath sounds from the right mid field to the base posteriorly and laterally with rhonchi at the base. The patient is treated in a left side-lying position and given a full treatment (as yesterday); the incentive spirometer is used in side-lying and sitting positions. Breath sounds are increased following a productive cough (thick, green secretions × 3). Ankle exercises are performed, and the incentive spirometer is used to 1500 milliliters in sitting.

Postoperative Day 3

The patient has been transferred to a semiprivate room. His temperature is 99.2 degrees F; his heart rate is 80 in normal sinus rhythm without ectopy. The report of the chest radiograph from the previous day shows significant atelectasis in the right lower lobe. All peripheral lines and one Jackson-Pratt drain have been removed. Auscultation indicates decreased breath sounds at the right base posteriorly. Treatment is given as previously, with lower extremity exercise and ambulation in the corridor added in a second (P.M.) treatment. Documentation of clinical findings (decreased breath sounds) and chest radiograph support further treatment. The goal is a return to preoperative status.

Postoperative Day 4

The patient's temperature is 98.8 degrees F; his heart rate is 80 in normal sinus rhythm. No new chest radiograph is available. The patient is ambulating for short distances with a nurse or his wife. His lungs are clear with decreased breath sounds at the right base. Breathing exercises are done in a sitting position. The lungs are clear with good aeration following treatment. The patient's cough is effective (but painful) and nonproductive. He is using an incentive spirometer to 2000 milliliters. The patient is taken off the physical therapy program but will continue incentive spirometry and ambulation. A return to preoperative pulmonary status has been achieved.

Summary of Treatment

Treatment of the surgical patient was geared to clear secretions, increase ventilation and respiration, decrease the work of breathing, and provide for early mobilization of the patient.

The patient was discharged from the hospital on postoperative day 7. Early aggressive intervention has helped this patient avoid serious pulmonary complications and helped ensure an early or timely discharge.

THE NONSURGICAL PATIENT

The Patient Population

Chronic Obstructive Pulmonary Disease

In the acute care setting, the patient with chronic obstructive pulmonary disease (COPD) has generally been hospitalized for either **exacerbation** of the condition or pneumonia. An exacerbation of COPD may follow a mild upper respiratory infection, a period of stress, or some prolonged, strenuous activity. The exacerbation is characterized by arterial blood gases that are altered beyond the individual's usual levels, moderate to severe shortness of breath at rest, respiratory muscle fatigue, and severely impaired functional abilities. In short, the patient is in respiratory distress with failure appearing imminent. Some of the same signs and symptoms may be present with pneumonia, but an active lower respiratory infection is responsible for the pneumonia. (See Chapter 6 for a discussion of the pathophysiology of the diseases that comprise COPD.)

An exacerbation of COPD may involve various types of symptoms that may be treated in different ways. Immediate medical management is essential to cure infection or to diminish brochospasm. Disturbances in arterial blood gases may require drug or oxygen therapy or both. If increased sputum production is part of the problem, postural drainage may be indicated. Auscultatory findings (e.g., **rhonchi** or wet rales) may also indicate the need for postural drainage.

The physical therapist may be called on to provide postural drainage with accompanying manual techniques. If the patient is receiving *nebulized* bronchodilator treatment, physical therapy should be coordinated to follow the treatment. The physical therapist should also instruct the patient in relaxation techniques and breathing retraining to decrease the rate and increase the depth of respiration as well as to decrease the use of accessory muscles when possible.

In many instances, the patient may have a very limited knowledge of the disease process (e.g., someone hospitalized for the first time with this condition). The physical therapist should be very familiar with the pathophysiology and progression of COPD. Patient education should be initiated regarding acceptance of the condition and understanding the implications on function in terms of activities of daily living and alterations in lifestyle that may be necessary. This is the optimal occasion to initiate a referral for pulmonary rehabilitation.

Restrictive Lung Disease of Pulmonary Etiology

Many conditions affect the interstitium of the lung (see Chapter 5). These include such conditions as diffuse interstitial pulmonary fibrosis, occupational diseases (e.g., asbestosis, silicosis, farmer's lung), and collagen disorders (e.g., rheumatoid arthritis, systemic lupus erythematosus). These patients generally derive benefit from breathing retraining and instruction in energy conservation techniques for activities of daily living. Intermittent positive-pressure breathing (IPPB) and self-assisted cough techniques may be indicated.

Pneumonia

There are approximately 6 million cases of pneumonia annually in the United States. Pneumonia may be community acquired or contracted in the hospital (nosocomial). The community-acquired infections may be viral, bacterial, or (less frequently) fungal or parasitic. Nosocomial pneumonias are primarily bacterial in origin and have the highest mortality rate of nosocomial infections.[11]

Many conditions predispose individuals to pneumonia. These include hospitalized patients who have adult respiratory distress syndrome. Seventy percent of these patients experience a secondary pneumonia with only 12% surviving.[11] Other risk factors for pneumonia include advanced age (pneumonia is the fourth leading cause of death in the elderly[11]), cardiac disease,

alcoholism, COPD, head injury, renal failure, or any immunosuppressive state caused by therapy or disease.

Bacterial pneumonia produces an **exudative infiltrate** in the air spaces, and postural drainage (as well as antibiotics) is indicated if the patient has difficulty with the mobilization of secretions. Other types of pneumonia are managed medically.

Musculoskeletal and Neuromuscular Disorders

Pathologic conditions such as polio, Guillain-Barré syndrome, amyotrophic lateral sclerosis, myasthenia gravis, muscular dystrophy, and quadriplegia or hemiplegia of any cause produce restrictive pulmonary conditions. Weakened or paralyzed accessory muscles result in shallow inspirations and markedly diminished lung volumes as well. Maintaining an adequate minute ventilation may not be possible, which results in respiratory muscle fatigue and often respiratory distress or even respiratory failure. Patients who are kept relatively bedbound may also develop retention and pooling of secretions. Pneumonia often ensues and becomes the cause for hospitalization.

Decreased lung volumes (secondary to increased secretions and inadequate inspirations) result in ineffective coughing. Intermittent positive-pressure breathing is one treatment that is utilized to provide a larger tidal volume than the patient is capable of achieving independently. Increased tidal volumes increase the effectiveness of the cough and assist in the mobilization and clearance of secretions.

Positioning to maximize the effectiveness of the cough is also an important component of treatment. The sitting position places the diaphragm in a higher position and assists the cough by helping to maintain a higher intra-abdominal pressure. If the cough is still ineffective, it can be assisted manually by the physical therapist. Specifics of IPPB treatment and assisted cough are discussed in the next section on treatment methods.

Treatment Methods and Progression

Postural Drainage

The indications for and principles of postural drainage are the same for all populations. All patients should be assessed initially for the presence of pulmonary secretions and the need for postural drainage as well as the need for restrictions on any of the positions. (See the section on the postoperative patient that appeared earlier in this chapter.)

Breathing Exercise and Retraining

Breathing exercise and retraining are vital elements of the treatment program for the nonsurgical patient. Initially relaxation may be needed before exercise or training can take place. Positioning for comfort, using visual imagery, and using reassuring verbal input are all aids to assist in the patient's relaxation.

The patient should be in a comfortable position with adequate supplemental oxygen (if needed). The patient is instructed to breathe in through the nose and exhale through pursed lips. Additionally, patients may be asked to count to themselves to time the phases of inhalation and exhalation. Exhalation should be roughly twice as long as inspiration. Generally a 3 to 6 or 4 to 8 ratio is comfortable. The therapist may use tactile cues to help facilitate the diaphragmatic breathing process. One hand may be placed lightly on the abdomen with the instruction to the patient to breathe into the hand or to move the hand by distending the abdomen on inhalation. This may facilitate diaphragmatic training. Gentle pressure on the upper chest with the therapist's other hand (during inspiration) inhibits thoracic excursion and decreases excessive use of the accessory musculature.

Rapid, shallow respirations may sometimes be altered by instruction in diaphragmatic breathing with pursed-lip expiration. Pursed-lip expiration is especially important to patients with COPD. Narrowing the external opening (the mouth) increases the resistance to airflow during exhalation. This creates a back pressure and retards collapse of the distal airways during exhalation.

Segmental expansions with tactile cuing are useful to aerate underventilated areas of the lungs (hands are placed on the rib cage over the area to be expanded). Upper extremity exercises, such as proprioceptive neuromuscular facilitation (PNF) patterns, coordinated with deep breathing also help to improve aeration. Gentle mobilization of the thorax produces relaxation by decreasing muscle tone. This, in turn, may also help to improve aeration in the underlying segments. Rib mobilization (both individually and in segments) and adversive trunk rotation (elongating the trunk by moving the shoulder anteriorly while rotating the pelvis posteriorly and then reversing hand placement and movements; Fig. 15–11) performed in the side-lying position are two of the most effective techniques. Ribs may be mobilized with the patient in various positions. Gentle pressure is placed on the more caudal rib or group of ribs. A downward force is exerted that gently stretches the intercostal muscles and increases rib cage mobility. For trunk rotation, the patient is placed in a side-lying position with the therapist's hands on the hip posteriorly and the shoulder anteriorly. Pressure is applied, pulling the hip forward and pushing the shoulder backward, thus slightly elongating the trunk. The patient inhales during this maneuver. Hand placements and pressure applications are reversed: the hip is pushed back and the shoulder forward as the patient exhales.

Bed Mobility, Transitions, and Transfers

For patients with COPD or with limited exercise or ventilatory capacity, transitions such as from supine to sitting or from sitting to standing tend to initiate or exacerbate **dyspnea**. The acute care setting is the ideal place to begin instruction in proper breath control and energy conservation during these movements. The patient should be instructed to avoid breath holding during activities and encouraged to coordinate exhalation during the exertive phase of any transition. For example, a patient may be instructed to "blow

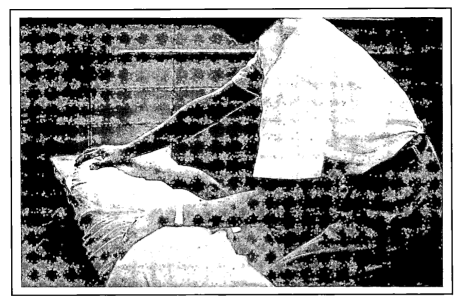

Figure 15-11.

Hand placement for adversive trunk rotation.

your breath out as you get out of the chair" while initiating standing.

In many instances, dyspnea or the apprehension of developing dyspnea has left these patients extremely anxious and impulsive. Instruction should also focus on decreasing the speed of movements as well as making slower transitions and avoiding unnecessary or excessive expenditures of energy.

Resistive Inspiratory Muscle Training

Resistive inspiratory (ventilatory) muscle training is a treatment designed to strengthen or improve the endurance of the inspiratory muscles. A plastic mouthpiece with a valve is used. The size of the port or opening of the valve is adjustable. The smaller the opening, the greater the resistance to inspiration. As the patient progresses, resistance is added by using a smaller port. Progress may be measured by increased ease of use of the device (patient's subjective report of less fatigue) and by a smaller change in the patient's vital signs during use. Two 15-minute sessions daily are recommended. Vital signs should be monitored during treatment. A heart rate increase beyond 20 beats per minute over the resting rate or excessive fatigue is an indication to stop the treatment session. (See Chapter 17 for more details on inspiratory muscle training in pulmonary rehabilitation.)

Intermittent Positive-Pressure Breathing

Intermittent positive-pressure breathing is a treatment method that provides a breath with positive pressure to supplement or assist the patient's inspiratory effort. Indications for use include

- providing hyperinflation to reverse atelectasis
- providing an additional volume of inspired air to make a cough more effective
- delivering medication

Intermittent positive-pressure breathing may be delivered by a ventilator but, more commonly, a machine designed specifically for this purpose is used (Fig. 15-12). One advantage of using this latter device is that it delivers a breath drawn from ambient (room) air, not from an oxygen source. This makes it a useful tool for delivering nebulized medications to selected patients with COPD who may demonstrate a decrease in respiratory drive and an increase in carbon dioxide retention when supplemental oxygen is provided.

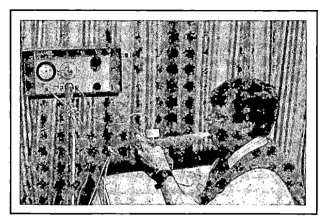

Figure 15–12.

Use of intermittent positive-pressure breathing unit.

Intermediate positive-pressure breathing is also useful in increasing the tidal volume in patients with neurologic or spinal cord injuries.

Before initiating IPPB treatment, the therapist should verify the positive pressure that is to be administered (the normal range is 10–15 cm H$_2$O) and be thoroughly familiar with the patient's history. This history alerts the therapist regarding any possible contraindications to use or conditions that may predispose the patient to complications. Complications that could result are

- pneumothorax
- increased intracranial pressure
- increased intrathoracic pressure that reduces venous return and thus cardiac output
- hyperventilation
- reduction of respiratory drive

Vital signs should also be monitored carefully (e.g., a drop in blood pressure during use may signal a decrease in cardiac output). Other complications to note are changes in respiratory rate, level of arousal, skin color **(cyanosis)**, sharp chest pain, or onset of headache.

Contraindications to use of the IPPB are

- **bullous emphysema**
- untreated **pneumothorax**
- recent open heart surgery
- cardiac compromise or hemodynamic instability

- recent lung resection
- recent craniotomy or head trauma

Assisted Cough

When the patient's cough is ineffective (especially with neurologic or neuromuscular disorders), the therapist may provide a manual assist to forced expiration. Various techniques are used to accomplish this assist. Choice of techniques depends on the disability involved, the position in which the cough is to be encouraged, and the level of the therapist's skill.

The most basic assisted cough is done with the patient in the supine position. The therapist places the heel of the hand on the upper abdomen about 1 inch above the umbilicus. The patient is asked to inhale, hold the breath, and then follow with a strong cough. As the patient coughs, the therapist quickly applies pressure under the diaphragm with the heel of the hand. This technique helps the patient expel the air more forcefully. It also uses a moderate amount of force over a small area and can be uncomfortable. It should not be done soon after meals because it may induce vomiting. The therapist should use the technique selectively on patients.

Exercise Training in the Hospital

Hospitalization and immobility quickly lead to a deconditioned state. The adverse effects of bedrest can be severe, and the cardiopulmonary responses to bedrest are the most serious of any system. These effects include

- orthostatic intolerance
- increased heart rate at rest and with exercise
- decrease in $\dot{V}o_{2max}$
- decrease in stroke volume
- reduction in lean body mass and total body calcium
- replacement of pliable connective tissue (in joints) with dense, less flexible tissue[12]

In people with chronic illness, the effects are even more devastating. Among the problems that the therapist may encounter are fatigue, weakness, orthostatic hypotension, stiffness, lack of coordination, and often depression.[12] Chronic illness and pain also affect posture. A habitually flexed posture is common, and gentle stretching should be incorporated with the exercise program.

Active range of motion should be done initially in bed in a supine or semi-Fowler's position and should progress to short sitting and standing. Large, proximal muscle groups should be addressed first, progressing distally. Bridging, straight-leg raises, and PNF patterns are useful in strengthening hips and knees. Stretching of the Achilles-gastroc-soleus complex may be necessary because tightness hinders balance. Stretching of the pectorals improves posture. As the duration of in-bed exercise increases, the patient should be able to tolerate activity in upright positions.

Heart rate (and rhythm) and blood pressure should be monitored before, during, and after each activity. Use of a simple blood pressure cuff and manual palpation of the patient's pulse are all that is necessary. When abnormal physiologic responses to exercise are detected (see Chapter 8), the activity should be stopped immediately and the patient returned to a sitting or recumbent position. Vital signs should be checked at 1-minute intervals until they return to baseline or until the nursing staff or physician is notified of the abnormality, or both.

Some contraindications to exercise are

● unstable angina
● resting systolic blood pressure higher than 200 mm Hg or resting diastolic blood pressure higher than 110 mm Hg
● uncontrolled atrial or ventricular arrhythmias
● suspected deep vein thrombosis[13]

Ambulation or Gait Training. The physician's order for ambulation may include a heart rate limit as well as a requirement for the use of supplemental oxygen. Before beginning ambulation, the patient's heart rate should be recorded and the rhythm noted (if telemetry is available). Blood pressure should be taken with the patient sitting and standing. Oxygen saturation at rest also should be noted. If necessary, the patient is first instructed in paced breathing with pursed-lip expiration. A chair should be placed within a reasonable distance from the patient's bedside. This enables the patient to rest when necessary. Positions for recovering from dyspnea should also be taught (Figs. 15–13 and 15–14). If the

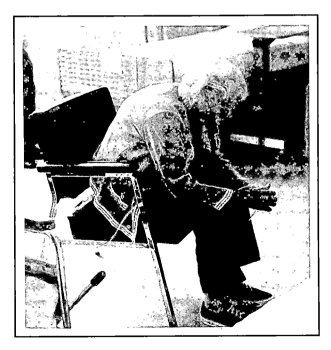

Figure 15–13.

One position for recovering from dyspnea.

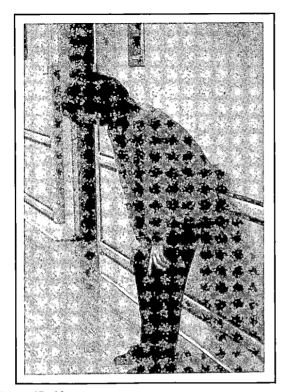

Figure 15-14.
One position for recovering from dyspnea.

patient is severely deconditioned, assistive devices such as a rolling walker may be used.

Pulse oximetry is very useful in patients with pulmonary dysfunction because it allows the therapist to judge instantaneously the patient's physiologic response to exercise. Generally, oxygen saturations of 90% or above are considered acceptable for patients at rest or performing light activities such as walking. When the saturation drops below 90% with minimal activity, supplemental oxygen may be ordered for exercise and ambulation.

Supplemental oxygen allows the patient to exercise at a slightly higher level or for a longer period of time than would be possible normally. The enhanced exercise capacity may produce a training effect, making the body more efficient in its utilization of oxygen and thus increasing endurance. If the patient responds favorably to the exercise, the oxygen may be withdrawn gradually. This may be determined by increased oxygen saturation and decreased heart rate at similar workloads.

The first step in withdrawing supplemental oxygen is to reduce the flow (e.g., from 2 L/min to 1 L/min). The training then resumes at the same level, and physiologic responses are again assessed. Exercise is stopped when the patient's oxygen saturation is consistently (as opposed to momentarily) below 90% (at the prescribed flow of oxygen and with proper breathing techniques). A heart rate of 30 beats per minute over resting or a drop in diastolic blood pressure greater than 20 mm Hg should also signal the therapist to stop or reduce the exercise. Subjective reports of fatigue or dyspnea should, of course, also be heeded.

A projected sequence or progression of treatment for a nonsurgical patient might include the following elements (in this order):

1. Evaluation
2. Postural drainage and breathing exercises
3. Breathing retraining
4. Active exercise of the extremities
5. Gait training

Initially the goals are to clear secretions and decrease the work of breathing. In the latter phase of acute care treatment, the focus should be on increasing mobility and function, as well as on monitoring for any abnormal or adverse responses.

CASE 3

Mrs. Bates is an 80-year-old woman who was found on the floor at home by a neighbor on 7/16/92. Breathing was labored; the patient was diaphoretic and somewhat incoherent, oriented only to person. Mrs. Bates was brought to the emergency department, where the following clinical picture was established.

Temperature:	102 degrees F
Pulse:	108 beats per minute
Respiration:	20 per minute
Blood pressure:	110/60
White blood	
cell count:	17,000 (normal = <12,000)

Arterial blood gases:	on room air: pH = 7.28; P_{O_2} = 40; P_{CO_2} = 74; HCO_3 = 34 (general notation is pH/P_{CO_2}/P_{O_2}/HCO_3 or 7.28/74/40/34)
Chest radiograph:	right middle and lower lobe infiltrate
Auscultation:	bronchial breath sounds right midfield to base; otherwise breath sounds were distant
Medical history:	osteoarthritis in both knees; COPD; congestive heart failure (provided by patient's physician)
Medications:	digoxin, furosemide (Lasix), potassium supplement, theophylline (Theo-Dur), albuterol (Proventil), and ipratropium bromide (Atrovent)

First Day

Mrs. Bates was given her first physical therapy treatment on 7/16/92. She was seen in the emergency department 3 hours after admission. Mrs. Bates was placed on supplementary oxygen via a nonrebreathing mask. She was very lethargic. The clinical picture at this time was as follows:

Temperature:	101.6 degrees F
Chest radiograph:	same as previous film
Respiration:	26 per minute
Arterial blood gases:	7.26/76/35/34
Auscultation:	bronchial breath sounds, right base laterally and posteriorly
Flat to percussion:	positive E to A egophony

Mrs. Bates was treated with percussion and vibration in the left side-lying, supine, and one quarter turn to prone from left side-lying positions. She was instructed in segmental expansion of the thorax and pursed-lip expiration. Mrs. Bates had a weak, ineffective cough and was suctioned for a large amount of thick, yellow secretions (sample sent for culture and sensitivity). Following treatment, her status deteriorated (arterial blood gases = 7.20/78/32/35). She was orally intubated and placed on mechanical ventilation (**synchronized intermittent mandatory ventilation** at 14 breaths per minute). Her FI_{O_2} was 50%; arterial blood gases were 7.30/50/80/26. Mrs. Bates was treated for the next 3 days with postural drainage and suctioning. The culture and sensitivity results showed evidence of bacterial pneumonia *(Escherichia coli)*. Antibiotics (gentamicin) were administered intravenously.

Fourth Day

Mrs. Bates was weaned from mechanical ventilation and extubated; postural drainage and percussion, vibration, and assisted cough were continued; and incentive spirometry, segmental expansion of the thorax, and breathing retraining were begun. She remained afebrile, and her chest radiograph showed resolving right lower lobe pneumonia. Her arterial blood gases were 7.32/48/87/24; oxygen saturation was 94%; auscultation indicated right base rhonchi; and her cough was productive of thick, green secretions.

Fifth through Eighth Days

Mrs. Bates was moved to a regular room. Her cough was clear and nonproductive by the eighth day. The chest radiograph on the eighth day was clear.

Ninth Day

Mrs. Bates began ambulation with a physical therapist with oxygen at 2 liters per minute via nasal cannula. Her heart rate at rest was 90 beats per minute; oxygen saturation was 97%. After 40 feet of ambulation with light contact guarding from the physical therapist, her heart rate was 112 beats per minute with an oxygen saturation of 91%. Mrs. Bates was short of breath and fatigued. She also performed active exercise in supine and sitting positions.

Tenth Day

Mrs. Bates ambulated 100 feet twice with oxygen at 2 liters per minute. Her maximum heart rate was 98 beats per minute with an oxygen saturation of 95% during ambulation.

Eleventh Day

Mrs. Bates's supplementary oxygen was lowered to 1 liter per minute. She ambulated 100 feet three times. Her heart rate was 96 beats per minute; oxygen saturation was 93%.

Twelfth through Fourteenth Days

Mrs. Bates continued active exercise and ambulation without supplementary oxygen. She consistently ambulated 200 feet with paced breathing and pursed-lip expiration. Her oxygen saturation was no lower than 91%.

Fifteenth Day

Mrs. Bates was discharged with a referral for visiting nurses and home physical therapy.

THE INTENSIVE CARE UNIT

Although there are many different kinds of ventilators in use, their basic function remains the same: to deliver sufficient volumes of air to adequately ventilate and oxygenate the patient who cannot breathe adequately without help (see earlier part of this chapter). Ensuring adequate ventilation does not guarantee that adequate respiration or gas exchange is taking place, however. Patients who require mechanical ventilation need careful physiologic monitoring as well as a great deal of attention. The primary purpose of

the intensive care unit is to provide a setting in which increased care may be provided.

The Mechanically Ventilated Patient

Patients with severe alterations in arterial blood gases require mechanical ventilation until the underlying problem (causing the abnormal arterial blood gases) is resolved. Generally speaking, patients who require an $F_{I_{O_2}}$ of 0.7 (70%) or greater to reverse hypoxemia and maintain adequate respiration are better served by an endotracheal tube and mechanical ventilation than by an external oxygen source. Other indications for mechanical ventilation include progressive alveolar hypoventilation with respiratory acidosis (insufficient ventilation to allow adequate gas exchange, resulting in retention of carbon dioxide); temporary prophylactic support following abdominal or thoracic surgery; barely adequate gas exchange in the face of high-energy expenditure (work of breathing); and, finally, assistance for patients who require heavy sedation, which depresses respiration.[14]

Alterations in Physiology Produced by Mechanical Ventilation

Positive-pressure ventilation increases intrathoracic pressure as it also increases alveolar ventilation. The work of breathing is reduced, and the respiratory muscles are rested to some degree with all modes of ventilation. Mucociliary clearance is also impaired.

In normal breathing there is a phasic variation in stroke volume of the two ventricles of the heart. During inspiration increased venous return results in increased pulmonary venous return to the left atrium associated with increased filling and stroke volume of the left ventricle. With mechanical ventilation inspiration becomes a positive-pressure event, and the phasic nature of breathing is altered. If venous return to the right ventricle is decreased or delayed, hypotension or diminished cardiac output may result. The amount of compromise depends on the patient's baseline cardiac status and the resultant mean airway pressure.

Artificial Airways

Mechanical ventilation also involves the introduction of an artificial airway. An **endotracheal** tube is optimally positioned when its distal tip is 1 or 2 centimeters above the carina.[6] The three routes for placement of this airway are through a nasal or oral pathway or through a **tracheostomy.** Nasal intubation is generally better tolerated than oral intubation.[14] It is more comfortable because the gag reflex is not stimulated as strongly. Also the position of the tube in oral intubation is not as stable as it is when placed through the nasal cavity.[14] An endotracheal (oral) tube is usually secured to the side of the mouth by tape (see Fig. 15–16). Although a tracheostomy with placement of an airway is an extremely invasive procedure, this tube is probably the most comfortable for the patient once it is in place. A tracheostomy tube is the choice when a patient is expected to be dependent on a ventilator for more than a few days. The tracheostomy tube is more comfortable; generally has a larger lumen (than that of a nasotracheal or endotracheal tube), which means less airway resistance; and allows less dead space. All of these factors make suctioning easier and more effective for the patient with a tracheostomy.

An inflatable cuff is positioned near the distal end of each artificial airway (in adults). It is made of soft plastic and inflates to create a seal against the tracheal wall (see Chapter 11). Externally there is a pilot tube through which the cuff may be inflated and a balloon that indicates whether the cuff is inflated. An artificial airway (e.g., a tracheostomy tube) should never be occluded or capped while the cuff is inflated.

Treatment Implications

The airways of mechanically ventilated patients should be kept clear to ensure optimal ventilation of all areas of the lung. For this reason postural drainage, huffing, and suctioning

are very important components of the physical therapy treatment. For the patient who is alert and capable, independent effort of inspiration, breathing exercises, and segmental expansion of the thorax should be utilized. Relaxation and positioning for comfort also help to diminish patient anxiety, slow spontaneous respirations, and generally conserve energy by decreasing the work of breathing.

Mechanical ventilation is not a contraindication to percussion and vibration. Percussion may be performed during all phases of the respiratory cycle, whereas vibration should be performed only on the expiratory phase (it is even more effective following a mechanical or assisted breath, which will have a larger volume).

Suctioning is more effective when performed by two people. One person bags and vibrates while the other suctions (see earlier section on suctioning). Passive or active range of motion is routinely performed on ventilated patients, with monitoring equipment being employed to judge whether the exercises are too strenuous. The therapist watches for increased heart rate greater than 20 beats per minute over the resting rate, blood pressure changes, and decreases in oxygen saturation. Transfers, standing, marching in place, and even ambulation may all be performed with the ventilated patient when appropriate safeguards are taken.

Patients on mechanical ventilation have more peripheral lines and monitoring devices attached than other patients, so great care must be taken not to dislodge or interrupt any of these systems in rolling them from side to side. The therapist should also be aware of the effects of position changes on the various monitoring devices and their readings. For example, rolling a patient onto the side into which a pulmonary artery catheter is inserted may advance the catheter and change the waveform, indicating that the patient should be returned to a resting position. In rolling a patient with many peripheral lines or devices, the therapist should assist the patient from the side from which the majority of the lines originate. Rolling the patient away from the therapist (with the side rail of the bed raised on the side toward which the patient is rolling) may be indicated, depending on the location of the monitoring devices. A therapist who is close to these devices can protect the lines from being dislodged or moved.

The therapist should consider the position of the artificial airway and its attachment to the ventilator tubing when rolling the patient. The ventilator tubing; the attachment to the external, rigid section of the airway; and the softer, heat-malleable internal portion of the airway can present a sort of crank-handle configuration. Turning the external segments can create a painful torsion on the inner part of the system that is in place in the trachea. This problem can be prevented by always allowing sufficient slack when rolling away from the ventilator and making sure that the tubing attachment (the circuit) is allowed to swivel freely (Fig. 15–15).

In addition, water from humidification collects in the ventilation tubing and should be cleared out at regular intervals and *always* before rolling the patient. When rolling the patient to the side away from the ventilator, the danger is always present that this water will move and be introduced into the trachea and smaller airways. To remove the water, the ventilator is detached from the patient at the juncture of the airway and tubing. The tubing is then stretched out (thus removing water from the corrugations in the tubing), and the water is allowed to drain into a bottle or container used for this purpose. Water is always emptied from the distal end of the tube, never back into the heater or humidification canister. This procedure should only take 10 to 20 seconds to complete and should not compromise the patient's respiratory status. If fear exists of respiratory compromise, the patient may be ventilated manually with an Ambu bag by a second person (Fig. 15–16).

Before beginning treatment, the therapist should reset the visual alarm on the ventilator. Alarm lights on most ventilators remain lit even after the cause for the alarm has been resolved. Many ventilators have a visual reset button. This button merely resets or primes the alarm system. By clearing the system, it is easier for the therapist to identify and rectify the problem when the alarm is activated during treatment. In general, a physical therapist should *never* adjust settings on the ventilator.

The therapist should also be aware of the complications or emergencies that can occur in a mechanically ventilated patient and the measures that can be implemented. Situations that trigger the high-pressure alarm of the ventilator may occur during huffing techniques, tracheal or bronchial obstruction by a mucous plug or blood

Figure 15–15.

Positioning a mechanically ventilated patient in a side-lying position, facing away from the ventilator. Note the roll to help the patient maintain position.

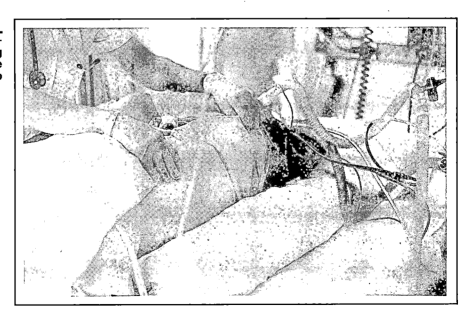

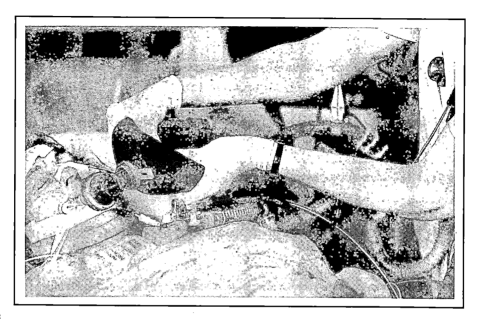

Figure 15-16.

Physical therapist preoxygenates a patient with an Ambu bag before suctioning.

clot, kinking or obstruction in the ventilator tubing, pneumothorax, or migration of the endotracheal tube into one of the mainstem bronchi. A leak in the ventilator tubing or around the cuff, a ventilator malfunction, or the development of a **tracheoesophageal fistula** triggers the low-pressure alarm. Obviously some of these situations can be remedied easily by the therapist whereas others are true medical emergencies. Physical examination of the patient and evaluation of the mechanical system help the therapist take appropriate action or summon assistance.

Considerations in Weaning from Mechanical Ventilation

Before removing a patient from a mechanical ventilator, a period of weaning or gradual diminution and withdrawal of the support system is necessary. The physician's decision to begin weaning is based on the attainment of certain physiologic and mechanical criteria.

One of the major criteria in determining if a patient is ready to begin weaning is when the problem necessitating mechanical ventilation is

resolved and the patient is medically stable. This may be determined by improvement in the patient's arterial blood gases. The patient should also be reasonably awake and alert.

Criteria for weaning that concern the mechanics of ventilation are

- a minute ventilation less than 10 liters per minute
- a respiratory rate between 12 and 20 per minute
- a vital capacity greater than 15 milliliters per kilogram of body weight
- an ability to generate a negative inspiratory force between -20 and -25 cm H_2O.[6,15,16]

In terms of oxygenation, the patient should have a Pa_{O_2} greater than 60 mm Hg with an FI_{O_2} no greater than 0.4, and the Pa_{CO_2} should be at or near normal levels for that patient[6,15,16] (patients with COPD have chronically elevated Pa_{CO_2} levels). Electrolyte and acid-base abnormalities should be resolved, and the patient's nutritional status should be optimal before beginning the process. In addition, the patient must be prepared psychologically for the process and must be reassured that mechanical ventilation is available if fatigue becomes a problem and spontaneous ventilation cannot be sustained.

Methods of Weaning

The process of weaning begins with gradual withdrawal of ventilatory support. This entails changing the mode of operation of the ventilator from more mechanical settings to a mode that allows the patient to breathe spontaneously with minimal support. An example of this would be changing the mode from **assist-control** to synchronized intermittent mandatory ventilation at a rate of 10 breaths per minute (this rate would be reduced to 4 breaths per minute over several hours), and finally placing the patient on **continuous positive airway pressure** (see Chapter 11 for explanations of these ventilator modes).

The patient who tolerates the initial weaning process well can then be removed from mechanical ventilation altogether for a short period of time with supplemental oxygen supplied through the endotracheal or tracheostomy tube. This may be done with a T-tube attachment (Fig. 15–17) for an endotracheal tube or a tracheostomy collar for a tracheostomy tube (Fig. 15–18). (A T-tube should not be used with a tracheostomy because T-tubes are too rigid, and movement by the patient can create torsion that is reflected back to the internal portion of the tracheostomy tube.)

The weaning process may proceed very quickly, particularly if the patient has been on mechanical ventilation for only a short period of time. Patients who take longer to wean may alternate periods of breathing spontaneously for progressively longer periods of time with rest periods on

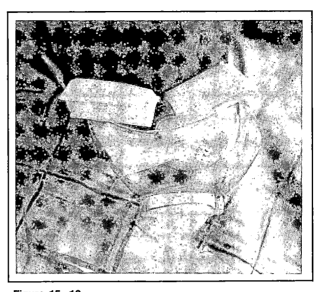

Figure 15–18.

A tracheostomy tube in place with a tracheostomy collar supplying supplemental oxygen.

a low synchronized intermittent mandatory ventilation setting or continuous positive airway pressure. In some cases pressure support or mandatory minute ventilation is employed as a weaning adjunct. Generally speaking, the longer a patient is dependent on mechanical ventilation, the longer and more involved the weaning process will be.

The airways must be kept free of secretions during the process, and the patient must be positioned comfortably. Incentive spirometry and breathing exercises may be incorporated into the process as the patient gains strength. These help build strength and endurance in the respiratory muscles.

Assessment of the Process

The patient's vital signs and arterial blood gases are monitored frequently during the weaning process. The patient is also observed for signs of fatigue or respiratory distress.

In the initial period of weaning, the patient's Pa_{CO_2} may increase because weaning involves hypoventilation (relative to mechanical ventilation). The Pa_{CO_2} should return to more normal levels as the process progresses.

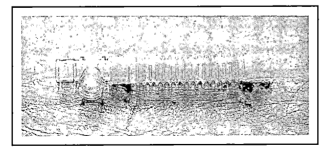

Figure 15–17.

A T-tube.

Complications that occur in weaning include right to left shunting and a drop in cardiac output. Atelectasis resulting from hypoventilation may cause right to left shunt (perfusion of unventilated areas of the lung indicated by an increasing $P(A-a)_{O_2}$). Cardiac output may drop because of the increased work on the cardiovascular system. Blood pressure must be carefully monitored during weaning. Oxygen consumption also increases because of this increased work of breathing. The FI_{O_2} may have to be increased accordingly.[6]

The Role of the Cardiopulmonary Physical Therapist in the Process of Weaning

The physical therapist is vital in helping to clear secretions during the weaning process. Breathing exercises taught by the physical therapist are helpful in gaining back strength and reexpanding atelectatic areas. In addition, the therapist helps to provide the reassurance and emotional support that are essential.

SPECIAL CONSIDERATIONS RELATED TO DIFFERENT AGE GROUPS

The cardiopulmonary physical therapist treats a wide range of pulmonary (and associated) problems in a population that encompasses all ages. Each age group, from neonate to geriatric, has unique characteristics that may predispose them to or may complicate pulmonary pathologic conditions. These characteristics may also necessitate changes and modifications in treatment plans and techniques.

Pediatric patients present different types of challenges. They are sometimes difficult to engage and to interest in treatment. Alternative strategies to accomplish the goals are needed. For example, for certain age groups or individuals blowing soap bubbles may be more fun than incentive spirometry; both increase ventilation. Some conditions common to pediatric patients are asthma, pneumonia, cystic fibrosis, and some

of the neuromuscular or restrictive conditions. The principles of treatment are basically the same as those for the adult surgical or nonsurgical patient, but treatment may also include instructing the parents or family members to provide certain parts of the patient's pulmonary care.

Considerations with geriatric patients range from precautions for physical conditions such as osteoporosis to strategies for dealing with dementia.

Care of the Neonate

The therapist may be called upon to treat patients in the neonatal intensive care unit. The physical therapist working in this area should be well trained in developmental theory and handling of infants as well as in the principles of cardiopulmonary physical therapy. Because of the size of the patient and the complexity of the monitoring and life-support equipment, rendering treatment to a neonate in the intensive care unit can be a complicated and anxiety-inducing task. The principles of treatment, however, remain the same for all patients.

The neonate differs anatomically and physiologically from the adult in ways that affect cardiopulmonary function (Table 15–3). Cardiopulmonary dysfunction in the neonate is associated with a variety of causes.

Immaturity

Idiopathic respiratory distress syndrome, also called **hyaline membrane disease,** is the most prevalent pulmonary pathologic condition in the newborn. It is caused by a deficiency in surfactant, which results in alveolar collapse. Oxygenation, thermal regulation, nutritional support, and continuous positive airway pressure are important elements of treatment. Postural drainage with manual techniques may also be indicated.

Adverse Events

Meconium aspiration syndrome results from aspiration of the dark, sticky fecal material that

TABLE 15–3. Anatomic and Physiologic Differences between the Neonatal and Adult Pulmonary System	
Anatomic	**Physiologic**
1. High larynx 2. Enlargement of lymphatic tissue 3. Five percent of the alveolar surface area of the adult 4. Decreased airway diameter and structural support 5. Decreased collateral ventilation 6. Circular rib cage configuration makes diaphragm inefficient	1. Decreased lung compliance 2. Irregular respiratory patterns are normal in neonates 3. Increase rate rather than depth of respiration in response to difficulty in respiration 4. Diaphragm more susceptible to fatigue because of the distribution of types of muscle fibers

accumulates in utero. Meconium aspiration may cause **pneumonitis** or airway obstruction. Suctioning and postural drainage with manual techniques are essential.

Perinatal Asphyxia

Perinatal asphyxia may result in central nervous system damage, which, in turn, may result in hypoventilation and airway obstruction. Some possible causes are umbilical cord compression, placental insufficiency, and excessive maternal anesthesia. Low **APGAR scores** (adaptability, partnership, growth, affection, resolve) at 1 minute following birth may indicate a problem. Treatment is supportive. Continuous positive airway pressure and postural drainage with manual techniques are important elements in management.

Surgery

The pulmonary complications of surgery have been discussed earlier in this chapter, and these same principles hold true for the infant. Because of the anatomic and physiologic differences and vulnerabilities in the neonate, the effects of those complications may be heightened. Postural drainage with manual techniques and positioning for comfort and to facilitate reexpansion of collapsed lung tissue are very important.

Iatrogenic Complications

Bronchopulmonary dysplasia is a condition strongly associated with the use of mechanical

ventilation with positive airway pressure and oxygen therapy (see Chapter 6). The child presents with signs and symptoms similar to those of idiopathic respiratory distress syndrome. A chronic stage results, with atelectasis, emphysema, and cystic changes being evident. Lower respiratory tract infections are common, and postural drainage with manual techniques as well as segmental expansion and breathing (retraining) exercises are often indicated.

Assessment of the Neonate

Assessment of the infant should include a complete history of labor and delivery and APGAR scores as well as all of the elements of the history and clinical condition applicable to the older child or adult. Some special considerations in assessing the neonate follow.

- Chest configuration—Barrel chest may be secondary to air trapping whereas funnel chest (pectus excavatum) or depression of the sternum may be due to prolonged periods of sternal retractions.
- Skin color—Cyanosis or pallor (mottling or webbing of the skin) may be associated with distress or hypoxemia.
- Breathing pattern—Keeping in mind that irregular patterns are normal, the therapist would look for tachypnea or apnea, which are signs of distress (40 breaths per minute is normal).
- Auscultation—This procedure should be done with the head in midline position when possible.
- Palpation—This technique has a limited application but may be useful in detecting subcutaneous emphysema.

● Percussion—This procedure may not be appropriate; when indicated it is done with one finger directly on the thorax.

Some clinical signs of respiratory distress that may be evident in the infant:

● Retractions—suprasternal, subcostal, substernal, or intercostal
● Nasal flaring
● Expiratory grunting
● **Stridor** (a high-pitched "crowing" sound heard on inspiration)
● Head bobbing
● Bulging of intercostal muscles

Treatment of the Neonate

Postural Drainage

Postural drainage with manual techniques and suctioning is the major element of bronchial hygiene for neonates. Because of the complexity of the situation and the fragility of the patient, treatment is not administered randomly, nor is it prescribed for all patients, because studies have shown that handling of infants and performance of routine tasks such as position changes and feedings can result in hypoxemia and increased oxygen consumption. The *need* for chest physical therapy must be clearly established and then weighed against precautions, contraindications, and possible complications.

Percussion

Percussion may be performed manually (by fitting and cupping one, three, or four fingers to the thorax) or with a percussor, medicine cup, or other device such as a rubber nipple that has been adapted for the purpose. Absolute contraindications to percussion for neonates include poor tolerance of treatment (as evidenced by decreased Po_2 measured transcutaneously), rib fracture, or hemoptysis. Precautions include presence of a chest tube, coagulopathy, poor skin condition, and cardiac arrhythmias.

Vibration

Vibration may be used more widely than percussion because it is generally better tolerated. Vibration may also be done manually or with devices adapted to the task (e.g., a padded electric toothbrush). Contraindications to treatment include untreated **tension pneumothorax,** intolerance of treatment (see earlier), and hemoptysis. Precautions include increased irritability during treatment, apnea, or bradycardia.

Positioning

Positioning of infants during treatment should also be considered on an individual basis, with the contraindications and precautions for each position strictly observed. The prone and head-down (Trendelenburg's) positions are contraindicated in certain situations such as untreated tension pneumothorax. Precautions for these positions include an abdominal incision or an anterior chest tube for the prone position and signs of acute respiratory distress (see earlier), heart failure, or cardiac dysrhythmias for the head-down position.

For a more detailed presentation of cardiopulmonary physical therapy for the neonate, the reader is referred to other references.[17,18]

SUMMARY

● Greater care must be taken in treating a patient with a pulmonary artery catheter. Chest percussion should be done cautiously, and waveform changes should be monitored.
● When pulmonary artery wedge pressure rises above 12 mm Hg, the patient should not be placed horizontal because this position increases venous return.
● The arterial line measures blood pressure and can be altered by the patient's position. Relative or absolute flexion of the wrist produces an erroneous reading.
● Rolling a patient with a central venous line to the side (particularly to the left) may advance the central venous line internally and trigger premature ventricular contractions.

- Chest percussion may produce artifact on the electrocardiographic telemetry and give false evidence of an elevated heart rate.
- A significant drop in arterial oxygen saturation may indicate that an activity is too strenuous for the patient or that the patient's cardiopulmonary function is inadequate to meet the demand.
- Atelectasis is often accompanied by a low-grade fever, whereas pneumonia or other infections may produce temperatures greater than 101 degrees F.
- The patient who has had upper abdominal or thoracic surgery is at increased risk for postoperative pulmonary complications, including atelectasis, pulmonary edema, lower respiratory tract infection, and ventilatory insufficiency.
- Inhaled anesthesia and high concentrations of oxygen temporarily alter the composition of surfactant as well as decrease the velocity of tracheal mucus.
- Preoperative teaching should begin with a brief discussion on the deleterious effects of anesthesia and the complications that physical therapy prevents, reverses, or both.
- One goal of treatment is to teach patients how to move themselves comfortably or to assist them in moving themselves.
- Significant changes in the rate and depth of respiration can be made simply by helping a patient become more comfortably positioned in the bed.
- The position of comfort for patients at highest risk for pulmonary complications is to have the head of the bed elevated 20 to 30 degrees and to place the knees and hips in a slightly flexed position.
- Treatments should be coordinated with the administration of pain medication.
- Percussion should be done cautiously in the presence of a pulmonary artery catheter and in patients with a history of prolonged corticosteroid treatment or with severe osteoporosis.
- Percussion is contraindicated in patients with platelet counts below 20,000 because of the risk of bleeding.
- As a general rule, any patient unable to clear secretions by coughing is a candidate for suctioning.
- Suctioning may be more effective when it is performed following postural drainage.
- The effectiveness of incentive spirometry is dependent on patient effort and correct usage of the device.
- There are five processes in the cough mechanism: deep inspiration, closure of glottis, contraction of chest and abdominal wall, opening of glottis, and forceful expulsion of air.
- Early mobility is stressed as a means of preventing postoperative complications such as atelectasis and pulmonary embolism.
- In the immediate postoperative period for coronary artery bypass graft surgery, percussion of the upper anterior thorax should be avoided.
- Ankle exercises are also important after coronary artery bypass graft surgery to prevent venostasis and help maintain an adequate cardiac output as well as to prevent deep venous thrombosis.
- Pulse oximetry is helpful in determining a need for supplemental oxygen or evaluating the efficacy of a system in use.
- When teaching breathing exercises, the exhalation should be roughly twice as long as the inspiration.
- Rapid, shallow respirations may sometimes be altered by instruction in diaphragmatic breathing with pursed-lip expiration.
- Dyspnea or the apprehension of developing dyspnea leaves pulmonary patients extremely anxious and impulsive.
- Resistive inspiratory muscle training is a treatment designed to strengthen and improve the endurance of the inspiratory muscles.
- Intermittent positive-pressure breathing provides a breath with positive pressure to supplement or assist the patient's inspiratory effort.
- When the patient's cough is ineffective, the therapist may provide a manual assist to forced expiration. The most basic assisted cough is done while the patient is supine.
- Before beginning ambulation, the patient's heart rate, rhythm, blood pressure, and oxygen saturation should be recorded.
- A projected sequence or progression of treatment for a nonsurgical patient may include the following elements: evaluation, postural drainage, breathing exercises, breathing retraining, active exercise of the extremities, and gait training.
- The airways of mechanically ventilated patients should be kept clear to ensure optimal ventilation of all areas of the lung.

- In general, a physical therapist should never adjust settings on the ventilator.
- Some clinical signs of respiratory distress that may be evident in the infant include retractions, nasal flaring, expiratory grunting, stridor, head bobbing, and bulging of intercostal muscles.

References

1. Jenkins SC. Pre-operative and post-operative physiotherapy—Are they necessary? In: Pryor JA (ed). International Perspectives in Physical Therapy 7: Respiratory Care. New York, Churchill Livingstone, 1991, pp 147–148.
2. Peper EA, Conrad SA. Respiratory complications of surgery and thoracic trauma. In: George RB, Light RW, Matthay MA, Matthay RA (eds). Chest Medicine: Essentials of Pulmonary and Critical Care Medicine. 2nd ed. Baltimore, Williams & Wilkins, 1990, pp 453–454.
3. Allen SJ. Respiratory considerations in the elderly patient. Clin Anesth 4:899–930, 1986.
4. Forshag MS, Cooper AD. Postoperative care of the thoracotomy patient. In: Buchalter SE, McElvein RB (eds). Clinics in Chest Medicine: Thoracic Surgical Considerations for the Pulmonologist. Philadelphia, WB Saunders, March 1992, pp 33–45.
5. Marfatia S, Donahue PK. Effect of dry and humidified gases on the respiratory epithelium in rabbits. J Paed Surj 10:583–592, 1975.
6. White GC. Basic Clinical Lab Competencies for Respiratory Care: An Integrated Approach. New York, Delmar Publishers, 1988.
7. O'Donahue WJ. National survey of the usage of lung expansion modalities for the prevention and treatment of postoperative atelectasis following abdominal and thoracic surgery. Chest 87(1):76–80, 1985.
8. Pryor JA. The forced expiration technique. In: Pryor JA (ed). International Perspectives in Physical Therapy 7: Respiratory Care. New York, Churchill Livingstone, 1991, pp 79–100.
9. Regan K, Kleinfeld ME, Castle Erik P. Physical therapy for patients with abdominal or thoracic surgery. In: Irwin S, Tecklin JS (eds). Cardiopulmonary Physical Therapy. 2nd ed. St. Louis, CV Mosby, 1990, p 341.
10. Villarino ME, Beck-Sague C, Jarvis WR. Aids, infection control, and employee health: Considerations in rehabilitation medicine. In: Mukand J (ed). Rehabilitation for Patients with HIV Disease. New York, McGraw-Hill, 1991, pp 371–392.
11. Neiderman MS, Sarosi GA. Respiratory tract infections. In: George RB, Light RW, Matthay MA, Matthay RA (eds). Chest Medicine: Essentials of Pulmonary and Critical Care Medicine. 2nd ed. Baltimore, Williams & Wilkins, 1991, pp 307–352.
12. Ellestad MM. Stress Testing: Principles and Practice. 3rd ed. Philadelphia, FA Davis, pp 56–57.
13. American Association of Cardiovascular and Pulmonary Rehabilitation. Guidelines for Cardiac Rehabilitation Programs. Champaign, Ill, Human Kinetics, 1991, p 12.
14. Tisi GM. The physiologic basis of ventilator use. In: Burton GG, Gee GN, Hodkin J (eds). Respiratory Care: A Guide to Clinical Practice. Philadelphia, JB Lippincott, 1977, pp 543–545.
15. Matthay MA, Hopewell PC. Acute respiratory failure. In: George RB, Light RW, Matthay MA, Matthay RA (eds). Chest Medicine: Essentials of Pulmonary and Critical Care Medicine. 2nd ed. Baltimore, Williams & Wilkins, 1990, pp 413–437.
16. Bowser MA, Hodgkin JE, Burton GG. Techniques of ventilator weaning. In: Burton GG, Gee GN, Hodgkin JE (eds). Respiratory Care: A Guide to Clinical Practice. Philadelphia, JB Lippincott, 1977, pp 664–671.
17. Crane LB, The neonate and child. In: Frownfelter DL (ed). Chest Physical Therapy and Pulmonary Rehabilitation: An Interdisciplinary Approach. 2nd ed. Chicago, Year Book Medical Publishers, 1987, pp 666–697.
18. Crane LD. Physical therapy for the neonate with respiratory disease. In: Irwin S, Tecklin JS (eds). Cardiopulmonary Physical Therapy. 2nd ed. St. Louis, CV Mosby, 1990, pp 389–415.

16 CARDIAC REHABILITATION

INTRODUCTION

In 1952, Levine and Lown demonstrated that early mobilization of the acute coronary patient to activity reduced complications and mortality.[1] Since then physicians have increasingly realized the benefits of early rehabilitative measures. Physical conditioning can improve heart rate response, arterial blood pressure response in hypertensives, myocardial oxygen uptake, and maximum cardiac output.[2] In addition, improvements in the peripheral circulation, the pulmonary ventilation, and the autonomic nervous system benefit one's tolerance for work. Accompanying these physical improvements are greater emotional stability and self-esteem.

Early mobilization of stable individuals after a cardiac event has become a well-established

633

practice. The time course of care for coronary disease is changing dramatically owing to early diagnostic testing and new interventions. Although rest is important to the impaired myocardium, optimal improvement of the patient requires redefinition of the degree and duration of rest. No longer is the patient lying in bed for weeks at a time. The average coronary artery bypass patient is ambulating on the unit by day 3 at the latest. After myocardial infarction, patients are usually moved out of the intensive care unit and into the stepdown unit within 72 hours and often are discharged 1 to 2 days later. Patients are no longer encouraged to seek alternative lifestyles or contemplate early retirement as a result of coronary disease. They are no longer spectators, but rather active participants, often more active and healthier in life after a cardiac event than before.

This chapter describes the various inpatient and outpatient phases of the cardiac rehabilitation program. It also identifies which patient groups are appropriate candidates for rehabilitation and under what conditions rehabilitation is most beneficial. Case studies exemplifying many of the concepts outlined in this chapter are also presented.

DEFINITIONS

Cardiac rehabilitation is a multidisciplinary program of education and exercise established to assist individuals with heart disease in achieving optimal physical, psychological, and functional status within the limits of their disease. This program includes

- education of the patient and family in the recognition, prevention, and treatment of cardiovascular disease
- amelioration or reduction of risk factors
- dealing with the psychological factors that influence recovery from heart disease
- structured, progressive physical activity, either in a rehabilitation setting or home program
- vocational counseling

The **cardiac rehabilitation center** is the facility in which an interdisciplinary team provides the planned and monitored program to promote physical, psychological, educational, and vocational improvement of the cardiac patient. Ideally, the center has classroom space for group patient education, private counseling facilities, and a library for educational materials. Exercise space should allow freedom of movement for warm-up and cool-down exercises and perhaps should have cameras to monitor patients in hallways and around blind corners. The facility should be easily accessible, pleasant, and clean —qualities that are important to boost morale and to support patient compliance. The facility may also be combined with a sports medicine or fitness facility to increase use and decrease costs. The following patient groups are referred to these facilities:

- **Uncomplicated myocardial infarction** (low-risk subset) usually refers to those patients with small to moderate size infarcts clinically. By the end of the fourth day post infarct, this group is defined by the absence of continuing ischemia, left ventricular failure, shock, serious arrhythmias, conduction disturbances, and other serious illness.[16] Approximately 75% of patients are in this category (Table 16–1).
- **Uncomplicated high risk** (moderate-risk subset) refers to patients who are considered uncomplicated and at low risk initially but later manifest poor ventricular function and cardiac reserve; or they have significant ischemia with low-level activity and require reclassifying as high risk.
- **Complicated myocardial infarction** (high-risk subset) is designated by the presence of one or more conditions listed as absent in uncomplicated myocardial infarction. In general, this occurs in patients who have large infarctions,

TABLE 16–1. Complicating Factors after Myocardial Infarction	
Low-risk subset	None by day 4
Moderate-risk subset (beyond day 4)	Poor ventricular function
	Significant ischemia with low-level activity
High-risk subset	Continued ischemia
	Left ventricular failure
	Shock
	Serious arrhythmias

high-grade subtotal occlusion proximally in two or three coronary vessels, or both. Some of these patients may stabilize after several days and warrant a change in management to uncomplicated status.

The previous classification of patient groups may also be used for patients who have undergone bypass surgery or have other cardiac disease that is not directly due to myocardial infarction. Several key features of exercise testing help to identify these moderate- and high-risk groups, including

- short test duration—inability to complete stage I of the Bruce protocol
- systolic blood pressure during exercise of less than 130 mm Hg[4]

- marked ST-T-segment depression at low workloads[5]
- serious life-threatening arrhythmia

Arrhythmias include ventricular tachycardia (four consecutive premature ventricular complexes); ventricular fibrillation; persistent atrial tachycardia or fibrillation; and multifocal, paired or R-on-T premature ventricular complexes.

Significant ischemia is indicated by 1.0- to 1.5-millimeter horizontal or downsloping ST depression, classic angina, or both (Fig. 16–1).

Exercise testing refers to a monitored, multilevel cardiovascular evaluation, usually performed using a treadmill or bicycle ergometer.

Exercise prescription refers to the instructions given to a patient to develop optimal physical

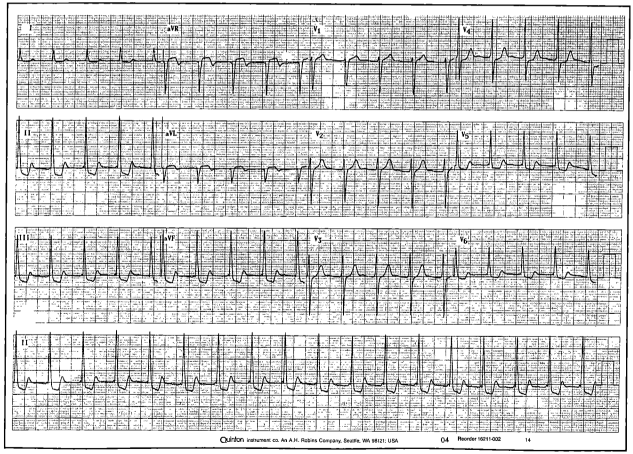

Figure 16–1.

Typical 12-lead electrocardiogram tracing. Tracings should be assessed for the presence of significant ischemia.

ability in daily living activities, work, and recreation. This prescription usually includes mode, intensity, frequency, and duration of activity. The data used to establish this prescription are from the results of the exercise test and are coordinated with findings from the laboratory tests and the patient's history and physical examination, activity requirements, and classification of risk status.

EQUIPMENT

The safe operation of any cardiac rehabilitation program relies on the proper maintenance of all basic and emergency equipment. All staff should be familiar with the proper use of all emergency equipment. The size and location of the facility may dictate the type and amount of exercise equipment that are available (Table 16–2).

THE CARDIAC REHABILITATION TEAM

Successful cardiac rehabilitation programs emphasize an interdisciplinary approach with team members contributing to all phases of patient assessment and direct patient care. Personnel and rehabilitative activities are under the direction of an advisory board and a medical director. The number of team members, as well as the role and function of each, may vary from center to center. Some facilities may have one person performing more than one function. In all cases, primary patient care remains the responsibility of the referring physician. Typical members of the cardiac rehabilitation program are the following:

- *Cardiac rehabilitation advisory board:* The role of this group is to establish all policy for the program. The board is usually composed of the medical staff representatives who have interest in rehabilitation and exercise, the medical and administrative directors, and the program coordinator.
- *Attending physician:* This individual is the long-term cardiac rehabilitation therapist for the patient and must carry on the work started by the rehabilitation team. The physician remains in charge of the patient during the program. This physician should receive reports from the team at successive stages of the program and is encouraged to participate within the structure of the program. Follow-up contact with the patient after the program is completed is another key function of this individual.
- *Medical director:* This individual, who is responsible for the overall effectiveness and safety of the program, is a physician with a special interest in exercise pathophysiology and training. The medical director works closely with the program coordinator and other members of the team and is available for consultation with team members, referring physicians, the media, and others.
- *Program coordinator:* A professional skilled in personnel and team management, the program coordinator oversees all team personnel and facilities. This individual develops and revises policy, procedures, and budgets; selects needed equipment; is responsible for coordinating and supervising staff; and works with other departments or facilities to evaluate the program needs. This individual may be a

TABLE 16–2. Basic and Emergency Equipment	
Basic Equipment	**Emergency Equipment**
Blood pressure cuffs and mercury sphygmomanometers (mercury sphygmomanometers are preferred owing to ease of calibration, accuracy, and long-lasting components) Dual-head (bell and diaphragm) stethoscopes Telemetry monitoring with strip chart recorder Exercise equipment—bicycle ergometers, treadmills, arm ergometers, rowing machines, pulleys, free weights, track, four-extremity ergometers Wall clock with second hand	Defibrillator with monitor Emergency medications, airway maintenance supplies, artificial respirator, suction machine, and the like (see American Heart Association, Advanced Cardiac Life Support, American College of Sports Medicine Guidelines) Oxygen and supplies for oxygen administration First aid equipment Communication system (telephone)

physical therapist, registered nurse, or other appropriate allied health professional with administrative leadership qualities.

- *Professional skilled in exercise training:* The person who fills this position is a professional knowledgeable in exercise physiology, pathology, exercise training techniques, monitoring equipment, arrhythmia recognition, cardiopulmonary resuscitation, and advanced cardiac life support (including defibrillation). Commitment to a healthy lifestyle is necessary because this person is a role model for patients and other staff members. The preparation and training of physical therapists make them the ideal professional group for this position. However, in many programs, registered nurses and exercise physiologists fill this role.
- *Dietitian:* A professional knowledgeable in nutrition assessment and counseling, a dietitian also is experienced in dietary planning and modification.
- *Behavior specialist:* This person must be a professional skilled in behavioral evaluation and counseling techniques who is familiar with coping mechanisms, family patterns of interaction, and available community resources. A psychologist or medical social worker usually fills this position.

Goals of the Team

1. To prevent the harmful effects of prolonged bedrest when a patient is hospitalized with heart disease.

2. To develop cardiovascular fitness after acute illness, with an emphasis on optimal ability for employment and leisure.

3. To identify patients whose psychological response to cardiac disease may require extra support and additional measures for successful rehabilitation.

4. To accomplish the first three goals through interdisciplinary efforts directed at discovering each patient's optimal activity level, diet, and ability to improve unfavorable risk factors.

CANDIDACY

Beyond the typical postinfarction and coronary bypass groups, the population base for cardiac rehabilitation has grown to include individuals who at one time were thought not to be good candidates for rehabilitation. Therapists must be flexible in program planning, must address each patient's needs on an individual basis, and must provide services through a patient-oriented rather than a program-oriented approach. This is particularly important with the following groups:

- *Patients with poor ventricular function:* This group includes patients who have had large infarctions and cardiomyopathies and, in general, those who have congestive heart failure. It has been demonstrated by a number of investigators that exercise training is safe for these patients with "sick ventricles." In fact, they may show significant changes in both physical and functional work capacity (perhaps more than other groups) because they usually function at such a low level.[6,7,8] Lee and colleagues reported improvement in mean functional aerobic impairment (decreased from 32% to 24%) along with significantly lower ($p < 0.01$ and < 0.05, respectively) resting and submaximal heart rates in 25 men with ejection fractions less than 40% who were followed for an average of 18.5 months.[7] Coates and associates demonstrated similar improvement in physical work capacity, rate pressure product, and symptom scores in a group of 11 coronary patients who had very low ejection fractions (mean ejection fraction of 19%).[8] Neither of these studies found that exercise was detrimental to cardiovascular health.
- *Patients with healthy ventricles:* With the advent of more aggressive initial intervention (e.g., thrombolytic therapy and percutaneous transluminal coronary angioplasty), the degree of ventricular impairment after cardiac events has been limited substantially. Some individuals with unstable angina pectoris can be admitted to the hospital in the morning, undergo percutaneous transluminal coronary angioplasty the same day, and be discharged within 48 hours. Unfortunately, many patients are left wondering which activities are appropriate and safe and how much exercise is too much. Included in this group with healthy ventricles may be patients who have known coronary artery disease but who have not had a myocardial infarction as well as those who have undergone coronary artery bypass surgery and had no previous myocardial damage.

- *Follow-up patients:* A group emerging in the cardiac rehabilitation arena includes those who return to a local hospital after having undergone a technical cardiac procedure at a different facility or regional center. This group consists of patients who underwent cardiac transplantation, implantation of a cardiac defibrillator, or another sophisticated procedure.
- *Elderly patients:* An increasingly elderly population that is often more debilitated is being referred for physical conditioning and risk modification programs.
- *Asymptomatic at-risk patients:* These individuals have no known coronary disease but do demonstrate multiple major or minor risk factors, or both. This group is referred for preventive modes of treatment. Individuals in this group may also include the offspring of patients with coronary artery disease who have elevated cholesterol, a multiple risk factor profile, or both.

Individuals who are not considered to be good candidates for rehabilitation include

- patients who have overt congestive heart failure (see Chapter 4), unstable angina pectoris (chest pain at rest), hemodynamic instability (falling blood pressure with exercise), serious arrhythmia, conduction defects, or impaired function of other organ systems
- patients who have uncontrolled hypertension
- patients who have other disease or illness that precludes exercise
- apparently healthy individuals (mixing healthy individuals with persons who have heart disease may inhibit the former and frustrate the latter)

Efficacy of Cardiac Rehabilitation

Medically prescribed and supervised exercise as part of a comprehensive rehabilitation program is a well-accepted standard of care throughout the world for cardiac patients, particularly following an acute myocardial infarction or coronary revascularization procedure. The degree of benefit from cardiac rehabilitation programs as documented in the literature varies considerably. However, exercise rehabilitation has made a positive impact on several risk factors, functional

capacity, cardiovascular efficiency, and to some degree on cardiac mortality.[9]

Risk factors have been shown to be favorably affected by exercise training in individuals with and without cardiac conditions.[10–13] The benefits of exercise training include

- loss of excess weight
- lowering of lipid levels, including total cholesterol and triglycerides
- elevation of levels of high-density lipoproteins (HDLs)
- reduction of elevated blood pressure levels
- improvement in glucose-insulin dynamics

Heart rate, systolic blood pressure, and the rate pressure product are generally lower during submaximal efforts following exercise conditioning, resulting in reduced myocardial oxygen demand.[14,15] This is particularly important to patients with exertional ischemia. Reported improvements in symptom-limited, maximal oxygen consumption for patients with angina pectoris range from 32% to 56%.[14]

Reduction of physical work capacity is thought to be the result of the degree of myocardial damage, myocardial ischemia, or both. Patients with acute myocardial infarction and coronary bypass surgery have been shown to demonstrate significant improvement in aerobic capacity following exercise conditioning, on the order of 11% to 66%. The greatest improvements were found in patients with the lowest initial maximal oxygen consumption levels.[14,16,17] The specific cardiovascular adaptations that occur in coronary patients vary depending on the training stimulus and the duration of the program. Eshani and colleagues demonstrated an increase in ejection fraction, stroke volume, and rate pressure product during maximal exercise in post–myocardial infarction patients who were trained at intensities of at least 85% of maximal heart rate for at least 1 year in duration.[18] However, no matter what mechanism or physiologic adaptation takes place in trained coronary patients, an increase of aerobic capacity means increased tolerance for daily life activities consisting of repeated submaximal physical exertion. This translates into a potential for an improved quality of life.

A definitive randomized clinical trial on the

independent effect of exercise in prevention of recurrent coronary events in patients recovering from myocardial infarction, coronary bypass surgery, or angina pectoris has not been conducted. The ability of a single study to test the hypothesis that exercise reduces mortality from coronary heart disease would require a randomized trial of more than 4000 patients. The ability to control all of the variables in a single study is nearly impossible and certainly improbable. Nonetheless, several reports have attempted to demonstrate a reduced cardiac mortality rate based on combined data from several larger studies (meta-analysis) and have in fact shown some interesting trends and statistical significance with a reduction in mortality similar to the salvage rate attributed to beta-blocking drugs in clinical trials following a myocardial infarction.[19]

PHASES OF RECOVERY

Cardiac rehabilitation is typically organized in progressive phases of programming to meet the specific needs of individuals and their families in the acute (phase I), subacute (phase II), intensive rehabilitation (phase III), and ongoing rehabilitation (phase IV) phases of recovery.

Acute Phase — Phase I

Inpatient cardiac rehabilitation usually begins when a patient arrives in the stepdown unit but may commence at the bedside in the intensive or coronary care unit, especially if the individual must remain there for an extended period of time. The ability of a patient management team (e.g., physician, surgeon, nurse, physical therapist, dietitian, respiratory therapist) to function as a coordinated and cohesive group is critical to the patient's and the family's experience following infarction, bypass surgery, or other life-threatening cardiac event.

Increasing the patient's knowledge about the disease process and prognosis and instilling the necessary confidence to perform safely in the home and community when discharged are primary objectives of the inpatient cardiac rehabili-

tation program. Each team member must be cognizant of the clinical and individual indications of the personality differences of patients and their families. Team members must take a practical approach to discharge preparation so as not to make their instructions too complicated or too simple for the patient. The allied health team must be flexible to deal with the differences in the clinical management techniques of many physicians. These complications often make the "stepdown ladder" approach to cardiac care difficult, if not impossible. The goals of inpatient cardiac rehabilitation are

- evaluation of individual physiologic responses to self-care and ambulation activities. In the stepdown unit, patients are usually closely monitored by electrocardiogram (ECG) while at rest. However, the hemodynamic changes that can take place with position change, self-care activities, toileting, and the like are potentially dangerous and usually go unobserved or are not closely monitored.
- provision of feedback to physicians and nurses regarding the patient's response to activity so that recommendations for activity in the stepdown unit can be made. The cardiac rehabilitation assessment is worthless unless the results can be applied practically on the unit. Information should be shared by all nursing shifts and with all physicians involved in the patient's care.
- provision of safe guidelines for progression of activity throughout convalescence. A day-to-day reassessment of function, as well as hemodynamic and ECG responses to progressive activity, provides further information to the physician. This is especially important because it relates to decisions on medication adjustments and on preparation for discharge. To facilitate the team's effectiveness, an overall activity plan can be used for progression in phase I. The use of a six-step functional level guide is recommended to communicate a patient's readiness for activity or discharge (Table 16–3).
- provision of patient and family education with reference to disease entity, risk factors and appropriate modification, self-monitoring techniques, and general activity guidelines. It is most important to instill a sense of confidence about what the patient can do safely and what

TABLE 16–3. Functional Classification Guide for Inpatient Activities

Functional Class I	Functional Class II	Functional Class III	Functional Class IV	Functional Class V	Functional Class VI
Sits up in bed with assistance Does own self-care activities— seated, or may need assistance Stands at bedside with assistance Sits up in chair 15–30 minutes 2–3 times per day	Sits up in bed independently Stands independently Does own self-care activities in bathroom— seated Walks in room and to bathroom (may need assistance)	Sits and stands independently Does own self-care activities in bathroom, seated or standing Walks in halls with assistance short distances (50–100 ft) as tolerated, up to 3 times per day	Does own self-care and bathes Walks in halls short distances (150–200 ft) with minimal assistance, 3–4 times per day	Walk in halls independently, moderate distances (250–500 ft), 3–4 times per day	Independent ambulation on unit 3–6 times per day vs. as desired

to expect the rate of recovery to be regarding activity.

Initial Assessment

The initial assessment is conducted as soon as possible by each team member involved in the patient's care, usually within a few hours of referral and certainly within 24 hours. A quick response is important to the patient who is anticipating resuming activity, as well as to the medical and allied health care team who have only a short amount of time to work with the patient and family during the inpatient stay. The assessment should include a thorough chart re-

view, patient-family interview, physical examination, and self-care and ambulation assessment or screening.

● *Chart review*—to obtain information, a review of pertinent medical history; physician admission report and subsequent chart notes; surgical report, including cardiac catheterization data; medications; laboratory studies (e.g., cardiac enzymes, hemoglobin/hematocrit, lipid analysis); noninvasive studies (e.g., echocardiography, ECG, exercise tests, nuclear studies); nurses notes; physician orders, including those for activity and special instructions for cardiac rehabilitation; and any other pertinent data (e.g., age, home town, insurance provider, height, weight).

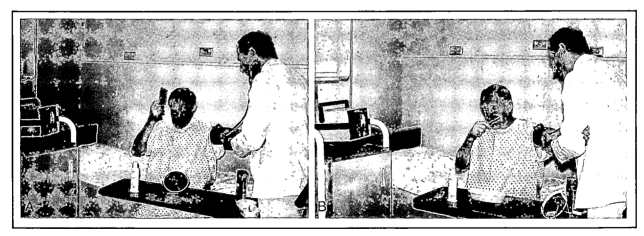

Figure 16–2.

The physical therapist monitors blood pressure responses while the patient performs typical activities of daily living.

● *Patient-family interview*—to gain a subjective description of symptoms and other problems; to assess the risk factor profile, diet profile, and patient-family goals; and to guide discharge disposition.

● *Physical examination*—to include assessment of vital signs (e.g., heart rate, blood pressure), auscultation of breath and heart sounds, chest wall inspection and palpation, examination of extremities (peripheral pulses, edema) and gross range of motion and strength.

● *Self-care and ambulation evaluation (activities of daily living [ADL] monitor)*—to monitor the patient's hemodynamic, symptomatic, and ECG response to typical self-care activities. This evaluation is performed one on one with a physical therapist and involves the use of a portable ECG monitor so the therapist can observe ECG changes as they occur when the patient becomes mobile (Fig. 16–2). Another option is to have a second person stationed at the central ECG monitors to observe any changes; however, a direct method of communication between therapist and observer must be available. Parameters to be measured during the evaluation include heart rate, blood pressure, ECG, and signs and symptoms. Each parameter is recorded at rest, with activity, immediately after the activity, and 1 to 3 minutes after the activity. Activities may include resting supine, sitting, standing, hygiene and grooming, Valsalva's maneuver (with nonsurgical patients), and lower and upper extremity dressing.

● *Ambulation activity*—to determine, in addition to the physiologic parameters, the patient's balance and coordination, level of independence, and distance traveled relative to normal ambulation velocity (Table 16–4). Response to stair climbing should be evaluated before discharge if the patient must negotiate stairs at home and is considered well enough to do so; however, this is not an activity to be performed early in the recovery phase (Fig. 16–3).

Activity Program Guidelines

Indications for an Unmodified Program. Patients who demonstrate appropriate hemodynamic, ECG, and symptomatic responses to the self-care and ambulation evaluation can have

their activity levels increased with the physician's approval. The rate of progression is individualized and adjusted to each patient's particular limitation, depending on many clinical and functional factors (e.g., complicated versus uncomplicated course, ventricular function, premorbid functional level, number of days on bedrest, philosophy of the referring physician). The physio-

TABLE 16–4. Normal Velocity 5-Meter Walk

		% Normal	
Seconds	Velocity m/min	Men (88.3 m/min)*	Women (80.1 m/min)*
3	100.0	113	125
3.5	85.7	97	107
4	75.0	85	94
4.5	66.6	76	83
5	60.0	68	75
5.5	54.6	62	68
6	50.0	57	62
6.5	46.2	52	58
7	42.9	49	54
7.5	40.0	45	50
8	37.5	43	47
9	33.3	38	42
10	30.0	34	37
11	27.3	31	34
12	25.0	28	31
13	23.1	26	29
14	21.4	24	27
15	20.0	23	25
16	18.8	21	23
17	17.7	20	22
18	16.7	19	21
19	15.8	18	20
20	15.0	17	19
21	14.3	16	18
22	13.6	15	17
23	13.0	15	16
24	12.5	14	16
25	12.0	13	15
26	11.5	13	14
27	11.1	13	14
28	10.7	12	13
29	10.3	12	13
30	10.0	11	12
31	10.0	11	12
32	9.4	11	12
33	9.1	10	11
34	8.8	10	11
35	8.6	10	11

* Normal velocity is based on data obtained in the Pathokinesiology Laboratory using footswitches. Distance: 6 meters; sample: 75 men, 107 women. (From Rancho Los Amigos Medical Center, Physical Therapy Department, Downey, Calif.)

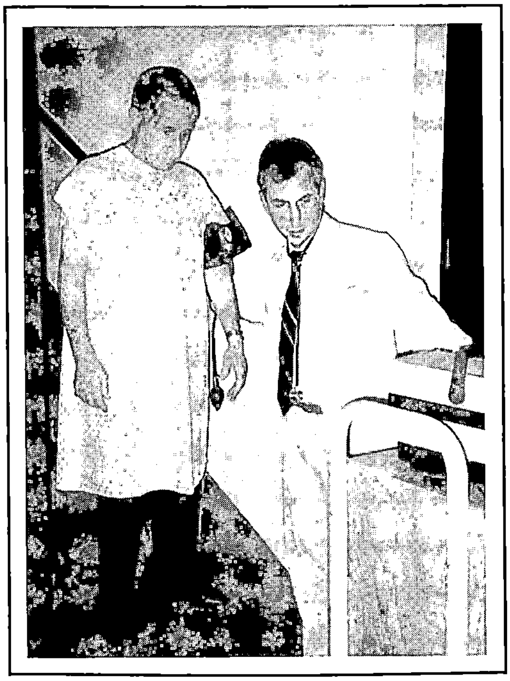

Figure 16-3.

Monitoring the electrocardiogram and blood pressure during stair climbing.

logic parameters of heart rate, blood pressure, signs and symptoms, ECG findings, and heart sounds continue to be monitored each session, with the results communicated when possible to the patient's nurse and always documented in the chart. Exercise periods are usually conducted twice daily, lasting approximately 10 minutes for patients on modified programs and 15 minutes for patients who have no limitations. Intensity of activity should be gauged by more than just heart rate limits and should be based on the patient's clinical status and medication regimen. Historically, heart rate levels up to 120 beats per minute (bpm) or 20 to 30 beats per minute above the resting rate have been used as guidelines; however, with the wide variety of rate-limiting medications, this method is not appropriate. It is the combination of all factors (hemodynamic, symptoms, and ECG findings) that must be considered in determining specific intensity parameters.

Indications for a Modified Program. Program parameters are modified for persons designated

as "complicated" for one or more of the following reasons:

● Large infarction clinically, although stable after 2 to 3 days
● Resting tachycardia (100 bpm) or inappropriate heart rate increase with self-care activities
● Blood pressure failing to rise or drop with self-care activities
● The ECG revealing more than 6 to 8 premature ventricular complexes per minute or progressive heart block with self-care activities
● Angina or undue fatigue with self-care activities
● Need for prolonged bedrest (more than 4 days)

Indications for Withholding a Program. The following are criteria to exclude patients from participation in the activity program:

● Severe pump failure (as evidenced by shortness of breath, peripheral edema, diaphoresis)
● Classification in a high-risk subset, described by
  ● recurrent malignant arrhythmias (ventricular tachycardia, four premature ventricular complexes in a row, ventricular fibrillation)
  ● angina at rest
  ● second- or third-degree heart block
  ● persistent hypotension (less than 90 mm Hg)
  ● rapid atrial rhythm
  ● unstable angina pectoris or change in symptoms in the preceding 24 hours

General Precautions

Before initiating each activity session, the patient's status should be reassessed. There *must* be a review of the patient's chart. The ECG monitor should be checked for any new changes and vital signs; cardiac rhythm, symptoms, and heart and lung sounds need to be rechecked. Activity sessions are not initiated within 1 hour after meals. This delay allows adequate digestion to occur without increased myocardial oxygen demand. It is also important to avoid isometric exercise, specifically breath holding with exercise, because it may produce dramatic changes in blood pressure and arrhythmias.

Relative Contraindications to Continuing Exercise

Whenever one of the following occurs, the event should be documented appropriately and the patient's nurse, physician, or both should be contacted immediately.

● Unusual heart rate increase—greater than 50 beats per minute increase with low-level activity
● Blood pressure indicative of hypertension—abnormally high systolic (greater than 210 mm Hg) or diastolic (greater than 110 mm Hg) pressure
● Drop in systolic blood pressure (greater than 20 mm Hg) with low-level exercise
● Symptoms with activity:
  ● angina (level 1 out of 4)—see Index of Anginal Levels (Table 16–5)
  ● undue dyspnea (level 2+/4+)—see Dyspnea Index (Table 16–6)
  ● excessive fatigue
  ● mental confusion or dizziness
  ● severe leg claudication—level 8/10 on a pain scale of 10/10
● Signs of pallor, cold sweat, ataxia
● Changing heart sounds with activity—new murmur or ventricular gallop
● An ECG abnormality, including marked ST changes (may be only a single event that requires notification, as well as a sustained event) or serious arrhythmias (development of coupled premature ventricular complexes or three in a row, second- or third-degree atrio-ventricular block, or intermittent rate–dependent conduction disturbance)

TABLE 16–6. Dyspnea Levels*

Level 0—Able to count to 15 easily (no additional breaths necessary)
Level 1—Able to count to 15 but must take one additional breath
Level 2—Must take two additional breaths to count to 15
Level 3—Must take three additional breaths to count to 15
Level 4—Unable to count

* The patient is asked to inhale normally and then to count out loud to 15 over a 7.5- to 8.0-second period. Any shortness of breath can be graded by levels, as shown in the table.
(From Physical Therapy Management of Patients with Pulmonary Disease, Ranchos Los Amigos Medical Center, Physical Therapy Department, Downey, Calif.)

Education Program Guidelines

The amount and type of information provided to patients and their families depend on a variety of factors, which include ability to follow directions, emotional stability after the cardiac event, and basic level of understanding and education. Considering the wealth of information they receive and the usual emotional fragility of the participants, it is best to keep information that patients and their families should retain in a neatly organized packet to which they can refer in the future. The instructions should be kept as simple as possible. It is particularly helpful to have the various team members coordinate their educational materials in one packet.

Any education plan should be specific to the individual's needs and particular risk factors. Almost all patients, and especially family members, are concerned about the prognosis of the disease, the foods they can or cannot eat, what to do in an emergency or if chest pain recurs, and what they can or cannot do physically when they get home. Concerns about acceptable activity usually include sexual activity, although many individuals do not verbalize this concern.

It is no one person's responsibility to provide all the information, but rather that of each team member within the particular specialty area. The educational component should include, but not be limited to, discussions about

TABLE 16–5. Angina Levels—An Individual's Subjective Response to Discomfort

Level 1—First perception of discomfort or pain in the chest area; this does not require one to stop physical activity
Level 2—Discomfort that increases in intensity, extends in distribution, or both, but is tolerable; patient slows activity in an attempt to decrease angina level
Level 3—Severe chest pain that increases to intolerable levels; patient must stop activity, take nitroglycerin, or both
Level 4—The most severe pain imaginable (infarction-like pain)

(From Physical Therapy Management of Cardiac Patients, Ranchos Los Amigos Medical Center, Physical Therapy Department, Downey, Calif.)

- the particular disease process and prognosis—usually discussed by the patient's physician and reinforced by nursing and other allied health team members
- the individual's risk factors and recommendations for behavior modification—usually performed by team members relative to their impact on the problem
- general activity guidelines and home exercise prescription—performed by the physical therapist with specific input from the physician
- the role of exercise—performed by the physical therapist and reinforced by other team members
- medications (especially the use of nitroglycerin)—performed by the physician, nurse, or pharmacist and reinforced by other team members
- nutrition and prescribed diet—performed by the physician and dietitian
- self-monitoring techniques—according to the patient's ability (usually based on symptom-limited response because heart rate may be difficult or inappropriate for patients to learn to monitor at this time) and performed by the physician, nurse, and physical therapist
- what to do in an emergency

Audiovisual aids (e.g., videos, books) are helpful for patients and family and may be left with them for a time when they are most alert, rested, and prepared to hear the message being presented. This is not always at the time when a team member comes by (Fig. 16–4).

Diet and Nutrition. Individual counseling by the dietitian with input from the attending physician usually begins during the inpatient stay. Specific problem areas such as hyperlipidemia, obesity, diabetes, and sodium restriction need to be addressed on an individual basis. Usually the person who prepares the meals at home wants to spend as much time as possible learning what they should or should not prepare. More specifics on this topic are discussed later in the chapter (Fig. 16–5).

Psychological Rehabilitation. Most patients experience some degree of fear, anxiety, depression, and anger that should be monitored. Psychologists, specialized clinical nurse practitioners, social workers, and others are often available to help patients deal with these problems. However, in day-to-day interactions with therapists, dietitians, and other cardiac rehabilitation team members, patients often more readily trust and look to these individuals for support in dealing with their disability. Patients need to be observed by all team members for any degree of denial or anxiety, which may be demonstrated in a variety of ways, such as anger, irritability, or conflict with different team members. Team

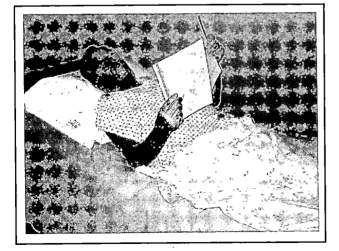

Figure 16–4.

A patient reviewing instructional materials.

Figure 16-5.

The dietitian giving instructions at the patient's bedside.

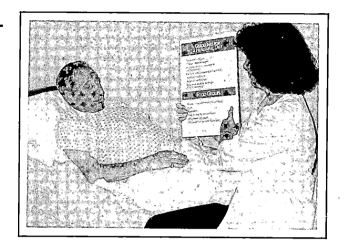

members should be alert for patients and family members who have a need for psychological intervention.

Discharge Planning

Patients and their families usually have some time to prepare for discharge, because discussions typically begin almost as soon as patients are admitted to the hospital. Certainly by the time patients reach the stepdown unit, the attending physician begins the process of planning for discharge. Cardiac rehabilitation team members should start presenting discharge information early rather than waiting until the day of discharge. This planning should include the following:

1. A review of general activity guidelines, exercise prescription, dietary regimen, medication regimen, and warning signs and symptoms and appropriate actions to be taken (Fig. 16-6).

2. A referral for the patient to the outpatient cardiac rehabilitation program for continued treatment, usually commencing within 2 to 3 days or as soon as possible. Patients who do not get referred immediately and do not have a date or time for return before discharge usually do not come back.

3. A low-level, symptom-limited exercise test for the patient before discharge. Most patients

can tolerate, and should undergo, an exercise tolerance test in a controlled environment to help identify those who are at high risk for repeat infarction or sudden death. The test also provides valuable information to the cardiac rehabilitation team in establishing discharge activity guidelines and prescription for exercise on return to the outpatient program (Fig. 16-7). It is also helpful to keep prepared "discharge packets"

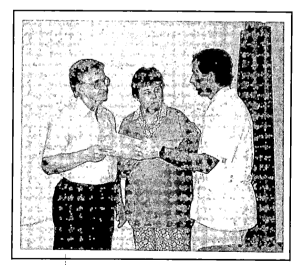

Figure 16-6.

The physical therapist reviews discharge recommendations with the patient (left) and spouse.

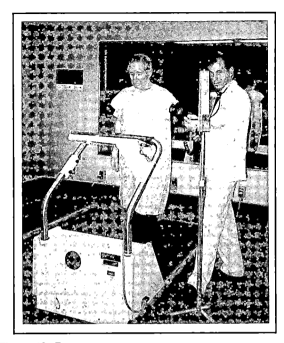

Figure 16–7.

A physical therapist conducting a low-level exercise test.

ready for distribution to patients when discharge is imminent. Table 16–7 summarizes the potential contents of such information packets.

OUTPATIENT PHASES—PHASES II, III, AND IV

Many approaches to outpatient cardiac rehabilitation exist, from large, multidisciplinary team approaches to smaller programs in which one person performs multiple functions. Although there are philosophic differences regarding frequency of activity, mode of exercise, monitoring,

TABLE 16–7. Discharge Packet Contents
Basic educational materials specific to the problem (e.g., basics of coronary artery disease, risk factors, angina pectoris)
Medication regimen
Activity guidelines
Dietary guidelines
Follow-up testing and physician appointments
Emergency procedures and phone numbers

and the like, the goals are generally the same. Ideally, the program begins within 48 to 72 hours following discharge from the hospital. Thus, problems that arise early after discharge can be sorted out, questions about care can be answered, and, most importantly, patients and their families can receive support from the staff and other patients. The goals of outpatient cardiac rehabilitation programs include

- provision of a flexible, individualized exercise program of the proper intensity to elicit improvement in the patient's cardiovascular fitness without exceeding the safe limits of exercise
- provision of a program that emphasizes patient education so that the individual can begin to understand the disease and to implement lifestyle changes
- provision of a program to enhance the confidence of patients with ischemic heart disease in their ability to work at safe, functional levels of activities
- provision of a program to aid the patient in personal risk factor reduction to help prevent new cardiovascular complications
- provision of a program that assists in and accelerates the return to work (most patients who have had an uncomplicated course should be able to return to work after no more than 2 months)
- promotion of psychological, behavioral, and educational improvement

The Essential Components of the Initial Assessment

The objective of the physical evaluation is to assess ventricular function (myocardial reserve, infarct size, or both; presence and severity of ischemia or serious arrhythmia, or both) as it relates to the ramifications of the disease state on the functional abilities of the patient. Components of the initial assessment include

- a thorough medical history
- a patient-family interview
- a physical examination
- an exercise test
- a blood chemistry panel

These are discussed in detail in Chapter 14 (Fig. 16–8).

Program Classification

For purposes of clarity, the initial or subacute outpatient period is classified as phase II; the higher level conditioning program as phase III; and the long-term conditioning program, sometimes referred to as a maintenance program, as phase IV. Phases II and III are usually based in a hospital because of the likelihood of dealing with higher risk patients and the potential need for emergency medical services; however, these services can be performed in independent practice settings with appropriate medical support systems. Reimbursement issues may dictate where these programs are carried out. Phase IV programs are often held outside the hospital setting in local YMCAs, community colleges, and the like. Recommendations are made regarding the usual length of time in each phase, but it must be stressed, especially for phase II and III programs, that they should last as long as the patient's symptoms indicate.

Subacute Phase of Rehabilitation — Phase II

This initial outpatient phase begins as early as 24 hours after discharge and lasts from 2 to 6 weeks. Frequency of visits depends on the patient's clinical needs, and most patients are seen twice a week and work on a 1 or 2 to 1 patient-to-staff ratio. During this phase, patients are monitored by ECG telemetry and are taught the basics of self-monitoring (e.g., heart rate, rating of perceived exertion [RPE], symptoms) , and proper exercise procedure (e.g., stretching, warm-ups, peak interval, and cool-down period). They also begin an activity program that becomes the basis for a home exercise program. Individual teaching regarding a patient's specific needs and a risk modification plan begins, with goals outlined by each team member. Any acute medical problems (e.g., change in symptoms, increased

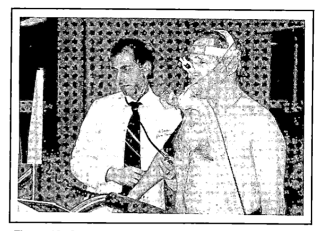

Figure 16–8.

Monitoring vital signs during an exercise test with expired gas analysis.

blood pressure, poor tolerance to medications) are reported immediately to the patient's physician. Only when patients demonstrate independence in performing self-monitoring techniques, are compliant with the home exercise program, are medically stable, and no longer require frequent ECG monitoring are they ready to begin phase III (Fig. 16–9).

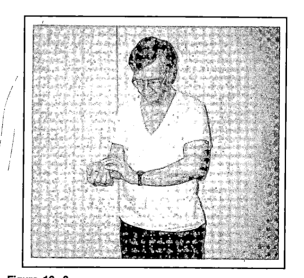

Figure 16–9.

A patient taking his own pulse as part of a self-monitoring instructional session.

TABLE 16–8. Patient Education Lectures —Phase III Rehabilitation
The heart and how it works
The role of exercise with heart disease
Low-fat and low-cholesterol diet
Modifying risk factors for heart disease
Stress and its effect on the heart
Medications
The role of sodium in the diet
Sexuality in patients with heart disease

Intensive Rehabilitation —Phase III

Patients are usually seen once a week, and phase III extends for approximately 6 to 8 weeks. Candidates are not only those completing the inpatient and subacute outpatient programs, but also other individuals who have heart disease or are at high risk for infarction and have the potential for more productive activity. Patients exercise in larger groups with a 3 or 4 to 1 patient-to-staff ratio and continue to progress in their exercise program, which often includes upper extremity and four-extremity exercise modes as well as light weight training. Patients and their families also attend a weekly education program given by the appropriate team member on various topics related to the basics of heart disease (Table 16–8; Fig. 16–10).

Patients are monitored for heart rate, blood pressure, weight, and symptoms on a regular basis. In addition, ECG telemetry is performed when there is a change in the symptoms, medications, or exercise program (e.g., beginning a jogging program, upper extremity weight training program) and when spot checking is advisable. On graduation from this phase of the program, and often before that time, most patients who were previously employed can return to work. It is important to try to keep these individuals involved in the program and to help support them as they return to their previous routines. Some patients are appropriate for phase IV at this time if their schedule does not permit completion of phase III.

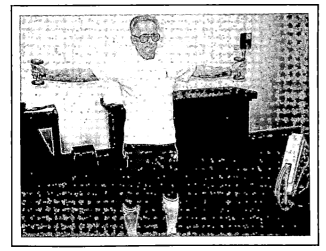

Figure 16–10.

A patient using weights while performing upper extremity exercises.

Ongoing Conditioning and Education — Phase IV

Some people refer to phase IV as the "maintenance phase"; however, patients are just beginning to scratch the surface of their physiologic potential at this point. There are different philosophies regarding how long this period of rehabilitation should extend. Most studies citing improved physiologic benefit from exercise conditioning report the need for at least 6 to 12 months of training, especially in patients with moderate to poor ventricular function.[7] Heart disease is not a short-term disease but rather a progressive process that requires active intervention for life. Ideally, all patients graduating from phase III continue with phase IV for another 6 months, but in reality, only a small percentage participate at this level. Possible reasons for lack of participation are limited insurance reimbursement for this phase of rehabilitation, conflicting work schedules, and the like. The more varied and stimulating this phase of the program (e.g., aerobic dance, weight training, track), the greater the likelihood of patient participation. Usually there is an 8 or 10 to 1 patient-to-staff ratio, with ECG monitoring available but infrequently performed except to spot check or note changes in symptoms or reactions to medications. Patients continue to monitor themselves while at rest and during activity, and blood pressure measurements are logged weekly. Spouses are encouraged to be as actively involved as possible and as space permits. Some appraisal of cardiovascular health should be made before active participation. Advanced education lectures on a variety of topics beyond the basics help to drive home and support earlier messages. Routine follow-up exercise tests help demonstrate to both patient and physician progress with regard to physical capacity and risk factor reduction. A reasonable routine of retesting every 6 to 12 months is recommended, although more frequent testing may be indicated for some patients.

Home-Based Cardiac Rehabilitation

A substantial number of uncomplicated (low-risk) patients with heart disease are considered to be candidates for cardiac rehabilitation but are unable to attend the outpatient program on a regular basis owing to the travel distance. For this group of patients, a different approach should be considered so that they benefit from the structure and support of this program. During the inpatient interview process, the therapist determines whether at-home therapy could be safely administered. Patients considered candidates for the program are given more extensive discharge instructions regarding self-monitoring techniques, exercise guidelines, dietary management, medications, and the like and are taught to keep an accurate daily activity log. A weekly telephone call is made by a member of the cardiac rehabilitation team to the patient to discuss progress or problems and to provide additional information or materials for program progression. Some programs also have the capability of having ECG information transmitted over the telephone lines while the patient exercises at home. When the patient returns for follow-up care with the physician or for exercise testing (3 to 6 weeks after discharge), a 2- to 3-hour follow-up session is arranged with the cardiac rehabilitation team members to review the individual's program. Follow-up telephone calls continue weekly for

the next month, and activity logs are sent by the patient every 2 weeks; thereafter monthly contacts are maintained for up to 6 to 12 months. Studies on this form of rehabilitation versus no program versus supervised exercise programs have been favorable; however physical work capacity improves most significantly in supervised programs.[20,21]

TREATMENT GUIDELINES FOR OUTPATIENT PROGRAMS

General Management Strategies

The maintenance of a safe and effective risk reduction program is paramount in establishing treatment-monitoring guidelines. The frequency of monitoring and the degree of direct supervision of an exercise treatment program must be determined for each patient based on prior clinical course (complicated or uncomplicated), exercise test results, degree of ventricular impairment, initial assessment, and the like. For some patients, direct monitoring and close supervision of each exercise session may be required and entirely appropriate for the first several weeks. However, for the majority of patients who have had a clinically uncomplicated course and an exercise test that was uneventful or that produced no negative findings, such close supervision and monitoring at each session can be counterproductive, implying more risk than is warranted. A number of studies have shown that the incidence of serious complications in the latter group is quite low.[22] For such patients an effective risk reduction program must concern itself with the development of self-confidence, the motivation for change, the sense of direct involvement of the patient with the management of the exercise program, and the development of skill in self-monitoring.

Some conditions should limit participation in an exercise program. Patients are not considered candidates for a cardiac rehabilitation program when they have

● unstable status — for example, recurrent ischemic pain, congestive heart failure, resting

tachycardia (greater than 100 bpm; slightly higher for postoperative patients), severe bradycardia (less than 50 bpm)
- uncontrolled hypertension
- other illness or disease that precludes exercise
- apparently good health (low risk for cardiac disease)

Exercise for the Coronary Patient — An Individualized Plan

A patient's exercise plan should be determined by objective assessment of clinical status, functional capacity, and personal need. What may be good for one person may prove to be detrimental to another. In addition to making a clinical evaluation, the therapist must determine the patient's exercise needs, interests, abilities, and previous habits. The exercise plan should also consider the facilities and equipment that are available as well as the climate and environmental factors that may affect whether the program can be carried out conveniently. These considerations are important in motivating the patient to be compliant with the program.

The Effects of Exercise

The specific demand of habitual physical exercise produces a biochemical change that ultimately enhances the functioning of skeletal muscle and the cardiovascular system. To a large degree the improvement made by the cardiac patient depends on the degree of ventricular impairment and function. Several studies have demonstrated that coronary patients can, in fact, improve not only the maximal aerobic capacity but the cardiac output as well.[23-26] Even patients with clinically large infarctions and poor ventricular function demonstrated significant improvement with regard to physical work capacity.[24] There are perhaps even greater functional consequences for them because their reserve is usually so low initially that simple, light household and ADL tasks are very difficult to perform. Persons with less impaired ventricular function (ejection fraction greater than 50%) often do not notice a very substantial difference in exercise tolerance

with usual activities unless they are stressed significantly (at which point they would probably slow down or stop).

Exercise training creates change specifically in the muscle groups that are challenged. This fact becomes important in selecting the most appropriate activity to produce the greatest functional gain. Nearly everyone needs to walk some distance. In addition, we all need to use our arms to some degree, some of us more than others. Why is it then that so many cardiac patients ride stationary bicycles? The exercise program should produce changes specific to the functional needs of the patient, especially those who have upper extremity demands. Upper extremity testing and training must be incorporated into the patients' plans, particularly if they will be returning to a vocation that requires a significant amount of arm work (e.g., maintenance workers, loggers, carpenters, plumbers).

The effects of conditioning last only as long as the individual continues to exercise. Cardiac patients must understand that exercise must be included as a lifetime process for the results to be lasting.

Types of Exercise: Aerobic and Anaerobic

Aerobic exercise involving moving large muscle groups in a dynamic manner has been shown to produce a substantial benefit in cardiorespiratory endurance. Static or isometric (anaerobic) exercise involving the development of tension but little or no change in muscle length or movement for short periods of time may improve strength but may also produce undesirable responses in the cardiac patient. Isometric exercise may, in fact, impose a pressure load on the left ventricle that is not tolerated well, increasing myocardial demand, especially in patients who have poor ventricular function.[27]

Aerobic forms of exercise can be performed continuously and can produce a training effect at workload intensities of 70% to 85% of maximal heart rate (as low as 40% to 50% in the elderly or in individuals with severe ventricular dysfunction) or 50% to 85% of maximal oxygen consumption.[9] Duration and frequency of exercise are also key elements in determining the correct formula for training.

Intensity. Training intensity is the key element in the exercise prescription for an individual starting an aerobic exercise program because if exertion is too intense, training can be compromised, hazardous, or both (Table 16–9). Heart rate is often a reliable indicator of myocardial and total oxygen requirement during exercise. Heart rate responses are commonly used to quantify and monitor endurance training.

Formulas used to predict appropriate training heart rates have been used in planning exercise programs for healthy individuals and for some patient groups, including those with coronary artery disease. The commonly accepted range of training heart rate is 70% to 85% of maximal heart rate or 50% to 85% of maximal oxygen consumption.[28,29] However, the effects of beta blockers, calcium channel blockers, surgical intervention, and pacemakers, among others, make it improbable that these methods would be accurate for cardiac patients who need more precise

---

TABLE 16–9. Abnormal Responses to Exercises

Exercise hypertension
  Systolic—greater than 240 mm Hg
  Diastolic—greater than 110 mm Hg, or until controlled
Systolic hypotension (greater than 20 mm Hg drop from upright resting blood pressure)
Unusual heart rate response—too rapid an increase, failure to increase, or a decrease with exercise
Symptoms
  Significant anginal response
  Undue dyspnea
  Excessive fatigue
  Mental confusion or dizziness
  Severe leg claudication
Signs
  Pallor
  Cold sweat
  Ataxia
  New murmur
  Pulmonary rales
  Onset of significant third heart sound
ECG abnormalities
  Serious arrhythmias
  Second- or third-degree heart block
  Onset of right or left bundle branch block
  Acute ST changes

(From Guidelines for Cardiac Rehabilitation Centers. 2nd ed. Los Angeles, American Heart Association, 1982.)

---

and effective measurements. Beta blockers and some calcium channel blockers decrease resting and exercising heart rate response. However, neither beta- nor calcium-blocking medications alter the relationship between the percentage of heart rate and the percentage of oxygen consumption.[30] The important implication is that, when exercise testing an individual before beginning exercise training, the individual should be taking the medication that will be used during the training program. The medication should not be discontinued for the exercise test. If medication that affects heart rate is started or discontinued or if the dosage is significantly altered after the initial test, a repeat exercise test should be performed to define the training heart rate. The key principle in determining a safe and appropriate intensity of exercise for individuals with heart disease is individualizing the prescription of exercise.

The importance of ventilatory threshold in exercise prescription has begun to be examined. This measurement, which is determined during exercise testing, is the level of exercise at which there is a nonlinear increase in the ventilation in relation to oxygen uptake. It is the estimated upper limit of aerobic exercise. Comparing heart rate relationships with the measured oxygen consumption and the ventilatory threshold provides a much more exact measurement of exertion levels and is a preferred noninvasive method of assessing training limitations. This method is particularly helpful in patients who have multisystem dysfunction, such as coronary artery disease with chronic obstructive pulmonary disease, coronary artery disease and diabetes, and ventricular pump dysfunction. In particular, patients on beta blockers and calcium channel blockers and those with pacemakers would benefit most from this type of assessment. Most testing, however, is done without metabolic analysis of exercise; therefore a combination of other intensity parameters should be examined in establishing a training heart rate.

Establishing a training heart rate by rating of perceived exertion. This method of measuring heart rate was first introduced in 1962 by Gunnar Borg (Table 16–10). It is a scale of subjective levels of exertion beginning with "very, very

TABLE 16–10. Borg Scale for Ratings of Perceived Exertion	
Rate	Description
6	
7	Very, very light
8	
9	Very light
10	
11	Fairly light
12	
13	Somewhat hard
14	
15	Hard
16	
17	Very hard
18	
19	Very, very hard
20	

(From Borg GV. Psychophysical basis of perceived exertion. Med Sci Sports Exerc 14[5]:377–381, 1982. © American College of Sports Medicine.)

light level," and advancing to "very, very hard level." This scale has been adapted several times to make it more easily understood. It has been shown to be a fairly accurate marker in some studies relating it to ventilatory threshold. Using it in conjunction with other markers of ischemia and arrhythmias and relative to maximal heart rate makes this a very valuable tool, especially for the individual who has difficulty in accurately measuring a pulse, such as in the presence of atrial fibrillation.

Establishing training heart rates using signs and symptoms. Patients may initially demonstrate symptoms of ischemia in the form of angina pectoris, dyspnea, or both. This should always be documented in relation to ECG changes and levels of myocardial oxygen consumption (heart rate times blood pressure). Usually this response has made itself evident in the testing laboratory, and precautions or limitations are documented before exercise training begins. However, changes can occur rapidly in this patient population, and it is often the therapist in the exercise area that first identifies this change. Levels of angina should be discussed with all patients before beginning exercise, with instructions as to appropriate responses. Cardiac pa-

tients are often allowed and even encouraged to exercise up to level 1 (see Table 16–5) as long as they are comfortable and recover well when they cool down. Some patients prefer to use nitroglycerin during exercise when symptoms begin or even during warm-up to prevent the onset of angina. Taking nitroglycerin often allows them to exercise at higher levels of intensity. Heart rate, blood pressure, and ECG changes must be monitored in these patients.[31]

Dyspnea is often another indication of exercise intolerance and may be used as a guide to limit intensity. Coronary patients with a smoking history and perhaps some degree of chronic obstructive pulmonary disease may find this particularly helpful (see Table 16–6).

Continuous Aerobic Training. Aerobic training involves three phases of exercise: a warm-up phase, a peak interval phase, and a cool-down phase. Each phase is important in the cardiac patient population because it allows certain physiologic adaptations to occur for the patient to exercise safely. The warm-up phase usually lasts 5 to 10 minutes and involves a form of stretching routine of the exercising muscles to be utilized and a period of slower performance of the same aerobic activity to be performed (e.g., walking before a walk/jog or before jogging). This allows time for the exercising muscles to achieve adequate stretch to the length they will be used during peak exercise, as well as time for the peripheral vasculature and coronary arteries to dilate to carry larger volumes of arterial blood. The peak interval usually lasts 15 to 45 minutes, depending on the level of conditioning, and is the period when the individual works at training intensity levels. Established parameters should be checked every 10 minutes or less to determine if the individual is exercising at, above, or below expected levels. The cool-down is a period of 5 to 15 minutes after the peak interval, during which time the exercising muscles are slowly brought to rest. Too abrupt an end or a cessation of exercise can reduce the return of blood to the myocardium, creating irritation and increased arrhythmia. Included in the cool-down period should be some stretching exercises for individuals who are extremely deconditioned or who have notable muscular inflexibility.

Circuit Training

Circuit training entails performing a series of activities one after another. At the end of the last activity, one starts from the beginning again and carries on until the entire series has been repeated several times. The advantage is that every individual undergoes a program adjusted to a personal level of fitness. Circuit training can also be performed in a limited space and produces a high degree of motivation.

Considerations with Exercise Prescription

Most patients entering cardiac rehabilitation programs have not in their recent past been involved in a regular exercise program. Since the large majority are also in the 40- to 70-year age group, the physical therapist should be concerned about the neuromuscular capability of this patient population. Exercise intensity, especially early on, should consider the patient's relative neuromuscular capability.

Silent ischemia is a phenomenon of changes that can be measured electrocardiographically (ST depression of more than 2 mm lasting longer than 3 min in recovery, T wave changes, arrhythmias) and hemodynamically (drops in systolic blood pressure and abnormal heart sounds [S4 gallop] in the absence of angina pectoris). Patients in this group are at high risk for ventricular tachycardia or ventricular fibrillation during exercise training.[32] Exercise intensity must be monitored closely and the patient counseled regarding the use of heart rate and rating of perceived exertion with this clinical picture.

Four- Versus Two-Extremity Exercise

Most exercise programs with coronary patients have emphasized dynamic leg exercise; however, activity patterns during daily life are more varied. Many tasks require static or isometric efforts, sometimes in combination with dynamic exercise and often involving more upper than lower extremity efforts. In prescribing exercises for conditioning, it is desirable to impose a large metabolic

load on the individual without causing cardiovascular or subjective strain. Spreading the work over greater muscle mass by using arms and legs together may allow a greater load to be tolerated with similar cardiac and subjective strain; however, the ability of the individual with left ventricular dysfunction to tolerate and benefit from this mode of training may vary. Combining upper and lower extremity exercise can produce a higher maximal oxygen consumption than that produced by either body segment alone.[33] A larger actively exercising skeletal muscle mass may explain this finding.

Gutin and colleagues have examined the physiologic response to arm and leg work with special attention to oxygen consumption and ventilatory threshold.[34] They found maximal oxygen consumption and heart rate significantly lower for exercise with arms alone but not for arms and legs combined or legs alone. The ventilatory threshold was significantly higher for arms alone than for legs alone, and even though adding arms to legs did not increase peak physiologic measures, it did not result in the ventilatory threshold occurring at a higher percentage of oxygen consumption. The rate pressure product and rating of perceived exertion were similar for all of these modes. None of the studies comparing two- and four-extremity ergometry included patients with coronary disease (Fig. 16–11).

Emphasis is increasing in exercise and rehabilitation centers on combined arm and leg work (e.g., use of the Schwinn Airdyne ergometer, Nordictrack cross-country ski machines, and hand weights while walking or jogging). In our experience, many coronary patients perceive work performance to be less taxing on four-extremity ergometers than treadmill walking at equivalent rate pressure products and tend to overexercise at unsafe levels. Patients with moderate to poor ventricular function should be monitored closely on this equipment.

Frequency and Duration of Exercise

Just as there is no best method to determine training heart rate, there is no standard exercise

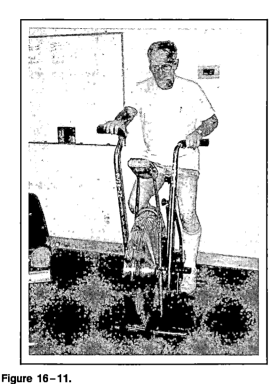

Figure 16–11.

A patient performing four-extremity exercise.

duration for all coronary patients. Exercise duration should be individualized and based on several factors:

● Length of disability
● Reduced activity as a result of the acute event
● Premorbid activity level and neuromuscular capability

Individuals who were quite active and who had good to moderate ventricular function usually can tolerate 20 to 30 minutes of exercise within 1 to 2 weeks of beginning the outpatient program, whereas individuals who have sustained considerable ventricular impairment or have a long-standing illness may have difficulty exercising for more than a few minutes before fatigue sets in. These patients usually do best with an intermittent activity program of low intensity, short duration, frequent rest periods, and progressing by systematically reducing periods of rest and increasing periods of exercise. In either case, it is important to remember that the exercising muscle needs time to recover before further activity can be tolerated comfortably. Some patients believe that if 30 minutes of exercise is good, 60 minutes is probably better, and 2 hours better still.

Understanding the way the body recovers from exercise and the need for modified activity patterns and rest periods, especially in phase II, is of utmost importance. Patients should learn that they are just beginning a process that, it is hoped, will last a lifetime and that a slow, systematic approach is not only safer but more enjoyable. The goal is to have the patient reach 45 minutes of continuous aerobic activity, including a warm-up and cool-down period, as soon as the patient can adjust and without exercising beyond the symptom limit. This may take 3 to 6 weeks or longer.

Most patients should be able to tolerate daily exercise. Some patients may find it difficult to maintain the same intensity or duration every day; however, they should be encouraged to work to their prescribed levels at least four times a week for the best conditioning effect. Initially, some patients with less than 20 minutes of exercise tolerance will be asked to work out two times per day and perhaps three times a day if tolerance is 10 minutes or less. Unless a patient is on bedrest or is hospitalized with restricted activity, independent exercise should be possible, even for most high-risk patients, as long as the patient understands how to monitor signs and symptoms and control activity levels. This should be an early lesson to enhance a patient's psychological outlook.

Other Considerations in Planning Exercise Programs

Altitude — Exercising Where the "Air Is Rare"

Below 3000 feet most patients find little discomfort exercising; however, above this level, and certainly above 5000 feet, the atmospheric pressure begins to drop, and the body adapts to achieve the same cardiac output by increasing the heart rate. Angina levels may be reached sooner in terms of exercise intensity and physically demanding activity that may not be a problem at sea level. Patients who enjoy skiing (especially cross-country) or who travel to destinations with an elevation above 3500 feet (e.g., Denver, Mexico City) should be counseled about activity guidelines at these levels.

Cold

Cold temperatures cause an increase in peripheral resistance at rest and with exercise. This peripheral vasoconstriction can subsequently cause an increase in arterial blood pressure and possibly create a situation for earlier ischemic changes with increased myocardial oxygen demands as well as cold-induced vasospasm. Patients exercising outdoors in cold weather should be counseled about the importance of wearing layers of clothing, a wool hat and gloves for body heat retention, and a scarf around the mouth to warm the air; and taking in an adequate amount of fluid despite the lack of noticeable perspiration.

Heat and Humidity

In response to higher temperatures and dilation of peripheral vasculature, heart rate increases to maintain adequate cardiac output. The ability of an individual to perform successfully in hot environments depends on the magnitude of heat, the existing humidity, the movement of air, and the intensity and duration of exercise. The amount of direct exposure as opposed to shade or cloud cover is also a critical factor. One of the primary concerns when exercising in the heat is dehydration. With high sweat rates, the body loses a large volume of water. Because a major portion of the water comes from blood volume, a serious condition exists unless rehydration is accomplished by consuming appropriate fluids (preferably water) both during and after exercise. Again, early symptoms of angina may occur. Avoidance of vigorous exercise or activity in temperatures above 75 degrees F or humidity greater than 65% to 70% is usually recommended. Wearing looser fitting and fewer clothes, protecting the skin by applying a sun screen, exercising at cooler times of the day, and staying in shaded areas as much as possible are recommended. Patients should consult with their physicians before using a steam bath or sauna.

Program Progression

Patients should be taught to pay attention to their bodies' responses to increasing activity and to progress in an orderly fashion based on acceptable evidence of tolerance of the activity. Patients should have their program goals reviewed on a regular basis (at least every 2 weeks initially) to reestablish guidelines for their exercise program (including contraindications to exercise) and risk reduction in general. Program progression can take several forms:

● Increasing the *intensity* of exercise
● Increasing the *duration* of exercise
● Changing the *mode* of exercise (e.g., including upper or combined upper and lower extremity exercise)

Many patients in phase II can progress to 85% to 95% or greater of the initial exercise test results, especially if the test was low level, was stopped before any limiting symptoms appeared, or both. A determination of the patient's safety of progression should be based on a daily observation and reassessment by the therapist. Cardiac bypass patients are often quite limited during the initial few weeks of the program owing to various medical factors, such as a low hemoglobin level and a healing sternum, but they demonstrate a rather quick turnaround and begin to work at much higher levels when these conditions normalize. Upper extremity stretching and strengthening are important with this population in particular and should be included in the exercise program when the sternum is well healed at approximately 6 weeks (Fig. 16–12). Some patients may also develop complications or problems that force them to discontinue their program for a period of time. When they resume, they must be cautioned about trying to catch up and progress too quickly. In general, if the individual becomes better conditioned, exercise intensity can be increased without significant increase in heart rate response, symptoms, or ECG changes. Most patients can be expected to in-

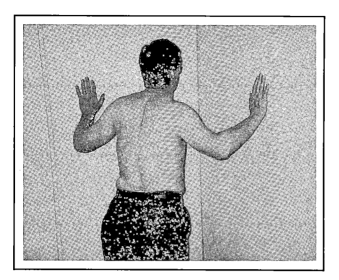

Figure 16-12.

A patient performing postoperative stretching exercises.

crease the peak interval period of exercise by at least 5 minutes a week barring medical complications.

Weight training, with emphasis on higher number of repetitions and low loads (approximately 40% of one repetition maximum), may be included after several weeks of training for low- and most moderate-risk patients. Heavy resistance exercises should be avoided to prevent Valsalva's maneuver; attention should be paid to coordinating inhalation and exhalation with exercise. Free weights or multistation weight systems may be used, and patients should be in-

structed in proper lifting techniques to avoid musculoskeletal injury. Other exercise modes may include cross-country skiing, rowing, sit-ups, and the like, again with initial instruction by a staff therapist and initially in a monitored situation (Fig. 16-13).

Safety in the Outpatient Cardiac Rehabilitation Setting

Safety in the outpatient cardiac rehabilitation exercise setting must be the number one priority

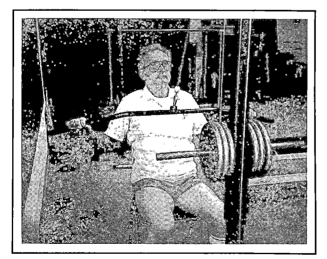

Figure 16-13.

A patient performing a resistance workout as part of a comprehensive cardiac rehabilitation program.

for any program. Even with the best precautions, major cardiovascular events may occur, the most frequent of which is sudden cardiac arrest.[9] Selection of appropriate patients who are adequately evaluated and deemed appropriate candidates for training (e.g., under medical supervision outside the program, screened via exercise test before entry to the program); who are cooperative, especially in understanding and use of heart rate and symptoms as limitations in exercise; and who are willing to follow the prescribed medical regimen is of critical importance.

The ability to deal with cardiac arrest and other medical emergencies depends on the immediate response of trained personnel in the exercise area, available emergency equipment, and availability of trained physicians. All professional exercise personnel must be trained to perform immediate basic cardiac life support in accordance with American Heart Association standards (advanced cardiac life support preferred), including defibrillation. All persons involved with the cardiac rehabilitation program must know their roles and be practiced in the various emergency procedures (Table 16–11).

Most data available demonstrate a relatively

TABLE 16–11. Emergency Procedures for Cardiac Rehabilitation

The following is instituted for persons who demonstrate cardiopulmonary distress and require emergency procedures during cardiac rehabilitation.

A. Nonmonitored Patient—Individual who is found unconscious or loses consciousness with no respiration or palpable pulse
  1. Person discovering victim
    a. Assess situation, determine need for CPR
    b. Call for help
    c. Initiate CPR
    d. Remain with patient until relieved
  2. Second person to respond
    a. Call for assistance
    b. Activate the E.M.S. (Call 911)
    c. Alert facility, front desk of emergency department, and person to inform medical director
    d. Assist with CPR
  3. Third person to respond
    a. Delivers crash cart to scene of code
  4. Exercise assistants
    a. Assist with CPR
    b. Escort other patients from the area and remain with them
    c. Direct ambulance personnel

If a code is called during cardiac rehabilitation, the cardiac rehabilitation coordinator is in charge of the code procedure. In the coordinator's absence, designated ACLS personnel will assume charge role and initiate ACLS standards of care until the emergency department personnel arrive or the paramedics, if program is held out of hospital.

B. Monitored arrest—The first available staff member who observes the emergency should immediately assess the patient's status and respond by performing the specific procedure that that staff member is authorized to deliver.

The second available staff member activates the emergency medical system and returns to assist the first rescuer. The third staff member delivers the crash cart to the code site and prepares it for use.
  1. Ventricular tachycardia (losing or lost consciousness), ventricular fibrillation
    a. If observed, administer precordial thump
    b. If no change in rhythm, defibrillate at 400 watts per sec
    c. Wait 10 seconds, check rhythm
    d. If no change, defibrillate again at 400 watts per sec
    e. If no response, initiate CPR
  2. Severe bradycardia, asystole, or other pulmonary emergency—initiate CPR and continue until directed to stop by physician
  3. Severe myocardial ischemia (with persistent symptoms and signs)
    a. Sitting or supine posture, check ECG
    b. Give oxygen and nitroglycerin
    c. Evaluate blood pressure and symptoms
    d. Notify the cardiologist covering the exercise class or the patient's attending physician

Emergency procedures vary according to established hospital and community standards.
CPR, cardiopulmonary resuscitation; E.M.S., Emergency Medical Service; ACLS, Advanced Cardiac Life Support.

low rate for cardiovascular complications during supervised cardiac rehabilitation programs. Van Camp and Peterson's survey of 167 cardiac rehabilitation programs suggests an incidence rate of 8 to 9 per 1 million patient hours of exercise for cardiac arrest, 3 to 4 per 1 million patient hours of exercise for myocardial infarction, and 1.3 per 1 million patient hours for fatalities.[35]

Other precautions with regard to safety in the cardiac rehabilitation setting include

- avoidance of exercise within 1 to 2 hours after meals
- avoidance of isometrics and breath holding with exercise
- adding warm-up and extended cool-off periods of 15 minutes or more with strenuous exercise
- keeping showers brief and not at a hot or cold temperature (keep legs active)

Special Patient Populations

The prescription of exercise for special patient populations requires the integration of clinical information and exercise physiology. The need for an appropriate exercise prescription in patients with noncardiac disease has been documented; however, patients with multiple system dysfunction may require special attention. The more we learn about exercise and disease, the more we find an influence of one on the other.

Patients with Peripheral Vascular Disease

Peripheral vascular disease is a fairly common disorder among individuals with coronary artery disease. The limiting factor to exercise is claudication — angina-like pain usually in the buttocks, the calf of one or both lower extremities, or both. Much like angina, claudication is related to exertional level. Exercise training has demonstrated significant functional improvement with reduction of symptoms at equivalent workloads.[36,37] Patients must be tolerant of working to various levels of discomfort, and the supervising therapist should use a symptom-limited approach with varying modes of exercise. One mode

should include walking because it is the most functional and usually limited activity for the individual to perform. Cigarette smokers must also agree to a smoking cessation program if they are serious about reducing their risk of disease progression.

Patients with Chronic Obstructive Pulmonary Disease

Many patients with coronary disease have a long-standing history of cigarette smoking with some degree of obstructive airway disease. Some individuals may be taking medications (e.g., theophylline) that are known to induce supraventricular arrhythmia with activity. Dyspnea levels, discussed earlier in this chapter (see Intensity), are most effective for determining an appropriate exercise intensity level. For patients with chronic obstructive pulmonary disease, pursed-lip breathing may enhance exercise performance because it helps control ventilation and oxygenation by reducing respiratory rate and increasing tidal volume, improving ventilation of previously underventilated areas. Use of upper extremity support with exercise, such as holding the bars of treadmills, stationary bikes, and rolling walkers, may assist the patient in stabilizing accessory muscles for improved ventilation. In more severe cases, supplemental oxygen may be of benefit. Blood saturation levels with exercise should be monitored, preferably with arterial blood gases and at least with oximetry. The supervising therapist should pay close attention to clinical signs of desaturation (e.g., blue nail beds and overall change in coloration).

Patients with Diabetes Mellitus

Diabetes is a risk factor for coronary disease, and diabetic patients are three times more likely to have coronary artery disease than nondiabetics.[38] In addition, type II diabetes (non–insulin-dependent type, which includes 80% to 90% of all diabetics) is associated with obesity. Research on the effect of exercise on the lives of patients with type II diabetes has been promising, demonstrating improvements in insulin activity and glucose tolerance, potential reductions in dosage and need of insulin or oral hypoglycemic medications, and reduction of body fat.[39] Patients should be cautious and aware of signs and symptoms of hypoglycemic episodes that can occur during or after the exercise session. Just before starting an exercise session each day, the patient should obtain a pre-exercise blood glucose reading. This reading is in addition to that for the daily fasting blood glucose value. If the pre-exercise blood glucose value is between 100 and 300 mg/dL, the person can engage in exercise. Because of the enhancement of insulin sensitivity with exercise, persons with diabetes should abstain from exercise during the peak activity of their insulin. If the pre-exercise value is equal to or greater than 300 mg/dL, exercise may induce a rise in blood glucose rather than a decline. Also, because of the major role of glucose as a fuel for exercise, there may not be enough energy to sustain the exercise if the pre-exercise blood glucose level is equal to or less than 100 mg/dL, and the person may become hypoglycemic. Some form of simple carbohydrate (e.g., juice, sugar, glucose) should be kept in the exercise area in case of such an emergency. As with anyone who exercises, persons with diabetes should begin the session with a 5- to 10-minute warm-up, which includes stretching and light calisthenics. At the end of the session, time must be allotted for a cool-down session. The exercise prescription for a person with diabetes is similar to the nondiabetic. Because of the postexercise recovery phase, a person may have a decrease in blood glucose values for up to 24 hours. Persons with diabetes must be told that on days they do not engage in exercise their blood glucose values may be higher.

Patients Who Have Had a Cerebral Vascular Accident

Some individuals present to the cardiac rehabilitation program with impaired ventricular function, having previously sustained a cerebral vascular accident. They therefore possess special medical and physical needs. Common sequelae of cerebral vascular accidents include weakness or neglect of one or more extremities, problems in communication, cognitive-perceptual dysfunc-tion, and dysphagia.[40] Inability to exercise weakened muscles or ones with excessive tone for prolonged periods may necessitate exercise of short duration. Despite unilateral limb dysfunction, the use of four-extremity ergometers such as the Schwinn Airdyne may allow for greater intensity of exercise. Blood pressure and heart rate responses to isometric and to upper and lower extremity ergometry have been found to be no greater in those who have had cerebral vascular accidents than in an age-matched control group[41]; however, with four-extremity ergometry and impaired ventricular function these patients are extremely important to monitor. The supervising therapist should be attuned especially to symptoms that exercising patients may have but cannot easily express because of a communication disorder.

Patients with Renal Disease

Patients with end-stage renal disease can benefit significantly from regular exercise training, although they may not exhibit the same responses to exercise as the patients usually seen in the cardiac rehabilitation program. Exercise tolerance in patients on hemodialysis has been found to be significantly below normal.[42,43] This low tolerance is probably due to lower arterial oxygen content because of

- lower hematocrit and hemoglobin values for oxygen transport
- altered stroke volume affected by the disease or its treatment
- peripheral factors as a result of autonomic dysfunction and metabolic acidosis

Exercise training has been found to increase physical work capacity, increase HDL cholesterol levels, and increase hematocrit values in this group. Improvements in glucose tolerance, blood pressure control, and physiologic profiles—important risk factors for heart disease—also result from exercise training.[44] Exercise sessions should be scheduled according to the patient's condition before and after dialysis and on the time requirements of the treatment. Often the day before and the day of dialysis are the patient's weakest days. Intermittent exercise, with work-to-rest ratios of 1 to 2 or 1 to 1, may be appropriate initially, although most patients can gradually increase to 30 to 45 minutes of continuous exercise over time. Training heart rates are difficult to use because of variable heart rate response, medication schedule, and physiologic changes that occur in these patients from day to day depending on their dialysis schedule. The Borg perceived exertion scale works well in evaluating these patients (see Table 16–10).

The Elderly Coronary Patient

Most elderly cardiac patients who have not exercised in their recent past probably have low expectations and possibly negative attitudes toward the rehabilitation process, participating only because their physicians told them they should. These same individuals may show the most improvement functionally. Exercise can promote a sense of well-being and heighten self-esteem, both of which are essential to independent living.

Regular physical activity can modify known coronary risk factors in the elderly. In a study of elderly Japanese men in Hawaii, higher levels of physical activity were associated with higher serum HDL and lower triglyceride levels.[45] Likewise, elderly athletic men have been shown to have higher HDL levels and lower total cholesterol–to-HDL ratios than elderly sedentary men.[46]

Many elderly patients present with multiple joint and musculoskeletal limitations. Therefore, a thorough mechanical assessment should be performed before initiating any exercise program. To achieve the greatest success early in the program and to diminish patient discouragement because "it hurts too much," light calisthenics and stretching exercises should be employed. Jarring activities such as jogging should be minimized to avoid musculoskeletal injury. Swimming is an excellent exercise; however, some weight-bearing activity should be encouraged, especially for women, to forestall the adverse effects of osteoporosis. A cool-down period is especially important for the elderly following aerobic activity and should actually be of slightly longer duration for adequate recovery. Frequency

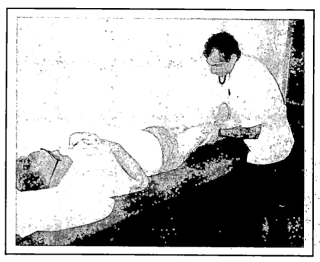

Figure 16–14.

A physical therapist conducts a musculoskeletal examination.

may need to be limited to every other day of exercise to give the musculoskeletal system a chance to rest (Fig. 16–14).

EDUCATION

Early Intervention

Educating the individual with heart disease about this problem plays a significant role in preventing further cardiovascular disease and in the rehabilitation process as a whole. Patients and their families must be informed about how to make lifestyle changes and kept up to date on current medical information as it pertains to the disease process. Many changes have occurred in the past 10 years that have had a profound effect on the management of cardiovascular disease, including exercise interventions, dietary modifications, and other lifestyle changes. Once through the crisis stage, and perhaps as early as the first or second day after the event (myocardial infarction, coronary artery bypass graft surgery, or other cardiovascular disorder), patients and their families are most receptive to learning about what they can do to reduce the risk of disease progression. It is at this time that, in addition to being supportive, the health care team (including the physician, nurse, physical therapist, dietitian) should begin the process of presenting specific information relating to the individual's particular risk factor profile. As patients progress through the hospitalization, small amounts of information in various forms prepare them to make educated choices about their cardiac health.

The Outpatient Setting

A patient's educational background should not be a limiting or predisposing factor in achieving an understanding of the disease and rehabilitative process or risk factor modification. There is no limit to the number of health care professionals, including physicians and nurses, whose level of understanding falls far short of what is necessary to make appropriate "heart healthy" choices. These individuals often need the most guidance and supervision because of the preconceived expectation that they will make all the correct decisions.

Basic education should be provided in both an individual encounter and in a group format. Initially, the patient and the family must understand their particular requirements regarding lifestyle modifications and a specific plan of action. The need to establish a specific time for follow-up should not be overlooked. Frequent checks of the level of understanding and progress being made should be performed by all team members with each visit. If a patient or family member seems to be having difficulty with the plan, for whatever reason, a team member should intervene to determine if goals were set too high, if certain points need to be clarified, or if some other problem mandates attention and program modification (e.g., problems related to the side effect of medications, new symptoms, or psychological problems).

Participation in group education programs is an excellent source of support for patients with similar cardiac diagnoses. Most programs include, and should encourage, spousal or family participation because their concerns and level of understanding play a vital role in the patient's

rehabilitation process. Sharing their cardiac experiences helps individuals adjust to their feelings and fears about the present and the future. Skilled, knowledgeable leaders are required for these education programs and should encompass a variety of disciplines because no single individual can address all aspects of care in the depth of expertise required.

Diet and Nutrition

Dietary management for the cardiac outpatient should be designed to fit that person's specific lipid abnormality, cultural background, and lifestyle. To determine specific needs for intervention, a nutritional assessment should be performed by a dietitian or physical therapist that includes the following anthropometric, biochemical, dietetic, and clinical parameters. Anthropometric parameters include height, weight, weight history, and skinfold measurements (when capable) to help determine the appropriate percentage of body fat. This information is useful in determining ideal weight and may show tendencies of the patient for a weight gain or loss (Fig. 16–15).

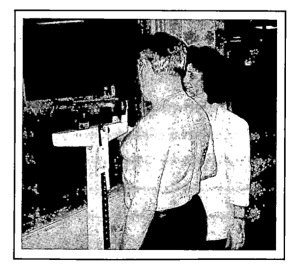

Figure 16–15.

The dietitian checks a patient's weight during a cardiac rehabilitation treatment session.

A biochemical analysis includes

- lipid profile (total serum cholesterol, HDL cholesterol, low-density lipoprotein [LDL] cholesterol, very low density lipoprotein [VLDL] cholesterol, and triglycerides)
- electrolyte panel (Na^+ and K^+)
- complete blood count (blood urea nitrogen, hemoglobin, hematocrit, and serum albumin)

The lipid profile is helpful when the ratio of total cholesterol to HDL cholesterol is calculated and compared with the data collected in the Framingham study.[47] Controversy exists about the values for normal total serum cholesterol. The Consensus Conference Report published in 1985 concluded that when an individual's total blood cholesterol is greater than the seventy-fifth percentile, treatment should be initiated (Table 16–12).[48] Total cholesterol values should be evaluated as well as values for LDL and HDL cholesterol, total cholesterol to HDL cholesterol, LDL to HDL cholesterol, apolipoproteins, and triglycerides. Optimal values for apolipoproteins are still under investigation. Even with an established normal cholesterol level, the validity of the values obtained during the analysis of lipids is questionable. Much discrepancy has been observed between laboratories when lipids are analyzed.[49]

To decrease the risk of coronary artery disease and its progression, it is necessary to increase

levels of HDL and decrease levels of LDL cholesterol, total cholesterol, and triglycerides. Studies indicate that for each 1% decrease in total cholesterol there is a corresponding 2% decrease in the risk of developing coronary disease.[50,51] Lipids may be altered through many methods, some of which offer better results than others (Table 16–13). There are many causes of hyperlipidemia, each of which must be identified and treated. If one method to alter lipids fails, other methods are available.

A complete blood count helps to identify patients, especially postoperative patients, who may be limited functionally because of poor oxygen-carrying capacity of the blood cells. Electrolyte panels determine deficiencies or abnormalities in other systems or organs.

Weight Loss

Obesity is a significant risk factor for coronary artery disease, and one reason is the effect that it has on serum lipid levels. Weight loss has been shown to reduce total cholesterol, LDL cholesterol, and triglycerides and to increase HDL cholesterol.[52,53]

A dietetic or clinical analysis should include a 24-hour recall of food eaten or a 3- to 7-day food diary and a nutritional history specific for coronary heart disease, including information on the use of fat, types of oils, cholesterol-rich foods, alcohol, caffeine, sucrose, sodium, and fiber. An individual diet prescription can be outlined, utilizing the patient's nutritional history and food preferences as well as estimating caloric needs by considering activity level and basal energy requirements.

Psychosocial Recovery

Readjustment after a cardiac event can be influenced by the degree of anxiety, depression, or denial each patient manifests on recovery from the acute stage. The more pronounced the symptoms at this point, the poorer the rehabilitation potential. The patients' perceptions of their health status are also influenced by previous ex-

TABLE 16–12. Lipid Values Indicative of Higher Risk

Total cholesterol (mg/dL)	>200	20–29 yr old
(>75th percentile)	>220	30–39 yr old
	>240	40 yr or older
Low-density lipoprotein	>100	
(LDL) (mg/dL)	>175	extremely high risk
High-density lipoprotein	<35	
(HDL) (mg/dL)		
LDL:HDL	3:1	
Triglycerides (mg/dL)	>250	

(Data from Lowering blood cholesterol to prevent heart disease. JAMA 253:2080–2090, 1985; Brown WV, Ginsberg H, Karmally W. Diet and the decrease of coronary heart disease. Am J Cardiol 54:27C–29C, 1984; Castelli WP, Garrison RD, Wilson PWF, et al. Incidence of coronary heart disease and lipoprotein cholesterol levels: The Framingham study. JAMA 256:2835–2838, 1986; Heiss G. Are triglycerides a risk factor for ischemic heart disease? An appraisal of evidence. Perspectives in Lipid Disorders 2:15–19, 1985.)

TABLE 16–13. A Comparison of the Various Methods to Alter Lipids: Effects (mg/dL or %)

Methods	Total Cholesterol	LDL	HDL	Triglycerides
Diet low in cholesterol and saturated fat, high in poly-unsaturated fat	−16 to −30% (−27 to −58 mg) (−12 mg per 100 mg decrease in dietary choles-terol)	−38% (−45 mg)	0 to −33% (−6 mg)	−13%
Fish consumption	−8 to −57% (88 mg)	−15% (−17 to −26 mg)	+4 to +18%	−35 to −79% (−237 mg)
Monounsaturated fats	−13 to −18%	−21%	—	—
Increased intake of beans, wheat, oats, and other grains	−10 to −30%	−14 to −24%	−5.6 to −12.7%	−8 to −41%
Vegetarian or modified vege-tarian diet	−30 to −58 mg	−20 to −45 mg	−4 to −7 mg	−27 mg
Weight loss	−5.5 to −57 mg	−11.1 to −13 mg	+2.3 to +5 mg	−21.5 to −503 mg
≤ Two cups of coffee/day	−20 mg	−20 mg	—	−10 to −20%
Exercise	−10 to −39.2 mg (−16.4%)	−5 to −8 mg (−13%)	+1.2 to +14 mg (0 to +25%)	−15.8 to −131 mg (−45%)
Smoking cessation	−3.45 to −23 mg	—	+2 to +6 mg	—
Stress reduction	−29 to −47 mg (−4 to −35%)	—	−8 mg	−29 mg
Lipid-lowering drugs	−28 to −48%	−24 to −42%	−9 to +21%	−5.8 to −18.4%

(From Cahalin LP. A comparison of various methods to alter lipids. Cardiopulmonary Physical Therapy 1:5, 1990.)

perience; premorbid health misconceptions; and body concerns, for example, an increased aware-ness of the chest region.

The support of the cardiac rehabilitation team and other patients can be a significant factor in reversing this state. Some patients need extra support and education, but exaggerated attention to the disease may be harmful to others. Foster-ing adequate communication and good relation-ships with patients promotes recovery by pre-cluding misunderstandings and correcting patients' misperceptions of their state of health. Relatives, neighbors, and friends should be made aware of the goals of the active rehabilitation program. Information must be provided to counteract re-strictive attitudes that can lead to psychological invalidism.

During this readjustment period, the patient increases self-confidence and improves self-image while learning an individual response to increasing levels of activity. Sexual activity is still of great interest in the age groups in which heart disease is prevalent. There may be problems due to physical load, effect of medications, or even fear of the partner. It is therefore worthwhile to focus on this point in discussions with both the patient and the partner.

It has been suggested that adequate social support is an important ingredient in recovery from the crisis of acute illness. Mumford and colleagues found that informational and emo-tional support to hospitalized heart patients can reduce their length of stay.[54] Successful rehabili-tation and return to a productive lifestyle are of interest from the standpoint of both economic benefit and improved quality of life. Another study addresses problems and interventions ger-mane to heart patients. In a controlled study of 46 patients who had experienced a myocardial infarction, researchers found that educational and counseling interventions produced better outcomes in measures of psychological dysfunc-tion, unhealthy lifestyle, and dependence on health care than educational interventions alone.[55] Social support literature is often vague about what specific ingredients or processes within supportive relationships lead to positive health outcomes. In a study of disaster survivors, Murphy addresses this issue and proposes that self-efficacy may be a key variable.[56] Self-efficacy is defined as the individual's expectation of capability to execute a specific behavior. The presence of supportive others seems to increase self-confidence in one's ability to carry out specific behavior. Self-efficacy theory also suggests that levels of self-efficacy can be enhanced by increasing social support generally and by breaking down the specific denied behavior into small manageable steps, which is referred to as goal scaling.[57]

Compliance

A major problem in all cardiac rehabilitation programs regardless of type or structure is compliance. Although the data are variable, only 20% to 50% of participants continue to exercise after 1 year.[58] The factors that promote poor compliance are rather complex and may include duration of rehabilitation, regimen complexity, nature of side effects, presence of symptoms, and social and environmental factors, as well as factors related to the therapist, such as patient-therapist interaction. Another key factor is physician encouragement, support, and effectiveness in the role of cardiac rehabilitation team leader.

Programs should include mechanisms to combat recidivism. Strategies generally involve education and behavioral measures, as well as attempts to remove barriers to participation. Such barriers begin with the convenience factor. Location, time of day, and facility amenities are among the determinants of convenience to the patient. Few patients will travel more than 10 miles to participate in an exercise program, especially if it is not in the same geographic area as their work. Programs should be scheduled to be convenient for employed and retired persons. Facilities and amenities, particularly parking and locker rooms, are other factors in the perception of convenience to the patient.[59]

The rehabilitation team plays a vital role in the long-term compliance of the patient. Strong leadership, enthusiasm, and development of a good relationship between therapist and patient can reinforce and motivate appropriate lifestyle change. The process begins with obtaining a history of the patient's previous exercise habits,

health beliefs, and perceptions of the need to make lifestyle changes. This helps in setting reasonable goals and in identifying potential problems. Special efforts should be made to improve patients' satisfaction with the care and attention they receive. At the same time their concept of self-management should be reinforced by encouraging them to take responsibility for their own health actions and providing techniques for self-monitoring, such as the rating of perceived exertion and heart rate limits. Patients can thus obtain more immediate feedback, which, in turn, becomes a powerful source of reinforcement for maintaining the exercise habit. Involving the family as much as possible, including allowing spouses to exercise with patients, is encouraged (Fig. 16–16).

Follow-up Assessment

Routine follow-up assessment by each team member should be performed and discussed with the patient at least twice a month during the subacute and intensive rehabilitation phases. At this time each team member should review the progress made by the patient since entering the program and any problems (risk factors) that still

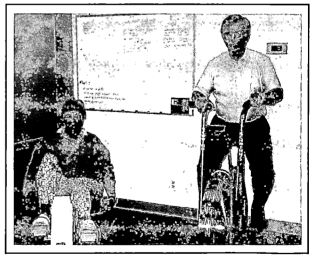

Figure 16–16.
Patient *(right)* and spouse enjoying an exercise session together.

need to be modified. New short-term goals and changes in the program should be established as patients increase their exercise performance and are cleared to resume various activities, for example, return to work. A copy of these assessments must be forwarded to the attending physician, who remains the primary physician throughout.

Discharge Criteria

When to discharge a patient from any program is a difficult decision to make, probably more so for cardiac patients because we are asking them to make lifelong changes, some of which require long-term support mechanisms from the appropriate sources. It is not easy for the patient and spouse to maintain a continuous awareness of the requirements of the program, and self-motivation is often hard to find. However, reimbursement agencies are requesting definitions of discharge criteria, and perhaps they are correct in trying to identify the point at which to say that the individual has completed the rehabilitation phase of recovery. Therefore, we need to become outcome oriented with our rehabilitation goals and plans. Some key points for discharge are

- achievement of goals
- failure to make reasonable progress toward goals, due to
  - nonadherence to the home program
  - failure to attend scheduled appointments
  - lack of willingness or ability to participate in the program

Records and Documentation

Records provide a method of retrieving information, evaluating the value and validity of the rehabilitation process, and analyzing cost effectiveness and quality assurance. Records should be kept thoroughly and accurately (Fig. 16–17), subject to periodic analysis, and include

- attending physician referral and authorization for treatment

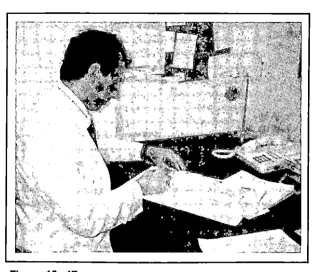

Figure 16–17.

The physical therapist documents the results of a cardiac rehabilitation session on a patient's chart.

- copies of pertinent medical data: results of ECG, echocardiogram, exercise tests, other noninvasive tests, cardiac catheterization report, results of cardiac surgery, and report from attending physician
- initial cardiac rehabilitation evaluation summary and goals listed by team members
- regular progress notes from each session that summarize the patient's performance, including resting and exercise heart rates, resting and exercise blood pressures, signs and symptoms, workload, peak interval time, ECG results, and any other pertinent data (e.g., medication changes, physician appointments, environmental conditions)
- monthly reports to attending physician as summarized by the medical director, program coordinator, and staff
- monthly log records—copies of patient's home records (e.g., exercise log, weight record, diet diary)
- discharge summary, including progress the patient has made regarding functional changes; physiologic and psychological changes; risk factor modifications achieved and those still needing further attention; compliance with home program; reasons for limited change, if that is the case; recommendations for follow-up testing or counseling; and reason the patient is being discharged

Medical and Legal Considerations

At times, certain legal and insurance considerations assume a very significant role in the rehabilitation of the cardiac patient. Possible legal problems stem from two aspects of this program:

- Adverse effects of medically prescribed exercise testing and fitness conditioning
- Consideration of disability pension and insurance benefits that may influence the patient's motivation to return to work and may affect the attitude of an employer toward a person with "a heart problem"

Exercise testing and recommendations to patients in the conditioning program by a physician constitute medical treatment. All medical personnel must be continuously alert to those aspects of testing and training that are eventually dangerous to each individual. They must pay special attention to recognize indications and contraindications to be sure that a thorough pre-exercise screening examination has been performed, that the exercise sessions are properly supervised and monitored, and that exercise is terminated when potentially dangerous situations arise. There must be adequate advance preparation for and training in emergency procedures in accordance with generally accepted medical standards. Patients also must be fully informed of the potential benefits, risks, and hazards associated with exercise conditioning programs and be given an opportunity to ask questions and withdraw from treatment without jeopardy of future medical care so that the informed consent document can be classified as legally valid. In addition, when a physician authorizes a return to work for the patient, the physician must understand the duties and potential hazards of the work for which clearance is being given.

Charges to Patients and Third-Party Carriers

Cardiac rehabilitation is not a major income producer in most facilities. In fact, cardiac rehabilitation often has difficulty breaking even in many settings in which both direct and indirect costs are factored, the latter being difficult to budget. Cardiac rehabilitation is considered by many administrations to be part of the total picture of cardiology care (product line) and can, to some degree, be carried by other subdepartments, given the positive influence a quality cardiac care program can have on the hospital and the community. The business structure and nature of each program and the overhead expenses dictate how fees are established. Although most insurance carriers reimburse part or all of the cardiac rehabilitation program, patients should take responsibility for understanding what the charges cover; therefore, the staff must understand these charges to explain them well. Fees should be kept reasonable and within the standards set for similar programs within the hospital and community. Since 1982, Medicare has reimbursed for up to 12 weeks or 36 visits of an approved outpatient cardiac rehabilitation program for patients who have undergone a myocardial infarction or bypass surgery or who have stable angina pectoris. Because a growing percentage of the cardiac patient population is covered by Medicare, it is important to have the program certified by Medicare. Many other insurance carriers follow Medicare's lead in coverage, and as Medicare changes, they will probably follow. Blue Cross–Blue Shield varies in coverage considerably from state to state; however, their national policy is to support and provide some degree of coverage (usually three visits). Patient education is felt to be the role of the physician and is not reimbursed. State-aid agencies rarely cover cardiac rehabilitation services. Nutrition counseling is rarely reimbursed as a separate service. Reimbursement for exercise testing depends on the policy; however, it is usually reimbursed as a procedure when ordered by the physician before commencing rehabilitation.

It is important to the financial success of the program to be familiar with reimbursement rates, company policies, and limitations in coverage of insurance companies in your area for inpatient and outpatient cardiac rehabilitation. Policies regarding treatment of uninsured or uncovered services must be established and understood by all team members and explained to the patient and family before commencing the rehabilitation program. Each individual should also be familiar with the program charges for each phase. Some programs take the position that it is the patient's responsibility to find out whether a particular insurance company covers cardiac rehabilitation. Having someone who can answer basic questions about insurance coverage can be helpful when the patient and family are going through a stressful time.

Pediatric Programs

As children with congenital cardiovascular disorders survive into their adult years, it becomes increasingly important to evaluate, train, and advise them and their families in activity and exercise prescription guidelines. Cardiac rehabilitation for children after cardiac surgery is emerging as an area of considerable interest. The Children's Hospital National Medical Center in Washington, D.C., has established a 12-week training program focusing on this specialty in an environment similar to that used in an elementary and secondary physical education class.[60] It is led by experienced physical education teachers who have expertise in current methodology and techniques of physical education and by other staff members, including exercise specialists and a pediatric cardiologist. Parents and siblings are encouraged to participate in the activity component of the program. These programs have demonstrated significant improvement in the child's physical work capacity as well as improved social interactions.

Screening of children for cardiovascular risk has become a topic of interest and some controversy. The American Academy of Pediatrics recommends screening children with a family history of premature coronary artery disease or hyperlipidemia; others support mass screenings of all children because some research has shown as many as two thirds of the children with elevated cholesterol levels would go undetected by use of the Academy's recommendations.[61,62] Several studies have noted a stronger relationship between several risk factors such as exercise and serum lipids and glucose intolerance and weight-height and skinfold thickness.[63] Advocates of mass screening also encourage aggressive early management of hyperlipidemia in this population

and point to school-based interventions as the best means of reaching the greatest number of children.[64]

CASE STUDIES

CASE 1 – Effect of cardiac rehabilitation on a young patient with idiopathic cardiomyopathy

Clinical History

On September 15, 1986, JS, a 22-year-old man, was admitted to the hospital from his doctor's office following a work-up for progressive dyspnea and orthopnea of 10-days' duration. The chest radiograph demonstrated cardiomegaly with pulmonary vascular engorgement and pulmonary venous hypertension. The ECG demonstrated left axis deviation, left ventricular hypertrophy, and diffuse Q waves anteriorly and inferiorly. Echocardiography demonstrated a dilated left ventricle with severe generalized hypokinesis and an estimated ejection fraction of 15% to 17%. On admission, his resting heart rate was 120, blood pressure 132/102, and respiratory rate 28; he had a loud S3 and S4 on auscultation.

JS was diagnosed as having a dilated cardiomyopathy of unknown origin, and he received conservative treatment for congestive heart failure, including high doses of furosemide (Lasix, 80–120 mg), captopril, continuous oxygen, and establishment of a 1-gram sodium diet. He was placed on strict bedrest and made a rather miraculous recovery during the next 7 days.

Cardiac Rehabilitation

On September 22, JS was referred to cardiac rehabilitation for monitoring during low-level activity, beginning with getting out of bed and into a chair. During the next several days his program was slowly advanced to include ADLs and progressive ambulation. He tolerated low-level activity well and had appropriate physiologic responses; however, it became difficult to restrain his activity as he began to feel stronger. Repeat echocardiography on September 29 still demonstrated severe left ventricular hypokinesis, not quite as sluggish, with an estimated ejection fraction of 20% to 25%. On September 30, JS was discharged from the hospital to his grandmother's house and given a 2-gram sodium diet and very low-level activity guidelines. He was told not to exceed household ambulation and to avoid climbing stairs.

JS was a 6-foot 1-inch well-built auto mechanic who lived in a second-floor apartment with his girlfriend. He had smoked cigarettes since he was 14 years old and consumed 4 to 6 cans of beer per day. He weighed 205 pounds on admission to the hospital and diuresed 17 pounds before his discharge.

Outpatient Program

JS underwent low-level treadmill testing on October 4 and began outpatient cardiac rehabilitation on October 6. Treadmill test results were very good considering his clinical status and degree of left ventricular dysfunction (see Exercise Tests). His training program results during the first 6 months were also very impressive.

dietary regimen; however, he refused to come in for a follow-up visit. In November 1987, JS was readmitted to the hospital's intensive care unit in overt congestive heart failure, his weight 211 pounds. Over the next 10 days he gradually improved. Nonetheless, the physician decided to have him evaluated for heart transplant at the University Hospital. Following a work-up by the heart transplant team, JS was declared to be a good candidate for transplantation; however, because of his limited finances and the scarcity of donor organs, JS was placed on a potential recipient list, and he was discharged home with high doses of Lasix, captopril, and digoxin, guidelines for low-level activity, and a beeper to signal when a donor organ was received. In the meantime, he was referred back to the cardiac rehabilitation program, where he worked closely with the rehabilitation team, especially with the dietitian, who helped JS and his girlfriend adopt a reasonable low-sodium diet plan.

As time progressed, JS demonstrated significant progress with his program. Four months after evaluation for cardiac transplantation, he decided to take himself off the list of potential recipients. Recent repeat echocardiography demonstrated marked global hypokinesis; however, in comparison with previous studies, left ventricular systolic function appeared to have improved. JS

Training Program

Date	Initial	1 month	2 months	3 months	6 months
Time (peak int)	3 × 5 min	5-20-5	5-30-5	5-30-5	5-40-5
Training heart rate (bpm)	120–126	132–138	132–144	132–150	150
Workload (treadmill, mph)	2	2.5–3.0	3.0	3.4	4–5
Weight (lbs)	190	192	188	194	196

JS moved back to his apartment in January 1987 and returned to part-time employment in April 1987, again working on cars. In May 1987 JS stopped coming to cardiac rehabilitation although we did keep in touch with him by telephone. He reported that he was doing well and complying with his home exercise program and

remains compliant with his home program of exercise and strict low-sodium diet and is reassessed regularly (at least monthly) in the phase IV program. His weight fluctuates within 6 pounds, and he is back in school studying computer programming.

Exercise Tests

Date	Initial	12/86	5/87	8/88	9/89
Protocol	Balke 2	Balke 3	Bruce	Bruce	Bruce
Time (min)	10	9	9	10	11
Heart rate (bpm)	87–170	89–187	90–185	66–188	74–186
Mean blood pressure	146/96	178/70	180/80	176/84	180/90
ECG	PACs	PAC, PVCs	PVCs	PVCs	PVCs
$\dot{V}O_{2max}$ (ml/kg/min)	18.8 (39%)	26.7 (56%)	24.4 (52%)	22.7 (48%)	26.2 (56%)
Heart rate at ventilatory threshold (bpm)	136	145	150	165	160
Weight (lbs)	189	191	194	192	187

CASE 2 – Effect of cardiac rehabilitation on an individual with an uncomplicated myocardial infarction and percutaneous transluminal coronary angioplasty

Clinical History

JH was a 51-year-old glazier when admitted to the emergency department on January 16, 1987, with a 2-hour duration of substernal discomfort after playing a vigorous game of basketball with his two sons. He had no previous history of chest discomfort; however, he had noticed some recent shortness of breath on the job. Echocardiography performed in the emergency department confirmed early ECG changes of anteroseptal infarction with a small area of akinesis. He was admitted to the intensive care unit and taken to the cardiac catheterization laboratory the next day for angiography. Selective coronary catheterization demonstrated proximal and mid left anterior descending artery (LAD) lesions of 80%, 75% to 80% lesions in the obtuse marginal branch of the circumflex, and a normal right coronary artery. It was decided to perform a percutaneous transluminal coronary angioplasty procedure on the 2 LAD lesions, which was done successfully with resultant 30% proximal stenosis. JH was placed on calcium antagonists (nifedipine 10 mg, three times a day) and was returned to the intensive care unit for the next 48 hours before being moved to the stepdown unit. Repeat echocardiography on January 20 confirmed a small area of

anteroseptal akinesis with good ventricular function.

Cardiac Rehabilitation

On January 20 JH was referred to cardiac rehabilitation for evaluation for appropriate activity guidelines. He demonstrated appropriate response to ADLs and ambulation except for slight tachycardia of 132 beats per minute with ambulation; however, no other symptoms or ECG changes occurred, and blood pressure response was appropriate.

JH's risk factor profile looked pretty good. He had a history of hypertension for the past 5 years that was controlled by diet; a family history of heart disease, with his father having had a myocardial infarction; and a slight problem with his weight (6 feet 6 inches, 230 pounds). His hobbies included fishing and watching sports, which are relatively sedentary. He was seen twice daily by the cardiac rehabilitation team for monitored ambulation, function on the stairs, and counseling by the dietitian; he was given discharge guidelines by the rehabilitation team. He also underwent a low-level treadmill test before discharge on January 22.

JH entered phase II of the cardiac rehabilitation program on January 24 and began a progressive ambulation training program at training heart rates of 126–138 and/or systolic blood pressure to 180, diastolic to 90. Unfortunately, his diastolic blood pressure was hard to maintain below 100 and it was elected to increase his nifedipine. JH's training program and exercise test results follow:

Training Program

Date	Initial	3 months	6 months	year 1	year 2	year 3
Time	5-20-5	5-45-5	5-60-5	5-60-5	5-60-5	5-60-5
Training heart rate (bpm)	126–132	140–150	150	150	150	150
Workload (treadmill and jogging)	3 mph (TM)	4–5 mph (TM)	9-min mile	8-min mile	7.5-min mile	7.5-min mile
Weight (lbs)	227	214	220	210	206	205

Exercise Tests

Date	Initial	5/87	6/88	4/90
Protocol	Mod. Bruce	Bruce	Bruce	Bruce
Time (min)	9	12	13	13.5
Heart rate (bpm)	78–152	72–145	63–146	48–155
Mean blood pressure	190/100	240/112	230/96	204/88
$\dot{V}O_{2max}$ (ml/kg/min)	Not tested	36.5	39.3	42.4
Heart rate at ventilatory threshold (bpm)	Not tested	128	123	130

JH returned to work within 4 weeks after his myocardial infarction and to full activity by week 6. Of significance is the continued improvement of his physical work capacity, lower resting heart rate, and improved blood pressure response. JH has participated in many 10-kilometer races and recently ran a sub 40-minute race. His wife and children have become avid exercisers as well.

CASE 3 – Effect of cardiac rehabilitation on an individual who had a complicated myocardial infarction course (moderate risk)

Clinical History

RK is a 63-year-old man who recently (4 months) retired from more than 30 years as a health and physical education instructor. He had no history of heart disease, chest pain, or shortness of breath with activity. He did have mild hypertension (systolic 160s, diastolic 80s) that was documented for the past 5 years, which was not treated medically. Other risk factors included a positive family history (mother and father having died of heart disease in their late sixties and a younger brother who had undergone coronary artery bypass graft surgery 2 years earlier at the age of 52). On October 12, 1987, he was admitted to the emergency department with a 1-hour history of chest pain. The ECG demonstrated evidence of acute injury pattern in the anterior leads. He was taken immediately to the cardiac catheterization laboratory where he was found to have a total occlusion of the mid LAD, a mid circumflex lesion of 50%, and a normal right coronary artery. A percutaneous transluminal coronary angioplasty was performed successfully (100% decreased to 40%) at that time. He spent the next 72 hours recovering in the intensive care unit with rhythm disturbances, including atrial fibrillation and multifocal premature ventricular complexes. Cardiac medications included low doses of verapamil.

Cardiac Rehabilitation

After being moved to the stepdown unit, cardiac rehabilitation was initiated on October 16 with instruction to move the patient slowly and assess cardiac rhythm. During self-care monitoring, he demonstrated several abnormal responses:

1. Resting heart rate: 98-supine, 110-sitting, 120-standing, 162-ADL (brushing teeth) at bedside
2. Blood pressure: 110/70-supine, 100/70-sitting, 90/60-standing, 85/50-ADL
3. Symptoms: fatigue and lightheadedness reported with ADLs
4. ECG: initially sinus rhythm, then atrial flutter (2:1) and atrial fibrillation with ADLs

Self-care monitoring was terminated, and RK returned to bed where his heart rate returned to the 90s, his symptoms improved, and his blood pressure returned to 110/70. His cardiologist was notified immediately of his poor response to low-level activity, so the verapamil dosage was increased and digoxin was added. Later that same day self-care monitoring was repeated, the results of which were an appropriate response to ADLs and ambulation of 600 feet.

RK progressed well the next 2 days with appropriate ECG and physiologic responses to activity, but on October 19, he notified nursing of right-sided chest pain at rest with accompanying hemoptysis. A lung scan revealed probable pulmonary embolus, and a chest radiograph demonstrated a moderate-sized pleural effusion. He was immediately started on anticoagulants (heparin) and was put on bedrest over the next few days until a chest radiograph confirmed clearing and his chest discomfort resolved some 72 hours later. Before his discharge on October 25, he underwent a low-level treadmill test and completed 4 minutes using a Bruce protocol, achieving a maximal heart rate of 100 and a maximal systolic blood pressure of 154 with multifocal premature ventricular complexes (<6 per min). No clinical or ECG changes indicated the presence of ischemia, and the test was stopped because of dyspnea and fatigue. Discharge guidelines were based on dyspnea levels (not to exceed 2+/4+) or an RPE level of 12 with any activity.

Outpatient Program

On October 27, RK returned to the hospital to begin phase II of the cardiac rehabilitation program. He reported no problems the first 2 days at home and tolerated low-level activity as prescribed. His program progression during the first 4 weeks (seen twice a week) was unremarkable, and he progressed to 25 minutes of continuous ambulation at a training heart rate of 96 beats per minute. At that time, however, his rhythm had changed from sinus to junctional, and he began having more frequent episodes of supraventricular tachycardia to rates of 160 to 180 beats per minute, along with multifocal premature ventricular contractions with occasional coupling. In addition, he experienced occasional bouts of lightheadedness not associated with position change or exercise. His cardiologist was notified, and he elected to increase his dosage of verapamil and add disopyramide phosphate (Norpace; antiarrhythmic). He was scheduled for a thallium treadmill test in 1 week. Forty-eight hours later, however, RK was brought to the emergency department with severe chest pain. He was taken immediately to the cardiac catheterization laboratory where it was determined that the original mid LAD lesion had narrowed again. It was redilated successfully and RK was taken to the intensive care unit, where he was monitored closely for the next 48 hours. Before discharge he underwent a thallium treadmill test, and metabolic data were also collected (see Exercise Tests). The thallium test demonstrated a small area of stress-induced ischemia of the anteroapical segment of the left ventricle.

RK returned to phase II for 2 more weeks and then moved to phase III, during which his program was slowly graduated to include 40 minutes of continuous ambulation at a training heart rate of 90 to 96 beats per minute, light weight training, and use of a four-extremity ergometer (Schwinn Airdyne). His home program included 15 minutes of warm-up stretching exercises (he placed a great deal of emphasis on flexibility owing to an old back problem), 35 to 45 minutes of fast walking or aerobics, and 10 to 15 minutes of cool-down exercises. He also did a series of exercises with 3- to 5-pound free weights for upper body conditioning. RK underwent repeat metabolic treadmill testing following completion of phase III and again 1 year later after participating in phase IV (see Exercise Tests). Of particular interest besides improvement in physical work capacity is the higher ventilatory threshold heart rates relative to maximal heart rates. Also of significance is the increased total time, lower resting heart rate, higher systolic blood pressure with exercise, and improved ECG response at maximal exercise. RK continues to do well despite bouts with supraventricular arrhythmia.

lateral ischemia. His creatine phosphokinase value on admission rose to a maximum of 452 (N = <150). BS had been a 1-pack-a-day smoker since he was 19. He had a history of mild hypertension that had not been treated and was physically inactive and overweight at 5 feet 11 inches and 192 pounds. His brother had elevated blood sugar levels and was on medication; otherwise there was no family history of heart disease. On admission BS's blood cholesterol level was 270, triglycerides 204, HDL 23, and LDL 149.

Exercise Tests

Date	10/25/87	12/3/87	4/7/88	6/16/89
Protocol	Bruce	Bruce	Bruce	Bruce
Time (min)	4.0	7.0	10.0	11.5
Heart rate (bpm)	58–108	57–122	49–133	47–128
Mean blood pressure	154/68	152/72	176/82	188/84
ECG	1 mm ST↓	1.5 mm ST↓	1.5 mm ST↓	<1 mm ST↓
$\dot{V}O_{2max}$ (ml/kg/min)		16.8	19.6	23.4
Heart rate at ventilatory threshold (bpm)		90	100	108
Weight (lbs)		152	155	159
RPE at ventilatory threshold		14	13	12

CASE 4 – Effect of cardiac rehabilitation for a patient who had a myocardial infarction followed by coronary bypass surgery

Clinical History

BS was a 40-year-old college administrator at the time of his admission to the hospital from the emergency department on January 20, 1986, following several episodes of nocturnal chest pain, nausea, and vomiting. He also had one episode of chest pain with nausea and vomiting the previous day while walking up a hill. In the emergency department his ECG tracing was suggestive of an old anteroseptal infarction and antero-

Cardiac catheterization was performed on January 22, which demonstrated a minimal impairment of left ventricular function inferiorly, a proximal LAD stenosis of 70%, a very large circumflex artery with 90% stenosis proximally, and a right coronary artery stenosis of 100% with retrograde filling of the posterior descending branch from collaterals of the left coronary system. On January 24, he underwent three-vessel bypass surgery, which included using the internal mammary artery as a graft to bypass the LAD lesion and two vein grafts to the obtuse marginal branch of the circumflex and posterior descending branches. Following a good postoperative recovery, which included phase I cardiac rehabilitation started on day 2 after the operation, and an appropriate response to progressive activity, he was discharged home 6 days after his surgery.

Outpatient Rehabilitation

BS was an ideal candidate for cardiac rehabilitation. He was well motivated, had three major and four minor risk factors, and experienced minimal ventricular dysfunction. Three days after discharge from the hospital, BS started phase II cardiac rehabilitation. He received an orientation to the program and began ambulation on the treadmill for 15 minutes at low level (2 mph, 0% grade) during his first visit. He was then referred for his initial low-level treadmill test (see Exercise Tests).

BS obviously made significant improvement in physical work capacity and in all exercise test parameters. Most noteworthy is a progressively lower resting heart rate, lower diastolic blood pressure values, and higher heart rate response before reaching ventilatory threshold. Most impressive is the change in BS's risk profile within 1 year after bypass surgery:

- Smoking — stopped
- Elevated cholesterol — normalized
- Hypertension — normalized
- Overweight — normalized
- Sedentary — became more active
- Stress — although hard to assess, BS reports that he now takes time to do the things he knew he should have been doing and enjoys life to the fullest.

Training Program

Date	Initial	3 mo	6 mo	yr 1	yr 2
Time	5-15-5	5-40-5	5-50-5	10-60-5	10-60-70-5
Training heart rate (bpm)	120	132–144	150	150	150+
Workload (treadmill, jogging)	2 mph	walk/jog	10-min mile	8-min mile	7.5-min mile
Weight (lbs)	193	181	175	166	167

Lipid Values

Cholesterol	204	225	185	197	152
Triglycerides	158	117	77	46	97
HDL	23	32	45	43	55
Chol: HDL	8.9:1	7:1	4:1	4.6:1	2.8:1
LDL	149	168	125	145	77

Exercise Tests

Date	2/2/86	4/5/86	11/11/86	5/9/87
Protocol	Mod. Bruce	Bruce	Bruce	Bruce
Time (min)	9	11	15	15
Heart rate (bpm)	75–135	80–188	62–177	54–178
Mean blood pressure	150/80	180/96	190/90	190/80
ECG			Premature atrial complexes	Occasional premature ventricular complexes
$\dot{V}O_{2max}$ (ml/kg/min)	Not tested	Not tested	39.14 (108% N)	42.18 (114% N)
Heart rate at ventilatory threshold (bpm)			145–150	160
RPE at ventilatory threshold			12	12

SUMMARY

- A growing number of patient populations are identified as appropriate candidates for exercise training.
- Longer duration and higher levels of intensity may produce the greatest change in exercise performance and risk factors across all patient populations.
- Stratification of patients as low, moderate, and high risk is an important element in the rehabilitation process to maintain a safe environment for all patients and to assist individuals who need a higher degree of support.
- Ways must be sought to keep individuals motivated to continue with their risk reduction programs.
- Programs that are patient oriented instead of facility oriented are most successful.
- Physical therapists should be acutely aware of the cardiovascular implications of the problems of all patient populations, especially when treating the elderly.
- One future problem in cardiac rehabilitation to be confronted is that of ensuring adequate reimbursement for all patients who choose to participate. This may in turn help to improve long-term patient compliance.

References

1. Levine SA, Lown B. "Armchair" treatment of acute coronary thrombosis. JAMA 148:1365, 1952.
2. Leon AS, Certo C, Comoss, P, et al. Position paper of the American Association of Cardiovascular and Pulmonary Rehabilitation: Scientific evidence of the value of cardiac rehabilitation services with emphasis on patients following myocardial infarction—section I: Exercise conditioning component. J Cardiopulmonary Rehab 10:79–87, 1990.
3. McNeer JF, Wallace AG, Wagner GS, et al. The course of acute myocardial infarction: Feasibility of early discharge of the uncomplicated patient. Circulation 51:410, 1975.
4. Hossack KF, Bruce RA. Prognostic value of exercise testing: The Seattle Heartwatch experience. J Cardiopulmonary Rehab 5:9–19, 1985.
5. Weiner DA, Ryan TJ, McCabe CH. The prognostic importance of a clinical profile and exercise test in medically treated patients with coronary heart disease. Am J Coll Cardiol 3:772–779, 1984.
6. Maskin C, Reddy H, Gulanick M, Perez L. Exercise training in chronic heart failure: Improvement in cardiac performance and maximum oxygen uptake. Circulation 74(suppl II):310, 1986.
7. Lee AP, Ice R, Blessey R, San Marco ME. Long term effects of physical training on coronary patients with impaired ventricular function. Circulation 60:1519–1526, 1979.
8. Coates AJ, Adamopoulos S, Meyer TE, et al. Effects of physical training in chronic heart failure. Lancet 335(8681):63–66, 1990.
9. Wenger NK, Hellerstein HK. Rehabilitation of the Coronary Patient. New York, John Wiley & Sons, 1984.
10. Garrow JS. Effects of exercise on obesity. Acta Med Scand 711(suppl):67–74, 1986.
11. Haskell WL. The influence of exercise training on plasma lipids and lipoproteins in health and disease. Acta Med Scand 711(suppl):25–38, 1986.
12. Hagberg JM, Seals DR. Exercise training and hypertension. Acta Med Scand 711(suppl):131–136, 1986.
13. Holloszy JO, Schultz J, Kusnierkiewicz J, et al. Glucose tolerance and insulin resistance. Acta Med Scand 711(suppl):67–73, 1986.
14. Clausen JP. Circulatory adjustments to dynamic exercise and physical training in normal subjects and in patients with coronary artery disease. In: Sonnenblick EH, Lesch M (eds). Exercise and the Heart. New York, Grune & Stratton, 1977, pp 39–75.
15. Detry J-MR, Rousseau M, Vandenbroucke G, et al. Increased arteriovenous oxygen difference after physical training in coronary heart disease. Circulation 64:109–118, 1971.
16. Pollack ML, Wilmore JH. Exercise in Health and Disease: Evaluation and Prescription for Prevention and Rehabilitation. 2nd ed. Philadelphia, WB Saunders, 1990, pp 1–750.
17. Thompson PD. The benefits and risks of exercise training in patients with chronic coronary artery disease. JAMA 259:1537–1540, 1988.
18. Ehsani AA, Biello DR, Schultz J, et al. Improvement of left ventricular contractile function in patients with coronary artery disease. Circulation 74:350–388, 1986.
19. May GS, Eberlein KA, Furberg CD, et al. Secondary prevention after myocardial infarction: A review of long term trials. Prog Cardiovasc Dis 24:331–362, 1982.
20. Heath GW, Malorey PM, Fure CW. Group exercise versus home exercise in coronary artery bypass graft patients: Effects on physical activity. J Cardiopulmonary Rehab 7:190–195, 1987.
21. Debusk RF, Haskell WL, Miller NH, et al. Medically directed at-home rehabilitation soon after clinically uncomplicated acute myocardial infarction. A new model for patient care. Am J Cardiol 55:251–257, 1985.
22. Wolfel EE, Hossack KF. Guidelines for exercise training of elderly healthy individuals and elderly patients with cardiac disease. J Cardiopulmonary Rehab 9:40–45, 1989.
23. Froelicher V, Jensen D, Genter F, et al. A randomized trial of exercise training in patients with coronary heart disease. JAMA 252:1291–1297, 1984.
24. Conn EH, Williams RS, Wallace AG. Exercise responses before and after physical conditioning in patients with severely depressed left ventricular function. Am J Cardiol 49:296–300, 1982.
25. Arvan S. Exercise performance of the high risk acute myocardial infarction patient after cardiac rehabilitation. Am J Cardiol 62(4):197–201, 1988.
26. Sullivan MJ, Cobb FR. The anaerobic threshold in chronic heart failure. Relation to blood lactate, ventilatory basis, reproducibility and response to exercise training. Circulation 81(suppl 2)II:47–58, 1990.

27. Naughton JP, Hellerstein HK. Exercise Testing and Exercise Training in Coronary Heart Disease. New York, Academic Press, 1973.

28. Goldberg L, Elliott DL, Kuehl KS, et al. Assessment of exercise intensity formulas by use of ventilatory threshold. Chest 94:95–98, 1988.

29. Gibbons E. The influence of anaerobic threshold in exercise prescription. Sports Med 27:357–361, 1987.

30. Dwyer J, Bybee R. Heart rate indices of the anaerobic threshold. Med Sci Sports Exerc 15:72–76, 1983.

31. Ades PA, Grunvald MH, Weiss RM, Hanson JS. Usefulness of myocardial ischemia as a predictor of training effect with cardiac rehabilitation after acute myocardial infarction or coronary artery bypass graft. Am J Cardiol 63(15):1032–1036, 1989.

32. Hossack VF, Hartwick R. Cardiac arrest associated with supervised cardiac rehabilitation. J Cardiopulmonary Rehab 2:402–408, 1982.

33. Bergh V, Kamstrup L, Ekblom B. Maximal oxygen uptake during exercise with various combinations of arm and leg work. J Appl Physiol 41:191–196, 1976.

34. Gutin B, Ang EK, Torrey MA. Cardiorespiratory and subjective responses to incremental and constant load ergometry with arms and legs. Arch Phys Med Rehabil 69:510–513, 1988.

35. Van Camp SP, Peterson RA. Cardiorespiratory complications of outpatient cardiac rehabilitation programs. JAMA 256(9):1160–1163, 1986.

36. Mannarino E, Pasqualini L, Menna M, et al. Effects of physical training on peripheral vascular disease: A controlled study. Angiology 40(1):5–10, 1989.

37. Johnson EC, Vogles WF, Atterbom HA, et al. Effects of exercise training on common femoral artery blood flow in patients with intermittent claudication. Circulation 80(5pt2):III59–72, 1989.

38. Kannel WB, McGee DL. Diabetes and cardiovascular risk factors: The Framingham study. Circulation 59:8, 1979.

39. American Diabetes Association. The Physicians Guide to Type II Diabetes (NIDMM): Diagnosis and Treatment. New York, American Diabetes Association, 1984.

40. Fowler RS, Fordyce WE. Stroke: Why Do They Behave That Way? Dallas, Texas, American Heart Association, 1974.

41. Monga TN, DeForge DA, Williams J, Wolfe LA. Cardiovascular responses to acute exercise in patients with cerebrovascular accidents. Arch Phys Med Rehabil 69:937–940, 1988.

42. Painter P, Hanson P. A model for clinical exercise prescription: Application to hemodialysis patients. J Cardiopulmonary Rehab 7:177–189, 1987.

43. Painter P, Messer-Rehale D, Hanson P, et al. Exercise capacity in hemodialysis, CAPD and renal transplant patients. Nephron 42:47–51, 1986.

44. Christie I, Pewen W. A 12 week trial of exercise training in patients on continuous ambulatory peritoneal dialysis (unpublished).

45. Seals DR, Allen WK, Hurley BF, et al. Elevated high density lipoprotein cholesterol levels in older endurance athletes. Am J Cardiol 54:390–393, 1984.

46. Lampman RM. Evaluating and prescribing exercise for elderly patients. Geriatrics 42(8):63–65, 1987.

47. Kannel WB, Castelli WP, Gordon T, et al. Serum cholesterol lipoproteins and risk of coronary heart diseases: The Framingham study. Ann Intern Med 74:1–12, 1971.

48. Lowering blood cholesterol to prevent heart disease. JAMA 253:2080–2090, 1985.

49. Blank DW, Hoeg JM, Kroll MH, et al. The method of determination must be considered in interpreting blood cholesterol levels. JAMA 256:2867–2870, 1986.

50. Lipid Research Clinics Program: The Lipid Research Clinics Coronary Primary Prevention Trial Results I. Reduction in incidence of coronary heart disease. JAMA 251:351–364, 1984.

51. Lipid Research Clinics Program: The Lipid Research Clinics Coronary Primary Prevention Trial Results II. The relationship of reduction in incidence of coronary heart disease to cholesterol lowering. JAMA 251:365–374, 1984.

52. Wood PD, Stefanick ML, Dreon DM, et al. Changes in plasma lipoproteins in overweight men during weight loss through dieting as compared with exercise. N Engl J Med 319:1173–1179, 1988.

53. Tran ZV, Weltman A. Differential effects of exercise on serum lipid and lipoprotein levels seen with changes in body weight. A meta-analysis. JAMA 254:919–924, 1985.

54. Mumford E, Schlessinger H, Glass G. The effects of psychological intervention on recovery from surgery and heart attacks: An analysis of the literature. Am J Public Health 72(2):141–151, 1982.

55. Oldenburg B, Perkins R, Andrews G. Controlled trial of psychological intervention in myocardial infarction. J Consult Clin Psychol 53:852–859, 1985.

56. Murphy S. Self efficacy and social support-mediators of stress on mental health following a natural disorder. West J Nurs Res 9(1):58–87, 1987.

57. Strecher V, McEvoy B, Becker M, Rosenstock I. The role of self efficacy in achieving behavior changes. Health Educ Q 13(1):73–91, 1986.

58. Oldridge NB. Cardiac rehabilitation exercise programme. Compliance and compliance-enhancing strategies. Sports Med 6(1):42–55, 1988.

59. Pashkow F, Pashkow P, Schafer M, Ferguson C. Successful Cardiac Rehabilitation. Loveland, Colo, The Heartwatchers Press, 1988.

60. Tomassoni TL, Galioto FM, Vaccaro P, et al. The pediatric cardiac rehabilitation program at Children's Hospital National Medical Center, Washington, D.C. J Cardiopulmonary Rehab 7:259–262, 1987.

61. American Academy of Pediatrics. Position statement on cholesterol screening. Pediatrics 83:141–142, 1989.

62. Blessey R, Blessey S. Hypercholesterolemia in children: Is it a problem requiring intervention? Cardiopulmonary Physical Therapy Journal 1:10–12, 1990.

63. Srinivasan SR. Biological determinants of serum lipoprotein. In: Berenson G (ed). Causation of Cardiovascular Risk Factors in Children. New York, Raven Press, 1986, pp 83–129.

64. Walter HJ, Hofman A, Vaughan RD, et al. Modification of risk factors for coronary heart disease: Five year results of a school based intervention trial. N Engl J Med 318:1093–1100, 1988.

17 PULMONARY REHABILITATION

HISTORICAL PERSPECTIVE

Rehabilitation programs for patients with chronic obstructive pulmonary disease (COPD) have existed for more than 25 years. The American College of Chest Physicians in 1974 defined pulmonary rehabilitation and described aspects of care for patients with respiratory impairments. These were incorporated into an official position statement by the American Thoracic Society in 1981.[1] Unfortunately, even though COPD is one of the leading causes of morbidity and mortality in the United States,[2,3] pulmonary rehabilitation programs have had less recognition and acceptance than rehabilitation programs for patients with cardiovascular, neuromuscular, or musculoskeletal disorders. The American Thoracic Society position paper and most of the research available

address the benefits of rehabilitation for patients with COPD while neglecting the rehabilitation of patients with other chronic respiratory diseases such as restrictive lung diseases, spinal and chest deformities, neuromuscular conditions that lead to respiratory failure, pulmonary vascular diseases, and those that affect the very obese.

Whether the patient derives any benefit from participation in pulmonary rehabilitation programs is still a matter of controversy (Table 17–1). Most of the research in the area of pulmonary rehabilitation has focused on the lack of improvement, as documented by pulmonary function testing, or the failure to reverse the natural progression of the disease process. Steadily deteriorating function and eventual death despite intervention is the accepted fate of patients with COPD. Consequently, rehabilitation intervention

677

TABLE 17–1. Outcomes of Pulmonary Rehabilitation	
Outcomes of Improvement	Outcomes without Accepted Improvements
Symptom-limited exercise capacity[4–22]	Lung function[6–8,10–12,14–21,24]
Functional level (ADL)[4,9,10,15–17,20,23]	Heart function[6,13,14,19]
Respiratory symptoms[5,9,15,16,18–20,23]	Maximal aerobic capacity[4,6,18]
Respiratory muscle function[8,10,24]	Mortality rate[23]
Psychological status[4,16,23]	
Quality of life[4,6,18,20,23]	
Frequency of hospitalization[15,16,23,25]	

has been considered maintenance activity, and **third-party payers** have often severely limited the benefits paid for pulmonary rehabilitation. These factors have hampered the growth of rehabilitation services for pulmonary patients.

Despite these adversities, many successful pulmonary rehabilitation programs exist. The need for early detection and treatment of respiratory dysfunction is widely accepted. Many cardiac rehabilitation programs are increasing their scope to include patients with other chronic diseases, such as respiratory diseases. Rehabilitation research is beginning to emphasize functional outcomes (see Table 17–1) as measures of efficacy instead of changes in physiologic parameters. This trend supports the benefits that pulmonary rehabilitation specialists have claimed for rehabilitation.

Many rehabilitation principles can be generalized to all patient populations, including pulmonary rehabilitation patients: the need for multidisciplinary programming; goals aimed at restoring optimal physical and psychological functioning; and components of exercise, education and counseling. Disease-specific aspects of rehabilitation include

- education
- medical management
- physiologic and symptomatic limitations to physical effort

In this chapter, the rehabilitation components important for the pulmonary patient, goals for rehabilitation, personnel and their qualifications, and specific exercise programming guidelines are presented.

GOALS OF PULMONARY REHABILITATION

Although the overall goals of a pulmonary rehabilitation program can be very general and applicable to a wide range of patients, the goals for an individual must be very specific and pertinent to the individual's lifestyle, needs, and interests. This is possible only after a thorough evaluation of the patient's disease state and clinical course, a patient-family interview, and a physical examination. These steps are reviewed in Chapter 14.

General program goals for pulmonary rehabilitation may include

- improvement in health status: the patient will stop tobacco use, stop drug or alcohol misuse, and comply with medical and rehabilitation treatments.
- improvement in respiratory symptoms: the patient will learn to mobilize respiratory secretions, employ strategies to relieve symptoms of shortness of breath and cough, recognize early signs of the need for medical intervention, decrease the frequency and severity of respiratory exacerbations, and obtain optimal **oxygen saturation** throughout the day and night.
- improvement in daily activity tolerance: the patient will gain sufficient strength, flexibility, and endurance to accomplish identified activities of daily living and requirements of employment and recreational tasks and will learn to employ strategies to manipulate the environment to maximize physical functioning.
- improvement in nutritional status: the patient will obtain and maintain optimal body weight and composition, demonstrate adequate growth and physical maturation, or both.
- improvement in self-reliance: the patient will become independent in all areas of care, know how to contact appropriate resources for assistance, and learn behaviors that are consistent with obtaining and maintaining goals.

PULMONARY REHABILITATION TEAM MEMBERS

The specific professionals involved in pulmonary rehabilitation vary from program to program. Their particular qualifications and interests are more important than the professional degree they hold. Optimally, the core of the pulmonary rehabilitation program team consists of at least three to four rehabilitation specialists with varied experience and academic backgrounds. Additional professionals may consult with patients on an "as needed" basis or serve as program advisers to meet the needs of a diverse patient population.

The Advisory Board

The function of an advisory board is to oversee the administration of the program, including approving policies and procedures, reviewing program costs and outcomes, and making recommendations for future directions of the program. The board consists of the medical and program directors and other hospital administrators, physicians, professionals, and consumers who are capable of supporting the program.

The Medical Director

The medical director should be a physician who is a **pulmonologist.** The medical director directs the rehabilitation program in matters of overall policy, procedures, and medical care, including specialized diagnostic test and medical treatments for pulmonary diseases.

The Program Director

The program director is the administrator or coordinator of services. This person is the team leader, directing day-to-day functions of the pulmonary rehabilitation program according to the established policies and procedures. A diverse background in respiratory care as well as in edu-

cation and administration are necessary for this individual. The program director is often a nurse, respiratory therapist, or physical therapist. In smaller programs, the program director also provides direct patient care services.

The Respiratory Care Specialist

The role of this team member, who may be a nurse, physical therapist, or respiratory therapist, is to provide patient care services and education regarding the management of respiratory symptoms and treatments aimed at optimizing respiratory function and oxygenation.

The Exercise Specialist

The exercise specialist plans and directs the exercise and functional training components of the program. Often this person is a physical, occupational, or respiratory therapist or a nurse or exercise physiologist. Qualifications should include an academic preparation in exercise and respiratory physiology and clinical experience in prescribing and leading exercise programs for respiratory patients.

The Nutritionist or Dietitian

The key role of the nutritionist or dietitian is to evaluate and monitor the over- and undernourished conditions of the participants in the program and to recommend dietary changes to maximize rehabilitation potential.

The Behavior Specialist

The **behavior specialist** may be a social worker or psychologist. This person should have skills in motivating patients and family members to adopt behaviors that support the lifestyle changes recommended by the rehabilitation team and to learn stress management. Screening for significant psychological conditions and referral for individual counseling are important responsibilities of the behavior specialist.

Other professionals who can provide rehabilitation services include the pharmacist, vocational rehabilitation counselor, and recreational therapist.

CANDIDATES FOR REHABILITATION

Ideally, any person with a primary or secondary pulmonary disease or anyone at risk for the development of pulmonary disease could be a candidate for rehabilitation (Table 17-2). Such a broad definition of candidacy would include very large numbers of people. The high cost of health care prohibits the inclusion of all potential rehabilitation candidates. Therefore, realistic priorities must be set so that the available health care dollars can be allocated to those who can derive the most benefit from them. Too frequently these priorities are determined by third-party payers. Generally, candidates for rehabilitation must meet the following criteria: a diagnosed respiratory disease and documented functional limitations. There are regional differences in reimbursement patterns for rehabilitation services. In some areas, patients are required to obtain approval from third-party payers before they can enter rehabilitation programs.

All patients with respiratory symptoms of wheezing, coughing, or dyspnea, with or without abnormal spirometry, and those who are identified as at risk for the development of COPD need medical therapeutic intervention and preventive care.[3] This care usually includes a recommendation of smoking cessation or medication, among others. Comprehensive rehabilitation services are usually reserved for those with moderate to moderately severe COPD.[1] However, even patients with very advanced disease who are extremely limited by respiratory symptoms can demonstrate important functional gains and should not be excluded from rehabilitation programs.[4]

PROGRAM COMPONENTS

According to the American Thoracic Society's position paper on pulmonary rehabilitation[1] and other sources,[9,26-28] a comprehensive pulmonary rehabilitation program should incorporate six primary components, including

- general care
- respiratory therapy
- physical therapy
- exercise conditioning
- education
- psychosocial management

For the purposes of this chapter, these components are renamed according to the type of service provided:

- General care
- Pulmonary care
- Exercise and functional training
- Education
- Psychosocial management

A physical therapist may participate in any or all of the pulmonary rehabilitation program com-

TABLE 17-2. Conditions That Produce Candidates for Pulmonary Rehabilitation

Obstructive Diseases	Restrictive Diseases	Exposure to Risks for COPD	Chest Wall Defects	Pulmonary Vascular Conditions
Emphysema	Idiopathic pulmonary fibrosis	Cigarette smoking	Neuromuscular weakness	Pulmonary emboli
Bronchitis		Occupational exposure		Idiopathic, occlusive conditions
Bronchiectasis	Sarcoidosis	Air pollution	Chest deformities	
Cystic fibrosis	Asbestosis	Infections of the lungs	Obesity	Pulmonary hypertension
Alpha-antitrypsin deficiency	Silicosis	Impaired immune defenses	Spinal deformities	
	Adult respiratory distress syndrome		Chest surgery	

ponents. A brief description of each component is presented, followed by a lengthy discussion of pulmonary care and exercise and functional training, because it is in these areas of the rehabilitation process that the physical therapist can make the greatest contributions.

General Care

General care includes an initial physical and medical diagnostic evaluation to determine a specific diagnosis and an assessment of the severity of disease.[29] After an assessment is made, therapeutic intervention often includes prescription of medication and possibly oxygen and recommendations for preventive care. Preventive care may include immunizations and vaccinations, smoking cessation, avoidance of environmental irritants, adequate hydration, and proper nutrition, including weight control.

Before initiating rehabilitation, the patient should be assessed carefully for activity- or sleep-related oxygen needs.[9,26,30-34] A **pulse oximeter** or serial arterial blood gas measurements are used to determine whether the patient requires supplemental oxygen during activity or exercise or at night while sleeping. Decisions can then be made on the need for continuous or intermittent oxygen, the most suitable delivery system, and the appropriate dosages. Third-party payers have set specific reimbursement guidelines for the prescription of home oxygen therapy. The partial cost of home oxygen that most patients are required to pay is sometimes prohibitive. Oxygen-saving devices and methods, which increase the oxygen delivered at lower flow rates, can offer significant cost savings and convenience for the patient.[35-39]

Pulmonary Care

Respiratory treatment techniques for clearing accumulated pulmonary secretions and relieving dyspnea include

- bronchial drainage
- breathing techniques
- cough facilitation

- postures to improve breathing
- relaxation techniques
- bronchodilators
- respiratory assistance devices to rest the breathing muscles at night or during exercise[40-46]

It is very important to try a variety of procedures while the patient is in the rehabilitation setting to evaluate which are most effective for the patient and can be instituted in the home environment. Patients whose production of mucus is **copious** may require two to four respiratory treatments each day, whereas other patients may require treatment only during an acute illness. These procedures are described in more detail in Chapter 15 and later in this chapter under Physical Therapy Management.

Exercise and Functional Training

Instruction in energy conservation, pacing, and the use of adaptive equipment may be necessary to optimize the patient's ability to carry out usual daily activities for home, work, and recreation. Exercise to improve strength, flexibility, and cardiopulmonary endurance, including respiratory muscle training, is a major component of rehabilitation. Specific guidelines for exercise for the pulmonary patient are addressed later in this chapter.

Education

Patient and family education are often provided in a group classroom format to facilitate questions and discussion. Topics may include anatomy and pathophysiology of disease, medical management, early detection and treatment of acute illness, use and misuse of oxygen, and practical solutions to incorporating diet reform and activity into daily lives.

Psychosocial Management

Psychosocial management is an integral component of pulmonary rehabilitation because chronic disease places stress on the whole family. Coping strategies, stress reduction and management techniques, and support systems are necessary.[26,47–49] Behavioral strategies for facilitating lifestyle changes and compliance with treatments should be incorporated to improve the outcome of rehabilitation. Patients may also need financial assistance, vocational rehabilitation services, or both.

PHYSICAL THERAPY MANAGEMENT

Because of regional differences in practice patterns, the role of the physical therapist in pulmonary rehabilitation varies widely among programs. Some programs do not have a physical therapist at all, whereas others consult with a physical therapist only for patients with complicated diagnoses, such as those who have musculoskeletal or neuromuscular conditions in addition to pulmonary disease.

Ideally, the physical therapist has expertise in pulmonary rehabilitation and is involved in all components of the program. In addition to leading exercise sessions, the physical therapist may also provide educational sessions, smoking cessation programs, weight control or reduction programs, and stress management and relaxation training. The physical therapist should also evaluate the patient's performance in rehabilitation by monitoring progress and assessing outcomes. The components of pulmonary care and exercise and functional training are discussed, including the physiologic basis for treatment, treatment strategies, and monitoring. Lastly, potential outcomes of treatment intervention are presented.

Pulmonary Care

The physiologic basis for treatment and descriptions of pulmonary hygiene (airway clearance) techniques are reviewed in Chapter 15. The main emphasis of pulmonary care in the rehabilitation setting is the removal of excessive secretions that obstruct airways, cause ventilatory defects and bothersome symptoms of cough, and

possibly lead to an increased incidence of respiratory infections and deterioration of lung function.[50–53] This is especially important for patients who have chronic, copious, or thick pulmonary secretions, such as those with cystic fibrosis, bronchiectasis, and chronic bronchitis.[47] Patients with severe neuromuscular weakness of the respiratory muscles may also benefit from airway clearance techniques because acute pulmonary infections often cause respiratory failure in this patient group.[54–57]

Following a thorough evaluation, the physical therapist should employ treatment techniques that offer the best therapeutic results and are most convenient for the patient to continue at home. It is essential to offer the patient and family a variety of treatment options to enhance compliance.[58] Treatment modifications may be necessary if the patient does not have assistance at home. Modifications in treatment that may allow for self-treatment include the following:

- Modified bronchial drainage positions to facilitate the ease of assuming the appropriate position independently and comfortably. Firm foam wedges or cushions may be used to assume the **Trendelenburg position.**
- If percussion or vibration is necessary for complete airway clearance and adequate assistance is not available, then **palm cups, mechanical percussors,**[59] or a self-administered, high-frequency **chest compression system** can be employed instead.[60,61]
- Performance of a series of deep breathing exercises, forced expirations, and coughing or use of a mask that provides positive expiratory pressure may be adequate without **bronchial drainage.**[62–68] The breathing and coughing exercises may be done after bronchodilator treatments, first thing in the morning to remove the secretions that have accumulated overnight or before and after each exercise session.
- Sustained exercise, if tolerated by the patient, can have very beneficial airway-clearing effects.[69–71]

Pulmonary rehabilitation should include assessing the patient's ability to perform treatments independently and effectively. The short-term effects of treatments, such as improved breath sounds, volume of pulmonary secretions produced, and subjective improvements in breathing ability are important to monitor immediately after treatments. Long-term benefits that are monitored over the rehabilitation period may include

- maintainance of baseline pulmonary function
- reduced frequency of respiratory exacerbations
- decreased number and length of hospitalizations

Functional Training

Functional training is especially important for patients who have end-stage disease or significant symptoms of weakness, fatigue, or severe dyspnea that limit activities. Treatment goals include

- adapting the environment to improve the ease of performing activities of daily living
- altering the performance of tasks to decrease energy costs
- incorporating methods to relieve symptoms associated with activity

Essential to rehabilitation is the reversal of deconditioning to improve the patient's ability to do work. However, once the disease has progressed to the point that a patient is unable to sustain a training exercise load, then functional activity training and energy conservation become major components of rehabilitation.[4,47,72]

Environmental Modifications

Identification of the activities of daily living that are most problematic for the patient is the first step in modifying the environment. Once identified, the areas in the home in which these activities are performed should be evaluated for modification. Adaptations are usually necessary in the bathroom, bedroom, and kitchen. Basic concepts include

- providing work areas with supported seating of appropriate height for tasks done on a counter or table
- placing equipment that is used most often in convenient locations so that bending, reaching, and lifting are minimized

- locating a table or counter at work stations on which one can slide heavy items instead of lifting and carrying them
- locating chairs at appropriate places when rests are needed, such as on the landing of stairs or beside the bathtub
- using adaptive equipment to simplify tasks and improve comfort, for instance, a bath seat and hand-held shower head, a wheeled cart for transporting laundry or items for the dinner table, a set of grab bars or booster seats to get up from a toilet or a low chair, a wheeled walker and hospital bed if necessary
- improving ventilation for the bathroom, kitchen, or other areas in which fumes, dust, smoke, or steam may cause respiratory symptoms

Task Modification

Tasks can be modified by including energy conservation techniques. Basic concepts include

- slowing down the pace
- minimizing large body movements such as moving the body weight up and down
- setting priorities and organizing activities to minimize wasted movement
- planning appropriate amounts of time to complete the task, including breaks for rest

Each activity can be broken down into smaller tasks and analyzed with regard to the most energy-efficient method to complete it.

Relief of Dyspnea

Simple procedures to minimize and relieve shortness of breath during activities of daily living can become incorporated into the functional training. Controlling the breathing pattern, altering postures to improve respiratory muscle function, and using relaxation techniques are some key principles of treatment.

An important principle in relieving dyspnea is that the patient should maintain an uninterrupted breathing pattern by avoiding breath holding, **Valsalva's maneuver,** or unnecessary talking during the task. Pursed-lip breathing may be useful for patients with obstructive lung disease whenever an increase in breathing effort is noticed. This naturally slows down respirations and decreases minute ventilation, relieving dyspnea in some patients.[47,73,74] Exhalations through pursed-lips during lifting, pushing, or pulling activities prevents breath holding and straining.

Patients with restrictive interstitial lung disease experience greater work of breathing when taking slower, deeper breaths owing to the increased elastic resistance in their respiratory systems. During effort, these patients demonstrate rapid, shallow breathing, which is more energy efficient for them.[75,76] With either obstructive or restrictive pulmonary dysfunction, patients naturally assume a breathing pattern that requires the least energy and delays respiratory muscle fatigue.[77-81]

Breathing retraining or teaching the patient to use a specific breathing strategy that is not automatic is a controversial component of pulmonary rehabilitation. Even if successfully retrained for a new breathing pattern, the patient is likely to maintain it only with conscious effort and to resume a natural breathing pattern when attention is diverted to a task. In addition, the patient often finds the new breathing pattern fatiguing or uncomfortable.[74,81,82]

Many patients with severe COPD have diaphragms flattened by lung hyperinflation. A leaning-forward position may offer postural relief from dyspnea by improving the function of a flattened diaphragm. This position increases the intra-abdominal pressure and pushes the diaphragm up into the thorax and into a more optimal position for contraction.[83-85] Leaning forward with upper extremity support (Fig. 17-1) has the additional benefit of fixing the distal attachments of respiratory accessory muscles (e.g., pectoralis major or sternocleidomastoid) and allowing the thoracic attachments to pull the chest into inspiration.[83] Supported leaning-forward postures along with a comfortable, controlled breathing pattern may be used between efforts to help relieve shortness of breath.

Relaxation of nonrespiratory muscles is another breathing technique that may decrease wasted energy consumption and hasten relief of dyspnea. Contraction-relaxation techniques or autogenic (mental imaging) relaxation can be employed for this purpose. In some cases, biofeedback may help the patient learn to relax specific muscle groups. By teaching the patient con-

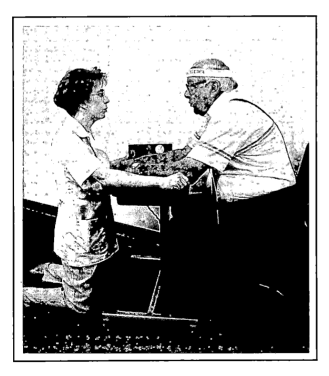

Figure 17-1.

Postures to relieve dyspnea. The physical therapist is instructing the patient in sitting in the leaning-forward position, using a table for upper extremity support, and doing pursed-lip breathing. The pulse oximeter with a forehead transducer, held securely with a headband, is used to monitor changes with the treatment technique.

trol of the relaxation response and breathing pattern, the anxiety associated with dyspnea can be reduced.[48,49]

Physiologic monitoring during functional training should be employed to ensure the safety and appropriateness of the exercises. Heart rate, blood pressure, respiratory rate, pulse oximetry, and dyspnea or effort scales, such as the **Borg scale** (Tables 17-3 and 17-4), are essential responses to monitor. The activity can be described in terms of intensity (percentage of maximum heart rate or degree of effort), duration (minutes of continuous or intermittent work), and frequency or number of repetitions of the activity carried out. Any symptoms (e.g., shortness of breath, fatigue, palpitations, chest discomfort) or a decrease of 3% to 5% on pulse oximetry should be noted. If the patient's level of desaturation is consistently below 85% on pulse oximetry, the physician should be contacted to prescribe supplemental oxygen or to increase the dosage of oxygen already in use.[9,32,33,86]

The physical therapist may advance functional training by

- increasing the patient's independence in performing a task
- decreasing the time to complete tasks
- decreasing the time or frequency of rest periods
- decreasing the dependence on adaptive equipment
- decreasing the need for supplemental oxygen

The ultimate goal is for the patient to be able to perform the necessary activity of daily living within a functional time frame, with as much independence as possible, and without undue fatigue or shortness of breath.

Progress in rehabilitation can be documented

TABLE 17-4. Ratings of Perceived Exertion Scale

6	
7	Very, very light
8	
9	Very light
10	
11	Fairly light
12	
13	Somewhat hard
14	
15	Hard
16	
17	Very hard
18	
19	Very, very hard
20	

(From Borg G. Psychophysical basis of perceived exertion. Med Sci Sports Exerc 14[5]:377-381, 1982. © American College of Sports Medicine.)

using a variety of measures, such as the quantity of work performed or the decrease in heart rate, respiratory rate, perceived exertion, or symptoms during performance of the functional task. Such changes seem to indicate that the patient is more efficient at performing the task. Improvement can also be documented by observing the patient apply the treatment concepts to new tasks or environments. The patient's report of improved quality of life and less reliance on help from others are still other ways to show that rehabilitation has increased the patient's ability to perform functional tasks.

Physical Conditioning

The goals of physical conditioning exercises are aimed at increasing cardiorespiratory endurance, maximal work capacity, strength, flexibility, and respiratory muscle function. Because it is not always possible to work on all of these areas at once, especially if the patient is very debilitated or deconditioned, priorities should be set for individualized goals based on the needs of the patient. It is optimal to prescribe exercises that accomplish more than one goal at a time and emphasize functional gains, such as increasing cardiorespiratory endurance for walking (Fig. 17-2).

TABLE 17-3. Dyspnea Scale

+1 Mild, noticeable to patient but not observer
+2 Mild, some difficulty, noticeable to observer
+3 Moderate difficulty, but can continue
+4 Severe difficulty, patient cannot continue

(From American College of Sports Medicine. Guidelines for Exercise Testing and Prescription. 4th ed. Philadelphia, Lea & Febiger, 1991. Reprinted with permission.)

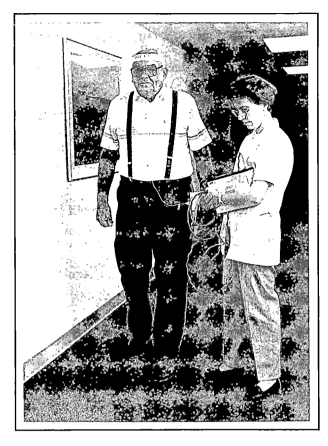

Figure 17-2.

Cardiovascular conditioning. The patient is using hall walking as the conditioning mode. The physical therapist monitors pulse and oxygen saturation changes continuously with the pulse oximeter.

Because exercise performance varies with the severity of disease, a discussion of the patient with mild, moderate, and severe respiratory disease is presented. Several classifications for describing clinical status are available, most of which use a combination of pulmonary function tests, symptoms, and exercise tolerance.[87-89]

Patients with Mild Lung Disease

Patients with mild lung disease usually have shortness of breath only with relatively heavy exercise, such as climbing hills and stairs, but may be asymptomatic with usual daily activities. Because respiratory symptoms are very mild, they do not often present to the physician for treatment of lung disease. The only indicating signs of mild disease may be symptoms with extreme effort, a chronic cough or sputum production, or a history of smoking or occupational exposure. Identifying the presence of lung disease at this early stage may be possible only through routine employment screenings and annual physical examinations.

Spirometry testing of the patient with mild disease shows values within 70% to 85% of predicted values for vital capacity (VC) and forced expiratory volume in 1 second (FEV_1). Ventilatory responses to exercise are normal and with sufficient ventilatory reserves during maximum effort. Arterial blood gas values are normal or with slight reductions in arterial oxygen levels.

Exercise for patients with mild disease can be prescribed using testing and training protocols that would be used for a normal population. Because exercise intensities associated with physiologic conditioning of the aerobic system should be easily attainable, the patient should do very well on an independent training program, and formal rehabilitation is not usually indicated.

Patients with Moderate Lung Disease

Patients with moderate lung disease usually present with an acute exacerbation of their disease or worsening symptoms of shortness of breath with normal daily activities. These patients may have shown a pattern of restricting or modifying their activity level to prevent respiratory symptoms. Still, they may attribute their symptoms to normal aging, to being out of shape or overweight, or to a smoking habit. Many seem to believe that their symptoms would be resolved with simple changes in lifestyle.

An episode of acute pneumonia or pulmonary complications following an elective surgery may be the appropriate time to identify the patient with moderate lung disease and initiate treatment. If the patient is rehabilitated at this stage of the disease process, further pulmonary complications may be prevented.

The patient with moderate lung disease has a VC and an FEV_1 between 55% and 70% of predicted values and an exercise tolerance that is limited by ventilation. That is, the ventilatory reserves are exhausted at peak exercise loads. The patient becomes short of breath with usual activities of daily living and with a moderate to fast walking pace (approximately 3 to 4 METs). Mild to moderate hypoxemia may be present at rest and may either improve or worsen with exercise.

Exercise tolerance evaluations for patients with moderate lung disease can be performed using progressive exercise protocols. However, the protocol should start at a very low MET level (1.5 METs) and advanced by 0.5 MET per stage.[87] Ideally, minute ventilation should be monitored, as well as the electrocardiogram (ECG), blood pressure (BP), heart rate (HR), and pulse oximetry.[87] Alternatively, a functional 12-minute walking test can be used.[90-92] See Chapters 8 and 10 for more information on evaluation procedures.

Exercise prescription should be aimed at increasing duration to a submaximum workload, one that taxes no more than 75% of the **ventilatory reserve.**[87] An alternative initial training workload can be estimated from the point on the exercise test at which the patient became noticeably but mildly dyspneic (level 2 to 3 on the dyspnea scale). The patient should first work to maintain this level for 20 to 30 minutes. Intermittent short bouts of slightly higher workloads can then be introduced gradually. Simple hand-held spirometers can be used to monitor minute ventilation during sustained steady-state exercise.

Because of ventilatory limitations during exercise, the intensity of the exercise and relative heart rate are lower than that usually prescribed for training the normal population. Therefore, the patient should exercise more frequently, at least 5 to 7 times weekly. The total dosage of the exercise stimulus may bring about modest increases in the symptom-limited maximum $\dot{V}O_2$ and decreases in the heart rate and minute ventilation responses to submaximum workloads.[4,86,93-95]

If the patient demonstrates arterial desaturation on pulse oximetry during exercise, supplemental oxygen may improve performance.[34] One training goal in this group of patients may be to reduce the supplemental oxygen dosage gradually, so that eventually only room air is available during exercise training.

Patients with Severe Lung Disease

Patients with severe lung disease usually are restricted by symptoms of shortness of breath during most daily activities. Even walking at a slow pace is limited. With spirometric testing, patients with severe lung disease demonstrate a VC and an FEV_1 below 55% of predicted values. The patient may require intermittent or continuous oxygen at rest and with activity and may have elevated arterial carbon dioxide levels. Some patients with severe disease show signs of right ventricular dysfunction during exercise, which seems to be related to oxygen desaturation, and improve with supplemental oxygen during exercise.[96]

Patients with severe lung disease require a modified approach to exercise testing. They should be given either low-level intermittent tests, in which they are given rests between work stages, or a steady-state endurance test at a 2 to 3 MET level.[97] Alternatively, a 6-, 3-, or even 2-minute functional walking test may be utilized.[91] Monitoring the patient closely for desaturation and exercise-induced arrhythmias is important during testing procedures. Supplemental oxygen dosages that maintain a saturation value higher than 85% should be identified and prescribed for patients who reach desaturation levels during exercise.[9,34,86,96]

The exercise prescription for patients with severe lung disease should be based on symptom-limited walking speeds and distances. Interval training programs are optimal, with very short exercise bouts and frequent rests initially. The prescription can be advanced gradually by increasing the number of bouts, lengthening the bouts, or decreasing the length of the rest periods. Because the initial training prescription (intensity and duration) is very low, the patient should exercise a minimum of one time per day. As the total exercise duration increases to 20 minutes continuously, the frequency may be reduced to 5 to 7 times per week. Even very *small* gains in exercise tolerance for the patient with severe lung disease can be significant for functional improvements and quality of life.[4,16,47,98,99]

Patients with severe lung disease need intensive monitoring and supervision, the degree of which depends on the severity of the disease. Therefore, a stratified approach to monitoring during rehabilitation sessions is most appropriate. Patients in the mild disease category may require only monitoring of exercise intensity through heart rate and perceived exertion determinations. Blood pressure, pulse oximetry, and ECG should be monitored only in patients who demonstrate hypertension or hypoxemia or who also have cardiac disease.[9,100,101]

Patients in the moderate disease category should be monitored more frequently with pulse oximetry and occasionally with ECG and exercise minute ventilation during the first 4 to 6 weeks of rehabilitation. Increased monitoring for patients with moderate disease assists in documenting improvement and establishing higher training workloads as they are tolerated.

Patients in the severe lung disease category need continuous monitoring of pulse oximetry and dyspnea or exertion scales. Patients with arrhythmias require ECG monitoring.[100,101] Intermittent blood pressure and minute ventilation checks are also appropriate. All patients should gradually require less supervision and monitoring

as rehabilitation goals are met and the patient develops independence in self-regulation and monitoring of the exercise intensity, duration, and frequency.

Strengthening

Patients with lung disease often suffer from appetite suppression, weight loss, and wasting of muscle mass.[47,102-104] For optimal rehabilitation, the patient's nutritional status must be determined regarding its adequacy for meeting the demands of increasing activity levels and replacing lost muscle. Increasing strength and local muscle endurance improves the patient's ability to perform functional activities, decrease local muscle fatigue, and enhance body image.[105]

Lower extremity strengthening can be accomplished through the aerobic training program if cycling, stair climbing, bench stepping, or aerobic dance are used as modes. If walking is the primary aerobic training mode, very little strengthening occurs unless hill climbing is included. As an alternative, the patient can use resistive weight training equipment, particularly if the equipment allows the patient to remain upright, or assume leaning forward postures to make breathing more comfortable, or both. The program should be started with low resistance and progress first by increasing repetitions, for example, 3 to 4 sets of 6 to 10 repetitions, before adding additional weight.

Upper body (trunk and upper extremity) training requires more ventilatory work, and patients are more likely to hold their breath, develop asynchronous breathing patterns, and become dyspneic.[106,107] However, clinical studies have demonstrated that patients with respiratory disorders can train successfully with upper body resistive work, which produces improvements in dyspnea, fatigue, and respiratory muscle function.[5,6,24] The strengthening program should start with very light weights (pulleys, TheraBand, wrist weights, weighted wands) and, again, advance first by increasing the number of repetitions. As the patient improves, light free weights or weight machines can be used. A 30-second bout of exercise with several minutes rest between bouts is a useful approach for patients with lung disease. Rotating between machines for upper extremity and lower extremity exercise may also improve tolerance for the strengthening program. Aerobic training modes of arm cranking and leg cycles that include arm work, rowing machines, or cross-country ski machines can also promote upper body strengthening and endurance (Fig. 17–3).

During resistive work, the physical therapist should monitor the breathing pattern, blood pressure, and pulse oximetry. The ECG should also be monitored if the patient has cardiovascular disease or demonstrates arrhythmias.

The results of standardized lifting tests or dynamometry or records of the resistive loads tolerated during training are objective ways to demonstrate the outcomes of a strengthening program. Improvement in muscle endurance can be shown by recording the increase in repetitions of an exercise per unit of time. Lastly, the measured or reported ability of the patient to carry out employment-specific, recreational, or daily activities should be documented.

Flexibility

Most patients with chronic respiratory disease have significant changes in posture and reduced mobility. These changes can be a result of inactivity or structural changes of the chest wall with hyperinflation and hypertrophy of the respiratory muscles. Flexibility exercises should be included to improve posture, increase joint range of motion, decrease stiffness, and prevent injury.

Gentle stretching with full body movements as occurs with dance, yoga, or calisthenics is appropriate for the pulmonary rehabilitation patient, especially if breathing exercises are coordinated with the movements. For instance, movements that bring full shoulder flexion, back extension, and inspiration can be performed together to increase trunk flexibility and facilitate breathing. Exercises with forward-reaching and trunk flexion or with unilateral or bilateral hip and lower trunk flexion may be combined with expiration.

The purpose of combined flexibility and breathing exercises is to teach the patient how

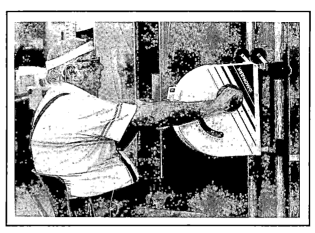

Figure 17–3.

Upper body strengthening. The patient is using intermittent arm cranking for both upper extremity strengthening and endurance training. The use of the forehead transducer for the pulse oximeter allows for stable measurements during vigorous arm movements.

body movements can influence and assist or resist ventilation. The flexibility or mobility exercises can be used as a warm-up or cool-down activity for aerobic conditioning or at any time to relieve muscle tension or anxiety.

Monitoring changes in posture, range of motion, and subjective ratings of stiffness can be used to document the effects of a flexibility program. Long-term outcomes of the program may be documented from a reduced incidence of back pain or joint injuries.

Respiratory Muscle Exercise

Exercises for improving respiratory muscle function are an important component of a pulmonary rehabilitation program. The increased work of breathing and chest wall changes that occur with chronic lung disease make respiratory muscle fatigue more likely to occur.[82] The fact that respiratory muscle fatigue is chronic may be significantly related to symptoms of shortness of breath. Two general approaches for improving respiratory muscle function are

● to rest the muscles with a device to assist breathing at night such as continuous positive airway pressure (CPAP)[40-43]

- to increase the performance capacity of the respiratory muscles through exercise training[108-111]

The work of breathing, or ventilatory work of moving air in and out of the lungs, is increased with most exercise or activity. Aerobic exercise training of the upper or lower extremities or both, that is moderate to high intensity may be an adequate stimulus to improve respiratory muscle endurance.[8,24,93] However, it is unlikely that older patients or those who have significant lung disease would be able to sustain high enough intensities to induce these changes.[5,6,7]

Training specific respiratory muscles with a resistive breathing device has been shown to improve respiratory muscle function in quadriplegics and in patients with COPD.[112-120] However, the presence of a carryover effect of improved respiratory muscle function to improved exercise tolerance, decreased dyspnea, and improved maximal work capacity has not been proved.[115,116,118-120] At least theoretically, the patient should be able to withstand more ventilatory work with less respiratory muscle fatigue so that exercise and pulmonary exacerbations are better tolerated.

For training the respiratory muscles, the patient is required to breathe against an added resistive load. This is accomplished by using one of several devices on the market that increases airway resistance (Fig. 17–4). The initial training prescription should include a resistance of 25% to 35% of the maximal negative inspiratory pressure measured at functional residual volume, a duration of up to 15 minutes, and a frequency of twice daily.[118-120] Alternatively, the patient can be started at an arbitrarily low resistance, that is, one that can be sustained for 15 minutes without fatigue, dyspnea, or oxygen desaturation. If the patient can complete two 15-minute sessions with a 20-minute rest between bouts, then the resistance can be increased to the next higher setting.[120]

Although most of the clinical studies on the efficacy of respiratory muscle training have included only patients with COPD or quadriplegia as subjects, the treatment may be applicable to other patient groups in whom respiratory muscle

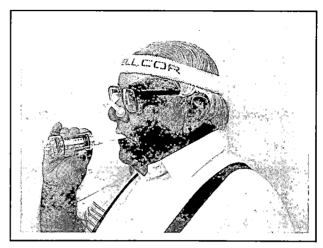

Figure 17–4.

Respiratory muscle exercise. A hand-held, single-patient use respiratory muscle exerciser is employed to offer added airway resistance and increase respiratory muscle strength and endurance.

weakness or fatigability is demonstrated: those who have neuromuscular syndromes, thoracic wall deformities such as kyphoscoliosis, and restrictive pulmonary diseases and those who are morbidly obese.

Outcomes of respiratory muscle training can be documented by recording increases in the training resistance and maximal inspiratory pressures. A change in the patient's breathing strategy (flow rate, breathing rate, and depth) may alter the effective resistive load. Therefore, these factors need to be controlled during training and evaluation sessions.[118-120] Improvements with exercise in carrying out activities of daily living and in exercise tolerance and decreased dyspnea may also be evidence of improvement with the training program.

CASE STUDIES

CASE 1 – The Patient with Chronic Restrictive Pulmonary Disease

CB is a 40-year-old woman with kyphoscoliosis, morbid obesity, chronic hypoventilation, and sleep apnea. Because of sleep deprivation at night, the patient experiences excessive daytime sleepiness. She has been treated with supplemental oxygen by nasal cannula, 1 liter per minute, and continuous positive airway pressure at night. She was also referred to pulmonary rehabilitation, to improve her exercise tolerance and to reduce her weight and percentage of body fat.

Tests

Chest roentgenogram:	Obesity, spinal deformity, no acute disease
Arterial blood gas (on room air):	Pa_{O_2}, 55; Pa_{CO_2}, 60; pH, 7.39; HCO_3^-, 36; base excess 10 (hypoxemia with mixed respiratory acidosis and metabolic alkalosis; compensated)
Electrocardiogram (rest, 12-lead):	normal sinus rhythm, left ventricular hypertrophy
Echocardiogram:	mild left ventricular hypertrophy, left ventricular ejection fraction (LVEF), 78%; right ventricular ejection fraction (RVEF), 54%
Pulmonary function tests:	VC, 0.8 liter; FEV_1, 0.78 liter; maximum voluntary ventilation (MVV), 24 L/min (severe restrictive lung disease)

Physical Therapy Evaluation

1. Patient interview: CB complained of right lower extremity pain at night and leg and foot pain and shortness of breath during walking. She reported being most comfortable pushing a cart while walking and could walk less than one block at a time. She had been confined to her home primarily, going out with assistance only. She wished to be able to go to the store or to a friend's house independently, to get off oxygen if possible, and to be less short of breath. She also wanted to be able to do some of her own housework and to climb stairs.

2. Resting evaluation: Relaxed breathing pattern on oxygen at 1 liter per minute by nasal prongs. Very short stature, very obese, and with a marked kyphoscoliosis. In sitting: heart rate (HR), 67 beats per minute (bpm); blood pressure (BP), 110/78; respiratory rate (RR), 20 bpm; oxygen saturation (So_2), 97%.

3. Cardiovascular evaluation: Test protocol was a single-stage walk at self-selected velocity on the treadmill: the treadmill speed was 2.5 miles per hour (mph), and the grade was 0%. CB walked a total of 2.0 minutes, stopping with shortness of breath. Peak HR, 101 bpm; BP, 124/80; RR, 42; So_2, 75%, minute ventilation ($\dot{V}E$), 18 liters per minute; rating of perceived exertion (RPE), 15. The patient recovered, returning to her baseline HR and So_2 within 1.0 to 1.5 minutes. She was able to repeat the same workload three more times. Her total exercise time was 7.5 minutes, and her total rest time was 6 minutes.

Upper extremity endurance test (upper extremity ergometer): At less than 5 watts at 50 revolutions per minute (rpm), the patient was able to exercise for less than 1 minute. She stopped with shortness of breath and arm fatigue. Peak HR, 96; BP, 130/84; So_2, 78%; RR, 45 bpm; $\dot{V}E$, 20.2; RPE, 17. CB recovered to her baseline within 2 minutes.

4. Functional evaluation: During a 6-minute walking test, CB walked 625 feet with three rest stops. She climbed up and down six steps in 3 minutes with two rest periods. She was limited by leg pain and shortness of breath. Peak HR, 105; BP, 118/80; RR, 45 bpm; So_2, 80%; RPE, 15 with walking and 17 with stair climbing.

Rehabilitation Goals

● Lose approximately 50 kilograms of body weight over the next 6 to 12 months or about 8 to 16 kilograms in the next 6 to 8 weeks.
● Increase endurance to 2.0 to 2.5 mph (walking) and to 20 to 40 minutes.

- Increase endurance for arm work to 5 watts for 10 minutes.
- Increase walking distance to more than 1000 feet in 6 minutes.
- Increase stair climbing to one flight (12 steps) within 2 minutes.

Training Program

Because the patient consistently became desaturated below 85%, the supplemental oxygen flow rate was increased to 1 to 3 liters per minute as needed during exercise sessions (based on protocol). Since weight loss was an important consideration, the exercise load was kept at a low to moderate intensity as tolerated. Increasing the total duration was emphasized to increase the caloric expenditure. Her severe pulmonary limitations made an interval program necessary. Functional activities of walking and stair climbing were the primary mode of training to accomplish the patient's identified goals.

Exercise Prescription

Modes:	Hall walking and treadmill walking, stair climbing, stationary cycling, and upper extremity ergometry
Intensity:	2.5 to 2.8 METs or a self-selected pace
Duration:	2-minute bouts with 2-minute rests; progress to 5-minute bouts with 1-minute rests as tolerated
Frequency:	Twice a day in physical therapy, once independently (three times a day total)

Monitoring and Ongoing Evaluations

Measured each session:	Workload, total exercise duration (minutes), total rest time, peak HR, RR, RPE, pulse oximetry, and signs and symptoms of exercise intolerance
Measured with increases in work intensity:	Peak $\dot{V}_E$, BP, and breathing pattern
Measured weekly for documenting outcomes:	Total body weight; ability to do activities of daily living independently, ability to self-monitor exercise performance, patient satisfaction; and subjective ratings of progress in symptoms, functional progress, and ability to sleep.

Rehabilitation Outcomes

CB was discharged after 8 weeks of inpatient rehabilitation, during which she increased her exercise tolerance from a 2.8 MET level to 4 METs and her exercise duration from 6 minutes to 45 minutes. She lost a total of 20 kilograms of body weight and became independent in all activities of daily living and in carrying out her exercise program. She required 1 to 2 liters of supplemental oxygen during her training sessions but could go portions of the day without oxygen. CB reported that she was feeling more confident in her abilities and that she was sleeping better during the night with less sleepiness during the day.

CASE 2 – The Patient with Cystic Fibrosis

SS is a 9-year-old girl with cystic fibrosis who is followed on an outpatient basis in the cystic fibrosis center, every 3 months. She has moderate COPD and pancreatic insufficiency as a result of her cystic fibrosis. For the past 4 years, SS has required hospitalization to treat pulmonary exacerbations with intravenous antibiotics and chest physical therapy. She has recently had a permanent central line placed for home antibiotic therapy. She has also had a jejunostomy placed for supplemental feedings at night. Current medications include methylprednisolone (Medrol), theophylline (Slo-bid), albuterol (metered-dose inhaler), oral dicloxacillin, and pancrelipase (Pancrease).

Tests

Chest roentgenogram: Bilateral hyperinflated lungs with peribronchial cuffing and chronic infiltrative changes; central line extends into the proximal aspect of the right atrium

Pulmonary function tests (pre- and postbronchodilator): FVC, 1.40/1.63 (liters); FEV_1, 0.79/1.03 (liters per minute); FEV_1/FVC, 56/63 (%)

Clinical microbiology report: Sputum quantification: 105,000,000 colony-forming units per milliliter of *Pseudomonas aeruginosa*

Physical Therapy Evaluation

1. Patient interview: SS stated that she had been feeling pretty well and attended school regularly. She occasionally has a cold that increases her cough and mucous production. She reported no problems in doing her home treatments but has been less energetic lately. SS has had some problems in physical education class because her teacher makes her sit down when she starts to cough. Her sports interests include skating, biking, and gymnastics and swimming in the summer.

2. Respiratory evaluation: SS's breathing pattern was slightly tachypneic (24 breaths per minute). A barrel chest and nail clubbing were evident, as were bilateral upper lobes with coarse inspiratory rales. Her cough was strong, effective, and productive of 5 to 10 milliliters of thick, tan mucus.

3. Cardiovascular Evaluation: Using a Bruce treadmill protocol, the following measurements were taken: resting HR, 127 bpm; resting So_2, 94%; peak HR, 180 bpm; peak So_2, 90%; peak METs, 10.0; peak RPE, 18. The reason for termination was leg fatigue and shortness of breath. Interpretation of results: Normal cardiovascular exercise response to 85% of age-predicted maximal heart rate; mild desaturation (4%) at peak exercise. SS's exercise tolerance was in the twenty-fifth percentile of the normal population for her age and sex.

Rehabilitation Goals

- Clearing of pulmonary rales on auscultation
- Decrease symptoms of cough and fatigue
- Improve leg strength and muscle endurance
- Increase exercise tolerance to the fiftieth percentile
- Increase participation in physical education class

Rehabilitation Program

1. Pulmonary treatments: SS and her mother have been performing postural drainage with percussion twice daily (before breakfast and at bedtime). SS's mother has been assisting with treatments, using a palm cup for percussion. Lower and middle lobes have been emphasized. SS coughed well after treatment at each position and cleared mucus easily. She uses her albuterol inhaler before each treatment. Her treatment techniques were superior.

Modifications in SS's pulmonary treatment regimen were as follows: Postural drainage positions for the upper lobes were reviewed. SS was shown how to do self-percussion for these positions. In addition, she was instructed in the forced expiratory maneuver to be performed for 5 minutes before physical education class and exercise. She was also issued and instructed in the operation of a positive expiratory pressure (PEP) mask, which was to be used independently after school each day. Her mother was shown how to use a stethoscope for monitoring breath sounds before and after pulmonary treatments.

2. Exercise training program: SS was encouraged to continue her gymnastics for whole body strengthening and flexibility training. Also for leg strengthening and endurance, she was instructed to continue her biking and to choose routes with an incline. Climbing stairs two at a time and jumping rope were other modes of leg strengthening.

Cardiovascular training guidelines were kept simple and emphasized her recreation. Running games (e.g., kickball, tag, dodgeball), biking, swimming, or jumping rope were listed as possible conditioning modes. She was instructed to exercise at an RPE rating of 13 to 15 or at a pace that induced breathing with moderate effort and coughing, a duration of 20 to 30 minutes without significant rest breaks, and a frequency of daily. She was also issued and instructed in the use of a dance videotape for children to be substituted for her regular exercise on rainy days or to supplement her conditioning play.

In addition, a letter with information on cystic fibrosis and treatment for pulmonary disease was sent to her physical education teacher, with a request for assistance in meeting SS's goals.

Monitoring and Measurements

Measured at each session:	Breath sounds, especially of the upper lobes, and volume of mucus produced were to be recorded by SS or her mother with each postural drainage treatment, or at least 3 days per week. A chart of her exercises was given to SS to record the activity, the length of play conditioning in minutes, the rating of perceived exertion, and the amount of mucus produced. She was encouraged to fill in this chart each evening and to bring it with her to her next physical therapy evaluation session.
Measured every 3 months:	At each follow-up evaluation, SS was monitored for changes in exercise tolerance, improved pulmonary function test results and breath sounds, ability to participate in school and play, compliance with home instructions, and growth in height and body weight.
Measured yearly:	The frequency of hospitalization and use of home antibiotics, school attendance, and changes in chest roentgenogram were evaluated annually.

Rehabilitation Outcomes

According to her home records, which she brought to the 3-month return visit, SS was compliant with her postural drainage sessions 80% of the time. She also maintained her exercise program an average of 5 days per week. She was able to demonstrate her postural drainage positions and percussion of the upper lobes and her forced cough technique with satisfaction. Her breath sounds were somewhat improved, with fine to medium rales in the upper lobes.

SS reported an improvement in her ability to participate in school physical education class and a better understanding of her coughing by her teacher.

On exercise testing, SS increased her peak work to 11.8 METs (25th to 50th percentile), with a maximal HR of 195 bpm, a peak RPE of 19, and pulse oximetry of 94%. She no longer demonstrated any desaturation with maximal exercise. The test was terminated with leg fatigue and no shortness of breath. Pulmonary function tests were unchanged, and she had gained about 2 kilograms of weight.

CASE 3 – The Patient with Emphysema

WS is a 48-year-old man with a history of progressive severe COPD and cor pulmonale. He was evaluated by the pulmonary medicine department and felt to be a good candidate for lung transplantation. He was referred to the pulmonary rehabilitation program to obtain an evaluation of his current physical capabilities and to increase his exercise tolerance and strength before transplantation.

WS is on the following supplements and medications: oxygen, 1½ liters per minute at night, and phenytoin (Dilantin) for a history of seizures.

Tests

Chest roentgen-ogram:	Hyperinflated lungs, with flattened diaphragms; increased anteroposterior diameter and bolus changes in the bases of the lungs. The pulmonary arteries appeared large.
Pulmonary function tests:	VC, 1.67 liters (39% predicted); inspiratory capacity, 1.22 liters (43% predicted); total lung capacity, 9.15 liters (133% predicted); FEV_1, 0.55 liters (15% predicted); FEV_1/VC, 33%; MVV, 35 L/min (25% predicted); DL_{CO}, 22 ml/mm Hg/min (69% predicted)
Resting ECG:	Normal sinus rhythm, with occasional supraventricular premature complexes; poor R wave progression
Hematology profile:	White blood cell count, 6.2; red blood cell count, 5.5; hemoglobin, 16.1; hematocrit, 49%; platelets, 262,000; reticulocytes, 0.3
Arterial blood gas:	Pa_{O_2}, 56 mm Hg; Pa_{CO_2}, 45 mm Hg; pH, 7.37; HCO_3^-, 28; S_{O_2}, 92% (on room air, at rest)
Cardiopulmonary exercise test (performed on a cycle ergometer):	Resting heart rate, 92 bpm; resting blood pressure, 169/106; peak heart rate, 138 bpm; peak blood pressure, 220/113; maximum $\dot{V}_{O_2}$, 0.86 L/min or 3.2 METs; maximum $\dot{V}_E$, 34 L/min. Arterial blood gases: Pa_{O_2}, 45; Pa_{CO_2}, 53; pH, 7.32; S_{O_2}, 80%. ECG, no changes in arrhythmia or ST segments. Test terminated with grade 4 dyspnea.

Interpretation: exercise capacity severely limited by ventilation deficits, with respiratory acidosis and arterial oxygen desaturation at peak exercise. Also resting and exercise hypertension.

Physical Therapy Evaluation

1. Patient interview: WS is currently working full time as an assistant director of a mental health center. His work tasks are primarily sedentary but include walking from a parking lot to the building, approximately a half-block walk. Other activities are some very light gardening, photography, traveling, and reading. He uses meditation and biofeedback for relaxation training. He is married and has two grown children. Family and friends are supportive.

WS reported symptoms of severe dyspnea that limit his activities of daily living, primarily shaving, showering, and dressing. Also he is unable to climb even one flight of stairs or walk more than one block without resting for relief of dyspnea. He wears his supplemental oxygen only at night. He has become quite limited in his ability to continue his current hobbies and reported interest in conditioning to improve his chances for a positive outcome of the lung transplantation.

2. Respiratory evaluation: WS's breathing pattern was moderately distressed at rest, with tachypnea (rate 28) and use of inspiratory accessory muscles. A barrel chest was noted. His breath sounds were decreased throughout, without adventitious sounds, and his cough was dry and nonproductive. The maximum negative inspiratory force was -48 cm H_2O; breathing endurance time at a load of -12 cm H_2O (25% max) was 5 minutes, limited by dyspnea.

3. Functional evaluation: Activities of daily living that require upper body and arm movement were the most difficult for WS to complete. During the assessment of shaving and dressing skills, he demonstrated increased dyspnea when his arms were held at face level for longer than 1 minute, when his arms were raised overhead, or when he leaned forward to reach his feet. During effort, he frequently held his breath and grunted on expiration. His pulse increased to 108 beats per minute, and pulse oximetry decreased to 88%. Time to complete each task was also recorded.

4. Cardiovascular endurance: WS's 6-minute walk test results were as follows: resting HR, 92 bpm; resting BP, 152/96; resting S_{O_2}, 92% (room air); peak HR, 121 bpm; peak BP, 198/102; peak S_{O_2} 82%; recovery time to return to baseline, 4

minutes; distance walked, 620 feet, with 3 stops for rest; peak RPE, 17; dyspnea rating, +3; $\dot{V}E$, 28 liters at peak exercise (80% MVV).

Rehabilitation Goals

● Increase walking endurance and distance
● Reduce dyspnea, if possible
● Increase tolerance for activities of daily living
● Improve respiratory muscle function
● Maintain or improve general health for upcoming surgery

Rehabilitation Program

1. Respiratory muscle training: WS was started at the lowest resistance setting (approximately −12 cm H_2O) for 5 minutes, twice daily at home. He was instructed to increase the duration by 1 to 2 minutes every 3 to 4 days as tolerated, until he reached 15 minutes. The resistance setting would then be increased gradually, as determined during weekly reassessments.

2. Exercise training: WS was started on a walking program at home and exercised on the treadmill and bicycle ergometer during the rehabilitation sessions. He was begun on an intermittent exercise training program, with incorporation of dyspnea relief skills. Emphasis was placed on pacing and control of a continuous breathing pattern while increasing the total exercise duration. Also, WS was placed on 1 liter of oxygen during his training session to keep the So_2 above 85%.

Modes:	Walking, treadmill, bicycling
Intensity:	RPE, 15; dyspnea, 2–3; HR, 110–120 bpm; 2.0–2.5 METs; $\dot{V}E$, 25 liters
Duration:	2-minute exercise; 2-minute rests; 4–5 bouts
Frequency:	Daily
Monitoring:	HR, BP, pulse oximetry, RPE, dyspnea ($\dot{V}E$ with increased workloads, or new modes)

3. Upper body training: WS was started on upper body calisthenics using an unweighted wand. Initially, two to three repetitions were performed on each exercise, which included overhead and reaching-forward movements with breathing techniques incorporated into the exercise. Repetitions were increased gradually to 20, then light weights were added in 0.25-pound increments. In addition, ball-handling exercises were performed with the rehabilitation group.

Measurements and Ongoing Evaluations

Measured at each session:	At each rehabilitation session, the patient was assessed for total walking time and distance, oxygen dosage, and So_2 at peak exercise. Resistance setting and duration of respiratory training, repetitions of upper body exercises, and maximum weight of resistance were also measured.
Measured weekly:	Measurements of maximal negative inspiratory force and endurance time at 25% maximum resistance, 6-minute walking distance, exercise $\dot{V}E$, and compliance with home programs were assessed weekly.

Rehabilitation Outcomes

WS increased his walking distance to 1150 feet in 6 minutes and his maximal negative inspiratory force to −62 cm H_2O. His upper body endurance increased to 20 repetitions of exercise, using 2 pounds. He also modified his activities of daily living with pacing and organizing so that he was less dyspneic. He completed his formal rehabilitation but continues to return for monthly reevaluations of his status and changes in his treatments until his lung transplantation.

SUMMARY

- Rehabilitation intervention has been considered maintenance activity, and third-party payers have often limited severely the benefits paid for pulmonary rehabilitation.
- Rehabilitation research is beginning to emphasize functional outcomes as measures of efficacy instead of changes in physiologic parameters.
- Goals for an individual must be very specific and pertinent to that individual's lifestyle, needs, and interests.
- Any person with a primary or secondary pulmonary disease or anyone at risk for the development of pulmonary disease is a potential candidate for rehabilitation.
- Candidates for rehabilitation must meet the following criteria: a diagnosed respiratory disease and documented functional limitations.
- A comprehensive pulmonary rehabilitation program should incorporate six primary components, including general care, respiratory therapy, physical therapy, exercise conditioning, education, and psychosocial management.
- After an assessment is made, therapeutic intervention often includes prescription of medication and possibly oxygen, preventive care such as immunizations and vaccinations, smoking cessation, avoidance of environmental irritants, adequate hydration, and proper nutrition including weight control.
- Respiratory treatment techniques for clearing accumulated pulmonary secretions and relieving dyspnea include bronchial drainage, breathing techniques, cough facilitation, postures to improve breathing, relaxation techniques, bronchodilators, and the use of respiratory assistance devices to rest the breathing muscles at night or during exercise.
- The main emphasis of pulmonary care in the rehabilitation setting is the removal of excessive secretions that obstruct airways and cause ventilatory defects, cause bothersome symptoms of cough, and possibly lead to an increased incidence of respiratory infections and deterioration of lung function.
- Treatment goals include adapting the environment to improve the ease of performing activities of daily living, altering the performance of tasks to decrease energy costs, and incorporating methods to relieve symptoms associated with activity.

- Identification of the activities of daily living that are most problematic for the patient is the first step in modifying the environment. Once identified, the areas in the home in which these activities are performed then need to be evaluated for modification.
- An important concept in relieving dyspnea is that the patient continues an uninterrupted breathing pattern by avoiding breath holding, Valsalva's maneuvers, or unnecessary talking during the task.
- Patients with restrictive interstitial lung disease experience greater work of breathing when taking slower, deeper breaths because of the increased elastic resistance in their respiratory system.
- Relaxation of nonrespiratory muscles is another breathing technique that may decrease wasted energy and hasten relief of dyspnea.
- Patients with severe lung disease require a modified approach to exercise testing. Tests should either be low-level intermittent tests, in which the patient is given rests between work stages, or a steady-state endurance test at a 2 to 3 MET level.
- Patients in the moderate disease category should be monitored more frequently with pulse oximetry and occasionally with ECG and exercise minute ventilation during the first 4 to 6 weeks of rehabilitation.
- Patients in the severe lung disease category need continuous monitoring of pulse oximetry and dyspnea-exertion scales. Some with arrhythmias require ECG monitoring. Intermittent blood pressure and minute ventilation checks are also appropriate.
- Patients with lung disease often have appetite suppression, weight loss, and wasting of muscle mass.
- Upper body (trunk and upper extremity) training requires more ventilatory work, and the patient is more likely to breath hold, develop an asynchronous breathing pattern, and become dyspneic.
- Most patients with chronic respiratory disease have significant changes in posture and reduced mobility.
- Two general approaches for improving respiratory muscle function are to rest the muscles with an assisted breathing device at night or to increase the performance capacity of the respiratory muscles through exercise training.
- For training the respiratory muscles, the pa-

tient is required to breathe against an added resistive load. The initial training prescription should include a resistance of 25% to 35% of the maximal negative inspiratory pressure measured at functional residual volume, a duration of up to 15 minutes, and a frequency of twice daily.

References

1. American Thoracic Society. Pulmonary rehabilitation: Official American Thoracic Society position statement. Am Rev Respir Dis 124:663–666, 1981.
2. Task Force Report: Epidemiology of respiratory diseases. US Department of Health and Human Services, Public Health Service. National Institutes of Health, Publication 81-2019, pp 13–25, 156–158, 1980.
3. Higgins M. Epidemiology of COPD, state of the art. Chest 85(6 suppl):3S–6S, 1984.
4. Niederman MS, Clemente PH, Fein AM, et al. Benefits of a multidisciplinary pulmonary rehabilitation program: Improvements are independent of lung function. Chest 19(4):798–804, 1991.
5. Ries AL, Ellis B, Hawkins RW. Upper extremity exercise training in chronic obstructive pulmonary disease. Chest 93(4):688–692, 1988.
6. Lake FR, Henderson K, Brifta T, et al. Upper-limb and lower-limb exercise training in patients with chronic airflow obstruction. Chest 97(5):1077–1082, 1990.
7. Belman MJ, Kendregan BA. Physical training fails to improve ventilatory muscle endurance in patients with chronic obstructive pulmonary disease. Chest 81(4):440–443, 1982.
8. Orenstein DM, Franklin BA, Doershuk CF, et al. Exercise conditioning and cardiorespiratory fitness in cystic fibrosis. Chest 80(4):392–398, 1981.
9. Moser KM, Bokinsky G, Savage RT, et al. Results of a comprehensive rehabilitation program: Physiologic and functional effects on patients with chronic obstructive pulmonary disease. Arch Intern Med 140:1596–1601, 1980.
10. Bass H, Whitcomb JF, Forman R. Exercise training: Therapy for patients with chronic obstructive pulmonary disease. Chest 57(2):116–121, 1970.
11. Swerts P, Kretzers L, Terpstra-Lindeman E, et al. Exercise reconditioning in the rehabilitation of patients with chronic obstructive pulmonary disease: A short- and long-term analysis. Arch Phys Med Rehabil 71:570–573, 1990.
12. Vyas MN, Banister EW, Morton JW, et al. Response to exercises in patients with chronic airway obstruction: Effects of exercise training. Am Rev Respir Dis 103:390–399, 1971.
13. Degre S, Sergysels R, Messin R, et al. Hemodynamic responses to physical training in patients with chronic lung disease. Am Rev Respir Dis 110:395–402, 1974.
14. Chester EH, Belman MJ, Bahler RC, et al. Multidisciplinary treatment of chronic pulmonary insufficiency. Chest 72(6):695–702, 1977.
15. Foster S, Thomas HM. Pulmonary rehabilitation in lung disease other than chronic obstructive pulmonary disease. Am Rev Respir Dis 141:601–604, 1990.
16. Brundin A. Physical training in severe chronic obstructive lung disease. Scand J Respir Dis 55:25–36, 1974.
17. Holden DA, Stelmach KD, Curtis PS, et al. The impact of a rehabilitation program on functional status of patients with chronic lung disease. Respir Care 35(4):332–341, 1990.
18. McGavin CR, Gupta SP, Lloyd EL, et al. Physical rehabilitation for the chronic bronchitic: Results of a controlled trial of exercises in the home. Thorax 32:307–311, 1977.
19. Mertens DJ, Shephard RJ, Kavanagh T. Long-term exercise therapy for chronic obstructive lung disease. Respiration 35:96–107, 1978.
20. Sinclair DJM, Ingram CG. Controlled trial of supervised exercise training in chronic bronchitis. Br Med J 280:519–521, 1980.
21. Unger LM, Moser KM, Hansen P. Selection of an exercise program for patients with chronic obstructive pulmonary disease. Heart Lung 9(1):68–76, 1980.
22. Ries AL, Archibald CJ. Endurance exercise training at maximal targets in patients with chronic obstructive pulmonary disease. J Cardiopulmonary Rehabil 7:594–601, 1987.
23. Sahn SA, Nett LM, Petty TL. Ten year follow-up of a comprehensive rehabilitation program for severe COPD. Chest 77(suppl 2):311–314, 1980.
24. Keens TG, Krastins RB, Wannamaker EM, et al. Ventilatory muscle endurance training in normal subjects and patients with cystic fibrosis. Am Rev Respir Dis 116:853–860, 1977.
25. Hudson LD, Tyler M, Petty TL. Hospitalization needs during an outpatient rehabilitation program for severe chronic airway obstruction. Chest 70(5):606–610, 1976.
26. Lertzman MM, Cherniack RM. Rehabilitation of patients with COPD. Am Rev Respir Dis 114:1145–1165, 1976.
27. Hudson LD, Pierson DJ. Rehabilitation of patients with chronic obstructive pulmonary disease. Med Clin North Am 65:629–644, 1981.
28. Hodgkin JE, Balchum OJ, Kass I, et al. Chronic obstructive airway diseases: Current concepts in diagnosis and comprehensive care. JAMA 232:1243–1260, 1975.
29. Burrows B. Differential diagnosis of chronic obstructive disease. Chest 97(suppl 2):165–185, 1990.
30. Timms RM, Kvale P, Anthonisen NR, et al. Selection of patients with chronic obstructive pulmonary disease for long-term O_2 therapy. JAMA 245:2514–2515, 1981.
31. Hughes RL, Davidson R. Limitations of exercise reconditioning in COPD. Chest 83(2):241–249, 1983.
32. Henke KG, Orenstein DM. Oxygen saturation during exercise in cystic fibrosis. Am Rev Respir Dis 129:708–711, 1984.
33. Versteegh FGA, Neijens HJ, Bogaard JM, et al. Relationship between pulmonary function, O_2 saturation during sleep and exercise, and exercise responses in children with cystic fibrosis. Adv Cardiol 35:151–155, 1986.
34. Lane R, Cockcroft A, Adams L, et al. Arterial oxygen saturation and breathlessness in patients with chronic obstructive airways disease. Clin Sci 72:693–698, 1987.
35. Leger P, Gerard M, Robert P. Simultaneous use of a pulsed dose demand valve with a transtracheal catheter; an optimal oxygen saving for long-term oxygen therapy. Am Rev Respir Dis 133:350, 1986.

36. Tiep BL, Nicotra B, Carter R, et al. Evaluation of a low-flow oxygen-conserving nasal cannula. Am Rev Respir Dis 130:500–502, 1984.

37. Soffer M, Tushkin DP, Shapiro BJ, et al. Conservation of oxygen supply using a reservoir nasal cannula in hypoxemic patients at rest and during exercise. Chest 88:663–668, 1985.

38. Tiep BL, Christopher KL, Spofford BT, et al. Pulsed nasal and transtracheal oxygen delivery. Chest 97(2):364–372, 1990.

39. Tiep BL, Lewis JI. Oxygen conservation and oxygen-conserving devices in chronic lung disease. Chest 92(2):263–272, 1987.

40. Scano G, Gigliotti F, Duranti R, et al. Changes in ventilatory muscle function with negative pressure ventilation in patients with severe COPD. Chest 97:322–327, 1990.

41. Goldstein RS, DeRosie JA, Avendano MA, et al. Influence of noninvasive positive pressure ventilation on inspiratory muscles. Chest 99:408–415, 1991.

42. Cropp A, Marco AF. Effects of intermittent negative pressure ventilation in respiratory muscle function in patients with severe chronic obstructive pulmonary disease. Am Rev Respir Dis 135:1056–1061, 1987.

43. Zibrak JD, Hill NS, Federman EC, et al. Evaluation of intermittent long-term negative pressure ventilation in patients with chronic obstructive pulmonary disease. Am Rev Respir Dis 138:1515–1518, 1988.

44. O'Donnell DE, Sani R, Younes M. Improvement in exercise endurance in patients with chronic airflow limitation using continuous positive airway pressure. Am Rev Respir Dis 138:1510–1514, 1988.

45. O'Donnell DE, Sani R, Giesbrecht G, et al. Effect of continuous positive airway pressure on respiration sensation in patients with chronic obstructive pulmonary disease during submaximal exercise. Am Rev Respir Dis 138:1185–1191, 1988.

46. Mahler DA, O'Donnell DE. Alternative modes of exercise training for pulmonary patients. J Cardiopulmonary Rehabil 11:58–63, 1991.

47. Paine R, Make BJ. Pulmonary rehabilitation for the elderly. Clin Geriatr Med 2:313–335, 1986.

48. Dudley DL, Glaser EM, Jorgenson BN, et al. Psychosocial concomitants to rehabilitation in chronic obstructive pulmonary disease. Part 1. Psychosocial and psychological considerations. Chest 77(3):413–420, 1980.

49. Dudley DL, Glaser EM, Jorgenson BN, et al. Psychosocial concomitants to rehabilitation in chronic obstructive pulmonary disease. Part 2. Psychosocial treatment. Chest 77(4):544–551, 1980.

50. Wanner A. The role of mucus in chronic obstructive pulmonary disease. Chest 92(2):11S–15S, 1990.

51. Desmond KJ, Schwenk WF, Thomas E, et al. Immediate and long-term effects of chest physiotherapy in patients with cystic fibrosis. J Pediatr 103:538–631, 1983.

52. Tecklin JS, Holsclaw DS. Evaluation of bronchial drainage in patients with cystic fibrosis. Phys Ther 55(10):1081–1084, 1975.

53. Selsby D, Jones JG. Some physiological and clinical aspects of chest physiotherapy. Br J Anaesth 64:621–631, 1990.

54. Carter RE. Respiratory aspects of spinal cord injury management. Paraplegia 25:262–266, 1987.

55. Mansel JK, Norman JR. Respiratory complications and management of spinal cord injuries. Chest 97(6):1446–1452, 1990.

56. Alvarez SE, Peterson M, Lansford BR. Respiratory treatment of the adult patient with spinal cord injury. Phys Ther 61(12):1737–1745, 1981.

57. Beigofsky EH. Respiratory failure in disorders of the thoracic cage. Am Rev Respir Dis 119:643–666, 1979.

58. Muszynski-Kwan AT, Perlman R, Rivington-Law BA. Compliance with and effectiveness of chest physiotherapy in cystic fibrosis: A review. Physiotherapy Canada 40(1):28–32, 1988.

59. Maxwell M, Redmond A. Comparative trial of manual and mechanical percussion technique with gravity-assisted bronchial drainage in patients with cystic fibrosis. Arch Dis Child 54:542–544, 1979.

60. Hansen LG, Warwick WJ. High-frequency chest compression system to aid in clearance of mucus from the lung. Biomed Instrum Technol 24:289–294, 1990.

61. Warwick WJ, Hansen LG. The long-term effect of high-frequency chest compression therapy on pulmonary complications of cystic fibrosis. Pediatr Pulmonol 11:265–271, 1991.

62. Rossman CM, Waldes R, Sampson D, et al. Effect of chest physiotherapy on the removal of mucus in patients with cystic fibrosis. Am Rev Respir Dis 126:131–135, 1982.

63. DeBoeck C, Zinman R. Cough versus chest physiotherapy. A Rev Respir Dis 129:182–184, 1984.

64. Sutton PP, Lopez-Vidriero MT, Pavia D, et al. Assessment of percussion, vibratory-shaking and breathing exercises in chest physiotherapy. Eur J Respir Dis 66:147–152, 1985.

65. Verboon JML, Bakker W, Sterk PJ. The value of the forced expiration technique with and without postural drainage in adults with cystic fibrosis. Eur J Respir Dis 69:169–174, 1986.

66. Van Hengstum M, Festen J, Bearskens C, et al. Conventional physiotherapy and forced expiration manoeuvres have similar effects on tracheobronchial clearance. Eur Respir J 1:758–761, 1988.

67. Falk M, Kelstrup M, Andersen JB, et al. Improving the ketchup bottle method with positive expiratory pressure, PEP, in cystic fibrosis. Eur J Respir Dis 65:423–432, 1984.

68. Oberwaldner B, Evans JC, Zach MS. Forced expirations against a variable resistance: A new chest physiotherapy method in cystic fibrosis. Pediatr Pulmonol 2:358–367, 1986.

69. Oldenburg FA, Dolovica MB, Montgomery JM, et al. Effects of postural drainage, exercise, and cough on mucus clearance in chronic bronchitis. Am Rev Respir Dis 120:739–745, 1979.

70. Zach MS, Oberwaldner B, Hausler F. Cystic fibrosis: Physical exercise versus chest physiotherapy. Arch Dis Child 57:587–589, 1982.

71. Salh W, Bilton D, Dodd M, et al. Effect of exercise and physiotherapy in aiding sputum expectoration in adults with cystic fibrosis. Thorax 44:1006–1008, 1989.

72. Hodgkin JE. Pulmonary rehabilitation. Clin Chest Med 11(3):447–454, 1990.

73. Mueller RE, Petty TL, Filley GF. Ventilation and arterial blood gas changes induced by pursed lips breathing. J Appl Physiol 28(6):784–789, 1970.

74. Paul G, Eldridge F, Mitchell J, et al. Some effects of slowing respiration rate in chronic emphysema and bronchitis. J Appl Physiol 21(3):877–882, 1966.

75. Chung F, Dean E. Pathophysiology and cardiorespiratory consequences of interstitial lung disease: Review and clinical implications. Phys Ther 69(11):956–966, 1989.
76. Jones JL, Killian KJ, Summers E, et al. Inspiratory muscle forces and endurance in maximum resistive loading. J Appl Physiol 58:1608–1621, 1985.
77. Meerhaeghe AV, Scano G, Sergysels R, et al. Respiratory drive and ventilatory pattern during exercise in interstitial lung disease. Bull Eur Physiopathol Respir 17:15–26, 1981.
78. Bradley GW, Crawford R. Regulation of breathing during exercise in normal subjects and in chronic lung disease. Clin Sci Mol Med 51:575–582, 1976.
79. Grassino A. A rationale for training respiratory muscles. Int Rehabil Med 6:175–178, 1984.
80. Bellemare F, Grassino A. Force reserve of the diaphragm in patients with COPD. J Appl Physiol 55:8–15, 1983.
81. Dodd DS, Brancatisano T, Engel LA. Chest wall mechanics during exercise in patients with severe chronic air flow obstruction. Am Rev Respir Dis 129:33–38, 1984.
82. Roussos C. Respiratory muscle fatigue and ventilatory failure. Chest 97 (suppl 3):89S–96S, 1990.
83. Sharp JT, Drutz WS, Molsan T, et al. Postural relief of dyspnea in severe chronic obstructive pulmonary disease. Am Rev Respir Dis 122:201–211, 1980.
84. Druz WS, Sharp JT. Electrical and mechanical activity of the diaphragm accompanying body position in severe chronic obstructive pulmonary disease. Am Rev Respir Dis 125:275–280, 1982.
85. Delgado HR, Braun SR, Skatrud JB, et al. Chest wall and abdominal motion during exercise in patients with chronic obstructive pulmonary disease. Am Rev Respir Dis 125:200–205, 1982.
86. Belman MJ. Exercise in chronic obstructive pulmonary disease. Clin Chest Med 7(4):585–596, 1986.
87. American College of Sports Medicine. Guidelines for Exercise Testing and Prescription. 4th ed. Philadelphia, Lea & Febiger, 1991.
88. Harber P. Alternative partial respiratory disability rating schemes. Am Rev Respir Dis 134:481–487, 1986.
89. Engelberg AL (ed). Guides to the Evaluation of Permanent Impairment. 3rd ed. Chicago, American Medical Association, 1988.
90. McGavin CR, Gupta SP, McHardy GJR. Twelve minute walking test for assessing disability in chronic bronchitis. Br Med J 1:822–823, 1976.
91. Butland RJA, Pany JA, Gross ER, et al. Two-, six-, and 12-minute walking tests in respiratory disease. Br Med J 284:1607–1608, 1982.
92. Upton CJ, Tyrrell JC, Hiller EJ. Two minute walking distance in cystic fibrosis. Arch Dis Child 63:1444–1448, 1988.
93. Gimenez M. Exercise training in patients with chronic airways obstruction. Eur Respir J 2(suppl 7):611S–617S, 1989.
94. Casaburi R, Wasserman K, Patessio A, et al. A new perspective in pulmonary rehabilitation: Anaerobic threshold as a discriminant in training. Eur Respir J 2(suppl 7):618S–623S, 1989.
95. Carter R, Coast JR, Idell S. Exercise training in patients with chronic obstructive pulmonary disease. Med Sci Sports Exerc 24(3):281–291, 1992.
96. MacNu W, Morgan AD, Wathen CG, et al. Right ventricular performance during exercise in chronic obstructive pulmonary disease: The effects of oxygen. Respiration 48:206–215, 1985.
97. Wasserman K, Hansen JE, Due DY, Whipp BJ. Protocols for exercise testing. In: Principles of Exercise Testing and Interpretation. Philadelphia, Lea & Febiger, 1986, Chap. 5.
98. Kaplan RM, Atkins CJ, Timms R. Validity of a quality of well-being scale as an outcome measure in chronic obstructive pulmonary disease. J Chron Dis 37(2):85–95, 1984.
99. Orenstein DM, Nixon PA, Ross EA, et al. The quality of well-being in cystic fibrosis. Chest 95:344–347, 1989.
100. Cheong TKH, Magder S, Shapiro S, et al. Cardiac arrhythmias during exercise in severe chronic obstructive pulmonary disease. Chest 97:973–977, 1990.
101. Incalzi RA, Pistelli R, Fuso L, et al. Cardiac arrhythmias and left ventricular function in respiratory failure from chronic obstructive pulmonary disease. Chest 97:1092–1097, 1990.
102. Hunter AMB, Carey MA, Larsh HW. The nutritional status of patients with chronic obstrucive pulmonary disease. A Rev Respir Dis 124:376–381, 1981.
103. Marcotte JE, Canny GJ, Grisdale R, et al. Effects of nutritional status on exercise performance in advanced cystic fibrosis. Chest 90(3):375–379, 1986.
104. Donahoe M, Roders RM. Nutritional assessment and support in chronic obstructive pulmonary disease. Clin Chest Med 11(3):487–495, 1990.
105. Strauss GD, Osher A, Wang CI, et al. Variable weight training in cystic fibrosis. Chest 92(2):273–276, 1987.
106. Tangri S, Woolf CR. The breathing pattern in chronic obstructive lung disease during the performance of some common daily activities. Chest 63:126–127, 1973.
107. Celli BR, Rassulo J, Make BJ. Dyssynchronous breathing during arm but not leg exercise in patients with chronic airflow obstruction. N Engl J Med 314(23):1485–1489, 1986.
108. Martin JG. Clinical intervention in chronic respiratory failure. Chest 97(suppl 3):105S–109S, 1990.
109. Shaffer TH, Wolfson MR, Bhutani VK. Respiratory muscle functions, assessment, and training. Phys Ther 61(12):1711–1723, 1981.
110. Grassino A. A rationale for training respiratory muscles. Int Rehabil Med 6:175–178, 1984.
111. Roussos C, Macklem PT. The respiratory muscles. N Engl J Med 307(13):786–797, 1982.
112. Leith DE, Bradley M. Ventilatory muscle strength and endurance training. J Appl Physiol 41(4):508–516, 1976.
113. Gross D, Ladd HW, Riley EJ, et al. The effect of training on strength and endurance of the diaphragm in quadriplegia. Am J Med 68:27–35, 1980.
114. Pardy RL, Rivington RN, Despas PJ, et al. The effects of inspiratory muscle training on exercise performance in chronic airflow limitation. Am Rev Respir Dis 123:426–433, 1981.
115. Belman MJ, Mittman C. Ventilatory muscle training improves exercise capacity in chronic obstructive pulmonary disease patients. Am Rev Respir Dis 121:273–280, 1980.
116. Levine S, Weiser P, Gillen J. Evaluation of a ventilatory

muscle endurance training program in the rehabilitation of patients with chronic obstructive pulmonary disease. Am Rev Respir Dis 133(3):400–406, 1986.

117. Belman MJ, Shadmehr R. Targeted resistive ventilatory muscle training in chronic obstructive pulmonary disease. J Appl Physiol 65(6):2726–2735, 1988.

118. Larson JL, Kim MJ, Sharp JT, et al. Inspiratory muscle training with a pressure threshold breathing device in patients with chronic obstructive pulmonary disease. Am Rev Respir Dis 138:689–696, 1988.

119. Harver A, Mahler DA, Daubenspeck JA. Targeted inspiratory muscle training improves respiratory muscle function and reduces dyspnea in patients with chronic obstructive pulmonary disease. Ann Int Med 111:117–124, 1989.

120. Flynn MG, Barter CE, Nosworthy JC, et al. Threshold pressure training, breathing pattern, and exercise performance in chronic airflow obstruction. Chest 95(3):535–540, 1989.

18 THE WELL INDIVIDUAL

A textbook on cardiopulmonary physical therapy would not be complete without a discussion of the well, or apparently well, individual. Well individuals are not appropriate candidates for traditional cardiopulmonary rehabilitation programs, but they may be candidates for conditioning or fitness programs or for instructional programs aimed at improving their exercise per-

formance. Typical instructional sessions focus on the effects of the environment, aging, and medications as well as training techniques and dietary considerations.

The many benefits of an exercise program are not known by all who begin an exercise program. Often individuals begin an exercise program for a particular reason, which may involve

703

weight loss, improvement of body build or physique, improvement of body image, stress reduction, and improvement of physical capabilities (fitness).

In recent years the value of strength training has become appreciated as an adjunct to aerobic training to assist in the performance of activities of daily living. One of the most visible and positive changes unique to strength training is increased muscle strength. Greater muscle strength makes the performance of regular activities of daily living easier, and performance in recreational activities improves as well. An additional benefit of strength training is the improved self-image associated with a change in physical appearance. Combined with aerobic exercise, strength training on a regular basis creates a balanced fitness. Strength training is now employed to improve endurance in runners and swimmers, whereas previously it was discouraged because of increased muscle bulk. A comprehensive list of the benefits of aerobic exercise and strength training exercise are presented in Table 18-1.

FITNESS EVALUATION

A fitness evaluation is used to determine baseline information before the development of an exercise prescription as well as to classify individuals based on their level of fitness. Controversy exists regarding the practice of assessing fitness because of the wide variety of operational definitions of fitness. Practically speaking, an individual should be assessed for fitness in a multitude of areas, including the existence of health problems and risk factors for problems, musculoskeletal integrity, body composition, psychological well-being, and cardiovascular status. In practice, however, fitness is more commonly associated with an individual's cardiovascular status and degree of training. The following discussion of fitness evaluation concentrates on physical assessments of fitness and refers the reader to other texts regarding psychological fitness (see the references listed under Additional Readings).

HEALTH RISK ASSESSMENT

Before initiating an exercise program, a complete fitness evaluation should be performed. Included in the fitness evaluation is an assessment of an individual's health status. In the population considered "well" (individuals without a *diagnosis* of any cardiopulmonary dysfunction), the most important assessment to be performed is the identification of the individual's risk for developing cardiopulmonary disease. Many apparently well individuals may not have a disease-related diagnosis but in fact may be at high risk for developing disease and, therefore, should not initiate an exercise program without undergoing a complete physical examination.

TABLE 18-1. Benefits of Aerobic Exercise and Strength Training Programs

Benefits of an Aerobic Exercise Program

Improvement in aerobic capacity
  Increased efficiency to extract oxygen in trained muscles
    increase in number of mitochondria
    increase in number and activity of succinate dehydrogenase enzymes
    increase in capillarization
    increase in amount of glycogen stored in muscles
  Increase in stroke volume
  Decrease in resting heart rate
  Decrease in submaximal heart rates
Changes in body composition (loss of fat)
Increase in fibrinolytic effect (decreased clotting)
Decrease in resting blood pressure in hypertensive individuals
Altered method of cholesterol transport
  Increase in high-density lipoproteins (HDLs)
  Slight decrease in low-density lipoproteins (LDLs)
Decrease in triglycerides
Increase in glucose utilization
  Decrease in blood glucose levels in diabetics
  Increase in sensitivity to insulin
Improvement in psychological well-being
  Improved response to stress
  Decrease in physiologic responsiveness to stimuli
  Improved self-image
Decrease in risk for developing heart disease owing to elimination of a number of the risk factors

Benefits of a Strength Training Program

Increase in strength of trained muscles
Increase in utilization of anaerobic metabolism
  Increase in phosphofructokinase stored in muscle
  Improved ease in performing many activities of daily living, especially with upper body strength training
Increase in bone mass
Increase in size, endurance, or both, of trained muscles
Improvement in body image and self-esteem

A risk factor profile can be used to screen persons who might be at risk for the development of cardiopulmonary disease. These profiles are often developed commercially, but they can be as simple as a series of questions to ascertain specific risk factor information. An example of a commercially prepared risk profile is presented in Figure 18–1 (*A* and *B*). This profile provides a classification of risk, from low to very high, that is based on the cumulative numeric value obtained from the answers to the questions. A less formal method of assessing the relative risk for cardiovascular disease is to ask questions about specific risk factors to determine the number of major and minor risk factors for disease. (See Chapter 3 for a more detailed discussion of the risk factors.) For example, in the black population a family history of sickle cell disease should be assessed because such a history increases significantly the risk for stroke and affects an individual's oxygen carrying capacity.

Unfortunately, stratification of risk for the development of pulmonary disease cannot be made from a risk factor profile as is done for cardiovascular disease. However, an inference of the risk for pulmonary disease can be ascertained from answers to questions regarding smoking history, occupational exposure to toxic chemicals, family history of disease, and social history. Information about smoking should include the number of cigarettes smoked per day and the number of years the individual smoked. Occupational exposure can be assessed by identifying the type of employment settings in which the individual worked and the kinds of toxins that might have been inhaled (e.g., sawdust, asbestos, coal dust, farm chemicals). In addition, family history should be evaluated for the presence of alpha$_1$-antitrypsin deficiency (i.e., determining if any nonsmoking male relatives died at a young age of emphysema), cystic fibrosis, tuberculosis, or asthma. Social history should be screened for exposure to tuberculosis or human immunodeficiency virus (HIV).

Clinical decisions about the continuance of the fitness evaluation or referral for further medical evaluation are assisted by the identification of an individual's risk for the development of cardiopulmonary disease. According to the latest guide-lines published by the American College of Sports Medicine, asymptomatic males older than 40 who have two or more major risk factors for coronary artery disease or who are sedentary and plan to begin *vigorous* exercise should be referred for a complete physical and for physician approval.[1] The individual may need to undergo a diagnostic exercise test before continuing with a fitness evaluation. Likewise, individuals who exhibit several risk factors for the development of pulmonary disease should probably be referred for baseline pulmonary studies, including pulmonary function tests and serial exercise arterial blood gases.

When the demonstrated risk for cardiopulmonary disease has been assessed as being low, an individual should then undergo a full fitness evaluation before initiating an exercise program of any sort. The components of a fitness evaluation include a personal interview to identify the individual's interests and goals, a medical history, a thorough physical evaluation of the musculoskeletal system, a body composition analysis, and an exercise tolerance test.

Medical History

Obtaining a good history is one of the most important aspects of the initial evaluation because preexisting injuries and dysfunction may become aggravated with increased activity. Included in the history taking should be a series of questions regarding sprains or strains, fractures, and surgery, as well as symptoms of instability, stiffness, pain, and swelling. If the individual reports a musculoskeletal problem, clarification of any precipitating factors should be obtained to prevent further injury or reinjury.

Musculoskeletal Evaluation

A thorough musculoskeletal evaluation should be performed before anyone begins an exercise program to screen for preexisting conditions, identify orthopedic abnormalities and dysfunction, determine baseline musculoskeletal data, and assist in developing a program to prevent

Heart Test for Women

Age
- 51 and over 5
- 35 - 50 2
- 34 and under 0

Family History
If you have parents, brothers, or sisters who have had a heart attack, stroke or heart bypass surgery at:
- Age 55 or before 5
- Age 56 or after 3
- None or don't know 0

Personal History
Have you had:
- A heart attack 20
- Angina, heart bypass surgery, angioplasty, stroke or blood vessel surgery 10
- None of the above 0

Smoking
Current smoker: how many cigarettes per day?
- 5 or more 20
- 4 or fewer 10

If you are a smoker currently taking oral contraceptives and are:
- Under 35 years old .... add 2
- 35 years old and over .... add 5

or

Previous smoker who quit less than 2 years ago: how many cigarettes did you smoke?
- 5 or more 10
- 4 or fewer 5

or

Never smoked or quit more than 2 years ago 0

Blood Pressure
If you have had your blood pressure taken in the last year, was it:
- Elevated or high (either or both readings above 160/95 mmHg) 6
- Borderline (between 140/90 and 160/95 mmHg) 3
- Normal (below 140/90 mmHg) or don't know 0

Hormone Status
If you have undergone natural menopause, your age at its start:
- 41 or older 1
- 40 or younger 2

If you have had a total hysterectomy, your age when it was done:
- 41 or older 1
- 40 or younger 3

If you take an oral estrogen supplement .... subtract 2
If you are still menstruating .... subtract 1

Exercise
Do you engage in any aerobic activity, such as brisk walking, jogging, bicycling or swimming for more than 20 minutes:
- Less than once a week 6
- 1 or 2 times a week 3
- 3 or more times a week 0

Blood Fats
If you have had your cholesterol and blood fat levels checked in the last year, score your risk here:
- Over 240 mg/dL 6
- 200 -240 mg/dL 3
- Cholesterol under 200 mg/dL 0
- If your HDLs are lower than 45 .... add 1

or

If you know your cholesterol to HDL ratio, use this section to score your risk:
- 7.1 and above 6
- 3.6 – 7.0 3
- 3.5 or below 0

or

If you do not know your blood fat levels, use this section to score your risk: Which of the following best describes your eating pattern?
- High fat: red meat, "fast" foods, and/or fried foods daily; more than 7 eggs per week; regular consumption of butter, whole milk, and cheese 6
- Moderate fat: red meat, "fast" foods, and/or fried foods 4-6 times per week; 4-7 eggs weekly; regular use of margarine, vegetable oils, and/or low-fat dairy products 3
- Low fat: poultry, fish, and little or no red meat, "fast" foods, fried foods, or saturated fats; fewer than 3 eggs per week; minimal margarine and vegetable oils; primarily non-fat dairy products 0

Use score from only one section above

Diabetes
If you have diabetes (blood sugar level above 140 mg/dL), your age when you found out:
- 40 or before 6
- 41 or older 4
- Do not have diabetes 0

Body Mass
Calculate your body mass index with the following formula:

Weight (pounds): _____ x 0.45 = _____ (W)

Height (inches): _____ x 0.025 = _____ (H)

Divide (W) by the square of (H) or W÷HxH = Body Mass Index (BMI).

(W)_____ ÷(HxH)_____ = _____ (BMI)

Example: a woman is 120 pounds and 5 feet 6 inches (66 inches) tall:

120 x 0.45 = 54 (W)   66 x 0.025 = 1.65 (H)

W÷H x H = 54÷1.65 x 1.65 = 54÷2.72 = 19.8 BMI

- If your BMI is 27 or greater 2
- If your BMI is below 27 0

Now measure your waist and hips and divide your waist measurement by your hip girth:

Example: your waist is 26 and your hips are 36: 26÷36 = 0.7

(waist)_____ ÷(hips)_____ = _____

- If your waist to hip ratio is 0.8 or greater 1
- If your ratio is 0.79 or less 0

Stress
Are you easily angered and frustrated:
- Most of the time 6
- Some of the time 3
- Rarely 0

Total Score

706

What Your Risk Factor Score Means...

15 points or below:
Low Risk

Congratulations! Maintain your heart-healthy status by watching your weight, blood pressure, and blood fat (cholesterol and HDL) levels; get regular check-ups and don't smoke. Retake this test every year to monitor your heart-health risk profile.

16 - 32 points:
Medium Risk

Our experience indicates that your medium risk level warrants attention. Personal factors or lifestyle habits may be increasing your vulnerability to heart disease. We strongly recommend you schedule an appointment with your doctor for an evaluation, and take this test with you to get advice on how you can improve your heart-health status.

33 points or above:
High Risk

Your potential for experiencing a heart attack or stroke is significant. Your must take action NOW. If you are not already being treated for heart disease, we urgently advise that you see your doctor immediately and take this test with you. You must seek ways to reduce your risk!

Figure 18-1.

Examples of risk factor profiles to assess the risk factors of heart disease. A, Heart test for women.

injury. The evaluation is typically performed before the initial exercise prescription and then is performed periodically throughout the exercise program. Periodic assessment provides the opportunity to reevaluate any abnormalities and assess the stretching and strengthening program.

The components of a musculoskeletal evaluation include assessment of the individual's medical and orthopedic history, posture and alignment, flexibility, strength, and stability.

Posture and Alignment

Posture and alignment should be assessed by simple observation of the individual in both the sagittal (side view) and frontal planes. Ideally, the evaluation is performed using a plumb line to provide visual feedback of correct alignment. Assessment of posture and alignment in the sagittal plane is performed to evaluate the position of the head (i.e., alignment of the midpoint of the ear with the shoulder), the integrity of the

lordotic curve of the cervical spine, the degree of curvature of the upper thoracic region (e.g., for kyphosis), the integrity of the lordotic curve of the lumbar spine, and the position of the knees in relation to that of the hips (e.g., for hyperextension of the knees) (Fig. 18-2A).

Assessment of posture and alignment in the frontal plane should consider the anterior and posterior views of the patient. Evaluation of alignment anteriorly includes checking for shoulder height to be equal bilaterally, for patellar position, and for genuvalgus (knock-kneed) or genuvarus (bowlegged) or other malalignment (Fig. 18-2B). Evaluation of alignment posteriorly involves observing the position of the scapulae and the degree of winging of the scapulae and checking the level of the pelvis bilaterally and the position of the calcaneus in relation to the tibia (Fig. 18-2C).

Abnormal findings from the assessment of posture and alignment provide information that is helpful in determining which modes of exercise should be avoided as well as in developing stretching and strengthening regimens. For example, individuals who exhibit a forward head or kyphotic posture, or both, are at increased risk of cervical and shoulder injury and may experience musculoskeletal breakdown with modes of exercise that aggravate the posture, such as rowing, biking, and swimming (using the crawl or breast stroke). The abnormal posture may be a reflection of tight pectoral musculature, weak and overstretched upper back and cervical muscles, or both. Individuals identified with an increased lordotic curve of the lumbar spine are also predisposed to injury and may demonstrate the abnormal posture as a result of weak abdominal muscles, tight hip flexors, or low back or hamstring muscle dysfunction. On identification of abnormal posture and alignment, the specific problem must be identified with flexibility and strength testing.

Flexibility

An assessment of flexibility is integral to any exercise program, be it strength training or aerobic exercise. Flexibility describes the range of motion available to a joint or series of joints.

Arizona Heart Institute & Foundation's

Heart Test for Men

Age
- 51 and over.....................................10
- 35 - 50 6
- 34 and under 1

Family History
If you have parents, brothers, or sisters who have had a heart attack, stroke or heart bypass surgery at:
- Age 55 or before 5
- Age 56 or after 3
- None or don't know 0

Personal History
Have you had:
- A heart attack 20
- Angina, heart bypass surgery, angioplasty, stroke or blood vessel surgery 10
- None of the above...........................0

Smoking
Current smoker: how many cigarettes per day?
- 5 or more 20
- 4 or fewer.......................................10

or

Previous smoker who quit less than 2 years ago: how many cigarettes did you smoke?
- 5 or more 10
- 4 or fewer...5

or

Never smoked or quit more than 2 years ago.......................0

Blood Pressure
If you have had your blood pressure taken in the last year, was it:
- Elevated or high (either or both readings above 160/95 mmHg) 6
- Borderline (between 140/90 and 160/95 mmHg) 3
- Normal (below 140/90 mmHg) or don't know 0

Exercise
Do you engage in any aerobic activity, such as brisk walking, jogging, bicycling or swimming for more than 20 minutes:
- Less than once a week 6
- 1 or 2 times a week 3
- 3 or more times a week 0

Diabetes
If you have diabetes (blood sugar level above 140 mg/dL), your age when you found out:
- 40 or before 3
- 41 or older 2
- Do not have diabetes 0

Blood Fats
If you have had your cholesterol and blood fat levels checked in the last year, score your risk here:
- Over 240 mg/dL 6
- 200 -240 mg/dL 3
- Cholesterol under 200 mg/dL 0
- If your HDLs are lower than 35 ....add 1

or

If you know your cholesterol to HDL ratio, use this section to score your risk:
- 7.1 and above 6
- 3.6 – 7.0...3
- 3.5 or below 0

or

If you do not know your blood fat levels, use this section to score your risk: Which of the following best describes your eating pattern?
- High fat: red meat, "fast" foods, and/or fried foods daily; more than 7 eggs per week; regular consumption of butter, whole milk, and cheese 6
- Moderate fat: red meat, "fast" foods, and/or fried foods 4-6 times per week; 4-7 eggs weekly; regular use of margarine, vegetable oils, and/or low-fat dairy products 3
- Low fat: poultry, fish, and little or no red meat, "fast" foods, fried foods, or saturated fats; fewer than 3 eggs per week; minimal margarine and vegetable oils; primarily non-fat dairy products 0

Use score from only one section above

Body Mass
Calculate your body mass index with the following formula:

Weight (pounds): _____ x 0.45= _____ (W)

Height (inches): _____ x 0.025= _____ (H)

Divide (W) by the square of (H) or W÷HxH = Body Mass Index (BMI).

(W)_____ ÷(HxH)_____ = _____ (BMI)

Example: a man is 170 pounds and 5 feet 10 inches (70 inches) tall:

170 x 0.45 = 76.5 (W)   70 x 0.025 = 1.75 (H)

W÷H x H= 76.5÷1.75 x 1.75 = 76.5÷3.06 = 25.0 BMI

- If your BMI is 27 or greater 2
- If your BMI is below 27 0

Now measure your waist and hips and divide your waist measurement by your hip girth:

Example: your waist is 30 and your hips are 34: 30÷34 = 0.88

(waist)_____ ÷(hips)_____ = _____

- If your waist to hip ratio is 0.96 or greater 1
- If your ratio is 0.95 or less 0

Stress
Are you easily angered and frustrated:
- Most of the time 6
- Some of the time 3
- Rarely 0

Total Score

What Your Risk Factor Score Means...

15 points or below:
Low Risk
Congratulations! Maintain your heart-healthy status by watching your weight, blood pressure, and blood fat (cholesterol and HDL) levels; get regular check-ups and don't smoke. Retake this test every year to monitor your heart-health risk profile.

16 - 32 points:
Medium Risk
Our experience indicates that your medium risk level warrants attention. Personal factors or lifestyle habits may be increasing your vulnerability to heart disease. We strongly recommend you schedule an appointment with your doctor for an evaluation, and take this test with you to get advice on how you can improve your heart-health status.

33 points or above:
High Risk
Your potential for experiencing a heart attack or stroke is significant. Your must take action NOW. If you are not already being treated for heart disease, we urgently advise that you see your doctor immediately and take this test with you. You must seek ways to reduce your risk!

Figure 18-1. ***(Continued)***

***B*, Heart test for men. (From Arizona Heart Institute & Foundation, Phoenix Ariz. © 1992.)**

Flexibility testing involves an assessment of both static and dynamic functions of the tissues surrounding the joint or joints. Static flexibility refers to the actual range of motion available, whereas dynamic flexibility refers to an individual's ability to move the associated limb segment through the available range of motion. Thus, flexibility consists of abilities that include both strength and control in addition to simple range of motion. Both static and dynamic flexibility are important aspects to be assessed for the establishment of baseline information and for the possible development of stretching or strengthening interventions.

The assessment of flexibility can be condensed to the testing of a series of specific muscles and joints to decrease the amount of time spent on the initial evaluation. The type of exercise the individual plans to do also determines how specific the assessment of flexibility should be. Individuals performing most weight-bearing exercises typically should have their lower extremities evaluated for limitations in normal range of motion, particularly the gastrocnemius-soleus group, the hamstrings, the hip flexors (including the rectus femoris), the hip abductors, and the hip adductors (Figs. 18-3 to 18-6).

All motions performed by the upper extremities can be assessed using Apley's maneuvers. First, the individual must flex and externally rotate the shoulder to its end range, bend the elbow, and then reach with the hand behind the head toward the top of the scapula (Fig. 18-7). The other maneuver involves extending the shoulder, rotating internally, and reaching behind the back with the hand to the bottom tip of the scapula (Fig. 18-8). If the individual is unable to reach either the top of the scapula with the shoulder flexion maneuver or the bottom of the scapula with the shoulder extension maneuver, limited flexibility is present in the upper extremity. Each joint should be assessed individually if limitations in flexibility are found in the gross assessment.

In addition, spinal flexibility should be assessed, including the cervical spine and the lumbar spine. Moving (or having the patient move) the patient's head through the normal cervical motions (lateral bending, rotation, and forward bending and extension) provides the necessary information regarding cervical flexibility. Limitations in range should be noted for all motions. Lumbar spine flexibility can be assessed by having the patient bend forward at the waist, reaching with the hands toward the floor. The curvature of the spine should be noted in the forward bent position, as well as the distance of the hands from the floor. A low back that appears very flat or with little curvature in the lumbar and lower thoracic region on forward bending is an abnormal sign and may be an indication of previous injury, joint restriction, or muscle tightness (Fig. 18-9).

Assessment of Strength

Assessment of strength does not require a full assessment of all muscles and muscle groups but rather can be streamlined for the individual without obvious musculoskeletal dysfunction. Assessment of strength should be focused on

Text continued on page 714

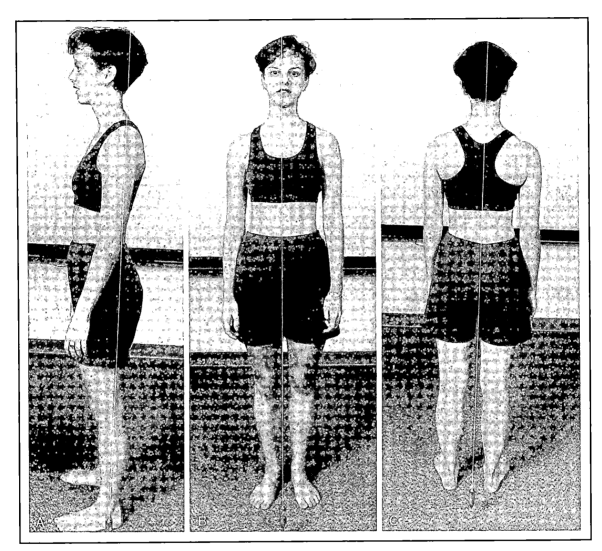

Figure 18-2.

A, Sagittal (side) view to assess posture and alignment. Particular areas to observe are (1) the position of the head in relation to the ears, (2) the curvature of the cervical spine, (3) the presence or absence of kyphosis, (4) the presence or absence of the normal lordotic curve or the degree of lordosis, and (5) the position of the knees. Note in this figure the individual's ear is far anterior to the plumb line. *B,* Frontal view to assess posture and alignment. Particular areas to observe include (1) the levelness of the shoulders, (2) the position of the patella, and (3) the alignment of the lower extremity. *C,* Posterior view to assess posture and alignment. Particular areas to observe include (1) the appearance of the scapula, (2) the levelness of the shoulders, (3) the levelness of the pelvis, and (4) the alignment of the calcaneus with the tibia.

Figure 18–3.

A, Evaluation of the tightness of the gastrocnemius-soleus group combined. Note the foot is in a position of dorsiflexion to the end of the passive range while the knee is fully extended. This technique particularly assesses the flexibility of the gastrocnemius muscle, a two-joint muscle. *B*, Evaluation of the flexibility of the soleus group. The gastrocnemius is relaxed by bending the knee, and then the foot is moved to a position of dorsiflexion to the end of the passive range.

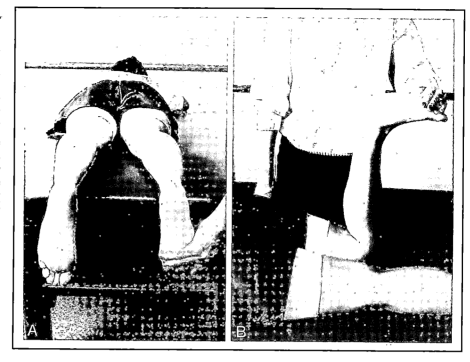

Figure 18–4.

Hamstring flexibility is optimally performed with one leg flat on the table, while the opposite hip is flexed to 90 degrees, starting with the knee bent at 90 degrees. The knee is then passively extended to the end of the passive range while maintaining the pelvis in neutral position.

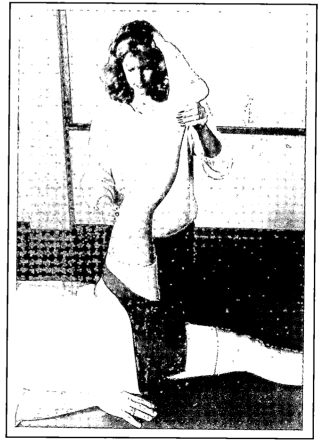

711

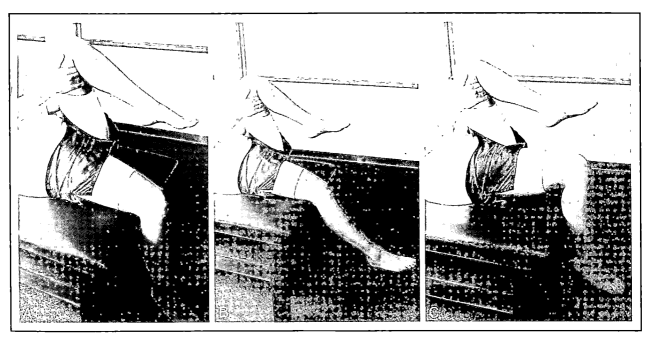

Figure 18–5.

The flexibility of the hip flexors is assessed while the patient lays supine on the plinth with the back flat and both knees flexed over the edge of the plinth. The patient slowly pulls one knee to the chest with the hands behind the thigh, pulling the thigh to the chest without raising the head off the plinth. Note the position of the opposite extremity. *A*, Normal hip flexor flexibility as the opposite thigh remains flat on the plinth while maintaining a 90-degree angle at the knee. *B*, The knee is unable to maintain a 90-degree angle, indicating rectus femoris tightness. *C*, The opposite thigh is unable to remain flat on the plinth, indicating iliopsoas tightness.

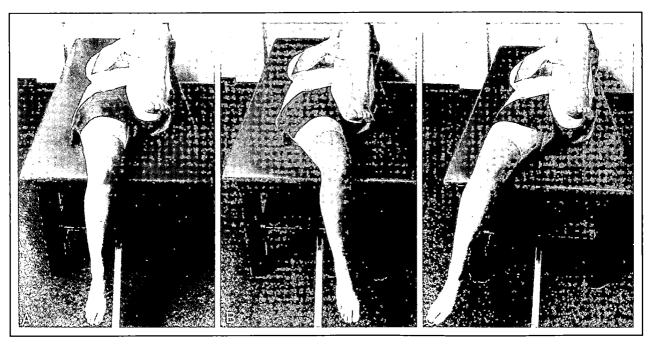

Figure 18–6.

Hip abductor-adductor flexibility can be assessed in the same positions as those of the hip flexors by observing the alignment of the opposite extremity. Alignment of the hips should be assessed as one leg is passively flexed. *A*, Normal alignment, which allows the assumption of normal abductor-adductor flexibility. *B*, The opposite hip is lying more medially, indicating hip adductor tightness. *C*, The opposite hip is lying more laterally, indicating hip abductor tightness.

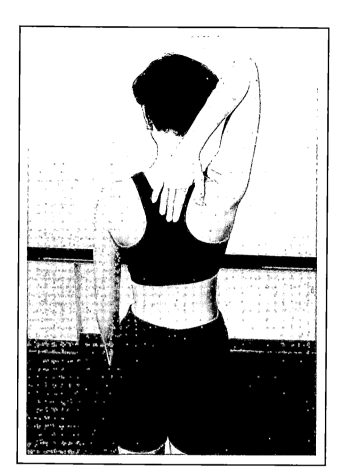

Figure 18-7.

Apley's flexion maneuver for gross evaluation of upper extremity flexibility. Note the right shoulder is flexed, externally rotated, and adducted with elbow flexion.

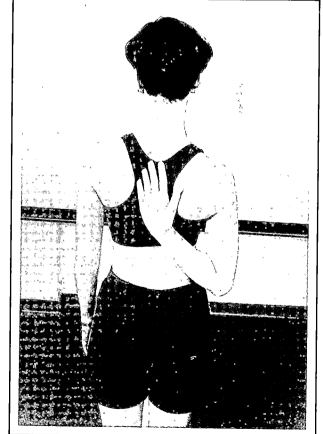

Figure 18-8.

Apley's extension maneuver for gross evaluation of upper extremity flexibility. Note the right shoulder is extended, internally rotated, and abducted with elbow flexion.

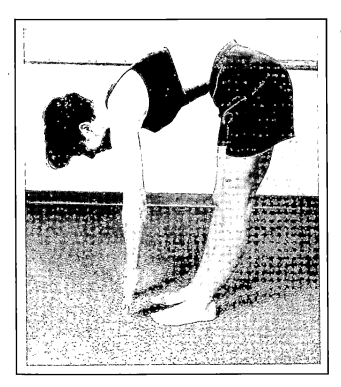

Figure 18-9.

Evaluation of spinal flexibility. Note the curvature of the lumbar and thoracic regions on forward bending.

those muscles that are most involved in the anticipated mode of exercise to be utilized in the exercise program. A break test is the easiest and the least time consuming and costly strength assessment tool. When the lower extremities are involved in exercising, the strength of the quadriceps, hamstrings, and gastrocnemius-soleus muscles should be assessed. Break tests for the gastrocnemius-soleus group are inappropriate; instead this muscle group should be assessed by having the individual push off and stand on the tips of the toes, one leg at a time (Fig. 18-10). When the upper extremities are involved in the exercise program, shoulder strength is the most important to assess. Break tests of shoulder flexion, extension, and abduction should be performed.

Assessment of Stability

An assessment of stability involves moving the extremities through the range of motion to assess for grinding, crepitus, pain, and ligament integrity. Instability might be suspected on learning of previous orthopedic history in a joint or extremity. For example, an individual with a history of arthroscopic knee surgery should have that knee evaluated for ligament integrity by performing the anterior and posterior drawer tests. Individuals wishing to initiate or resume a swimming program should have the shoulder assessed for capsular tightness or restriction as well as shoulder stability. The older individual may demonstrate grinding, crepitus, or pain during hip motion evaluation and may therefore develop problems in any weight-bearing activities. Therefore, a stationary bicycle riding program may be more appropriate for this individual to prevent musculoskeletal breakdown in the future and lack of compliance with an exercise program due to the development of pain.

The assessment of joint stability, ligamentous integrity, and the like provides valuable information that can help prevent future injury by indicating whether a specific strengthening program is necessary to protect the unstable joint. In addition, the musculoskeletal evaluation provides information that may be helpful in avoiding

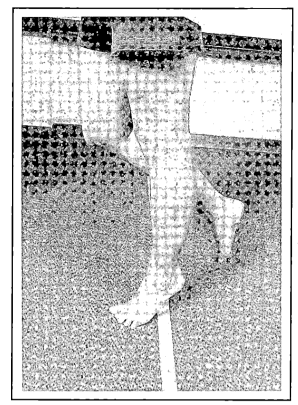

Figure 18-10.

Strength assessment of the gastrocnemius-soleus muscle group. Individuals should be able to elevate body weight on one leg at a time for normal strength.

modes of exercise that might further aggravate an instability or lead to injury. Further information on specific musculoskeletal evaluation techniques and interpretation can be obtained from other sources.[2-5]

BODY COMPOSITION ANALYSIS

The assessment of body composition (percentage of body fat versus percentage of lean mass) is an important component of the fitness evaluation, particularly for those who wish to lose weight in an exercise program. The general public is overly concerned about scales and pounds and should instead be oriented to the percentage of body fat and the fit of their clothes.

Body composition is typically assessed clinically via three methods:

- Hydrostatic weighing
- Electrical impedance
- Anthropometric measurement

There are advantages and disadvantages to all three methods. Other methods of body composition analysis are used in the laboratory situation but are not practical for the clinician. The most recent advancement in technology for soft tissue measurements involves the use of a roentgen ray source. Dual photon absorptiometry (DPA) using gadolinium 153 or dual energy x-ray absorptiometry (DEXA) have proved to be the most accurate for the measurement of body fat. These two procedures also provide information on bone mineral density and bone mineral content. Table 18-2 presents a summary of the advantages and disadvantages of body composition analysis.

Hydrostatic Weighing

Hydrostatic (underwater) weighing is considered to be the optimal clinical method for the assessment of body composition because it is believed to be the most accurate.[6,7] The literature estimates approximately 2% to 3% variation due to error with this method.[6,7] Hydrostatic weighing involves placing an individual on a chair-swing attached to a scale overhead in a tank of water, having the individual exhale all possible air, then submerging the whole body under water and recording the weight. The principle involved in hydrostatic weighing is Archimedes' principle, which relates mass to volume: the density of bone and muscle is greater than water, whereas that of fat is less than water. Therefore, if two individuals weigh the same amount "dry," the one with more muscle and bone (lean mass) weighs heavier in water and has a greater body density than the one with more fat. The weight in water is measured and compared with the land weight, and both weights are used in an equation to determine the relative density and thereby the percentage of body fat.

The disadvantages of using hydrostatic weighing include the amount of space required, the

TABLE 18–2. Advantages and Disadvantages of Clinical Measurement Techniques for Body Composition

	Hydrostatic Weighing	Electrical Impedance	Skinfold Calipers
Advantages	Most reliable Gold standard of clinical use	Easy to use Portable Relatively inexpensive Gives information as percentage of total body water as well as percentage of body fat	Easy to use Portable Inexpensive Provides percentage of body fat as well as specific site measurements
Disadvantages	Error with measuring or estimating residual volume Expensive and takes up space Requires considerable evaluation time Only gives percentage of body fat	Least reliable (5%–20% error in measurement) Does not give specific site measurements—only gives percentage of body fat Day-to-day fluctuations in body fat due to hydration, sweating, electrolyte loss, etc.	Equations used to determine body fat are population specific Measurement error is high in the unskilled

expense, the difficulty of accurately measuring residual volume, and the inconvenience of the procedure. The underwater weighing tank must be approximately 4 feet × 4 feet × 5 feet and can cost up to $5000. In addition, underwater weighing takes a considerable amount of time (to measure the residual volume, to fill the tank, and then to weigh the individual) and effort from both the therapist and the individual being weighed.

Electrical Impedance

Bioelectrical impedance is relatively new to the field of body composition analysis, being in common use only in the past 20 years. The principle of bioelectrical impedance involves the electrolyte content of different types of tissue and the detection of changes in electrolyte levels, lean tissue having greater electrolyte content than fat tissue. Electrical conduction occurs across body fluids and electrolytes, with fat tissue having low amounts of fluid as well as decreased electrolyte content.

Bioelectrical impedance is relatively simple to use, as it basically requires only good preparation of the skin (cleansing the area with alcohol and then drying it) where the electrodes are placed. Electrode placement differs according to the manufacturer of the bioelectrical impedance equipment; each has a somewhat different procedure. Most commonly the electrodes are placed on the dorsum of the hands or wrists and sometimes on the dorsal aspects of the feet. Once the electrodes are in place and after specific information about the individual is given to the computer, the machine can provide information on the percentage of body fat as well as the total amount of body water. The body composition assessment can be performed within a matter of minutes, and the cost of the machine (and electrodes) is the only cost of bioelectrical impedance testing.

The major disadvantage of bioelectrical impedance is the unreliability of the results.[8,9] The literature reports a variance in error of 5% to 20%,[10] making this method extremely unreliable. The problem with this technique is that daily fluctuations in body water and diet (e.g., sweating, eating, drinking, dehydration, medications that affect diuresis) affect impedance testing because these affect the various electrolyte concentrations. For example, lean individuals have had their percentage of body fat overestimated, and obese individuals have had their percentage of body fat underestimated. When individuals follow a specific protocol before body composition assessment (Table 18–3), reliability appears to improve.[11,12] The newer equipment on the mar-

TABLE 18–3. Bioelectrical Impedance Measurement Protocol

1. Measurement should be no less than 2 hours after eating.
2. Measurement should be within 30 minutes after voiding.
3. Previous day's intake of fluid and sodium should be of normal values.
4. Strenuous exercise should be avoided before the measurement.
5. Measurement should be taken in well-ventilated or air-conditioned room to prevent excessive sweating.
6. Skin should be cleansed with alcohol.

ket may prove to be more reliable if it is used with standardized pretest protocols. Unfortunately, until the reliability improves, bioelectrical impedance cannot be supported for medical use.[9,10,12] In the meantime, bioelectrical impedance is more often used for its assessment of total body water, which appears to be reliable, than for its assessment of body fat.

Anthropometric Measurement

Anthropometric measurement for body composition analysis involves the use of skinfold measurements and girth measurements. However, because girth measurements (measurement with tapes involves the assessment of muscle, fat, and water, not just fat), are not as accurate as skinfold measurements, girth measurements are used for individuals who are too large and therefore inappropriate for skinfold assessment (because the amount of fat is greater than the width of the skinfold caliper jaws). The girth measurements that have been found to be the most accurate are the waist and gluteal regions for women and the waist only for men.[12]

The skinfold method of body fat assessment has three great advantages that are responsible for its widespread use. The first is that skinfold calipers are easy to use and portable. They are only slightly larger and no heavier than a textbook (Fig. 18–11). Second, skinfold calipers are inexpensive, with the most expensive ones costing less than $500. Finally, the error involved in assessment with calipers is minimal. The literature reports a 3% to 4% error in body fat assessment with the use of skinfold calipers.[9] The amount of error is related to the amount of experience of the individual performing the body fat assessment with the calipers; the more experienced the individual, the less the percentage of error.

Seven sites for measurement of body composition with the skinfold calipers have been consistently identified in the literature,[13] yet different groupings of the skinfold measurements may be

Figure 18–11.

The Harpenden skinfold caliper.

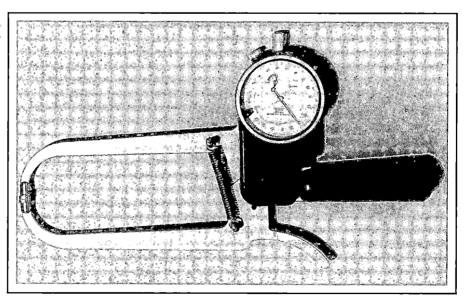

TABLE 18–4. Anatomic Sites for Body Fat Measurement

Chest—diagonal fold taken one half the distance between the anterior axillary line and the nipple in men or one third the distance from the anterior axillary line in women

Abdomen—vertical fold taken at a lateral distance of 2 cm from the umbilicus

Suprailiac—diagonal fold above the crest of the ilium where an imaginery line from the anterior axillary line would meet

Subscapular—fold taken on diagonal line coming from the vertebral border to 1–2 cm from the inferior angle of the scapula

Triceps—vertical fold on posterior midline of the upper arm halfway between the acromion and the olecranon processes

Thigh—vertical fold on the anterior aspect of the thigh, midway between the hip and knee joints

Midaxillary (axilla)—vertical fold on the midaxillary line at the level of the xiphoid process of the sternum

utilized in equations to determine an individual's percentage of body fat (Table 18–4). Table 18–5 provides a few examples of equations used for determining percentage of body fat from various skinfold sites. Table 18–6 provides normative values for percentage of body fat that are widely accepted.[14,15] The reader should see Pollock and Wilmore[13] or the American College of Sports Medicine guidelines for exercise testing and exercise prescription[1] for further use of the skinfold sites for determining body fat percentage.

Although the various equations to determine percentage of body fat, do not all use measurements from all seven sites, the sites can be reevaluated regularly throughout the exercise program to provide feedback and motivation to the individual. Skinfold measurement is performed before initiating an exercise program and then again for reevaluation no earlier than 6 to 8 weeks later.

EXERCISE EVALUATION

Any patient initiating an exercise program should be evaluated with an exercise tolerance test. Ideally, the individual undertakes a submaximal or maximal exercise test on the stationary bicycle or treadmill, but this is not always practical or even cost effective. However, some

sort of evaluation of the individual's exercise performance should be undertaken. A 6- or 12-minute walk test, a 1.5-mile run for time, a Harvard step test, or some other protocol may be used depending on the individual's health risk appraisal and other limiting factors to exercise. It is recommended that individuals assessed as being at moderate risk for the development of cardiac disease have a physical and physician consent before undergoing a progressively increased workload test, whereas individuals with high risk for heart disease need a diagnostic exercise evaluation to rule out ischemic heart disease (see Chapter 8). The essential reason for an

TABLE 18–5. Examples of Equations for Determining Body Fat and Body Density from Various Skinfold Sites

Method 1

Males

Body density = 1.1093800 − 0.0008267 (A) + 0.0000016 (A)
2.0 − 0.0002574 (B)

  A = Sum of chest, abdomen, and thigh skinfolds (in mm)

  B = Age (in years)

Females

Body density = 1.0994921 − 0.0009929 (C) + 0.0000023 (C)
2.0 − 0.0001392 (B)

  B = Age (in years)

  C = Sum of triceps, suprailium, and thigh skinfolds (in mm)

Method 2

Young Women − Age 17–26

%Fat = 0.55(A) = 0.31(B) + 6.13

  A = Triceps fatfold (in mm)

  B = Subscapula fatfold (in mm)

Young Men − Age 17–26

%Fat = 0.43(A) + 0.58(B) + 1.47

  A = Triceps fatfold (in mm)

  B = Subscapula fatfold (in mm)

Method 3

Men

Body density: 1.1043 − (0.00133 × thigh skinfold) − (0.00131 × subscapular skinfold)

Women

Body density = 1.0764 − (0.00081 × suprailiac skinfold) − (0.00088 × triceps skinfold)

Fat percentage = 4.570/body density − 4.142 × 100.0

(Method 2 from McArdle WD, Katch FI, Katch VL. Exercise Physiology: Energy Nutrition and Human Performance. Philadelphia, Lea & Febiger, 1991. Used with permission. Method 3 from Sloan AW, Weir JB. Nomograms for prediction of body density and total body fat from skinfold measurements. J Appl Physiol 28:221–222, 1970.)

TABLE 18–6. Body Fat Norms

Standards of Fatness for Men and Women in Percentage of Body Fat

	Men	Women
Essential fat	0–5	0–8
Minimal weight	5	15
Most athletes	5–13	12–22
Optimal health	10–25	18–30
Optimal fitness	10–18	16–15
Obesity	>25	>30

Body Fat Norms

Classification	Men (%)	Women (%)
Very low fat (skinny)	7.0–9.9	14.0–16.9
Low fat (trim)	10.0–12.9	17.0–19.0
Average (normal)	13.0–16.9	20.0–23.9
Above normal (plump)	17.0–19.9	24.0–26.9
Very high fat (fat)	20.0–24.9	27.0–29.9
Obese	>25	>30

exercise test is to evaluate the individual's responses to exercise, including heart rate response, blood pressure response, symptoms, perceived exertion, and other variables (e.g., respiratory rate, electrocardiogram [ECG] for arrhythmia). For example, an individual with a history of diabetes or hypertension who is deemed to be at low to moderate risk for the development of heart disease should be monitored for blood pressure response as well as heart rate and perceived exertion. Individuals with palpable arrhythmia or with a history of arrhythmia should be monitored with ECG via telemetry at the very minimum.

The American College of Sports Medicine identifies other specifics with regard to who should be tested as well as protocols that should be followed.[1] These guidelines should be referred to for more specific information regarding testing.

THE EXERCISE PRESCRIPTION

A good exercise prescription is one that is individualized and based on the results of an exercise test. The degree of aggressiveness versus conservativeness that is incorporated into the prescription depends on the findings of the fitness evaluation. Key variables for an individualized exercise prescription include

● age
● percentage of body fat
● previous exercise history
● musculoskeletal abnormalities that could affect performance of exercise on a certain mode of exercise
● risk factors that could affect performance (e.g., smoking) or that require close monitoring (e.g., diabetes—blood sugars; hypertension—blood pressure)

Four parameters that are regularly involved in the exercise prescription include

● mode of exercise
● intensity
● frequency of participation
● duration

These parameters are used in all aspects of physical therapy from getting a patient out of bed to strength training, from functional activity training to home exercise programs. An exercise prescription should provide guidelines for each of these four parameters.

Another consideration that should not be overlooked in the development of an exercise prescription is the compliance factor. Only 10% to 20% of American adults participate in fitness activities to meet conventional training guidelines.[16] In addition, Oldridge in 1982 reported that approximately one half of the participants in supervised exercise programs for preventive medicine drop out prematurely, and between 30% and 80% comply with the provisions of their exercise prescriptions.[17] Part of the problem may be that the existing fitness standards and exercise prescriptions are excessive and may create behavioral problems that lead to noncompliance.

Mode

When developing an exercise prescription for an aerobic exercise program, the mode chosen should be one that uses a large amount of muscle mass, is rhythmic in nature, can be performed in a continuous manner, and, most important, is enjoyable for the individual. Modes of exercise that are routinely used for aerobic exercise prescription are

- swimming
- walking
- running
- bicycling
- skating
- bench stepping
- aerobic dance
- cross-country skiing
- stair stepping

To be truly aerobic, the exercise must be performed for longer than 5 minutes in duration. The choice of mode should conform to the abilities and goals of the individual but should be realistic to enhance the compliance factor.

Frequency

The frequency of participation in exercise initially depends on the individual's age, musculoskeletal limitations, and fitness level. Individuals who are older, who have a musculoskeletal dysfunction that limits performance, or who are extremely deconditioned should start with a frequency of three to four times per week, allowing one day of rest between the exercise days (unless the duration of the exercise performed by the individual in each session is less than 15 minutes). The individual who is older or deconditioned is limited by musculoskeletal dysfunction rather than by cardiovascular limitations and is more likely to incur injury if pushed to exercise on a daily basis. If, however, the individual's duration of exercise is extremely low, the frequency of sessions per day and per week can be increased until a sufficient continuous duration of exercise can be achieved (15 to 20 minutes).

When older and deconditioned individuals have been performing their exercise program without musculoskeletal discomfort or breakdown, the frequency can be increased slowly up to 6 days per week but never 7 days. The incidence of injury escalates once the individual does not have a day of rest for the musculoskeletal system and especially when the intensity and duration are relatively high. The recommended frequency of participation is between four and six times per week to make an effective change on cholesterol level and fitness and body composition. When an individual has reached the desired level of fitness (attained a maintenance intensity level), the frequency may be cut to two to three times per week to achieve maintenance.

Duration

The *initial* duration for the exercise to be performed is set in relation to the individual's fitness level and previous medical history. Deconditioned individuals experience difficulty performing exercise for longer than 20 minutes continuously without developing musculoskeletal dysfunction (soreness, fatigue or pain) either acutely or at a later time. The length of time (in years) that an individual has been inactive or has had exercise limitations also affects the initial duration prescribed. For example, an individual who has been relatively sedentary until the age of 60 experiences greater limitations with performance of exercise and should be given an initial exercise prescription of 10 minutes in duration, whereas a younger sedentary or active older individual may be able to tolerate up to 20 minutes initially.

Duration may be set at 5 to 10 minutes initially and performed a few times per day to increase the patient's tolerance to exercise. Once the individual can exercise continuously for 15 to 20 minutes (or more), the frequency of the exercise sessions should be cut to one time per day. However, the goal should be to increase the duration beyond 20 minutes but no longer than 60 minutes. Research has demonstrated that both fitness and body composition changes increase as the duration of exercise increases beyond 20 minutes. If the individual's goal is to lose body fat and weight, then the duration of the exercise should be increased until a minimum of 40 minutes (walking or biking) is achieved with the intensity maintained between 60% and 75% maximal consumption of oxygen ($\dot{V}O_2$). However, for the individual who has an extremely busy schedule, 40 minutes (even 20 or 30 minutes) at one time may be too much to ask. Blair and colleagues studied exercise duration as it relates to an individual's achieved level of fitness. Three 10-minute sessions throughout the day produced an increased level of fitness but probably not as great a change as for those who exercised continually for 30 minutes. The three 10-minute bouts may help more for overall fitness, including improvements in bone density and flexibility.[18]

Duration is the parameter that should be continuously increased until a minimum of 20 to 30 minutes is attained before altering any of the other parameters.

Intensity

The intensity level to be used in the exercise prescription can be monitored in several ways. Chief among these methods of monitoring are

- determining a target heart rate and teaching the individual to count the pulse
- determining an appropriate rate of perceived exertion
- performing a "talking test"
- defining a specific distance to be covered in a prescribed amount of time

Each of these methods has its advantages and disadvantages and should be chosen after due consideration has been given to the individual's capability of using the method with the particular mode of exercise to be employed.

Identification of a target heart rate and instruction in pulse counting is probably the most frequently recommended method of prescribing exercise intensity, but this method is also probably the most difficult to utilize by individuals who are not regular exercisers or familiar with counting a pulse. For most individuals who are not used to exercising, pulse counting at rest, let alone during or after exercise, is not an easy task. Therefore, practice should be built into the exercise program for taking pulses both at rest and during exercise.

$$\boxed{\text{Target HR} = (\text{MHR} - \text{RHR})\ \% + \text{RHR}}$$

Figure 18–12.

Development of a target heart rate (HR) using the Karvonen method.

Development of a target heart rate requires some mathematic calculations (Fig. 18–12), but a target rate can easily be determined if the resting heart rate is known; the maximal heart rate is known (or else is calculated); and data on the patient's history, age, previous exercise history, and body fat are available. The *true* maximal heart rate is that which was achieved at the peak of exercise or just before the onset of symptoms (e.g., a demonstration of ischemia on the ECG or an abnormal blood pressure response). The American College of Sports Medicine advocates the use of a target heart rate in the range of 60% to 90% of the maximal heart rate for the individual to experience the true effects of training.[1] However, some literature has documented that target heart rates in the range of 40% to 60% of maximal heart rate can elicit training effects in certain populations.[1] The populations with whom the lower target heart rates (in the range of 40% to 60%) should be used include the elderly, the markedly obese or deconditioned, and those with acute cardiac dysfunction or other severe cardiac limitations.

The patient's history is pertinent to the development of a target heart rate, particularly if the history entails one of cardiac dysfunction or some other dysfunction that requires limitation in intensity (e.g., multiple sclerosis). The patient's age is pertinent to the identification of predicted maximal heart rate (Fig. 18–13). Previous exercise history is important information for determining an initial intensity at which to work the individual. If the individual has been extremely sedentary, then 40% may be the number inserted in the formula (see Fig. 18–12) to determine a target heart rate; an individual who has been active or who exercises regularly could probably use 75% in the target heart rate formula. Also, body fat is considered when determining initial intensity because an individual with excess body

| A | PMHR = 220 − AGE |
| B | PMHR = 205 − 1/2 AGE |

Figure 18–13.

Two formulas for the determination of the predicted maximal heart rate (PMHR) for *(A)* **the general population and** *(B)* **fit individuals older than 40.** *Note:* **These formulas should** *not* **be used when the true maximal heart rate can be determined or the patient is taking medications that would affect the resting and exercise heart rate (e.g., beta-blocking medications).**

fat demonstrates less tolerance to exercise owing to inability to effectively dissipate heat that has accumulated as a result of exercise.

Although exercise testing is highly recommended before the development of an exercise prescription, in some cases an individual will not be required to perform an exercise test. Examples include an individual with extremely limited exercise tolerance whom the physician believed could not tolerate an exercise test or an individual with an orthopedic or a neurologic injury that may limit performance on a standard exercise evaluation. Only in such circumstances should a predicted maximal heart rate (see Fig. 18–13 for predicted heart rate formulas) be used in the target heart rate formula and then only in the absence of medications that affect the heart rate (e.g., beta-blocking medications). In addition, reducing the maximum heart rate obtained from the treadmill exercise or predicted by age by 12 beats per minute provides a more accurate estimate of the maximum heart rate for swimming and should be used in the formula for the target heart rate during swimming.[19]

Identification of a perceived level of exertion that can be utilized for exercise intensity is a subjective means of limiting exercise intensity based on the individual's own sense of physiologic response to exercise. The use of a rating of perceived exertion (RPE), as developed by Borg (Fig. 18–14), has been demonstrated to correspond with energy expenditure and physiologic strain.[20-22] Therefore, individuals may be taught to exercise at a particular RPE based on their subjective feelings about exertion. The RPE coincides with objective measures of exercise intensity.

Clinical experience has shown that a "talking test," although subjective, may be employed with success in the older and more deconditioned population for guiding exercise intensity. Individuals who have difficulty taking their pulse or understanding the perceived exertion scale find they can adhere to prescribed intensity levels once instructed to exercise comfortably so that they are still able to carry on a conversation without becoming winded while talking. This tool for setting intensity is extremely helpful when initiating an exercise program for the de-

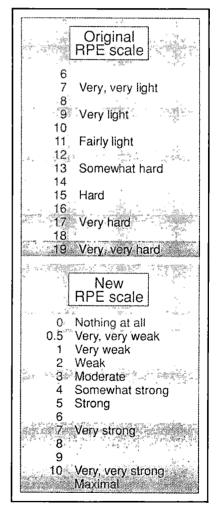

Figure 18–14.

Scales used for ratings of perceived exertion (RPE). (From Borg GA. Psychophysical bases of perceived exertion. Med Sci Sports Exerc 14:377–381, 1982. © Private Practice Section of the APTA.)

conditioned or older populations, because these individuals have more musculoskeletal limitations than cardiovascular limitations and are thereby more attuned to how they feel rather than to physiologic limitations. *Windedness* is therefore a subjective but useful tool for the lay person unfamiliar with exercise.

In addition, setting a specific distance and a specific time in which to cover this distance is a method of guiding exercise intensity. For example, if the intensity desired is 2 miles per hour and the individual is supposed to walk for 30 minutes, then the intensity set for the home program would be to walk 1 mile in 30 minutes on a fairly flat terrain. If a track is inconvenient to perform the walking exercise, the individual can measure the distance using an automobile's odometer or can purchase a pedometer. Pedometers can be very useful for measuring distance if they have been set accurately for the individual's stride length. If the exercise program includes a stationary bicycle, the prescription can be set for miles (or kilometers) registered on the odometer in the time desired. However, with stationary cycling exercise a specific pedaling speed should also be prescribed (50 to 70 revolutions per minute is standard on European bicycles; 10 to 20 miles per hour on American bicycles).[1]

Intensity prescriptions that do not adequately consider the patient's desires and capabilities may lead to noncompliance and may create barriers to motivation. Studies using behavior modification techniques to increase physical activity have focused more on frequency or duration than on intensity.[23]

Specificity

The principle of specificity of exercise should be understood and stated as it relates to the exercise prescription. Specific adaptations in the body's responses to training (e.g., in the muscles and the cardiovascular system) can be related directly to the type of training employed. Therefore, if the goal of the training is to improve an individual's performance in some particular activity, the muscles involved in that activity should be trained in the same manner in which

they will be used. For example, if an individual's goal is to improve walking performance and endurance, arm exercises probably are not the best kind of activity for achieving that goal; walking is more likely to enhance walking performance. By the same token, individuals who wish to improve their ability to perform activities of daily living should be involved in an exercise program that trains the muscles that are used in those activities in a brief but increasingly intense exercise program. It may be less obvious, however, that the individual who performs activities from a wheelchair should be trained in wheelchair propulsion, with an emphasis on increasing the duration of wheelchair propulsion and functional activities from the wheelchair level, rather than in upper extremity training with arm ergometry. The muscle groups that are used in the activity are the ones that need to undergo the training.

Principle of Overload

To improve physiologic performance and demonstrate a training effect, all exercise prescriptions must take into consideration the principle of overload. By manipulating frequency, intensity, duration, or mode, progressive overload can be applied to the individual performing the exercise prescription to increase the amount of energy expenditure or work, with the goal of improving the physiologic state. An initial exercise prescription should have mild overload built in, as the goal is to increase the work on the individual but not enough to create pain, soreness, or musculoskeletal dysfunction. However, all exercise prescriptions should include progression to continually overload the individual, after the initial exercise prescription becomes "easy," to develop the optimal physiologic state.

Progression

An initial exercise prescription provides overload to the individual for the first few sessions or few weeks of the exercise program, but eventually the individual becomes conditioned to that level. To demonstrate continual improvement in cardiovascular fitness, progression must be built into the prescription. Progression can be easily determined if the individual returns to the clinic on an intermittent or infrequent basis for reevaluation of the exercise prescription and readjustment. However, health maintenance visits and exercise prescriptions for individuals who do not have a diagnosed disease are often not covered for reimbursement by most insurance companies, which increases the out-of-pocket cost to the individual. Frequently the progression of exercise is created for the individual when the initial exercise prescription is developed in case the individual does not return for further treatment.

Progression of the exercise program should be based on the individual's goals for the exercise program. Weight loss, lowering of cholesterol, and lowering of blood pressure in individuals who have hypertension are three goals accomplished by increasing the duration (minimum of 40 to 60 minutes if walking, 20 to 30 minutes if jogging). Therefore, duration should be the first parameter that is slowly progressed in an exercise program until the optimal exercise duration is achieved. One consideration that should be included is the amount of time the individual can actually devote to the exercise, either on a daily or a weekly basis. Compliance may decline sharply with increasing duration if the individual is not capable of devoting the amount of time necessary (e.g., 40 minutes if the goal is to decrease body fat and weight). Semiretired or retired individuals may have the amount of time to devote to exercise and should be encouraged to exercise at longer durations; however, the busy executive, the working mother, or the active single individual may find it difficult to adhere to a program of 40 minutes per day.

Once a minimum of 20 to 30 minutes of continuous exercise has been achieved, the individual should be encouraged to increase the intensity of the exercise. Increasing the intensity of the exercise may involve working toward achieving a higher target heart rate or exertion level or a longer distance in a shorter amount of time. If increasing the intensity causes musculoskeletal discomfort or dysfunction, intensity should be maintained at the individual's comfort level, and instead frequency should be the parameter that is increased—up to 6 days per week. In addition, the individual should be reevaluated to determine the cause of the musculoskeletal dysfunction or discomfort.

Compliance

Approximately 30% to 60% of the population is sedentary in its leisure time activities,[16] and only approximately 10% of all American adults participate in vigorous and frequent activity.[24-26] Estimates of the degree of sedentary leisure behavior in the American population have not varied in the past 15 years. The typical dropout rate from supervised exercise programs is approximately 50%.[27] Understanding the factors that affect an individual's level of physical activity as well as understanding the interventions aimed at changing behavior assist the therapist in developing exercise prescriptions to improve the chances of patient compliance.

Factors that affect an individual's level of physical activity include

● personal attributes
● medical status
● past and present behaviors
● psychological traits and states
● environment

Table 18-7 provides a summary of variables that may determine the probability of an individual's engaging in physical activity. Of the aforementioned factors, activity history has the greatest significance for predicting future participation in activities.[28] Oldridge performed one of the most systematic prospective studies of patients enrolled in the Ontario Exercise Heart Collaborative study and found dropouts from cardiac rehabilitation programs were characterized as blue-collar workers, smokers, individuals who were inactive in their leisure time, and those who held a job that required a low expenditure of energy.[29]

Part of the problem of achieving compliance may be that existing fitness standards and exercise prescriptions are excessive and may be creating behavioral problems. Higher compliance with exercise prescriptions was found in the obese and middle- to older-aged subjects who were given low-intensity exercise prescriptions.[28]

TABLE 18–7. Summary of Variables That May Determine Probability of Physical Activity

Determinant	Changes in Probability		Determinant	Changes in Probability	
	Supervised Program	Free-living Activity		Supervised Program	Free-living Activity
Personal Attributes			*Environmental Factors and Interventions*		
Past program participation	++	+(≠)	Spouse support	++	+
Past free-living activity	+	+	Perceived lack of time	--	-(≠)
Contemporary program activity		0	Facilities access or convenience	++	0
School sports	0	0	Disruptions in routine	-	
Health behaviors	00	+(≠)	Social reinforcement or support	+	
Blue-collar occupation	--	-	(staff, exercise partner)		
Smoking	--	0	Past family influences		+(≠)
Overweight (fatness or body mass	-	-	Peer influence (past or present)		+(≠)
index)			Physician influence		+
High risk for coronary heart dis-			School programs	+	+(≠)
ease*	-	-	Cost	0	0
Type A behavior pattern	-	+	Medical screening or fitness test-	0	0
Health and exercise knowledge	0	0	ing		
Health locus of control	+	+	Climate (or geographical region)*	-	-
Attitudes	0	0	Contracts, agreements, contingen-	++	+(≠)
Enjoyment of activity	+	+(≠)	cies		
Perceived health or fitness	++	-(≠)	Stimulus control and reinforce-	++	
Mood disturbance	-	-	ment control		
Education (yr)*	+	++	Benefit and cost decision analysis	++	
Age*	00	-	Relapse prevention training	++	+(≠)
Expect personal health benefit	0	+(≠)	*Physical Activity Characteristics*		
Value exercise outcomes	0	0	Activity intensity	-	-
Self-efficacy for exercise	+	+	Choice of activity type (perceived)	+	
Intention to be active	0	+	Perceived effort	--(≠)	-(≠)
Active self-schemata		+			
Self-motivation	+	++			
Behavioral skills (goal setting,		+			
self-monitoring, self-reinforce-					
ment, relapse planning)					

* Likely a selection bias, not a causal determinant.

Note. ++, Repeatedly documented increased probability; +, weak or mixed documentation of increased probability; 00, repeatedly documented that there is no change in probability; 0, weak or mixed documentation of no change in probability; -, weak or mixed documentation of decreased probability; --, repeatedly documented decreased probability; (≠) indicates unknown validity of measures employed. Blank spaces indicate no data. (From Dishman RK, Sallis JF, Orenstein D. The determinants of physical activity and exercise. Public Health Rep 100(2):162, 1985. Adapted by permission.)

The challenge is to find the optimal exercise prescription to achieve compliance and health gains.

Exercise prescriptions that incorporate goal orientation and planning, as well as self-monitoring and self-reward, increase the tendency to continue to maintain physically active behavior.[30] Goal setting and reinforcement skills have been used to increase involvement in physical activity behaviors (over a short term of between 4 and 10 weeks). In addition, evidence from self-reports indicate that individuals' perceptions of internal rewards (e.g., feeling better or feeling positive about achieving goals) increase the probability that they will continue to perform their prescribed exercise.[23]

FACTORS THAT AFFECT EXERCISE PERFORMANCE

Because environmental conditions influence exercise performance, they must be considered when prescribing exercise for the apparently healthy population. Temperature, wind, altitude, air pollution, and terrain affect exercise performance and are discussed here. Nutrition, pharmacologic agents, and blood products are discussed later, along with the controversies associated with them.

Heat and Cold

As the ideal temperature for exercise (40 to 70 degrees F) is not often the reality in most climates, the effect of heat and cold on individuals and their performance is best understood by understanding the thermoregulatory system.

Thermoregulation

The thermoregulatory system consists of the hypothalamus, which is the regulatory center for temperature control; the thermal receptors; and the thermal effectors. The thermal receptors include the skin, which senses the changes in temperature in the external environment, and the hypothalamus, which senses the changes in the temperature of the internal environment (via the blood). The thermal effectors include the skeletal muscles, which respond to cold more than heat; the sweat glands, which assist in getting rid of the heat; the arterioles, which respond by constricting or dilating the vessels in response to temperature changes; and the endocrine glands, which respond on a long-term basis (over a period of days) to environmental changes in temperature.

The core temperature of the body remains in dynamic equilibrium, balancing the mechanisms that alter heat transfer, regulating evaporative cooling, and varying the rate of heat production. When the body gains more heat than it loses (as can occur in vigorous exercise or in an excessively warm environment), the core temperature rises. Heat is gained from reactions of energy metabolism (the burning or oxidation of food materials for energy allows for heat to be liberated and therefore made available), such as in muscle activity from exercise or shivering, in digestion, and in infection. For example, shivering alone can increase the total metabolic rate three to five times.[31] In addition, the metabolic rate may increase up to 25 times the basal level and core temperature may rise by as much as 1.8

degrees F every 5 minutes with sustained vigorous exercise.[32]

The skin perceives changes in the temperature of the external environment. However, these changes must be of a magnitude of 2 to 3 degrees. When large changes occur in the external environment (e.g., walking from a hot yard into a cool, air-conditioned room), the thermoregulatory system responds with increased expediency to adapt to the environment. The hypothalamus, which detects changes in the internal environment, perceives differences in temperature of 0.1 to 0.2 degrees. Factors that affect changes in internal temperature include

- exercise
- infection
- extreme changes in external temperature (e.g., jumping into a lake of extremely cold water)

Messages from the thermal receptors are transmitted to the thermoregulatory center in the brain, which in turn sends afferent messages to the effectors to initiate a response to maintain homeostasis at a body temperature of approximately 98.6 degrees F.

The thermal effectors respond to messages from the thermoregulatory center depending on whether the environment has been perceived as hot or cold. When heat has been detected, the response is a withdrawal of stimulation to the arterioles, causing vasodilation and shunting of the blood to the skin as well as increasing sweat production. The conscious act that also occurs in warm environments is to remove excess clothing. When a cold environment or situation is detected, the response is to stimulate the arterioles to constrict, shunting blood from the periphery and the areas close to the skin, and to increase muscular activity by shivering to increase metabolic activity. The conscious act that also occurs in cold situations is to increase the amount of clothing that is worn, possibly adding a hat or gloves, and to attempt to remove oneself from the cold environment.

When the individual remains in the cold or hot environment for a period of days to weeks (as in spring or fall when the temperature is changing), the endocrine system is activated to assist in the body's acclimatization to the environment. During prolonged cold exposure two hormones from the adrenal medulla (epinephrine and norepinephrine) assist in increasing heat production. In addition, thyroxine is released, which leads to sustained elevation in the resting metabolism. With prolonged heat stress the body attempts to conserve salts and fluid via hormonal input.[33,34] Antidiuretic hormone is released from the pituitary gland to increase the water reabsorption from the kidneys, causing the urine to become more concentrated. In addition, aldosterone is released from the adrenal cortex, acting on the renal tubules to increase the reabsorption of sodium. The sodium concentration in the sweat is also decreased during repeated exposure to the heat, but the mechanism of this action remains unknown at this time.

Heat

The mechanisms for thermoregulation are primarily geared to protect against overheating.[35] During exercise heat is generated from the contracting muscles of the body. Consequently, heat must be lost to the environment if the body is to function optimally. Heat may be lost by convection, conduction, radiation, or evaporation, or by some combination of these. Heat loss by convection is via air or water movement, such as the currents of air on a windy day, the breeze from a fan, and movement when running or swimming. Heat loss by conduction involves the transfer of heat through solid, liquid, or gas from one molecule to another. Examples of heat loss by conduction include touching a piece of ice with a warm hand and watching the ice melt and the hand cool. The rate of conductive heat loss is related to the temperature gradient between the skin and the surface with which it is in contact. Water, for example, can absorb several times more heat than air and can conduct it away from the body, which can result in the same temperature of water feeling much colder than that of air.

Heat loss by radiation is via the emission of electromagnetic heat waves given off from the body, which typically is warmer than the surrounding environment. Heat may be gained by thermal radiation from solar energy (the sun's

rays) when an individual is standing or exercising in the sun rather than the shade.

In addition, heat loss can occur by evaporation, which is the major physiologic defense the body has available to prevent overheating. Heat is transferred to the environment via vaporized water from the upper respiratory passages and from the skin. There are approximately 2 to 4 million sweat glands that are distributed throughout the body, and these are controlled by cholinergic sympathetic nerve fibers.[36] For an individual acclimatized to a hot environment, water loss through sweating can achieve 500 milliliters per hour during moderate work or 3 liters per hour during hard work. In addition, approximately 300 milliliters of water vaporize from the respiratory passages each day. Heat loss in high environmental temperatures is dependent solely on sweat evaporation to keep the body cool.

Sweat evaporation depends on the surface that is exposed to the environment, the temperature and humidity of the environment, and the convective air currents. The most important factor, however, is the relative humidity (the ratio of water in the environmental air to the total quantity of moisture that can be carried in air at a particular temperature, expressed as a percentage). Therefore, the higher the relative humidity, the greater the amount of moisture in the air, and the less the chance to lose heat via sweat evaporation. High temperatures are tolerated better than high humidity.

The cardiovascular system responds to heat by means of changes in heart rate, stroke volume, vasomotor tone, and endurance in the heat. As a result of an elevated external or internal temperature, vasodilation to the peripheral areas of the body (e.g., subcutaneous tissue, skin) occurs that ultimately lowers the preload to the heart. Therefore, stroke volume is decreased based on a decreased available preload. In addition, more work is performed to maintain a normal core temperature; therefore, the heart rate is elevated at rest in the heat. Furthermore, the heart rate may demonstrate increases throughout exercise that are greater than normal and may not reach a previously demonstrated plateau when steady state exercise has been reached. Vasoconstriction in the vessels that supply blood to the viscera allows for shunting of blood to the areas where it is needed. Blood pressure is usually maintained and does not decrease.

Problems arise with prolonged exposure to heat. Excessive water loss as a result of profuse sweating can lead to dehydration and can severely compromise cardiovascular function. Without adequate rehydration during times of increased water loss, the blood volume decreases, as does the preload on the heart. As a consequence, stroke volume is decreased, necessitating an elevated heart rate to attempt to maintain an adequate cardiac output. With a diminishing cardiac output, signs and symptoms of disorientation and confusion occur that are due to inadequate brain perfusion. In addition, the skin may begin to feel cold and clammy and may take on an ashen color.

With the decreased blood volume, the supply of water to use for heat dissipation becomes inadequate, so the core temperature begins to climb. Core temperatures higher than 104 degrees F are critical and require fast action in treatment with fluids (possibly even intravenous) and ice packs or ice baths to cool the periphery.

Oral fluid replacement should occur throughout any activity in a hot environment. The primary aim of fluid replacement is the maintenance of adequate plasma volume to ensure optimal cardiac output as well as sweat production. Therefore, the key fluid to replace is water. Changes in the body mass should be used to indicate the amount of water loss with exercise and to determine the amount of rehydration that should occur following the exercise. (The easiest mechanism is to weigh the individual before and after exercising.) Fallacies exist regarding the amount of electrolyte replacement that should be given to individuals who sweat large amounts in the heat. In the normal individual, sodium can easily be replenished over time by adding slightly increasing amounts of salt to food over a period of days. Sodium losses during endurance exercise are usually regulated by the kidney.[37]

Problems arise in individuals who may be on sodium-restricted diets or in those who take prescribed diuretics. For persons on sodium-restricted diets, a dietary supplement of sodium may be necessary in extremely hot environments on a regular basis or when partaking in excessive exercise and sweating large amounts of fluid. The individual who is taking prescribed diuretics may need to supplement the diet with electrolytes on a regular basis, with increases in the supplement when excessive sweating is induced either by the hot environment or the exercise.

Exertional dehydration can be compounded if an individual is taking medication to reduce the plasma volume, as is the case with diuretics, which are typically prescribed for persons with hypertension as well as for those who are trying to lose weight quickly. In any situation involving reduced plasma volume, the blood volume that is available is often shunted from the working muscles to be used for heat dissipation peripherally at the skin. What ensues as a result of this dehydration is a decrease in performance due to lack of oxygen to the working muscles. Individuals taking these medications should be educated in the importance of fluid replacement whenever an exercise prescription is developed.

A key factor influencing the efficiency of fluid replacement is the rate of gastric emptying. Cold fluids are emptied from the stomach at a faster rate than fluids at body temperature.[38,39] The volume of fluid ingested is also of importance, as gastric emptying speeds up for each 100-milliliter increase in volume up to 600 milliliters taken in at 15 minute intervals (although 250 milliliters or 8.5 ounces is probably a more realistic goal).[40] However, during vigorous exercise only about 800 milliliters of fluid can be emptied from the stomach each hour, an amount that is insufficient to match the amount of water loss (approximately 2 liters per hour).[32]

Gastric emptying is retarded when the fluid contains increased levels of sugar in the form of glucose, fructose, or sucrose.[41] The addition of salt to the fluid can further depress the emptying of the stomach. Drinks containing glucose polymer of 7.5% or less concentration do not appear to retard gastric emptying when ingested in small amounts over 15 minutes.[42] As replacement fluids are typically chosen on the basis of marketing appeal to the consumer and not on scientific evidence of true benefit, the therapist involved in developing exercise prescriptions is the most appropriate person to provide this information to the individual. Therefore, the replacement fluid of choice for most individuals who are not performing vigorous exercise should be water.

Acclimatization to the heat as well as to the level of training are two factors that modify an individual's heat tolerance. The major acclimatization to heat occurs during the first week of exposure to the heat and is completed by the end of 10 days.[43,44] The physiologic adjustments to the heat and the training include peripheral vasodilation, development of a lower threshold for sweating, lower core temperature, lower heart rate response, and less salt lost in the sweat. The physiologic responses to training include an increase in the sensitivity and response time of sweating and a dilution of the sweat produced due to adaptations in the sweat glands.[45]

Cold

Cold does not produce the extreme reactions of heat, but the physiologic strain imposed depends on the temperature of the environment, the individual's level of metabolism, and the resistance to heat flow (conductance) provided by body fat.[46] Depending on the environment (e.g., cold water induces much greater heat loss than cold air), additional oxygen uptake may be required to perform exercise in the cold owing to the added energy cost of shivering as the body attempts to combat heat loss. Typically this additional oxygen uptake occurs only when the individual is at rest and early during exercise in cold air. The body does have warning signs that cold injury is developing, such as a tingling and numbness in the fingers and toes or a burning sensation of the nose and ears. However, the major problem the cold environment imposes on running performance is that no one has set any endurance event records in the cold environment. Some researchers have theorized that the cold has an effect on coordination and may in fact alter the activity of the muscle spindle.[47]

Again, acclimatization increases the individual's capacity to adapt to the cold. Individuals develop a lower rectal temperature in response to the cold and develop peripheral adaptations such as peripheral vasoconstriction.[48]

Cold air is particularly detrimental for some individuals owing to its effect on the respiratory tract when inhaled through the mouth. The nose functions to filter and humidify as well as warm the incoming air, but if the air is breathed in directly through the mouth this "warming effect" does not happen. As a result, air is colder on inspiration through the mouth. Two complications are often mentioned with the inhalation of cold air: bronchospasm and dry or irritated mouth. Individuals who have these complications in the cold air are often encouraged to use a scarf over their mouth when exercising to warm the air and cut down on the heat and water loss.

A problem in evaluating the effect of the temperature on performance is the "wind" factor. The air currents magnify heat loss as well as sweat loss, and an individual can actually feel colder or become dehydrated. The wind can increase or decrease the work on the individual, depending on whether the individual is working with (resulting in a decrease in work) or against (resulting in an increase in work) the wind.

Altitude

The effects of medium- and high-altitude environments on exercise performance have been studied for years. However, they have received intensified scrutiny after athletes who trained at high altitudes (e.g., in Kenya) began winning Olympic endurance events consistently. The altitude effects are related to the decreased partial pressure of oxygen in the inspired air. The barometric pressure and the weight of the atmosphere are decreased at high altitudes, but the percentage of oxygen is the same; therefore, the number of molecules of oxygen per unit volume inspired is decreased. As a result, with increased elevation the partial pressure of alveolar oxygen decreases as does the oxygen saturation. With this decrease in partial pressure of oxygen is an increased desire to breathe in more air, so the respiratory rate increases, resulting in hyperventilation. Stroke volume does not increase, but the submaximal heart rate and cardiac output increase to compensate for the reduced arterial oxygen saturation.[49-51] As a result, submaximal work requires greater oxygen consumption at high altitudes as compared with that of sea level, yet the oxygen consumption for maximal work is reduced (the maximal oxygen capacity is reached earlier, or approximately at one fourth of normal maximal work).

Some individuals experience altitude sickness owing to the stress of the altitude in the first few days of exposure. The most common symptoms are headache (due to cerebral vasodilation), nausea, dizziness, vomiting, and generalized weakness. Approximately 2% of those who visit altitudes higher than 10,000 feet experience a severe form of altitude sickness termed *high-altitude pulmonary edema*, which is a life-threatening condition associated with fluid in the lungs and brain.[52] Immediate return to a sea level environment is the best treatment.

Acclimatization to higher altitudes results in physiologic and metabolic adjustments over a period of time. The adjustments that occur involve readjustment of the acid-base balance, hematologic changes, and changes in local circulation and cellular function. The amount of time required to become acclimatized is dependent on the altitude. In general, the higher the altitude, the longer the time it takes to become acclimatized to the environment.

The acid-base adjustments that occur owing to acclimatization involve an altered blood pH that develops as a result of hyperventilation. With increased amounts of CO_2 "blown off" by the lungs, the blood pH becomes more alkalotic (pH greater than 7.45). Normally the kidneys control the amount of bicarbonate (HCO_3^-) that is maintained in the blood to act as a buffer to maintain the pH in the normal range. (Normal HCO_3^- blood levels range between 22–26 mg/dL.) In response to the hyperventilation at high altitudes (and the resultant alkalosis), the kidneys increase the excretion of bicarbonate (HCO_3^-) through the renal tubules, providing for a normal pH to be maintained.

The second long-term adaptation to elevated altitude is the increase in the blood's oxygen carrying capacity. Both a decrease in plasma volume and an increase in production of erythrocytes and hemoglobin (stimulated by the hypoxic situation created at high altitudes) occurs, creating a polycythemia. In addition, iron supplementation can increase the prealtitude values for hematocrit and hemoglobin.[53]

The third adjustment to high altitude appears to be the local circulatory and cellular adaptations to extreme hypoxia. Capillaries appear to be more concentrated in skeletal muscle of animals born and raised at high altitudes.[54] Natives of high altitudes also demonstrate an increase in the concentration of 2,3-diphosphoglycerate in the red blood cells, causing a slight shift to the right of the oxyhemoglobin dissociation curve (see Chapter 10).[55] In combination with increased circulating hemoglobin, an increase in 2,3-diphosphoglycerate increases the supply of oxygen to active tissue during strenuous exercise and increases performance.

Acclimatization at higher altitudes does improve one's capacity to perform work at higher altitudes, but some of the physiologic changes that occur as a result of prolonged altitude exposure can also cause a decrease in performance on return to sea level.[56] In fact, the changes in the breathing (hyperventilation) that cause a situation of alkalosis in the blood, the increased bicarbonate excretion to normalize the blood pH, and the reduced maximal heart rate diminish the improvement that could be gained with the increased oxygen carrying capacity that develops at high altitudes.

Air Pollution

Caution needs to be observed when exercising in environments with elevated air pollution levels. The effect of air pollution on performance depends on the nature of the pollutants. Primary pollutants include carbon monoxide, nitrogen oxides and sulfur dioxides (from the combustion of fossil fuels), and particulates (from incinerators or forest fires). Secondary pollutants occur as the result of chemical reactions with the primary pollutants (ozone being the most widely known).

The site of action of the pollutants depends on their solubility within the respiratory tree.[57,58] The sulfur dioxides are soluble and act primarily on the upper respiratory airways. Ozone and carbon monoxide, which are insoluble, act on the smaller airways. Ozone acts on the small airways and changes pulmonary function, as noted by the measurement of forced vital capacity and forced expiratory flow. Carbon monoxide demonstrates an even greater effect on the body than ozone, as carbon monoxide penetrates the alveoli and actually diffuses into the circulatory system, binding with hemoglobin. Carbon monoxide has a stronger affinity for hemoglobin than does oxygen or even carbon dioxide and therefore monopolizes the binding sites on the hemoglobin molecule. As a result, an individual exposed to carbon monoxide pollution has a decreased oxygen carrying capacity until the carbon monoxide is eliminated from the body.

Carbon monoxide, unlike ozone, may remain in an individual's circulatory system for up to 3 hours after the exposure. Exposure to carbon monoxide can be a result of primary exposure (e.g., smoking a cigarette or inhaling automobile exhaust fumes) or secondary exposure (e.g., inhaling someone else's cigarette smoke). The carbon monoxide decreases an individual's performance by decreasing maximal oxygen consumption and increasing submaximal oxygen consumption with activity.

Athletes and individuals who exercise tend to have greater exposure to pollution owing to their breathing patterns during exercise.[13,57] During moderate or vigorous exercise, individuals tend to breathe through the mouth, which decreases the filtration normally performed by the nose and increases the amount of pollutants that can be inhaled at one time. As a result, individuals who exercise in areas with increased levels of air pollution may demonstrate the manifestations of air pollution, which include chest pain with deep inspirations, substernal soreness, dry cough, dryness of the upper airways, or eye irritation. Individuals who exercise in areas of high air pollution should be cautioned of the potential hazards. Acclimatization to air pollution should never be encouraged, because air pollution only hurts performance. In addition, there may be a correlation between exposure to air pollution and risk for lung cancer.

Exercise Surfaces

The type of surface that an individual exercises on can affect performance and has the potential to cause injury. The types of surfaces that are of concern include hills, uneven surfaces, banked tracks, and hard surfaces.

Hills can create problems because the intensity of exercise varies when an individual ascends and descends the hill. Intensity of exercise is difficult to determine on hills; therefore, a prescription for exercising in hilly areas needs to be based on perceived exertion and heart rate. In addition, walking and running down hills often precipitates injury in the form of shin splints.[59–61] Shin splints can develop owing to the excessive eccentric contraction of the anterior tibialis when descending a hill. Individuals may have to alter their exercise route if they develop shin splints. In addition, an exercise program to work on strengthening the anterior tibialis with eccentric activity built into the program should be initiated.

Caution should be taken whenever an individual exercises on any uneven surfaces, because these surfaces can contribute to the development of sprains and strains, particularly involving the ankle. Exercising on streets whose edges are canted may cause undue strain of the muscles on the side of the lowermost extremity. If individuals plan to exercise on such terrain, they should be told to exercise on one side of the road when they begin their program and to return on the same side so that the imbalances are the same for both lower extremities. Running or walking on indoor tracks can lead to similar kinds of imbalances to the lower extremity musculature.

Hard surfaces also pose a potential problem as a result of shock being transmitted up the lower extremity from the surface. Good shoes with sufficient shock absorbability and foot support are essential, and all individuals should be told this, whether or not they are exercising on hard surfaces.

Medications

Many medications have potential effects on performance, but only a few are mentioned in this section. Further information on medications can be obtained from Chapters 12 and 13. The medications that are most important for consideration when prescribing exercise include beta-blocking medications, diuretics, and insulin.

Beta-blocking medications—including propranolol (Inderal), metoprolol tartrate (Lopressor), labetalol (Normodyne), atenolol (Tenormin), to name a few—affect the resting as well as the exercising heart rate and blood pressure. Consequently, the intensity portion of an exercise prescription should not be based on a target heart rate. Instead intensity determinations should be based on observed performance, perceived exertion, or symptoms. Recommendations for exercising should be given with caution unless the individual has been observed while exercising or has undergone a formal exercise evaluation (preferably using the mode of exercise to be employed in their regular exercise program, such as a treadmill or bicycle).

Diuretics—including furosemide (Lasix), bumetenide (Bumex), methyclothiazide (Enduron), hydrochlorothiazide (HydroDIURIL), triamterene (Dyazide), to name a few—decrease the plasma volume via the kidneys. Diuretics may elicit an adverse exercise response as a result of dehydration. During exercise the core temperature may increase, resulting in a physiologic shunting of blood to the skin to dissipate the internal heat, with the consequence that less volume is shunted to the muscles. Given a decreased plasma volume, particularly when exercising in warm environments, even less volume is available to be used by the working muscles.[57] The activation of this physiologic mechanism can decrease the individual's performance and may also create a situation of dehydration. In addition, some of the diuretics are not potassium sparing, and therefore an increased amount of potassium may be excreted with the water via the kidney. Low levels of potassium in the blood can create a critical situation, increasing the chance of arrhythmias.

Diabetics who use the injectable form of insulin (e.g., NPH, lente) require supervision when initiating an exercise program and when altering a program. The amount of insulin injected, the diet consumed, the time of the insulin injection, the peak effect of the insulin, and the site of the injection all must be considered when these individuals exercise.

Levels of insulin above the required amount can create a situation of hypoglycemia. Elevated insulin levels can develop when increased amounts of glucose are required as a result of exercise and when no cutbacks in the insulin injected have occurred. Hypoglycemic individuals may feel weak and dizzy and may even develop palpitations. Therefore, levels of insulin as well as diet should be altered when developing exercise prescriptions for diabetics. (See Chapters 7 and 16 for further discussion of exercise for individuals with diabetes.)

The insulin should never be injected into the exercising muscle, particularly before the exercise. In addition, the individual should be educated to exercise at times when the insulin is not having its peak effect, because the risk for hypoglycemia is greatly increased.

CONTROVERSIAL SUBSTANCES THAT AFFECT EXERCISE PERFORMANCE

Anabolic Steroids

Anabolic steroids are drugs that function in a manner similar to the male hormone testosterone and as a result have played a major role in competitive sports. These drugs bind with special receptor sites on the muscle and other tissues and act to increase muscle mass and strength, as does the male hormone at the onset of puberty. The original steroid drugs typically had masculinizing effects associated with them; however, the newer derivatives have been chemically manipulated and produce fewer masculine side effects and more muscular growth.

Steroids are typically taken for strength training or power building and then stopped before competition because it is illegal to use these drugs in athletic competition. Drug screening via urinalysis is performed to detect the use of illicit drugs. The American College of Sports Medicine has developed a position statement regarding anabolic-androgenic steroids that includes the following: "The use of anabolic-androgenic steroids by athletes is contrary to the rules and ethical principles of athletic competition as set forth by many of the sports governing bodies."[58]

The ergogenic effectiveness of steroids has not been clearly proved with research on humans owing to the variations in specific drugs, experimental design, dosage, treatment duration, specific training, measurement techniques, and nutritional supplementation. However, when research with steroids was performed on animals it was concluded that anabolic steroids, with exercise and protein supplementation, stimulated protein synthesis and increased the skeletal muscle protein content.[59] The human studies that have been performed demonstrate conflicting results with body mass, muscular strength, and the like.[60,61] In addition, the possibility of harmful side effects exists, including liver disease, interference with the body's immune system, elevation of low-density lipoprotein cholesterol and total cholesterol, and sterility in both males and females.[62-66]

Growth Hormone

The latest training aid appears to be human growth hormone—a hormone that is produced by the pituitary gland but is currently used in the synthetic form. Growth hormone in the human body stimulates amino acid uptake and protein synthesis and is often given to children who lack this hormone to achieve a normal size. In the athlete, fat-free weight has been demonstrated to increase and body fat to decrease with the use of human growth hormone. Growth hormone also stimulates the use of fat as an energy source, thereby sparing the amount of carbohydrate that is required.[67] As this hormone is normally produced by the body, no way is known at this time to detect its use for performance enhancement.

Amphetamines

Amphetamines, otherwise known as "pep pills" are often used to improve performance, because they mimic the sympathetic hormones epinephrine and norepinephrine and decrease the sensation of muscle fatigue.[68] Amphetamines have a profound effect on the cardiopulmonary system because they increase blood pressure, heart rate, cardiac output, ventilation, metabo-lism, and use of blood sugar. Amphetamines are often used for their stimulant effect and for the psychological lift they provide before an athletic event. The side effects are similar to those with increased sympathetic stimulation and include headaches, tremulousness, agitation, fever, and confusion. In addition, research has shown that amphetamines do not enhance athletic performance. The International Olympic Committee as well as other athletic governing groups have rules disqualifying athletes who use these pills.

Caffeine

Caffeine is probably the only stimulant that is not considered an illicit drug, and therefore caffeine is used by some individuals for performance enhancement. The International Olympic Committee has banned its use by competitors in the Olympic games.[69]

The literature regarding caffeine is not without controversy, and, therefore, the conclusions regarding the effects of caffeine on performance are inconsistent. Caffeine consumed 60 minutes before exercise (an amount equal to 2.5 cups of coffee or 330 milligrams) extended endurance significantly in persons performing moderately strenuous exercise.[70] The improvement in endurance is associated with an increase in free fatty acid concentration.[71] Caffeine has also been shown to elevate glycerol levels and, along with the rise in free fatty acids, to cause a decreased rate of glycolysis and conservation of muscle glycogen.[71] Therefore, it is likely that the improvement is due to the facilitated use of fat as a fuel and the sparing of the carbohydrate reserves.[72] Another effect appears to be a lessening of perceived effort due to a possible analgesic effect of caffeine or, possibly, a lowering of the threshold for motor unit recruitment and transmission of nerve conduction.[70] Caffeine may act directly on the muscle by increasing the rate at which force is developed but without causing a change in the maximal force.[73]

Caffeine is not without negative effects, as has been found in studies of laboratory mice that have ingested caffeine on a long-term basis. Habitual use of caffeine diminished the animals' ability to perform exhaustive work under stressful conditions.[74] In addition, noticeable rises in plasma noradrenalin and adrenalin accompanied by an associated tachycardia have been documented with ingestion of caffeine.[75] This finding was attributed to a possible hypersensitivity to caffeine. Other side effects of caffeine are headaches, insomnia, and nervous irritability. Excess coffee consumption has also been associated with lipoprotein profiles suggestive of an increased risk of cardiovascular problems.[76] Finally, caffeine acts as a potent diuretic and may affect hydration and thermoregulation with exercise. The current consensus is that the diuretic effect (a negative effect for exercise) of caffeine probably far outweighs the ergogenic potential, so that individuals who exercise should be discouraged from using caffeine for improving performance.

Blood Doping

Blood doping or blood boosting involves the withdrawal of and then reinfusion of red blood cells before an endurance event to increase the hemoglobin concentration and therefore improve performance. The procedure involves the withdrawal of 1 to 4 units of an individual's blood (each unit withdrawn every 3 to 8 weeks), followed by reinfusion of the packed frozen red blood cells anywhere from 1 to 7 days before an endurance event. The increase in red blood cells has been demonstrated to be as much as 20% (rise in hemoglobin level from 15 g per 100 ml to 19 g per 100 ml) and appears to remain for approximately 14 days.[77]

Blood doping appears to increase aerobic capacity (anywhere from 5% to 13%), decrease submaximal heart rate and blood lactate accumulation, and improve sweating responses, depending on the blood storage method before reinfusion.[78,79] The downside of blood doping is that it does increase the blood viscosity and can in turn decrease the cardiac output. As a result, new methods of blood boosting are under investigation, including hormonal boosting with erythropoietin, a hormone that is normally produced by the kidneys. Erythropoietin stimulates the production of red blood cells by the bone marrow. The problem with the current use of

erythropoietin is that it has not been monitored or regulated, and hematocrit levels have been elevated to excessively dangerous levels. More research is required with this new controversial practice.[80]

DIETARY CONSIDERATIONS

Carbohydrate Modification

Carbohydrate loading or glycogen supercompensation is probably the most popular method of nutritional modification used for enhancement of performance. Sensations of extreme muscle fatigue and pain experienced by marathon runners, also known as "hitting the wall," describe the physiologic considerations that limit prolonged endurance exercise. The fatigue is related to the depletion of muscle glycogen even though sufficient oxygen is available to the muscles and potential energy is available in the form of stored fat. Diets modified to include consumption of a greater percentage of calories from carbohydrates before an event have been shown to increase the amount of glycogen stored in the muscle and therefore improve performance in endurance events.[80,81]

The classic approach to carbohydrate loading begins with complete depletion of all glycogen stores approximately 1 week before an event. This involves consuming a diet that is high in protein and fat and extremely low in carbohydrates and, in addition, engaging in strenuous aerobic training. This stage is termed the stripping phase of carbohydrate loading to deplete all stores of glycogen. It is initiated approximately 6 days before an endurance event and spans approximately 4 days. The individual then switches to a diet that is extremely high in carbohydrates (the packing phase) and changes to tapered, light workouts to supercompensate the stripped muscles.[82] The problems with the classic approach involved the extreme side effects experienced (lightheadedness and lethargy) especially during the carbohydrate stripping phase. A modified regimen was designed by Sherman and colleagues whereby athletes train at approximately

75% of their maximal oxygen consumption for 1.5 hours and gradually taper the duration of the exercise while consuming their usual 50% carbohydrate diet. After 3 days, the diet is then changed to a 70% carbohydrate diet. The modified regimen demonstrated an increase in glycogen storage equivalent to that found after the classic carbohydrate loading method.[81]

One of the most negative aspects of carbohydrate loading is the heaviness that the athlete perceives as a result of water retention (2.7 g of water are stored with each gram of muscle glycogen). Body mass may increase considerably and make the individual feel heavy and uncomfortable. However, the additional water that is stored with the glycogen may assist with thermoregulation and hydration.

Other types of dietary intervention, particularly those aimed at reducing weight, may actually interfere with performance. The prevalence of fad diets in American culture is primarily due to the obsession with an improved body image and the need to change it immediately with a "quick fix." Most fad diets to induce rapid weight loss are primarily low in carbohydrates and high in protein. This combination itself decreases performance capability because the individual is deficient in energy, lethargic, and lightheaded and may not feel like exercising.[83] Therefore, it is wisest *not* to implement dietary restrictions, particularly restrictions of carbohydrates, when initiating an exercise program. Dietary modification should be made only after an individual has been exercising for a few weeks.

IMPROVING THE PERFORMANCE OF A TRAINED ATHLETE

Techniques and tools to improve the performance of a trained athlete include ventilatory threshold training, nutrition assessment, and biomechanical analysis.

Ventilatory Threshold

During steady state exercise, sufficient oxygen is available to the working muscles so that lactic acid production does not exceed lactic acid uptake, resulting in no accumulation of blood lactate. However, at some level of oxygen consumption that is unique to each individual, depending on training, genetics, and the like, the threshold of the onset of blood lactate accumulation (OBLA), or the anaerobic threshold occurs. The terms *anaerobic threshold* and *OBLA* are controversial owing to the existence of individual patterns in the kinetics of lactate production and removal.[84] This threshold is difficult to determine (with as much as 16% variability) owing to speed of movement and nutritional state as well as method of measurement.[85]

An alternative method to establish the anaerobic threshold is to determine at what rate of exercise or oxygen uptake a nonlinear increase in pulmonary ventilation is observed. The physiologic basis for this phenomenon exists in the alteration in the pH with the increase in lactic acid in the blood. In untrained individuals, this threshold occurs at approximately 50% to 60% of the maximal oxygen consumption ($\dot{V}o_2$). In highly trained endurance athletes, this threshold may be more than 80% of the maximal $\dot{V}o_2$. When excess lactic acid accumulates as a result of anaerobic metabolism supplementing the aerobic metabolism for energy, a mechanism occurs in the blood to buffer the excess acid.

$$\text{Lactic acid} + NaHCO_3 \rightarrow \text{Na lactate} + H_2CO_3$$
$$\rightarrow H_2O + CO_2$$

With the increase in CO_2 produced, an increase in pulmonary ventilation occurs to exhale the increased CO_2. This is where the term *ventilatory threshold* comes from. However, the controversy over the ventilatory threshold and the OBLA exists in the measurement technique, which is an assessment of the lactate levels in the blood and not necessarily that in the muscle. A current belief is that everyone possesses an individual lactate shuttle whereby the lactate is shuttled to be converted to pyruvate, which then can be used in Krebs's cycle to generate energy. When the production of lactate exceeds the conversion of lactate via the lactate shuttle to pyruvate, accumulation of lactate occurs in the blood, thereby known as OBLA.[86]

Training to improve an individual's aerobic capacity is usually centered around training just above or below the ventilatory threshold. The point of OBLA has been shown to increase with training, even without showing an increase in $\dot{V}o_{2max}$.[87] In fact, changes in performance with training are more often associated with changes in the intensity of exercise that brings on OBLA than in changes in $\dot{V}o_{2max}$. The exercise intensity at the point of OBLA is a more powerful predictor of performance in aerobic exercise.[88,89] Training should therefore be centered around increasing the OBLA via aerobic endurance training as well as anaerobic endurance training.

Nutrition Assessment

Optimal nutrition for exercise requires an evaluation of an individual's regular activity level to assess the amount of energy expended. On the basis of regular energy expenditure, caloric intake can be assessed, and nutrient intake can be prescribed. In general, approximately 15% of caloric intake should be in the form of protein; no greater than 30% in the form of fat (of which 70% should be unsaturated); and approximately 50% to 60% in the form of carbohydrates, predominantly complex carbohydrates.[80] In addition, the fluid intake should be evaluated to prevent possible dehydration.

Many athletes still believe that more than 15% of calories from protein is necessary to build muscle. A meal high in protein, fat, or both before an event may actually affect performance in a negative manner, because digestion and absorption of protein increase the metabolic rate more than carbohydrates do, resulting in increased metabolic heat being produced. When increased metabolic heat is produced, more work must be performed by the body to dissipate the heat.

Biomechanical Analysis

An evaluation of an individual's biomechanics when performing a specific activity is used both to improve mechanical economy as well as to decrease the risk of injury from overuse. Biome-chanics combines engineering with biology and physiology.

Measuring $\dot{V}o_2$ while performing a particular activity is the simplest way to establish economy of physical effort. An individual with greater economy of movement consumes less oxygen when performing a specific task at submaximal work levels. Any adjustment in training that improves the economy of effort improves the performance. Economy with the activity improves with training and may improve with biomechanical adjustments.

FACTORS THAT AFFECT OLDER WELL INDIVIDUALS

Although in terms of epidemiology exercise has not been shown to improve overall longevity, it does decrease the incidence of premature death.[90,91] In the MRFIT study, the risk of any mortality was significantly lower in the moderately active man compared with that in the least active man.[92]

Individuals who exercised more had an improved health profile. In contrast, lack of regular activity was found to increase an individual's risk of developing heart disease almost twofold compared with that of active individuals.[93] Because the older population is the fastest growing segment of the American population, and the average life expectancy of men and women is in the mid seventies, reducing chronic disease and improving the health status of this growing group of individuals would have a significant impact on health care economics. Therefore, activity should be encouraged for this population.

The *well older population* is the term assigned to individuals who have no evidence of disease, nor are at high risk for disease; nonetheless, these individuals may not be considered to be *fit*. Physiologic decline is not as rapid in individuals without disease and is even less in those who continue to remain active into and throughout their older years. Previously it was reported that after age 25, the $\dot{V}o_{2max}$ declined at about 1% per year, so that by age 55 an individual's $\dot{V}o_{2max}$ should be approximately 27% below that of a 20 year old.[80] Current literature reports that one's activity level is more a determinant of aerobic capacity than of chronologic age.[94] For true physiologic changes with aging the reader should refer back to Chapter 2.

Regular physical activity produces physiologic improvements regardless of age. However, the magnitude of the changes and the speed at which the changes occur depend on factors that include initial fitness status, age, and specific type of training. The exercise program should be comprehensive and based on the functional needs of the patient. Specific attention should be given to including exercises to improve muscle strength, flexibility, and endurance.

In general, some of the factors that should be considered in exercise prescription for the older population include the effects of heat, the intensity and frequency of exercise and other parameters of exercise prescription, and the incidence of musculoskeletal injuries associated with older adults.

Heat

Older individuals tend to be less tolerant of heat than younger individuals. This finding appears to be related to a decrease in peripheral blood flow and sweating rate as well as an increase in subcutaneous fat that occurs in the older population.[95] Older individuals should be cautioned regarding exercise in the heat and should be observed for signs and symptoms of heat stress. Education regarding the importance of adequate fluid intake should also be a component of the exercise prescription.

Parameters for Exercise Prescription

Exercise prescription parameters should stress all components of the exercise, including a very thorough cardiovascular and stretching warm-up and cool-down. Nontrained older individuals may require a longer time to stretch to increase flexibility before exercise owing to changes in the collagen as a result of aging.[96,97] In addition, a longer time is often needed to achieve a physiologic steady state and to recover from exercise. Slower adjustment to the exercise and the recov-

ery from exercise may be due to a decreased responsiveness of the cardiovascular system to catecholamines, to the decreased fitness level or to both.[98]

Initially, the frequency of exercise bouts for the older population should allow a day of rest in between bouts of exercise. Injury is the second most common barrier to participation in sports or other activities in the older age groups.[99] Therefore, decreasing the frequency in the early stages of an exercise program decreases the risk of injury, particularly the risk of overuse injuries that may develop from doing too much too soon. A minimum frequency of three sessions per week is recommended.[100] Aerobic training could be alternated with strength and flexibility training during the week, thereby increasing the frequency of total exercise to 6 days per week.

The intensity of the training should be adjusted for the older population. Suggestions for intensity should be lower than that recommended for the younger population, with even 40% of maximal heart rate reserve demonstrating aerobic and functional training adaptations. Target heart rates alone should not be used for the exercise prescription (see the earlier discussion under Intensity) because the use of perceived exertion with target heart rate is an extremely useful tool that includes subjective information. In addition, progression should be slow, particularly in light of the tendency of older individuals to be more prone to injury.[101]

In addition, duration should be increased slowly until 30 minutes of continuous exercise is achieved, at which time the intensity can then be progressively increased according to the individual's tolerance.

MUSCULOSKELETAL INJURIES

Although both aging and inactivity tend to reduce flexibility and joint range of motion, it appears that inactivity is the dominant factor in the deterioration of flexibility. Both the changes due to age and the loss of flexibility associated with inactivity place the older individual at an increased risk for injury.[96,97]

There also appear to be age-dependent differences in the process of wound healing.[102] In the older individual the inflammatory response to injury is dampened; the proliferative phase, cell migration, and maturation are all delayed; and in the remodeling phase the collagen is laid down less rapidly, in smaller volumes, and with an altered binding pattern.[102] Therefore, older individuals not only are at an increased risk for injury but also recover more slowly from injuries than younger individuals, and their injuries tend to become more long term in nature.[96] Anatomically, injury was found to be more common in the foot in the older group, including metatarsalgia and plantarfasciitis.[103] An increase in frequency of osteoarthritis has been found to be more common with increasing age; yet, little evidence indicates that exercise per se is deleterious to joints that have not been injured previously.[104]

In general, the literature as well as clinical practice seems to support the assertion that the older population is an excellent group in whom to see improvement in functional capacity and activities of daily living by increasing their activity. Modifications in the exercise prescription and adequate guidance of the older individual when initiating an exercise program will decrease the incidence of musculoskeletal injuries and increase compliance with the exercise program.

SUMMARY

- In the population considered to be well (individuals without a diagnosis of any cardiopulmonary dysfunction), the most important assessment to be performed is identification of the individual's risk for developing cardiopulmonary disease.
- An assessment of risk for cardiopulmonary disease can be ascertained from answers to questions on smoking history, occupational exposure to toxic chemicals, and family history of disease.
- The components of a fitness evaluation include a thorough physical evaluation of the musculoskeletal system, a body composition analysis, an exercise test, and a personal interview to identify the individual's interests and goals.
- A thorough musculoskeletal evaluation is performed before initiating an exercise program to

screen for preexisting conditions, identify orthopaedic abnormalities and dysfunction, determine baseline musculoskeletal data, and assist in developing a program to prevent injury.
- Abnormal findings noted during the assessment of posture and alignment provide information to assist in determining modes of exercise to avoid as well as to assist in developing a stretching and strengthening program.
- Static flexibility is the actual available range of motion when the individual is in a stretched position, whereas dynamic flexibility is the ability to move certain components of the musculoskeletal system through the available range of motion quickly.
- Assessment of strength does not require a full assessment of each muscle and muscle group but rather can be streamlined for the individual who is without obvious musculoskeletal dysfunction or any other pathology that might weaken the musculoskeletal system.
- Assessment of stability involves moving the extremities through the range of motion to assess for grinding, pain, and ligament integrity.
- Body composition can be assessed clinically via three methods: anthropometry, hydrostatic weighing, and electrical impedance.
- Hydrostatic weighing (underwater weighing) is considered to be the optimal method for body fat assessment because this method is the most accurate.
- Four parameters involved in the exercise prescription that are regularly modified include mode of exercise, intensity, frequency of participation, and duration.
- When developing an exercise prescription for an aerobic exercise program, the mode chosen should be one that utilizes a large amount of muscle mass, is rhythmic in nature, and can be performed on a continuous basis.
- The frequency of participation that is set initially depends on the individual's age, musculoskeletal limitations, and initial fitness level.
- Deconditioned individuals will have difficulty performing exercise for more than 20 minutes continuously without developing musculoskeletal dysfunction (soreness, fatigue or pain) either at the time of exercise or later.
- Studies using behavior modification techniques to increase physical activity have focused more on frequency or duration than on intensity.
- To improve physiologic performance and demonstrate a training effect, all exercise pre-

scriptions must have the principle of overload built in.

- Understanding the known determinants of physical activity as well as the interventions that can be aimed at changing behavior helps those who develop exercise prescriptions improve the chances of patient compliance.
- Part of the compliance problem may be that existing fitness standards and exercise prescriptions are excessive.
- The environmental temperature, wind, altitude, air pollution level, type of terrain and surface for exercising, nutrition, pharmacologic agents, and blood products may affect exercise performance.
- The cardiovascular system demonstrates changes in heart rate, stroke volume, vasomotor tone, and endurance in the heat.
- The primary aim of fluid replacement is to maintain adequate plasma volume to ensure adequate cardiac output and sweat production.
- Dehydration is increased if an individual is taking medications to reduce plasma volume, for example, diuretics, which typically are prescribed for individuals with hypertension and for those trying to lose weight quickly. With the plasma volume reduced because of the diuretics, the blood volume that is available is often shunted from the working muscles to the surface of the skin to be used for heat dissipation.
- Cold does not produce as extreme effects as heat, but the physiologic strain imposed on the individual depends on the environmental temperature, the level of metabolism, and the resistance to heat flow provided by body fat.
- Cold air is particularly detrimental for some individuals owing to the effect it has on the respiratory tract when inhaled through the mouth.
- Acclimatization at higher altitudes does improve capacity to perform work at higher altitudes, but some of the physiologic changes that occur during prolonged altitude exposure may cause a decrease in performance on return to sea level.
- Carbon monoxide, unlike ozone, may remain in an individual's circulatory system for up to 3 hours after the exposure. Exposure to carbon monoxide may vary from first-hand smoke (smoking a cigarette); to second-hand smoke (being in the environment of a smoker); to inhalation of car exhaust.

- Shin splints develop owing to the excessive eccentric contraction of the anterior tibialis when descending the hills.
- Diabetics who are involved in using the injectable form of insulin (e.g., NPH, lente) require supervision when initiating an exercise program and when altering a program. The amount of insulin injected, the diet consumed, the time of the insulin injection, the peak effect of the insulin, and the site of the injection all must be considered when planning exercise programs for these individuals.
- The possibility of harmful side effects with the use of anabolic steroids includes liver disease, interference with the body's immune system, elevation of low-density lipoprotein cholesterol and total cholesterol, and sterility in both males and females.
- Caffeine consumed 60 minutes before exercise (an amount equivalent to 2.5 cups of coffee or 330 mg) significantly extended endurance in those performing moderately strenuous exercise.
- At some level of oxygen consumption that is unique to each individual and is dependent on their training, genetics, and the like, the threshold of the OBLA occurs.
- In general, approximately 15% of the caloric intake should be in the form of protein, no more than 30% in the form of fat (of which 70% should be unsaturated), and approximately 50% to 60% in the form of carbohydrates, predominantly complex carbohydrates.
- In general, some of the factors that should be considered in exercise prescriptions for older adults include the effects of heat, the intensity of exercise and other parameters of the exercise prescription, and the incidence of musculoskeletal injuries associated with older adults.
- Although both aging and inactivity tend to reduce flexibility and joint range of motion, it appears that inactivity is the dominant factor in the deterioration of flexibility.

References

1. American College of Sports Medicine. Guidelines for Exercise Testing and Prescription. 4th ed. Philadelphia, Lea & Febiger, 1991.
2. Norkin C, LeVingie PK. Joint Structure and Function. Philadelphia, FA Davis, 1992.

3. Magee DJ. Orthopedic Physical Assessment. Philadelphia, WB Saunders, 1992.
4. Salter R. Textbook of Disorders and Injuries of the Musculoskeletal System. 2nd ed. Baltimore, Williams & Wilkins, 1983.
5. Hertling D, Nessler RM. Management of Common Musculoskeletal Disorders. 2nd ed. Philadelphia, JB Lippincott, 1990.
6. Behnke AR, Wilmore JH. Evaluation and Regulation of Body Build and Composition. Englewood Cliffs, NJ, Prentice-Hall, 1974.
7. Lukaski HC. Methods for the assessment of human body composition: Traditional and new. Am J Clin Nutr 46:537–556, 1987.
8. Katch FI. Assessment of lean body tissues by radiography and by bioelectric impedance. In: Roche AS (ed). Body Composition Assessments and Use in Adults. Report of the Sixth Ross Conference on Medical Research. Columbus, Ohio, 1985.
9. Jackson AS, Pollock ML, Graves JE, Mahar M. Comparison of the reliability and validity of total body bioelectrical impedance and anthropometry in determining body composition. J Appl Physiol 62:529–534, 1988.
10. Van Loan M, Mayolin P. Bioelectrical impedance analysis: Is it a reliable estimator of lean body mass and total body water? Hum Biol 59:299–309, 1987.
11. Segal KR, Gutin B, Presta E, et al. Estimation of human body composition by electrical impedance methods: A comparative study. J Appl Physiol 58:1565–1571, 1985.
12. Malina RM. Bioelectric methods for estimating body composition: An overview and discussion. Hum Biol 59:392–435, 1987.
13. Pollock ML, Wilmore JH. Exercise in Health and Disease. 2nd ed. Philadelphia, WB Saunders, 1990.
14. Jackson AS, Pollock ML. Practical assessment of body composition. Physician and Sportsmedicine 13:76–90, 1985.
15. Buskirk ER. Underwater weighing and body density. In: Brozek J, Henschel A (eds). Techniques for Measuring Body Composition. Washington, DC, National Academy of Sciences, 1961, pp 90–105.
16. Centers for Disease Control. Sex, age and region specific prevalence for sedentary lifestyle in selected states in 85—the Behavioral Risk Factor Surveillance System. MWR 36:195–198, 1987.
17. Oldridge NB. Compliance and exercise in primary and secondary prevention of coronary heart disease: A review. Prev Med 11:56–70, 1982.
18. Blair SN, Kohl HW, Paffenbarger RS, et al. Physical fitness and all-cause mortality: A prospective study of healthy men and women. JAMA 262:2395–2401, 1989.
19. DiCarlo LJ, Sparling PB, Millard-Stafford ML, Rupp JC. Peak heart rates during maximal running and swimming: Implications for exercise prescription. Int J Sports Med 12(3):309–312, 1991.
20. Borg GAV. Psychophysical bases of perceived exertion. Med Sci Sports Ex 14:377–381, 1982.
21. Noble BJ. Clinical applications of perceived exertion. Med Sci Sports Exerc 14:406–411, 1982.
22. Pollock ML, Jackson AS, Foster C. The use of the perception scale for exercise prescription. In: Borg G, Ottoson D (eds). The Perception of Exertion in Physical Work. London, The MacMillan Press, 1986.

23. Dishman RK, Holl RG, Schelegle E. Psychometric, perceptual and metabolic predictors of self-limited maximal and submaximal treadmill performance. Med Sci Sports Exerc 17:198, 1985.
24. Centers for Disease Control. Guidelines for fitness—CDC 1985 status of the 1990 physical fitness and exercise objectives. MWR 34:521–524, 529–531.
25. Brooks CM. Leisure time physical activity assessment of American adults through an analysis of time diaries collected in 1981. Am J Public Health 77:455–460, 1987.
26. Brooks CM. Adult participation in physical activities requiring moderate to high levels of energy expenditure. Physician and Sportsmedicine 15:119, 1987.
27. Dishman RK (ed). Exercise Adherence: Its Impact on Public Health. Champaign, Ill, Human Kinetics, 1988.
28. Dishman RK, Sallis JF, Orenstein D. The determinants of physical activity and exercise. Public Health Rep 100:158–171, 1985.
29. Oldridge NB, Donner A, Buck CW, et al. Predictive indices for drop-out: The Ontario Exercise Heart Collaborative Study Experience. Am J Cardiol 51:70–74, 1983.
30. Knapp DN. Behavioral management techniques and exercise promotion. In: Dishman RK (ed). Exercise Adherence: Its Impact on Public Health. Champaign, Ill, Human Kinetics, 1988, pp 203–208.
31. Hemingway A. Shivering. Physiol Rev 43:397, 1963.
32. Gisolfi CV, Copping JR. Thermal effects of prolonged treadmill exercise in the heat. Med Sci Sports 6:108, 1974.
33. DeSouza MJ, Maresh CM, Maguire MS, et al. Menstrual status and plasma vasopressin, renin and aldosterone exercise responses. J Appl Physiol 67:736, 1989.
34. Francesconi RP. Endocrine logical responses to exercise in stressful environments. In: Pandolf KB (ed). Exercise and Sport Sciences Reviews, Vol 16. New York, Macmillan, 1988.
35. Sawka MN, Wegner CB. Physiological responses to acute exercise heat stress. In: Pandolf KB, Sawka MN, Gonzales RR (eds). Human Performance Physiology and Environmental Medicine at Terrestrial Extremes. Indianapolis, Ind, Benchmark Press, 1988.
36. Lockhart RD, Hamilton GF, Fyfe FW. Anatomy of the Human Body. Philadelphia, JB Lippincott, 1974.
37. Irving RA, Noakes TD, Irving GA, et al. The immediate and delayed effects of marathon running on renal function. J Urol 136:1176, 1986.
38. Costill DL, Saltin B. Factors limiting gastric emptying during rest and exercise. J Appl Physiol 37:679, 1974.
39. Costill DL, Coté R, Miller E, et al. Water and electrolyte replacement during repeated days of work in the heat. Aviat Space Environ Med 46:795, 1975.
40. Fordtran JS, Saltin B. Gastric emptying and intestinal absorption during prolonged severe exercise. J Appl Physiol 23:331, 1967.
41. Coyle EF. Gastric emptying rates for selected athletic drinks. Res Q 49:119, 1978.
42. Mitchell JB, Costill DL, Hoummard JA, et al. Effects of carbohydrate ingestion on gastric emptying and exercise performance. Med Sci Sports Exerc 20:110, 1988.
43. Lind AR, Bass DE. Optimal exposure time for development of acclimatization to heat. Fed Proc 22:704, 1963.
44. Taylor HL, Buskirk E, Henschel A. Cardiovascular adjustments of man at rest and work during exposure to dry heat. Am J Physiol 139:583, 1955.

45. Buono MJ, Sjoholm NT. Effect of physical training on peripheral sweat production. J Appl Physiol 65:1984, 1988.

46. Toner MM, Sawka MN, Holden WL, et al. Thermal responses during arm and leg and combined arm-leg exercise in water. J Appl Physiol 56:1355, 1984.

47. Irving L. Adaptations to cold. Sci Am 214(1):94, 1966.

48. LeBlanc J. Factors affecting cold acclimation and thermogenesis in man. Med Sci Sports Exerc 20:S193, 1988.

49. Dempsey JA. Effects of acute through life-long hypoxic exposure on exercise pulmonary gas exchange. Respir Physiol 13:62, 1971.

50. Schoene RB, Lahiri S, Hackett PH, et al. Relationship of hypoxic ventilatory response to exercise performance on Mount Everest. J Appl Physiol 56:1478, 1984.

51. Vogel JA, Hansen JE, Harris CW. Cardiovascular responses in man during exhaustive work at sea level and high altitude. J Appl Physiol 523:531, 1967.

52. Schoene RB. High altitude pulmonary edema: The disguised killer. Physician and Sportsmedicine 16:103, 1988.

53. Hannon JP, Shields JL, Harris CW. Effects of altitude acclimatization on blood composition of women. J Appl Physiol 26:540, 1969.

54. Valdivia E. Total capillary bed in striated muscle of guinea pigs native to Peruvian mountains. Am J Physiol 194:585, 1958.

55. Eaton JW, Brewer GJ, Grover RF, et al. Role of red cell 2,3 diphosphoglycerate (DPG) in adaptation of men to altitude. J Lab Clin Med 73:603, 1969.

56. Faulkner JA, Kollias J, Favour C, et al. Maximum aerobic capacity and running performance at altitude. J Appl Physiol 24:658, 1968.

57. Claremont AD, Costill AD, Fink W, Van Handel P. Heat tolerance following diuretic induced dehydration. Med Sci Sports 8(4):239–243, 1976.

58. American College of Sports Medicine. The use of anabolic-androgenic steroids in sports. Sports Med Bull 19:13, 1984.

59. Rogozkin V. Metabolic effects of anabolic steroids on skeletal muscle. Med Sci Sports 11:160, 1979.

60. Hervey GR, Knibbs AV, Burkinshaw L, et al. Effects of methandienone on the performance and body composition of men undergoing athletic training. Clin Sci 60:457, 1981.

61. Wilson JD. Androgen abuse by athletes. Endocr Rev 9:181, 1988.

62. Alén M, Reinilä M, Vihko R. Response of serum hormones to androgen administration in power athletes. Med Sci Sports Exerc 17:354, 1985.

63. Calabrese LH, Kleiner SM, Barna BP, et al. The effects of anabolic steroids and strength training on the human immune response. Med Sci Sports Exerc 21:386, 1989.

64. Johnson FL. The association of oral androgenic steroids and life-threatening disease. Med Sci Sports 7:285, 1975.

65. Hurley BF, Seals DR, Hagberg JM, et al. High density lipoprotein cholesterol in body builders vs. power lifters. Negative effects of androgen use. JAMA 252:4, 1984.

66. Kantor MA, Binchini A, Bernier D, et al. Androgens reduce HDL-26 cholesterol and increase hepatic triglyceride lipase activity. Med Sci Sports Exerc 17(4):462, 1985.

67. Rogol AD. Growth hormone: Physiology, therapeutic use, and potential for abuse. In: Exercise and Sport Sciences Review. Vol 17. New York, Macmillan, 1989.

68. Chandler JV, Blair SN. The effect of amphetamines on selected physiological components related to athletic success. Med Sci Sports 12:65, 1980.

69. Duthel JM, Vallon JJ, Martin G, et al. Caffeine and sport: Role of physical exercise upon elimination. Med Sci Sports Exerc 23:980–984, 1991.

70. Costill DL, Dalsky GP, Fink WJ. Effects of caffeine ingestion on metabolism and exercise performance. Med Sci Sports 10:155, 1978.

71. Doubt TJ, Hsieh SS. Additive effects of caffeine and cold water during submaximal leg exercise. Med Sci Sports Exerc 23:435–441, 1991.

72. LeBlanc J, Jobin M, Côté J, et al. Enhanced metabolic response to caffeine in exercise trained human subjects. J Appl Physiol 59:832, 1985.

73. Lopes JM, Aubier M, Jardim J, et al. Effect of caffeine on skeletal muscle function before and after fatigue. J Appl Physiol 54:1303, 1983.

74. Estler J, Ammon HPT, Herzog C. Swimming capacity of mice after prolonged treatment with psychostimulants. Psychopharmacology 58:161–166, 1978.

75. Jung RT, Shetty, James WPT, et al. Caffeine: Its effect on catecholamines and metabolism in lean and obese humans. Clin Sci 60:527–535, 1981.

76. Williams PT, Wood PD, Vranizan KM, et al. Coffee intake and elevated cholesterol and apoliproprotein B levels in men. JAMA 253:1407, 1985.

77. Gledhill N. Blood doping and related issues: A brief review. Med Sci Sports Exerc 14:183, 1982.

78. Sawka MN, Dennis RC, Gonzalez RR, et al. Influence of polycythemia on blood volume and thermoregulation during exercise heat stress. J Appl Physiol 62:912, 1987.

79. Sawka MN, Gonzalez RR, Young AJ, et al. Polycythemia and hydration: Effects on thermoregulation on blood volume during exercise-heat stress. Am J Physiol 255:456, 1988.

80. McArdle WD, Katch FI, Katch VL. Exercise Physiology: Energy Nutrition and Human Performance. Philadelphia, Lea & Febiger, 1991.

81. Sherman WM, Costill DL, Fink WJ, et al. Effect of exercise-diet manipulation on muscle glycogen and its subsequent utilization during performance. Int J Sports Med 2(2):114, 1981.

82. Thornton JS. Carboloading and endurance: A new look. Physician and Sportsmedicine 17(10):149, 1989.

83. Pavlou KN, Steffee WP, Lerman RH, Burrows BA. Effects of dieting and exercise on lean body mass, oxygen uptake and strength. Med Sci Sports Exerc 17(4):466, 1985.

84. Jones N, Ehrsam RE. The anaerobic threshold. In: Terjung R (ed). Exercise and Sports Sciences Reviews 10:49, 1982.

85. Yeh MP, Gardner M, Adams TD, et al. Anaerobic threshold: Problems of determination and validation. J Appl Physiol 55:1178, 1983.

86. Brooks GA, Brauner KE, Cassens RG. Glycogen synthesis and metabolism of lactic acid after exercise. Am J Physiol 224:1162, 1973.

87. Denis C, Fouquer R, Poty P, et al. Effect of 40 weeks of endurance training on anaerobic threshold. Int J Sports Med 3:208, 1982.

88. Fay L, Londeree BR, Lafontaine TP, et al. Physiological

parameters related to distance running performance in female athletes. Med Sci Sports Exerc 21:319, 1989.

89. Kumagi S, Tanaka K, Matsoura Y, et al. Relationship of the anaerobic threshold with the 5 km, 10 km, and 10 mile races. Eur J Appl Physiol 49:13, 1982.

90. Heyden S, Fodor GJ. Does regular exercise prolong life expectancy? Sports Med 6:63–71, 1988.

91. Paffenbarger RS Jr, Hyde RT, Wing AL, et al. Physical activity, all-cause mortality and longevity of college alumni. N Engl J Med 314:605, 1986.

92. Leon AS, Connett J, Jacobs DR, Rauramas R. Leisure-time physical activity levels and risk of coronary heart disease and death. JAMA 258:2388–2395, 1987.

93. Powell KE, Thompson PD, Caspersen CJ, et al. Physical activity and the incidence of coronary heart disease. Annu Rev Public Health 8:253, 1987.

94. Upton SJ, Hagan RD, Lease B, et al. Comparative physiological profiles among young and middle-aged female distance runners. Med Sci Sports Exerc 16:67, 1984.

95. Tankersley CG, Smolander J, Kenney WL, Fortney SM. Sweating and skin blood flow during exercise: Effects of age and maximal oxygen uptake. J Appl Physiol 71(1):236–242, 1991.

96. Menard D. The aging athlete. Topics in Geriatric Rehabilitation 6(4):1–16, 1991.

97. Alnaqeeb MA, Alzrid NS, Eoldspink E. Connective tissue changes and physical properties of developing and aging skeletal muscle. J Anat 139:677–689, 1984.

98. Peel C. Cardiopulmonary changes with aging. In: Irwin S, Techlin J (eds). Cardiopulmonary Physical Therapy. St. Louis, CV Mosby, 1990.

99. Canada Fitness Survey. Fitness and aging. Ottawa: Fitness Canada, Government of Canada, 1983.

100. Landin RJ, Linnemeier TJ, Rothbaum DA. Exercise testing and training of the elderly patient. In: Wenger NK (ed). Exercise and the Heart. 2nd ed. Philadelphia, FA Davis, 1985.

101. Skinner JS. Importance of aging for exercise testing and exercise prescription. In: Skinner JS (ed). Exercise Testing and Exercise Prescription for Special Cases. Philadelphia, Lea & Febiger, 1987.

102. Eaglestein WH. Wound healing and aging. Clin Geriatr Med 5:183–188, 1989.

103. Matheson GO, Macintyre JG, Taunton JE, et al. Musculoskeletal injuries associated with physical activity in older adults. Med Sci Sports Exerc 221(4):379, 1989.

104. Puranen J, Ala-Ketola L, Peltokallio P, Saarela J. Running and primary osteoarthritis of the hip. Br Med J 424–425, 1975.

Additional Readings

Morgan WP, Goldston SE. Exercise and Mental Health. Washington, DC, Hemisphere Publishing Co, 1987.

Pelletier KR. Healthy People in Unhealthy Places: Stress and Fitness at Work. New York, Delacorte Press, 1984.

Diamont L. Psychology of Sports, Exercise and Fitness: Social and Personal Issues. Washington, DC, Hemisphere Publishing Co, 1991.

GLOSSARY

a wave
the rise in the atrial pressure curve caused by the contraction of the atria during atrial systole

accessory atrioventricular tracts or bundles
the fine terminal branches of the internodal tracts that are postulated to "bypass" the atrioventricular node; their existence and function is controversial

acebutolol (Sectral, Monitan, Prent, Neptall)
a beta-adrenoceptor blocking agent

acellular hyaline membrane
a layer of nearly translucent material (formerly eosinophilic) that lines the bronchioles, alveolar ducts, and alveoli of premature infants with respiratory distress

acetylcholine
an acetic acid ester of choline; it is liberated from the preganglionic and postganglionic endings of parasympathetic fibers and from the preganglionic endings of the sympathetic fibers where it acts as a transmitter on the effector organ; causes cardiac inhibition, vasodilation, gastrointestinal peristalsis, and other parasympathetic effects

acetylcholinesterase
an enzyme that catalyzes the hydrolysis of acetylcholine to form acetic acid and choline

acidemia
a condition of increased hydrogen ion concentration (decreased pH) in the blood

acidosis
a pathologic condition arising from the accumulation of acid in (or loss of base from) the body

acromegaly
an enlargement of the head, face, hands, feet, and internal organs that results from the hypersecretion of growth hormone from an abnormal pituitary gland after maturity

action potential
the rapid sequence of changes in electrical potential that takes place across a cell membrane during depolarization and repolarization

activation gate
the manner in which flux is controlled through an ionic channel in a cell membrane; as the membrane potential becomes less negative, this "gate" opens, allowing ions to pass along the channel

active transport
the utilization of energy to move ions against an electrochemical gradient

acute respiratory acidosis
a pathologic condition typified by a lower than normal pH and a higher than normal Pa_{CO_2}

acute ventilatory failure
a pathologic condition typified by a pH below 7.30 and a Pa_{CO_2} greater than 50 mm Hg

acyclovir (Zovirax)
an antiviral agent that is effective against herpes virus infections

adenosine triphosphate (ATP)
a nucleotide composed of a nitrogenous base, *adenine*; a pentose sugar, *ribose*; and three *phosphate radicals*. The last two phosphate radicals are bound to the main portion of the molecule by so-called *high-energy phosphate bonds*, which may be broken easily to release energy for bodily needs

adenylate cyclase
one of the many catalytic units within a cell that may be activated by G proteins when a receptor site is stimulated; adenylate cyclase catalyzes the conversion of adenosine triphosphate (ATP) to cyclic adenosine monophosphate (cAMP)

adipocytes
fat cells

adipose
of or related to fat

adrenergic
nerve fibers of the sympathetic division of the autonomic nervous system that secrete norepinephrine

adrenoceptors
the sites on an effector organ innervated by postganglionic adrenergic fibers of the sympathetic division of the autonomic nervous system

advanced cardiac life support (ACLS)
the electrical, pharmacologic, vascular and airway access techniques used to resuscitate or sustain life in addition to those associated with the basic life support measures of cardiopulmonary resuscitation

adventitia
the outermost layer of connective tissue of an artery or vein; tunica adventitia

adventitious breath sounds
abnormal sounds heard during auscultation of the lung fields

aerosol
liquid or solid particles suspended in a gas

aerosol mask
a device used to facilitate the delivery of an aerosol to a patient

afterload
the force against which the muscular wall of the ventricle exerts its contraction

agenesis
an abnormal development or absence of a part

agonist
a drug that interacts with receptors to initiate a response

airway reactivity
the alteration in bronchomotor tone in response to noxious stimuli

airway resistance (Raw)
the force opposing the flow of gases during ventilation; results from obstruction or turbulent flow in the upper and lower airways

albumin
one of the most common plasma proteins

alcoholic cardiomyopathy
cardiac muscle disease that is associated with chronic alcohol abuse

aldosterone
a steroid hormone produced in the adrenal cortex; it causes resorption of sodium and excretion of hydrogen and potassium in the distal renal tubules

aldosteronism
an intrinsic disorder of the adrenal cortex that results in the excessive secretion of aldosterone

alkalemia
an increase in the pH of the blood; a decrease in the hydrogen ion concentration of the blood

alkalosis
a pathologic condition arising from the accumulation of base in (or loss of acid from) the body

alkalotic
referring to the condition of alkalosis

allergic angiitis
an inflammation of the small (dermal) blood vessels with polymorphonuclear infiltrate; cutaneous vasculitis

alpha-adrenergic receptor
a subclass of neuroreceptor located at the norepinephrine synapses of the sympathetic (adrenergic) division of the autonomic nervous system; further divided into alpha$_1$ and alpha$_2$ categories

alpha₁-acid-glycoprotein
a subgroup of the α_1-globulin fraction of blood; one of the most common plasma proteins

alpha₁-antitrypsin deficiency
a genetically determined (autosomal recessive) disorder in which the glycoprotein alpha₁-antitrypsin (the major protease inhibitor of human serum) is deficient; persons with the disorder are predisposed to juvenile hepatic cirrhosis and pulmonary emphysema

alpha₁ (α_1) receptor
alpha-adrenergic neuroreceptors that are located primarily in the vascular and intestinal smooth muscle, where they elicit contraction or relaxation, respectively

alpha₂ (α_2) receptor
alpha-adrenergic neuroreceptors that are located primarily on the presynaptic terminals of certain adrenergic receptors, where they elicit a reduction in norepinephrine release; postsynaptically on fat cells, where they decrease lipolysis; and postsynaptically on certain central nervous system adrenergic receptors, where they elicit a reduction in sympathetic output from the brain stem

alpha sympatholytic
a drug that inhibits alpha-adrenergic receptors of the autonomic nervous system

alteplase recombinant tPA
a tissue plasminogen activator (tPA; Activase)

alveolar-arterial defects
an imperfection or absence of the alveolar arterial blood supply

alveolar ducts
the part of the respiratory passages that connects the respiratory bronchioles and the alveolar sacs

alveolar hemorrhage
the escape of blood through pulmonary blood vessels into the alveolar spaces

alveolar hyperventilation
increased alveolar ventilation to the extent that arterial carbon dioxide levels are decreased below normal; Pa_{CO_2} less than 30 mm Hg; respiratory alkalemia

alveolar pattern
one of two main roentgenographic patterns; radiopaque confluent densities that may have a localized, diffuse, or centralized distribution depending on the disease process; likened to "fluffy clouds"

alveolar sacs
the terminal dilation of the alveolar ducts

alveolar surfaces
the combined area of the alveoli

alveolar ventilation
the alveolar gas flow

alveolitis
inflammation of the alveoli

alveolus
one of the terminal saclike dilations of the alveolar ducts in the lungs

amantadine (Symadine, Symmetrel)
an antiviral agent; used in the prevention and treatment of influenza A infection (also used in the treatment of parkinsonism)

amenorrhea
the absence of menstruation

amiodarone (Cordarone)
a coronary vasodilator used in the treatment of symptomatic supraventricular and ventricular arrhythmias

amrinone (Inocor)
an inotropic agent with vasodilator action; used in the treatment of congestive heart failure

amyotrophic lateral sclerosis (ALS)
a disease of the motor tracts of the lateral columns and anterior horns of the spinal cord; associated with progressive muscular atrophy and fibrillation and hyperreflexia

anaerobic threshold (AT)
the limit of the ability of the blood to buffer the by-products of anaerobiosis (e.g., lactic acid); the onset of plasma lactate accumulation (OPLA); an indirect measure of an individual's endurance

analeptic
a central nervous system stimulant; used in the treatment of depressed central nervous system function

anatomic dead space volume
the volume of gas that occupies the nonrespiratory conducting airways

anemia
a condition in which the number of red blood cells per cubic millimeter or the volume of packed red blood cells per 100 milliliters of blood is less than normal (also when the amount of hemoglobin per 100 milliliters of blood is less than normal)

aneurysm
a circumscribed dilation, especially of an artery or a chamber of the heart

angina
angina pectoris

angina pectoris
severe constricting pain in the chest, often radiating from the precordium to the left shoulder and down the arm, due to ischemia of the heart muscle, which is usually caused by coronary disease

angioblastic tissue
the primordial mesenchymal tissue that develops into embryonic blood cells and vascular endothelium

angiotensin converting enzyme (ACE)
a dipeptidyl-carboxypeptidase that splits off histidyl-leucine from angiotensin I to form angiotensin II; located in endothelial cells; most of the conversion occurs as blood passes through the lungs

ACE inhibitors
a group of antihypertensive drugs that works by inhibiting the action of angiotensin converting enzyme, thus blocking the conversion of angiotensin I to angiotensin II

angiotensin I
a decapeptide formed by the splitting of the tetradecapeptide angiotensinogen in the presence of renin; physiologically inactive

angiotensin II
a potent vasopressor; an octapeptide formed by the splitting off of histidyl-leucine from angiotensin I, it is the greatest stimulus to the adrenal gland for the production and release of aldosterone

angiotensinogen
a tetradecapeptide formed by the liver (formerly considered to be a portion of the α_2-globulin fraction of the proteins in the circulating plasma) that is converted to angiotensin I by renin

anisoylated plasminogen streptokinase activator complex (ASPAC, Eminase)
a form of streptokinase to which a methoxybenzene has been added

ankylosing spondylitis
arthritis of the spine, progressing to bony fixation with lipping of the vertebral margins; Marie-Strümpell disease

anorexia nervosa
a psychological disorder in which an individual exhibits an aversion to food owing to an extreme fear of becoming obese

antagonist
a drug that interacts with receptors to block or inhibit a response

anterior basal segmental bronchus
the portion of the tracheobronchial tree arising from the right lower lobe bronchus that is distributed to the anterior basal segment

anterior cardiac veins
three or four small veins receiving blood from the right ventricle

anterior interventricular artery
the anterior interventricular branch of the left coronary artery; left anterior descending artery

anterior interventricular sulcus
a groove on the anterosuperior surface of the heart that marks the location of the interventricular septum

anterior leaflet of the mitral valve
the larger of the two cusps of the mitral valve; it has no basal zone; also called the anteromedial, aortic, or septal leaflet

anterior papillary muscles
arise from the inferior border of the moderator band in the right ventricle and from the sternocostal wall of the left ventricle

anterior pulmonary plexus
a network of nerves formed by branches of the vagus nerves and the deep cardiac plexus supplying anterior branches of the bronchi and the pulmonary and bronchial vessels

anterior segmental bronchus
the portion of the tracheobronchial tree arising from the right or left upper lobe bronchus that is distributed to the anterior segment

anterolateral thoracotomy
an incision into the anterolateral aspect of the chest wall

anteromedial basal segmental bronchus
the portion of the tracheobronchial tree arising from the left lower lobe bronchus that is distributed to the anteromedial basal segment

anteroposterior (AP) view
describes the direction of the roentgen ray beam through the patient from anterior to posterior

anthracycline
an antineoplastic agent; a glycoside antibiotic used in the treatment of solid tumors (e.g., breast, ovarian, small cell bronchogenic cancers), it is believed to intercalate between the base pairs of DNA, thus inhibiting its synthesis; cardiac cells are especially sensitive to the chemotoxic effects of anthracycline glycosides

anthracycline toxicity
refers to the two types of cardiotoxicity generally associated with anthracycline: an acute, transient type characterized by abnormal ECG findings (e.g., ST and T wave changes, tachy arrhythmias);

and a chronic, cumulative, dose-dependent type characterized by congestive heart failure and cardiorespiratory decompensation

antibiotic
a substance that inhibits the growth of a microorganism; derived from a mold or bacterium

antibody
a class of immunoglobulins that results from an antigenic stimulus

anticholinesterase
a drug that inhibits or inactivates acetylcholinesterase

anticoagulant
an agent that prevents coagulation

antidiuretic hormone (ADH)
a nonpeptide hormone that causes contraction of vascular smooth muscle; vasopressin

antigen
any substance capable of causing the production of antibodies

antigen-antibody reaction
the combination of an antibody with an antigen of the type that initially stimulated the formation of the antibody, causing the agglutination, precipitation, fixation, or phagocytosis of the antigen

antihistamine
a drug that inhibits the action of histamine

antilymphocyte globulin (ALG)
an immunosuppressant; used to suppress the cell-mediated immune response to transplanted tissue (e.g., liver, heart)

antimicrobial
a substance that destroys or prevents the development or action of microbes

antithymocyte globulin (ATG)
an immunosuppressant; used to suppress the cell-mediated immune response to transplanted tissue (e.g., liver, heart)

antitussive
a drug that relieves coughing

aorta
the main trunk of the systemic arterial system arising from the left ventricle

aortic aneurysm
a circumscribed dilation of the aorta

aortic area (space)
the region of the chest (second intercostal space along the right sternal border) where the normal and pathologic sounds made by the aortic valve are traditionally said to be best appreciated

aortic sinuses
three dilations above the attached mar-

gins of the cusps of the aortic valve at the root of the aorta

aortic stenosis
a pathologic narrowing of the orifice of the aortic valve

aortic vestibule
the portion of the left ventricle immediately below the aortic orifice

aorticopulmonary septum
the spiral septum formed from the bulbar and truncal ridges that separates the bulbus cordis and the truncus arteriosus into a ventral pulmonary trunk and dorsal aorta

apex of the heart
the conical extremity of the heart formed by the left ventricle

APGAR score
numerical scale (0 to 2) assigned to each of five criteria (heart rate, respiratory effort, muscle tone, response to stimulation, and skin color); used in assessment of the status of newborn infants at 1 and 5 minutes following birth

apical segmental bronchus
the portion of the tracheobronchial tree arising from the right upper lobe bronchus that is distributed to the apical segment

apicoposterior segmental bronchus
the portion of the tracheobronchial tree arising from the left upper lobe bronchus that is distributed to the apicoposterior segment ·

aplasia
abnormal development or congenital absence of an organ or tissue

aplastic anemia
a condition of less than the normal amount of erythrocytes and hemoglobin as a result of defective bone marrow; usually associated with granulocytopenia and thrombocytopenia

Arantius's nodules
nodular, fibrous thickenings at the midpoints of the free edges of the semilunar cusps of the aortic valve

arch of the aorta
the curved portion of the aorta between the ascending and descending portions of the aorta

arm ergometry
upper extremity exercise performed on a crank dynamometer

arrhythmogenic
capable of producing cardiac arrhythmias

arterial catheter
a hollow, tubular device placed intra-arterially to allow the passage of fluid into or out of the artery

arteries
blood vessels conveying blood in a direction away from the heart

arterioles
a minute artery with a muscular wall; a terminal artery continuous with the capillary networks

aryepiglottic folds
the posterior boundary of the laryngeal inlet formed by the ligamentous and muscular fibers between the epiglottis and arytenoid apex

ascending aorta
the first part of the aorta between its origin from the heart and the arch of the aorta

aspartate aminotransferase (AST)
an enzyme released into the blood as the result of myocardial injury; formerly serum glutamic-oxaloacetic transaminase (SGOT)

asphyxia
impaired or absent oxygen and carbon dioxide exchange

aspiration pneumonia
inflammation of the lung parenchyma resulting from the entrance of oral or gastric contents into the bronchi congenital absence of the spleen

asplenia
congenital absence of the spleen

assist-control mode
a method of mechanical ventilatory assistance in which a set volume of gas is delivered each time the inspiratory phase is triggered

asthma
bronchoconstriction, mucosal edema, and mucous plugging of the airways in response to some noxious stimulus

Åstrand exercise protocol
a graded exercise test protocol for treadmill or bicycle ergometers; treadmill: constant 5 mph speed; after 3 minutes at 0% grade, the grade is increased 2.5% every 2 minutes; bicycle: constant 50 or 60 rpm, after 3 minutes at 0 W resistance, the resistance is increased by 25 W every 2 minutes

atelectasis
the absence of gas in part or all of a lung

atelectatic
relating to atelectasis

atenolol (Tenormin)
a beta-adrenergic blocking agent

atherosclerotic heart disease
the blockage of coronary blood vessels owing to the formation of atherosclerotic plaque

atherosclerotic occlusive disease
the blockage of blood vessels as the result of atherosclerotic plaque formation

atherosis
lipid deposits in the intima of arteries that produce a yellow swelling on the endothelial surface

atria
a chamber or cavity to which are connected several chambers or passageways

atrial fibrillation
rapid twitching of the atrial walls

atrial flutter
rapid atrial contraction, usually at rates between 250 and 400 per minute

atrial gallop
the triple cadence of heart sounds heard by auscultation and characterized by an audible sound (fourth heart sound) occurring in late diastole in addition to the normal first and second heart sounds; presystolic gallop

atrial kick
the increased ventricular stroke volume resulting from the priming force of atrial contraction immediately before ventricular contraction

atrial septal defect (ASD)
opening in the septum between the two atria as the result of a failure of the septum primum or secundum to close normally during development

atrial tachycardia
depolarization of the atria at a rate in excess of 100 per minute

atrioventricular canals
the left and right halves of the atrioventricular canal of the heart tube; formed by the union of the dorsal and ventral endocardial cushions

atrioventricular nodal artery
a branch of the right coronary artery proximal to the posterior interventricular artery that supplies the atrioventricular node in 80% of hearts

atrioventricular (AV) node
an accumulation of specialized myocytes located near the ostium of the coronary sinus

atrium
the division of the heart tube between the ventricle and the sinus venosus

atypical chest pain
angina that does not conform to the typical or normal form

auscultatory gap
the fading away, and the reappearance at a lower point, of the sounds that indicate systolic blood pressure; in hy-

pertensive patients this may lead to the recording of falsely low (as much as 25 mm Hg) systolic blood pressure values (it may be avoided by pumping the sphygmomanometer 30 mm Hg beyond palpable systolic pressure)

autacoid
hormone; an obsolete term

autoantibody response
the formation of antibodies in response to antigenic constituents of one's own tissue

autogenic relaxation
self-directed lessening of tension

autoimmunity
a condition in which one's own tissues are the object of the immune system

automaticity
a cell's ability to initiate its own depolarization

autonomic dysreflexia (hyperreflexia)
exaggerated autonomic nervous system responses

autonomic nervous system
comprises all the afferent and efferent nerves through which the viscera is innervated

autonomic neuropathy
any disease that affects the autonomic nervous system

autosomal dominant trait
any genetic characteristic transmitted to the exclusion of a contrasting allele

axillary-femoral bypass
a surgical procedure that circumvents flow-limiting stenoses or occlusions of the infrarenal aorta and iliac arteries by creating a tunnel from the axillary artery, beneath the pectoralis major, into the subcutaneous tissue of the lateral chest wall, passing medial to the anterior superior iliac spine to reach the ipsilateral femoral artery; axillofemoral bypass

axillary thoracotomy
an incision into the chest wall in the region of the axilla

azathioprine (Imuran)
an immunosuppressive agent used in organ transplantation; a cytotoxic agent used in the treatment of autoimmune hemolytic anemias, systemic lupus erythematosus, and rheumatoid arthritis

azotemia
retention of nitrogen as the result of some process other than renal failure

Bachmann's bundle
the portion of the specialized conduction system of the heart that is a con-

tinuation of the right atrial anterior internodal tract into the left atrium

bactericidal
having the ability to cause the death of bacteria

bacteriostatic
having the ability to inhibit or retard the growth of bacteria

Bainbridge's reflex
an atrial stretch reflex that causes changes in heart rate; it is elicited when the right atrial pressure rises sufficiently to distend the right atrium

Balke exercise protocol
a graded treadmill exercise test protocol consisting of stages of variable (tester choice) duration with incremental speed and grade change at each stage

baroreceptors
sensory nerve endings in the walls of the auricles of the heart, vena cavae, aortic arch, and carotid sinuses that are sensitive to stretch (resulting from increased pressure from within)

barotrauma
injury caused by too much or too little pressure

basal cells
undifferentiated cells in parts of the airway lined by pseudostratified epithelium; basal cells mature to replace other epithelial types

basal chordae
chordae tendineae that arise directly from the ventricular wall to attach to the basal regions of the leaflets of the valves of the heart

base excess (BE)
a measure of the metabolic acid-base status; if a positive value, a measure of metabolic alkalosis; if a negative value (base deficit), a measure of metabolic acidosis; the amount of acid or alkali that would have to be added per unit volume of whole blood (at 37 degrees C and at a partial pressure for CO_2 of 40 mm Hg) to achieve a pH of 7.40

base of the heart
that portion of the heart bounded by the bifurcation of the pulmonary trunk superiorly, the coronary sulcus inferiorly, the sulcus terminalis on the right, and the oblique vein of the left atrium on the left

basic cardiac life support (BCLS)
the emergency procedures of establishing an airway, providing breathing, and performing cardiac compressions as needed; cardiopulmonary resuscitation (CPR)

behavior specialist
a member of a multidisciplinary cardiac or pulmonary rehabilitation team; a mental health professional (e.g., social worker, psychologist)

beriberi
a specific type of polyneuropathy resulting principally from a vitamin B_1 deficiency

beta-adrenergic blocker
any substance that results in the selective inhibition of the responses of effector cells to beta-adrenergic stimuli

beta-adrenergic receptor
a specific subclass of neuroreceptor located at the norepinephrine synapses of the sympathetic (adrenergic) division of the autonomic nervous system; further divided into beta$_1$ and beta$_2$ categories

beta blockade
selective inhibition of the responses of effector cells to beta-adrenergic stimuli

beta$_1$ (β_1) receptor
distributed predominantly in cardiac smooth muscle (where they increase heart rate and contractility), kidney (where they increase renin secretion), and fat cells (where they increase lipolysis)

beta$_2$ (β_2) receptor
distributed predominantly in bronchiolar smooth muscle (where they elicit bronchodilation), peripheral and hepatic vascular smooth muscle (where they cause vasodilation), gastrointestinal smooth muscle (where they decrease motility), and skeletal muscle and liver cells (where they cause increased cellular metabolism)

bigeminal
paired; especially, the occurrence of heart beats in pairs

bioavailability
the physiologic availability of a particular amount of a drug

bioelectrical impedance
the estimation of body composition or changes in volume by measuring the resistance to the flow of electrons (electrical impedance) between two electrodes placed on distant parts of the body

bipolar pacing system
a type of cardiac pacemaker that employs electrodes that have two poles

biventricular hypertrophy
thickening of the walls of both ventricles of the heart in response to an obstructed outflow

bleb
a sac containing fluid or gas; refers to

the coalescent alveolar sacs formed from the destruction of alveolar septa as the result of pulmonary disease (e.g., emphysema)

blood islands
clusters of mesodermal cells on the outer surface of the yolk sac that differentiate into the first blood cells

blood urea nitrogen (BUN)
the most prevalent nonprotein nitrogenous compound in the blood; normally about 10 to 15 mg of urea per 100 ml of blood

blunted heart rate response
a less than anticipated heart rate for the amount of work being performed

body of the sternum
the middle segment of the sternum

body plethysmography
the measurement and recording of changes in volume (usually lung volumes) obtained by placing the body in a chamber that surrounds it completely

Borg scale
a numerical scale for the rating of perceived exertion

brachiocephalic trunk
the largest branch of the arch of the aorta; innominate artery; gives off the right common carotid and right subclavian arteries

bradycardia
heart rate of less than 60 beats per minute

bretylium tosylate (Bretylol)
a sympatholytic agent that inhibits the release of norepinephrine from nerve endings

bronchial breath sounds
the sounds normally heard over the large bronchi on auscultation of the chest; the inspiration to expiration ratio is typically 1 to 1; an abnormal sound when heard over the peripheral lung tissue

bronchial buds
outgrowths of the primordial bronchus of the fetus from which the bronchi and lungs eventually form

bronchial drainage
the removal of fluids (e.g., secretions) from the bronchi; postural drainage

bronchial glands
mucous and seromucous glands, the secretory units of which lie outside the muscular layer of the bronchi

bronchiectasis
dilation of the bronchial and bronchiolar walls as the result of chronic inflammation or obstruction

bronchioles
a subdivision of the bronchi that are less than 1 millimeter in diameter and have no cartilage in their walls

bronchiolitis
an inflammation of the bronchioles

bronchoconstriction
a reduction in the luminal caliber of a bronchus or bronchi

bronchogenic carcinoma
squamous or oat cell cancer arising in the mucosa of the bronchi

bronchogram
the radiographic image obtained following the injection of a radiopaque material into the tracheobronchial tree

bronchography
the radiographic examination of the tracheobronchial tree after the injection of a radiopaque material

bronchophony
the increased intensity and clarity of vocal sounds heard over a region of consolidated lung tissue

bronchopneumonia
acute inflammation of the walls of the small bronchi and bronchioles

bronchopulmonary dysplasia (BPD)
chronic pulmonary insufficiency associated with long-term positive-pressure mechanical ventilatory support, especially in premature infants

bronchopulmonary segments
the largest subdivisions of a lobe of the lung; each is fed by a direct branch from a lobar bronchus

bronchospasm
involuntary contraction of the smooth muscle of the bronchi and bronchioles

bronchovesicular breath sounds
a mixture of bronchial and vesicular breath sounds normally heard in the region of the mainstem bronchi (anteriorly, in the first and second intercostal spaces; posteriorly, between the scapulae); the duration of the inspiratory and expiratory phases is about equal

Bruce exercise test protocol
a graded treadmill exercise test protocol consisting of stages of 3-minutes duration with incremental speed (1.7, 2.5, 3.4, 4.3, 5.0, 5.5, 6.0, 6.5 mph) and grade (2%) change at each stage

brush cells
nonciliated epithelial cells in the trachea that have a distinct luminal border of microvilli; probably play a role in absorption

buccal
adjacent to the cheek (wall)

bulbar
relating to the hindbrain (rhombencephalon)

bulbar ridges
the spiral epithelial outgrowths from the walls of the bulbus cordis that combine with the truncal ridges to form the aorticopulmonary septum

bulbous cordis
the division of the heart tube between the truncus arteriosus and the ventricle

bulboventricular loop
the bend formed in the developing heart tube as its length increases more rapidly than that of the surrounding pericardium

bulimia nervosa
a chronic disorder characterized by repeated bouts of eating, followed by self-induced vomiting and anorexia

bullous emphysema
the destruction of alveolar septa and the reduction in the number of alveoli, creating thin-walled cavities (bullae)

cachectic
relating to cachexia

cachexia
weight loss and wasting as the result of a chronic disease or an emotional disturbance

calcium pump
a biologic mechanism that uses energy from ATP to actively transport calcium across the cell membrane

capacitance vessels
the large venules and veins that form a large, variable-volume, and low-pressure reservoir

capillaries
the smallest vessels at the junction of the arteriole with the venous vascular beds; resembling a hair; fine; minute; a capillary vessel

capillary stasis
stagnation of blood in the capillaries

captopril (Capoten)
an antihypertensive agent; an angiotension converting enzyme inhibitor

carbonaceous
containing or composed of carbon

carbonic anhydrase
an enzyme in red blood cells that catalyzes the conversion of carbon dioxide into carbonic acid or vice versa

carboxyhemoglobin
the result of the union of carbon monoxide with hemoglobin

cardiac cirrhosis
the fibrotic reaction that occurs within

the liver as the result of prolonged congestive heart failure

cardiac cycle
the period from the beginning of one heart beat to the beginning of the next

cardiac impression
the indentations on the inner surfaces of the lungs that outline the contact areas of the heart

cardiac index
a relative measure of cardiac output based on body size; expressed in terms of liters per square meter per unit of time

cardiac jelly
the noncellular material between the endothelial lining and the myocardial layer of the early embryonic heart

cardiac muscle dysfunction (CMD)
a term that has gained popularity in describing an apparently common finding in patients with heart and lung disease

cardiac notch
a roughly V-shaped depression in the anterior border of the left lung at the level of the fourth costal cartilage

cardiac output
the amount of blood ejected into the aorta each minute

cardiac plexus
the anastomosing network of sympathetic and parasympathetic (vagus) nerves that surround the arch of the aorta and the pulmonary artery before continuing to the atria, ventricles, and coronary vessels

cardiac rehabilitation
a multidisciplinary program designed to assist patients with cardiac disease to achieve their optimal physiologic, psychological, and functional status through the use of education and exercise

cardiac rehabilitation center
a facility in which cardiac rehabilitation is conducted

cardiac silhouette
the outline of the heart seen on a radiographic image of the chest

cardiac tamponade
compression of the heart resulting from accumulation of fluid within the pericardial sac

cardiogenic
of cardiac origin

cardiogenic area
the region of the coelom of the presomite embryo in which mesenchymal cells begin to migrate and proliferate

between the layers of the splanchnic mesoderm and endoderm

cardiogenic cords
strands of mesenchymal cells that develop in the cardiogenic area of the presomite embryo

cardiogenic shock
a condition arising when the blood supply to the body tissues is insufficient because of inadequate cardiac output

cardiomyopathy
any disease of the myocardium; a classification of diseases of the myocardium that have no known underlying etiology

cardiothymic silhouette
the line of demarcation between the thymus gland and the heart in the superior mediastinum; sometimes visible in radiographic images of the chest

cardiotoxic
having a deleterious or detrimental effect on the action of the heart

cardioversion
the restoration of the normal rhythm of the heart by electrical countershock

carina
the ridge separating the openings of the right and left main bronchi at their junction with the trachea

carotid endarterectomy
the excision of occluding material (e.g., thrombus) from the carotid artery

carotid massage
the manual rhythmic compression of the carotid sinuses at the bifurcation of the common into the internal and external carotid arteries in an effort to slow the heart rate

carotid sinuses
slight dilations of the common carotid arteries at their bifurcation into the internal and external carotid arteries that contain baroreceptors; cause slowing of the heart rate, vasodilation, and reduction of blood pressure

catecholamine
a pyrocatechol with an alkylamine side chain; examples are epinephrine, norepinephrine, and dopamine

catechol-*o*-methyl transferase (COMT)
the enzyme that catalyzes the degradation of the catecholamines norepinephrine and epinephrine at the synaptic junction

cavitation
the formation of a cavity

central fibrous body
a part of the fibroskeleton of the heart

located between the annulus of the aortic valve and the atrioventricular annuli; right fibrous trigone

central venous catheter
a hollow, tubular instrument passed through a peripheral vein into the vena cava immediately proximal to the right atrium; used for the measurement of right atrial pressure or the infusion of fluids and medications

centriacinar emphysema
a condition resulting from the destruction of the septal walls of the alveoli surrounding the central terminal bronchioles; centrilobular emphysema

cervical pleura
the serous membrane that covers the uppermost aspect of the lung in the neck

channels
macromolecular protein pathways that cross the lipid bilayer of a cell's membrane

chemoreceptor reflex
an increase in the depth and rate of ventilation in response to a lack of oxygen; it also influences heart rate

chest compression system
a mechanical device that applies pressure in such a way to decrease the anteroposterior dimension of the body, thus squeezing the contents of the thoracic cage between the vertebrae and the sternum

Cheyne-Stokes respiration
the pattern of breathing with gradual increase in depth and sometimes in rate to a maximum, followed by a decrease resulting in apnea; the cycles ordinarily are 30 seconds to a minute in length; characteristically seen in coma from alteration in the nervous centers of respiration

cholinergic
nerve fibers that secrete acetylcholine

cholinoceptors
an alternative name for cholinergic adrenoceptors

chordae tendineae
small, delicate fibrous cords attaching to the leaflets (cusps) of the valves of the heart

chronic airflow obstruction
a blockage or impediment to the flow of air that is of long duration

chronic interstitial lung disease
a disease that affects the connective tissue framework of the lung

chronic obstructive pulmonary disease (COPD)
a general descriptive term used for

those diseases in which forced expiratory flow rates are decreased

chronic renal failure (CRF)
an insufficiency or nonperformance of the kidney(s) of long duration

chronotropic
affecting the rate of the rhythm of the heart

chronotropic incompetence
failure of the normal rate regulating mechanisms of the heart

chronotropy
relating to the rate or timing of an event

ciliated cell
the most abundant type of cell found in the bronchial epithelium

circuit
the tubing that connects a mechanical ventilator to a patient's endotracheal or tracheostomy tube

circumflex artery
a branch of the left coronary artery that passes to the diaphragmatic surface of the left ventricle

cirrhosis
a progressive liver disease characterized by nodular regeneration, fibrosis, and alteration of hepatic parenchymal structure

Clara's cells
nonciliated epithelial cells that are most prevalent in the terminal airways; Clara's cells are believed to play a secondary role in the production of surfactant

clear region
the middle portion of the valve leaflet of the mitral and tricuspid valves; it is smooth and translucent, receives few chordae, and has a thinner lamina fibrosa than the other parts of the leaflet; clear zone

closing volume
the lung volume at which airway closure begins during expiration; an index of the status of the small airways

clubbing
a proliferative change in the soft tissues of the distal fingers and toes (especially the nail beds), resulting in a broadening of their ends; the nails are abnormally curved

coagulation
the process of clotting, especially of the blood

coagulopathy
any condition that affects coagulability, especially of the blood

coal workers' pneumoconiosis (CWP)
an inflammation, typically leading to fibrosis of the lungs, caused by the inhalation of coal dust

coalescent opacities
the blending or fusing together of opaque regions in a radiographic image

coarctation of the aorta
a deformity of the media of the aorta at the level of the ductus arteriosus that causes stricture or stenosis of the lumen

collateral vessels
secondary or accessory branches of blood vessels

colonized
the presence of a group or groups of microorganisms

commensal
pertaining to a relationship between two organisms in which one organism benefits and the other is unharmed

commissural chordae
chordae tendinae that attach at the corners of adjacent valve leaflets (commisures)

commissurotomy
a surgical division of the junction between adjacent cusps of a valve of the heart

common atrioventricular bundle
the collection of specialized myocytes that begins at the atrioventricular node and passes through the annulus of the right atrioventricular valve to the membranous portion of the interventricular septum where it splits into two branches; bundle of His; His-Kent bundle

compensatory acid-base disorder
a normal or anticipated attempt to restore the acid-base balance that occurs in response to some disruptive factor

compensatory pause
the suspension or delay of myocardial electrical activity that may occur following an extrasystole

compliance (C)
a measure of the distensibility of a material; the reciprocal of elastance

complicated myocardial infarction
a myocardial infarction of such severity that there is evidence of continued ischemia, left ventricular failure, shock, serious arrhythmia or other conduction disturbance, or other serious illness persisting beyond the fourth day after the infarction; constitutes a high-risk subset of patients

computed tomography (CT)
produces a computer-generated cross-sectional image that is derived from the synthesis of roentgen-ray transmission data obtained in several different directions through a given plane

conductivity
the property of transmitting or conveying electrical impulses

consolidation
solidification of a normally aerated portion of a lung due to the presence of cellular exudate in the alveolar spaces

continuous ambulatory peritoneal dialysis (CAPD)
a method for the removal of soluble substances and water by means of the intermittent introduction of a dialysis solution into, and subsequently removal of it from, the peritoneal cavity

continuous arteriovenous hemofiltration (CAVH)
a method for the removal of soluble substances and water from the blood by filtering arterial blood through a semipermeable membrane (ultrafiltration) and simultaneously reinfusing venous blood

continuous postive airway pressure (CPAP)
an airway maneuver, in spontaneously breathing patients, in which airway pressure is maintained above atmospheric pressure throughout the respiratory cycle (inspiratory and expiratory phases)

continuous subcutaneous insulin infusion (CSII)
a method for the controlled introduction of insulin beneath the skin

contractility
an ill-defined concept that represents muscular performance at any given preload and afterload

contraindication
a circumstance or condition that, because of associated risk, makes the use of a particular intervention inadvisable

conus arteriosus
the outflow tract of the right ventricle; infundibulum

copious
a large amount

cor pulmonale
right-sided heart failure arising from disease of the lungs; chronic cor pulmonale is characterized by right ventricular hypertrophy; acute cor pulmonale is characterized by right ventricular dilation

coronary angiography
radiographic imaging of the vessels of the heart

coronary artery bypass graft (CABG)
a surgical procedure in which flow-limiting stenoses or occlusions of the coronary arteries are circumvented

coronary artery disease
the presence of a flow-limiting obstruction in the coronary arteries that has not yet produced the signs and symptoms of ischemic myocardial damage

coronary artery spasm
an involuntary constriction of the smooth muscle of the coronary arteries

coronary atherosclerosis
arteriosclerosis characterized by lipid deposits in the intima; irregularly distributed in large and medium-sized arteries of the heart

coronary heart disease (CHD)
the signs and symptoms of ischemic myocardial damage as the result of a flow-limiting obstruction in the coronary arteries

coronary sinus
the left horn of the sinus venosus, forming a short trunk that receives most of the veins of the heart

coronary sulcus
the groove on the outer surface of the heart that marks the division between the atria and the ventricles

corticosteroid-related myopathy
any abnormal condition that affects the muscular tissues

cortisol
a steroid hormone secreted by the adrenal cortex; hydrocortisone

costal groove of the rib
the groove along the inferior border of the rib dorsally that changes to the internal surface of the rib where it bends

costophrenic angle
the junction of the costal and diaphragmatic pleurae

costovertebral pleura
the serous membrane that lines the ribs and vertebrae

couplet
two consecutive atrial or ventricular extrasystoles; paired extrasystoles

crackles
adventitious breath sounds heard on auscultation of the parenchymal tissues of the lungs when fluid has accumulated in the distal airways or when air sacs are collapsed and partially reopening (during inspiration)

crash cart
slang term describing the container that holds the emergency medications and equipment used as part of advanced cardiac life support techniques

creatine phosphokinase (CPK)
an enzyme that catalyzes the transfer of a high-energy phosphate from phosphocreatinine to ADP; creatine kinase

creatinine
a component of urine and the final product of creatine catabolism

crista terminalis
a muscular ridge that separates the right atrium into two parts

cromolyn sodium (Intal, Aarane)
a prophylactic antiasthmatic agent

crush injuries
the damage or wounds that result from being squeezed between two hard objects

cryptogenic fibrosing alveolitis
an alveolar inflammatory process of indeterminate etiology that leads to fibrosis of the lungs

crystalline silicon dioxide
the primary constituent of sand; silica

cuirass
a type of negative pressure mechanical ventilator that covers the anterior surface of the thorax

Cushing's syndrome
a condition that arises from increased adrenocortical secretion of cortisone or as a side-effect of steroid therapy; characterized by trunkal obesity, moon face, acne, hypertension, decreased carbohydrate tolerance, protein catabolism, hirsutism (especially in females), and psychiatric disturbances; pituitary basophilism

cusps
the leaflets of the heart's valves

cyanosis
a bluish or purplish coloration of the skin and mucous membranes as a result of insufficient oxygenation; when reduced hemoglobin exceeds 5 grams per 100 milliliters of blood

cyanotic
pertaining to cyanosis

cyclic adenosine monophosphate (cAMP)
the "second messenger" created by the catalytic interaction of ATP with adenylate cyclase following activation by G proteins at enzymatic receptor sites in the cell surface; one of the primary effects of cAMP is to change the degree of phosphorylation of several enzymes involved in muscle contraction

cyclic nucleotide phosphodiesterase
an enzyme that breaks the bonds between the diesterified orthophosphoric acids that constitute the components of nucleic acids

cyclosporine (cyclosporin, cyclosporin A)
an immunosuppressive agent; a cyclic oligopeptide produced by the fungus *Tolypolcladium inflatum Gams*

cylindric bronchiectasis
a dilation, of uniform caliber, of the bronchi and bronchioles that results from chronic inflammation or obstruction

cystic lesion
an injury or wound caused by the formation of cysts

cystinuria
the presence of cystine in the urine; results from a defect in renal tubular reabsorption of amino acids, especially cystine

cytomegalovirus (CMV)
a herpetovirus that causes an enlargement of the cells of various organs and the development of characteristic intranuclear inclusion bodies

cytosol
cytoplasm, with the exception of the mitochondria and endoplasmic reticular components

cytosolic
pertaining to cytosol

cytotoxic
destructive to cells

decongestant
an agent that possesses the property of reducing congestion

decubitis views
refers to radiographic images obtained while the patient is lying down

deep (distal) bronchial veins
an intrapulmonary bronchiolar plexus of veins that communicates freely with the pulmonary veins and eventually coalesces into a single trunk that ends in a main pulmonary vein or in the left atrium

deep cardiac plexus
the dorsal part of the network of nerves that constitutes the cardiac plexus; formed by branches from the cervical and upper thoracic sympathetic ganglia and from the vagus and recurrent laryngeal nerves; located anterior to the tracheal bifurcation, superior to the division of the pulmonary trunk, and posterior to the arch of the aorta

deep chordae
chordae tendineae that attach to the more peripheral aspects of the rough region of a valve leaflet

defibrillate
the act of stopping fibrillation of either atrial or ventricular muscle

defibrillation
cessation of fibrillation of either atrial or ventricular muscle, with restoration of a normal rhythm

defibrillator
anything that stops fibrillation of either atrial or ventricular muscle and restores a normal rhythm

demyelinating
refers to the destruction or loss of myelin

depolarization
the loss of a negative charge in the myocardial cells

depressor muscle of the septum of the nose
muscle running from the maxilla above the central incisor tooth to the nasal septum (flares the nostrils)

desaturate
the act of desaturating; an increase in the percentage of total oxygen-binding sites on the hemoglobin molecule that is unfilled

descending aorta
the part of the aorta between the arch and the bifurcation into the iliac arteries; it includes the thoracic and abdominal aortae

diabetes mellitus (DM)
a disease in which carbohydrate utilization is reduced while lipid and protein utilization is enhanced as the result of a relative deficiency in the amount of insulin

diabetic cardiomyopathy
myocardial dysfunction attributable to the effects of diabetes

diagonal artery
the first, and generally largest, of the left anterior ventricular branches of the anterior interventricular (left anterior descending) coronary artery; it sometimes arises directly from the trunk of the left coronary artery

dialysate
the portion of a solution that can pass through a dialyzing membrane; diffusate

dialysis
a form of filtration that separates smaller molecules from larger ones in a solution by placing a semipermeable membrane between the solution and water

diaphoresis
perspiration, often profuse

diaphragm
the musculotendinous dome that forms the floor of the thorax

diaphragmatic paralysis
loss of function of the diaphragm or hemidiaphragm as the result of a disease or injury to the nerve supply

diaphragmatic pleura
the serous membrane lining the diaphragm

diastasis
the late portion of diastole when blood is entering the ventricles slowly and the venous pressure tends to rise

diastole
the period of ventricular relaxation

diastolic blood pressure (DBP)
the lowest arterial blood pressure reached during a given ventricular cycle

diffusing capacity (DL_{CO})
the amount of gas (typically carbon monoxide or oxygen) taken up by the pulmonary capillary blood per unit of time per unit of average pressure gradient between the alveolar gas and the pulmonary capillary blood; expressed in terms of milliliters/minute/mm Hg

diffusion
the passive tendency of molecules to move from an area of high concentration to an area of lower concentration

digital clubbing
a proliferative change in the soft tissues of the distal fingers and toes (especially the nail beds), resulting in a broadening of their ends; the nails are abnormally curved

digitalis
the dried leaf of *Digitalis purpurea*, a genus of perennial flowering plants that are the main source of cardioactive steroid glycosides used in the treatment of certain heart diseases, especially heart failure

digitoxin (Crystodigin)
one of the primary digitalislike drugs used in the treatment of congestive heart failure; a secondary derivative of the leaves of *Digitalis purpurea*; it is better absorbed from the gastrointestinal tract than digitalis

digoxin (Lanoxin, Lanoxicaps)
one of the primary digitalislike drugs used in the treatment of congestive heart failure; a derivative of *Digitalis lanata*

1,25-dihydroxycholecalciferol
the most active known derivative of vitamin D

dilated cardiomyopathy
a disease of the myocardium characterized by ventricular dilation and cardiac muscle contractile dysfunction

diplopia
double vision; the perception of one object as two objects

dipyridamole (Persantine)
an agent that reduces platelet aggregation and causes coronary vasodilation

directional coronary atherectomy (DCA)
a procedure in which atherosclerotic plaque is removed from the lumen of a coronary artery

dissecting aneurysm
the splitting of an arterial wall by interstitial hemorrhage or by blood that enters from an intimal tear

distributing vessels
the elastic and muscular arteries

diuresis
the excretion of urine; commonly denotes production of unusually large volumes of urine

dobutamine (Dobutrex)
a synthetic derivative of dopamine; possesses strong inotropic but weak chronotropic properties

dopamine (Intropin)
a neural transmitter substance and an intermediate in the biosynthesis of norepinephrine and epinephrine; used at low dosages to enhance renal perfusion and at high dosages as a vassopressor agent

dopaminergic
relating to those nerves or receptor sites that employ dopamine as their neurotransmitter

Doppler velocimetry
the use of Doppler ultrasonography techniques to determine both direction and velocity of blood flow

dromotropic
possessing the ability to influence the conduction velocity of a nerve or muscle fiber

ductus venosus
the continuation of the umbilical vein through the liver to the inferior vena cava in the fetus

dysarthria
a disturbance of articulation

dysphagia
difficulty in swallowing; aphagia

dyspnea
a subjective difficulty or distress in breathing

dyspneic
relating to or suffering from dyspnea

echocardiography
the use of ultrasound in the assessment of the heart and great vessels

ectopic foci
multiple aberrant points of origin; the locations from which abnormal myocardial depolarizations originate

ectopic pacemakers
any center of rhythmic depolarization other than the sinus node

egophony
an auscultatory finding denoting an increased density of the underlying lung tissue; demonstrated when the vowel sound "e" is spoken but is heard through the stethoscope as "a"

Ehlers-Danlos syndrome
a generalized connective tissue disorder that results from a deficient quality or quantity of collagen; characterized by overelasticity and friability of the skin, hypermobility of the joints, and fragility of the superficial vasculature

ejection fraction (EF)
the portion of the stroke volume pumped from the left ventricle

elastance
a measure of an object's tendency to return to its normal shape after removal of the force that distorted it

elastase
a serine proteinase that hydrolyzes elastin

elastin
a fibrous mucoprotein that constitutes the primary connective tissue protein of elastic structures

electrocardiogram (ECG)
a graphic record of the electrical activity of the heart

electroencephalograph (EEG)
a graphic record of the electrical activity of the brain or the apparatus used to obtain it

electrolyte
any substance that, when placed in solution, conducts and is decomposed by electricity

electromyographic
pertaining to the graphic record of the electrical activity of active muscle or the apparatus used to obtain it

electron transport chain
the series of oxidation-reduction reactions through which electrons are accepted from reduced compounds and eventually transferred to oxygen, liberating energy and forming water; respiratory chain

embolectomy
the removal of an embolus

emboli
the plural of embolus; multiple plugs that occlude a vessel; composed of de-

tached thrombus, bacterial mass, vegetation, or other foreign bodies

emphysematous changes
relating to the pathologic alterations arising from emphysema; characterized by undue breathlessness with exertion, abnormal enlargement of the airways distal to the terminal bronchioles, destruction of the walls of the alveoli, and reduction in the number of alveoli

enalapril (Vasotec)
an antihypertensive agent; an angiotensin converting enzyme inhibitor

encephalopathy
any disease of the brain

end-stage renal disease (ESRD)
any condition that impairs the function of the kidneys to such an extent that the patient exhibits kidney failure, hypertension, excessive glomerular permeability to proteins, and other specific tubular abnormalities

endocardial cushions
the epithelial outgrowths of the dorsal and ventral walls of the atrioventricular divisions of the heart tube

endocardial fibroelastosis
a congenital disorder characterized by thickening of the endothelium and subendothelial layer of connective tissue of the left ventricle, thickening and malformation of the cardiac valves, and hypertrophy of the heart; endocardial sclerosis

endocardial heart tubes
canalized extensions of the cardiogenic cords that form the primitive lateral hearts where the first contractions occur

endocardial leads
electrical connection, usually of a pacemaker, attached to the innermost epithelial lining of the heart

endocarditis
inflammation of the innermost epithelial lining of the heart

endocardium
the innermost epithelial lining of the heart; formed from the inner endocardial tube

endogenous
a substance produced in the body

endoluminal stent
a thin coil, wire, or thread placed within the lumen of a blood vessel or other tubular structure; used to maintain the patency of an intact but constricted lumen

endothelial-derived relaxation factor (EDRF)
a substance released from the endothelial cells of the arterioles in response to histamine; postulated to remove calcium ions from myosin-ATPase sites, thus returning muscle fibrils to the resting state

endotracheal tube
a flexible, hollow cylinder inserted nasally or orally into the trachea to provide an airway

enteral
via an intestinal route, referring to one of the routes by which a medication is administered

epicardial lead
electrical connection, usually of a pacemaker, attached to the innermost epithelial lining of the heart

epicardium
the outermost layer of the heart; the visceral layer of the pericardium; formed from the outer layer of the myoepicardial mantle

epinephrine (Adrenalin Chloride)
a sympathomimetic agent; the most potent stimulant of alpha- and beta-adrenergic receptors

ergonovine stimulation
a test of cardiac performance in which a pharmacologic stimulant (ergonovine) is administered to the patient; ergonovine is an alkaloid of ergot used as a stimulant of smooth muscle

erythrocyte sedimentation rate (ESR)
the rate of sedimentation of red blood cells in anticoagulated blood; measured by mixing venous blood with a solution of sodium citrate and allowing it to stand for an hour in a calibrated pipet; an above normal rate (>15 mm for men; >20 mm for women) is associated with anemia or inflammation

erythropoietin
a protein secreted by the kidney that stimulates the formation of red blood cells from bone marrow

eschar
the thick, coagulated crust that forms after a chemical or thermal burn

Escherichia coli
a species of aerobic, facultatively anaerobic bacteria that contains gram-negative rods; occurs normally in the intestines

esophagus
the portion of the foregut that connects the pharynx and the stomach

essential (primary) hypertension
abnormally high blood pressure that has no discernible cause; accounts for approximately 90% of cases of hypertension

eukaryote
a cell containing a membrane-bound nucleus with DNA and RNA chromosomes

Ewing's sarcoma
a malignant neoplasm of the bones of the extremities; endothelial myeloma

exacerbation
an increase in severity of the signs and symptoms of a disease

exchange vessels
the capillaries, sinusoids, and postcapillary venules where the exchange of gases, nutrients, and metabolic products occurs

excitation-contraction coupling
the mechanism by which the action potential causes myofibrillar contraction

exercise prescription
the instruction given to a patient or client regarding the mode, intensity, duration, and frequency of exercise to be performed

exercise testing
monitored, multilevel cardiovascular or pulmonary (or both) evaluation of a patient's responses to controlled stress (exercise)

exocrine glands
the secretory or excretory organs from which the secretions reach a free surface of the body by way of ducts

exogenous
substance produced outside the body

expectorant
anything that promotes bronchial secretion and facilitates its expulsion

expiratory reserve volume (ERV)
the additional volume of air that can be let out beyond the normal tidal exhalation

expiratory retard
an orificial resistance applied during exhalation that permits the ventilatory circuit pressure to drop slowly to atmospheric pressure as the flow of expiratory gas ceases

external elastic lamina
a fenestrated layer of elastic connective tissue that covers the tunica media

external intercostal muscles
11 pair of muscles; each attaching from the inferior border of a rib to the superior border of the rib below; acts to pull the ribs together

extracellular parasite
an organism that lives in and derives nourishment from another organism without invading the host's cells

extracorporeal ultrafiltration
a process by which large molecules are separated from small molecules in a solution outside the body

extrapyramidal
outside or other than the pyramidal (corticospinal) tract

extrinsic asthma
a narrowing of the bronchial airways as the result of an allergic reaction to foreign substances

exudate
any fluid that gradually passes (oozes) out of a body tissue, usually as the result of inflammation

exudative infiltrate
fluid that has permeated or penetrated into the tissues

facioscapulohumeral muscular dystrophy
a genetically transmitted (autosomal dominant inheritance) abnormality of the muscle characterized by wasting of the muscles of the face, shoulder girdle, and arms

facultative parasite
an organism that lives in and derives nourishment from another organism under more than one specific set of environmental factors

false chordae
a fibrous collagenous cord passing from the papillary muscles to one another or to the ventricular walls

false-negative
a test result that erroneously excludes an individual from a particular reference group because of insufficiently stringent testing criteria

false ribs
the five lower ribs on either side of the thorax that do not articulate directly with the sternum

fan-shaped chordae
chordae with radiating branches projecting outward from a single stem to attach to the margins of the interleaflet commissures

fasciculations
involuntary contractions of groups of muscle fibers; a coarser type of muscular contraction than fibrillation

fecal impaction
a collection of compressed or hardened feces in the colon or rectum that cannot be moved voluntarily

femoral-popliteal bypass
a surgical procedure in which a vascular prosthesis is placed to bypass an occlusion of the distal femoral artery or proximal popliteal artery, or both

fetid breath
foul-smelling breath

fibrin
a filamentous elastic protein derived from fibrinogen in the presence of thrombin

fibroplastic
producing fibrous tissue

fibrosis
the reactive or preparative process in which fibrous tissue is formed

fibroskeleton of the heart
an intricate, malleable, three-dimensional continuum of dense and membranous collagen forming the annuli of the principal valvular orifices

fibrous pericardium
outer sac of the pericardial sac consisting of collagenous fibrous tissue

filum coronarium
the anterolateral arm of the mitral annulus

FiO_2
the fraction of inspired oxygen; the portion of an inhaled mixture of gases that is oxygen

first-degree atrioventricular block
an impairment of the normal conduction between the atria and the ventricles; characterized by a prolongation of the P–R interval (atrioventricular conduction time)

first heart sound (S_1)
a sound heard during auscultation of the heart; occurs at the onset of ventricular systole (just preceding the normally palpable pulse in a peripheral artery); produced primarily by closure of the atrioventricular valves

first pass effect
the partial inactivation of a drug as the result of metabolic processes

flux
the number of moles of a substance crossing through a unit area of a membrane per unit time

foam cells
cells that have accumulated or ingested material that dissolves during the tissue preparation, usually lipids; lipophage

focal biliary cirrhosis
damage to hepatic parenchymal cells as the result of bile duct obstruction

foramen ovale
an oval opening in the dorsal part of the septum secundum

foramen secundum
an opening in the dorsal part of the septum primum that forms before the septum fuses with the endocardial cushions

forced expiratory flow, 200–1200 ($FEF_{200-1200}$)
the mean flow rate of gas measured between two expired volumes (200 ml and 1200 ml) during a forced vital capacity maneuver

forced expiratory volume in 1 second (FEV_1)
the maximal volume that can be expired in 1 second, starting from a maximal inspiratory effort

forced midexpiratory flow (FEF_{25-75})
the mean flow rate of gas measured between two expired volumes (25% of FVC and 75% of FVC) during a forced vital capacity maneuver

forced vital capacity (FVC)
the largest volume of gas that can be forcefully exhaled from the lungs after a maximal inspiratory effort

fossa ovalis
an ovoid depression above and to the left of the inferior vena cava orifice on the lower central portion of the septal wall of the right atrium

fourth heart sound (S_4)
a sound heard in late diastole on auscultation over the heart; corresponds with atrial contraction; is rarely heard in normal hearts

Fowler's position
a supine-lying position in which the head of the bed is elevated approximately 2 feet

fractionation
separation of the components of a mixture

free-edge chordae
single strands arising from the papillary muscle and attaching near the middle of the free margin of a valve leaflet

free fatty acids (FFAs)
the product obtained when fatty acids (from the hydrolysis of triglycerides) are bound to proteins in the plasma

fremitus
a vibration imparted to the hand resting on the chest or other part of the body

Friedreich's ataxia
uncoordinated voluntary movement of the extremities, with eventual paralysis, as the result of sclerosis of the lateral and posterior columns of the spinal cord; an autosomal recessive trait; hereditary spinal ataxia

fulminant
suddenly occurring

functional capacity
ability or power to perform necessary activities

functional residual capacity (FRC)
the sum of the expiratory reserve and residual volumes; it is the amount of air remaining in the lungs at the end of a normal tidal exhalation

furosemide (Lasix)
a diuretic agent

ganglioside
a glycosphingolipid (fatty acid derivative) that contains one or more sialic acid residues; found primarily in nerve tissue and in the spleen

gas transport system
the combination of musculoskeletal, cardiovascular, and respiratory systems, which together function to deliver and eliminate gases

globin
the protein molecule of hemoglobin

globular leukocytes
migratory cells of the tracheobronchial epithelia, possibly derived from mast cells; postulated to play a role in the immunologic process

glomerular filtration rate (GFR)
the volume of water filtered out of the plasma through the glomerular capillaries into Bowman's capsule per unit time

glottis
the fissure between the vocal folds; also called the rima glottidis

glucagon
a pancreatic hormone that initiates the release of glycogen from the liver

gluconeogenesis
the formation of glycogen from noncarbohydrates

glucose tolerance test
a test of the liver's ability to absorb and store excess amounts of glucose; normally, after ingestion of 100 grams of glucose, the blood sugar level rises and returns to normal within 2 hours; in diabetic patients, the rise is greater and the return to normal is prolonged or absent

glycogenolysis
the hydrolysis of glycogen to glucose

glycosylated hemoglobin (Hb A_{1c})
hemoglobin to which glucose and related monosaccharides bind

granulation
the formation of very small, rounded connective tissue projections that form on healing surfaces

granulomatosis
any condition characterized by the formation of nodular inflammatory lesions

granulomatous uveitis
an inflammation of the vascular (middle) coat of the eye

Graves's disease
diffuse hyperplasia of the thyroid gland, a form of hyperthyroidism

great cardiac vein
vein that runs from the apex of the heart to the base of the ventricles in the anterior interventricular sulcus, before turning to the left in the coronary sulcus to reach the back of the heart

growth hormone
a protein hormone from the anterior lobe of the pituitary that promotes bodily growth, fat mobilization, and inhibition of glucose utilization; somatotropin

Guillain-Barré syndrome
a neuromuscular disorder characterized by paresthesia of the limbs, muscular weakness or flaccid paralysis; acute idiopathic polyneuritis; probably an immune-mediated disorder

half-life
the time it takes for the plasma concentration of a drug to be reduced to 50% of its peak value

Hamman-Rich syndrome
interstitial fibrosis of the lung, leading to severe right ventricular failure and cor pulmonale

head of the rib
the end of the rib that articulates with the vertebrae

helium dilution method
one of the most commonly used methods for the measurement of static lung volumes

hematocrit
the percentage of the volume of a sample of blood occupied by cells

heme
a ferrous ion covalently bound to four nitrogens on the pyrole groups of a porphyrin ring

hemidiaphragm
one of the two domes of the diaphragm

hemiplegia
paralysis of one side of the body

hemochromatosis
a disorder of iron metabolism

hemolytic
destructive to blood cells

hemoptysis
expectoration of blood derived from the lungs as a result of pulmonary or bronchial hemorrhage

hemostasis
stagnation of blood; stoppage of bleeding

hemothorax
the presence of blood in the pleural cavity

heparin (Liquaemin Sodium)
an anticoagulant; prevents platelet agglutination and subsequent thrombus formation

hepatitis
inflammation of the liver; usually in response to a viral infection but may also be from toxic agents

hepatomegaly
abnormally enlarged liver

herpes simplex
a group of infections caused by one of the two types of herpes simplex virus; type 1, the pathogen of herpes simplex in humans; type 2, the cause of genital herpes

heterologous
pertains to a substance derived from an animal of a different species

high-density lipoprotein (HDL)
one of the major classes of lipoproteins, containing about 50% protein and much smaller concentrations of phospholipids than either VLDL or LDL; has a flotation fraction (density) between 1.063 and 1.21

high-risk patient
patients, who by nature of their cardiovascular or pulmonary disease, demonstrate markedly abnormal signs and symptoms during activity

hilus
the point at which the nerves, vessels, and primary bronchi penetrate the parenchyma of each lung

histochemistry
pertaining to the composition of the tissues

Hodgkin's disease
a malignant neoplasm of lymphoid cells of uncertain origin; associated with inflammatory infiltration of lymphocytes and eosinophilic leukocytes and fibrosis

Holter monitoring
a technique of long-term recording of ECG activity to screen for arrhythmias or ischemia

homocystinuria
an autosomal recessive trait resulting in a defect in the enzyme cystathionine synthetase; that when exhibited is characterized by excessive excretion of homocystine in the urine

homologous
alike in specific ways

horizontal fissure
the secondary groove that separates the

middle from the upper lobe of the right lung

huffing
a technique to assist in the expectoration of secretions; a cough assistance technique

humoral
pertaining to any clear fluid or semifluid hyaline anatomic substance

hyaline membrane disease
a disease of the neonate associated with decreased amounts of surfactant characterized by atelectasis and alveolar ducts lined by an eosinophilic membrane

hyaline membrane
an eosinophilic membrane lining the alveolar ducts of infants suffering from respiratory distress syndrome

hydralazine (Apresoline)
a vasodilating antihypertensive agent

hyperalimentation
the administration of nutrients beyond the normal minimum requirement

hyperbilirubinemia
an abnormally high amount of bilirubin in the circulating blood, resulting in clinically apparent icterus or jaundice when the concentration is sufficient

hypercapnia
hypercarbia; the presence of an abnormally large amount of carbon dioxide in the circulating blood

hypercholesterolemia
the presence of abnormally large amounts of cholesterol in the circulating blood

hyperglycemia
the presence of abnormally high concentrations of glucose in the circulating blood

hyperinflated
distended beyond the normal extent

hyperkalemia
a greater than normal concentration of potassium ions in the circulating blood that may be due to tissue destruction, renal failure, and Addison's disease; may cause bradycardia with hypotension and changes in the electrocardiogram, including elevating the T wave, and muscle weakness

hyperlipidemia
the presence of an abnormally high level of lipids in the circulating blood; lipemia

hyperlucent lung syndrome
a variant of panacinar (panlobular) emphysema

hypernatremia
an abnormally high concentration of sodium ions in the plasma

hyperosmolality
an increase in the osmotic concentration of a solution

hyperparathyroidism
a condition due to an increase in the secretion of the parathyroid glands; characterized by elevated serum calcium levels and decreased serum phosphorus

hyperplasia
an increase in the number of cells in an organ or tissue; hypertrophy

hyperplastic
pertaining to hyperplasia

hypersomnolence
a condition of drowsiness approaching coma

hypertension (HTN)
an arterial blood pressure in excess of 140/90 (American Heart Association) or 160/95 (World Health Organization)

hypertensive heart disease
myocardial dysfunction as a result of abnormally high blood pressure

hyperthyroidism
an abnormality of the thyroid gland in which thyroid hormone secretion is increased

hypertriglyceridemia
a condition in which the triglyceride concentration in the blood is greater than normal

hypertrophic cardiomyopathy
a disease of the myocardium characterized by inappropriate and excessive left ventricular hypertrophy and normal or even enhanced cardiac muscle contractile function

hypertrophy
a general increase in the size or bulk of an organ or tissue, unrelated to tumor formation

hyperuricemia
a greater than normal concentration of uric acid in the blood

hyperventilation
an arterial carbon dioxide level that is below normal as a result of increased alveolar ventilation relative to metabolic carbon dioxide production

hypoadaptive
a failure in the occurrence of expected or anticipated results

hypogammaglobulinemia
a less than normal amount of the gamma fraction of serum globulin

hypokalemia
an abnormally low concentration of potassium ions in the circulating blood

hyponatremia
an abnormally low concentration of sodium ions in the circulating blood

hypophosphatemia
a less than normal concentration of alkaline phosphatase in the blood; hypophosphatasia

hypoplasia
the underdevelopment of an organ or tissue

hyposthenia
weakness

hypothalamic
pertaining to the hypothalamus (the ventromedial region of the diencephalon forming the walls of the ventral portion of the third ventricle); the hypothalamus is intimately involved in autonomic nervous system and endocrine functioning

hypothalamic dysfunction
an abnormal function of the hypothalamus

hypothyroidism
a condition in which the production of thyroid hormone is below normal; characterized by low metabolic rate, tendency for weight gain, somnolence

hypovolemic
pertaining to hypovolemia (decreased amount of blood in the body)

hypoxemia
a condition in which arterial oxygenation is below normal

hypoxia
a condition in which the level of oxygen in the arterial blood or tissue is below normal

idiopathic
of unknown origin

idiopathic congestive cardiomyopathy
a myocardial dysfunction that has no discernible cause

idiopathic hypertrophic subaortic stenosis (IHSS)
an obstruction of the left ventricular outflow tract due to hypertrophy of the left ventricular septum; of unknown origin

idiopathic pulmonary fibrosis
the formation of tissue containing fibroblasts, and the fibers and fibrils they form, in the lungs for no known reason

iliocostalis cervicis muscle
an accessory inspiratory muscle arising from the angles of the upper six ribs, medial to the iliocostalis thoracis, and

inserting into the transverse processes of the fourth, fifth, and sixth cervical vertebrae

iliocostalis lumborum muscle
an accessory inspiratory muscle arising from the sacrum, the iliac crest, and the spinous processes of most of the lumbar and the lower two thoracic vertebrae upward to the lower borders of the last six or seven ribs as far laterally as their angles

iliocostalis muscles
accessory inspiratory muscles that are the most lateral division of the erector spinae group

iliocostalis thoracis muscle
an accessory inspiratory muscle arising from the upper borders of the lower six ribs medial to the insertion of the iliocostalis lumborum up to the upper six ribs

immune system
a complex of interrelated cellular, molecular, and genetic components that provide a defense against foreign organisms or substances and abnormal native cells

immunodeficiency
a condition in which some component of the immune system is lacking

immunoglobulin (Ig)
a protein consisting of two pairs of polypeptide chains, one pair of low molecular weight chains, and one pair of high (relatively) molecular weight chains linked together by disulfide bonds

immunosuppression
the prevention or interference with the development of an immunologic response

immunosuppressive
any agent that prevents or interferes with the development of an immunologic response

inactivation gate
the chemical (e.g., neurotransmitter) or electrical (e.g., membrane potential) action that closes an ion channel after it has been opened

incentive spirometer
a flow- or volume-dependent device that is used to facilitate slow, deep, sustained inspiratory efforts in patients who might otherwise be disposed to breathe shallowly

incubator
a container in which controlled environmental conditions (e.g., temperature, pressure, gas composition) may be maintained

infarction
the sudden venous or arterial insufficiency that produces an area of macroscopic necrosis

inferior pulmonary vein
the vein returning blood from right or left lower lobes of the lungs to the left atrium

inferior vena cava
the blood vessel that receives blood from the lower limbs and the greater part of the pelvic and abdominal organs; it begins at the level of the fifth lumbar vertebra on the right side, pierces the diaphragm at the level of the eighth thoracic vertebra, and empties into the back part of the right atrium of the heart

inflammation
a complex of histologic and cytologic reactions that occur in response to an injury or abnormal stimulus caused by a biologic, chemical, or physical agent

infundibulum
the outflow tract of the right ventricle, conus arteriosus

innermost intercostal muscles
11 pairs of muscles, each attaching from the superior border of a rib to the inferior border of the rib above; acts to pull the ribs together

inoculum
the causative agent (microorganism or other material) that is introduced into the body

inotrope
an agent that influences the contractility of muscular tissue

inotropic
influencing the contractility of muscular tissue

inotropy
the characteristic contractile state of muscular tissue

inspiratory capacity (IC)
the sum of the tidal and inspiratory reserve volumes; the maximum amount of air that can be inhaled after a normal tidal exhalation

inspiratory hold
a mechanical ventilatory maneuver in which either the preset pressure or predetermined volume is reached and held for some period of time before exhalation is initiated

inspiratory reserve volume (IRV)
the additional volume of air that can be taken into the lungs beyond the normal tidal inhalation

insulin-dependent diabetes mellitus (IDDM)
a metabolic disease that requires insulin

therapy in which lipid and protein utilization are increased and carbohydrate utilization is decreased as the result of a relative or absolute insulin deficiency; juvenile diabetes; type I diabetes

integumentary
relating to the covering of a body or body part

interalveolar septum
the tissue between two adjacent alveoli; comprises the alveolar epithelium, the capillary epithelium, and the interstitial space

interatrial atrioventricular tracts or bundles
specialized paths for interatrial conduction of the depolarization wave

interatrial septum
the wall separating the right and left atria

intercostal muscles
the three sets of 11 pairs of muscles occupying the intercostal spaces and connecting the adjoining ribs; external, internal, and innermost intercostal muscles

intercurrent
occurring during the course of an existing process

intermediate cells
may be undifferentiated forms of ciliated or secretory cells in the tracheal epithelium

intermittent claudication
an attack of lameness and pain caused by ischemia, chiefly of the calf muscles, that is brought on by walking and is due to atherosclerotic lesions in peripheral arteries

intermittent mandatory ventilation (IMV)
a mode of mechanical ventilatory assistance; the mandatory (preset) ventilator breath is delivered at a preset interval regardless of the phase of the patient's breathing efforts

internal elastic lamina
a fenestrated layer of elastic connective tissue that covers the tunica intima

internal intercostal muscles
11 pairs of muscles, each attaching from the superior border of a rib to the inferior border of the rib above; acts to pull the ribs together

internodal atrioventricular tracts or bundles
specialized conduction pathways between the sinoatrial and atrioventricular nodes

interpolated
to occur, or be inserted, between other things

interstitial pattern
one of two main roentgenographic patterns characterized by interstitial thickening and the formation of thin-walled cystic spaces less than 10 mm in diameter, generally divided into three subcategories (fine, medium, coarse) based on the degree of interstitial thickening and the size of the cystic spaces; reticular pattern

interstitial pneumonitis
an inflammation involving the spaces within an organ or tissue (excluding body spaces or cavities)

interventricular foramen
the opening that separates the interventricular septum from the endocardial cushions

interventricular septum
the septum that develops from the ventricular apex, growing toward the fused dorsal and ventral endocardial cushions, and separating the ventricle into left and right halves

intima
the innermost coat of a vessel, tunica intima

intra-aortic balloon counterpulsation (IABC)
a means of assisting ventricular ejection by reducing aortic pressure just before and during ventricular systole with an intra-aortic balloon pump activated by an automatic mechanism triggered by the ECG

intra-aortic balloon pump (IABP)
a pump connected to a balloon catheter that is inserted into the descending aorta to provide temporary cardiac assistance by means of counterpulsation

intrapleural drainage tube
a hollow cylinder inserted through the chest wall into the pleural space

intrapulmonary shunt
the passage of blood from the right side of the heart through the lungs to the left side of the heart without participation in gas exchange; perfusion in excess of ventilation

intrinsic asthma
a condition of the lungs in which there is widespread bronchial and bronchiolar constriction due to varying degrees of smooth muscle spasm, mucosal edema, and mucous plugging that has no identifiable extrinsic cause

intubated
the condition of having a hollow cylindric device inserted through the nose or mouth into the trachea

intubation
the insertion of a hollow cylindric de-

vice through the nose or mouth into the trachea

intussusception
the infolding of one segment of the intestine within another

irregular emphysema
atypical emphysema

ischemia
a condition of having an inadequate supply of arterial blood

ischemic
relating to ischemia

islets of Langerhans
cellular masses in the interstitial tissue of the pancreas that produce insulin and glucagon

isoenzymes
enzymes that are very similar in catalytic properties but can be differentiated by variations in their physical properties

isoproterenol (Isuprel)
a sympathomimetic beta-receptor stimulant; similar to epinephrine but does not share its vasoconstricting properties

isovolumic contraction
the action of the ventricular muscle fibers in early systole, when they initially increase their tension without shortening and thus without an associated alteration of ventricular volume

isovolumic relaxation
the phase immediately following aortic valve closure and continuing until the mitral valve opens when ventricular pressure falls below atrial pressure

isthmus
a constriction connecting two larger parts of an organ or other anatomic structure

J-type receptors
stretch receptors in the interstitium

Jackson-Pratt drain
a flexible silicon rubber suction drain with small intraluminal ridges that prevent its collapse

jaundice
icterus; a yellowish staining of the integument, sclerae, and deeper tissues and the excretions with bile pigment

jugular venous distension (JVD)
stretching or overfilling of the jugular vein

junctional rhythm
the rhythm of the heart when the atrioventricular node initiates the depolarization wave; nodal rhythm; atrioventricular junctional rhythm

junctional tachycardia
a junctional rhythm in which the rate exceeds 100 per minute

juxtaglomerular
in close proximity to a renal glomerulus

Kaposi's sarcoma
a multiform malignant neoplasm occurring in the skin, consisting of spindle cells and irregular small vascular spaces

Kawasaki's disease
a polymorphous erythematous febrile disease of unknown origin; characterized by a desquamation of fingers and toes and a furrowing depression of the nails; mucocutaneous lymph node syndrome

Kerley B lines
fine horizontal lines a few centimeters above the costophrenic angle in chest radiographs; postulated to be caused by distention of interlobular lymphatics with edema fluid

ketoacidosis
acidosis resulting from the formation of excessive ketone bodies (a group of ketones containing acetone)

ketogenesis
the production of ketones

ketone
a substance with the carbonyl group linking two carbon atoms

ketosis
a condition (e.g., diabetes, starvation) in which the production of ketone bodies is enhanced

Kohn's pores
interalveolar foramina

Korotkoff's sounds
sounds heard over an artery when pressure over it is reduced during the determination of blood pressure by the auscultatory method

Kulchitsky's cells
the rarest type of bronchial epithelial cell; Kulchitsky's cells are neurosecretory cells believed to play a role in the regulation of lobular growth

kyphoscoliosis
a deformity of the spine characterized by excessive flexion and lateral curvature

labetalol (Normodyne, Trandate)
an antihypertensive agent; an alpha- and a beta-adrenergic blocking agent

lactate
a salt or an ester of lactic acid

lactic dehydrogenase (LDH)
an enzyme (actually four) that acts in the oxidation of lactate to pyruvate; the L-isomer transfers H ions to ferricytochrome c, and the D-isomer carries H ions to NAD$^+$

Lambert's canals
collateral interalveolar ducts

Lanoxin
a brand name of digoxin preparation

laryngospasm
an involuntary muscular contraction that results in closure of the glottic aperture

laryngotracheal diverticulum
the pouch that develops from the laryngotracheal groove as a precursor of the laryngotracheal tube

laryngotracheal groove
the depression in the posterior wall of the pharynx from which the lower larynx and the trachea, bronchi, and lungs eventually develop

laryngotracheal tube
the tube that develops from the laryngotracheal diverticulum as a precursor of the bronchi and lungs

larynx
the organ of voice production; formed from the proximal end of the laryngotracheal tube and the fourth and sixth pairs of branchial arches

lateral basal segmental bronchus
the portion of the tracheobroncheal tree arising from the right or left lower lobe bronchus that is distributed to the lateral basal segment

lateral segmental bronchus
the portion of the tracheobroncheal tree arising from the right middle lobe bronchus that is distributed to the lateral segment

lateral thoracotomy
a surgical incision into the lateral chest wall

latissimus dorsi muscle
an accessory inspiratory muscle arising from the spinous process of the lower six thoracic, the lumbar, and the upper sacral vertebrae; from the posterior aspect of the iliac crest; and slips from the lower three or four ribs to attach to the intertubercular groove of the humerus

leaflet chordae of the anterior leaflet of the mitral valve
specialized variants of rough zone chordae; strut chordae

left atrioventricular orifice
the opening leading from the left atrium into the left ventricle

left atrium
the chamber of the heart that receives blood from the pulmonary veins

left auricle
the small conical projection from the left atrium; remnant of the left portion of the primitive atrium

left bundle branches
the left crus of the atrioventricular (His) bundle of specialized myocytes that ramifies in the subendocardium of the left ventricle; part of the specialized conduction system of the heart

left common carotid artery
arises from the highest part of the arch of the aorta to the left of the brachiocephalic trunk

left coronary artery
originates in the left posterior aortic sinus, passing between the pulmonary trunk and the left auricle, as it proceeds to the atrioventricular sulcus, where it typically divides into two branches: the anterior interventricular (descending) ramus and the circumflex ramus; usually supplies almost all of the left ventricle and atrium and most of the interventricular septum

left coronary plexus
primarily an extension of the left half of the deep part of the cardiac plexus, although it does receive some fibers from the right half; it follows the distribution of the left coronary artery, supplying the left atrium and ventricle

left dominant coronary arterial system
the majority of the blood supply to the heart is provided via the left coronary artery; occurs in about 20% of the population

left fibrous trigone
the part of the fibroskeleton of the heart that is located between the left side of the left annulus of the mitral valve and the aortic annulus

left inferior pulmonary vein
the vein that returns blood from the lower lobe of the left lung to the left atrium

left lateral view
refers to the preferred view for a lateral radiograph of the chest; taken with the left side of the chest against the film cassette

left (obtuse) margin of the heart
the left border of the heart, descending obliquely (convex toward the left) from the left auricle to the cardiac apex; formed mainly by the left ventricle, separates the sternocostal and the left surfaces of the heart

left (pulmonary) surface of the heart
the surface of the heart, consisting almost entirely of the left ventricle, that faces upward, back, and toward the left; it is convex and widest above, narrowing toward the cardiac apex

left marginal artery
a large ventricular branch of the cir-

cumflex artery, occurring in about 90% of cases

left marginal vein
one of the larger tributaries to the great cardiac vein; delivers blood from the left ventricle

left pulmonary artery
the left branch of the pulmonary artery distributed to the left lung; runs in front of the descending aorta and the left primary bronchus to the root of the lung

left subclavian artery
the last branch from the arch of the aorta

left superior pulmonary vein
the vein that returns blood from the upper lobe of the left lung to the left atrium

left ventricle
one of the four chambers of the heart; receives arterialized blood from the left atrium, propelling it by contraction of its muscular walls into the aorta

left ventricular end-diastolic pressure (LVEDP)
the pressure in the left ventricle at the end of the diastolic phase of the cardiac cycle

leukocytosis
an abnormally large number (usually $>$ 10,000/mm^3) of white blood cells

leukotriene
a product of arachidonic acid metabolism; postulated to have a role as a mediator in inflammatory and allergic reactions

lidocaine (Xylocaine)
a local anesthetic with significant antiarrhythmic properties

ligamentum arteriosum
the remains of the ductus arteriosus of the fetus; between the left pulmonary artery and the arch of the aorta

ligamentum teres
the remains of the umbilical vein of the fetus

ligamentum venosum
the remains of the ductus venosus of the fetus

limb-girdle muscular dystrophy
a genetically transmitted (autosomal recessive) progressive abnormality of the muscle that usually begins in the preadolescent period; characterized by enlarged, weakened, and inelastic muscles; commonly affects the pelvic girdle predominantly

limbus marginalis
the line of demarcation between the muscular septum and a thin, rounded,

collagenous area immediately below the right and posterior cusps of the aortic valve

limen nasi
the upper limit of the lower nasal cartilage

lingula
the anteroinferior area of the left upper lobe corresponding to the right middle lobe

lipolysis
the hydrolysis of fat

lisinopril (Zestril)
an antihypertensive agent; an angiotensin converting enzyme inhibitor

lobar
relating to a lobe (in this case, of a lung)

lobectomy
the excision of a lobe (in this case, of a lung)

lobular bronchiole
the bronchiole that enters the secondary lobules of the lung; each lobular bronchiole gives off about six terminal bronchioles

loop diuretic
one of a group of agents that enhances the excretion of urine; acts by inhibiting sodium and chloride reabsorption not only in the proximal and distal tubules but also in Henle's loop

lordotic view
a posteroanterior or anteroposterior upright radiograph in which the roentgen-ray beam is aimed at an oblique angle

lovastatin
an antihyperlipidemic agent; reduces both normal and elevated serum cholesterol levels

low-density lipoprotein (LDL)
one of the major classes of lipoproteins, having a relatively large molecular weight and containing proportionally less protein and more cholesterol and triglycerides than HDL; has a flotation fraction (density) of between 1.019 and 1.063

lower lobe bronchus
the portion of the tracheobronchial tree that gives off the segmental and subsegmental bronchi of the lower lobe of the lung

lung abscess
a circumscribed collection of pus, associated with tissue destruction, within the lung

lung bud
the endodermal origin of the bronchi and lungs in the fetus

lunulae
the thin lamina fibrosa on either side of Arantius's nodules of the semilunar cusps of the aortic valve

lymphadenopathy
any disease process that affects the lymph nodes

lymphatic space
a tissue or vessel filled with lymph

lymphocyte
a white blood cell formed in lymphoid tissue throughout the body; a nonnative cell found in the mucosa of the tracheobronchial tree

lymphokines
soluble substances that stimulate the activity of monocytes and macrophages; released by sensitized lymphocytes on contact with specific antigens as part of the cellular immune response

lymphoma
a general term for malignant neoplasms of the lymphoid tissues

macular
pertaining to a small, discolored patch or spot on the skin that is neither elevated above nor depressed below the surface

magnetic resonance imaging (MRI)
an imaging modality in which the patient's body is placed in a magnetic field and its hydrogen nuclei are excited by radiofrequency pulses at varying angles to the field's axis; nuclear magnetic resonance (NMR)

malaise
a general feeling of discomfort or uneasiness

manubrium
the upper segment of the sternum

Marfan's syndrome
a congenital disorder (autosomal dominant) of the mesodermal and ectodermal tissues; characterized by arachnodactyly, excessively long extremities, laxness of the joints, bilateral ectopia lentis, and vascular defects (especially aortic aneurysm)

maximal expiratory flow-volume (MEFV) curve
the expiratory portion of the flow-volume curve generated during a forced expiratory maneuver

maximal oxygen consumption ($\dot{V}O_{2max}$)
the rate at which oxygen enters the blood from alveolar gas, equal in the steady state to the consumption of oxygen by tissue metabolism throughout the body during maximal exercise; units: milliliters of oxygen (STPD) used per minute

maximum voluntary ventilation (MVV)
the volume of air breathed when an individual breathes as fast and as deeply as possible for a given time (e.g., 12 or 15 seconds)

mean arterial pressure (MAP)
the average pressure within the cardiovascular system throughout the cardiac cycle

mechanical percussor
an apparatus used to perform repeated blows or taps to the external chest wall in an effort to mobilize secretions in the underlying lungs

meconium aspiration
the act of sucking into the airways, by the fetus in utero, amniotic fluid contaminated with the first intestinal discharges

meconium ileus
an intestinal obstruction in the newborn following the thickening of meconium due to a lack of trypsin

media
middle; denoting an anatomic structure that is between two other similar structures or that is midway in position

medial basal segmental bronchus
the portion of the tracheobronchial tree arising from the right lower lobe bronchus that is distributed to the medial basal segment

medial or septal papillary muscles
muscles that are variable in their origin from the wall of the right ventricle

medial segmental bronchus
the portion of the tracheobronchial tree arising from the right middle lobe bronchus that is distributed to the medial segment

medial umbilical ligaments
the remains of the intra-abdominal umbilical arteries of the fetus

median sternotomy
a form of thoracotomy in which the chest wall is entered via a midline incision through the sternum

mediastinal drainage tube
a hollow catheter introduced into the mediastinum to facilitate removal of fluid

mediastinal pleura
the serous membrane overlying the mediastinum

mediastinal shift
a deviation of the mediastinum as the result of an intrathoracic pathologic condition (e.g., movement toward the opposite side of the thoracic cavity due to a tension pneumothorax)

mediastinum
the median portion of the thoracic cavity; divided into superior and inferior divisions

mediastinum, anterior compartment of the inferior division of the
that portion of the mediastinum bounded by the sternum anteriorly, the pericardium posteriorly, the superior division cranially, and the diaphragm inferiorly; contains the ascending aorta

mediastinum, inferior division of the
the part of the mediastinum that extends from a line passing from the fourth thoracic vertebra to the lower border of the manubrium downward to the diaphragm; subdivided into anterior, middle, and posterior compartments

mediastinum, middle compartment of the inferior division of the
that portion of the mediastinum bounded by the pericardium anteriorly and posteriorly, the superior division superiorly, and the diaphragm inferiorly; contains the heart and great vessels

mediastinum, posterior compartment of the inferior division of the
that portion of the mediastinum bounded by the bodies of the fifth through the twelfth thoracic vertebrae posteriorly, the pericardium anteriorly, the diaphragm inferiorly, and the superior division cranially; contains the esophagus and thoracic aorta

mediate percussion
the act of tapping on the surface of the chest to evaluate the condition of underlying structures, to identify the resting levels of the hemidiaphragms posteriorly, or to measure diaphragmatic excursion during breathing

membranous septum
a thin, rounded, collagenous area immediately below the right and posterior cusps of the aortic valve in the interventricular septum just below the limbus marginalis

meningioencephalitis
an inflammation of the brain and its membranes

meningitis
an inflammation of the membranes of the brain or spinal cord

mesothelioma
a rare neoplasm derived from the cells lining the pleura and peritoneum

MET
the abbreviation for metabolic equivalent; the cost, in terms of oxygen consumption, of energy expenditure (e.g., 3

to 5 METs for light work; more than 9 METs for heavy work)

metabolic acidosis
decreased arterial plasma pH and bicarbonate concentration as the result of metabolic pathology

metabolic alkalosis
an increase in the concentration of arterial plasma bicarbonate as the result of metabolic pathology

metastasize
the spread of a disease process from one part of the body to another

methylxanthines
a class of drugs (e.g., aminophylline) that have diuretic, vasodilator, and cardiac stimulant properties

microatelectasis
the absence of gas in a very small part of the lungs due to resorption of the gas from the alveoli

microgallbladder
a very small receptacle on the inferior surface of the liver for the storage of bile

middle cardiac vein
a vein that receives blood from tributaries from both ventricles; runs in the posterior interventricular sulcus

minoxidil (Loniten)
an antihypertensive agent

minute ventilation (V̇E)
the amount of air moved into or out of the lungs per unit time

mitochondrial enzyme
enzyme (e.g., pyruvate dehydrogenase, lactate dehydrogenase) involved in the exhange and transport of energy within the mitochondrion

mitral area
the region of the chest (at the cardiac apex) where the normal and pathologic sounds made by the mitral valve are traditionally said to be best appreciated

mitral valve prolapse
the excessive retrograde movement of the mitral valve into the left atrium during left ventricular systole

monoamine oxidase (MAO)
an oxidoreductase, containing flavin, that oxidizes amines to aldehydes or ketones, releasing NH_3 and H_2O_2

morphine
the major alkaloid of opium; used as an analgesic, a sedative, and an anxiolytic

mucociliary transport
the action of the cilia in mobilizing the mucus overlying the mucosa of the tracheobronchial tree

mucokinetic
an agent capable of enhancing the mobilization of mucus

mucolytic
an agent capable of dissolving, digesting, or liquifying mucus

mucopolysaccharidoses
a group of lysosomal storage diseases that are characterized by a disorder in metabolism of glycosaminoglycans (mucopolysaccharides)

mucopurulent
containing both mucus and pus

mucous cells
bronchial epithelial cells that secrete mucus; sometimes called *goblet cells*

multifocal
having more than one point of origin

multigated acquisition or angiogram (MUGA) imaging
a process by which a radioisotope is injected as a bolus and allowed to equilibrate within the vasculature, the cardiac cycle is divided into 12 to 28 frames (with the R wave as the reference point), and several hundred cardiac cycles are imaged; radionuclide angiography; gated equilibrium blood-pool imaging

muscarinic
characterizes the effects of muscarine on cholinergic receptors located at the interfaces between the postganglionic neurons and the effector cells of all parasympathetic terminal synapses and some specialized sympathetic postganglionic cholinergic branches

myalgia
muscular pain

myasthenia gravis
a chronic progressive muscular weakness unaccompanied by atrophy; usually begins in the muscles of the face and throat

Mycobacterium avium-intracellulare
an aerobic, nonmotile bacteria containing gram-positive, acid-fast, straight, or slightly curved rods

Mycobacterium tuberculosis
an aerobic, nonmotile bacteria containing gram-positive, acid-fast, straight, or slightly curved rods that causes tuberculosis; tubercle bacillus

myocardial infarction
a local arrest or sudden insufficiency of arterial blood supply that produces a macroscopic area of necrosis in the heart

myocarditis
an inflammation of the muscular walls of the heart

myocardium
the muscular middle layer of tissue in the heart; formed from the inner layer of the myoepicardial mantle; also used in general reference to the heart as a whole

myocytes
muscle cells

myoepicardial mantle
a thickening of the splanchnic mesenchyme around the outside of the endocardial heart tube

myofibrillar
pertaining to the fine longitudinal fibrils occurring in skeletal or cardiac muscle fibers

myofilaments
the ultramicroscopic threads of filamentous proteins making up myofibrils in striated muscle; thick myofilaments contain myosin, and thin myofilaments contain actin

myogenic
beginning in or starting from muscle

myogenic rhythm
the intrinsic, spontaneous rhythm possessed by each cardiac myocyte

myopathy
any condition or disease that hinders or impairs the function of muscle cells

myotonic muscular dystrophy
a slowly progressive disease, with onset typically in the third decade, inherited by autosomal dominant transmission; characterized by muscular atrophy and generalized weakness, deterioration of vision, lenticular opacities, ptosis, and slurred speech

myxoma
a benign neoplasm derived from connective tissue

nares
nostrils

nasal cannula
a device for the delivery of low-flow supplemental oxygen; generally a tube with two prongs that fit into the nostrils

nasal cavity
the irregularly shaped space bounded by the nares anteriorly, the buccal roof inferiorly, the cranial base superiorly, and the oropharynx posteriorly; divided into three regions: vestibular, olfactory, and respiratory

nasal cavity, olfactory region of the
the superior nasal concha, the intervening septum and roof of the nasal cavity

nasal cavity, respiratory region of the
the inferoposterior portion of the nasal cavity bounded by the olfactory region

superiorly, the vestibular region anteriorly, and the posterior nasal apertures posteriorly

nasal cavity, vestibular region (vestibule) of the
the area extending from the nares backward and upward about two thirds of an inch to the limen nasi

nasal conchae
shell-shaped structures projecting into the nasal cavity from the lateral wall toward the medial wall

nasal endotrachael tube
a flexible, hollow cylinder, inserted through the nose and into the trachea to provide an airway

nasal pharyngeal airway
a short rubber tube inserted through the nares into the hypopharynx that is used to maintain airway patency

nasal septum
the medial wall that separates the nasal cavity into two chambers

nasalis muscle
the muscle arising lateral to the nasal notch of the maxilla spreading into an aponeurosis from its opposite-side counterpart over the bridge of the nose and an aponeurosis from the procerus, as well as attaching to the alar cartilages (muscle that flares the anterior nasal aperture)

natriuresis
the urinary excretion of sodium; commonly designates enhanced sodium excretion, which may occur in certain diseases or as a result of the administration of diuretic drugs

natriuretic
a chemical compound that may be used as a means of retarding the tubular reabsorption of sodium ions from glomerular filtrate, thereby resulting in greater amounts of that ion in the urine

Naughton exercise test protocol
a graded treadmill exercise test protocol consisting of stages of variable (tester choice) duration with incremental speed and grade change at each stage

neck of the rib
the portion of the rib that extends from the head to the body or shaft of the rib

necrotizing
any pathologic condition that causes the death of cells

neonate
a newborn infant; usually refers to the infant in the first 28 days of life

nephron
a portion of the kidney; consists of the renal corpuscle, the proximal convo-

luted tubule, both limbs of Henle's loop, the distal convoluted tubule, and the collecting tubule

nephrotoxicity
the quality of being toxic to the cells of the kidney

neuroblastoma
a malignant neoplasm that is characterized by immature, poorly differentiated nerve cells of embryonic type

neurogenic
anything that originates in, starts from, or is caused by the nervous system or nerve impulses

neurotoxin
an antibody that causes destruction of ganglion and cortical cells

neurotropic
something that has an affinity for the nervous system

neutropenia
the condition of having too few neutrophils in the circulating blood

nicotinic
characterizes the effect of nicotine on cholinergic receptors found at the junctions between the preganglionic and postganglionic neurons of both branches of the autonomic nervous system and at the neuromuscular junctions of skeletal muscle fibers

nifedipine (Procardia)
a calcium channel-blocking and vasodilating agent

nitrogen washout method
a pulmonary function test used to measure lung volumes and gas distribution within the lungs; the subject breathes 100% oxygen for 7 minutes, and then the concentration of N_2 in the alveolar gas at the end of a forced expiration is measured

nitroglycerin
a vasodilating agent

nodal myocytes
specialized cardiac muscle cells that contain few myofibrils and an atypical sacrotubular system; primarily located in clusters in both the sinoatrial and atrioventricular nodes; have a faster myogenic rhythm than all other myocytes; have an impulse conduction rate that is slower than Purkinje's but faster than transitional or working myocytes

Nomina Anatomica
the system of anatomic nomenclature adopted by the International Congress of Anatomists

non-Hodgkin's lymphoma
a neoplasm of the lymphoid tissue other than Hodgkin's disease

non-insulin-dependent diabetes mellitus (NIDDM)
a metabolic disease that does not require insulin therapy in which lipid and protein utilization are increased and carbohydrate utilization is decreased as the result of a relative or absolute insulin deficiency; type II diabetes

noncaseating
a type of coagulation necrosis in which the necrotic material contains a mixture of protein and fat (resembling cheese) that is absorbed very slowly; typically occurs in tuberculosis

norepinephrine (Levophed)
a catecholamine hormone that possesses the excitatory actions of epinephrine but has minimal inhibitory effects; it has feeble effects on bronchial smooth muscle and metabolic processes and differs from epinephrine in its cardiovascular action, chiefly vasoconstriction, exerting little effect on cardiac output

normal flora
the population of microorganisms that normally inhabit the internal or external surfaces of healthy individuals

normal sinus rhythm
the cardiac rhythm of depolarization that originates in and proceeds from the sinoatrial node

nosocomial
pertains to or originates in the hospital; usually refers to a hospital-acquired infection

obesity
the condition of abnormal amounts of fat in the subcutaneous connective tissues

obesity hypoventilation syndrome
a condition of acidemia and hypercarbia associated with reduced alveolar ventilation secondary to obesity; the chest wall is too heavy to move in the reclined position

obligate intracellular parasite
an organism that must live within the cells of its host to survive

oblique fissure
the main or primary groove separating the upper and middle lobes from the lower lobe of the right lung and the upper and lower lobes of the left lung

oblique sinus
a cul-de-sac formed behind the left atrium by the epicardial coverings of the venae cavae and pulmonary veins

oblique view
a frontal radiograph in which the patient stands diagonally at an angle of 45 to 60 degrees to the film cassette

obliterating bronchitis
an inflammation of the mucosal lining of the bronchi in which the exudate is not expectorated but becomes organized, obliterating the affected bronchial lumen; bronchitis obliterans

obstructive jaundice
the yellowish staining of the skin and sclerae by bile pigments that results from an obstruction to the flow of bile into the duodenum

opportunistic infection
the multiplication of parasitic organisms in individuals whose immune systems have become compromised

oral endotracheal tube
a flexible, hollow cylinder that is inserted through the mouth into the trachea to provide an airway

oral pharyngeal airway
a short rubber or plastic device inserted into the mouth to maintain the patency of the airway to the hypopharynx

orthopnea
a discomfort on breathing in any but the erect sitting or standing position

orthostatic hypotension
the low blood pressure that occurs with rapid changes in upright posture

orthotopic
the normal or usual position

orthotopic heart transplantation
transplantation of the heart in which the native heart is removed and the donor heart is placed in its position

osmolality
the osmotic concentration; the number of osmoles of a solute per kilogram of solvent

ossification
the formation of bone

osteodystrophy
the formation of abnormal or defective bone

osteogenesis imperfecta
a condition of abnormal fragility and plasticity of the bones

osteoporosis
a reduction in the amount of bone or the atrophy of skeletal tissue

oversew
to close or join with sutures

overshoot
the momentary reversal of membrane potential of a cell during an action potential

oxidative capacity
the potential to combine elements or radicals with oxygen or to lose electrons

oxidative phosphorylation
the formation of high-energy phosphoric bonds from the energy released by the dehydrogenation of various substrates

oximeter
an instrument that determines the oxygen saturation of a blood sample photoelectrically

oxygen hood
a supplemental oxygen delivery device that covers the entire head; generally used in the neonatal setting

oxygen pulse
the volume of oxygen extracted by the peripheral tissues or the volume of oxygen added to the pulmonary blood per heart beat

oxygen saturation
refers to the percentage of hemoglobin that is bound with oxygen

oxygen tent
a supplementary oxygen delivery device that covers the upper torso

oxygen toxicity
the impairment of normal bodily functions (e.g., visual and hearing abnormalities, dyspnea, muscular twitching, anxiety, confusion, incoordination, and convulsions) as a result of breathing concentrations of oxygen that are too high

palliative
mitigating; reducing the severity of; denoting a method of treatment of a disease or of its symptoms

pallor
paleness of the skin

palm cup
an adjunctive aid to the performance of chest percussion used in efforts to mobilize excessive pulmonary secretions

palpitation
a pulsation of the heart that is perceptible to the patient

panacinar emphysema
the diffuse, generalized destruction of alveolar structural components

pancarditis
an inflammation of all the structures of the heart

pancreatitis
an inflammation of the pancreas

papillary muscles
projections of cardiac muscle that terminate in the chordae tendineae

paradoxical
other than that which normally occurs

paranasal sinuses
the frontal, ethmoidal, sphenoidal, and maxillary sinuses

paraseptal emphysema
the destruction of alveolar septa and the reduction in the number of alveoli involving the periphery of the pulmonary lobules

parasympathetic nervous system
one of two parts of the autonomic nervous system; the innervation pathway is composed of two motor neurons: the preganglionic neurons compose the visceral efferent nuclei of the brain stem and the lateral columns of the second through fourth sacral segments of the spinal cord; the ganglia are either intramural ganglia within the organ to be innervated or lie nearby; the pre- and postganglionic neural transmitter is traditionally said to be acetylcholine

parasympatholytic
a drug that inhibits cholinergic receptors of the autonomic nervous system

parasympathomimetic
a drug that stimulates cholinergic receptors of the autonomic nervous system

parathyroid hormone
a peptide substance formed in the parathyroid glands that plays a role in calcium deposition and resorption in bone

parenchyma
the specific cells of a gland or organ contained in and supported by the connective tissue framework or stroma

parenteral
via other than an intestinal route; referring to the means by which a medication may be administered (e.g., subcutaneous, intramuscular, intravenous)

parenteral nutrition
the administration of nutritive material by other than an intestinal route; usually via an intravenous or subcutaneous route

paresis
partial or incomplete paralysis

parietal layer
the outer portion of the serous pericardium that is supported by the fibrous pericardium

parietal pleura
the serous membrane that covers the inner surface of the chest wall, the exposed part of the diaphragm and the mediastinum

paroxysmal atrial tachycardia (PAT)
recurrent episodes of rapid heart rate (in excess of 100 beats per minute), with abrupt onset and cessation, originating from an ectopic focus in the atria

paroxysmal supraventricular tachycardia
recurrent episodes of rapid heart rate

(in excess of 100 beats per minute), with abrupt onset and cessation, originating from an ectopic focus in the atria or atrioventricular node

partial expiratory flow volume (PEFV)
a pulmonary function test that may be used to reveal low forced expiratory rates in children

partial thromboplastin time (PTT)
the time it takes for a fibrin clot to form after calcium and a phospholipid have been added to a blood sample; a test of the intrinsic clotting system; activated partial prothrombin time

patent ductus arteriosus (PDA)
a condition in which the vessel that connects the pulmonary artery with the descending aorta in the fetus does not close after birth

pathogenic
anything that causes disease or abnormality

peak expiratory flow (PEF)
the maximum flow of gas at the beginning of a forced expiratory maneuver

peak expiratory flow rate (PEFR)
the highest point on the expiratory curve of a flow-volume loop

pectinate muscles
muscular ridges running across the walls of the auricula of the atria

pectoralis major muscle
an accessory inspiratory muscle arising from the medial third of the clavicle, from the lateral part of the anterior surface of the manubrium and body of the sternum, and from the costal cartilages of the first six ribs to insert onto the lateral lip of the crest of the greater tubercle of the humerus

pectoralis minor muscle
an accessory inspiratory muscle arising from the second to fifth or the third to sixth ribs to insert onto the medial side of the coracoid process

pectus carinatum
a forward projection (much like the keel of a boat) of the sternum; pigeon breast

pectus excavatum
a posterior displacement of the sternum; funnel chest

penetrating wound
trauma that results in disruption of the continuity of the tissue at the surface of the body and extends into the underlying tissue or body cavity

peptic ulcer
a lesion of the alimentary mucosal surface, usually in the stomach or duodenum

percutaneous transluminal coronary angioplasty (PTCA)
a procedure for enlarging the lumen of a narrowed artery; a balloon-tipped catheter is introduced into the artery to be dilated, inflated, and removed

perfusate
the fluid used for perfusion

perfusion
the transporting of dissolved and bound gases to and from the lungs and the cells in the blood

peribronchial
in close proximity to or surrounding a bronchus or the bronchi

pericardial effusion
the escape of fluid (e.g., vascular fluid) into the pericardial space

pericardial friction rub; pericardial rub
a creaking sound caused by the rubbing together of the inflamed pericardial surfaces as the heart contracts and relaxes

pericardial sac
the fibroserous membrane consisting of mesothelium and submesothelium connective tissue covering the heart and the beginning of the great vessels

pericardial tamponade
a reduction of the venous return to the heart as the result of fluid in the pericardial space

pericardiocentesis
the drainage of fluid from the pericardium by insertion of a hollow needle into the pericardial space

pericarditis
an inflammation of the pericardial sac surrounding the heart

pericardium
the fibroserous membrane covering the heart and the beginning of the great vessels; forms the boundaries of the anterior, middle, and posterior compartments of the mediastinum

perinatal asphyxia
the impairment or absence of gas exchange (oxygen and carbon dioxide) as the result of ventilatory impairment at any time in the period from the twenty-eighth week of gestation through the seventh day after delivery

peripheral neuropathy
any disease involving the peripheral nerves

peripheral vascular disease
any occlusive process involving the vascular beds of the peripheral tissues

peritoneal hemodialysis
the removal of soluble substances and

water from the body by intermittently introducing and removing a dialysate into and from the peritoneal cavity

peritonitis
the inflammation of the peritoneum

persistent fetal circulation
a condition in which the vascular shunts (e.g., foramen ovale, ductus arteriosus) that are present in the fetus fail to close following birth

pertussis
an acute inflammation of the larynx, trachea, and bronchi characterized by recurrent bouts of exhaustive spasmodic coughing that ends in stridor; whooping cough

phagocytosis
the ingestion and digestion of solid substances by cells

pharmacodynamics
the study of the mechanism by which a drug achieves its effect within the body

pharmacokinetics
the study of the movement of a drug within the body; particularly the uptake, distribution, elimination, and transformation of a drug within the body after it has been administered

pharyngeal isthmus
the space between the free edge of the soft palate and the posterior wall of the pharynx; the juncture of the nasopharynx and oropharynx

phase I cardiac rehabilitation
the program of education and exercise established to assist an individual with heart disease achieve optimal physical and psychological functioning that begins in the acute phase of recovery; typically begins in the coronary critical care unit or the cardiac stepdown unit

phase II cardiac rehabilitation
the program of education and exercise established to assist an individual with heart disease achieve optimal physical and psychological functioning that begins in the subacute phase of recovery; typically the initial outpatient phase of rehabilitation

phase III cardiac rehabilitation
the continuing program of education and exercise established to assist an individual with heart disease achieve optimal physical and psychological functioning that begins in the acute phase of recovery; typically when intensive, high-intensity rehabilitation occurs

phase IV cardiac rehabilitation
the ongoing or maintenance program of education and exercise established to assist an individual with heart disease

achieve optimal physical and psychological functioning

phenylalanine-hydroxylase pathway
an intrahepatic intermediary amino acid metabolic pathway

pheochromocytoma
a typically benign neoplasm derived from cells in the adrenal medulla, characterized by the secretion of catecholamines

phonation
the creation of sounds by means of the vocal cords

phosphocreatinine
a compound of creatinine with phosphoric acid; an intermediary energy source, that provides phosphate for the resynthesis of ATP from ADP

phosphodiesterase
an enzyme that splits the phosphodiester bonds of some nucleotides

photophobia
an abnormal sensitivity to or fear of light

physiologic dead space
parts of the lung that are ventilated although they receive no blood supply and therefore cannot participate in gas exchange

pindolol (Visken)
a beta-adrenergic blocking agent used in the treatment of hypertension

plasmapheresis
the removal of whole blood from the body, followed by centrifugal separation into its cellular components and their reinfusion in a saline suspension, thereby reducing the plasma volume without depleting the cell volume

platelet-derived growth factor (PDGF)
a substance derived from platelets that causes the proliferation of endothelial tissue at the site of an arterial sclerotic lesion

pleura
the serous membrane enveloping the lungs and lining the walls of the pleural cavity

pleural abrasion
the excoriation of the mucous membrane of the pleura

pleural effusion
the escape of fluid (e.g., vascular exudate) into the pleural space

pleural pressure
the pressure within the pleural space between the visceral and parietal pleurae

pleural rub
a friction sound created by the rubbing

together of the roughened surfaces of the parietal and visceral pleurae

pleural space
the potential space between the parietal and visceral pleura

pleurectomy
the excision of the pleura, usually the parietal pleura

pleurisy
the inflammation of the pleura; pleuritis

pneumatocele
a thin-walled cavity within the lung; characteristic of staphylococcal pneumonia

pneumococcal pneumonia
an inflammation of the lungs due to infection with *Streptococcus pneumoniae* bacteria

pneumoconiosis
an inflammatory fibrosis of the lungs as the result of inhaling dust particles incidental to occupational exposure

***Pneumocystis carinii* pneumonia**
a cystic infection of the lungs caused by the protozoan *Pneumocystis carinii;* pneumocystosis

pneumomediastinum
air within the mediastinal tissues

pneumonectomy
the surgical removal of a single lung

pneumonia
an inflammation of the lungs, particularly as the result of a pathogen

pneumonitis
an inflammation of the lungs

pneumotaxic center
the region of the medulla oblongata concerned with respiration

pneumothorax
air in the pleural cavity

poliomyelitis
an inflammation of the gray matter of the spinal cord

polyarteritis nodosa
an inflammation, with eosinophilic infiltration, of the small or medium-sized arteries

polycythemia
an excessive amount of red corpuscles in the blood

polymyositis
the simultaneous inflammation of several voluntary muscles

polyneuritis
the simultaneous inflammation of several spinal nerves

polyp
any mass of tissue that bulges or pro-

jects outward from the normal surface level

porphyrin
four pyrrole groups cyclically linked by methylene bridges

portopulmonary shunting
a potential complication of liver disease

positive end-expiratory pressure (PEEP)
a mechanical ventilatory maneuver in which a thresholdlike resistance applied at the end of exhalation permits the pressure in the ventilator circuit to drop only to a set level above atmospheric pressure

positive expiratory pressure (PEP) mask
a device used to increase the functional residual volume and enhance oxygenation in the treatment of some pulmonary disorders

positive inotropic
the property of being able to enhance the contractility of a muscle

positron emission tomography (PET)
tomographic imaging of tissues formed by tracing the path of photons created by the collision of positrons emitted by a radioactive biochemical (previously administered to the patient) with the electrons normally present in the cells

posterior basal segmental bronchus
the portion of the tracheobronchial tree arising from the right or left lower lobe bronchus that is distributed to the posterior basal segment

posterior interventricular artery
the continuation of the right coronary artery on the posterior surface of the heart

posterior leaflet of the mitral valve
the smaller of the two cusps of the mitral valve; also called the ventricular, mural, or posterolateral leaflet

posterior papillary muscles
muscles that arise at the apical ventriculoseptal juncture in the right ventricle; from the diaphragmatic wall of the left ventricle

posterior pulmonary plexus
a network of nerves formed by branches from the vagus nerves, the deep cardiac plexus and the second and fifth thoracic sympathetic ganglia, and the left recurrent laryngeal nerve supplying posterior branches of the bronchi and the pulmonary and bronchial vessels

posterior segmental bronchus
the portion of the tracheobronchial tree arising from the right upper lobe bron-

chus that is distributed to the posterior segment

posterior vein of the left ventricle
vein that accompanies the circumflex branch of the left coronary artery across the diaphragmatic surface of the left ventricle

posteroanterior (PA) view
the image produced by the roentgen-ray beam as it passes through the patient from posterior to anterior

posterolateral thoracotomy
a surgical incision into the posterolateral aspect of the chest wall that provides access to the underlying tissues

postperfusion syndrome
a condition of decreased cardiac output in conjunction with other cardiovascular symptoms that arise following the use of a perfusion pump in cardiovascular surgical procedures

postpericardiotomy syndrome
the occurrence, often repeatedly, of the symptoms of pericarditis (with or without febrile episodes) weeks to months after cardiac surgery

postural drainage
the use of gravity to assist or facilitate the removal of fluids or secretions from the lungs by positioning the body in such a manner as to place the involved segment or segments perpendicular to the forces of gravity

postural hypotension
a form of low blood pressure that occurs on the assumption of upright postures; orthostatic hypotension

pravastatin
an antihyperlipidemic agent; acts by inhibiting cholesterol synthesis

prazosin (Minipress)
an antihypertensive agent

prediabetic
a state of potential diabetes mellitus, with normal glucose tolerence but with increased risk of developing diabetes

prednisone
a dehydrogenated analogue of cortisone, having the same uses and actions

preinfarction angina
a severe constricting chest pain, often radiating from the precordium, that frequently precedes a myocardial infarction

preload
the amount of tension on the muscular wall of the ventricle before it contracts

premature atrial complex (PAC, APC)
an extrasystole arising from an ectopic atrial focus that occurs before the usual

or expected time of the normal depolarization wave

premature junctional complex
an extrasystole arising from an ectopic atrioventricular nodal focus that occurs before the usual or expected time of the normal depolarization wave

premature ventricular complex (PVC, VPC)
an extrasystole arising from an ectopic ventricular focus that occurs before the usual or expected time of the normal depolarization wave

preprandial
before a meal

pressor
an agent that enhances vasomotor tone and increases blood pressure

pressoreceptors
pressosensitive; capable of receiving as stimuli changes in pressure, especially in blood pressure

pressure support ventilation (PSV)
a mode of mechanical ventilatory assistance in which a preselected positive pressure is delivered each time the ventilator is triggered by the patient's spontaneous inspiratory effort

primary acid-base disorder
a disturbance of the normal acid-base balance to which other complications are attributable

primary bronchi
the main bronchi arising from the bifurcation of the trachea; right and left

primitive pulmonary vein
the small venous conduit between the nonfunctioning lungs and the left atrium

Prinzmetal's angina
a form of angina that is not precipitated by cardiac exertion; generally is of longer duration, more severe, and associated with unusual ECG manifestations (e.g., ST segment elevation) when compared with typical angina pectoris

procainamide (Pronestyl)
an antiarrhythmic agent that depresses the irritability of cardiac muscle; used in the treatment of ventricular arrhythmias

procerus muscle
a small slip of muscle originating as a continuation of the occipitofrontalis and attaching to the fascia covering the lower part of the nasal bone and the upper part of the lateral nasal cartilage (muscle that wrinkles the skin of the nose)

prodromal
an early or premonitory symptom of a disease

professorial position
a standing posture in which the trunk is forward leaning, with the upper body supported on extended arms

progressive systemic sclerosis
a progressive disease characterized by the formation of hyalinized and thickened collagenous fibrous tissues, thickening of the skin and adhesion to the underlying tissues, submucosal fibrosis of the esophagus, pulmonary and myocardial fibrosis, renal vascular changes, Raynaud's phenomenon, atrophy of the soft tissues, and osteoporosis of the distal phalanges; scleroderma

prokaryote
a single-cell organ that lacks nuclear organization, mitotic capacity, or complex organelles

prophylactically
in a manner to prevent disease

propranolol (Inderal)
a beta-adrenergic blocking agent

prostaglandin
a class of physiologically active substances capable of effecting vasodilation, vasoconstriction, stimulation of intestinal or bronchial smooth muscle, uterine stimulation, and lipid metabolism

protein-calorie deficiency
the primary nutritional abnormality contributing to malnutrition

proteinuria
the presence of urinary protein in concentrations greater than 0.3 gram in 24-hour urine collection or in concentrations greater than 1 gram per liter in a random urine collection on two or more occasions

prothrombin
a glycoprotein in the blood that is converted to thrombin in the presence of thromboplastin and calcium ions

prothrombin time (PT)
the time it takes for a clot to form after thromboplastin and calcium are added to the blood; the greater the time it takes, the lower the level of prothrombin

pseudohypertrophy
the increase in the size of an organ due to an increase of some tissue other than itself

psittacosis
an infectious disease caused by *Chlamydia psittaci*; characterized by flulike (in mild cases) or bronchopneumonia-like (in severe cases) symptoms

ptosis
the prolapse of an organ or tissue

pulmonary alveoli
the final saclike dilatations of the terminal sacs in the lung

pulmonary arterial hypertension
a condition of abnormally high pulmonary arterial blood pressure

pulmonary arterioles
the smallest subdivision of the pulmonary arterial tree before the pulmonary capillary bed

pulmonary artery balloon counterpulsation (PABC)
a means of assisting right ventricular ejection by reducing pulmonary artery pressure just before and during ventricular systole with an intrapulmonary-arterial balloon pump activated by an automatic mechanism triggered by the ECG

pulmonary artery catheter
a thin, flexible, flow-directed, balloon-tipped catheter introduced into the pulmonary artery used to monitor cardiovascular pressures

pulmonary artery pressure
the blood pressure in the pulmonary artery

pulmonary artery wedge pressure
the pressure obtained by wedging a flow-directed, balloon-tipped catheter into a small branch of the pulmonary artery so that the flow of blood from behind is blocked and the pressure beyond can be sampled; normally not greater than 12 mm Hg; pulmonary wedge pressure; pulmonary capillary wedge pressure

pulmonary capillaries
an intermeshed network of blood vessels, whose walls consist of a single layer of cells, in the septa and walls of the alveolar ducts and alveoli; the bridge between pulmonary arterioles and venules

pulmonary congestion
the presence of an abnormal amount of fluid in the interstitial spaces of the lungs

pulmonary edema
the accumulation of an excessive amount of fluid in the alveolar spaces of the lungs

pulmonary emboli
a detached piece of thrombus occluding a blood vessel in the lungs

pulmonary fibroplasia
an abnormal increase of nonneoplastic fibrous tissue in the lungs

pulmonary insufficiency
failure of the pulmonic valve to close

completely, allowing regurgitation of blood

pulmonary interstitial edema
the presence of an abnormal amount of fluid in the interstitial spaces of the lungs; pulmonary congestion

pulmonary ligament
the extension of the pleural covering below and behind the hilus from the root of the lung

pulmonary perfusion
the pulmonary blood flow

pulmonary trunk
the common conduit of the pulmonary artery before its bifurcation into right and left branches

pulmonary veins
the four veins returning oxygenated blood from the lungs to the left atrium

pulmonic area (space)
the region of the chest (second intercostal space, along the left sternal border) where the normal and pathologic sounds made by the pulmonic valve are traditionally said to be best appreciated

pulmonic stenosis
a narrowing of the pulmonary valvular orifice or the right ventricular outflow tract

pulmonologist
a physician specializing in pulmonary medicine

pulse oximeter
an instrument that photoelectrically determines the oxygen saturation of arterial blood as it courses through the peripheral arteries with each pulse

pulsus alternans
the mechanical alteration of the pulse typified by a regular rhythm and alternating strong and weak pulses; characteristic of significant myocardial disease

pulsus paradoxus
a marked variation in the cardiac stroke volume with respiratory effort, such that the pulse becomes stronger with expiration and weaker with inspiration; characteristic of pericardial effusion or restrictive pericarditis

Purkinje's fibers
the terminal projections of the specialized conduction system of the heart, spread in an interlaced network throughout the endocardium of the ventricles

Purkinje's myocytes
the specialized cardiac muscle cells that are wider and shorter, contain fewer myofibrils and more mitochondria, and have larger intercalated discs than working myocytes; primarily located in

terminal branches of the conduction system of the heart; have a myogenic rhythm that is slower than nodal myocytes but faster than working or transitional myocytes; have an impulse conduction rate that is faster than all other myocytes

purulent
containing or forming pus

quadratus lumborum muscle
an accessory inspiratory muscle arising from the iliac crest and transverse processes of the lumbar vertebrae upward to attach to the twelfth rib

quantitative pilocarpine iontophoresis
the introduction of a parasympathomimetic agent into the tissues by means of an electric current for the purpose of determining the amount of salt in the sweat

quinidine (Duraquin, Cardioquin)
an alkaloid of cinchona, a stereoisomer of quinine; used in the treatment of atrial fibrillation and flutter

R on T phenomenon
the occurrence of an effective premature ventricular depolarization (R wave) during the relative refractory period of the preceding normal complex (T wave)

radiolucency
the characteristic of being relatively penetrable by roentgen rays

radiopacity
the condition of being relatively impenetrable by roentgen rays

rales
an adventitious sound heard on auscultation of breath sounds; characteristically an inspiratory sound; postulated to be caused by the mixing of air with thin secretions in the distal, small airways, or the popping open of collapsed alveoli

rapid-filling phase
the phase that occurs once the mitral valve opens and the ventricular volume begins rising as the ventricle passively fills

rate-pressure product (RPP)
the product of the multiplication of the heart rate by the systolic blood pressure; a parameter used to monitor the onset of angina in some patients

rating of perceived exertion (RPE)
a subjective scale of exercise intensity

Raynaud's phenomenon
the paroxysmal cyanosis of the digits due to contraction of the digital arteries and arterioles

receptor-G protein
guanine nucleotide-binding regulatory proteins (G proteins) are the links between the many different receptors on a cell's surface and their catalytic units or other effectors within the cell

refractory period
the time following effective myocardial stimulation during which the myocytes fail to respond to a stimulus of threshold intensity

renal failure
the state of insufficiency or nonperformance of the kidneys

renal transplantation
the implantation of a kidney from a compatible donor to restore kidney function in a recipient suffering from renal failure

renin
the enzyme that converts angiotensinogen to angiotensin

reperfusion
the reestablishment of blood flow to a tissue

repolarization
the process of repolarizing the cell, fiber, or membrane after depolarization

residual volume (RV)
the volume of air that remains in the lungs after a forceful expiratory effort

resistance to flow
the force acting in opposition to the movement of a fluid or gas

resistance vessels
the arterioles and precapillary sphincters that provide peripheral resistance to blood flow

resistive inspiratory muscle training
a technique of repeatedly inhaling through progressively smaller orifices in an effort to increase the strength and endurance of the inspiratory musculature

resonance
the sound produced by percussing on a part that can vibrate freely

respiration
breathing; taking in of oxygen and throwing off the products of oxidation in the tissues, mainly carbon dioxide and water

respiratory acidosis
inadequate pulmonary ventilation that results in the retention of carbon dioxide and the decrease in blood pH

respiratory alkalosis
hyperventilation that results in an abnormal loss of CO_2 and an increase in blood pH

respiratory bronchioles
the part of the respiratory passages after the terminal bronchioles; the first level at which gas exchange may occur

respiratory center
the region of the medulla oblongata concerned with the control of respiration

respiratory depressant
any agent that acts to reduce the activity of the respiratory center or otherwise retard pulmonary ventilation

respiratory distress syndrome (RDS)
a condition of acute lung injury from a variety of causes; characterized by interstitial or alveolar edema, or both, and hemorrhage associated with hyaline membrane, proliferation of collagen fibers, and epithelial swelling

respiratory failure
the inability of the respiratory system to ventilate the alveoli

respiratory stimulant
any agent that enhances the activity of the respiratory center

respiratory syncytial virus
a paramyxovirus that forms a multinucleated protoplasmic mass in tissue culture; causes mild respiratory infection in adults but can cause bronchitis and bronchopneumonia in children

resting membrane potential
the electrical potential inside a cell membrane, relative to the extracellular fluid when there is no action potential

restrictive
any condition that limits the normal capacity of an organ system

restrictive cardiomyopathy
a disease of the myocardium characterized by marked endocardial scarring of the ventricles with resulting impaired diastolic filling

restrictive changes
the fibrosis and scarring that are typically associated with restrictive diseases

restrictive lung dysfunction
an abnormal reduction in pulmonary ventilation

reticulation
the formation of a fine network formed by specific structures with cells, formed by cells themselves, or formed by the connective tissue fibers between cells

reticulogranular pattern
a network of granulelike shadows in a radiograph of an infant with infant respiratory distress syndrome (IRDS); the radiographic presentation of IRDS

reticulonodular pattern
a network of nodulelike shadows throughout both lungs; the typical ra-

diographic presentation of idiopathic pulmonary fibrosis

retinopathy
a noninflammatory degenerative disease of the retina

rhabdomyolysis
an acute, fulminating disease that destroys skeletal muscle

rhabdomyosarcoma
a malignant neoplasm derived from skeletal muscle

rheumatoid arthritis (RA)
a systemic disease that affects the connective tissues of the body; characterized by extension of synovial tissue over the articular cartilages with cartilaginous thickening and erosion in multiple joints

rhinorrhea
a discharge from the nasal mucosal lining

rhinovirus
a genus of acid-labile viruses (of which there are more than 100 antigenic types) associated with the common cold in humans and foot-and-mouth disease in cattle

rhonchi
adventitious sounds occurring during inspiration or expiration, heard on auscultation of the lungs, and caused by turbulence created when air passing through the midsized and larger bronchi reaches the secretions in the lumen

rhythmicity
the cadence or pattern of recurrence of a phenomenon

ribavirin (tribavirin, Virazole)
an antiviral agent used to treat respiratory syncytial virus

right anterior ventricular rami
branches to the right ventricle from the right coronary artery

right atrial pressure
the blood pressure in the right atrium

right atrium
the chamber of the heart that receives blood from the venae cavae

right auricle
the small conical projection from the right atrium; remnant of the right portion of the primitive atrium

right bundle branches
offshoots of the right division of His's bundle in the right ventricle

right coronary artery
the artery that arises from the right anterolateral surface of the aorta and passes between the auricular appendage

of the right atrium and the pulmonary trunk

right coronary plexus
formed from contributions of both the deep and superficial parts of the cardiac plexus; follows the distribution of the right coronary artery, supplying the right atrium and ventricle

right dominant coronary arterial system
a condition in which the majority of the blood supply to the heart is provided via the right coronary artery; occurs in approximately 50% of the population

right inferior pulmonary vein
the vein that returns blood from the lower lobe of the right lung to the left atrium

right marginal artery
a branch of the right coronary artery

right marginal vein
the vein that receives blood from the right margin of the heart, sometimes emptying directly into the right atrium or joining the small cardiac vein in the coronary sulcus

right pulmonary artery
the right branch of the pulmonary artery distributed to the right lung; runs behind the ascending aorta, superior vena cava, and upper pulmonary vein but in front of the esophagus and right primary bronchus to the root of the lung

right superior pulmonary vein
the vein that returns blood from the upper and middle lobes of the right lung to the left atrium

right (pulmonary) surface
the right side of the heart that is in contact with the right lung

right-to-left shunt
when blood passes from the right to the left side of the heart without participating in gas exchange; intrapulmonary shunt

right ventricle
one of the two lower chambers of the heart

right ventricular hypertrophy
a condition of increased bulk, but not number, of working myocytes in the right ventricle as the result of an increased resistance to right ventricular outflow

rima glottidis
the fissure between the vocal folds commonly called the glottis

rima vestibuli
the fissure between the vestibular folds

roentgenogram
a radiograph

rotation
the misalignment of the body with respect to the film cassette, which can distort the image represented in a radiograph

rough zone chordae
chordae that arise from a single stem but split into three filaments: one attaches to the free margin of the leaflet, another attaches to the ventricular aspect of the rough zone of the leaflet, and the third attaches to some intermediate position

saccular bronchiectasis
a type of chronic dilation of the bronchi or bronchioles that appear to have a pouchlike shape

saccule of the larynx
a small pouch extending upward from the anterior aspect of the sinus of the larynx

salicylic acid (aspirin)
an analgesic and anti-inflammatory agent

sarcoidosis
a systemic granulomatous disease that predominantly affects the lungs with resulting fibrosis

scaleni muscles
a group of three muscles (anterior, medial, and posterior scalenes) acting as accessory inspiratory muscles to elevate the first and second ribs

scapuloperoneal myopathy
Emery-Dreifuss muscular dystrophy

scintillography
a diagnostic procedure in which a radionuclide is injected intravenously, and a photographic recording of its distribution is made

scoliosis
a condition of lateral curvature of the spine

second-degree atrioventricular block
two types of atrioventricular arrhythmias in which some but not all atrial impulses fail to reach the ventricle, and thus some ventricular depolarizations are dropped; in type I (Wenckebach's), there is progressive lengthening of the atrioventricular conduction time until a ventricular depolarization is dropped; after the dropped cycle the P–R interval returns to normal; in type II, there is a dropped ventricular cycle with or without an alteration in the preceding atrioventricular conduction time

second heart sound (S₂)
the sound created by the closure of the

semilunar valves of the heart; signifies the end of ventricular systole

secondary bronchi
the initial divisions off the primary bronchi; the lobar bronchi: three from the right primary bronchus; two from the left primary bronchus

secondary hypertension
a condition of abnormally high blood pressure that is the result of some directly identifiable cause

secondary lobule
an outmoded term describing a functional unit of the lung; anatomically, the secondary lobules contain as many as fifty primary lobules

selectivity
the ability of a drug to interact with specific receptors on the target tissue and not with other receptors or other tissues

semilunar cusps
the crescentic leaflets of the aortic valve

sensitivity
the probability that, given the presence of a disease, an abnormal test result will indicate the presence of the disease

septomarginal trabecula
the anteroinferior boundary between the inflow and outflow tracts of the right ventricle near the apex

septum primum
the crescent-shaped membrane arising from the dorsocephalic wall of the primitive atrium that initiates the partitioning of the atrium into two chambers; the ends of the septum eventually fuse with the dorsal endocardial cushions of the atrioventricular canal

septum secundum
the crescent-shaped membrane arising from the ventrocranial wall of the atrium on the right side of the septum primum; the ends of the septum reach dorsally toward the sinus venosus

serotype
the antigenic character that distinguishes a subdivision of a species from other strains

serous cavities
hollow spaces filled with serum or a substance having a watery consistency

serous cells
bronchial epithelial cells that secrete mucus

serous pericardium
the inner sac of the pericardial sac consisting of a visceral layer and a parietal layer

serratus anterior muscle
an accessory inspiratory muscle arising from the outer surfaces of the upper eight or nine ribs to attach along the costal aspect of the medial border of the scapula

serratus posterior superior
an accessory inspiratory muscle arising from the lower part of the ligamentum nuchae and the spinous processes of the seventh cervical and the first two or three thoracic vertebrae downward into the upper borders of the second to fourth or fifth ribs

shaft of the rib
the central portion of the rib

shock
a state of profound physical depression subsequent to a severe physical injury or impairment

sick sinus syndrome
a condition of continual, chaotic changes in the configuration of the P wave on ECG; characterized by bradycardia alternating with recurrent ectopic extrasystoles and supraventricular tachycardia

sickle cell disease
an anemic disorder of the red blood cells characterized by crescent- or sickle-shaped erythrocytes and by accelerated hemolysis

silent ischemia
a condition of inadequate blood circulation to the myocardium without the typical accompanying signs or symptoms

silhouette sign
a radiographic finding (demonstrated when the normal line of demarcation between two structures is partially or completely obliterated) used to localize lesions within the lung fields

silicosis
a type of pneumoconiosis that results from occupational exposure (over a period of years) to or inhalation of silica dust; characterized by slow, progressive fibrosis of the lungs

simple mask
a type of supplemental oxygen delivery device

single-chain urokinase plasminogen activator (SCU-PA, pro-urokinase)
a proteinase that converts plasminogen to plasmin

sinoatrial (SA) node
the mass of specialized myocytes that normally acts as the "pacemaker" for the specialized conduction system of the heart

sinus arrhythmia
an extrasystole having an ectopic focus within the atrial tissues of the heart (other than the sinoatrial node)

sinus block
failure of an impulse, generated in the sinoatrial node, to get out of the sinoatrial node

sinus bradycardia
a slow heart rate (less than 60 beats per minute) that has its origin in the sinoatrial node

sinus of the larynx
a fusiform recess between the vestibular and vocal folds

sinus venosus
the dilatation of the heart tube inferior to the atrium that is formed by the proximal portions of the veins

sinusoid
a blood channel in certain organs that is lined by reticuloendothelium

sleep apnea
an absence of breathing caused by an upper airway obstruction during sleep

small cardiac vein
a vein that receives blood from the back of the right atrium and ventricle; runs between the right atrium and ventricle in the coronary sulcus

sodium-calcium antiporter
a carrier mechanism that carries sodium and calcium ions through a membrane in opposite directions; the energy for the transport of the ions is derived from the potential energy of the ions being transported

sodium nitroprusside (Nipride)
a potent intravenous antihypertensive agent

sodium-potassium pump
a biochemical mechanism that uses metabolic energy from ATP to achieve the transport of sodium and potassium ions in opposite directions through a membrane

spasmodic cough
an involuntary, uncontrollable sudden explosive forcing of air through the glottis

specificity
the probability that, given the absence of a disease, a normal test result excludes the disease

sphygmomanometer
an instrument used to determine blood pressure

sphygmomanometry
the determination of blood pressure by means of auscultation and a blood pressure cuff (sphygmomanometer)

spinal cord injury
the damage resulting from trauma to the spinal cord

spinocerebellar
refers to all parts of the cerebellum rostral to the primary fissure; corresponds to the region of distribution of the spinocerebellar tracts

spirogram
a tracing or graphic representation of the depth and rapidity of respiratory movements

spirometric measurement
the determination of pulmonary volumes using a spirometer (a counterbalanced cylindric bell sealed by dipping into a trough of water)

sputum
expectorated matter

squamous metaplasia
the transformation of glandular or mucosal epithelium into stratified squamous epithelium

Starling's forces
the force tending to move or retard a substance across a membrane as the result of the differences between hydrostatic and oncotic pressures

Starling's hypothesis
the idea that net filtration through a capillary is proportional to the transmembrane hydrostatic pressure difference minus the transmembrane oncotic pressure difference

static volumes
pulmonary volumes measured at rest without chest wall movement (e.g., residual volume, functional residual volume)

status asthmaticus
severe, prolonged asthma

steatorrhea
the presence of large amounts of fat in the feces

sternocleidomastoid muscle
an accessory inspiratory muscle that arises by two heads (sternal and clavicular) that unite to extend obliquely upward and laterally across the neck to the mastoid process

sternocostal (anterior)
the surface of the heart in contact with the sternum and ribs

sternotomy
a surgical incision through the sternum

sternum
the breast bone; the tripartite flat bone forming the middle part of the anterior chest wall

steroids
a family of chemical substances that

make up many hormones and vitamin D

streptokinase (Kabikinase, Streptase)
an extracellular metalloenzyme from hemolytic streptococci that disrupts plasminogen, producing plasmin and causing the liquefaction of fibrin

stress
refers to the psychological stimuli that impinge on an individual to produce strain or disequilibrium

stridor
a high-pitched inspiratory or expiratory sound created by an obstruction to air flow, especially an obstruction occurring in the trachea or larynx

stroke volume
the amount of blood ejected from the ventricles with each systolic contraction

strut chordae
the specialized variants of rough zone chordae of the anterior leaflet of the mitral valve; leaflet chordae

subacute
the course of a disease that has moderate severity or duration; denotes a distinction in time between acute and chronic

subepithelial fibrosis
fibrosis occurring beneath the epithelium

sublingual
under the tongue, referring to a parenteral route of drug administration; also subglossal or hypoglossal

submaximal
denoting less than the maximum potential

sudden cardiac death
death within 1 hour of the onset of cardiac symptoms

sulfonamide diuretic
a sulfa-containing agent that increases the amount of urine excreted

summation effect
the normal blending together of the various densities of the soft tissues that overlie one another in a radiograph

superficial (proximal) bronchial veins
an extrapulmonary plexus of veins that communicates freely with the pulmonary veins, ending on the left in either the left superior intercostal vein or the accessory hemiazygos veins and on the right in the azygos vein

superficial cardiac plexus
the ventral part of the network of nerves that make up the cardiac plexus; formed by a branch from the left superior cervical sympathetic ganglion and the lower of the two cervical cardiac

branches of the left vagus nerve; located anterior to the right pulmonary artery, below the arch of the aorta

superior pulmonary veins
the veins that return blood from the left upper, right upper, and middle lobes of the lungs to the left atrium

superior segmental bronchus
the portion of the tracheobronchial tree arising from the right or left lower lobe bronchus that is distributed to the superior segment

superior vena cava
the conduit of blood from the head and neck, upper limbs, and thorax to the right atrium

superior vesical arteries
the remains of the proximal portions of the umbilical arteries of the fetus; supplies the superior portion of the bladder

suppuration
the formation of pus

supravalvular ridges
a linear elevation of tissue in the wall of the aorta that marks the limit of the free borders of the cusps of the aortic valve

supraventricular crest
the boundary between the posteroanterior inflow tract and the anterosuperior outflow tract of the right ventricle

surface-active agent
an agent that acts to reduce the alveolar surface tension

surface tension
the force that results from the interactions of the pressures tending to collapse the alveoli and those tending to expand them

surfactant
a surface-active agent forming a layer over the pulmonary alveolar surfaces that reduces surface tension and alters the relationship between surface tension and surface area, stablizing alveolar volume

symbiotic
any intimate relationship between two species

sympathetic nervous system
one of two parts of the autonomic nervous system; the innervation pathway is composed of two motor neurons: the preganglionic neurons comprise the visceral efferent nuclei of the brain stem and the lateral columns of the thoracic and upper two lumbar segments of the spinal cord; the ganglia are the paravertebral ganglia of the sympathetic trunk and the prevertebral ganglia; the preganglionic neural transmitter is traditionally said to be acetylcholine, and

the postganglionic transmitter is norepinephrine

sympatholytic
a drug that inhibits adrenergic receptors of the autonomic nervous system

sympathomimetic
a drug that stimulates adrenergic receptors of the autonomic nervous system

synchronized intermittent mandatory ventilation (SIMV)
a mode of mechanical ventilatory assistance; the mandatory (preset) ventilator breath is synchronized with the patient's breathing efforts

syncope
temporary loss of consciousness due to generalized cerebral ischemia

systemic lupus erythematosus (SLE)
a generalized connective tissue disorder, characterized by skin eruptions, arthralgia, leukopenia, visceral lesions, and fever; affects mostly middle-aged females

systole
the period of ventricular contraction

systolic blood pressure (SBP)
the maximum pressure of the blood on the walls of the arteries; occurs near the end of the stroke output of the left ventricle

systolic murmur
a periodic sound occurring during the systolic phase of the cardiac cycle and heard during auscultation of the heart; usually attributable to mitral or tricuspid regurgitation or to aortic or pulmonary obstruction

tachypnea
very rapid breathing; polypnea

tamponade
compression of the heart as the result of fluid accumulating within the pericardial sac

tendon of the infundibulum
a fibrous band connecting aortic and pulmonary annuli

tension pneumothorax
the air within the pleural cavity as the result of a communication between the lung and the pleural space in which a valve effect exists; air enters the pleural space on inspiration but is trapped during expiration

terazosin (Hytrin)
an antihypertensive agent; an alpha$_1$-antagonist with actions similar to prazosin but with a longer half-life

terminal bronchioles
the final part of the conducting airways

terminal sacs
the part of the respiratory passages that

develops from the alveolar ducts at the end of the canalicular period of lung development; alveolar sacs

tetralogy of Fallot
the most common cyanosis-producing congenital heart defect consisting of pulmonary stenosis, ventricular septal defect, dextroposition of the aorta, and right ventricular hypertrophy

tetraplegia
paralysis of all four extremities; quadriplegia

thallium exercise stress test
radionuclear perfusion scintigraphy exercise test in which thallium-201 (a radionuclide) is rapidly injected into the blood at near maximal exercise; either treadmill or bicycle ergometer protocols may be used

thebesian veins
a number of minute veins arising in the walls of the heart, most emptying directly into the atria, but a few ending in the ventricles; smallest cardiac veins

thermodilution method
a means of determining the cardiac output; a cold bolus of saline is injected into the right atrium via the proximal lumen of a flow-directed, thermal-sensitive catheter; the resultant temperature change is sensed by a thermistor near the tip of the catheter located in the pulmonary artery

third-degree (complete) atrioventricular block
the pathologic loss of conduction through the atrioventricular junctional tissues; atrioventricular dissociation in which atrial or sinus foci elicit depolarization of the atria, while an idioventricular focus stimulates the ventricles

third heart sound (S₃)
a weak, low-pitched sound occurring in early diastole, soon after the second heart sound; believed to be caused by vibrations of the poorly compliant ventricular wall as it is distended during filling

third-party payer
the source of reimbursement (e.g., an insurance carrier) for services received (e.g., physical therapy) that is different from the individual who received the services

thoracentesis
insertion of a hollow needle into the pleural cavity

thoracic inlet
the upper margin of the thorax; formed by the first thoracic vertebra posteriorly, the superior border of the manubrium anteriorly, and the first ribs laterally

thoracic outlet
the lower margin of the thorax; formed by the twelfth thoracic vertebra posteriorly, the seventh through tenth costal cartilages anteriorly, and the eleventh and twelfth ribs laterally

thoracoabdominal incision
a cut into the abdomen and thorax

thrombin
the enzyme derived from prothrombin (factor II) that converts fibrinogen into fibrin

thrombocytopenia
an abnormally small number of platelets in the blood

thromboembolism
an embolism from a venous thrombus

thrombolysis
the dissolving of a thrombus

thrombophlebitis
the formation of a thrombus as the result of inflammation of a vein

thromboplastin
a substance necessary for the coagulation of blood; catalyzed by calcium, it converts prothrombin to thrombin

thyrotoxicosis
the state produced by excessive quantities of endogenous and exogenous thyroid hormone

tidal volume (VT)
the volume of air normally inhaled and exhaled with each breath during quiet breathing

tissue plasminogen activator (tPA; Activase)
a genetically engineered thrombolytic agent used in conjunction with heparin for the limitation of infarct size following myocardial infarction due to the blockage of coronary arteries by thrombi

titration
a means of adjusting a drug's dosage by repeatedly increasing or decreasing the dose administered until the desired effect is achieved or the undesired effect is eliminated

Todaro's tendon
a tendonous structure extending from the right fibrous trigone of the heart toward the valve of the inferior vena cava

torsades de pointes
paroxysmal ventricular tachycardia; characterized on ECG by runs of 5 to 20 complexes with an undulating QRS axis that progressively changes direction

total lung capacity (TLC)
the maximum volume to which the

lungs can be expanded; it is the sum of all the pulmonary volumes

total peripheral resistance (TPR)
the force opposing the flow of blood in the systemic circulatory bed; derived by dividing the mean arterial pressure by the cardiac output

trabeculae carneae
irregular muscular ridges or bundles of variable thickness, lining the walls of the ventricles

trachea
the tube extending from the larynx into the lungs; formed from the central portion of the laryngotracheal tube

tracheitis
inflammation of the mucosal lining of the trachea

tracheoesophageal fistula
a congenital abnormality in which the trachea and esophagus freely communicate; frequently associated with esophageal atresia; may also be acquired in later life

tracheostomy
an opening into the trachea; the creation of an opening into the trachea

tracheostomy button
a capped, hollow tube inserted through an opening into the trachea

tracheostomy tube
a curved tube inserted through an opening and projecting into the trachea

transesophageal echocardiography
the use of ultrasound in the investigation of the heart and great vessels and the diagnosis of cardiovascular lesions using a transducer within the esophagus

transitional myocytes
specialized cardiac muscle cells that have a structure similar to regular working myocytes but are less wide; have a myogenic rhythm that is slower than nodal but faster than Purkinje's or working myocytes; have an impulse conduction rate that is faster than working but slower than nodal or Purkinje's myocytes

translation
the motion of a roentgen-ray source parallel to, and at the same distance from, a film cassette that is moved about a target

transmural
across a wall

transmural pressures
the pressure difference across the wall of a container; the difference between the pressure inside and that outside

transpulmonary pressure
the difference between the pressure of the gas at the mouth (atmospheric pressure) and the pressure within the pleural space (pleural pressure)

transsulfuration pathway
an intrahepatic intermediary amino acid metabolic pathway

transudate
the material that passes through a membrane (e.g., capillary walls, alveoli) as a result of a difference in hydrostatic pressures on either side of the membrane

transverse myelitis
an inflammation of the spinal cord (its complete thickness)

transverse sinus
a cul-de-sac formed by the epicardial coverings of the aorta and the pulmonary trunk

trapezius muscle
an accessory inspiratory muscle, the upper fibers of the trapezius arise from the superior nuchal line on the occiput and the ligamentum nuchae to insert onto the distal third of the clavicle

Trendelenburg position
a supine position with the bed inclined at an angle of 45 degrees so that the hips are higher than the head

tricarboxylic acid cycle
Krebs's cycle

tricuspid space (area)
the region of the chest (fourth and fifth intercostal spaces) where the normal and pathologic sounds made by the tricuspid valve are traditionally said to be best appreciated

triglyceride
a molecule of glycerol bound to three long chain fatty acid molecules

triplet
three consecutive atrial or ventricular extrasystoles

troponin
a protein molecule attached to the tropomyosin molecule of an actin filament

true chordae
a fibrous collagenous cord spanning the gap between the papillary muscles and the valve leaflets

true ribs
the first seven ribs on either side of the thorax whose cartilages articulate directly with the sternum

truncal ridges
the spiral epithelial outgrowths from the walls of the truncus arteriosus that combine with the bulbar ridges to form the aorticopulmonary septum

truncus arteriosus
the primitive ascending aorta that opens from both ventricles in the early stages of fetal development

tubercle of the rib
the junction of the neck and the shaft of the rib; an articular portion of tubercle articulates with transverse process of the inferiormost vertebra to which the head is connected

tympany
a low-pitched, drumlike resonance produced by percussing (mediate percussion) the chest wall or other hollow structure

type I (Wenckebach's) second-degree block
a progressive lengthening of the P–R interval until a cardiac cycle is dropped; after the dropped cycle the P–R interval is shortened again

type II (Mobitz II) second-degree block
a dropped cardiac cycle with or without alteration in the conduction of preceding intervals

type I (squamous) pneumocytes
the cells covering approximately 93% of the alveolar surface; accounts for about 8.3% of the total cells of the parenchyma of the lungs

type II (granular) pneumocytes
the cells covering approximately 7% of the alveolar surface; accounts for about 16% of the total cells comprising the parenchyma of the lungs

umbilical vein
the vein that returns the blood from the placenta to the fetus

uncompensated metabolic alkalosis
any condition that causes the arterial pH to rise above 7.40 and the partial pressure of arterial carbon dioxide to rise above 40mm Hg without eliciting a compensatory alveolar hypoventilation

uncomplicated myocardial infarction
a myocardial infarction in which there is no evidence of continued ischemia, left ventricular failure, shock, serious arrhythmia or other conduction disturbance, or other serious illness persisting beyond the fourth day after the infarction; constitutes a low-risk subset of patients

uncomplicated, high-risk myocardial infarction
a myocardial infarction that is initially considered to be uncomplicated but later manifests poor ventricular function, poor cardiac reserve, or significant ischemia at low levels of exertion; constitutes a moderate-risk subset of patients

unipolar pacing system
a type of cardiac pacemaker

unstable angina
a constricting chest pain that occurs now at rest when previously it occurred with exertion associated with myocardial ischemia, injury, and necrosis

upper lobe bronchus
that portion of the tracheobronchial tree that gives off the segmental and subsegmental bronchi of the upper lobe of the lung

uremia
the excessive concentration of urinary retention products in the blood (e.g., creatinine, uric acid, phenols, guanidine bases, sulfates, phosphates, nitrates, urea, and other nonprotein nitrogenous wastes)

uremic syndrome
the symptoms of renal failure (e.g., water retention and edema, acidosis, excessive concentrations of urinary retention products)

urokinase (abbokinase)
a proteinase that coverts plasminogen to plasmin; plasminogen activator

v wave
the rise in the atrial pressure curve near the end of ventricular contraction that results from the gradual accumulation of blood in the atria while the atrioventricular valves are closed during ventricular contraction

Valsalva's maneuver
contraction of the muscles of the abdomen, chest wall, and diaphragm in a forced expiratory effort against the closed glottis

Valsalva's sinuses
three dilations in the aortic wall that correspond to the cusps of the aortic valve

valve leaflets
the cusps of the cardiac valves

valve of the coronary sinus
a semicircular fold of the lining of the right atrium attached to the right and inferior margins of the orifice of the coronary sinus; the remnant of the lower part of the right venous valve of the fetus; thebesian valve

valve of the foramen ovale
a fold of tissue from the margin of the foramen ovale that projects into the left atrium of the fetus; at birth, left atrial blood pressure increases and closes the valve

valve of the inferior vena cava
a crescent-shaped fold attached to the left ventral aspect of the orifice of the inferior vena cava; the remnant of the upper part of the right venous valve of the fetus; eustachian valve

valvular insufficiency
the inadequate closure of one of the valves of the heart, allowing regurgitant flow of blood through the closed valve

valvular stenosis
the narrowing of a valvular orifice

valvuloplasty
the surgical reconstruction of a deformed valve or valve leaflet to relieve an incompetence or stenosis

valvulotomy
a surgical incision through a stenosed valve or valve leaflet to relieve an obstruction

variant angina
atypical angina

varicella zoster
chickenpox; herpes zoster virus

varicose bronchiectasis
the tortuous dilation of the bronchial or bronchiolar airways

vasa vasorum
the blood vessels of the blood vessels; small nutrient blood vessels that supply the larger blood vessels

vascular markings
the shadows produced on a radiographic image of the chest by the pulmonary vasculature

vasculitis
the inflammation of a blood vessel

vasomotor tone (VMT)
the balance between vasoconstriction and dilation

vasopressor
a substance that produces vasoconstriction or an increase in blood pressure

veins
a blood vessel carrying blood toward the heart

venous return
the amount of blood flowing from the veins into the right atrium per minute

ventilation
the replacement of the air or gas in a space by fresh air or gas; movement of gas to and from the alveoli

ventilation-perfusion mismatching
an inequality between the amount of air breathed per unit of time and the amount of blood pumped through the pulmonary vasculature per unit of time; normally a ratio of about 0.8

ventilatory failure
a mechanical inadequacy of the respiratory musculature to move air into and out of the lungs; inability of the lungs to adequately exchange carbon dioxide ($Paco_2$ in excess of 50 mm Hg); pulmonary insufficiency

ventilatory reserve
the difference between the amount of air normally breathed (tidal volume) and that which can be maximally breathed (maximal voluntary ventilation)

ventricle
the division of the heart tube between the bulbus cordis and the atrium

ventricular ejection phase
the portion of the cardiac cycle in which blood is driven out of the ventricles

ventricular fibrillation (VF)
a life-threatening arrhythmia originating from an ectopic focus in the ventricles that results in a twitching of individual fibrils

ventricular gallop
the triple cadence of heart sounds heard on auscultation and characterized by an audible sound (third heart sound) occurring in early diastole in addition to the normal first and second heart sounds; protodiastolic gallop

ventricular septal defect (VSD)
a cogenital defect (opening) in the wall between the ventricles; the most prevalent congenital cardiac defect

ventricular tachycardia (VT)
a life-threatening arrhythmia originating from an ectopic focus in the ventricles; ventricular depolarization at a rate in excess of 100 times per minute

ventriculography
the radiographic visualization of the ventricles by the injection of a radiopaque material into them

Venturi mask
a supplemental oxygen delivery device that can be adjusted to deliver a specific fraction of inspired oxygen at relatively high flow rates

venule
a minute vein

verapamil (Calan, Isoptin)
a calcium channel blocking agent

very low density lipoproteins (VLDL)
one of the major classes of lipoproteins, containing high concentrations of triglycerides and moderate concentrations of cholesterol and phospholipids; has a flotation fraction (density) between 1.006 and 1.019

virus
a group of microbes composed of a

protein coat over a central nucleic acid core

visceral
pertaining to the internal organs of the body

visceral pleura
the serous membrane covering the surface of each lung

viscosity
resistance to flow resulting from molecular cohesion

vital capacity (VC)
the sum of the inspiratory reserve, tidal, and expiratory reserve volumes; it is the maximum amount of air that can be exhaled following a maximum inhalation

vocal ligament
a continuation of the cricothyroid ligament

vocational rehabilitation
training, following disease or injury, for an occupation or profession, taking into account the special physical or mental capabilities of the patient

volvulus
an obstruction of the intestine caused by twisting

wandering pacemaker
an abnormal cardiac rhythm in which the site of the controlling focus of depolarization shifts from depolarization to depolarization, usually between the sinus and atrioventricular nodes

warfarin (Coumadin)
an anticoagulant agent that inhibits the formation of prothrombin in the liver

wedge resection
the excision of a wedge-shaped portion of the lung

Wegener's granulomatosis
a rare, progressive, and fatal ulcerative disease of the upper respiratory tract; occurs in young to middle-aged men and is characterized by necrotizing arteritis

wetting agent
a surface-active agent (e.g., surfactant) that forms a monomolecular layer over the pulmonary alveolar surfaces

wheeze
the high-pitched sound made by air passing through narrowed tracheobronchial airways

whispered pectoriloquy
an auscultatory technique; the whispered voice is transmitted through the lungs and chest wall in the same manner as the normal voice; it indicates an increase in the density of the underlying lung tissue

Wilson's disease
exfoliative dermatitis

Wolff-Parkinson-White (WPW) syndrome
tachyarrhythmia characterized by a short P–R interval ($\geq$ 0.1 second) and a prolonged QRS duration; preexcitation syndrome

working myocytes
the cardiac muscle cells that comprise the bulk of the heart; to be distinguished from conducting myocytes

xiphoid process
the lower segment of the sternum

Index

777

ISBN 0-7216-3609-8

90069